The
Amygdala

The Amygdala

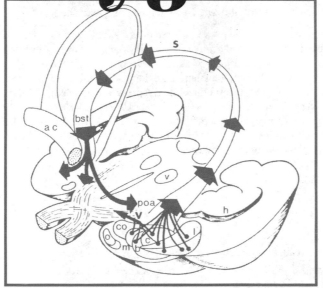

Neurobiological Aspects of Emotion, Memory, and Mental Dysfunction

Edited by John P. Aggleton

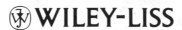 WILEY-LISS

A JOHN WILEY & SONS, INC., PUBLICATION

New York • Chichester • Brisbane • Toronto • Singapore

Address all Inquiries to the Publisher
Wiley-Liss, Inc., 605 Third Avenue, New York, NY 10158-0012

Copyright © 1992 Wiley-Liss, Inc.

Printed in the United States of America.

Library of Congress Cataloging-in-Publication Data

The Amygdala: neurobiological aspects of emotion, memory, and
    mental dysfunction
        p.   cm.
    Includes bibliographical references and index.
    ISBN 0-471-56129-0 (hardcover); ISBN 0-471-30825-0 (paperback)
    1. Amygdaloid body. I. Aggleton, John P.
    [DNLM: 1. Amygdaloid Body—Physiology. 2. Amygdaloid Body—
physiopathology. 3. Emotions—physiology. 4. Memory—physiology.
WL 314 A531]
QP382.T4A49   1992
612.8'25—dc20
DNLM/DLC   91-27869
for Library of Congress   CIP

The text of this book is printed on acid-free paper.

10 9 8 7 6 5 4

To JEA 1923–1990

Contents

Contents

Contributors

John P. Aggleton
Department of Psychology, University of Durham, Durham DH1 3LE, United Kingdom [xi,485]

David G. Amaral
The Salk Institute, San Diego, CA 92186-5800 [1]

Leslie A. Brothers
Psychiatry Service, Sepulveda Veterans Affairs Medical Center, Sepulveda, CA 91343 [353]

Larry Cahill
Center for the Neurobiology of Learning and Memory and Department of Psycho-biology, University of California, Irvine, CA 92717 [431]

Donald P. Cain
Department of Psychology, University of Western Ontario, London, Ontario N6A 5C2, Canada [539]

S. Thomas Carmichael
Department of Anatomy and Neurobiology, Washington University School of Medicine, St. Louis, MO 63110 [1]

Philippe Ciofi
Department of Anatomy and Neurobiology, University of California at Irvine, Irvine, CA 92717 [97]

Michael Davis
Department of Psychiatry, Connecticut Mental Heatlh Center, Yale University School of Medicine, New Haven, CT 06508 [255]

Barry J. Everitt
Department of Anatomy, University of Cambridge, Cambridge CB2 3DY, United Kingdom [401]

James H. Fallon
Department of Anatomy and Neurobiology, University of California at Irvine, Irvine, CA 92717 [97]

David Gaffan
Department of Experimental Psychology, Oxford University, Oxford OX1 3UD, United Kingdom [471]

Michela Gallagher
Department of Psychology, University of North Carolina, Chapel Hill, NC 27599 [307]

P. Gloor
Montreal Neurological Institute and Department of Neurology and Neurosurgery, McGill University, Montreal Quebec, Canada H3A 2B4 [505]

Eric Halgren
VA Wadsworth Medical Center, Los Angeles, CA 90073 [191]

Peter G. Henke
Department of Psychology, St. Francis Xavier University, Antigonish, Nova Scotia, Canada B2G 1CO [323]

Peter C. Holland
Department of Psychology, Duke University, Durham, NC 27710 [307]

The numbers in brackets are the opening page numbers of the contributors' articles.

Ines B. Introini-Collison
Center for the Neurobiology of Learning and Memory and Department of Psychobiology, University of California, Irvine, CA 92717 [431]

Bruce S. Kapp
Department of Psychology, University of Vermont, Burlington, VT 05405 [229]

Raymond P. Kesner
Department of Psychology, University of Utah, Salt Lake City, UT 84112 [379]

Munsoo Kim
Center for the Neurobiology of Learning and Memory and Department of Psychobiology, University of California, Irvine, CA 92717 [431]

Arthur S. Kling
Psychiatry Service, Veterans Affairs Medical Center, Sepulveda, CA 91343 [353]

Joseph E. LeDoux
Center for Neural Science, New York University, New York, NY 10003 [339]

K.C. Liang
Department of Psychology, National Taiwan University, Taipei, Taiwan [431]

D.M.A. Mann
Department of Pathological Sciences, Division of Molecular Pathology, University of Manchester, Manchester, M13 9PT, United Kingdom [575]

Alexander J. McDonald
Department of Anatomy, Cell Biology, and Neurosciences, University of South Carolina, Columbia, SC 29208 [67]

James L. McGaugh
Center for the Neurobiology of Learning and Memory and Department of Psychobiology, University of California, Irvine, CA 92717 [431]

Elisabeth A. Murray
Laboratory of Neuropsychology, National Institute of Mental Health, Bethesda, MD 20892 [453]

Hisao Nishijo
Department of Physiology, Faculty of Medicine, Toyama Medical and Pharmaceutical University, Toyama 930-01, Japan [167]

Taketoshi Ono
Department of Physiology, Faculty of Medicine, Toyama Medical and Pharmaceutical University, Toyama 930-01, Japan [167]

Jeffrey P. Pascoe
Department of Psychology, University of Vermont, Burlington, VT 05405 [229]

Asla Pitkänen
Department of Neurology, University of Kuopio, F-70 211 Kuopio, Finland [1]

Joseph L. Price
Department of Anatomy and Neurobiology, Washington University School of Medicine, St. Louis, MO 63110 [1]

Gavin P. Reynolds
Department of Biomedical Science, The University of Sheffield, Sheffield S10 2TN, United Kingdom [561]

Trevor W. Robbins
Department of Experimental Psychology, University of Cambridge, Cambridge CB2 3DY, United Kingdom [401]

Gareth Wyn Roberts
Department of Anatomy and Cell Biology, St. Mary's Hospital Medical School, London W2 1PG, United Kingdom [115]

Edmund T. Rolls
Department of Experimental Psychology, University of Oxford, Oxford OX1 3UD, United Kingdom [143]

William F. Supple
Department of Psychology, University of Vermont, Burlington, VT 05405 [229]

Paul J. Whalen
Department of Psychology, University of Vermont, Burlington, VT 05405 [229]

Preface

There can be few greater challenges in neuroscience than uncovering the neural mechanisms of emotion and memory. It is now becoming clear that in order to understand these mechanisms we will have to understand the aymgdala. Furthermore, recent research has linked this structure with senile dementia, amnesia, epilepsy, and schizophrenia. It is therefore remarkable that, in spite of the many recent advances, this is the first book on the amygdala to be published for a decade. That there is a real need to provide an up-to-date account of current findings on the amygdala is reflected by the willingness of the leading researchers all over the world to contribute to this volume. *The Amygdala: Neurobiological Aspects of Emotion, Memory, and Mental Dysfunction* brings together many new findings and many new ideas into a single integrated volume, a volume that not only provides comprehensive reviews of current research into this fascinating brain region but will, I hope, also promote future research. In this way *The Amygdala* will be of value both to the expert and to the newcomer interested in the neural basis of emotion and memory.

The amygdala, so named for its fanciful resemblance to an almond, lies in the medial wall of the temporal lobes. It forms a key component of the "limbic system" of the brain. The involvement of the amygdala in emotion, motivation, learning, and memory has been suspected for many years, but the last decade has seen a tremendous acceleration in research uncovering the fine details of its functions. Much of this has been stimulated by remarkable advances in our understanding of the neuroanatomy and neurochemistry of the amygdala. Although the clinical significance of this region has often been underestimated, important new findings mean that the need to understand the detailed workings of this region is more vital than ever.

The opening chapters of the book review current knowledge concerning the neuroanatomy and neurochemistry of the amygdala. Later chapters describe different, but often complementary, studies into the function of this structure. Last, a number of chapters concentrate on the involvement of the amygdala in various clinical conditions. In spite of the ordering of the chapters, there has been no attempt to section the book. This is to help emphasize the fact that these bodies of information should not be seen as separate islands of knowledge, but rather as integrated pieces of a larger (and very complex) puzzle. Where possible, a standard nomenclature for the amygdala has been adopted (see Amaral et al., Chapter 1).

I would like to thank the following for all of their help and support in compiling this volume: Jane Aggleton, Peter Brown, Margaret Hall, Paula Nesbitt, and all of the contributing authors.

John P. Aggleton

The Amygdala: Neurobiological Aspects of Emotion,
Memory, and Mental Dysfunction, pages 1–66

1
Anatomical Organization of the Primate Amygdaloid Complex

DAVID G. AMARAL, JOSEPH L. PRICE, ASLA PITKÄNEN, AND
S. THOMAS CARMICHAEL

*The Salk Institute, San Diego, California (D.G.A., A.P.); Department of
Neurology, University of Kuopio, Kuopio, Finland (A.P.); and Department
of Anatomy and Neurobiology, Washington University School of Medicine,
St. Louis, Missouri (J.L.P., S.T.C.)*

INTRODUCTION

The amygdaloid complex remains an enigma. It is a prominent component of the medial temporal lobe in primates, including man, and has undergone progressive phylogenetic development (Stephan et al., 1987). Yet, the precise role of the amygdaloid complex in primate behavior is not much clearer today than it was in 1956, when Weiskrantz demonstrated that the dramatic Klüver-Bucy (1939) syndrome could be obtained in monkeys subjected to relatively discrete, bilateral ablations of the amygdaloid complex and medial temporal polar cortex. He concluded that "the effect of amygdalectomy ... is to make it difficult for reinforcing stimuli, whether positive or negative, to become established or to be recognized as such ... According to this notion AM (amygdaloid) operates should not be hyperphagic or hypersexual, but indiscriminately phagic and sexual." As Geschwind (1965) later suggested, many of the symptoms of the Klüver-Bucy syndrome, such as the monkeys' apparent lack of normal fear of their keepers or their inability to visually discriminate normal food objects from nonfood items, can be explained on the assumption that the amygdaloid complex is disconnected from visual information relayed from the temporal neocortex. In particular, Geschwind suggested that sensory percepts processed in visual areas of the temporal lobe must interact with the amygdaloid complex in order for them to be tagged with an appropriate affective or motivational label. The notion has thus arisen that the amygdaloid complex plays a central role in allowing an organism to appreciate the species-specific significance of environmental stimuli. If this general idea is substantially correct, it is easy to appreciate how the amygdaloid complex might have widespread

Address correspondence to: Dr. David G. Amaral, The Salk Institute, P.O. Box 85800, San Diego, CA 92186-5800.

and varied roles in the day-to-day existence of the behaving organism. These might range from facilitating the selection of an appropriate food or mate, to insuring the avoidance of dangerous situations or substances, to facilitating the aesthetic appreciation of art or music. A major unresolved issue in this scenario is what happens once the amygdala has been successful in forging the linkage between the sensory experience and its motivational significance, i.e., through which mechanisms and via what routes does the amygdala affect ongoing behavior? As we review, some of the amygdaloid nuclei project directly to autonomic and visceral centers in the diencephalon and brain stem. These projections presumably mediate fairly direct alterations of cardiac, respiratory, and visceral function. But what is the role of the substantial projections to frontal neocortex and to the visual regions of the inferotemporal cortex? Do the prominent projections to the striatum have a role in initiating an appropriate motor response to a motivating stimulus or might they be related to more cognitive functions such as skill learning? And to what extent do the heavy projections to the cholinergic basal forebrain provide another route for amygdaloid modulation of cortical function? While there are many unanswered questions concerning the anatomy of the primate amygdaloid complex, it is quite clear that the design of behavioral and physiological analyses directed at unraveling the functional correlates of the amygdala must take the richness of its anatomical organization into consideration.

In this chapter we provide a selective overview of the anatomical organization of the primate amygdaloid complex, focusing primarily on the organization and connections observed in the old world monkey. We point out that the amygdaloid complex comprises a heterogeneous group of cytoarchitectonically, histochemically, and connectionally distinct nuclear and cortical structures. We also point out that the extrinsic connectivity of the monkey amygdaloid complex provides myriad routes for it to affect behavior or modulate information processing in widespread regions of the brain. It is precisely the richness of these interrelationships with other brain regions that is most predictive of functional diverse roles the amygdala.

INTRINSIC ORGANIZATION OF THE
MONKEY AMYGDALOID COMPLEX

In this first section we summarize several aspects of the intrinsic organization of the monkey amygdaloid complex. Because of the confusing use in the literature of multiple terminologies for the nuclei and cortical regions of the primate amygdala, we shall begin with a fairly detailed description of the position of each of the nuclei and cortical regions that we have differentiated, with occasional comments concerning the history of terminology for these areas (Figs. 1, 2; Table I). It should be pointed out that because of the complexity of the primate amygdala and the relatively meager anatomical attention that it has received, the delimitation and subdivision of nuclei is an ongoing process that will ultimately lead to the adoption of a standardized nomenclature for the various amygdaloid regions. The nuclei we describe are essentially similar to those outlined by Price et al. (1987) with slight modification. The description begins with the deep nuclei (lateral, basal, and accessory basal), followed by the superficial nuclei and areas (anterior cortical nucleus, medial nucleus, nucleus of the lateral olfactory tract, periamygdaloid cortex, posterior nucleus), followed by the central nucleus and the remaining amygdaloid nuclei (anterior amygdaloid area, amygdalohippocampal area, and intercalated nuclei).

The Major Fiber Bundles of the Amygdaloid Complex

The amygdaloid complex is generally considered to have two major extrinsic fiber systems: the ventral amygdalofugal pathway and the stria terminalis. The ventral amygdalofugal system comprises fibers which enter or leave the amygdala through its dorsomedial edge, especially at rostral levels. The stria terminalis, in contrast, is composed of fibers that collect at the ventromedial portion of the caudal amygdala and continue caudally just above the lateral ventricle. Price and Amaral (1981) pointed out that these two bundles do not carry distinct complements of fibers. Fibers from one bundle appear to join fibers in the other bundle throughout their trajectories. Fibers which initially run in the ventral amygdalofugal pathway, for example, have been observed to run through the internal capsule to join the stria terminalis. It is also clear that efferent fibers from most of the amygdaloid nuclei generally exit the amygdala via both the stria terminalis and the ventral amygdalofugal pathway. While the ventral amygdalofugal pathway and the stria terminalis are both primarily subcortical fiber systems, in the primate there are also numerous connections between the amygdala and the neocortex. Both the amygdalofugal and amygdalopetal connections with the cortex travel via the external capsule, which is laterally and ventrally adjacent to the amygdaloid complex. In the monkey brain, this fiber system is equal to, or perhaps even more prominent than, the other subcortically directed fiber bundles.

The amygdala also contains a number of prominent intrinsic fiber bundles (Fig. 1). In fiber stained preparations, the major fiber bundles respect the cytoarchitectonic boundaries of the major amygdaloid nuclei. For simplicity of description, we shall name four of these bundles (Fig. 1). The "medial bundle" (Fig. 1C, arrow 5) separates the medial nucleus from the central and accessory basal nuclei. The "intermediate bundle" (Fig. 1C, arrow 6) separates the basal nucleus from the accessory basal nucleus and the "lateral bundle" (Fig. 1C, arrow 7) separates the basal nucleus from the lateral nucleus. These bundles are, in part, components of what Johnston (1923) described as "longitudinal association bundles." At anterior levels of the amygdala, there is a prominent fiber bundle running along the medial border of the parvicellular portion of the basal nucleus, which we will refer to as the "ventral bundle" (Fig. 1B, arrow 2). The central nucleus is surrounded by thick fiber bundles; a component of these fibers also subdivides the central nucleus into medial and lateral divisions (Fig. 1D, arrows 8, 9). These fibers appear to coalesce just ventral to the central nucleus (Fig. 1D, asterisk) and probably contribute to the stria terminalis.

Position, Nomenclature, and Cytoarchitectonic Organization of Amygdaloid Nuclei and Cortical Regions

Deep Nuclei

Lateral nucleus.

Position and nomenclature. The lateral nucleus is the most laterally situated of the amygdaloid nuclei (Fig. 1). It is bordered laterally by the external capsule

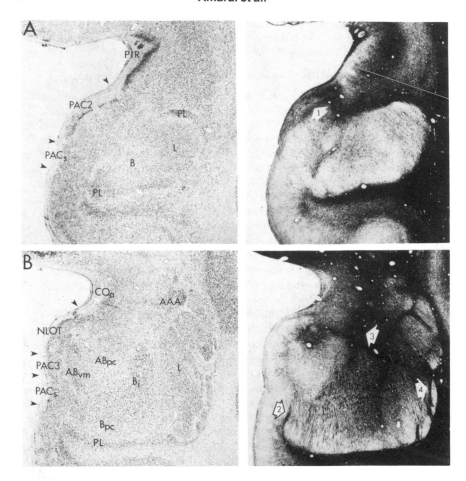

Fig. 1. A series of coronal sections through the monkey amygdaloid complex stained by the Nissl method (**left**) or by a method for the demonstration of myelinated fibers (**right**). The sections are arranged from rostral (**A**) to caudal (**D**). Numbered arrows on

ABBREVIATIONS IN FIGURES

AAA	anterior amygdaloid area
AB	accessory basal nucleus of the amygdala
ABmc	accessory basal nucleus, magnocellular division
ABpc	accessory basal nucleus, parvicellular division
ABvm	accessory basal nucleus, ventromedial division
Acc	nucleus accumbens
AChE	acetylcholinesterase
AHA	amygdalohippocampal area

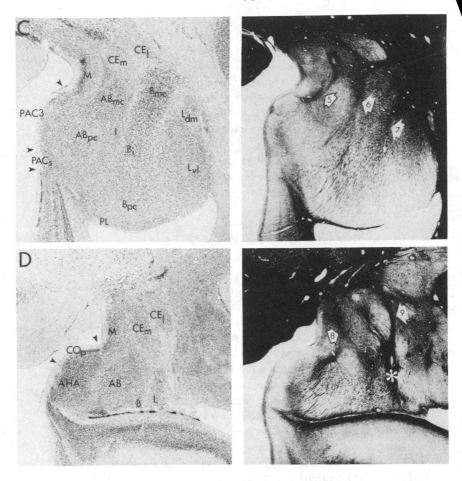

the fiber stained sections indicate prominent fiber bundles which are discussed in the text. Asterisk (D) indicates confluence of stained fibers just ventral to the central nucleus. These fibers appear to contribute to the stria terminalis. Bar = 1 mm.

AON	anterior olfactory nucleus
B	basal nucleus of the amygdala
Bi	basal nucleus, intermediate division
Bmc	basal nucleus, magnocellular division
Bpc	basal nucleus, parvicellular division
BZ/GABA$_A$	benzodiazepine/GABA$_A$ receptor
Ca	caudate nucleus
CCK-r	cholecystokinin receptor binding

(continued)

(continued)

CE	central nucleus of the amygdala
CEl	central nucleus, lateral division
CEm	central nucleus, medial division
ChAT	choline acetyltransferase
COa	anterior cortical nucleus of the amygdala
COp	posterior cortical nucleus of the amygdala
CRF	corticotropin-releasing factor
cs	cingulate sulcus
DBH	dopamine-β-hydroxylase
DNX	dorsal motor nucleus of the vagus
E1	estrone
EC	entorhinal cortex
GABA	γ-aminobutyric acid
Galanin-r	galanin receptor binding
G	gustatory cortex
HRP	horseradish peroxidase
5-HT	5-hydroxytryptamine (serotonin)
5-HT1-r	5-hydroxytryptamine receptor, type 1 binding
I	intercalated nucleus of the amygdala
Iad	insula, agranular dorsal subdivision
Ial	insula, agranular lateral subdivision
Iap	insula, agranular posterior subdivision
Ias	insula, agranular sulcal subdivision
Iav	insula, agranular ventral subdivision
Id	insula, dysgranular subdivision
L	lateral nucleus of the amygdala
LAMP	limbic system associated membrane protein
l-m	stratum lacunosum-moleculare of the hippocampus
LHA	lateral hypothalamic area
LTN	lateral tuberal nucleus of the hypothalamus
M	medial nucleus of the amygdala
M1-r	muscarinic receptor, type 1 binding
MDm	mediodorsal nucleus of the thalamus, medial part
Met-ENK	methionin-enkephalin
MGmc	medial geniculate nucleus of the thalamus, magnocellular part
NADPH-d	reduced nicotinamide adenine dinucleotide phosphate diaphorase
NBM	nucleus basalis of Meynert (basal nucleus of Meynert)
NLOT	nucleus of the lateral olfactory tract
NPY	neuropeptide Y
NTS	nucleus of the solitary tract
o	stratum oriens of the hippocampus
OT	olfactory tubercle
p	pyramidal cell layer of the hippocampus

P	putamen
PAC	periamygdaloid cortex
PAC2	periamygdaloid cortex 2
PAC3	periamygdaloid cortex 3
PACs	periamygdaloid cortex, sulcal division
PAG	periaqueductal grey
PB	parabrachial nucleus
PFC	prefrontal cortex
pl	posterolateral part (of area 36)
PL	paralaminar nucleus
pm	posteromedial part (of area 36)
PIR	piriform cortex
PO	posterior nuclear complex of the thalamus
PP	peripeduncular nucleus
PrCO	precentral operculum
RF	reticular formation
rs	rostral sulcus
S	subiculum
SG	suprageniculate nucleus of the thalamus
SN	substantia nigra
SPf	subparafascicular nucleus
TH	tyrosine hydroxylase
VMH	ventromedial hypothalamic nucleus
VPMpc	ventroposteromedial nucleus (parvicellular part) of the thalamus
VTA	ventral tegmental area
VP	ventral pallidum

except at its caudal pole, where it adjoins the putamen and the ventral horn of the lateral ventricle. A lateral extension of the paralaminar nucleus and the sub-amygdaloid white matter form the ventral border of the lateral nucleus rostrally. These structures are replaced by the lateral ventricle and the hippocampus caudally. Medially, the "lateral bundle" of fibers separates the lateral nucleus from the basal nucleus. The rostral pole of the lateral nucleus is surrounded by the paralaminar nucleus. The caudal third of the lateral nucleus is bordered dorsally by the "dogleg part" of the magnocellular division of the basal nucleus (Fig. 1C) and then, at more caudal levels, by the central nucleus (Fig. 1D).

Even a cursory survey of a Nissl-stained section through the lateral nucleus amply demonstrates that it is a cytoarchitectonically heterogeneous region. As many as six and as few as one subdivisions have been attributed to the primate lateral nucleus (Fig. 2; Johnston, 1923; Lauer, 1945; Jimenez-Castellanos, 1949; Koikegami, 1963). In this chapter, we use the nomenclature of Price et al. (1987) as slightly modified by Amaral and Bassett (1989). Thus, the lateral nucleus of the *Macaca fascicularis* monkey has been subdivided into dorsomedial and ventrolateral divisions (Table I, Fig. 1C) based largely on differences in Nissl and acetylcholinesterase (AChE) staining (Amaral and Bassett, 1989).

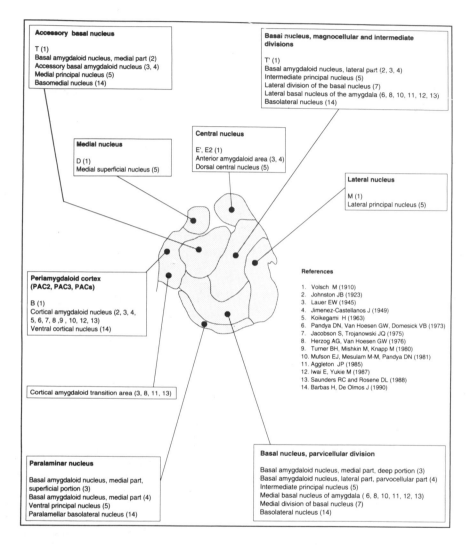

Accessory basal nucleus

T (1)
Basal amygdaloid nucleus, medial part (2)
Accessory basal amygdaloid nucleus (3, 4)
Medial principal nucleus (5)
Basomedial nucleus (14)

Basai nucleus, magnocellular and intermediate divisions

T' (1)
Basal amygdaloid nucleus, lateral part (2, 3, 4)
Intermediate principal nucleus (5)
Lateral division of the basal nucleus (7)
Lateral basal nucleus of the amygdala (6, 8, 10, 11, 12, 13)
Basolateral nucleus (14)

Medial nucleus

D (1)
Medial superficial nucleus (5)

Central nucleus

E', E2 (1)
Anterior amygdaloid area (3, 4)
Dorsal central nucleus (5)

Lateral nucleus

M (1)
Lateral principal nucleus (5)

Periamygdaloid cortex (PAC2, PAC3, PACs)

B (1)
Cortical amygdaloid nucleus (2, 3, 4, 5, 6, 7, 8 ,9 , 10, 12, 13)
Ventral cortical nucleus (14)

References

1. Volsch M (1910)
2. Johnston JB (1923)
3. Lauer EW (1945)
4. Jimenez-Castellanos J (1949)
5. Koikegami H (1963)
6. Pandya DN, Van Hoesen GW, Domesick VB (1973)
7. Jacobson S, Trojanowski JQ (1975)
8. Herzog AG, Van Hoesen GW (1976)
9. Turner BH, Mishkin M, Knapp M (1980)
10. Mufson EJ, Mesulam M-M, Pandya DN (1981)
11. Aggleton JP (1985)
12. Iwai E, Yukie M (1987)
13. Saunders RC and Rosene DL (1988)
14. Barbas H, De Olmos J (1990)

Cortical amygdaloid transition area (3, 8, 11, 13)

Paralaminar nucleus

Basal amygdaloid nucleus, medial part, superficial portion (3)
Basal amygdaloid nucleus, medial part (4)
Ventral principal nucleus (5)
Paralamellar basolateral nucleus (14)

Basal nucleus, parvicellular division

Basal amygdaloid nucleus, medial part, deep portion (3)
Basal amygdaloid nucleus, lateral part, parvocellular part (4)
Intermediate principal nucleus (5)
Medial basal nucleus of amygdala (6, 8, 10, 11, 12, 13)
Medial division of basal nucleus (7)
Basolateral nucleus (14)

Fig. 2. A prototypical coronal section through the monkey amygdala with outlines around the major nuclei and cortical regions. For each area, a window indicates the term used in this chapter (in bold lettering) and then several additional terms used by others to label similar regions. The number after each alternative item indicates the reference from which the term was taken; the references are listed at the right side of the illustration. The list of alternative terms is not intended to be comprehensive but rather indicates those terms that are significant for historical reasons or because they are commonly used in current literature.

TABLE I. Classification of Amygdaloid Subnuclei in the Monkey[a]

Lateral nucleus (L)	Nucleus of the lateral olfactory tract (NLOT)
Dorsomedial division (Ldm)	
Ventrolateral division (Lvl)	Periamygdaloid cortex (PAC)
	PAC2
Basal nucleus (B)	PAC3
Magnocellular division (Bmc)	PACs
Intermediate division (Bi)	(PAC, PAC 0)
Parvicellular division (Bpc)	Anterior amygdaloid area (AAA)
Accessory basal nucleus (AB)	Central nucleus (CE)
Magnocellular division (ABmc)	Medial division (CEm)
Parvicellular division (ABpc)	Lateral division (CEl)
Ventromedial division (ABvm)	
	Posterior cortical nucleus (COp)
Paralaminar nucleus (PL)	
	Amygdalohippocampal area (AHA)
Anterior cortical nucleus (COa)	
	Intercalated nuclei (I)
Medial nucleus (M)	

[a]The locations of the various nuclei are shown in Figure 1.

Cytoarchitectonic organization. In Nissl-stained material, the lateral nucleus is composed of small to medium-sized cells which stain moderately and distinctly lighter than cells in the medially adjacent basal nucleus. Neurons in the *ventrolateral* division, which is only found in the caudal part of the lateral nucleus, are more densely packed and more darkly stained than cells in the *dorsomedial* division (Fig. 1C). The dorsomedial division stains weakly for the presence of AChE, whereas the ventrolateral division stains moderately.

Along the lateral edge of the lateral nucleus there are occasionally patches of tightly packed, small neurons which are encapsulated by fiber bundles emanating from the external capsule. These cell groups were called the *lateral capsular* nuclei by Amaral and Bassett (1989) and stained intensely for AChE and choline acetyltransferase (ChAT). In fiber stained preparations (Fig. 1B, arrow 4), there are very prominent fiber bundles in the dorsal half of the lateral nucleus. These enter the lateral nucleus from the external capsule and cross the nucleus (laterally to medially) in an oblique direction. At least some of these fibers arise in the entorhinal cortex and appear to take this path through the lateral nucleus en route to terminations in the basal forebrain and striatum (Amaral, unpublished observation).

Basal nucleus.

Position and nomenclature. The basal nucleus is the largest nucleus in the monkey amygdala (Figs. 1A–C). The "lateral bundle" and "intermediate bundle" of fibers separate it, respectively, from the laterally adjacent lateral nucleus and from the medially adjacent accessory basal nucleus (Fig. 1C). The basal nucleus extends nearly to the ventral limit of the amygdala and is separated from the subamygdaloid white matter by the distinctive paralaminar nucleus.

The nomenclature and delimitation of the basal nucleus has historically been rather variable and even to this day, different authors use one of several common terminologies for this region (Fig. 2). Modern terminology began with the description of Johnston (1923), who called what we have labeled the basal nucleus "the lateral, large-celled part of the basal amygdaloid nucleus." Johnston's basal nucleus actually comprised both the basal nucleus and the accessory basal nucleus as we have defined it. The accessory basal nucleus in our description was included in his "medial, small-celled part of the basal amygdaloid nucleus." Lauer (1945) departed from Johnston's nomenclature and used the term basal nucleus much as we have done to refer to the lateral, large-celled part of Johnston's basal nucleus. Lauer further subdivided the basal nucleus into a dorsally located, lateral, large-celled part (which corresponds to the magnocellular division of Price et al., 1987) and a ventrally located, medial, small-celled part (equivalent to the parvicellular division of Price et al., 1987). Lauer noted that the most ventral aspect of his medial, small-celled part of the basal nucleus was distinct from the remainder of the nucleus and he called this area the "superficial portion of medial part of basal amygdaloid nucleus." This area corresponds to what we have called the paralaminar nucleus. There are still a variety of names applied to the monkey basal nucleus (Fig. 2). One common variant uses the terms "lateral basal" or "basolateral" when referring to the magnocellular division of the basal nucleus and the terms "medial basal" or "basomedial" when referring to the parvicellular division. This situation is made all the more confusing by the use, in many biochemical studies, of the more general term "basolateral nuclei," which typically encompasses all of the deep nuclei.

Cytoarchitectonic organization. The largest portion of the basal nucleus is the *parvicellular* division (from the Latin *parvus*, meaning small), which extends throughout the whole rostrocaudal extent of the basal nucleus (Fig. 1). While the cells of the parvicellular division are small relative to those in other parts of the nucleus, they are nonetheless relatively large compared to cells in other parts of the amygdala. The parvicellular portion of the basal nucleus is sometimes difficult to delimit, especially from the lateral nucleus. The cells in the parvicellular basal nucleus are more darkly stained, however, and not quite as densely packed as those in the lateral nucleus. Medially, the parvicellular division of the basal nucleus apposes the sulcal portion of the periamygdaloid cortex, which has a distinctly higher cellular packing density than the parvicellular basal nucleus. Fibers of the "intermediate bundle" separate the parvicellular division of the basal nucleus from the dorsomedially located accessory basal nucleus.

Dorsal to the parvicellular division of the basal nucleus is the *intermediate division*. The cells here are larger, more densely packed, and more darkly stained than in the parvicellular division. The dorsoventral border between the parvicellular and intermediate divisions of the basal nucleus extend further dorsally on the lateral and medial edges of the nucleus. Price et al. (1987) did not distinguish the intermediate division. The intermediate division contains higher levels of the cholinergic markers than the parvicellular division but lower levels than in the magnocellular division (Amaral and Basset, 1989).

The most dorsal part of the basal nucleus is the *magnocellular division*, which is located only in approximately the caudal third to half of the amygdala. In

Nissl preparations, it contains the largest and most darkly stained cells of the amygdala. It also has an extremely high density of ChAT-positive fibers (Amaral and Bassett, 1989).

In fiber stained preparations, the basal nucleus has prominent bundles of fibers running dorsoventrally through the parvicellular and intermediate divisions (Fig. 1B,C). The fiber plexus is especially dense at rostral levels of the nucleus. Many of these fibers appear to coalesce just dorsal to the basal nucleus (Fig. 1B, arrow 3). Many individual fibers, which typically have a mediolateral orientation as they cross through the nucleus, form a dense plexus in the magnocellular division of the nucleus.

Accessory basal nucleus.

Position and nomenclature. The accessory basal nucleus is the most medial of the deep amygdaloid nuclei. It first appears about 1 mm caudal to the rostral pole of the amygdala and continues nearly to the caudal pole. Laterally, it is bordered by the basal nucleus, from which it is separated by the "intermediate fiber bundle." The accessory basal nucleus is bordered medially by the periamygdaloid cortex and the nucleus of the lateral olfactory tract. In caudal sections, the "medial fiber bundle" separates it from the medial nucleus (Fig. 1C, arrow 5). In the most caudal sections, the amygdalohippocampal area is located ventromedial to the accessory basal nucleus.

Terminology for the accessory basal nucleus has been somewhat less variable than for the basal nucleus* (Fig. 2). Johnston (1923) included the area that we have labeled the accessory basal nucleus in his "small-celled, medial part of the basal nucleus." Lauer (1945), however, named this area the accessory basal nucleus and divided it into a lateral, large-celled portion and a medial, smaller-celled portion. These regions closely correspond to the magnocellular and parvicellular divisions, respectively, described by Price et al. (1987) and used in this chapter. Price et al. (1987) described an additional "superficial division" of the accessory basal nucleus and Amaral and Bassett (1989) described a fourth division, the ventromedial division, which had distinctly higher levels of cholinergic markers. More recently, Pitkänen and Amaral (1991b) have evaluated the pattern of labeling of this region in preparations stained for the enzyme NADPH-diaphorase (NADPH-d). It became clear in this analysis that the region formerly called the superficial division of the accessory basal nucleus is more likely to be a rostral extension of the amygdalohippocampal area, and in this chapter the term superficial division of the accessory basal nucleus has been eliminated.

Cytoarchitectonic organization. The *parvicellular* division (Fig. 1B,C) accounts for the major portion of the rostral part of the accessory basal nucleus and continues throughout almost its full rostrocaudal extent. The parvicellular division is composed of small, lightly stained cells and the intensity of AChE

---

*In subprimates, the accessory basal nucleus has often been termed the basomedial nucleus (see Price et al., 1987), and this nomenclature has recently been applied to the monkey (Barbas and deOlmos, 1990) and the human (deOlmos, 1990). In primates, unfortunately, this usage may be confusing because many investigators have used the term basomedial (or mediobasal) for the parvicellular division of the basal nucleus.

and ChAT staining is very low. The *ventromedial* division is located along the medial border of the nucleus at a mid-rostrocaudal level of the amygdala (Fig. 1B). It is generally seen as a dorsoventrally elongated group of cells which are slightly darker and more densely packed than the cells in the parvicellular division. The ventromedial division is most easily distinguished in histological preparations for the demonstration of ChAT or AChE, in which it is darkly stained. The *magnocellular* division of the accessory basal nucleus (Fig. 1C,D) first appears at about the mid-rostrocaudal level of the nucleus and is located dorsolateral to the parvicellular division. It is composed of medium- to large-sized cells which stain more darkly in Nissl preparations than the cells in the parvicellular portion; this division contains moderate to high levels of cholinergic markers.

Paralaminar nucleus.

Position and nomenclature. The paralaminar nucleus is a relatively narrow sheet of darkly stained and densely packed cells that forms much of the ventral surface of the amygdala. The sheet continues rostrally and dorsally to cover the amygdala's rostral pole. The paralaminar nucleus is observed for about three-quarters of the rostrocaudal extent of the amygdala (Fig. 1A–C).

Cytoarchitectonic organization. In Nissl-stained sections, the paralaminar nucleus is composed of densely packed, medium-sized, darkly stained neurons. These characteristics allow the paralaminar nucleus to be easily differentiated from the less-densely packed, lightly stained cells in the dorsally adjacent parvicellular division of the basal nucleus. The paralaminar nucleus contains a particularly prominent investiture of glial cells which makes the neuropil even darker than the surrounding areas. Staining for cholinergic markers in the paralaminar nucleus is similar to that in the parvicellular division of the basal nucleus.

Superficial Nuclei

Anterior cortical nucleus.

Position and nomenclature. The anterior cortical nucleus is located in the rostral half of the amygdala (Fig. 1B). It borders the piriform cortex rostrally, the medial nucleus caudally, and the nucleus of the lateral olfactory tract ventrally. In the older literature, the area corresponding to the anterior cortical nucleus was often included in the rostral part of the medial nucleus. The term "cortical nucleus" has also often been used to designate the area that we have labeled the periamygdaloid cortex (Fig. 2; Johnston, 1923; Lauer, 1945; Jimenez-Castellanos, 1949; Koikegami, 1963).

Cytoarchitectonic organization. The anterior cortical nucleus has three layers: a broad layer I, a thick layer II that is populated by lightly stained and diffusely scattered, small to medium-sized cells, and a layer III in which the cell density is slightly lower than in layer II. The anterior cortical nucleus has the very lowest levels of cholinergic markers in the amygdala, which helps to distinguish it from the rostrally located piriform cortex that has moderate levels of AChE and ChAT staining.

Medial nucleus.

Position and nomenclature. The medial nucleus is located just caudal to the anterior cortical nucleus and extends to the caudal pole of the amygdaloid complex (Fig. 1C,D). Compared to the anterior cortical nucleus, the medial nucleus has a denser, narrower, and more darkly stained layer II. The transition between the two nuclei is gradual, however. Rostrally, the medial nucleus is located dorsal to the nucleus of the lateral olfactory tract and caudally it is just dorsal to the posterior cortical nucleus. The accessory basal nucleus and the central nucleus are located ventrolaterally and laterally, respectively.

Cytoarchitectonic organization. The medial nucleus has three layers: a cell-free layer I, a cell dense layer II containing small to medium-sized cells, and a more diffusely cellular layer III containing somewhat more lightly stained neurons. The medial nucleus, like the anterior cortical nucleus, demonstrates extremely low levels of staining for cholinergic markers. In fiber stained material, the medial nucleus is separated from the rest of the amygdala by the "medial fiber bundle" (Fig. 1C, arrow 5).

Nucleus of the lateral olfactory tract.

Position and nomenclature. The nucleus of the lateral olfactory tract is relatively smaller in primates than in nonprimate species such as the rat and cat. In standard Nissl preparations, it is very difficult to identify and even more difficult to define its borders. It could easily be mistakenly included in the periamygdaloid cortex. The nucleus of the lateral olfactory tract, however, contains high levels of ChAT staining which is distributed in distinctive pericellular plexuses (Amaral and Bassett, 1989). This characteristic has proven to be very helpful in defining the location of the nucleus. Rostrally, it is located on the medial surface of the amygdala just ventral to the piriform cortex and anterior cortical nucleus and dorsal to the periamygdaloid cortex (Fig. 1B). At more caudal levels, its cells are no longer situated on the surface of the brain but move laterally to lie among fibers situated between the medial nucleus and the magnocellular division of the accessory basal nucleus. The nucleus of the lateral olfactory tract is mostly located in the rostral half of the amygdaloid complex.

Cytoarchitectonic organization. Layer II is populated by neurons that are slightly more darkly stained than the cells in the periamygdaloid cortex and they sometimes form small clusters. The cells in layer III are diffusely scattered.

Periamygdaloid cortex.

Position and nomenclature. The periamygdaloid cortex forms much of the medial or superficial surface of the amygdaloid complex and it extends for about two-thirds of the rostrocaudal length of the amygdala (Fig. 1A–C). The dorsal boundary is formed by the piriform cortex, the nucleus of the lateral olfactory tract, or the medial nucleus. Ventrally, the periamygdaloid cortex borders the olfactory portion of the entorhinal cortex. The ventral limit is roughly coincident with a minor sulcus usually called the sulcus semiannularis or the amygdaloid sulcus. Laterally, the deep layer of the periamygdaloid cortex borders the accessory basal nucleus and the parvicellular division of the basal nucleus.

Historically, the nomenclature for the periamygdaloid cortex is perhaps the most variable of any amygdaloid area. There are still several different terminologies commonly used (Fig. 2). Johnston (1923) named the periamygdaloid cortex the "cortical nucleus," a term that is perhaps even now most commonly applied to this region (see Fig. 2). Lauer (1945) also used the term cortical nucleus and divided it into dorsal and ventral divisions. He mentioned that the radial dimension of the cortex varied along its dorsoventral extent mainly due to changes in the width of layer III. He also noted that layer II was not continuous throughout the extent of the field. Jimenez-Castellanos (1949) divided the cortical nucleus into superficial or "periamygdaloid" regions and deep or "amygdaloid" regions. Taken together, he identified approximately 10 divisions in the general area that we have labeled as the periamygdaloid cortex. Attempting to acknowledge the regional differences in the organization of the periamygdaloid cortex, Price et al. (1987) divided it into four subdivisions: PAC1, PAC2, PAC3, and PACs. Because the distinction between PAC1 and PACs was tenuous in some animals and because the two regions had very similar staining patterns for cholinergic markers, Amaral and Bassett (1989) used the term PACs to encompass PACs and PAC1; this modification is followed in this chapter.*

Cytoarchitectonic organization. The periamygdaloid cortex has a rudimentary cortical organization consisting of three layers.

PAC2 is located in the rostral part of the amygdaloid complex just dorsal to PACs (Fig. 1A). Its rostrocaudal length is often less than 1 mm in the *Macaca fascicularis* monkey. In Nissl-stained material, layer II of PAC2 is thin and composed of darkly stained, densely packed, medium-sized cells; layer III has relatively few scattered pale cells. There is often a cell-free space between layers II and III. As illustrated in Figure 1A (arrow 1), there is a prominent band of fibers located throughout PAC2 but more densely in layers I and III. PAC2 also stains intensely for cholinergic markers, and in part, the fibers mentioned above are coincident with ChAT immunoreactive fibers that innervate PAC2 (Amaral and Bassett, 1989).

PAC3 is located caudal to PAC2 and forms the largest portion of the periamygdaloid cortex (Fig. 1B,C). It is located ventral to the nucleus of the lateral olfactory tract and, at caudal levels, ventral to the medial nucleus. PAC3 is bordered ventrally by PACs and its lateral border is formed by the accessory basal nucleus. In PAC3, layer II is wider, but the cells are not as darkly stained as the cells of layer II in PAC2. Relative to the nucleus of the lateral olfactory tract, layers II and III in PAC3 are more homogeneous and the cells in layer II are not as darkly stained. Compared to PACs, there is a clearer laminar pattern of the cell layers in PAC3. PAC3 has the lowest level of cholinergic markers of the three periamygdaloid regions.

PACs (formerly PAC1 and PACs) begins near the rostral pole of the amygdaloid complex and continues until the beginning of the amygdalohippocampal

---

*It should be noted, however, that the regions formerly indicated as PAC1 and PACs do not have identical appearances. The more rostrally situated PAC1 is thicker than PACs. The cell layer (layer II) is well formed but without obvious sublamination. The cell layer in PACs is less substantial. The PAC1 has a distinctive fiber bundle (the ventral bundle) located deep to its cell layer. In addition, PAC1 is reciprocally interconnected with the olfactory bulb, while PACs does not appear to be (Price 1990, Price and Carmichael, unpublished observations). We should also point out that Price (1990) has distinguished an additional subregion of the periamygdaloid cortex, called PACo, that lies rostral to the rest of the amygdala. PACo is located ventral to the piriform cortex and is characterized by a layer II that is broken up into prominent cell islands and a relatively thick layer III.

area (Fig. 1A–C). Layers II and III are not distinct from each other, although the cells located more superficially are more densely packed. Through caudal levels of the amygdala, PACs surrounds the sulcus semiannularis in a crescentlike fashion. Compared to the cells in the medially located parvicellular division of the basal nucleus, the cells in the PACs are darker. PACs also demonstrates a higher level of cholinergic markers. In the literature, some variable portion of the most ventral part of PACs is often referred to as the corticoamygdaloid transition area (see Fig. 2).

Posterior cortical nucleus.

Position and nomenclature. The posterior cortical nucleus is located in the caudal one-third of the amygdaloid complex (Fig. 1D). It is bordered dorsally by the medial nucleus and laterally and ventrally by the amygdalohippocampal area.

Cytoarchitectonic organization. The posterior cortical nucleus is composed of two layers: a narrow layer I and a thicker layer II, which is composed of medium-sized, palely stained cells. The layer II cells are slightly more densely packed in the upper portion of the layer. It is often difficult to set the boundary between the posterior cortical nucleus and the amygdalohippocampal area.

Central nucleus.

Position and nomenclature. The central nucleus is located in the caudal third of the amygdala and continues almost to the caudal pole of the amygdaloid complex (Fig. 1C,D). The most rostral part lies dorsal to the "dogleg" of the magnocellular division of the basal nucleus and medial to the external capsule. More caudally, the size of the nucleus increases so that it encompasses much of the areal extent of the caudal pole of the amygdala. At the most caudal levels, it lies medial to the putamen and lateral to the medial nucleus.

Both Lauer (1945) and Jimenez-Castellanos (1949) described a central nucleus which corresponds only to what we have called the lateral division of the central nucleus (Fig. 2). These authors considered what we have called the medial division of the central nucleus to be a caudal extension of the anterior amygdaloid area (which, in their descriptions, extended nearly to the caudal pole of the amygdala).

Cytoarchitectonic organization. The central nucleus can be partitioned into medial and lateral divisions. The *medial* division is composed of small to medium-sized pale cells with a lower packing density than in the lateral division. The *lateral* division contains darker cells that are more densely and homogeneously packed. As many authors have noted, the cytoarchitectonic organization of the lateral division of the central nucleus has some similarities with the putamen. In fiber stained material, thick fiber bundles surround the central nucleus both medially and laterally (Fig. 1D, arrows 8, 9) and a band of fibers also separates the two divisions of the nucleus (asterisk in Fig. 1D).

Remaining Nuclei

Anterior amygdaloid area.

Position and nomenclature. The anterior amygdaloid area is relatively less prominent in the monkey than in the rat. In the monkey, it is located in the rostral half of the amygdaloid complex (Fig. 1B). At rostral levels, its cells lie in close proximity to the endopiriform nucleus, which makes delimitation of the area difficult. The anterior amygdaloid area extends for about 1.5 mm rostrocaudally.

Cytoarchitectonic organization. The anterior amygdaloid area is composed of small to medium-sized neurons which stain darkly in Nissl material and contain very low levels of cholinergic markers.

Amygdalohippocampal area.

Position and nomenclature. The amygdalohippocampal area is located in the caudal third of the amygdaloid complex and forms the caudal pole of the amygdala (Fig. 1D). Rostrally, it is bordered dorsally by the posterior cortical nucleus and laterally by the accessory basal nucleus and the medial part of the parvicellular division of the basal nucleus. The term amygdalohippocampal area was first used by Krettek and Price (1978b) in the rat and cat amygdala and was later applied to the nomenclature of the monkey amygdaloid complex (Price et al., 1987). Few other authors have provided a distinct name for this region; many incorporate it into either the "cortical nucleus" or into the "cortical amygdaloid transition area."

Cytoarchitectonic organization. The nuclear boundaries of the amygdalohippocampal area have been difficult to delineate based solely on Nissl-stained preparations. The caudal half of the amygdalohippocampal area comprises darkly stained and densely packed cells that form a fairly distinct elliptical mass. More rostrally, however, the packing density decreases and the cells are more lightly stained (see Pitkänen and Amaral, 1991b, for a description of this region and its correlation with NADPH-d histochemistry). The anterior portion of the amygdalohippocampal area was previously named the superficial portion of the accessory basal nucleus (Price et al., 1987). However, histochemical characteristics, such as the distribution of AChE and NAHDP-d, indicate that it is more closely associated with the amygdalohippocampal area than with the accessory basal nucleus.

Intercalated nuclei.

Position and nomenclature. The intercalated nuclei are small, separate cell groups that are found in different areas of the monkey amygdala (Fig. 1C). They are typically found embedded in the white matter between the basal and accessory basal nuclei or between the basal and lateral nuclei or just below the central nucleus. While the intercalated nuclei look basically similar in Nissl preparations, several studies have indicated that they may not all share similar staining patterns for neuroactive substances. It is possible, therefore, that subsets of the intercalated nuclei are quite different from each other.

Cytoarchitectonic organization. In Nissl-stained material, the intercalated nuclei appear to be densely packed clusters of small, darkly stained cells.

Chemoarchitectonic Organization

While there is a fairly substantial and growing literature concerning the distribution of neuroactive substances in the rat amygdala (summarized in Price et al., 1987), there is far less known about the monkey amygdala. Nonetheless, in the following section we provide an overview of currently available information on the chemical neuroanatomy of the monkey amygdala. The density and location of various neuroactive substances is listed in Table II and, where anatomical information is not available, the relative level of biochemically detected substances is indicated in Table III.

Amino Acids

The monkey amygdala contains high concentrations of the inhibitory neurotransmitter γ-aminobutyric acid (GABA; Singh and Malhotra, 1962). However, we are not aware of any comprehensive study of the distribution of GABA or glutamic acid decarboxylase (GAD) containing cells and fibers in the monkey amygdala. Nor has the distribution of other markers of GABAergic systems, such as the calcium-binding protein parvalbumin, been reported. From work carried out in the rat, one would expect a dense terminal plexus in the central and medial nuclei, and in the anterior amygdaloid area. The accessory basal nucleus would have an intermediate level of GABA immunoreactivity and much lower levels of GABAergic markers would be found in the basal and lateral nuclei and the periamygdaloid cortical areas (Ottersen et al., 1986). In the rat amygdala, GABA immunoreactivity is associated with fibers, terminals, and cell bodies. GAD or GABA-immunoreactive cell bodies are scattered throughout all of the amygdaloid nuclei, with a somewhat higher concentration in the lateral, basal, and cortical nuclei (McDonald, 1985; Ottersen et al., 1986).

The therapeutic effects of the most widely used anxiolytic benzodiazepines are mediated by their selective binding with benzodiazepine receptor sites that interact allosterically with $GABA_A$ receptors (Costa et al., 1975). Recently, Dennis et al. (1988) surveyed the distribution of benzodiazepine receptors ($\omega1$ and $\omega2$ subtypes) in the monkey brain. Using ligands such as tritiated flunitrazepam, which binds both to the $\omega1$ and $\omega2$ sites, and tritiated zolpidem, which binds more selectively to $\omega1$ sites, they found that the amygdala contains more $\omega2$ binding sites than $\omega1$ binding sites. Stroessner et al. (1989) used antibodies to the benzodiazepine/$GABA_A$ receptor complex to characterize its regional distribution in the monkey amygdaloid complex. Benzodiazepine/$GABA_A$ immunoreactivity was particularly prominent in the lateral and accessory basal nuclei.

Singh and Malhotra (1962) found that the monkey amygdala had high levels of glutamate/glutamine (the two amino acids were not separated by the method used), aspartate, glycine, and taurine. Unfortunately, the nuclear distribution of the excitatory amino acid receptors in the monkey brain is not known. In the rat, Ottersen and colleagues (1986) have studied the pattern of $D-[^3H]$-aspartate uptake (which is primarily mediated by the high-affinity uptake system for glutamate and aspartate). The highest activity is seen in the lateral and basal nuclei, and in the anterior cortical nucleus and periamygdaloid cortex, while somewhat lower levels of uptake are found in the more medially situated nuclei (Ottersen et al., 1986). Much of this uptake may be mediated by terminals of corticoamygdaloid fibers which use glutamate and/or aspartate as neurotransmitters. Injection of $D-[^3H]$-aspartate into the lateral and basal nuclei of the amygdala leads to retrogradely labeled cells in neocortex, hippocampal formation, and subcortical regions such as the peripeduncular nucleus (Amaral and Insausti, unpublished observations). While a detailed description of the distribution of glutamate receptors has not yet been established either for the monkey or rat, a survey in the rat brain indicates that the amygdala has high levels of glutamate receptors. High levels of binding were demonstrated with ligands for N-methyl-D-aspartate, kainate, and quisqualate (Miller et al., 1990; Insel et al., 1990).

TABLE II. Distribution of the Markers of Different Neurotransmitter and Neuromodulator Systems in the Monkey Amygdaloid Complex

Marker		L	B	AB	PL	COa	ME	COp	AHA	PAC	NLOT	CE	AAA	I	Reference
ChAT	fibers	f	fff	ff	ff	f	f	ff	fff	ff	fff	ff	f	ff	Amaral and Bassett (1989)
AChE	cells	c	ccc	c	–	ccc	ccc	c	c	c	–	cc	ccc	ccc	Amaral and Bassett
	fibers	f	fff	ff	ff	f	f	ff	fff	ff	fff	ff	f	ff	(1989)
M1-r	binding	+++	++	+++						+++					Marsh et al. (1988)
NADPH-d	cells	ccc	ccc	ccc	cc	cc	cc	–	ccc	c	ccc	c	cc	cc	Pitkänen and
	fibers	fff	f	ff	f	f	f	f	–	f	ff	f	fff	–	Amaral (1991b)
BZ/GABA$_A$	neuropil	nnn	n	nnn						n	nnn				Stroessner
	cells		ccc							ccc					et al. (1989)
TH	fibers	fff	ff	f		f	f		–	f	f	fff	f	fff	Sadikot and Parent (1990)
5-HT	fibers	fff	ff	f		f	f		fff	ff	f	fff	f	f`	Sadikot and Parent (1990)
5-HT1-r	binding	++	++							+++					Stuart et al. (1986)
DBH	fibers	f	f	f		ff	ff		f	ff	f	ff	f	ff	Sadikot and Parent (1990)
Somatostatin	cells	ccc	c	ccc	ccc	cc	cc	c	cc	ccc	cc	ccc	c	c	Amaral et al.
	fibers	fff	ff	fff	fff	ff	fff	ff	ff	ff	f	fff	f	ff	(1989)

	1	2	3	4	5	6	7	Reference
NPY cells	cc	cc	c		c	cc	–	Smith et al. (1985)
NPY fibers	fff	f	ff		fff	fff	ff	
Met-ENK cells	c	c	c		c	cc	c	Inagaki and Parent (1985)
Met-ENK fibers	f	f	f		f	ff	ff	Haber and Elde (1982)
Vasopressin cells	–	–	–		–	–	–	Caffé et al. (1989)
Vasopressin fibers	–	–	ff		ff	fff	–	Caffé et al. (1989)
Oxytocin fibers	–	–	–		f	fff	f	Caffé et al. (1989)
CRF cells	ccc	ccc	c		c	c	c	Bassett and Foote (1990)
CRF fibers	fff	fff	ff		ff	fff	ff	
Neurotensin cells	cc	cc	ccc		ccc		ccc	Chen et al. (1988)
Neurotensin fibers	f	ff	ff		fff	fff	fff	Chen et al. (1988)
CCK-r binding	+++	+++	+++		+	+	+	Kritzer et al. (1988)
Galanin-r binding	+++	+++	+++	++	+++	+++	+++	Köhler et al. (1989)
LAMP neuropil	n	nn	nn	n	n	nn	nn	Carmichael and Price, unpublished

Abbreviations: Fiber density: fff, high; ff, medium; f, low; –, not found. Number of cells: ccc, high; cc, medium; c, low; –, not found. Density of receptor binding: +++, high; ++, medium; +, low. Neuropil staining: nnn, high; nn, medium; n, low. Empty area: data not available.

TABLE III. Neurochemical Substances Analyzed in the Monkey Amygdaloid Complex

Substance	Method	Amount	Reference
Neurotransmitters			
GABA	Paper chromatography	High	Singh and Malhotra (1962)
Aspartate	Paper chromatography	High	Singh and Malhotra (1962)
Glutamate/glutamine	Paper chromatography	High	Singh and Malhotra (1962)
Dopamine	Spectrophotofluorometry	Intermediate	Brown et al. (1979)
Noradrenaline	Spectrophotofluorometry	Intermediate	Brown et al. (1979)
Serotonin	Spectrophotofluorometry	Intermediate	Brown et al. (1979)
Peptides			
Somatostatin	Radioimmunoassay	High	Hayashi and Oshima (1986), Beal et al. (1987)
Neuropeptide Y	Radioimmunoassay	High	Beal et al. (1987)
Substance P	Radioimmunoassay	High	Hayashi and Oshima (1986)
Vasoactive intestinal polypeptide	Radioimmunoassay	Intermediate	Hayashi and Oshima (1986)
Nerve growth factor	Enzymeimmunoassay	High	Hayashi et al. (1990)
Enkephalin	Inhibition of opiate binding	Intermediate/low	Simantov et al. (1976)
Neurophysin	Immunohistochemistry	High	Sofroniew et al. (1981)
Somatostatin binding	Radioligand binding	Intermediate	Beal et al. (1986)
	Radioligand binding	High	Kuhar et al. (1973)
	Radioligand binding	High	LaMotte et al. (1978)
Opiate binding	Autoradiography	High	Wamsley et al. (1982)

Vasoactive intestinal polypeptide binding	Autoradiography	High	Dietl et al. (1990)
Neurotensin binding	Autoradiography	Intermediate/high	Quirion et al. (1987)
Corticotropin releasing factor binding	Radioligand binding	High	Millan et al. (1986)
Nerve growth factor binding	Immunohistochemistry	Low	Kordower et al. (1988)
Dynorphin binding	Autoradiography	Low	Slater and Cross (1986)
Hormones			
Dihydrotestosterone concentrating cells	Autoradiography	High	Michael and Rees (1982)
Estrogen concentrating cells	Autoradiography	High	Pfaff et al. (1976), Bonsall et al. (1986)
Aromatase	E1 formation	High	Clark et al. (1988)
5-alpha-reductase	Dihydrotestosterone formation	High	Roselli et al. (1987), Sholl et al. (1989)
Androgen receptors	Radioligand binding	High	Clark et al. (1988)
Estrogen receptors	Radioligand binding	Medium	Sholl and Kim (1989)
Estrone sulphatase	Enzyme assay	Medium	Lakshmi and Balasubramanian (1981)
Dehydroepiandrosterone sulphatase	Enzyme assay	Medium	Lakshmi and Balasubramanian (1981)
Arylsulphatase	Enzyme assay	Medium	Lakshmi and Balasubramanian (1981)
Luteinizing hormone releasing hormone	Immunohistochemistry	Low	Silverman et al. (1982)
Other			
Protein kinase	Immunoblotting	High	Huang et al. (1987)
Benzodiazepine receptors ω_1	Radioligand binding	Low	Dennis et al. (1988)
ω_2	Radioligand binding	Intermediate	Dennis et al. (1988)

Noradrenaline, Serotonin, and Dopamine

Noradrenaline. The monkey amygdala contains intermediate levels of noradrenaline when assayed from tissue homogenate (Brown et al., 1979). Immunohistochemical localization of dopamine-β-hydroxylase (the enzyme that converts dopamine to noradrenaline) demonstrated that the central nucleus, medial nucleus, intercalated nuclei, and periamygdaloid cortex have an intermediate level of fiber staining. In contrast, the deep nuclei contain relatively few labeled fibers (Sadikot and Parent, 1990). There is substantial intranuclear variability, however, within several of the amygdaloid nuclei. For example, the density of fiber and terminal staining in the parvicellular division of the basal nucleus is moderate, whereas labeling in the magnocellular division is very light. Similarly, the medial division of the central nucleus contains a higher density of labeled fibers than the lateral part. The noradrenergic projection to the monkey amygdala arises primarily from the locus coeruleus and perhaps, in part, from the lateral tegmental area (Mehler, 1980; Norita and Kawamura, 1980). Immunohistochemical analysis of phenylethanolamine-N-methyltransferase (the enzyme that converts noradrenaline to adrenaline and is a selective marker for adrenergic neuronal terminals) demonstrates a very sparse system of immunoreactive fibers in the central nucleus of the monkey amygdala (Sadikot and Parent, 1990).

Serotonin. The levels of serotonin and its deaminated metabolite, 5-hydroxyindoleacetic acid, in the monkey amygdala are intermediate to high, relative to the other brain regions (Brown et al., 1979; Azmitia and Gannon, 1986). Moreover, the demonstrated high levels of synthesis and synaptosomal uptake of serotonin (Azmitia and Gannon, 1986) are consistent with substantial serotonergic neurotransmission.

Using an antibody directed against serotonin, Sadikot and Parent (1990) reported fairly dense immunoreactive fibers plexuses in the lateral nucleus, parvicellular division of the basal nucleus, magnocellular division of the accessory basal nucleus, central nucleus, and amygdalohippocampal area. Importantly, the density of serotonin immunoreactive fibers in the monkey amygdala was reported to be relatively high compared to noradrenergic and dopaminergic markers. The serotonergic input to amygdala probably originates in the dorsal raphe nucleus with perhaps an additional contribution from the median raphe nucleus (Mehler, 1980; Norita and Kawamura, 1980). Serotonin receptors (5-HT$_1$ subtype) are abundant in the lateral nucleus, basal nucleus, and in the periamygdaloid cortex (Stuart et al., 1986).

Dopamine. The dopamine content of the monkey amygdala is intermediate compared to the other brain areas studied by Brown et al. (1979). Sadikot and Parent (1990) stained the monkey amygdala using an antibody raised against tyrosine hydroxylase (TH), the rate-limiting enzyme for catecholamine synthesis. For reasons beyond the scope of this review, TH is believed to be a relatively selective marker for dopaminergic fiber systems. The highest levels of TH labeling are found in the lateral nucleus, central nucleus, and in the intercalated nuclei. In the basal nucleus, the highest level of immunoreactivity is seen in the lateral part of the parvicellular division. The dopaminergic innervation of the amygdala originates from the ventral tegmental area and the dorsal substantia nigra (Mehler, 1980; Norita and Kawamura, 1980).

Cholinergic System

The monkey amygdaloid complex contains high levels of the cholinergic enzymes ChAT and AChE. There is marked variation in the levels of these substances in different amygdaloid regions (Amaral and Bassett, 1989). The distribution of ChAT provides the most selective marker for cholinergic processes in the amygdala. A high density of ChAT immunoreactive fibers and terminals is observed in the basal nucleus, parvicellular division of the accessory basal nucleus, amygdalohippocampal area, and the nucleus of the lateral olfactory tract.

The cholinergic fibers that innervate the amygdala originate in the basal nucleus of Meynert (Mesulam et al., 1983). Most of the cholinergic cells that project to the amygdala are specifically located in the anterolateral portion of the basal nucleus of Meynert (Kordower et al., 1989). A smaller number of neurons in the anteromedial and intermediate portions of the basal nucleus of Meynert and in the nucleus of the horizontal limb of the diagonal band project to the amygdala.

High-affinity choline uptake sites are thought to be labeled by $[^3H]$hemicholinium. The distribution of these binding sites correlates fairly closely with the known distribution of the cholinergic enzymatic markers. There are high levels of $[^3H]$hemicholinium, for example, in the basal nucleus of the monkey amygdala (Quirion, 1987). Mash et al. (1988) determined the distribution of cholinergic muscarinic receptors, M1 and M2, in the monkey brain using in vitro autoradiography. Neither subclass of muscarinic receptors matched the pattern of presynaptic cholinergic markers. For example, the magnocellular division of the basal nucleus, which has a very high level of ChAT immunoreactive fiber and terminal labeling, had very low M1 and M2 binding. The parvicellular division of the basal nucleus, in contrast, had higher M1 receptor binding intensity but substantially lower ChAT fiber and terminal labeling. The M2 binding in general was very low in the monkey amygdaloid complex.

Peptides

Somatostatin. High levels of somatostatin have been reported in the monkey amygdala when analyzed by radioimmunoassay of tissue homogenates (Hayashi and Oshima, 1986; Beal et al., 1987). Specific, high-affinity somatostatin receptor binding (using $^{125}I[Leu^8, D\text{-}Trp^{22}, Tyr^{25}]SS\text{-}28$ as a ligand) has been reported in the amygdala although the amount of binding was only 45% of the level observed in the frontal cortex (Beal et al., 1986). The distribution of somatostatin immunoreactive cells and fibers has been evaluated using polyclonal antibodies to different fragments of the prosomatostatin peptide (Amaral et al., 1989; Table II). The distribution of immunoreactivity shows both internuclear and intranuclear variability. In the lateral nucleus, the density of immunoreactive fibers is highest in the ventrolateral part, whereas the number of immunoreactive cells was highest in the dorsomedial portion. In the basal nucleus, there is a decreasing gradient of fiber density running from ventral to dorsal within the nucleus. In the central nucleus, the lateral division contains more somatostatin immunoreactive cells and fibers than the medial division.

Neuropeptide Y. The monkey amygdala contains high levels of neuropeptide Y (Beal et al., 1987). The distribution of neuropeptide Y immunoreactive cell bodies and fibers is similar to that for somatostatin (Smith et al., 1985). Since somatostatin and neuropeptide Y have been shown to colocalize in the monkey cortex (Hendry et al., 1984), it is likely, though not currently demonstrated, that at least some of the same cells and fiber systems contain the two peptides in the amygdala.

Vasopressin, neurophysin, and oxytocin. The medial nucleus of the amygdala contains vasopressin immunoreactive fibers and cell bodies (Caffé et al., 1989). Sofroniew et al. (1981) found that the "medial amygdala" receives a projection containing vasopressin/neurophysin from the suprachiasmatic nucleus of the hypothalamus, while the "central amygdala" receives some vasopressin/neurophysin and oxytocin immunoreactive fibers arising from the paraventricular nucleus.

Opiate peptides. Simantov et al. (1976) assayed the monkey amygdaloid complex for enkephalin content from tissue homogenates and found only moderate-to-low levels. Subsequently, Haber and Elde (1982) found heavy Met-enkephalin immunoreactive fiber and terminal labeling in the central nucleus, especially in its lateral part. This finding was later confirmed by Inagaki and Parent (1985) and Sadikot et al. (1988). Only occasional fibers were found in the lateral and basal nuclei. There are also Met-enkephalin immunoreactive cell bodies in the central nucleus which are small to medium in size and mostly fusiform in shape. Only occasional immunoreactive cells were found in the deep nuclei.

Kuhar et al. (1973) studied opiate binding in the monkey amygdala using [^{3}H] dihydromorphine as a ligand and found that it had the highest level of binding in the monkey brain. Later, LaMotte et al. (1978), using [^{3}H]naloxone as a ligand, also reported very high levels of binding in tissue homogenate taken from the "basolateral" and "corticomedial" portions of the amygdala. The autoradiographic study of Wamsley et al. (1982), using [^{3}H]diprenorphine as a ligand, confirmed that there were high levels of opiate binding sites in the central, medial, basal, and lateral nuclei and the periamygdaloid cortex. Slater and Cross (1986) used [^{3}H]dynorphin$_{1-9}$ as a ligand to recognize the κ subtype of opiate receptors. Only low levels of binding were observed in the "basolateral" region, though more binding was found in the medial nucleus and in the periamygdaloid cortex. In general, therefore, there appears to be relatively few opiate-related neurons or fibers in the monkey amygdaloid complex but relatively high levels of opiate binding sites.

Other peptides. Homogenates of monkey amygdala contain an intermediate level of *vasoactive intestinal polypeptide* (VIP) compared to the other brain regions studied (Hayashi and Oshima, 1986). The number of VIP binding sites, however, is high (Dietl et al., 1990), using M-^{125}I-VIP as ligand.

The monkey amygdaloid complex contains *corticotropin-releasing factor* immunoreactive cell bodies and fibers (see Table II) (Bassett and Foote, 1990) as well as receptor binding sites (Millan et al., 1986). The amygdala also contains binding sites for *cholecystokinin* (Kritzer et al., 1988), *galanin* (Köhler et al., 1989), and *neurotensin* (Quirion, 1987) (Table II).

Hormones

The amygdala contains numerous estrogen-concentrating cells in the medial nucleus, the mediodorsal part of the accessory basal nucleus, the periamygdaloid cortex, and particularly in the posterior cortical nucleus and the amygdalo-hippocampal area. Fewer estrogen-concentrating cells are found in the basal nucleus, lateral nucleus, and in the anterior amygdaloid area (Pfaff et al., 1976; Bonsal et al., 1986).

Cells concentrating [^{3}H]dihydrotestosterone (the 5α-reduced metabolite of testosterone which, unlike testosterone, is not aromatizable to estrogens in the brain) are found mainly in the medial nucleus but also scattered throughout the accessory basal nucleus, parvicellular division of the basal nucleus, lateral nucleus, and periamygdaloid cortex (Michael and Rees, 1982). The activity of aromatase, an enzyme that converts testosterone to estrogens, is high in homogenates taken from the monkey amygdala, as is the activity of 5α-reductase, which converts testosterone to dihydrotestosterone. The high level of aromatase activity in the amygdala suggests that testosterone is converted to estrogens in the amygdala, and the effect of testosterone is thus mostly mediated via estrogen receptors. The enzymatic activity of sulphatases, which desulphates steroid sulphates to free steroids, is also high in the monkey amygdala (Lakshmi and Balasubramanian, 1981). Homogenates taken from the monkey amygdaloid complex were also found to contain a moderate number of estrogen binding sites (Sholl and Kim, 1989) and high numbers of androgen binding sites (Clark et al., 1988). The regional distribution fo these receptors, however, has not been investigated in the monkey amygdala.

Other Substances

The monkey amygdaloid complex contains a high number of NADPH-d positive cell bodies and fibers with clear-cut regional differences in distribution (Pitkänen and Amaral, 1991b) (Table II). Positively labeled cell bodies can be divided into three categories on the basis of cytosolic staining intensity, which probably reflects the level of intracellular enzymatic activity. Darkly stained cells are common in the accessory basal nucleus. Cells with medium cytosolic intensity for NADPH-d staining are widely distributed in the deep nuclei of the monkey amygdala. The third cell type, which stained only slightly for NADPH-d, is found in the anterior cortical nucleus, medial nucleus, and in the paralaminar nucleus. The highest density of NADPH-d positive fibers is found in the lateral nucleus and in the accessory basal nucleus. Interestingly, Hope et al. (1991) recently found that NADPH-d is a nitric oxide synthase that produces nitric oxide in response to changes in intracellular free calcium levels. In addition, NADPH-d positive cells are relatively resistant to N-methyl-D-aspartate (NMDA) receptor mediated neurotoxicity (Koh and Choi, 1988).

Trophic factors. The monkey amygdala contains relatively high concentrations of nerve growth factor (Hayashi et al., 1990). In contrast, when antibodies to the nerve growth factor receptor (NGFr) were used to stain the amygdala, only a very sparse immunopositive fiber network is found (Kordower et al., 1988). These fibers are preferentially located close to blood vessels and no correlation is found between the NGFr immunoreactivity and the distribution of cholinergic markers.

Intrinsic Connections of the Monkey Amygdala

Historically, the analysis of intrinsic connections of the amygdaloid complex has been hampered by the fiber of passage problem, which plagued degeneration techniques and certain of the retrograde tracer methods such as horseradish peroxidase (HRP). This problem has been largely eliminated by more selective and and discrete anterograde tracing techniques such as [^{3}H]-amino acid autoradiography and especially the newly developed lectin tracer *Phaseolus vulgaris* leucoagglutinin (PHA-L). While these, and other techniques, provide the means for conducting detailed analyses of the intrinsic circuitry of the amygdala, there is surprisingly little published information on these connections in the monkey. It is likely that the description provided below substantially underestimates the extent of inter- and intranuclear connectivity in the monkey amygdala.

In the monkey, as in nonprimate species, there is general agreement that the major intra-amygdaloid connections arise in the lateral and basal nuclei and terminate in the more medial nuclei. The accessory basal nucleus also projects to the central, medial, and cortical nuclei and the amygdalohippocampal area. Since there are only weak projections from the medial, cortical, or central nuclei, or the amygdalohippocampal area back to the lateral and basal nuclei, the intrinsic flow of information through the amygdala is primarily unidirectional and follows a lateral to medial direction.

Lateral Nucleus

Efferents. The lateral nucleus projects to all subdivisions of the basal nucleus (Pitkänen and Amaral, 1991a), the accessory basal nucleus (especially its parvicellular portion), paralaminar nucleus, anterior cortical nucleus, medial nucleus, and the PAC3 (Fig. 3A). It projects more lightly to PAC2, the nucleus of the lateral olfactory tract, central nucleus, and anterior amygdaloid area (Price and Amaral, 1981; Aggleton, 1985; Pitkänen and Amaral, unpublished). Some of these intrinsic connections, such as the lateral nucleus projection to the accessory basal nucleus, have been reported previously in a number of species including the monkey. Others, however, such as the lateral nucleus projection to the basal nucleus, have only recently been identified in the monkey (Pitkänen and Amaral, 1991a).

Afferents. While the lateral nucleus originates many of the major intrinsic amygdaloid connections, it actually receives rather few inputs from other amygdaloid nuclei. Aggleton (1985) observed a very small number of retrogradely labeled cells in the accessory basal and basal nuclei following an HRP injection focused in the lateral nucleus (see also Price and Amaral, 1981). The central nucleus may also contribute a minor projection to the lateral nucleus (Aggleton, 1985).

Intranuclear connections. There appear to be complex intranuclear connections within the lateral nucleus (Pitkänen and Amaral, unpublished observations). In general, the dorsal part of the nucleus appears to send projections to the ventral part.

Basal Nucleus

Efferents. The magnocellular and intermediate divisions of the basal nucleus project to the accessory basal nucleus, central nucleus (more heavily to its medial

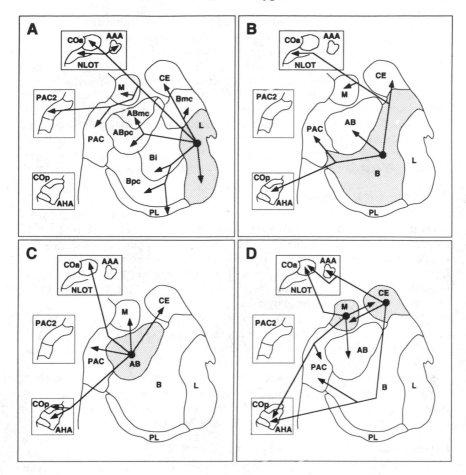

Fig. 3. Line drawings of prototypical coronal section through the amygdala to illustrate the organization of the *major* efferent intrinsic connections of the monkey amygdala. Windows around the left side of the amygdala indicate additional regions that are not usually observed at the mid-rostrocaudal level portrayed in the prototypical section. **A:** Instrinsic efferent connections of the lateral nucleus. Note that the arrow which ends within the nucleus indicates that there are significant intranuclear connections. **B:** Intrinsic efferent connections of the basal nucleus. **C:** Intrinsic efferent connections of the accessory basal nucleus. **D:** Intrinsic efferent connections of the central and medial nuclei.

part), medial nucleus, nucleus of the lateral olfactory tract, periamygdaloid cortex, and amygdalohippocampal area (Fig. 3B; Price and Amaral, 1981; Aggleton, 1985). The parvicellular division of the basal nucleus projects to the accessory basal nucleus, the central nucleus, the caudal part of the medial nucleus, the periamygdaloid cortex, and to the amygdalohippocampal area (Aggleton, 1985).

Afferents. The basal nucleus receives a major projection from the lateral nucleus (Pitkänen and Amaral, 1991a). It receives less substantial projections from the accessory basal nucleus, central nucleus (which projects more heavily to the parvicellular division), and from the periamygdaloid cortex (which projects to the medial portion of the parvicellular division) (Van Hoesen, 1981; Price and Amaral, 1981; Aggleton, 1985).

Intranuclear connections. The magnocellular and intermediate divisions of the basal nucleus project ventrally to the parvicellular division of the nucleus (Price and Amaral, unpublished observations; Pitkänen and Amaral, unpublished observations). The parvicellular division of the basal nucleus, in turn, contributes projections to the more dorsal divisions of the nucleus (Price et al., 1987).

Accessory Basal Nucleus

Efferents. The accessory basal nucleus sends a dense projection to the central nucleus, which is heaviest to its medial division (Fig. 3C). It also projects to the medial nucleus, periamygdaloid cortex, anterior and posterior cortical nuclei, amygdalohippocampal area, and intercalated nuclei. There is some indication that the accessory basal nucleus might also originate a light projection to the basal and lateral nuclei (Price and Amaral, 1981; Aggleton, 1985), though this must be confirmed by more discrete tracer methods.

Afferents. The accessory basal nucleus receives a major input from the lateral nucleus (to all portions but especially to the parvicellular division). Lighter projections originate in the basal nucleus, central nucleus, and medial nucleus (that project to the dorsal third of the accessory basal nucleus) (Price and Amaral, 1981, unpublished observations; Aggleton, 1985; Pitkänen and Amaral, 1990).

Intranuclear connections. There appear to be reciprocal connections between the magnocellular and parvicellular divisions of the accessory basal nucleus (Amaral and Price, unpublished observations).

Paralaminar Nucleus

Not much is known about the intra-amygdaloid connections of the paralaminar nucleus. Injections of retrograde tracers into the basal nucleus lead to numerous labeled cells in the paralaminar nucleus (Amaral and Insausti, unpublished observation). This indicates that either the paralaminar nucleus provides the basal nucleus with a fairly substantial input or that the paralaminar nucleus originates fibers that travel through the basal nucleus to another location. PHA-L studies have shown that it receives a dense projection from different parts of the lateral nucleus, especially its lateral part (Pitkänen and Amaral, unpublished observations).

Anterior Cortical Nucleus

The intrinsic efferent connections of the anterior cortical nucleus are unknown. The anterior cortical nucleus receives projections from the lateral nucleus, the accessory basal nucleus, central nucleus, and medial nucleus (Price et al., 1987; Pitkänen and Amaral, unpublished observations).

Medial Nucleus

Efferents. The medial nucleus sends projections to the dorsal third of the accessory basal nucleus, anterior cortical nucleus, periamygdaloid cortex, amygdalohippocampal area, and central nucleus (Fig. 3D; Aggleton, 1985).

Afferents. The superficial layer of the medial nucleus receives a relatively heavy projection from the lateral nucleus. The medial nucleus also receives inputs from the basal nucleus, the accessory basal nucleus, and the periamygdaloid cortex (Van Hoesen, 1981; Price and Amaral, 1981; Aggleton, 1985; Pitkänen and Amaral, unpublished observations).

Periamygdaloid Cortex

Since data concerning the intrinsic connectivity of the different parts of the periamygdaloid cortex are very limited, we shall not attempt to separately describe projections to or from each of the subdivisions.

Efferents. The periamygdaloid cortex projects to the parvicellular division of the basal nucleus, the accessory basal nucleus, the medial nucleus, the central nucleus, and the posterior cortical nucleus (Van Hoesen, 1981; Price and Amaral, 1981, unpublished observations).

Afferents. The periamygdaloid cortex receives projections from the lateral nucleus (which projects most heavily to PAC3 but also to PAC2), basal nucleus, accessory basal nucleus, medial nucleus, and central nucleus (Price and Amaral, 1981; Aggleton, 1985; Pitkänen and Amaral, 1990).

Central Nucleus

Efferents. The central nucleus projects to the anterior cortical nucleus, periamygdaloid cortex, amygdalohippocampal area, and anterior amygdaloid area (Fig. 3D). There appear to be very light projections to the lateral nucleus, parvicellular portion of the basal nucleus, and accessory basal nucleus (Price and Amaral, 1981; Aggleton, 1985).

Afferents. The central nucleus is the focus of many of the intrinsic amygdaloid projections. It receives projections from all divisions of the basal nucleus (which projects more heavily to the medial division of the nucleus) and the accessory basal nucleus (which also projects more heavily to the medial division); a light projection to the central nucleus arises from the lateral nucleus, the periamygdaloid cortex, and the medial nucleus (Van Hoesen, 1981; Price and Amaral, 1981, unpublished observations; Aggleton, 1985; Pitkänen and Amaral, 1990).

Posterior Cortical Nucleus and Amygdalohippocampal Area

Efferents. Because of the close proximity of the posterior cortical nucleus and the amygdalohippocampal area, the differentiation of their intrinsic connections has been difficult. There appears to be a projection to the medial nucleus, and a lighter projection to the periamygdaloid cortex (Price and Amaral, unpublished observation).

Afferents. The posterior cortical nucleus receives projections from the accessory basal nucleus and from the periamygdaloid cortex. The amygdalohippocampal area appears to receive projections from the rostroventral lateral nucleus, basal nucleus, accessory basal nucleus, medial nucleus, and central nucleus (Price and Amaral, 1981; Aggleton, 1985).

Other Nuclei

The anterior amygdaloid area. The intrinsic connections of the anterior amygdaloid area are mostly unknown. There do appear, however, to be inputs from the lateral and central nuclei (Aggleton, 1985; Pitkänen and Amaral, unpublished observations). The *intercalated nuclei* receive projections from the lateral nucleus and from the accessory basal nucleus (Aggleton, 1985).

SUBCORTICAL CONNECTIONS OF THE AMYGDALA

In the following sections we review the extrinsic connections of the amygdaloid complex with subcortical structures. We first describe amygdalostriatal connections, followed by sections on the basal forebrain, diencephalon, and finally the brain stem. In this section, more than in the others, we must resort to descriptions provided by data obtained in nonprimate species. Several important projections have simply not been evaluated in the monkey and we felt that for the sake of completeness, the organization of these connections should be reported.

Striatum

It has been known for some time that there is a substantial amygdaloid projection to the ventral parts of the striatum, especially the nucleus accumbens and olfactory tubercle (see summary in Fig. 11; Nauta, 1962; DeOlmos and Ingram, 1972; Krettek and Price, 1978a; Groenewegen et al., 1980; Newman and Winans, 1980; Hemphell et al., 1981). The amygdala also projects, however, to more dorsal and caudal parts of the striatum (Kelly et al., 1982; Russchen and Price, 1984; Parent et al., 1983; Russchen et al., 1985b; Ragsdale and Graybiel, 1988). Some of the amygdaloid projections terminate in the ventral and medial parts of the caudate nucleus and putamen that border the nucleus accumbens, but many amygdalostriatal fibers extend to the caudal part of the ventral putamen, dorsal to the amygdala, and to the entire extent of the body and tail of the caudate nucleus, bordering the stria terminalis (Russchen et al., 1985b). In terms of its extent and density, the amygdalostriatal projection must be considered as one of the most substantial efferents of the amygdala.

The amygdalostriatal projection originates predominantly from the basal and accessory basal nuclei; the central and lateral nuclei provide essentially no projections to the striatum (Parent et al., 1983; Russchen et al., 1985b). The parvicellular division of the basal nucleus projects preferentially to the medial part of the nucleus accumbens, while the magnocellular division of the basal nucleus projects more extensively to the body and tail of the caudate nucleus and to the ventral putamen. Fibers from both divisions overlap in the lateral part of the nucleus accumbens (Russchen et al., 1985b).

In the cat, the amygdaloid fibers are preferentially distributed to specific histochemical compartments within the striatum (Ragsdale and Graybiel, 1988). In the caudate nucleus, for example, the amygdaloid fibers preferentially terminate in the acetylcholinesterase-poor striosomes. These striosomes are not readily visible in the nucleus accumbens, but similar butyrylcholinesterase-rich patches are apparent in the dorsal part of this nucleus, and amygdaloid fibers preferentially end among these patches as well. In addition to the striosomal labeling, there is also a lighter innervation of the matrix compartment. In fact, there are places in the dorsal caudate nucleus where amygdaloid fibers appear to avoid terminating in striosomes.

The amygdala also projects to the ventral pallidum, although this projection is relatively light compared to projections to ventral striatal areas (Russschen et al., 1985a). The nucleus accumbens (which receives a strong amygdaloid input), however, has a substantial projection to the ventral pallidum. Since the ventral pallidum projects to the mediodorsal thalamic nucleus (Russschen et al., 1987), the ventral striato-pallidal system provides another pathway in addition to the direct projection from the amygdala to the mediodorsal nucleus (page 51), by which the amygdala may interact with the mediodorsal nucleus and thereby with the prefrontal cortex.

Basal Forebrain

One aspect of the neuroanatomy of the primate amygdaloid complex that is not widely appreciated is that it provides a major input to the basal forebrain and receives an equally substantial return projection (Figs. 4, 5; Mesulam et al., 1983; Russschen et al., 1985a). The amygdaloid projection is directed heavily, though not exclusively, to the major components of the magnocellular basal forebrain nuclei MBNF (the basal nucleus of Meynert and the nucleus of the horizontal limb of the diagonal band). The projection to the amygdala arises primarily from the anterolateral part of the nucleus basalis. The termination of these fibers is concentrated in the magnocellular division of the basal nucleus, with somewhat lower densities in other areas such as the magnocellular and ventromedial divisions of the accessory basal nuclei (Amaral and Bassett, 1989). As judged by the concentration of the cholinergic marker enzyme choline acetyltransferase, the magnocellular division of the basal nucleus of the amygdala receives perhaps the most substantial cholinergic projection of any forebrain region (Hellendall et al., 1986).

The efferent projection from the amygdala to the magnocellular basal forebrain originates primarily in the parvicellular division of the basal nucleus, the magnocellular division of the accessory basal nucleus, and the central nucleus, although the origin of the projection is not restricted to these nuclei (Russschen et al., 1985a). It is important to emphasize that very few cells that project to the cholinergic basal forebrain are located in the magnocellular division of the basal nucleus, which receives the largest input from the basal forebrain.

The fibers which innervate the cholinergic nuclei sweep through the basal forebrain, and apparently continue on to the thalamus, hypothalamus, and brain stem (Russschen et al., 1985a). While they do not, therefore, terminate within the basal forebrain, the fibers form *en passant* synapses with cells of the magnocellular nuclei (Zaborszky et al., 1984). Most of the fibers are distributed diffusely around and among the magnocellular cell groups, while those originating from the central nucleus tend to be concentrated around, rather than among, the large cell bodies of the cholinergic cell groups (Russschen et al., 1985a).

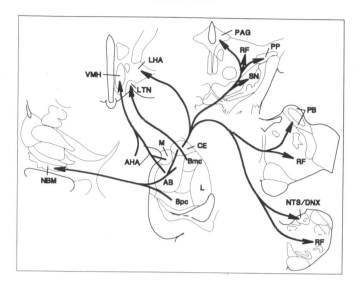

Fig. 4. Summary diagram of the subcortical efferent connections of the monkey amygdala. The source of connections is indicated by the origin of arrows from the prototypical coronal section through the amygdala in the center of the illustration. Terminal zones are indicated by the regional icons arranged around the amygdala section. Moving clockwise from left to right, the icons represent the basal forebrain, hypothalamus, midbrain, pons, and medulla.

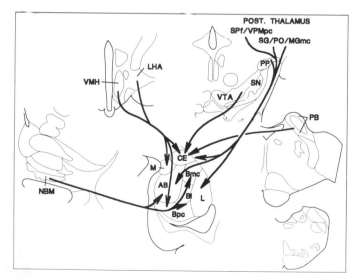

Fig. 5. Summary diagram of the subcortical afferents to the monkey amygdala. The same icons used in Figure 4 are used here as well. The main sites of termination are indicated with arrows in the amygdala.

Diencephalon

Thalamus

Projections to the thalamus. The projections from the amygdala to the mediodorsal nucleus of the thalamus are described in a later section dealing with amygdalocortical connections. In this section we describe projections to thalamic nuclei, especially the midline nuclei, that arise from the central and medial nuclei of the amygdala (Fig. 11).

The central and medial nuclei project to the midline thalamic nuclei, including the superior, inferior, and densocellular parts of the nucleus centralis of Olszewski (1952; Price and Amaral, 1981). Because these nuclei lie immediately medial to the mediodorsal nucleus of the thalamus, experiments with injections of retrograde tracers into the medial part of the mediodorsal nucleus (with likely diffusion of the tracer into the midline nuclei) have often labeled cells in the medial and central nuclei (e.g., Aggleton and Mishkin, 1984; McDonald, 1987). Anterograde tracing experiments indicate, however, that fibers from the central and medial nuclei are restricted to the midline nuclei and do not enter the mediodorsal nucleus. In fact, these projections terminate preferentially rostral to the mediodorsal nucleus within nucleus reuniens and in the caudal part of the centralis nuclear complex (Price and Amaral, 1981; Aggleton and Mishkin, 1984). A light projection to the medial pulvinar nucleus from the central amygdaloid nucleus has also been identified in the monkey (Price and Amaral, 1981).

Thalamic projections to the amygdala. One unusual aspect of amygdaloid neuroanatomy in the primate is that the main thalamic recipient of amygdala projections, the mediodorsal nucleus, does not reciprocate the projection. Other thalamic nuclei, however, do project to the amygdala. These projections have been studied most thoroughly in the rat and cat (Veening, 1978; Ottersen and Ben-Ari, 1979; Russchen, 1982; Yasui et al., 1987; LeDoux et al., 1990a), although there is evidence that similar projections are present in the monkey (Mehler, 1980). Much of the thalamoamygdaloid projection arises in the midline thalamic nuclei that themselves receive fibers from the central and medial amygdaloid nuclei. These fibers end primarily in the central nucleus and adjacent parts of the basal nucleus. In the rat and cat, the parvicellular part of the ventroposterior medial nucleus also projects to the amygdala. This thalamic nucleus is a relay for gustatory/visceral information from the brain stem and is also connected with the gustatory/visceral regions of cortex (Ottersen and Ben-Ari, 1979; Yasui et al., 1987). These thalamoamygdaloid fibers end in a portion of the lateral nucleus that, in the cat, is itself connected with the gustatory/visceral cortex.

Work in the rat and cat indicates that a substantial input to the amygdala originates from cells in the posterior thalamus situated in and around the medial geniculate nucleus. This projection ends in the lateral, accessory basal, medial, and central nuclei (Ottersen and Ben-Ari, 1979; Russchen, 1982; Mehler, 1980; LeDoux et al., 1990a). These posterior thalamic areas receive auditory inputs from the inferior colliculus and the pathway to the amygdala has been implicated in conditioned emotional responses to auditory stimuli (LeDoux et al., 1990b).

Hypothalamus

Projections from the amygdala to the bed nucleus of the stria terminalis and hypothalamus. The bed nucleus of the stria terminalis has many striking anatomical similarities to the central and medial nuclei of the amygdala and is considered by many to be an extension of these nuclei drawn out along the stria terminalis (see Price et al., 1987). Like the central and medial nuclei, the bed nucleus provides a relay for projections from the amygdala to the hypothalamus and brain stem (e.g., Holstege et al., 1985). Most amygdaloid fibers reach the bed nucleus through the stria terminalis, but others run through the ventral amygdalofugal pathway. The amygdaloid projection is organized such that the central and basal nuclei project to the lateral part of the bed nucleus, while the medial and posterior cortical nuclei and the amygdalohippocampal area project to the medial bed nucleus (Krettek and Price, 1978a,b; Weller and Smith, 1982). Other nuclei, including the accessory basal and parvicellular basal nuclei, project to both medial and lateral parts of the bed nucleus.

Medial hypothalamus. Caudal to the bed nucleus, amygdaloid fibers continue into and through the anterior hypothalamus. Fibers originating in the anterior cortical and medial nuclei appear to terminate in the anterior hypothalamus (Price et al., 1991). Some of the fibers may also terminate on dendrites of cells in the supraoptic and paraventricular nuclei (Oldfield and Silverman, 1985).

A more substantial amygdaloid projection terminates in and around the ventromedial hypothalamic nucleus and the premammillary nuclei (Fig. 4). The projection to the ventromedial nucleus can be divided into two components. The first originates in the amygdalohippocampal area and the adjacent ventral subiculum and terminates in the cell-sparse "shell" around the ventromedial nucleus, while the second originates in the medial and accessory basal amygdaloid nuclei and terminates in the cellular "core" of the ventromedial nucleus (Heimer and Nauta, 1969; DeOlmos and Ingram, 1972; McBride and Sutin, 1977; Krettek and Price, 1978a). The fibers to the premammillary nuclei originate in the same nuclei that project to the ventromedial nucleus.

Lateral hypothalamus. The amygdala projects to the full rostrocaudal extent of the lateral hypothalamus (Fig. 4; Krettek and Price, 1978a; Price and Amaral, 1981). This projection originates mainly in the central nucleus, with minor additional contributions from the medial and anterior cortical nuclei (Price et al., 1991). Most of these fibers reach the hypothalamus through the ventral amygdalofugal pathway, but some also run in the stria terminalis. Projections from the central nucleus penetrate the internal capsule from the stria terminalis to enter the lateral hypothalamus (Price and Amaral, 1981). Fibers from the central nucleus also innervate the paramammillary, tuberomammillary, and supramammillary nuclei, before continuing into the ventral midbrain.

The basal nucleus does not contribute substantially to the overall hypothalamic projection but, in the monkey, it does send a heavy, and discrete, projection to the small lateral tuberal nucleus. This projection is complementary to the projection from the central nucleus, which avoids the cell-dense portion of the lateral tuberal nucleus (Price, 1986) and generates a terminal plexus all around the nucleus.

Projections from the hypothalamus to the amygdala. The hypothalamus originates return projections to the amygdala, which appear meager in relation to the density of the amygdalohypothalamic projections. Most of these arise in the ventromedial hypothalamic nucleus and the more caudal parts of the lateral hypothalamic area, and terminate in the central, medial, and accessory basal nuclei and parvicellular division of the basal nucleus (Fig. 5, Amaral et al., 1982; Price et al., 1987).

Brain Stem

Caudal to the hypothalamus, fibers from the central nucleus of the amygdala descend into and through the midbrain, pons, and medulla; some even extend into cervical levels of the spinal cord (Hopkins, 1975; Krettek and Price, 1978a; Price and Amaral, 1981; Mizuno et al., 1985). None of the other amygdaloid nuclei contribute to this projection, but the bed nucleus of the stria terminalis has an essentially similar projection (Holstege et al., 1985). Throughout their course, the fibers innervate a number of structures that have been implicated in autonomic control, including the periaqueductal gray, the parabrachial nucleus, the dorsal vagal nuclei, and the reticular formation. Many of these structures also send ascending fibers to the amygdala (Fig. 4; Mehler, 1980; Norita and Kakamura, 1980).

In the midbrain, the central nucleus projects to the ventral tegmental area and substantia nigra, particularly to the lateral part of the pars compacta of the substantia nigra. Caudal to this, the projection extends into the peripeduncular nucleus and tegmental reticular formation, and then dorsomedially into the periaqueductal gray. In the periaqueductal gray, terminal areas are focused in the ventrolateral and dorsomedial portions, leaving the dorsolateral part relatively free (Price and Amaral, 1981).

The central nucleus projection continues through the pontine reticular formation, and terminates heavily in the parabrachial nuclei located around the superior cerebellar peduncle. A few fibers also extend medially into the nucleus raphe magnus. In the medulla, the projection is distributed to the lateral part of the reticular formation, most heavily to the nucleus of the solitary tract and the dorsal motor nucleus of the vagus (Price and Amaral, 1981).

The amygdaloid projection to the dorsal pons is reciprocated by fibers from the parabrachial nucleus which end in the central nucleus (Norgren, 1976; Nomura et al., 1979; Mehler, 1980; Norita and Kawamura, 1980; Ottersen, 1981; Russchen, 1982). As mentioned earlier, the amygdala also receives a substantial noradrenergic input that terminates in the central and basal amygdaloid nuclei (Fallon et al., 1978) and arises mainly from the locus coeruleus. In the rat, the nucleus of the solitary tract projects directly to the central nucleus (Ricardo and Koh, 1978), but this projection has not been demonstrated in the cat or monkey (Beckstead et al., 1980; Russchen, 1982). However, the primate nucleus of the solitary tract does project to the parabrachial nuclei which, in turn, project to the amygdaloid complex (Fig. 5; Beckstead et al., 1980).

CONNECTIONS WITH THE OLFACTORY SYSTEM
Inputs From the Olfactory Bulb

Although the amygdala in primates is clearly not dominated by olfaction as in some lower animals, it nonetheless has substantial interconnections with several parts of the olfactory system. In particular, there are direct projections from the olfactory bulb to the nucleus of the lateral olfactory tract, anterior cortical nucleus, and most parts of the periamygdaloid cortex (except PACs) (Turner et al., 1978; Price, 1990). As in the piriform cortex and other areas that receive a projection from the olfactory bulb, the fibers end in the superficial portion of layer I (i.e., layer Ia). The nucleus of the lateral olfactory tract and the periamygdaloid cortex also project back to the olfactory bulb (DeOlmos et al., 1978, 1985; Carmichael and Price, unpublished observations in the monkey).

Connections With Primary Olfactory Cortex

In addition to the direct connections between the amygdala and the main or accessory olfactory bulbs, there are substantial associational connections between all parts of the primary olfactory cortex, including the piriform cortex and the superficial amygdaloid structures. These have been best defined in the rat (Price, 1973; Krettek and Price, 1978a; Luskin and Price, 1983), but projections have been demonstrated in the monkey from the piriform cortices to the nucleus of the lateral olfactory tract, anterior cortical nucleus, and the periamygdaloid cortex (Carmichael and Price, unpublished observations). These fibers end in the deep part of layer I (layer Ib) in a position complementary to the fibers from the main and accessory olfactory bulbs. Cells in the deep layers of the piriform cortex also project to the medial and posterior cortical amygdaloid nuclei (Krettek and Price, 1978a; Ottersen, 1982).

THE HIPPOCAMPAL FORMATION

The hippocampal formation* and amygdaloid complex are the most prominent components of the primate medial temporal lobe. Both regions have been implicated in functions such as memory and emotion, and the relative contribution of these structures to such functions remains a matter of intense controversy (see Chapter 17, Murray, this volume). Despite the close physical proximity of the amygdaloid complex and the hippocampal formation, there has been relatively little evidence obtained of anatomical interconnections between the two regions until recently. The first modern experimental demonstration of amygdaloid projections to the hippocampal formation was reported by Krettek and Price (1974, 1978a) in the rat and cat. Thereafter, several papers have appeared that document amygdalohippocampal interconnections in the monkey brain (Rosene and Van Hoesen, 1977; Amaral and Cowan, 1980; Amaral and Price, 1984; Aggleton, 1986; Amaral, 1986; Saunders and Rosene, 1988; Saunders et al., 1988). While many of the connections in the monkey appear to be similar to those reported for nonprimate species, a few projections observed

---

*In this section, the term hippocampal formation refers to a group of cytoarchitectonically distinct but closely anatomically linked regions. The hippocampal formation includes the dentate gyrus, the hippocampus (which is subdivided into fields CA3, CA2, and CA1), the subicular complex (which is divided into the subiculum, presubiculum, and parasubiculum), and the entorhinal cortex [which has been divided into seven cytoarchitectonic divisions (Amaral et al., 1987), which need not be distinguished for the present discussion].

in the monkey have not been reported for the rat or cat. In particular, the accessory basal nucleus of the monkey originates a substantial component of the hippocampally directed projection, and this projection has not been described in the rat.

Projections From the Amygdaloid Complex to the Hippocampal Formation

The Entorhinal Cortex

The predominant interaction between the amygdaloid complex and the hippocampal formation is mediated via the entorhinal cortex (Fig. 6). Within the hippocampal circuit, the entorhinal cortex is the main recipient of extrinsic sensory information arriving from several polysensory neocortical regions (Insausti et al., 1987) and this is then relayed to all of the other hippocampal fields via the perforant path projection (Witter and Amaral, 1991). From the amygdaloid complex, the entorhinal cortex receives projections from the lateral nucleus, accessory basal nucleus, periamygdaloid cortex, anterior cortical and medial nuclei, and the paralaminar nucleus (Insausti et al., 1987; Saunders

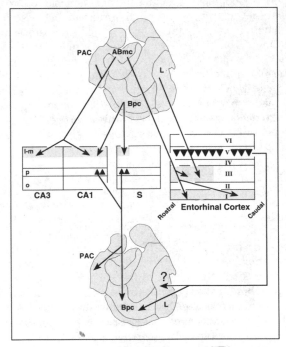

Fig. 6. Summary diagram of the interconnections between the amygdaloid complex and the hippocampal formation. The amygdalohippocampal projections are illustrated at the top and terminal regions are indicated by shading in the boxes representing the hippocampal regions. The projections from the hippocampal formation to the amygdala are illustrated in the bottom portion of the diagram. Cells of origin for these projections are indicated as triangles in the hippocampal boxes.

and Rosene, 1988). A very minor and diffuse projection originates from the basal nucleus. Only the rostral portion of the entorhinal cortex (roughly equivalent to the lateral entorhinal cortex of the rat) receives a prominent amygdaloid projection (Insausti et al., 1987; Saunders and Rosene, 1988).

The largest input to the entorhinal cortex originates in the lateral nucleus, though not all regions of the lateral nucleus contribute to this projection. The main pathway arises from cells located roughly in the caudal half to two-thirds of the lateral nucleus that are situated in a mid to ventral position (dorsoventrally) within the nucleus (see Fig. 1 in Insausti et al., 1987; Fig. 15 in Saunders and Rosene, 1988). The lateral nucleus projection terminates mainly in layer III of the rostral entorhinal cortex, and particularly heavily in the deep half of the layer. Some radially oriented fibers extend through the superficial half of layer III and into the cell-sparse regions of layer II. A more modest projection is directed to layer I (Amaral and Price, 1984; Amaral, 1986; Saunders and Rosene, 1988). As noted by Saunders and Rosene (1988), the lateral nucleus projection to layer III of the rostral entorhinal cortex is complementary to the similar projection which arises from the presubiculum and terminates in layer III of the caudal entorhinal cortex.

The accessory basal nucleus provides the next largest input to the entorhinal cortex. At rostral levels of the entorhinal cortex, the accessory basal projection is directed both to layer III and to layer I. Unlike the lateral nucleus projection, however, fibers from the accessory nucleus also innervate caudal levels of the entorhinal cortex but this projection is preferentially directed to layer I. The laminar termination of the other amygdaloid projections to the entorhinal cortex is not presently clear, although their density is far less than those from the lateral and accessory basal nuclei. The medial nucleus apparently projects to layer I of rostromedial portions of the entorhinal cortex (Saunders and Rosene, 1988) and the periamygdaloid cortex provides a light input to layers II and III of the rostral entorhinal cortex (Amaral, 1986).

The Subicular Complex and Hippocampus

Of the remaining fields of the hippocampal formation, the dentate gyrus does not appear to receive an input from the amygdala. The hippocampus and the subicular complex, however, do receive substantial amygdaloid inputs.

Cells located primarily in the magnocellular division of the accessory basal nucleus give rise to a projection that travels ventrally, through the region of the amygdalohippocampal area and ultimately enters the hippocampal formation through its dorsomedial attachment to the amygdala. The fibers then form a relatively compact bundle that occupies stratum lacunosum-moleculare of the hippocampus (Amaral, 1986, see Fig. 2; Saunders et al., 1988). The bundle travels medially through the dorsomedially situated components of CA1 and subiculum† and ventrally to ultimately innervate CA3, CA2, and CA1. These fibers

---

†It is possible and even likely that fibers passing through the dorsomedial subiculum and CA1 form contacts with the cells in this region. If the subicular cells are contacted, they may be homologous with the ventral subicular region that, in the rat and cat, is preferentially innervated by amygdaloid fibers (Krettek and Price, 1974, 1977).

do not appear to be en route to some other nonhippocampal terminal regions and are presumably, therefore, terminating on the distal apical dendrites of hippocampal pyramidal cells. However, it should be pointed out that there is currently no electron microscopic evidence to confirm whether these fibers are terminating on cells in all of the hippocampal fields or, for example, traveling through CA3 and CA2 to terminate on cells in CA1. This projection extends throughout virtually the full rostrocaudal length of the hippocampus.

A second amygdaloid projection, arising mainly from the parvicellular division of the basal nucleus (Amaral and Cowan, 1980) and from the periamygdaloid cortex, terminates in a narrow zone at the border of CA1 and the subiculum (Amaral, 1986; Saunders et al., 1988). In this region, the pyramidal cell layers of CA1 and the subiculum partially overlap in a mitered fashion, with the CA1 cells lying superficially to the subicular cells. The projection from the basal nucleus and periamygdaloid cortex terminates among the CA1 cell bodies and in the deep portion of the overlying molecular layer. It should be noted tht this projection involves a relatively narrow extent of CA1 and the subiculum [a region that Rosene and colleagues (Rosene and Van Hoesen, 1987) label the prosubiculum]. While cells in the remainder of the CA1 field are potentially innervated by fibers originating in the accessory basal nucleus (described above), it is important to emphasize that most of the subiculum is devoid of an amygdaloid input. Moreover, while our own autoradiographic preparations have indicated that the presubiculum and parasubiculum may receive a light amygdaloid projection (Amaral, 1986), the origin of these fibers is unknown and they are undoubtedly few in number.

Projections of the Hippocampal Formation to the Amygdala

The projections from the hippocampal formation to the amygdala are clearly not reciprocal (Fig. 6). In fact, judging from standard indices of anatomical connectivity, i.e., the density of anterogradely labeled fibers or the numbers of retrogradely labeled cells, the hippocampal projection to the amygdala would be considered substantially weaker than the projections in the opposite direction.

Entorhinal Cortex

If an injection of a retrograde tracer is placed into the lateral nucleus of the amygdala, large numbers of retrogradely labeled cells are observed in layer V of most of the transverse and rostrocaudal extent of the entorhinal cortex (Pitkänen and Amaral, unpublished observations). However, when the converse experiment is attempted and an anterograde tracer is injected into the entorhinal cortex, a strange pattern of labeling is observed in the lateral nucleus. Fibers from the entorhinal cortex join the subamygdaloid white matter that separates the amygdala from the entorhinal cortex and travel to the lateral aspect of the amygdala. The fibers then form various-sized fascicles that pierce the lateral nucleus en route to the substantia innominata and other basal forebrain regions. Thus, fibers from the entorhinal cortex pass through much of the lateral nucleus and would therefore have the potential of forming *en passant* contacts with cells in the nucleus. However, the fibers are relatively coarse, mainly smooth, and certainly do not contribute a diffuse terminal plexus to the lateral nucleus.

It is difficult to conclude, therefore, whether the entorhinal fibers form synaptic contacts with cells of the lateral nucleus or simply pass through the nucleus. Since there are alternative routes for the entorhinal cortex fibers to take to the basal forebrain, it would be surprising if these fibers only coincidentally travel through the lateral nucleus without forming any synaptic contacts. The entorhinal cortex also contributes a more standard, though light, terminal plexus to the basal nucleus that is situated mainly in its parvicellular division.

Subicular Complex and Hippocampus

The projection to the amygdala from the subicular complex and hippocampus arises from a relatively limited region of these fields (Saunders et al., 1988). Throughout most of the rostrocaudal extent of the hippocampus, the only cells that give rise to projections to the amygdala are situated along the border of the subiculum and CA1. Cells in this region project to the parvicellular division of the basal nucleus and to the periamygdaloid cortex (Rosene and Van Hoesen, 1977; Saunders et al., 1988). Since these CA1/subiculum cells are located in the region which also receives a projection from the parvicellular division of the basal nucleus and the periamygdaloid cortex, this connection is potentially a reciprocal one.

An additional projection to the amygdala originates from a population of cells in the most rostral portion of the hippocampal formation that are located dorsally and medially. These cells are likely to be the most rostral extension of CA1 and/ or the subiculum which, due to the complex geometry of the uncal hippocampal formation, are separated from the main portion of the field. In addition to the other projections from CA1 and the subiculum, these cells may also innervate the parvicellular division of the basal nucleus (Saunders et al., 1988).

Summary

Several amygdaloid nuclei, but most prominently the lateral nucleus, magnocellular division of the accessory basal nucleus, and the parvicellular division of the basal nucleus, contribute projections to the hippocampal formation. The main projection, coming from the lateral nucleus, is to the rostral entorhinal cortex, but significant projections are directed to the hippocampus and at least to the most proximal portion of the subiculum. The hippocampal projection back to the amygdala, by comparison, seems rather meager. The main recipient of hippocampal innervation is the parvicellular division of the basal nucleus, which receives inputs from the CA1/subiculum border zone and the entorhinal cortex. The same regions also project to the periamygdaloid cortex and perhaps lightly to the parvicellular division of the basal nucleus. While many fibers from the entorhinal cortex travel through the lateral nucleus of the amygdala, they have the morphological appearance of fibers of passage. Since there is no clear terminal plexus generated by these fibers, the extent to which the entorhinal cortex communicates with cells of the lateral nucleus is unclear at this time. Thus, there appears to be a polarity to the amygdalohippocampal interconnection. The amygdala is in a position to have substantially greater influence on the hippocampal formation than vice versa.

AMYGDALOCORTICAL INTERACTIONS

Despite the fact that it has been over 35 years since Whitlock and Nauta (1956) demonstrated that the anterior temporal neocortex of the monkey projects directly to the amygdala, and many subsequent papers have convincingly demonstrated the widespread interconnections of the monkey amygdala with much of the neocortical mantle (Pandya et al., 1973; Leichnetz and Astruc, 1977; Herzog and Van Hoesen, 1976; Turner et al., 1980; Aggleton et al., 1980; Van Hoesen, 1981; Avendaño et al., 1983; Amaral and Price, 1984; Tigges et al., 1983; Friedman et al., 1986; Iwai and Yukie, 1987), there is little or no available information on the contribution of the amygdala to neocortical function. Moreover, the mistaken view that projections from the amygdala are mainly directed to subcortical structures such as the hypothalamus is still prevalent in texts. As will become clear in the following section, in the primate (and presumably in the human), much of the amygdala's input arrives from various unimodal and polymodal regions of the frontal, cingulate, insular, and temporal neocortex. Similarly, much of the output of the primate amygdala is directed to an even broader expanse of the neocortex. Thus, it is reasonable to predict that the amygdaloid complex might influence both early stages of sensory processing as well as higher level cognitive processing.

There are a number of ways that the amygdalocortical anatomy can be presented. We have chosen to organize our description according to cortical regions. Embedded within these descriptions are discussions of unimodal sensory versus polymodal sensory innervation and issues of topographic distribution of these systems within the amygdala. At the end of the section, we summarize the major organizational principles of the amygdalocortical system.

Temporal and Occipital Cortical Connections

The amygdaloid complex is reciprocally interconnected with large portions of the temporal lobe (Fig. 7). Connections are established with unimodal sensory cortices such as the visually related area TE of the inferotemporal cortex, as well as with a variety of polysensory regions such as the perirhinal cortex and the cortex lining the dorsal bank of the superior temporal sulcus.

Amygdolopetal Connections

When large injections of HRP are focused in the lateral nucleus of the amygdala (Aggleton et al., 1980), retrogradely labeled cells are observed in the anterior half of the inferotemporal cortex (area TE). Since area TE is a region of unimodal visual processing (Pandya and Yeterian, 1985), this connection appears to be the major route of entry for unimodal visual information to the amygdala. Unfortunately, it is not clear whether all portions of TE project to the amygdala. Taking together all of the descriptions of anterograde degeneration after lesions of the temporal lobe or of anterograde transport of tracer following injections of HRP or [³H]-amino acids into the inferotemporal cortex, it would appear that most of the inferior temporal cortex located anterior to the rostral limit of the occipital temporal sulcus (from about the level of the uncus of the

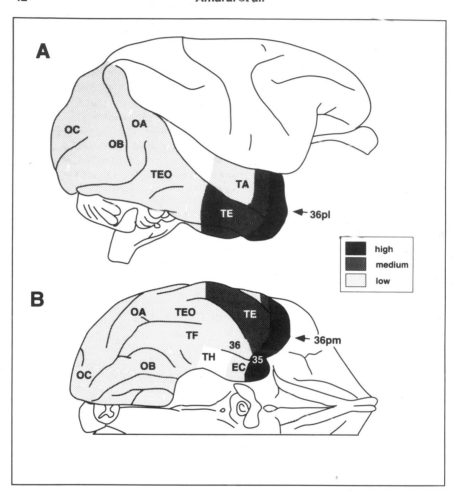

Fig. 7. Line drawings of the macaque monkey brain showing the lateral surface (**top**) and the ventral surface (**bottom**). The shading patterns indicate the regions within the temporal and occipital lobes that receive direct amygdaloid input; the denser the shading pattern, the heavier the terminal labeling (key at middle right). Note that in the caudal part of area TA and in the caudal part of the entorhinal cortex (EC) and throughout TH, the projections are extremely light or lacking altogether.

hippocampus) does contribute to the amygdaloid projection (Herzog and Van Hoesen, 1976; Van Hoesen, 1981; Turner et al., 1980; Iwai and Yukie, 1987).

The TE projection, and most of the other cortical projections, originate mainly from cells located in layer III; some variable amount of the projection also arises in layer V. Projections from caudal levels of TE terminate exclusively in the dorsal half of the lateral nucleus. Projections from more rostral levels of TE, however, especially the ventromedial portion of the field, may also terminate in the dorsal tip of the magnocellular division of the basal nucleus.

The connections between the auditory regions of the temporal lobe and the amygdala are not as well defined as visual connections. Primary auditory cortex is situated in the caudal portion of the superior temporal gyrus and is ringed by unimodal association areas (Pandya and Yeterian, 1985). Aggleton et al. (1980) found no retrogradely labeled cells in primary auditory cortex or immediately adjacent association cortex even after large injections of HRP into the amygdala. Similarly, Turner et al. (1980) found no degeneration in the amygdala following selective lesions of primary auditory and surrounding cortex. These lesions did lead, however, to projections to more rostral levels of the superior temporal gyrus. These rostral levels of the superior temporal gyrus project, in turn, to the ventrolateral portion of the lateral nucleus (Turner et al., 1980; see also Van Hoesen, 1981). While there is little physiological evidence dealing with the functional characterization of the rostral portion of the superior temporal gyrus, on anatomical grounds it appears that it may function, in part, as unimodal auditory association cortex (Pandya and Yeterian, 1985). Thus, projections from this region may provide the major auditory input to the amygdala and the projection terminates in a portion of the lateral nucleus that is distinct, at least in part, from the terminal field for the visual input.

The amygdaloid complex receives additional projections from so-called "polysensory" association cortices of the temporal lobe. The justification for calling these regions polysensory is that they have been consistently shown to receive projections from two or more unimodal association areas, or from several other polysensory areas (Pandya and Kuypers, 1969; Jones and Powell, 1970; Seltzer and Pandya, 1976; Van Hoesen et al., 1975; Turner et al., 1980; Mufson and Mesulam, 1982; Galaburda and Pandya, 1983). These areas include the perirhinal cortex (areas 35 and 36) located lateral to the rhinal sulcus, the parahippocampal cortex (areas TF and TH), which forms the caudal half of the parahippocampal gyrus, the cortex forming the dorsal bank of the superior temporal sulcus (areas TPO, POa, etc., of Seltzer and Pandya, 1978) and the cortex of the temporal pole. The temporal polar region is poorly understood anatomically and functionally. Insausti et al. (1987) have pointed out that the medial aspect of the temporal pole has cytoarchitectonic characteristics similar to those of the perirhinal cortex and have labeled this region area 36pm (medial polar division of area 36).

Both the medial and lateral portions of the temporal pole contribute heavy projections to the amygdala (Turner et al., 1980; Van Hoesen, 1981; Pitkänen and Amaral, unpublished observations). The projection is heaviest to the lateral nucleus and focused in the ventromedial portion of the nucleus. The accessory basal nucleus, especially the magnocellular division, also receives a prominent projection and the parvicellular division of the basal nucleus appears to receive a more modest input. From progressively more caudal levels of the perirhinal cortex (areas 36r and 36c of Insausti et al., 1987) the projection to the amygdala decreases in size and is more exclusively distributed to the lateral nucleus (Pitkänen and Amaral, unpublished observations). Areas TF and TH of the parahippocampal cortex contribute relatively meager projections to the amygdala. Unlike area TE, most of the cells of origin for the parahippocampal cortex projections are located in layer V (Aggleton et al., 1980). The projection does not terminate in the lateral nucleus but ends almost exclusively in the basal nucleus.

The cortex forming the dorsal bank of the superior temporal sulcus, especially in the anterior half of the temporal lobe, contributes a strong projection to the amygdala (Turner et al., 1980; Van Hoesen, 1981; Aggleton et al., 1980; Amaral et al., 1983). The projection is heaviest to the lateral nucleus with additional termination in the magnocellular division of the accessory basal nucleus and lighter projections to the remainder of the accessory basal and basal nuclei.

Amygdalofugal Projections

Perhaps one of the most surprising anatomical findings concerning the monkey amygdala is that it projects to virtually all levels of the visual cortex (Fig. 7). Early studies by Mizuno et al. (1981) and Tigges et al. (1982, 1983) demonstrated retrogradely labeled cells in the magnocellular division of the basal nucleus following large injections of retrograde tracers such as HRP into primary visual cortex (area 17, V1) or prestriate cortex of the macaque monkey, chimpanzee, or squirrel monkey. Subsequently, Amaral and Price (1984) demonstrated with the anterograde autoradiographic technique that the magnocellular division of the basal nucleus gives rise to projections to much of the inferior temporal cortex which continue into the prestriate and striate cortex of the macaque monkey. These findings have been confirmed by Iwai and Yukie (1987), who placed retrograde tracer injections into many visually related cortices of the temporal and occipital lobes. Moreover, in a recent series of studies (Amaral, unpublished observations) we placed pairs of fluorescent tracer injections into different levels of the temporal and occipital cortices. The results of all of these studies are consistent with the following conclusions. First, the amygdala appears to project to all portions of the visually related temporal and occipital neocortex (Fig. 7). Second, the projection is distributed in a gradient fashion, with the heaviest projections going to the anterior temporal lobe and progressively lighter projections going to more caudal levels of the visual cortex. Third, the projections to caudal levels of the visual cortex (to area TEO and caudally) originate exclusively from the basal nucleus, especially from the magnocellular division of the nucleus. Projections to rostral levels of the inferior temporal cortex, however, also originate in the accessory basal nucleus. Fourth, the cells of origin for the visual cortex projection are topographically organized. Cells projecting to TE, for example, are located rostral to cells projecting to TEO. Fifth, by using two distinct tracers in each experiment, it has been determined that largely independent populations of cells in the basal nucleus project to different parts of the visual cortex, i.e., double-labeled cells were an infrequent occurrence so the amygdaloid projection to the visual cortex does not appear to be diffusely distributed.

Two points concerning the organization of these projections should be emphasized. The first is that the amygdala projects to a far greater extent of the visual cortex than from which it receives a projection. The second point is that the cells of the lateral nucleus, which receive the bulk of the visual input, do not originate the return projection to visual cortex. The cells of the basal nucleus which project to visual cortex receive either no direct visual input (those in

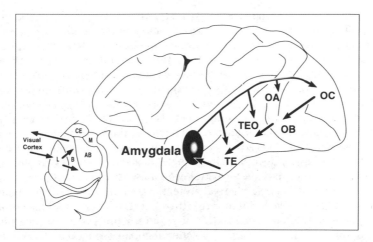

Fig. 8. Schematic illustration showing the relationship of the amygdala with the visually related cortices of the temporal and occipital lobes. Visual information is processed in a hierarchical fashion in cortical regions at progressively greater distances (OB OA TEO TE) from the primary visual cortex (OC). The amygdaloid complex receives a substantial input from the highest level of the hierarchy (area TE). This information enters the amygdala via the lateral nucleus (see the drawing of the amygdaloid complex at lower left). A projection back to the visual cortex originates in the basal nucleus and this projection extends to all levels of the visually related cortex in the temporal and occipital lobes. Within the amygdala, prominent projections between the lateral and basal nuclei potentially "close the loop" on amygdaloid interconnections with the visual cortex.

the intermediate and parvicellular divisions of the nucleus) or only minor input from the most rostral levels of the temporal lobe (the dorsally located cells in the magnocellular division). Closing the loop between the amygdala and visual cortex, therefore, requires one or more stages of intrinsic processing within the amygdala (Fig. 8).

The amygdala's projection to auditory cortex has not been studied using retrograde tracers. However, the amygdala does project to the rostral half of the superior temporal gyrus and these projections extend back, albeit very lightly, into primary auditory cortex and immediately adjacent association cortex (Amaral and Price, 1984). As in the visual system, however, a much heavier projection is directed to more rostral levels of the superior temporal gyrus than to the caudal periauditory regions. While the amount of data is very limited, it would appear that the interactions of the amygdala with visual regions of the temporal lobe are substantially greater than with auditory-related regions.

Amygdalofugal projections to the polysensory regions of the temporal lobe reciprocate, in large part, the polysensory inputs directed to the amygdala. Thus, the amygdala projects heavily to the temporal polar cortex (Amaral and Price, 1984). Moreover, the amygdaloid projection to the medial, perirhinal portion of the temporal pole (area 36pm of Insausti et al., 1987) is much heavier than the projection to the lateral component (Morán et al., 1987). Interestingly, the projections to the temporal pole originate mainly from the lateral and accessory basal nuclei (Morán et al., 1987). Unlike the projection to area TE, little or none of the temporal polar projection originates in the basal nucleus. Thus, the amygdaloid projection to the temporal polar cortex is more reminiscent of the projection to the entorhinal cortex (which also originates in the lateral and accessory basal nuclei) than the amygdala's projections to sensory neocortex (which arise predominantly from the basal nucleus).

The amygdaloid projection to the temporal polar portion of perirhinal cortex continues caudally into rostroventral levels of the perirhinal cortex that lie deep to the amygdala and adjacent to rostral levels of the entorhinal cortex. The projection rapidly decreases in strength at more caudal levels of the perirhinal cortex. The projection to rostral area 35 originates in the lateral, basal, and accessory basal nuclei, whereas projections to area 36 originate mainly in the basal and accessory basal nuclei (Suzuki and Amaral, unpublished observations). The amygdala contributes a very minor projection to area TF and almost nothing to TH of the parahippocampal cortex (Amaral and Price, 1984). This projection originates exclusively in the basal nucleus (Suzuki and Amaral, unpublished observations). The amygdala also contributes a projection to the polysensory regions located along the dorsal bank of the superior temporal sulcus (Amaral and Price, 1984). However, the projection appears to be relatively minor and directed mainly to the rostral half of the temporal lobe.

The amygdalocortical fibers directed to temporal lobe regions terminate most heavily along the border of layers I and II. Although in regions with particularly heavy inputs, such as the temporal polar portion of perirhinal cortex, there is additional lighter labeling in layers V and VI.

Frontal, Insular, and Cingulate Connections

Amygdalofugal Projections

The amygdala has a widespread projection to frontal, insular, and cingulate cortices. Within this larger territory, four regions receive the heaviest amygdaloid projection: the agranular insular cortex, the lateral orbital cortex, the medial orbital cortex, and the medial wall of the frontal lobe (Amaral and Price, 1984).

The agranular insula extends rostrally to occupy the caudal part of the orbital cortex, and can be subdivided into four areas based on cytoarchitectonic and connectional differences: Iav, Iad, Iap, and Ias (Carmichael and Price, 1991b). All of these areas are densely innervated by the amygdala, although from different amygdaloid nuclei.

The lateral orbital cortex, according to the terminology of Walker (1940), consists mostly of area 12 (see Carmichael and Price, 1991a,b). The medial orbital cortex contains Walker's area 14 and part of area 13. Walker's original area 13 has been subdivided into three regions (Fig. 10A): areas 13a and 13b, which are situated medially and receive a substantial amygdaloid projection, and a more laterally positioned area 13 proper, which receives very little amygdaloid input.

The region on the medial wall of the hemisphere that receives amygdaloid input consists of areas 24, 25, and 32, located rostral and ventral to the corpus callosum, and area 24 of the anterior cingulate gyrus (Vogt et al., 1987).

Moving away from the four heavily innervated regions described above, the density of the amygdaloid projection falls off gradually in all directions (Fig. 9). In the insula, the projection fades out caudally through the dysgranular and granular fields. The projection to the orbital cortex and medial wall diminishes over rostral parts of areas 12, 14, 24, and 32 and also fades laterally toward the principal sulcus. The projection to the cingulate gyrus decreases caudally toward area 23. It is important to emphasize that several areas of the frontal cortex receive little or no amygdaloid input. Since the area of innervation fades out before the frontal pole, for example, area 10 appears to be completely devoid of a projection from the amygdala. In the central part of the orbital cortex, areas 11 and 13 receive only a light and patchy input. This contrasts with the much heavier innervation of regions that virtually surround areas 11 and 13. Dorsolateral regions of the prefrontal cortex (areas 8, 9, 45, 46, and the premotor cortex, area 6) also receive only a patchy and insubstantial projection.

The distinction of heavily and lightly innervated cortical regions is also highlighted by the pattern of laminar termination of amygdaloid fibers. As in the temporal lobe, all areas that receive an amygdaloid input receive terminations at the border of layers I and II. In those four regions that receive a dense amygdalocortical projection, however, fibers also terminate in layer V and VI (Amaral and Price, 1984).

The location of the cells of origin for the amygdalofugal projections (Fig. 10) can be summarized from the findings of several studies in which injections of retrograde tracers have been placed into frontal, insular, or cingulate areas (Mufson et al., 1981; Friedman et al., 1986; Carmichael and Price, 1989; Barbas and DeOlmos, 1990). The basal nucleus projects to all of the frontal, cingulate, and insular areas in receipt of an amygdaloid input (Mufson et al., 1981; Friedman et al., 1986; Carmichael and Price, 1989; Barbas and DeOlmos, 1990). The cells giving rise to different components of this projection form partially overlapping clusters within the basal nucleus. The clusters are organized, however, to reflect a topographic organization with respect to the innervated regions (Carmichael and Price, 1989; Barbas and DeOlmos, 1990). Thus, the agranular insular cortex receives a projection from the most ventromedial part of the basal nucleus and progressively more rostral orbital areas receive projections from progressively more dorsal parts of the basal nucleus; the light projection to prefrontal areas 46 and 8 originates from the extreme dorsal part of the nucleus (Barbas and DeOlmos, 1990; Carmichael and Price, unpublished observations). There is also a mediolateral dimension to the topography. Thus, the medial portion of orbital cortex receives a projection from medial parts of the basal nucleus and projections to the lateral orbital areas originate in the lateral portion of the basal nucleus. Finally, cells projecting to the medial wall of the frontal cortex or to the orbital cortex are situated in the mid-dorsoventral part of the basal nucleus. But those projecting to the medial wall tend to lie caudal to those projecting to the orbital cortex (Carmichael and Price, 1989; Barbas and DeOlmos, 1990).

The accessory basal nucleus also contributes projections to the frontal and cingulate cortices and cells located in the magnocellular, parvicellular, and ventromedial subdivisions of the nucleus project to different cortical areas (Fig.

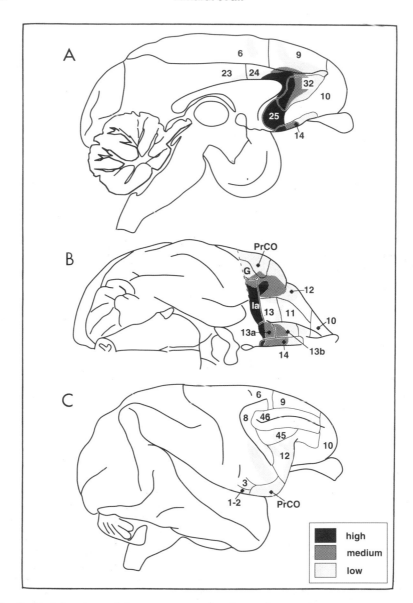

Fig. 9. Line drawings of the macaque monkey brain showing the medial surface (**A**), ventral surface (**B**), and lateral surface (**C**). The dashed line at the temporal pole in panel B indicates that the temporal polar region has been shortened to allow visualization of the insular cortex. The regions of the frontal, insular, and cingulate cortex that receive amygdaloid projections are indicated by shading patterns. The relative strength of projections to the various cortical regions is indicated by the three different gray levels used for shading (key at bottom right).

10). The magnocellular division of the accessory basal nucleus originates most of the cortical projections and these are distributed widely to several regions, including the agranular insula, the medial orbital cortex, and the ventromedial portion of the medial wall of the prefrontal cortex (Mufson et al., 1981; Porrino et al., 1981; Carmichael and Price, 1989; Barbas and DeOlmos, 1990). The parvicellular division of the accessory basal nucleus projects to area 14 (Carmichael and Price, 1989, unpublished observations) and the ventromedial division of the accessory basal nucleus projects only to areas 14, Iap, and area 12 (Carmichael and Price, unpublished observations).

The lateral nucleus projects to a band of cortex stretching from the medial orbital areas 13a and 13b, to the caudal orbital cortex, and all divisions of the insula (Fig. 10; Mufson et al., 1981; Barbas and DeOlmos, 1990; Carmichael and Price, unpublished observations). The cells giving rise to this projection are located in the dorsomedial part of the lateral nucleus. The projection is heaviest to the rostral insular cortex and tapers off both caudally and rostrally, with the medial orbital areas 13a and 13b receiving a minor input.

The medial and anterior cortical nuclei and periamygdaloid cortex project most heavily to the agranular insula (Mufson et al., 1981), particularly Iap (Carmichael and Price, unpublished observations).

Amygdalopetal Connections

In general, projections from the frontal, cingulate, and insular cortices appear to reciprocate the amygdalocortical projections (Aggleton et al., 1980; Mufson et al., 1981; Van Hoesen, 1981). However, the topographic organization of the corticoamygdaloid projections has not yet been precisely defined and it remains unclear whether the amygdaloid cells which originate the amygdalocortical projections are the same that receive cortical inputs; there are some good examples in the literature where this is clearly not the case (see below).

Within the insula, the rostral insula projects heavily to the dorsomedial part of the lateral nucleus, the parvicellular division of the basal nucleus, and the medial nucleus. The posterior insula projects almost exclusively to the lateral nucleus (Mufson et al., 1981; Van Hoesen, 1981). The caudal insular projection deserves further comment because it may provide the major route for somatosensory information to reach the amygdala. As Friedman et al. (1986) have pointed out, the second somatosensory area is reciprocally connected with both the granular and dysgranular insular cortices. Since these regions both project to the lateral nucleus, they provide the most direct route for somatosensory information to reach the amygdala. Friedman et al. (1986) further observed that the regions of the lateral nucleus, which receive inputs from the somatosensory portions of the insula, do not give rise to projections back to the insula. Rather, cells located primarily in the parvicellular division of the basal nucleus actually originated the return projection to the insula.

The caudal orbital cortex projects to the basal nucleus, magnocellular division of the accessory basal nucleus, and dorsomedial portion of the lateral nucleus (Van Hoesen, 1981; Carmichael and Price, unpublished observations). There is some evidence that the rostral insula and caudal orbital cortex may project to the central nucleus (Mufson et al., 1981; Van Hoesen, 1981). The cin-

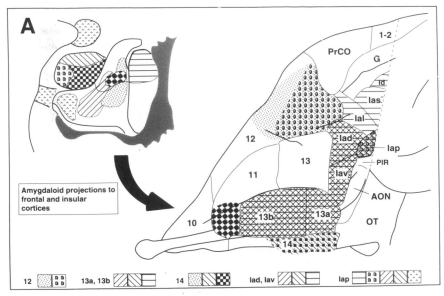

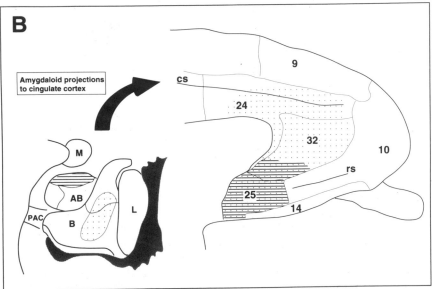

Fig. 10. A,B: These illustrations demonstrate the amygdaloid origin of projections to different portions of the orbitofrontal cortex (A) or to the cingulate cortex (B) and were generated by combining data from numerous experiments in which retrograde tracers were injected into individual frontal cortical regions. We should point out that such experiments provide a clear indication of the origin of the projections but may not demonstrate the full extent of their terminations. **A:** The origin and termination of amygdaloid projections to frontal and insular cortical areas is indicated by similar shading patterns in the two diagrams. When a retrograde tracer was injected into area 14, for example, retrogradely

gulate gyrus projects to the magnocellular division of the basal nucleus (Pandya et al., 1973), whereas the medial wall of the prefrontal cortex projects to both the magnocellular divisions of the basal and accessory basal nuclei (Van Hoesen, 1981). Finally, area 46 projects to the magnocellular division of the basal nucleus (Van Hoesen, 1981).

Amygdalocortical Interactions Mediated Through the Mediodorsal Thalamic Nucleus

In addition to the extensive direct interconnections between the amygdala and the prefrontal cortex, the amygdala can also influence the frontal cortex through connections via the thalamus (Fig. 11). The amygdala projects to the mediodorsal thalamic nucleus (MD), which in turn projects to the prefrontal cortex. These projections were first described from axonal degeneration experiments (Fox, 1940; Nauta, 1961, 1972) and have been extensively studied with axonal transport methods (Krettek and Price, 1977; Porrino et al., 1981; Aggleton and Mishkin, 1984; Russchen et al., 1987). Although the amygdaloid cells that project to MD appear to be different from those that project to the frontal cortex (see below), the two sets of cells are interspersed within several of the amygdaloid nuclei.

The projection to MD arises from almost all of the amygdaloid nuclei but especially the lateral, basal, and accessory basal nuclei and the periamygdaloid cortex. The only possible exceptions are the central and medial nuclei. [As noted earlier, these nuclei do project to the medial thalamus but most, if not all, of the fibers end in the midline thalamic nuclei located medial to MD (Price and Amaral, 1981; Russchen et al., 1987)]. The amygdaloid projection to MD originates from large cells that are scattered throughout the amygdaloid complex. The transmitter used by these cells is unknown, although it is probably not glutamate (McDonald, 1987; Ray et al., 1991). This is unlike the cells that give rise to the amygdalocortical projections, which do appear to be glutamatergic (Carnes and Price, 1991).

Within MD, the amygdaloid fibers terminate in the medial, magnocellular part of the nucleus, which, in turn, projects to the same orbital and medial prefrontal cortical areas that receive direct projections from the amygdala (Porrino et al., 1981; Goldman-Rakic and Porrino, 1985; Aggleton and Mishkin, 1984; Russchen et al., 1987). There is a broad and somewhat overlapping organization in the amygdalothalamic projection such that cells situated dorsally in the amygdala project to ventral parts of MD and ventrally situated cells project dorsally in the thalamus. The amygdala projection terminates predominantly in the rostral half of MD, although some fibers extend into the caudal part of the

---

labeled cells were mainly observed in the parvicellular division of the accessory basal nucleus. Several cortical regions received input from two or more amygdaloid nuclei. Because it is difficult to distinguish the overlying shading patterns, a key is presented below. Injections of tracer into area 13a or 13b, for example, result in retrogradely labeled cells in the mid-portion of the basal nucleus, the dorsal portion of the lateral nucleus, and the magnocellular division of the accessory basal nucleus. **B:** The origin of projections to the cingulate cortex are demonstrated in the same way.

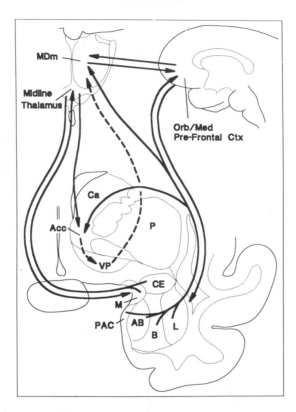

Fig. 11. Various routes through which the amygdaloid complex can influence the function of the frontal lobe are demonstrated. First, the amygdala has direct reciprocal connections with various regions of the orbital and medial frontal lobe. Second, the amygdala projects to the mediodorsal nucleus of the thalamus which, in turn, projects to the same regions of the frontal lobe that receive a direct amygdaloid input. Third, many amygdaloid nuclei project to the nucleus accumbens either directly or via the midline thalamus. The nucleus accumbens projects heavily to the ventral pallidum which, in turn, projects to the mediodorsal nucleus of the thalamus.

nucleus. Fibers from subregions of the amygdala tend to be distributed in two to four discontinuous zones situated at different rostrocaudal levels of the nucleus (Aggleton and Mishkin, 1984; Russchen et al., 1987). Within these zones, the fibers generate terminal fields that are concentrated in smaller patches.

Because the amygdalothalamic, amygdalocortical, and thalamocortical projections involving MD and the prefrontal cortex are all topographically organized, an important question is whether the direct and transthalamic pathways are closely correlated with each other, i.e., does an area of the amygdala that projects to a given region of the cortex also project to the part of MD that projects to the same region of cortex? Experiments in which several of these projections were demonstrated in the same animal with different axonal tracers indicate that the direct and transthalamic pathways from the amygdala to the orbital cortex are in register with each other. However, projections to the medial prefrontal cortex (including the prelimbic and anterior cingulate areas) arise from the most caudal and dorsal part of MD, which does not receive fibers from the amygdala (Ray and Price, 1990). Therefore, although these medial prefrontal cortical areas receive a substantial direct amygdaloid projection, there is apparently little or no indirect communications with them via the amygdala to MD to frontal cortex pathway.

Summary of Cortical Connections

The primate amygdala is massively interconnected with the neocortex. It receives unimodal sensory input from the visual, auditory, and somatosensory systems from relatively advanced levels in the hierarchy of unimodal sensory processing [the olfactory input is organized in a different fashion since it origi-nates from very early stages in olfactory processing (e.g., the olfactory bulb) and the projections terminate in superficial structures such as the periamygdaloid cortex rather than the deep nuclei]. Thus, in the visual system, the amygdala does not receive input from the primary visual cortex or even from the prestriate areas but receives inputs primarily from anterior portions of area TE.

The monkey amygdala also originates projections that are directed to unimodal sensory cortices. The surprising aspect of the return projection is that the amyg-dala projects to much more of the cortical mantle than from which it receives inputs. In the visual system there is substantial evidence that the amygdala pro-jects to virtually all visually related areas of the temporal and occipital cortex. Thus, the amygdala potentially can modulate sensory processing at a very early stage in the cortical hierarchy.

Where appropriate experiments have been conducted, it appears quite clear that the projections from sensory cortex terminate on cells in the lateral nucleus which do not originate the return projection to cortex. This again is most clear in the visual system, where the major portion of the visual input to the amyg-dala terminates in the lateral nucleus but the projection back to visual cortex originates mainly in the basal nucleus. Thus, one or more stages of intrinsic processing must take place in the amygdala before the amygdalocortical loop can be closed.

There are also very substantial connections between the amygdala and polysensory regions of the temporal, insular, cingulate, and frontal lobes. Inter-estingly, while the lateral nucleus does not project to unimodal sensory corti-ces, it does project to many of the polysensory regions such as the agranular insula and orbital cortex. These polysensory regions also receive inputs from the basal nucleus and it will be of interest to learn whether the neurons that originate projections to unimodal cortices also contribute to the polysensory cortex projections.

FINAL COMMENTS

It is hoped that the reader will come away from this chapter with the per-spective that the amygdala has myriad routes through which it can influence behavior. Unfortunately, the precise function or functions of the primate amygdala remains a matter of conjecture. This contrasts with the rather rapid progress that has taken place in the last two decades on the function of the closely related temporal lobe structure, the hippocampal formation. The link between the hippocampal formation and memory function was forged initially on the basis of clinical observations demonstrating that bilateral removal of the hippocampus and associated cortical regions eliminates the ability to form new declarative or episodic memories (Scoville and Milner, 1957). This deficit is obtained even in patients with selective damage of portions of the hippocampal formation (Zola-Morgan et al., 1986). In a very real sense, the functional analysis of the amygdaloid complex has been hampered by the lack of neuropsychologically evaluated patients with circumscribed and complete bilateral damage of the amygdala, i.e., a human model of amygdaloid dysfunction. What sorts of behavioral impairments would a patient with this type of damage display? Despite recent intriguing clinicopathological case studies in which portions of the amygdala have been damaged by disease (Tranel and Hyman, 1990) or intentional ablation (Lee et al., 1988), the literature does not provide a satisfying answer to this question. We are left, therefore, to speculate on primate amygdaloid function from the context of animal research.

A logical starting place in a discussion of amygdaloid function is to consider whether the amygdala performs an elemental operation that leads, depending on the result, to appropriate modulation of activity in all, or many, of the brain regions to which it is connected. One might surmise from the disturbances associated with the Klüver-Bucy syndrome, that the fundamental task of the amygdala is to interpret incoming sensory information in the context of species-specific objectives. A concomitant function might then be the evocation or potentiation of visceral and behavioral responses appropriate to this interpretation.

For the amygdaloid complex to adequately assess the species-specific significance of current experience, it must receive sophisticated sensory information. As we have reviewed, the primate amygdala is reciprocally connected with brain regions representing all sensory modalities. It receives input from visually related areas in the rostral inferior temporal cortex, auditory-related areas in the superior temporal cortex, and somatic sensory-related areas in the posterior insula (Turner et al., 1980; Aggleton et al., 1980; Van Hoesen, 1981; Friedman et al., 1986; Iwai and Yukie, 1987). All of these cortical regions are fairly advanced in the cortical hierarchy of sensory processing and are presumably involved with complex perceptual and other "higher order" cognitive functions. Cells in the rostral inferotemporal cortex, for example, respond to complex visual stimuli such as faces (Rolls, 1984; Desimone et al., 1984). The amygdala is also privy to olfactory information through direct olfactory inputs from the olfactory bulb and cortex (Price, 1990) and taste and visceral information via inputs from the parabrachial nucleus (Mehler, 1980). Taken together, these sensory inputs to the amygdala provide it with rather high-level information concerning potentially all aspects of ongoing sensory experiences.

Much of the sensory information to the amygdala is directed to the lateral nucleus, which then has intrinsic projections to the basal nucleus, accessory basal nucleus, periamygdaloid cortex, and other regions. An interesting question is whether these connections reflect an obligatory serial processing sequence for information transfer through the amygdala. Would it be the case, for example, that a selective lesion of the lateral nucleus would be sufficient to disrupt all functioning of the amygdala or are there sufficient inputs to the basal and accessory basal nuclei to maintain some level of amygdaloid function? (But see Aggleton and Passingham, 1981). If there is serial processing within the amygdala, it would be of substantial interest to determine what operations are performed on sensory information at different stages in the amygdaloid circuit. This question is best approached by electrophysiological studies of the behaving monkey.

While the electrophysiological analysis of the primate amygdaloid complex has not been extensive (see Chapter 5, by Rolls, and Chapter 6, by Ono and Nishijo, this volume), there are indications that its neurons are both responsive to sensory and polysensory information and that neuronal activity can be modulated by the affective valence of the stimulus. As noted by Rolls (1984) and Nishijo et al. (1988), individual amygdaloid neurons respond to visual or auditory stimuli or ingestion of food, or to a combination of these different stimulus modalities. Furthermore, many cells respond to complex stimuli such as faces, or they may be selective for multimodal stimuli such as the sight and ingestion of a slice of watermelon while giving little response to similar stimuli such as an apple. Although it is difficult at present to correlate these response patterns with patterns of axonal connections, it is notable that many of the unimodal neurons are located in the lateral and accessory basal nuclei, while the multimodal and selective cells tend to be concentrated in the basal nucleus (Nishijo et al., 1988).

Nishijo (1988) also made the important observation that the response of many amygdaloid neurons does in fact appear to be dependent on the affective significance of the stimulus. For example, a neuron may respond to the visual presentation of a slice of watermelon, but not to watermelon that has been salted and thereby made aversive. While appreciation of the affective attributes of sensory stimuli may be an operation performed within the intrinsic circuitry of the amygdala, there are other equally plausible alternatives. One possibility is that this function is dependent on the interconnections between the amygdala and basal forebrain or the orbital prefrontal cortex, since neurons in those areas also respond to stimuli based on their affective qualities (Rosenkilde et al., 1981; Thorpe et al., 1983; Wilson and Rolls, 1990). Hopefully, future electrophysiological studies will more precisely define the response properties of amygdaloid neurons and attempt to correlate their responsivity with the known anatomy of the amygdala. In particular, it will be of interest to determine whether the response characteristics of amygdaloid neurons to, for example, visual stimuli are qualitatively different from cells in regions such as area TE, from which the amygdala receives most of its visual input, and the degree to which amygdaloid neurons are tuned to the affective qualities of the test stimuli.

If, as portrayed in the scenario developed above, the elemental assessment of species-specific relevance of a sensory stimulus is accomplished by the amygdala, then what role might it play in enabling the organism to mount a concerted effort to carry out whatever behaviors are appropriate for the situation. The behavioral response would most certainly involve adaptation of bodily state through visceral and autonomic mechanisms. In this respect, some of the best-studied outputs of the amygdala are the projections from the central nucleus to the lateral hypothalamus and brain stem, and from the medial and accessory basal nuclei and the amygdalohippocampal area to the medial hypothalamus. Together with the similar projections of the bed nucleus of the stria terminalis, these subcortically directed projections can affect both the hypothalamo-pituitary system and all levels of the parasympathetic and sympathetic systems, as well as other brain stem reflexes. It has been known for some time, in fact, that stimulation of the amygdala can cause changes in several autonomic functions, including pupillary dilation, piloerection, micturition, blood pressure and heart rate, respiratory rate, and gastric motility and secretion (Kaada, 1972).

For the organism to respond maximally to a challenging situation, the sensory processing apparatus of the organism would also need to be focused, perhaps through modulation of attentional mechanisms. This is perhaps one of the functions of the robust amygdaloid projections back to the neocortex. While the projections to, for example, primary visual cortex might at first seem somewhat surprising from a "limbic" entity such as the amygdala, it may not be far-fetched to think that the emotional state of an organism can influence sensory processing at even very early stages in the process.

To this point, our comments have dealt primarily with putative real-time functions of the amygdala. But it is highly likely that the amygdaloid complex also has a tonic influence on behavior. One possibility is that the amygdala is influential in setting the emotional set point, or mood, of the organism. As we have already mentioned, the amygdala contains a very high level of $GABA_A$/benzodiazepine receptors and may be a strong candidate region for the mediation of anxiolytic effects of the benzodiazepine drugs. Since the highest level of these receptors is located in the lateral nucleus, which receives most of the sensory information directed to the amygdala, it is plausible that the benzodiazepine drugs might act upon the lateral nucleus to prevent the linkage of emotional significance to sensory stimuli.

Similarly, recent experiments using positron emission tomography (PET) to monitor local synaptic activity (reflected as regional cerebral blood flow, rCBF) support the involvement of the amygdala in the psychopathology of mood seen in the affective disorders. Thus, in studies of patients with severe unipolar depression, significant increases in rCBF were found in the amygdala and in areas to which it is closely connected in the ventrolateral and medial prefrontal cortex (Drevets et al., 1991). Increases in blood flow were also found in the substantia innominata/ventral pallidum region, and in the medial thalamus. While it is still difficult to assess the role of each of these areas in mood, it is striking that they largely correspond to many of the forebrain circuits connecting the amygdala and related parts of the prefrontal cortex (Fig. 11).

A similar interaction of the amygdala and many of the regions to which it is connected may underlie the phenomenon of panic disorder. Patients experiencing severe anxiety as part of a panic attack show increased rCBF in the cortex of the temporal pole, a region that is extensively interconnected with the amygdala (Reiman et al., 1989). Similar patterns of rCBF were seen in normal subjects experiencing anticipatory anxiety in expectation of a mild aversive shock. For technical reasons the amygdala was not sampled in this study, but subsequent preliminary measurements have indicated that the amygdala also shows increased rCBF in these conditions (Raichle, 1990).

To conclude, the amygdala is an important nodal point in the adaptive neural response to an environment with constantly changing affective contingencies. For this reason, the amygdala undoubtedly plays an influential role in a wide range of behaviors. While the notion that the amygdala is influential in affective behavior has been discussed for many decades, the challenges for the future are to establish how the structure, physiology, and pharmacology of the amygdala enables it to participate in the normal appreciation of emotion and to further determine whether dysfunction of the amygdala is an important contributor to the etiology of affective illness.

ACKNOWLEDGMENTS

The original work reported in this chapter was supported by NIMH grant R37 MH41479, NIH grant NS 16980 (to D.G.A.), and NIH grant DC 00093 (to J.L.P.). Dr. Pitkänen is supported by a Fogarty International fellowship (1 F05 TW04343) and by the Academy of Finland, Medical Council. Mr. Carmichael is supported by NIH training grant 5T32 NS 07057.

REFERENCES

Aggleton JP (1985): A description of intra-amygdaloid connections in old world monkeys. Exp Brain Res 57:390–399.

Aggleton JP, Burton MJ, Passingham RE (1980): Cortical and subcortical afferents to the amygdala of the rhesus monkey (Macaca mulatta). Brain Res 190:347–368.

Aggleton JP, Mishkin M (1984): Projections of the amygdala to the thalamus in the cynomolgus monkey. J Comp Neurol 222:56–68.

Aggleton JP, Passingham RE (1981): Syndrome produced by lesions of the amygdala in monkeys (Macaca mulatta). J Comp Physiol Psych 95:961–977.

Aggleton JP (1986): Description of the amygdalo-hippocampal interconnections in the macaque monkey. Exp Brain Res 64:515–526.

Amaral DG, Cowan WM (1980): Subcortical afferents to the hippocampal formation in the monkey. J Comp Neurol 189:573–591.

Amaral DG, Veazey RB, Cowan WM (1982): Some observations on hypothalamo-amygdaloid connections in the monkey. Brain Res 252:13–27.

Amaral DG, Insausti R, Cowan WM (1983): Evidence for a direct projection from the superior temporal gyrus to the entorhinal cortex in the monkey. Brain Res 275:263–277.

Amaral DG, Price JL (1984): Amygdalo-cortical projections in the monkey (Macaca fascicularis). J Comp Neurol 230:465–496.

Amaral DG (1986): Amygdalohippocampal and amygdalocortical projections in the primate brain. In Schwarcz R, Ben-Ari Y (eds): "Excitatory Amino Acids and Epilepsy." New York: Plenum Press, pp 3–17.

Amaral DG, Insausti R, Cowan WM (1987): The entorhinal cortex of the monkey. I. Cytoarchitectonic organization. J Comp Neurol 264:326–355.

Amaral DG, Bassett JL (1989): Cholinergic innervation of the monkey amygdala: An immunohistochemical analysis with antisera to choline acetyltransferase. J Comp Neurol 281:337–361.

Amaral DG, Avendaño C, Benoit R (1989): Distribution of somatostatin-like immunoreactivity in the monkey amygdala. J Comp Neurol 284:294–313.

Avendaño C, Price JL, Amaral DG (1983): Evidence for an amygdaloid projection to premotor cortex but not to motor cortex in the monkey. Brain Res 264:111–117.

Azmitia EC, Gannon PJ (1986): The primate serotonergic system: A review of human and animal studies and a report on *Macaca fascicularis*. Adv Neurol 43:407.

Barbas H, DeOlmos J (1990): Projections from the amygdala to basoventral and mediodorsal prefrontal regions in the rhesus monkey. J Comp Neurol 300:549–571.

Bassett JL, Foote SL (1990): Localization of corticotropin-releasing factor (CRF)-like immunoreactivity in monkey amygdala. Soc Neurosci Abstr 16:430.

Beal MF, Tran VT, Mazurek MF, Chattha G, Martin JB (1986): Somatostatin binding sites in human and monkey brain: Localization and characterization. J Neurochem 46:359–365.

Beal MD, Mazurek MF, Martin JB (1987): A comparison of somatostatin and neuropeptide Y distribution in monkey brain. Brain Res 405:213–219.

Beckstead RM, Morse JR, Norgren R (1980): The nucleus of the solitary tract in the monkey: Projections to the thalamus and brainstem. J Comp Neurol 190:259–282.

Bonsall RW, Rees HD, Michael RP (1986): [^{3}H]Estradiol and its metabolites in the brain, pituitary gland, and reproductive tract of the male rhesus monkey. Neuroendocrinology 43:98–109.

Brown RM, Crane AM, Goldman PS (1979): Regional distribution of monoamines in the cerebral cortex and subcortical structures of the rhesus monkey: Concentrations and in vivo synthesis rates. Brain Res 168:133–150.

Caffé AR, Van Ryen PC, Vand Der Woude TP, Van Leeuwen FW (1989): Vasopressin and oxytocin systems in the brain and upper spinal cord of *Macaca fascicularis*. J Comp Neurol 287:302–325.

Carmichael ST, Price JL (1989): Corticocortical and other telencephalic connections of the orbital and medial prefrontal cortex in the monkey. Soc Neurosci Abstr 15:70.

Carmichael ST, Price JL (1991a): Compartmentalization of the lateral orbital cortex of the monkey. IBRO Cong (in press).

Carmichael ST, Price JL (1991b): Orbital prefrontal cortex in the monkey: Structurally distinct areas with sensory and limbic inputs, connected by parallel networks. Soc Neurosci Abstr (in press).

Carnes KM, Price JL (1991): Sources of presumptive glutamatergic/aspartatergic afferents to limbic-related cortex in the rat. (In preparation.)

Chen S-T, Tsai M-S, Shen C-L (1988): Distribution of neurotensin-like immunoreactivity in the central nervous system of the Formosan monkey. Proc Natl Sci Counc B ROC 12:163–173.

Clark AS, MacLusky NJ, Goldman-Rakic PS (1988): Androgen binding and metabolism in the cerebral cortex of the developing rhesus monkey. Endocrinology 123:932–940.

Costa E, Guidotti A, Mao C, Suria A (1975): New concepts in the mechanisms of action of benzodiazepines. Life Sci 17:167–186.

Dennis T, Dubois A, Benavides J, Scatton B (1988): Distribution of central ω_1 (benzodiazepine$_1$) and ω_2 (benzodiazepine$_2$) receptor subtypes in the monkey and human brain. An autoradiographic study with [^{3}H]flunitrazepam and the ω_1 selective ligand [^{3}H]zolpidem. J Pharmacol Exp Therapeutics 247:309–322.

DeOlmos JS, Ingram WR (1972): The projection field of the stria terminalis in the rat brain. An experimental study. J Neurol 146:303–334.

DeOlmos JS, Hardy H, Heimer L (1978): The afferent connections of the main and the accessory olfactory bulb formations in the rat: An experimental HRP study. J Comp Neurol 181:213–244.

DeOlmos JS, Alheid GF, Beltramino CA (1985): Amygdala. In Paxinos G (ed): "The Rat Nervous System," Vol 1. New York: Academic Press, pp 223–334.

DeOlmos J (1990): Amygdala. In Paxinos G (ed): "The Human Nervous System." Sidney, Australia: Academic Press, pp 583–710.

Desimone R, Albright TD, Gross RG, Bruce CTI (1984): Stimulus-selective properties of inferior temporal neurons in the macaque. J Neurosci 4:2051–2062.

Dietl MM, Hof PR, Martin J-L, Magistretti PJ, Palacios JM (1990): Autoradiographic analysis of the distribution of vasoactive intestinal peptide binding sites in the vertebrate central nervous system: A phylogenetic study. Brain Res 520:14–26.

Drevets WC, Videen TO, Preskorn SH, Price JL, Carmichael ST, Raichle ME (1991): A functional anatomical study of unipolar depression. (Submitted.)

Fallon JH, Koziell DA, Moore RY (1978): Catecholamine innervation of the basal forebrain: II. Amygdala, suprarhinal cortex and entorhinal cortex. J Comp Neurol 180:509–532.

Fox CA (1940): Certain basal telencephalic centers in the cat. J Comp Neurol 72:1–62.

Friedman DP, Murray EA, O'Neill JB, Mishkin M (1986): Cortical connections of the somatosensory fields on the lateral sulcus of macaques: Evidence for a corticolimbic pathway for touch. J Comp Neurol 252:323–347.

Galaburda AM, Pandya DN (1983): The intrinsic architectonic and connectional organization of the superior temporal region of the rhesus monkey. J Comp Neurol 221:169–184.

Geschwind N (1965): Disconnection syndromes in animals and man. Brain 88:237–294.

Goldman-Rakic PS, Porrino LJ (1985): The primate mediodorsal nucleus and its projection to the frontal lobe. J Comp Neurol 242:535–560.

Groenewegen HJ, Becker NE, Lohman AH (1980): Subcortical afferents of the nucleus accumbens septi in the cat, studied with retrograde axonal transport of horseradish peroxidase and bisbenzimid. Neuroscience 5:1903–1916.

Haber S, Elde R (1982): The distribution of enkephalin immunoreactive fibers and terminals in the monkey central nervous system: An immunohistochemical study. Neuroscience 7:1049–1095.

Hayashi M, Oshima K (1986): Neuropeptides in cerebral cortex of macaque monkey (*Macaca fuscata fuscata*): Regional distribution and ontogeny. Brain Res 364:360–368.

Hayashi M, Yamashita A, Shimizu K (1990): Nerve growth factor in the primate central nervous system: Regional distribution and ontogeny. Neuroscience 36:683–689.

Heimer L, Nauta WJH (1969): The hypothalamic distribution of the stria terminalis in the rat. Brain Res 115:57–69.

Hellendall RP, Godfrey DA, Ross CD, Armstrong DM, Price JL (1986): The distribution of choline acetyltransferase in the rat amygdaloid complex and adjacent cortical areas, as determined by quantitative micro-assay and immunohistochemistry. J Comp Neurol 249:486–498.

Hemphill M, Holm G, Crutcher M, DeLong M, Hedreen J (1981): Afferent connections of the nucleus accumbens in the monkey. In Chronister RB, France JF (eds): "The Neurobiology of the Nucleus Accumbens." Brunswick, ME: Haer Institute, pp 75–81.

Hendry SHC, Jones EG, Emson PC (1984): Morphology, distribution and synaptic relations of somatostatin- and neuropeptide Y-immunoreactive neurons in rat and monkey neocortex. J Neurosci 4:2497–2512.

Herzog AG, Van Hoesen GW (1976): Temporal neocortical afferent connections to the amygdala in the rhesus monkey. Brain Res 115:57–69.

Holstege G, Meiners L, Tan K (1985): Projections of the bed nucleus of the stria terminalis to the mesencephalon, pons, and medulla oblongata in the cat. Exp Brain Res 58:370–391.

Hope BT, Michael GJ, Knigge KM, Vincent SR (1991): Neuronal NADPH diaphorase is a nitric oxide synthase. Proc Natl Acad Sci USA 88:2811–2814.

Hopkins DA (1975): Amygdalotegmental projections in the rat, cat and rhesus monkey. Neurosci Lett 1:263–270.

Huang FL, Yoshida Y, Nakabayashi H, Huang K-P (1987): Differential distribution of protein kinase C isozymes in the various regions of brain. J Bio Chem 262:15714–15720.

Inagaki S, Parent A (1985): Distribution of enkephalin-immunoreactive neurons in the forebrain and upper brainstem of the squirrel monkey. Brain Res 359:267–280.

Insausti R, Amaral DG, Cowan WM (1987): The entorhinal cortex of the monkey. III. Subcortical afferents. J Comp Neurol 264:396–408.

Insel TR, Miller LP, Gelhard RE (1990): The ontogeny of excitatory amino acid receptors in rat forebrain. I. N-methyl-d-aspartate and quisqualate receptors. Neuroscience 35:31–43.

Iwai E, Yukie M (1987): Amygdalofugal and amygdalopetal connections with modality-specific visual cortical areas in Macaques (Macaca fuscata, M. mulatta, and M. fascicularis). J Comp Neurol 261:362–387.

Jimenez-Castellanos J (1949): The amygdaloid complex in monkey studied by reconstructional methods. J Comp Neurol 91:507–526.

Johnston JB (1923): Further contributions to the study of the evolution of the forebrain. J Comp Neurol 35:337–481.

Jones EG, Powell TPS (1970): An anatomical study on converging sensory pathways within the cerebral cortex of the monkey. Brain Res 83:793–820.

Kaada B (1972): Stimulation and regional ablation of the amygdaloid complex with reference to functional representation. In Eleftheriou BE (ed): "The Neurobiology of the Amygdala." New York: Plenum Press, pp 145–204.

Kelly AE, Domesick VB, Nauta WJ (1982): The amygdalostriatal projection in the cat—an anatomical study by anterograde and retrograde tracing methods. Neuroscience 7:615–630.

Klüver H, Bucy PC (1939): Preliminary analysis of functions of the temporal lobes in monkeys. Arch Neurol Psychiatry 42:979–997.

Koh J-Y, Choi DW (1988): Vulnerability of cultured cortical neurons to damage by excitotoxins: Differential susceptibility of neurons containing NADPH-diaphorase. J Neurosci 8:2153–2163.

Köhler C, Hallman H, Melander T, Hökfelt T, Norheim E (1989): Autoradiographic mapping of galanin receptors in the monkey brain. J Chem Neuroanat 2:269–284.

Koikegami H (1963): Amygdala and other related limbic structures; experimental studies on the anatomy and function. Acta Med Biol 10:161–277.

Kordower JH, Bartus RT, Bothwell M, Schatteman G, Gash DM (1988): Nerve growth factor receptor immunoreactivity in the nonhuman primate (Cebus appella): Distribution, morphology, and colocalization with cholinergic enzymes. J Comp Neurol 277:465–486.

Kordower JH, Bartus RT, Marciano FF, Gash DM (1989): Telencephalic cholinergic system of the new world monkey (Cebus appella): Morphological and cytoarchitectonic assessment and analysis of the projection to the amygdala. J Comp Neurol 279:528–545.

Krettek JE, Price JL (1974): A direct input from the amygdala to the thalamus and the cerebral cortex. Brain Res 67:169–174.

Krettek JE, Price JL (1977): Projections from the amygdaloid complex and adjacent olfactory structures to the entorhinal cortex and to the subiculum in the rat and cat. J Comp Neurol 172:723–752.

Krettek JE, Price JL (1978a): Amygdaloid projections to subcortical structures within the basal forebrain and brainstem in the rat and cat. J Comp Neurol 178:225–253.

Krettek JE, Price JL (1978b): A description of the amygdaloid complex in the rat and cat with observations on intra-amygdaloid axonal connections. J Comp Neurol 178:255–280.

Kritzer MF, Innis RB, Goldman-Rakic PS (1988): Regional distribution of cholecystokinin receptors in macaque medial temporal lobe determined by in vitro receptor autoradiography. J Comp Neurol 276:219–230.

Kuhar MJ, Pert CB, Snyder SH (1973): Regional distribution of opiate receptor binding in monkey and human brain. Nature 245:447–450.

Lakshmi S, Balasubramanian AS (1981): The distribution of estrone sulphatase, dehydroepiandrosterone sulphatase, and arylsulphatase C in the primate (Macaca radiata) brain and pituitary. J Neurochem 37:358–362.

LaMotte CC, Snowman A, Pert CB, Snyder SH (1978): Opiate receptor binding in rhesus monkey brain: Association with limbic structures. Brain Res 155:374–379.

Lauer EW (1945): The nuclear pattern and fiber connections of certain basal telencephalic centers in the Macaque. J Comp Neurol 82:215–254.

LeDoux JE, Farb C, Ruggiero DA (1990a): Topographic organization of neurons in the acoustic thalamus that project to the amygdala. J Neurosci 10:1043–1054.

LeDoux JE, Cicchetti P, Xagoraris A, Romanski LM (1990b): The lateral amygdaloid nucleus: Sensory interface of the amygdala in fear conditioning. J Neurosci 10:1062–1069.

Lee GP, Meador KJ, Smith JR, Loring DW, Flanigan HF (1988): Preserved crossmodal association following bilateral amygdalotomy in man. Intern J Neurosci 40:47–55.

Leichnetz GR, Astruc J (1977): The course of some prefrontal corticofugals to the pallidum, substantia innominata, and amygdaloid complex in monkeys. Exp Neurol 54:104–109.

Luskin MB, Price JL (1983): The topographic organization of associational fibers of the olfactory system in the rat including centrifugal fibers to the olfactory bulb. J Comp Neurol 216:284–291.

Mash DC, White WF, Mesulam M-M (1988): Distribution of muscarinic receptor subtypes within architectonic subregions of the primate cerebral cortex. J Comp Neurol 278:265–274.

McBride RL, Sutin J (1977): Amygdaloid and pontine projections to the ventromedial nucleus of the hypothalamus. J Comp Neurol 174:377–396.

McDonald AJ (1985): Immunohistochemical identification of gamma-aminobutyric acid-containing neurons in the rat basolateral amygdala. Neurosci Lett 53:203–207.

Mehler WR (1980): Subcortical afferent connections of the amygdala in the monkey. J Comp Neurol 190:733–762.

Mesulam M-M, Mufson EJ, Levey AI, Wainer BH (1983): Cholinergic innervation of cortex by the basal forebrain: Cytochemistry and cortical connections of the septal area, diagonal band nuclei, nucleus basalis (substantia innominata) and hypothalamus in the rhesus monkey. J Comp Neurol 214:170–197.

Michael RP, Rees HD (1982): Autoradiographic localization of ^{3}H-dihydrotestosterone in the preoptic area, hypothalamus, and amygdala of a male rhesus monkey. Life Sci 30:2087–2093.

Millan MA, Jacobowitz DM, Hauger RL, Catt KJ, Aguilera G (1986): Distribution of corticotropin-releasing factor receptors in primate brain. Proc Natl Acad Sci USA 83:1921–1925.

Miller LP, Johnson AE, Gelhard RE, Insel TR (1990): The ontogeny of excitatory amino acid receptors in the rat forebrain. II. Kainic acid receptors. Neuroscience 35:45–51.

Mizuno N, Uchida K, Nomura S, Nakamura Y, Sugimoto T, Uemura-Sumi M (1981): Extrageniculate projections to the visual cortex in the macaque monkey: An HRP study. Brain Res 212:454–459.

Mizuno N, Takahashi O, Satoda T, Matsushima R (1985): Amygdalospinal projections in the macaque monkey. Neurosci Lett 53:327–330.

Morán MA, Mufson EJ, Mesulam M-M (1987): Neural inputs into the temporopolar cortex of the rhesus monkey. J Comp Neurol 256:88–103.

Mufson EJ, Mesulam M-M, Pandya DN (1981): Insular interconnections with the amygdala in the rhesus monkey. Neuroscience 6:1231–1248.

Mufson EJ, Mesulam M-M (1982): Insula of the old world monkey. II. Afferent cortical input and comments of the claustrum. J Comp Neurol 212:23–37.

Murray EA, Mishkin M (1985): Amygdalectomy impairs crossmodal association in monkeys. Science 228:604–606.

Nauta WJH (1961): Fibre degeneration following lesions of the amygdaloid complex in the monkey. J Anat 95:515–532.

Nauta WJH (1962): Neural associations of the amygdaloid complex in the monkey. Brain 85:505–520.

Nauta WJH (1972): Neural associations of the frontal cortex. Acta Neurobiol Exp 32:125–140.

Newman R, Winans SS (1980): An experimental study of the ventral striatum of the golden hamster. I. Neuronal connections of the nucleus accumbens. J Comp Neurol 191:167–192.

Nishijo H, Ono T, Nishino H (1988): Topographic distribution of modality-specific amygdalar neurons in alert monkey. J Neurosci 8:3556–3569.

Nishijo H (1988): Single neuron responses in amygdala of alert monkey during complex sensory stimulation of affective significance. J Neurosci 8:3570–3583.

Nomura S, Mizuno N, Itoh K, Matsuda K, Sugimoto T, Nakamura Y (1979): Localization of parabrachial nucleus neurons projecting to the thalamus or the amygdala in the cat using horseradish peroxidase. Exp Neurol 64:375–385.

Norgren R (1976): Taste pathways to hypothalamus and amygdala. J Comp Neurol 166:17–30.

Norita M, Kawamura K (1980): Subcortical afferents to the monkey amygdala: An HRP study. Brain Res 190:225–230.

Oldfield BJ, Silverman AJ (1985): A light microscopic HRP study of limbic projections to the vasopressin-containing nuclear groups of the hypothalamus. Brain Res Bull 14:143–157.

Olszewski J (1952): "The Thalamus of *Macaca mulatta*. An Atlas for Use with the Stereotaxic Instrument." New York: S. Karger.

Ottersen OP, Ben-Ari Y (1979): Afferent connections to the amygdaloid complex in the rat and cat: I. Projections from the thalamus. J Comp Neurol 187:401–424.

Ottersen OP (1981): Afferent connections to the amygdaloid complex of the rat with some observations in the cat. III. Afferents from the lower brain stem. J Comp Neurol 202:335–356.

Ottersen OP (1982): Connections of the amygdala of the rat. IV. Corticoamygdaloid and intraamygdaloid connections as studied with axonal transport of horseradish peroxidase. J Comp Neurol 205:30–48.

Ottersen OP, Fischer BO, Rinvik E, Storm-Mathisen J (1986): Putative amino acid transmitters in the amygdala. In Schwarcz R, Ben-Ari Y (eds): "Excitatory Amino Acids and Epilepsy." New York: Plenum Press, pp 53–66.

Pandya DN, Kuypers HGJM (1969): Cortico-cortical connections in the rhesus monkey. Brain Res 13:13–36.

Pandya DN, Van Hoesen GW, Domesick VB (1973): A cingulo-amygdaloid projection in the rhesus monkey. Brain Res 61:369–373.

Pandya DN, Yeterian EH (1985): Architecture and connections of cortical association areas. In Peters A, Jones EG (eds): "Cerebral Cortex," Vol. 4. New York: Plenum Press, pp 3–55.

Parent A, Mackey A, DeBellefeuille L (1983): The subcortical afferents to caudate nucleus and putamen in primate: A fluorescence retrograde double labelling study. Neuroscience 10:1137–1150.

Pfaff DW, Gerlach JL, McEwen BS, Ferin M, Carmael P, Zimmerman EA (1976): Autoradiographic localization of hormone-concentrating cells in the brain of the female rhesus monkey. J Comp Neurol 170:279–294.

Pitkänen A, Amaral DG (1990): Intrinsic connections of the monkey amygdala: A PHA-L analysis of projections originating in the lateral nucleus. Soc Neurosci Abstr 16:122.

Pitkänen A, Amaral DG (1991a): Demonstration of projections from the lateral nucleus to the basal nucleus of the amygdala: A PHA-L study in the monkey. Exp Brain Res 83:465–470.

Pitkänen A, Amaral DG (1991b): Distribution of reduced nicotinamide adenine dinucleotide phosphate diaphorase (NADPH-d) cells and fibers in the monkey amygdaloid complex. J Comp Neurol (In press).

Porrino LJ, Crane AM, Goldman-Rakic PS (1981): Direct and indirect pathways from the amygdala to the frontal lobe in the rhesus monkey. J Comp Neurol 198:121–136.

Price JL (1973): An autoradiographic study of complementary laminar patterns of termination of afferent fibers to the olfactory cortex. J Comp Neurol 150:87–108.

Price JL, Amaral DG (1981): An autoradiographic study of the projections of the central nucleus of the monkey amygdala. J Neurosci 1:1242–1259.

Price JL (1986): Subcortical projections from the amygdaloid complex. In Ben-Ari Y, Schwarcz R (eds): "Excitatory Amino Acids and Epilepsy." New York: Plenum Press, pp 19–33.

Price JL, Russchen FT, Amaral DG (1987): The limbic region. II. The amygdaloid complex. In Björkland A, Hökfelt T, Swanson LW (eds): "Handbook of Chemical Neuroanatomy," Vol 5, "Integrated Systems of the CNS," Part I. Amsterdam: Elsevier, pp 279–381.

Price JL (1990): Olfactory system. In Paxinos G (ed): "The Human Nervous System." San Diego: Academic Press, pp 979–998.

Price JL, Slotnick BM, Revial MF (1991): Olfactory projections to the hypothalamus. J Comp Neurol 306:447–461.

Quirion R (1987): Characterization and autoradiographic distribution of hemicholinium-3 high-affinity choline uptake sites in mammalian brain. Synapse 1:293–303.

Quirion R, Welner S, Gauthier S, Bedard P (1987): Neurotensin receptor binding sites in monkey and human brain: Autoradiographic distribution and effects of 1-methyl-4-phenyl-1,2,3,6-tetrahydropyridine treatment. Synapse 1:559–566.

Ragsdale CW, Graybiel AM (1988): Fibers from the basolateral nucleus of the amygdala selectively innervate striosomes in the caudate nucleus of the cat. J Comp Neurol 269:506–522.

Raichle M (1990): Exploring the mind with dynamic imaging. Seminars in the Neurosciences 2:307–315.

Ray JP, Price JL (1990): The organization of projections from the mediodorsal nucleus of the thalamus to orbital and medial prefrontal cortex in the monkey. Soc Neurosci Abstr 16:1093.

Ray JP, Russchen FT, Fuller TA, Price JL (1991): Sources of presumptive glutamatergic/aspartatergic afferents to the mediodorsal nucleus of the thalamus in the rat. (In preparation.)

Ricardo JA, Koh ET (1978): Anatomical evidence of direct projections from the nucleus of the solitary tract to the hypothalamus, amygdala and other forebrain structures in the rat. Brain Res 153:1–26.

Reiman EM, Raichle ME, Robins E, Mintun E, Fusselman MJ, Fox PT, Price JL, Hackman KA (1989): Neuroanatomical correlates of a lactate-induced anxiety attack. Arch Gen Psychiat 46:493–500.

Rolls ET (1984): Neurons in the cortex of the temporal lobe and in the amygdala of the monkey with responses selective for faces. Human Neurobiol 3:209–222.

Roselli CE, Stadelman H, Horton LE, Resko JA (1987): Regulation of androgen metabolism and luteinizing hormone-releasing hormone content in discrete hypothalamic and limbic areas of male rhesus macaques. Endocrinology 120:97–106.

Rosene DL, Van Hoesen GW (1977): Hippocampal efferents reach widespread regions of the cerebral cortex and amygdala in the rhesus monkey. Science 198:315–317.

Rosene DL, Van Hoesen GW (1987): The hippocampal formation of the primate brain. A review of some comparative aspects of cytoarchitecture and connections. In Jones EG, Peters A (eds): "Cerebral Cortex," Vol 6. New York: Plenum Press, pp 345–456.

Rosenkilde CE, Bauer RH, Fuster JM (1981): Single cell activity in ventral prefrontal cortex of behaving monkeys. Brain Res 209:375–394.

Russchen FT (1982): Amygdalopetal projections in the cat: II. Subcortical afferent connections. A study with retrograde tracing techniques. J Comp Neurol 207:157–176.

Russchen FT, Price JL (1984): Amygdalostriatal projections in the rat. Topographical organization and fiber morphology shown using the lectin PHA-L as anterograde tracer. Neurosci Lett 47:15–22.

Russchen FT, Amaral DG, Price JL (1985a): The afferent connections of the substantia innominata in the monkey, *Macaca fascicularis*. J Comp Neurol 242:1–27.

Russchen FT, Bakst I, Amaral DG, Price J (1985b): The amygdalostriatal projections in the monkey. An anterograde tracing study. Brain Res 329:241–257.

Russchen FT, Amaral DG, Price JL (1987): The afferent input to the magnocellular division of the mediodorsal thalamic nucleus in the monkey, *Macaca fascicularis*. J Comp Neurol 256:175–210.

Sadikot AF, Smith Y, Parent A (1988): Chemical anatomy of the amygdala in primate. Soc Neurosci Abstr 14:860.

Sadikot AF, Parent A (1990): The monoaminergic innervation of the amygdala in the squirrel monkey: An immunohistochemical study. Neuroscience 36:431–447.

Saunders RC, Rosene DL (1988): A comparison of the efferents of the amygdala and the hippocampal formation in the rhesus monkey: I. Convergence in the entorhinal, prorhinal, and perirhinal cortices. J Comp Neurol 271:153–184.

Saunders RC, Rosene DL, Van Hoesen GW (1988): Comparison of the efferents of the amygdala and the hippocampal formation in the rhesus monkey: II. Reciprocal and non-reciprocal connections. J Comp Neurol 271:185–207.

Scoville WB, Milner B (1957): Loss of recent memory after bilateral hippocampal lesions. J Neurol Neurosurg Psychiatry 20:11–21.

Seltzer B, Pandya DN (1976): Some cortical projections to the parahippocampal area in the rhesus monkey. Exp Neurol 50:146–160.

Seltzer B, Pandya DN (1978): Afferent cortical connections and architectonics of the superior temporal sulcus and surrounding cortex in the rhesus monkey. Brain Res 149:1–24.

Sholl SA, Goy RW, Kim KL (1989): 5α-reductase, aromatase, and androgen receptor levels in the monkey brain during fetal development. Endocrinology 124:627–634.

Sholl SA, Kim KL (1989): Estrogen receptors in the rhesus monkey brain during fetal development. Dev Brain Res 50:189–196.

Silverman AJ, Antunes JL, Abrams GM, Nilaver G, Thau R, Robinson JA, Ferin M, Krey LC (1982): The luteinizing hormone-releasing hormone pathways in rhesus (*Macaca mulatta*) and pigtailed (*Macaca nemestrina*) monkeys: New observations on thick, unembedded sections. J Comp Neurol 211:309–317.

Simantov R, Kuhar MJ, Pasternak GW, Snyder SH (1976): The regional distribution of a morphine-like factor enkephalin in monkey brain. Brain Res 106:189–197.

Singh SI, Malhotra CL (1962): Amino acid content of monkey brain. I. General pattern and quantitative value of glutamic acid/glutamine, γ-aminobutyric acid and aspartic acid. J Neurochem 9:37–42.

Slater P, Cross AJ (1986): Autoradiographic distribution of dynorphin$_{1-9}$ binding sites in primate brain. Neuropeptides 8:71–76.

Smith Y, Parent A, Kerkérian L, Pelletier (1985): Distribution of neuropeptide Y immunoreactivity in the basal forebrain and upper brainstem of the squirrel monkey (*Saimiri sciureus*). J Comp Neurol 236:71–89.

Sofroniew MV, Weindl A, Schrell U, Wetzstein R (1981): Immunohistochemistry of vasopressin, oxytocin and neurophysin in the hypothalamus and estrahypothalamic regions of the human and primate brain. Acta Histochem (Suppl Band XXIV) S79–95.

Stephan H, Frahm HD, Baron G (1987): Comparison of brain structure volumes in insectivora and primates. VII. Amygdaloid components. J Hirnforsch 28:571–581.

Stroessner HM, Houser CR, Richards JG, Amaral DG (1989): Distribution of benzodiazepine/GABA$_A$ receptors in the monkey medial temporal lobe: An immunohistochemical analysis. Soc Neurosci Abstr 15:1154.

Stuart AM, Mitchell IJ, Slater P, Unwin HLP, Crossman AR (1986): A semi-quantitative atlas of 5-hydroxytryptamine-1 receptors in the primate brain. Neuroscience 18:619–639.

Thorpe SJ, Rolls ET, Maddison S (1983): The orbitofrontal cortex: Neuronal activity in the behaving monkey. Exp Brain Res 490:93–115.

Tigges J, Tigges M, Cross NA, McBride RL, Letbetter WT, Anschel S (1982): Subcortical structures projecting to visual cortical areas in squirrel monkey. J Comp Neurol 209:29–40.

Tigges J, Walker LC, Tigges M (1983): Subcortical projections to the occipital and parietal lobes of the chimpanzee brain. J Comp Neurol 220:106–115.

Tranel D, Hyman BT (1990): Neuropsychological correlates of bilateral amygdala damage. Arch Neurol 47:349–355.

Turner BH, Gupta KC, Mishkin M (1978): The locus and cytoarchitecture of the projection areas of the olfactory bulb in *Macaca mulatta*. J Comp Neurol 177:381–396.

Turner BH, Mishkin M, Knapp M (1980): Organization of the amygdalopetal projections from modality-specific cortical association areas in the monkey. J Comp Neurol 191:515–543.

Van Hoesen GW, Pandya ND, Butters N (1975): Some connections of the entorhinal (area 28) and perirhinal (area 35) cortices of the rhesus monkey. II. Frontal lobe afferents. Brain Res 95:25–38.

Van Hoesen GW (1981): The differential distribution, diversity and sprouting of cortical projections to the amygdala in the rhesus monkey. In Ben-Ari Y (ed): "The Amygdaloid Complex." Amsterdam: Elsevier/North Holland Press, pp 77–90.

Veening JG (1978): Subcortical afferents to the amygdaloid complex in the rat: An HRP study. Neurosci Lett 8:196–202.

Vogt BA, Pandya DN, Rosene DL (1987): Cingulate cortex of the rhesus monkey: I. Cytoarchitecture and thalamic afferents. J Comp Neurol 262:256–270.

Völsch M (1910): Zur vergleichenden anatomie des mandelkerns und seiner nachbargebilde. Arch Mikrosk Anat Entwick 76:373–523.

Walker AE (1940): A cytoarchitectural study of the prefrontal area of the macaque monkey. J Comp Neurol 98:59–86.

Wamsley JK, Zarbin MA, Young WS, Kuhar MJ (1982): Distribution of opiate receptors in the monkey brain: An autoradiographic study. Neuroscience 7:595–613.

Weller KL, Smith DA (1982): Afferent connections to the bed nucleus of the stria terminalis. Brain Res 232:51–77.

Weiskrantz L (1956): Behavioral changes associated with ablation of the amygdaloid complex in monkeys. JCPP 49:381–391.

Whitlock DG, Nauta WJH (1956): Subcortical projections from the temporal neocortex in macaca mulatta. J Comp Neurol 106:183–212.

Wilson FA, Rolls ET (1990): Neuronal responses related to the novelty and familiarity of visual stimuli in the substantia innominata, diagonal band of Broca and periventricular region of the primate basal forebrain. Exp Brain Res 80:104–120.

Witter MP, Amaral DG (1991): Entorhinal cortex of the monkey: V. Projections to the dentate gyrus, hippocampus, and subicular complex. J Comp Neurol 307:1–23.

Yasui Y, Itoh K, Sugimoto T, Mizuno N (1987): Thalamocortical and thalamo-amygdaloid projections form the parvicellular division of the posteromedial ventral nucleus in the cat. J Comp Neurol 257:253–268.

Zaborszky L, Leranth C, Heimer L (1984): Ultrastructural evidence of amygdalofugal axons terminating on cholinergic cells of the rostral forebrain. Neurosci Lett 52:219–225.

Zola-Morgan S, Squire LR, Amaral DG (1986): Human amnesia and the medial temporal region: Enduring memory impairment following a bilateral lesion limited to field CA1 of the hippocampus. J Neurosci 6:2950–2967.

The Amygdala: Neurobiological Aspects of Emotion,
Memory, and Mental Dysfunction, pages 67–96
© 1992 Wiley-Liss, Inc.

2
Cell Types and Intrinsic Connections of the Amygdala

ALEXANDER J. MCDONALD

*Department of Anatomy, Cell Biology and Neurosciences, University of
South Carolina, Columbia, South Carolina*

INTRODUCTION

The amygdala is involved in some of the most complex functions of the brain, including emotion and memory. Not surprisingly, the functional complexity of the amygdala is paralleled by its structural complexity; in all mammals the amygdala consists of numerous nuclei and subnuclei that have distinct connections and that may participate in discrete functions. Comparative neuroanatomical studies conducted in the first half of this century revealed considerable variation in the cytoarchitecture of the amygdala in different species, such that it was often difficult to establish exact nuclear homologies (see reviews by Koikegami, 1963, and Hall, 1972). Nevertheless, it was possible to recognize two major subdivisions in the mammalian amygdala: a superficially located corticomedial nuclear group and a more deeply situated basolateral nuclear group (Johnston, 1923; Humphrey, 1936).

The corticomedial amygdala consists of the cortical nucleus (located just medial to the piriform cortex), medial nucleus (medially adjacent to the cortical nucleus), central nucleus (located between the medial nucleus and caudatoputamen), and nucleus of the lateral olfactory tract (located anteromedial to the cortical nucleus). Price and coworkers divided the cortical nucleus into three parts termed the anterior cortical nucleus, posterior cortical nucleus, and the periamygdaloid cortex (Krettek and Price, 1978b; Price et al., 1987). The anterior amygdaloid area (a diffuse region near the rostral pole of the amygdala that blends with the central nucleus) and the amygdalohippocampal area (located caudal to the medial nucleus) are also often included in the corticomedial amygdala. The basolateral amygdala consists of the accessory basal nucleus (located deep to the periamygdaloid cortex; termed the basomedial nucleus by Krettek and Price, 1978b), magnocellular and parvicellular basal nuclei (located deep to the accessory basal nucleus; termed, respectively, the anterior and posterior subdivisions of the basolateral nucleus by Krettek and Price, 1978b), and a more laterally and dorsally situated lateral nucleus. Subsequent cytoarchitectural and histochemical studies in a variety of species have demonstrated that each of the amygdaloid nuclei may exhibit several subdivisions.

A thorough understanding of the anatomy and physiology of the amygdala will ultimately require a detailed knowledge of the specific cell types contained in individual amygdaloid nuclei. This aspect of the amygdala received little attention prior to 1970. During the last two decades, however, there have been several detailed studies of the neuronal morphology in the amygdala using the Golgi technique. This technique, when successful, stains all portions (cell body, axon, and dendrites) of a small percentage of the neurons contained in any brain region. It is the method of choice for the initial identification and characterization of the major players in the information processing of any brain area. In the first part of this chapter, the neuronal morphology of each of the amygdaloid nuclei is reviewed.

There have been numerous investigations of the connections of the amygdala using a variety of tract tracing techniques. These studies have demonstrated that each nucleus of the amygdala has a distinctive set of connections with extrinsic brain regions. Often overlooked, however, are the rich array of interconnections between individual amygdaloid nuclei. These intra-amygdaloid connections, which are undoubtedly crucial for normal amygdaloid functioning, are reviewed in the second part of this chapter.

CELL TYPES OF THE AMYGDALA
Basolateral Amygdala

In his seminal paper on the comparative neuroanatomy of the vertebrate amygdala, Johnston (1923) noted that the basolateral amygdala was continuous with the piriform cortex in the region of the amygdaloid fissure. In fact, in the caudal portion of the amygdala of nonprimate mammals, the posterior portion of the basal nucleus (i.e., the parvicellular basal nucleus) appears to be an infolding of cortex that is continuous with the piriform cortex laterally and the entorhinal cortex caudally. At the caudal pole of the amygdala the amygdaloid fissure curves medially around the posterior aspect of the posterior cortical nucleus; the amygdalohippocampal area appears as an infolding of cortex associated with this medial extension of the amygdaloid fissure.

Gurdjian (1928) studied the rat amygdala using Nissl and Golgi techniques and noted that the cells of the basolateral amygdala were very similar to those of adjacent cortical regions (piriform cortex and hippocampal formation) and the claustrum. In a more extensive Golgi analysis of the cat amygdala, Hall (1972) demonstrated that the basolateral nuclei exhibited two major cell classes: spiny pyramidal-like neurons (type P cells) and spine-sparse stellate neurons (type S cells). She noted that these cells closely resembled, respectively, the pyramidal and stellate (nonpyramidal) neurons of the cerebral cortex. Subsequent studies have revealed that the ultrastructure, synaptology, and neurotransmitter immunohistochemistry of the pyramidal and nonpyramidal amygdaloid neurons are very similar to their cortical counterparts (McDonald, 1985a,b, 1989b; McDonald and Pearson, 1989; McDonald et al., 1989; McDonald and Baimbridge, 1990; Carlsen, 1989; Carlsen et al., 1985; Carlsen and Heimer, 1986, 1988). These two major cell types of the basolateral amygdala have been found in all species investigated, including the opossum (McDonald and Culberson, 1981), rat (McDonald, 1982b, 1984; Millhouse and DeOlmos, 1983), cat (Hall, 1972; Tömböl and Szafranska-Kosmal, 1972; Kamal and Tömböl, 1975); dog (Mukhina and Leontovich, 1970), monkey (Herzog, 1982) and human (Braak and Braak, 1983). Since the morphology of these neurons has been described and illustrated in the most detail in the rat basolateral amygdala (McDonald, 1982b, 1984; Millhouse and DeOlmos, 1983), the following account is based primarily on this species.

Pyramidal Neurons

Amygdaloid pyramidal neurons (P cells of Hall, 1972; class I cells of McDonald and Culberson, 1981 and McDonald, 1982b; pyramidal neurons of Millhouse and DeOlmos, 1983) constitute the predominant cell type in the basal, accessory basal, and lateral nuclei. They are also the principal neurons in the amygdalo-hippocampal area (DeOlmos et al., '85; personal observations). These neurons have pyramidal or piriform somata that vary in size depending on the nucleus. For example, in the rat magnocellular basal nucleus the cell bodies average 20 × 16 μm (Fig. 1) while in the lateral nucleus the average size is 16 × 12 μm. The

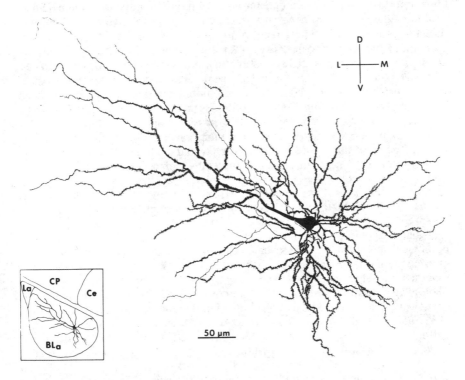

Fig. 1. A Golgi-impregnated pyramidal neuron in the magnocellular basal nucleus of the rat (anterior division of the basolateral nucleus of Krettek and Price, 1978b). Note pyramidal shape of the cell and the presence of one apical dendrite and numerous basal dendrites. Arrow indicates axon in this and all subsequent figures. **Inset** shows position of cell. Cross indicates orientation. Reprint from McDonald (1982b) with permission.

cell bodies of these neurons are larger in the cat (Tömböl and Szafranska-Kosmal, 1972) and monkey (personal observations). Although the exact dendritic aborization pattern of amygdaloid pyramidal cells varies in different nuclei and in different neurons of the same nucleus (see below), all pyramidal neurons are characterized by the presence of a dense covering of dendritic spines on secondary dendrites and more distal dendritic branches (Fig. 1). Most of these spines have thin stalks (1.0–1.5 μm long) with small terminal swellings. Primary dendrites have only a few spines, many of which are sessile.

The pyramidal neurons in nuclei adjacent to the amygdaloid fissure (amygdalohippocampal area and parvicellular basal nucleus) most closely resemble cortical pyramidal neurons (McDonald, 1982b, 1984; Millhouse and DeOlmos, 1983). The pyramidal cells in these nuclei usually have one thick apical dendrite that arises from the superficial pole of the cell body and several thinner basal dendrites that arise from the opposite side of the cell; the apical dendrites extend toward the pial surface and tend to parallel one another. The apical dendrites are longer than the basal dendrites and have more branches. In deeper portions of the basolateral amygdala (e.g., lateral nucleus, magnocellular basal nucleus, and basal accessory nucleus) some of the amygdaloid pyramidal cells have a marked pyramidal morphology, with clear differentiation of apical and basal dendrites, while other spiny neurons of this type may be semipyramidal neurons with less distinction between apical and basal dendrites. Although apical dendrites in these deeper nuclei may exhibit a preferred orientation in certain regions, they are far more randomly organized than in the nuclei bordering the amygdaloid fissure (Millhouse and DeOlmos, 1983; McDonald, 1984). In some cases pyramidal cells may have two apical dendrites or exhibit apical dendrites that bifurcate into two robust branches. In addition, some spiny neurons have primary dendrites of roughly equal caliber with no obvious apical dendrite; these neurons resemble the spiny stellate neurons of the cortex. In the present account, the spiny semipyramidal neurons and spiny stellate neurons in the basolateral amygdala (and also in the amygdalohippocampal area, cortical nuclei, and nucleus of the lateral olfactory tract) are considered to represent modified pyramidal neurons.

Thus, amygdaloid "pyramidal neurons" constitute a broad, continuous morphological spectrum. At one extreme are neurons that are virtually identical to cortical pyramidal neurons, while at the other end of the spectrum are neurons that more closely resemble cortical spiny stellate cells. Actually, this same morphological variability also exists in the cortex itself. Recent investigations of cortical ultrastructure and synaptology (Lund, 1984; Saint Marie and Peters, 1985), as well as electrophysiological studies of intrinsic action potential firing patterns (Conners and Gutnick, 1990), suggest that pyramidal cells, star pyramids, and spiny stellate cells are all part of a continuum of spiny cortical neurons. Like their counterparts in the cerebral cortex, amygdaloid pyramidal cells are intensely immunoreactive for glutamate and aspartate (McDonald et al., 1989; McDonald, 1989b).

The axons of amygdaloid pyramidal cells arise from the cell body or proximal portion of a primary dendrite (Fig. 1). The axon hillock and initial segment of pyramidal neurons in the rat (McDonald, 1982b; Millhouse and DeOlmos,

1983), opossum (McDonald and Culberson, 1981), and cat (personal observations) frequently have several spines, most of which are sessile. There is evidence that these spines, and the shaft of the initial segment, are postsynaptic to the axons of a particular type of nonpyramidal neuron (amygdaloid chandelier cell, see below). Axons of pyramidal cells give rise to several beaded collaterals that arborize modestly in the vicinity of the parent cell. These collaterals frequently contact the spiny dendrites of the parent cell or neighboring pyramidal neurons. The axons of pyramidal neurons can sometimes be seen exiting the amygdala and projecting toward the stria terminalis or external capsule, suggesting that these cells are projection neurons. Consistent with this suggestion is the finding that injections of retrograde tracers into the cortical targets of the basolateral amygdala label numerous cells with pyramidal somata (Sripanidkulchai et al., 1984; McDonald, 1987).

Nonpyramidal Neurons

Nonpyramidal neurons of the basolateral amygdala are characterized by spine-sparse dendrites. These cells are situated among the pyramidal neurons in all parts of the basolateral amygdala but are found in far fewer numbers. Like their counterparts in the cerebral cortex, amygdaloid nonpyramidal neurons are morphologically heterogeneous (Fig. 2). In the cerebral cortex, the dendritic and axonal arborizations of distinct subclasses of nonpyramidal neurons often exhibit characteristic orientations in relation to cortical laminae and columns. Perhaps because of the more loosely organized cytoarchitecture of the basolateral amygdala, it has been more difficult to recognize distinct subtypes in this region purely on the basis of morphology. Like the nonpyramidal cells of the cortex, amygdaloid nonpyramidal cells contain GABA, choline acetyltransferase (the synthetic enzyme for acetylcholine), calcium binding proteins, and a variety of peptides, including somatostatin, vasoactive intestinal peptide (VIP), cholecystokinin (CCK), and neuropeptide Y (McDonald, 1985a,b; McDonald and Baimbridge, 1990; Carlsen and Heimer, 1986; Gustafson et al., 1986). The colocalization patterns of these substances in individual neurons of the cortex are also repeated in the basolateral amygdala (McDonald, 1989a; McDonald and Pearson, 1989; McDonald and Baimbridge, 1990).

Although the perikarya of most nonpyramidal neurons are small (10–14 μm in diameter) and ovoid, some cells are as large as pyramidal neurons (Fig. 2). Most nonpyramidal neurons have 2–6 primary dendrites that branch modestly and exhibit few spines. The larger neurons generally have stout primary dendrites which distort the perikarya into pyramidal or irregular shapes (Fig. 2, neuron D). The diameter of the dendritic arborization is usually proportional to perikaryal size and varies from 100–700 μm. The terminal portions of the dendrites of some nonpyramidal cells, particularly the larger ones, sometimes give rise to a tuft of tortuous branches that exhibit varicosities and long beaded appendages (McDonald, 1982b). There are also spine-sparse neurons in the external capsule whose dendrites extend into the basolateral amygdala and exhibit similar "gnarled" dendritic terminal segments (Millhouse and DeOlmos, 1983; personal observations). These dendritic endings resemble the growing or involuting dendrites seen in fetal and early postnatal brains.

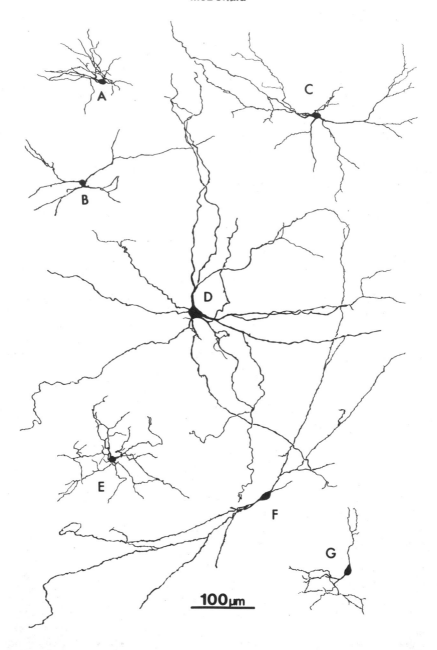

Fig. 2. Drawings of Golgi-impregnated nonpyramidal cells that best illustrate the morphological variation of these neurons in the rat basolateral amygdala. Only cell bodies and dendrites of these neurons are illustrated. **A:** Small bitufted neuron of the lateral

Axons of nonpyramidal neurons originate from the cell body or the proximal portion of a primary dendrite. Usually only the initial segment of the axon is impregnated by the Golgi technique. When more distal portions of the axon are stained, they are seen to branch several times and give off numerous beaded collaterals (Fig. 3). Collaterals branch to form a moderate-to-dense axonal arborization in the vicinity of the parent cell. Axonal varicosities have frequently been seen forming delicate synapselike contacts with the dendrites of amygdaloid pyramidal neurons (McDonald, 1982b; Millhouse and DeOlmos, 1983). The dense local axonal arborization exhibited by nonpyramidal cells suggests that most are local circuit neurons like their counterparts in the cerebral cortex. Recent studies conducted in the author's laboratory, however, indicate that a small percentage of the somatostatin and neuropeptide Y containing nonpyramidal cells may have axons that project to the cerebral cortex or striatum (McDonald, 1986). In addition, the neuronal population in the basolateral nuclei projecting to the mediodorsal thalamic nucleus consists entirely of large, and some medium-sized, nonpyramidal neurons (McDonald, 1987). The latter cells may be a special subclass of nonpyramidal neurons since they appear to be part of an array of similar polymorphic neurons of the basal forebrain that provide the projection to the mediodorsal nucleus (Russchen et al., 1987).

As in the cerebral cortex (Feldman and Peters, 1978), it is possible to recognize *multipolar, bitufted,* and *bipolar* varieties of nonpyramidal cells on the basis of dendritic patterns (McDonald, 1982b). In addition, several specific subpopulations of amygdaloid nonpyramidal neurons can be identified because they exhibit distinctive axonal or dendritic features. These latter cell types include chandelier cells, neurogliaform cells, cone cells, and extended neurons.

Amygdaloid chandelier cells, which closely resemble the chandelier cells of the cerebral cortex (Peters, 1984), have been observed in the opossum (McDonald and Culberson, 1981) and rat (McDonald, 1982b) basolateral amygdala. The axonal varicosities, presumed to be axon terminals, tend to be clustered rather than diffusely distributed, as in most nonpyramidal cells. These "axonal clusters" usually consist of 4–7 varicosities located along a 15-μm-long axon segment. These terminal specializations have been observed to form intimate contacts with the initial segments, including axonic spines, of amygdaloid pyramidal neurons (McDonald and Culberson, 1981; McDonald, 1982b). Likewise, the chandelier cells of the cerebral cortex have similar contacts with cortical pyramidal cells and there is evidence that these synapses in the cortex are inhibitory (Peters, 1984). Since the output of the basolateral amygdala depends on action potential generation at the initial segments of amygdaloid pyramidal cell axons, amygdaloid chandelier cells could have a powerful influence on the ability of

---

nucleus. **B:** Small multipolar neuron of the basal parvicellular nucleus. **C:** Medium-sized bitufted neuron of the parvicellular basal nucleus. **D:** Large multipolar neuron of the magnocellular basal nucleus. **E:** Small multipolar neuron of the magnocellular basal nucleus. **F:** Large bipolar neuron of the magnocellular basal nucleus. **G:** Medium-sized bipolar neuron of the magnocellular basal nucleus. Reprint from McDonald (1982b) with permission.

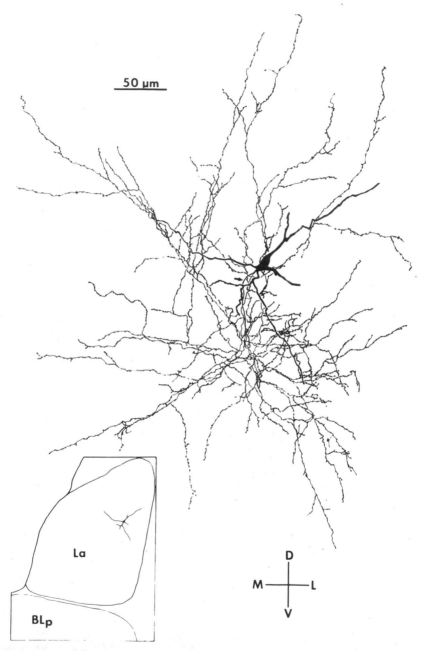

50 μm

La

BLp

D
M——L
V

Fig. 3. Drawing of a Golgi-impregnated nonpyramidal neuron in the rat lateral nucleus. Note the dense local axonal arborization, including the numerous varicosities (presumptive axon terminals). Reprint from McDonald (1982b) with permission.

the amygdala to activate other brain regions. One chandelier cell could simultaneously modulate the activity of numerous pyramidal cells in its vicinity.

Amygdaloid neurogliaform neurons, which resemble their counterparts in the cerebral cortex, have been observed in the basolateral amygdala of the cat (Tömböl and Szafranska-Kosmal, 1972; Kamal and Tömböl, 1975), rat (McDonald, 1982b), opossum (McDonald and Culberson, 1981) and monkey (personal observations). They have small (9–12 μm diameter), spherical cell bodies, and 6–10 primary dendrites which branch profusely to form a small, spherical dendritic field that averages 100 μm in diameter. Axons branch profusely to form a dense tangle of collaterals that only extends slightly beyond the confines of the dendritic field. Axonal collaterals, as well as distal dendritic branches, make numerous intimate contacts with dendrites of neighboring pyramidal neurons, but never with their own dendrites. These cells appear to be local circuit neurons with a very small sphere of influence.

The "cone cells" described by Millhouse and DeOlmos (1983) in the rat lateral nucleus have large cell bodies and spine-sparse dendrites that consist of numerous irregular varicosities. These cells have not been observed in other species. The "extended neurons" of Millhouse and DeOlmos (1983) are large nonpyramidal cells with long spine-sparse dendrites which branch very sparingly. They closely resemble the "reticular" neurons described by Mukhina and Leontovich (1970) in the dog and may correspond to the large nonpyramidal neurons that project to the mediodorsal thalamic nucleus (see above). In the author's opinion the so-called "modified pyramidal neurons" of Millhouse and DeOlmos (1983), which have spine-sparse dendrites, should be classified as large nonpyramidal cells.

CORTICAL NUCLEUS

The cortical nucleus, which can be divided into several subdivisions (anterior cortical nucleus, posterior cortical nucleus, and periamygdaloid cortex), is continuous with the piriform cortex along the inferior surface of the brain. Its deeper layers merge imperceptibly with the basolateral amygdala. As pointed out by Hall (1972), the cells of the cortical nucleus of the cat closely resemble those of the adjacent piriform cortex and basolateral amygdala. The majority of the neurons are spiny pyramidal and semipyramidal neurons. In addition, there are scattered, spine-sparse, nonpyramidal cells that often have beaded dendrites. Similar observations have been made in the rat (Yu, 1969) and opossum (McDonald, 1978). The following description of the cell types of the cortical nucleus is based primarily on the observations by Hall (1972) in the cat, but applies equally well to the rat and opossum. Figure 4 illustrates the neuronal morphology of the posterior cortical nucleus of the opossum. Hall (1972) did not identify discrete subdivisions in the cat cortical nucleus.

The cortical nucleus consists of a superficial molecular layer that contains few neurons (layer I of Hall, 1972) and a deeper cell-rich region (layers II–IV of Hall, 1972). The most superficial zone of the cell-rich portion of the nucleus (layer II) has a higher neuronal density than the deeper portions of the nucleus (layers III and IV). The principal neurons of the cortical nucleus are spiny pyram-

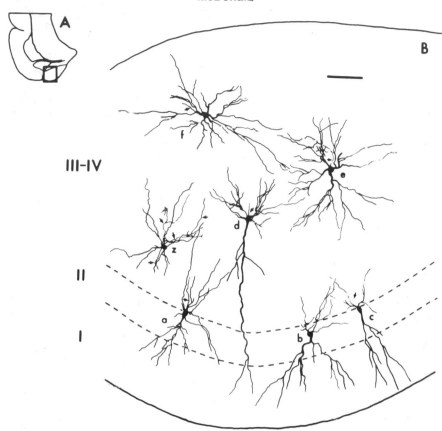

Fig. 4. Composite drawing of Golgi-impregnated neurons in the posterior cortical nucleus of the opossum (**Inset A** shows the location of the field illustrated in **B**). Dendritic spines are not illustrated. Roman numerals indicate layers. Cell z is a spine-sparse nonpyramidal neuron with a modest local axonal arborization. The remaining cells are spiny "pyramidal neurons". Scale = 100 μm.

idal neurons whose apical dendrites often extend into the superficial plexiform layer (Fig. 4, neurons c, d), where most of their branches arise (Hall, 1972). Some of these apical dendrites are oriented perpendicular to the pial surface while others are oriented obliquely, or even horizontally. The degree to which apical dendrites are oriented perpendicular to the pial surface varies in different subdivisions of the nucleus. Other spiny neurons do not have easily distinguishable apical and basal dendrites and have been termed modified pyramidal cells (Fig. 4, neurons e, f). Some spiny neurons exhibit polygonal or fusiform configurations (Fig. 4, neuron a); the latter cells were seen primarily in layer II. The axons of the various forms of spiny neurons arise from the cell body or the proximal portion of one of the basal dendrites. These axons course toward the stria terminalis and give off collaterals to deeper portions of the nucleus.

The spine-sparse neurons of the cortical nucleus (Fig. 4, neuron z) closely resemble their counterparts in the basolateral amygdala (Hall, 1972). Their axons arborize in the vicinity of the cell of origin, which suggests that they are local circuit neurons (Szafranska-Kosmal and Tömböl, 1972; Kamal and Tömböl, 1975).

From the description above it is quite clear that the neurons of the cortical nucleus are very similar to those of the basolateral amygdala (and the adjacent piriform cortex). Since there is extensive dendritic overlap in the region where the cortical nucleus merges with the basolateral amygdala, and also at the borders between many of the individual nuclei of the basolateral amygdala, the cortical nucleus and basolateral amygdala appear to form an anatomical continuum (Hall, 1972). On the other hand, it is important to remember that each of the nuclei of the basolateral amygdala and subnuclei of the cortical nucleus have distinct connections and, undoubtedly, distinct functions.

Nucleus of the Lateral Olfactory Tract

The nucleus of the lateral olfactory tract (NLOT) is a very conspicuous structure located rostromedial to the anterior cortical nucleus. NLOT consists of three layers and is less than 1 mm in diameter (Fig. 5). Layer I is a superficial plexiform layer that contains very few neurons. Layer II is a well-circumscribed cell-dense layer that consists primarily of medium-sized pyramidal neurons. Layer III is an aggregation of large neurons deep to layer II that caps the nucleus. Deep to layer III caudally is a compact fiber bundle, the commissural bundle of the stria terminalis, which arises from NLOT and joins the stria terminalis.

Perhaps because of its compelling architecture, there have been two separate investigations of the neuronal morphology of this small nucleus in the rat (McDonald, 1983b; Millhouse and Uemura-Sumi, 1985). In addition, the cell types in the cat have been described as part of more comprehensive Golgi studies of the amygdala in this species (Hall, 1972; Tömböl and Szafranska-Kosmal, 1972; Kamal and Tömböl, 1975). The cytoarchitecture of NLOT appears to be virtually identical in both rat and cat. There are two main cell classes which closely resemble the two cell classes in the basolateral and cortical nuclei. Most of the neurons in NLOT are spiny neurons that may exhibit pyramidal, semipyramidal, or stellate morphologies (class A neurons of McDonald, 1983b). The remaining cells constitute a heterogeneous population of spine-sparse nonpyramidal cells (classes B and C of McDonald, 1983b; stellate and nonspiny cells of Millhouse and Uemura-Sumi, 1985).

Layer II consists primarily of spiny pyramidal neurons that resemble those of the cortical nucleus (Fig. 5, neurons 5–8). The basal dendrites are relatively short and arborize in the vicinity of the cell body, whereas the apical dendrite extends into layer I, where it gives rise to several branches. The axons of these cells give off several collaterals which arborize in layer II. Most pyramidal cells have axons that course dorsally and enter the commissural bundle of the stria terminalis. Other axons or axonal branches course medially, laterally, rostrally, or caudally from the nucleus (Millhouse and Uemura-Sumi, 1985), presumably

McDonald

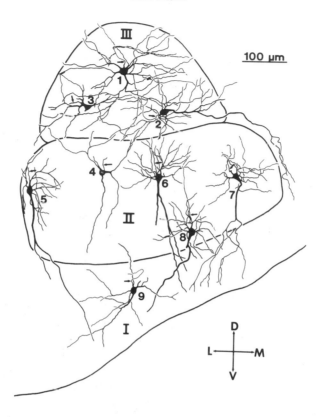

Fig. 5. Composite drawing of Golgi-impregnated neurons in the nucleus of the lateral olfactory tract of the rat that best illustrate the cytoarchitecture of the nucleus. Dendritic spines are not illustrated. All cells are spiny pyramidal or semipyramidal neurons except cells 3 and 4, which are spine-sparse nonpyramidal neurons. Reprint from McDonald (1983b) with permission from Pergamon Press.

to project to various regions in the basal forebrain. The spiny neuronal population in layer I and the most superficial portion of layer II consists of pyramidal and semipyramidal neurons with obliquely oriented apical dendrites (Fig. 5, neurons 8, 9), as well as spiny stellate cells.

Most of the neurons in layer III are large spiny stellate cells (Fig. 5, neuron 1). In addition, there are some pyramidal neurons with apical dendrites that course along one of the borders of layer II (Fig. 5, neuron 2), or even through layer II (Millhouse and Uemuri-Sumi, 1985), and give rise to branches that extend into layer I. The axons of the spiny neurons in layer III give off collaterals that arborize mainly within layer III. The main axon courses dorsally and some have been seen entering the commissural bundle of the stria terminalis (McDonald, 1983b).

All three layers contain spine-sparse nonpyramidal neurons that vary in morphology (Fig. 5, neurons 3, 4). In both rat (McDonald, 1983b; Millhouse and Uemura-Sumi, 1985) and cat (Tömböl and Szafranska-Kosmal, 1972) some of these cells exhibit dense local axonal arborizations typical of local circuit neurons. One type of nonpyramidal cell observed only in the most dorsal part of layer III resembles a neurogliaform neuron (class C neuron of McDonald, 1983b; small aspiny neuron of Millhouse and Uemura-Sumi, 1985).

NLOT is replaced caudally and medially by the bed nucleus of the accessory olfactory tract (BNAOT). Like NLOT, the BNAOT is fairly well circumscribed. The principal neurons in BNAOT are pyramidal and modified pyramidal cells with apical dendrites that are oriented obliquely and horizontally as well as vertically.

Central Nucleus

The central nucleus has recently attracted considerable attention because it has been found to contain a vast array of different neuropeptides and is unique among amygdaloid nuclei in its extensive connections with visceral and monoaminergic nuclei of the brain stem. Cytoarchitectural studies of the central nucleus have been conducted in a variety of species using Nissl and Golgi techniques; these investigations have revealed that the central nucleus in all species consists of several subdivisions. Detailed hodological and immunohistochemical studies, conducted primarily in the rat, have demonstrated that each subdivision exhibits a characteristic set of connections and neuropeptides (for a review see DeOlmos et al., 1985). In virtually all mammals it is possible to recognize a medial subdivision of the central nucleus located just lateral to the medial amygdaloid nucleus, and a lateral portion located just medial to the caudoventral caudatoputamen (Koikegami, 1963). In the rat the lateral portion can be divided into two subdivisions: (1) a lateral subdivision proper (CL) located just lateral to the medial subdivision; and (2) a lateral capsular subdivision (CLC) that encapsulates the lateral half of CL (McDonald, 1982a). The CLC merges laterally with the caudoventral caudatoputamen. In addition, two further subdivisions of the central nucleus, located between the medial and lateral portions of the nucleus, have been identified in the rat (intermediate subdivision of McDonald, 1982a, and the ventral subdivision of Cassell et al., 1986). Since the latter two subdivisions appear to be unique to the rat, they are not discussed in the present account.

The principal neurons in the medial subdivision of the central nucleus of the rat (Fig. 6, neuron A) have ovoid or fusiform cell bodies that are approximately $18 \times 12 \ \mu m$ (McDonald, 1982a; Cassell and Gray, 1989). These cells have three to four primary dendrites that branch sparingly and have a moderate-to-sparse density of dendritic spines. Axons give off several thin, beaded collaterals with few branches before leaving the nucleus by crossing its dorsal or medial boundaries. Similar neurons have been observed in the medial subdivision of the cat central nucleus, but these cells are larger in this species (Hall, 1972; Tömböl and Szafranska-Kosmal, 1972; Kamal and Tömböl, 1975).

The medial subdivision of the rat central nucleus also contains a small number of cells with virtually no dendritic spines (McDonald, 1982a; Cassell and Gray, 1989). The cell bodies of these neurons are slightly larger than those of the

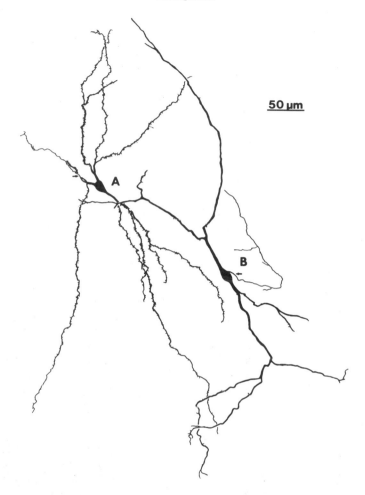

50 µm

Fig. 6. Golgi-impregnated neurons of the medial subdivision of the central nucleus in the rat. Dendrites of cell **A** are thin and have a moderate covering of spines, while cell **B** has thick dendrites with virtually no dendritic spines. Reprint from McDonald (1982a) with permission.

principal cell type (Fig. 6, neuron B). These cells have two to four primary dendrites that are quite thick (3–4 µm) and give rise to several large-caliber branches that are very long. Their axons are similar to those of the principal cells. This second cell type has not been described in the cat.

As first pointed out by Hall (1972), the principal cell type in the lateral portion of the central nucleus of the cat resembles the medium spiny neurons of the laterally adjacent putamen (see also Tömböl and Szafranska-Kosmal, 1972, and Kamal and Tömböl, 1975). Similar medium-sized spiny neurons have been

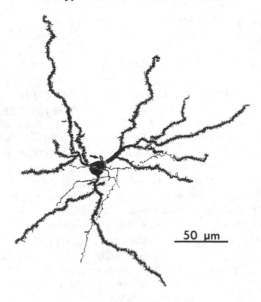

50 µm

Fig. 7. Golgi-impregnated medium-sized spiny neuron of the lateral subdivision of the central nucleus in the rat. Reprint from McDonald (1982a) with permission.

observed in both the CL and CLC of the rat central nucleus (medium-sized spiny neurons of McDonald, 1982a; Cassell and Gray, 1989). The cell bodies of these cells in the rat are ovoid and average 16 × 12 µm (Fig. 7). They have three to five primary dendrites, each of which forms a dendritic arborization with three to six branch points. Frequently a number of branches are given off in rapid succession, giving the dendritic arborization a tufted appearance. The secondary and more distal dendritic branches have the highest density of dendritic spines of any cells in the amygdaloid complex. Neurons near the borders of CL in the rat often have dendrites that are oriented tangential to the border of the subdivision so as not to enter the adjacent subdivisions of the central nucleus. The axons of medium-sized spiny neurons extend for 25–150 µm before their impregnation ceases. These axons give off several beaded collaterals that arborize modestly in the region of the cell; they have been observed forming intimate contacts with the dendrites of other medium-sized spiny neurons and their own dendrites (McDonald, 1982a).

In addition to the medium-sized spiny neurons, the lateral portions of the central nucleus of the rat also contain a small number of spine-sparse neurons whose cell bodies vary from medium-sized to small (McDonald, 1982a; Cassell and Gray, 1989). The main axon was only impregnated for a short distance but in some instances was seen to give rise to several beaded collaterals which branched modestly in the region of the cell. Similar spine-sparse neurons have also been described in the lateral part of the central nucleus of the cat (Tömböl and Szafranska-Kosmal, 1972; Kamal and Tömböl, 1975). In addition, Hall (1972) observed a small number of large spine-sparse neurons with large-caliber primary dendrites in the lateral subdivision of the cat central nucleus. McDonald described similar cells located adjacent to the CLC of the rat but considered them to be constituents of a medially directed extension of the putamen which appeared to merge with the central amygdaloid nucleus (McDonald, 1982a). These large neurons resemble the large cholinergic neurons of the striatum (Bolam et al., 1984) as well as the large spine-sparse neurons of the medial subdivision of the rat central nucleus.

Thus, not only does the lateral portion of the central nucleus blend with the laterally adjacent striatum, but the cytology of the two regions is also very similar. The medium-sized spiny neurons of the central nucleus resemble their counterparts in the striatum (Hall, 1972; McDonald, 1982a; Chang et al., 1982). In addition, the morphology and relative numbers of spine-sparse neurons of the central nucleus (McDonald, 1982a) are comparable to those of the striatum (Chang et al., 1982). Since the connections of the central nucleus also bear a close resemblance to those of certain parts of the striatum, especially the nucleus accumbens, it would appear that anatomically, and perhaps functionally, the central nucleus should be considered a striatumlike structure (McDonald, 1982a; Fallon and Loughlin, 1987; Heimer et al., 1985; DeOlmos et al., 1985; Alheid and Heimer, 1988). On the other hand, the neuropeptide chemistry of the central nucleus is quite different from that of most parts of the striatum (DeOlmos et al., 1985).

Medial Nucleus

The medial amygdaloid nucleus, located along the medial surface of the amygdala just medial to the central nucleus, has been studied using Golgi methods in the cat (Hall, 1972; Tömböl and Szafranska-Kosmal, 1972; Kamal and Tömböl, 1975), dog (Mukina and Leontovich, 1970) and rat (Yu, 1969; Millhouse and DeOlmos, 1981). Its neuronal organization, which appears to be relatively simple, is very similar in all species. In most studies only one cell type was observed; these cells are very similar to the principal cell type found in the adjacent medial subdivision of the central nucleus (see above). These neurons have oval cell bodies which vary from small to medium-sized and have only two to four primary dendrites. These primary dendrites give rise to only a few branches which extend for fairly long distances within the nucleus. The dendritic spine density varies among neurons from moderate to fairly sparse. Some neurons in the rat medial nucleus have thick dendrites that exhibit a very dense covering of spines (Millhouse and DeOlmos, 1981; personal observations); the spine density of these latter neurons is equivalent to that of the lateral portion of the central nucleus (personal observations).

Most dendrites extend toward the pial surface in either an oblique or perpendicular manner (personal observations in the rat). Some dendrites located in the deep part of the nucleus are oriented parallel to the fibers of the adjacent stria. In addition, some superficially located neurons have dendrites oriented parallel to the pial surface (Millhouse and DeOlmos, 1981). In all species studied, only the initial portion of the axon was impregnated; these axons coursed medially toward the basal nucleus or dorsomedially toward the stria terminalis (Tömböl and Szafranska-Kosmal, 1972; Kamal and Tömböl, 1975). In some cases the axons were seen to give rise to a few sparsely branched collaterals that were confined to the medial nucleus (Kamal and Tömböl, 1975). Thus, there is no evidence for the existence of local circuit neurons in the medial nucleus. However, Hall (1972) observed a small number of neurons with beaded dendrites and no dendritic spines; although it is possible that these cells could function as local circuit neurons, there is no information concerning their axonal morphology.

Hall (1972) noted that the border separating the medial and cortical nuclei in the cat was easily discernible in Golgi preparations due to the differences in neuronal morphology in the two nuclei. The pyramidal and semipyramidal morphology of cortical nucleus neurons was quite distinct from the sparsely branched, extended dendritic arborizations typical of medial nucleus neurons. This distinction is also evident in the rat (personal observations). Likewise, the border separating the medial nucleus from the caudoventrally adjacent amygdalohippocampal area is also very evident because the principal cells of the latter nucleus, like the cortical nucleus, are pyramidal neurons (personal observations in the rat). On the other hand, the exact borders separating the medial nucleus from the substantia innominata, anterior amygdaloid area, and medial subdivision of the central nucleus are not evident in Golgi preparations because the neurons in these various areas are similar and there is extensive dendritic overlap (personal observations).

Bed Nucleus of the Stria Terminalis

It was Johnston (1923) who first pointed out that the bed nucleus of the stria terminalis (BNST) was actually a rostral extension of the amygdala. Johnston provided evidence that, both ontogenetically and phylogenetically, the BNST and the central and medial amygdaloid nuclei develop from the same rudiment. Thus, in nonmammalian vertebrates and fetal mammals the centromedial amygdala and BNST are found at opposite ends of a sagittally oriented gray column in which the stria terminalis is embedded. The expansion of the internal capsule (both ontogenetically and phylogenetically) divides this column into rostral and caudal parts, the BNST and centromedial amygdala, respectively, which remain interconnected by the stria terminalis. In most species there are scattered cells associated with the stria that are remnants of the intermediate portions of the original cell column. Recent hodological and immunohistochemical studies have provided evidence that there are additional cell bridges connecting the BNST and amygdala that are located just ventral to the internal capsule in the substantia innominata (for reviews see DeOlmos et al., 1985, and Alheid and Heimer, 1988). The BNST, substantia innominata, and centromedial amygdala have been called the "extended amygdala" by Alheid and Heimer (1988).

A Golgi study of the rat BNST conducted in the author's laboratory demonstrated that the cell types of the centromedial amygdala and BNST were virtually identical (McDonald, 1983a). This investigation revealed that in the anterodorsal part of the lateral subdivision of the BNST there exists a fairly well-circumscribed

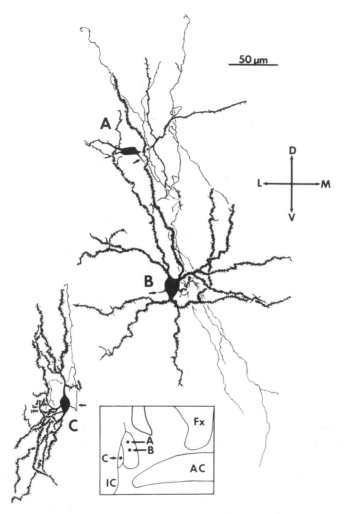

Fig. 8. Golgi-impregnated neurons in the bed nucleus of the stria terminalis of the rat at the level of the anterior commissure (AC) that were drawn from two adjacent sections. **Inset** shows location of neurons A, B, and C (IC, internal capsule; Fx, fornix). Cell **A** is a spine-sparse neuron in the anterodorsal part of the lateral BNST. Cell **B** is a medium-sized spiny neuron in this same part of the BNST. Cell **C** is a typical neuron of the juxtacapsular subdivision of the nucleus. Reprint from McDonald (1983a) with permission.

region that closely resembles the CL of the central amygdaloid nucleus. The predominant cell type in this region is a medium-sized spiny neuron with a stellate dendritic configuration (Fig. 8, neuron B). In addition, a small number of spine-sparse neurons were observed (Fig. 8, neuron A). Both of these cell types are identical to their counterparts in CL (e.g., compare neuron B in Fig. 8 with the neuron in Fig. 7). The medium-sized spiny neurons of the anterodorsal part of the lateral BNST, like their counterparts in CL, resemble medium spiny neurons of the striatum.

The principal cell type in more ventral and posterior parts of the lateral subdivision of the BNST is a moderately spiny neuron with two to three sparsely branched extended dendrites (personal observations). These neurons closely resemble those of the medial subdivision of the central nucleus. Likewise, comparisons of the brain stem projections and peptide immunohistochemistry of the central amygdaloid nucleus and BNST also suggest that the anterodorsal and ventroposterior parts of the lateral BNST are homologous with, respectively, the lateral and medial subdivisions of the central amygdaloid nucleus (Moga and Gray, 1985; Gray and Magnuson, 1987; Moga et al., 1989). It remains to be determined whether there is a portion of the BNST that corresponds to the lateral capsular subdivision of the central nucleus.

Neurons in the medial subdivision of the BNST are medium-sized cells with 2–3 primary dendrites that branch modestly (Fig. 9). These dendrites, whose spine density varies from sparse to dense depending on the exact location of

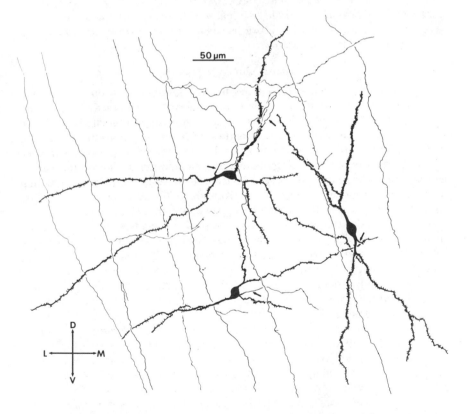

Fig. 9. Composite drawing of Golgi-impregnated neurons in the posterior portion of the medial subdivision of the rat BNST. The fibers running through this field appeared to be derived from the stria terminalis. Reprint from McDonald (1982a) with permission.

the cell, extend for 200–400 μm. Thus, the morphology of the neurons in the medial subdivision of the BNST, including their dendritic arborization pattern and variability in dendritic spine density, is virtually identical to that seen in the medial amygdaloid nucleus. In addition to these morphological findings, there is also hodological and immunohistochemical evidence which suggests that the medial amygdaloid nucleus and medial BNST are homologous structures (see DeOlmos et al., 1985, for a review).

An additional subdivision of the BNST can be found between the internal capsule and the lateral BNST. This small lens-shaped region, termed the juxtacapsular subdivision of the BNST (McDonald, 1983a), contains small neurons whose spiny dendrites tend to remain confined to the subdivision (Fig. 8, neuron C). Both the morphology (McDonald, 1983a) and developmental origins (Bayer, 1987) of the neurons of the juxtacapsular subdivision suggest that it may be homologous to the intercalated masses of the amygdala.

Recent detailed cytoarchitectural and immunohistochemical studies have identified many additional subdivisions in the bed nucleus of the stria terminalis (DeOlmos et al., 1985; Moga et al., 1989; Ju and Swanson, 1989; Ju et al., 1989). Although the neuronal morphology in each of these subdivisions has not yet been studied in detail, initial indications suggest that they may exhibit cytological differences (Shi et al., 1990).

Intercalated Masses

The intercalated masses of the amygdala are a more-or-less continuous network of neurons that is associated with the borders of the central and basolateral nuclei. In the rat this network thickens to form substantial cell clusters located ventral, anterior, and medial to the rostral portion of the basal magnocellular nucleus. Similar intercalated masses have been identified in all species investigated. The neuronal morphology of the intercalated masses has been studied with the Golgi technique in rat (Millhouse, 1986), cat (Hall, 1972; Tömböl and Szafranska-Kosmal, 1972; Kamal and Tömböl, 1975) and dog (Mukhina and Leontovich, 1970); the main cell types are very similar in all of these species.

The great majority of neurons in the intercalated masses of all species are small ovoid cells with very spiny dendrites. These neurons are virtually identical to those of the juxtacapsular portion of the BNST and resemble smaller versions of the medium-sized spiny neurons of the striatum and lateral portions of the central nucleus. The initial portion of the axon of these cells usually gives off several short collaterals that arborize in the vicinity of the cell. The more distal portions of the axon have been observed to provide collaterals to the basolateral or central amygdaloid nuclei (Tömböl and Szafranska-Kosmal, 1972; Millhouse, 1986). Immunohistochemical studies indicate that these neurons are GABAergic (Nitecka and Ben-Ari, 1987). In addition to the small spiny neurons, Millhouse (1986) has observed a few small spine-sparse neurons that have well-arborized axons typical of local circuit neurons.

The other major cell type seen in the intercalated masses is a large neuron. These cells, which have been observed in all species investigated, tend to be found along the borders of the intercalated masses and make up a small percentage of the constituent neurons. These neurons have two to four robust primary dendrites that influence the shape of the cell body and branch rather modestly. The cell bodies of these neurons are very large for the amygdala—up to 40–60 μm in diameter in the rat (Millhouse, 1986) and 90 × 30 μm in the dog (Mukhina and Leontovich, 1970). The dendritic branches, which tend to parallel the borders of the adjacent basal, lateral, and central nuclei, extend for long distances from the cell body—up to 800 μm in the cat (Tömböl and Szafranska-Kosmal, 1972). Two major subclasses of large neurons can be identified on the basis of dendritic spine density: spiny and spine-sparse. Both types were observed in the rat, with the spine-sparse variety comprising the majority (Millhouse, 1986). Only spine-sparse cells were described in the dog (Mukhina and Leontovich, 1970), whereas only spiny cells were observed in the cat (Tömböl and Szafranska-Kosmal, 1972; Kamal and Tömböl, 1975). Only the initial portions of the axons of these cells were impregnated.

The terminal dendritic segments of the large intercalated neurons are frequently contorted, varicose, and spiny (Millhouse, 1986). In this respect, as well as in cell size and dendritic arborization pattern, they resemble the neurons of the globus pallidus (Millhouse, 1986) and some of the large nonpyramidal neurons of the basolateral amygdala. Since immunohistochemical studies have found large neurons in the intercalated masses that contain choline acetyltransferase, it appears that at least some of the large neurons are cholinergic (Nitecka and Frotscher, 1989).

Anterior Amygdaloid Area

The anterior amygdaloid area (AAA) is a diffuse region that surrounds the NLOT. Hall (1972) found that most of the cells in the cat AAA have medium-sized ovoid cell bodies that give rise to three to four primary dendrites. These dendrites branch sparingly and have a sparse-to-moderate density of dendritic spines. Other medium-sized neurons have beaded dendrites and few spines. Hall (1972) noted that the neuronal morphology of the AAA was very similar to that of the medial subdivision of the central nucleus and the medial amygdaloid nucleus. Likewise, Johnston (1923) did not distinguish the AAA from the anterior part of the central nucleus in his original Nissl studies of the mammalian amygdala. Price and coworkers have recently changed the nomenclature used to describe a cell-dense region located lateral to the caudal part of the substantia innominata in the rat; although this region was initially considered the anterior part of the central nucleus (Krettek and Price, 1978b), it is now considered a dorsal part of the AAA (Price et al., 1987). Observations in the author's laboratory indicate that the morphology of the medium-sized cells in the AAA, substantia innominata, medial nucleus, and medial subdivision of the central nucleus in the rat are similar (personal observations; Yu, 1969; DeOlmos et al., 1985). Hall (1972) and Yu (1969) provided no information on the axons of the medium-sized cells in AAA. Only the initial portions of the axons were observed in the material available in the author's laboratory.

In addition to the medium-sized cells in the cat AAA, there were also a small number of large neurons that were scattered between the diagonal band of Broca and the globus pallidus (Hall, 1972); only the cell bodies and the initial portions of the dendrites were impregnated. Similar cells have been observed in the rat AAA (personal observations, DeOlmos et al., 1985). These neurons in the rat have a small number of primary dendrites that branch sparingly. The dendritic branches extend for long distances and have few spines. Only the initial portions of the axons were observed. These cells appear to correspond to the large cholinergic neurons observed in the AAA in immunohistochemical preparations (Carlsen et al., 1985; Nitecka and Frotscher, 1989).

INTRINSIC CONNECTIONS OF THE AMYGDALA
Significance and Relationship to Amygdaloid Cytology

Because each of the amygdaloid nuclei exhibits distinctive connections with numerous extrinsic areas, the hodology of the amygdala is very complex. However, in addition to these extrinsic connections, there is an elaborate array of intrinsic connections between amygdaloid nuclei. These intra-amygdaloid circuits allow the integration and association of information from some of the highest brain centers to occur within the amygdala, and to subsequently influence amygdaloid output to CNS regions modulating visceral, endocrine, affective, and mnemonic activities.

The intrinsic connections of the amygdala have been studied with modern tract-tracing techniques in the rat (Nitecka et al., 1981a; Ottersen, 1982; DeOlmos et al., 1985), cat (Krettek and Price, 1978b; Wakefield, 1979; Russchen, 1982) and monkey (Aggleton, 1985). Because of the close proximity of the nuclei to each other, these intra-amygdaloid connections are more easily investigated in the larger-brained species. Although there appear to be some species differences, the overall organization of connections is basically similar in the rat, cat, and monkey (for a review see Price et al., 1987). These connections, and their relationship to the cytological configuration of the amygdala, are illustrated in Figure 10.

The morphological studies reviewed in the first part of this chapter reveal that the nuclei of the amygdala can be divided into at least two major groups on the basis of cytology: cortexlike nuclei and noncortexlike nuclei. The cortexlike nuclei include the basal, lateral, accessory basal, and cortical nuclei, as well as the periamygdaloid cortex, amygdalohippocampal area, and nucleus of the lateral olfactory tract. Like the cerebral cortex, these nuclei contain two main cell types: (1) spiny pyramidal (or modified pyramidal) projection neurons that constitute the majority of the constituent neurons, and (2) spine-sparse nonpyramidal neurons that are found in smaller numbers and function primarily as local circuit neurons. The remaining (noncortexlike) nuclei include the central and medial nuclei (and their counterparts in the bed nucleus of the stria terminalis and substantia innominata), and the anterior amygdaloid area. In addition, the intercalated masses constitute a special group of noncortexlike nuclei. The principal neurons in the noncortexlike nuclei, by definition, do not have a pyramidallike configuration. As illustrated in Figure 10, these two cytologically defined amygdaloid nuclear groups play different roles in the intrinsic circuitry of the amygdala. The cortexlike nuclei have extensive connections with each other and

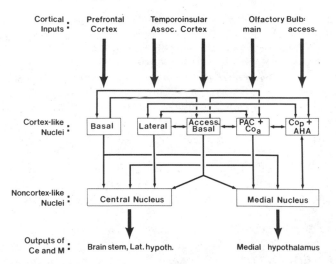

Fig. 10. Diagram illustrating the intrinsic connections and certain extrinsic connections of the amygdala in relation to the cytological configuration of its nuclei. For diagrammatic simplicity the anterior cortical nucleus (Co_a) and periamygdaloid nucleus (PAC), as well as the posterior cortical nucleus (Co_p) and amygdalohippocampal area (AHA), have been grouped together. Many of the connections illustrated have been demonstrated in at least two species (see Price et al., 1987, and DeOlmos et al., 1985 for detailed reviews). The projection from the lateral nucleus to the medial nucleus, demonstrated only in the monkey, is not indicated. Although the majority of the cortical inputs are directed to cortexlike nuclei, there are also some cortical inputs to the noncortexlike nuclei as well (not illustrated). Likewise, the connections of the cortexlike nuclei to the hypothalamus are not illustrated.

also project to the noncortexlike nuclei, whereas the latter have few projections back to the cortexlike portions of the amygdala.

Cortexlike Nuclei

In Figure 10, the cortexlike nuclei are illustrated so that the deeper nuclei are on the left and the more superficial nuclei are on the right. As illustrated in the diagram, there are extensive interconnections among these nuclei. One noteworthy exception to this rule, however, is the lack of connections between the basal and lateral nuclei [although there is very recent evidence that there may be such a connection in the monkey (Pitkänen and Amaral, 1990)]. In general, the projections of the deep nuclei (left side) to the superficial nuclei (right side) are more robust than the projections in the opposite direction. The projections of the lateral nucleus to the accessory basal nucleus and periamygdaloid cortex (PAC) are especially strong. As illustrated in Figure 10, these interconnections of the cortexlike nuclei suggest that complex information received from the frontal and temporoinsular cortices—including highly processed visual, auditory, somesthetic, and multimodal sensory information from sensory association cortices (Russchen, 1986)—is transmitted via intra-amygdaloid connections from the basolateral nuclei to the olfactory receiving areas of the superficial amygdala. The PAC and accessory basal nucleus may be important sites for this type of olfactory-nonolfactory sensory integration.

There is evidence from retrograde tract tracing studies that the connections between the lateral and accessory basal nuclei are subserved mainly by pyramidal and modified pyramidal cells (Wakefield, 1979; Aggleton, 1985). The finding that the neurons of the lateral nucleus are retrogradely labeled by injections of tritiated D-aspartate into the accessory basal nucleus suggests that these cells may use the excitatory amino acids glutamate and/or aspartate as neurotransmitters (Price et al., 1987). It is of interest in this regard that the pyramidal and modified pyramidal neurons of the cortexlike nuclei are intensely immunoreactive for glutamate and aspartate (McDonald et al., 1989; McDonald, 1989b).

The cortexlike nuclei also have extensive connections with the central and medial (noncortexlike) amygdaloid nuclei. The deeper cortexlike nuclei project mainly to the central nucleus, whereas the superficial nuclei project mainly to the medial nucleus. This is an important distinction since the central and medial nuclei influence different subcortical structures via their efferent projections (Fig. 10).

Noncortexlike Nuclei

Although the central and medial nuclei receive extensive projections from the cortexlike nuclei, they have only very weak projections back to these amygdaloid regions. There is evidence that the portions of the BNST that are analogous to the central and medial nuclei (i.e., the lateral and medial subdivisions of the BNST, respectively) have connections with the amygdala that are similar to those of the central and medial nuclei (DeOlmos et al., 1985; Grove, 1988a). It has been difficult to determine whether the central and medial amygdaloid nuclei are interconnected since these nuclei are adjacent to each other and there are problems distinguishing labeled projections from diffusion of injected tracer in tract tracing experiments. Nevertheless, interconnections between the two nuclei are indicated in the monkey (Price et al., 1987).

There is evidence that the central and medial nuclei have reciprocal connections with their analogues in the BNST and substantia innominata (DeOlmos et al., 1985; Grove, 1988a,b; Krettek and Price, 1978a). Thus the central amygdaloid nucleus, lateral BNST, and dorsal substantia innominata exhibit reciprocal interconnections with one another. Likewise, the medial amygdaloid nucleus, medial BNST, and ventral substantia innominata are reciprocally interconnected. The substantia innominata is different from other portions of the "extended" centromedial amygdala, however, since in addition to receiving projections from the cortexlike amygdaloid nuclei, it also has extensive efferent projections back to these nuclei (Ottersen, 1980; Grove, 1988b). It should also be mentioned in this regard that the anterior amygdaloid area, which constitutes another noncortexlike portion of the amygdala, has extensive reciprocal connections with all portions of the amygdala and extended amygdala, including the cortexlike amygdaloid nuclei, central and medial nuclei, BNST, and substantia innominata (Krettek and Price, 1978a; Ottersen, 1980; DeOlmos et al., 1985; Grove, 1988a,b).

Nucleus of the Lateral Olfactory Tract and Commissural Connections

NLOT is a cortexlike nucleus of the amygdala that exhibits very distinctive intrinsic, as well as extrinsic, connections. Amygdaloid inputs to NLOT arise from the periamygdaloid cortex and anterior cortical nucleus (i.e., the amygdaloid nuclei receiving inputs from the main olfactory bulb) and terminate mainly in the deep portion of the molecular layer (Krettek and Price, 1978b; Luskin and Price, 1983). Additional amygdaloid inputs from the basal nuclei terminate mainly in layer II (Krettek and Price, 1978b). NLOT has a glutamatergic projection to the basal nuclei that arises from layer III (Ottersen et al., 1985) as well as a projection to the contralateral NLOT (Krettek and Price, 1978b; Luskin and Price, 1983).

A number of additional commissural interamygdaloid connections have been described. The posterior part of the cortical nucleus projects to its contralateral homologue (Krettek and Price, 1978b; Nitecka et al., 1981b; Ottersen, 1982) as well as to the contralateral medial nucleus (Ottersen, 1982). Nitecka and coworkers (1981b) have described projections from the basal and accessory basal nuclei to the contralateral central, medial, and lateral nuclei.

CONCLUSIONS

Each of the amygdaloid nuclei contains two or more morphologically distinct cell types. The principal neurons in every amygdaloid nucleus are projection neurons whose dendrites exhibit a moderate-to-dense covering of dendritic spines. In most nuclei there is a second cell type observed in far fewer numbers whose dendrites are spine-sparse. In some nuclei these spine-sparse cells appear to be local circuit neurons. The neuronal morphology in the nucleus of the lateral olfactory tract, intercalated masses, and the basal, lateral, and central nuclei of nonprimate species have been investigated in the most detail. There is clearly a need to study the cell types of the primate amygdala and to examine the remaining nuclei of nonprimates more thoroughly. In addition, there have been few investigations that have sought to determine the ultrastructure, synaptology, hodology, or electrophysiology of identified cell types in any of the amygdaloid nuclei. This information is essential to understanding amygdaloid function at the neuronal level.

Different investigators have grouped the amygdaloid nuclei in various ways using different criteria. On the basis of neuronal morphology, amygdaloid nuclei can be lumped into two major groups: (1) cortexlike nuclei (which exhibit pyramidal or modified pyramidal neurons); and (2) noncortexlike nuclei (which do not contain pyramidal-like neurons). The cortexlike nuclei are contiguous with each other and exhibit dendritic overlap at most of their mutual borders. The nuclei near the brain surface more closely resemble the cortex than the more deeply situated nuclei. The borders separating the cortexlike nuclei from the noncortexlike nuclei are sharply drawn; there is little or no dendritic overlap between the two groups.

Like the cortexlike nuclei, the noncortexlike nuclei are contiguous with each other and exhibit significant dendritic overlap at their mutual borders. The noncortexlike nuclear group is more centrally placed than the cortexlike group and abuts the striatum. In fact, the nuclei in direct contact with the striatum (e.g., the lateral subdivision of the central nucleus, which is adjacent to the caudoventral striatum, and the anterodorsal part of the lateral BNST, which is adjacent to the nucleus accumbens) have neurons that resemble the medium spiny neurons of the striatum. In general, however, these striatumlike amygdaloid neurons tend to have fewer, and less tortuous, dendrites than their striatal counterparts. This trend is continued in the noncortexlike nuclei that are more distant from the striatum. Thus the spiny neurons of the medial subdivision of the central nucleus and the medial amygdaloid nucleus have fewer dendrites than those of the lateral subdivision of the central nucleus. In addition, their dendrites are more rectilinear and have fewer spines. Although it could be argued that these cells may represent highly modified striatumlike neurons, it has been suggested that some parts of the more medial regions of the noncortexlike group may be pallidumlike structures (Fallon and Loughlin, 1987; Turner and Zimmer, 1984; Alheid and Heimer, 1988).

In conclusion, it appears that the cortexlike nuclei and some of the noncortexlike nuclei exhibit features characteristic of the cortex and corpus striatum, respectively. It has also been suggested that the intra-amygdaloid connections of certain of these two amygdaloid groups resemble the connections of the cortex with the corpus striatum (Fallon and Loughlin, 1987). Thus the cortexlike nuclei project to the noncortexlike nuclei, but there is no significant projection of the latter to the former. The hypothesis that these two amygdaloid groups are modeled after the cerebral cortex and corpus striatum may be of heuristic value for directing future research on the amygdala.

ACKNOWLEDGMENTS

The author is grateful for the continued support from the National Institutes of Health (grant NS19733). The technical assistance provided by Ms. Peggy Sullivan and Patricia Knecht is greatly appreciated. I would also like to thank Drs. George Alheid, Lennart Heimer, and Jose DeOlmos for their valuable comments on an earlier version of this chapter.

REFERENCES

Aggleton JP (1985): A description of intra-amygdaloid connections in old world monkeys. Exp Brain Res 57:390–399.

Alheid GF, Heimer L (1988): New perspectives in basal forebrain organization of special relevance for neuropsychiatric disorders: The striatopallidal, amygdaloid, and corticopetal components of substantia innominata. Neuroscience 1:1–39.

Bayer SA (1987): Neurogenetic and morphogenetic heterogeneity in the bed nucleus of the stria terminalis. J Comp Neurol 265:47–64.

Bolam JP, Wainer BH, Smith AD (1984): Characterization of cholinergic neurons in the rat neostriatum. A combination of choline acetyltransferase immunocytochemistry, Golgi-impregnation and electron microscopy. Neuroscience 3:711–718.

Braak H, Braak E (1983): Neuronal types in the basolateral amygdaloid nuclei of man. Brain Res Bull 11:349–365.

Carlsen J (1989): New perspectives on the functional anatomical organization of the basolateral amygdala. Acta Neurol Scand (Suppl 122) 79:5–27.

Carlsen J, Heimer L (1986): A correlated light and electron microscopic immunocyto-chemical study of cholinergic terminals and neurons in the rat amygdaloid body with special emphasis on the basolateral amygdaloid nucleus. J Comp Neurol 244:121–136.

Carlsen J, Heimer L (1988): The basolateral amygdaloid complex as a cortical-like structure. Brain Res 441:377–380.

Carlsen J, Zaborszky L, Heimer L (1985): Cholinergic projections from the basal forebrain to the basolateral amygdaloid complex: A combined retrograde fluorescent and immunohistochemical study. J Comp Neurol 234:155–167.

Cassell MD, Gray TS, Kiss JZ (1986): Neuronal architecture in the rat central nucleus of the amygdala: A cytological, hodological and immunocytochemical study. J Comp Neurol 264:478–499.

Cassell MD, Gray TS (1989): Morphology of peptide-immunoreactive neurons in the rat central nucleus of the amygdala. J Comp Neurol 231:320–333.

Chang HT, Wilson CJ, Kitai ST (1982): A Golgi study of rat neostriatal neurons: Light microscopic analysis. J Comp Neurol 208:107–126.

Connors BW, Gutnick MJ (1990): Intrinsic firing patterns of diverse neocortical neurons. Trends in Neurosciences 13:99–104.

DeOlmos JS, Alheid GF, Beltramino CA (1985): Amygdala. In Paxinos G (ed): "The Rat Nervous System." Orlando, FL: Academic Press, pp 223–334.

Fallon JH, Loughlin SE (1987): Monoamine innervation of cerebral cortex and a theory of the role of monoamines in cerebral cortex and basal ganglia. In Jones EG, Peters A (eds): "Cerebral Cortex: Further Aspects of Cortical Function, Including Hippocampus." New York, Plenum Press pp. 41–127.

Feldman M, Peters A (1978): The forms of nonpyramidal neurons in the visual cortex of the rat. J Comp Neurol 179:761–794.

Gray TS, Magnuson DJ (1987): Neuropeptide neuronal efferents from the bed nucleus of the stria terminalis and central amygdaloid nucleus to the dorsal vagal complex in the rat. J Comp Neurol 262:365–374.

Grove EA (1988a): Neural associations of the substantia innominata in the rat: Afferent connections. J Comp Neurol 277:315–346.

Grove EA (1988b): Efferent connections of the substantia innominata in the rat. J Comp Neurol 277:347–364.

Gurdjian ES (1928): The corpus striatum of the rat. J Comp Neurol 45:249–281.

Gustafson EL, Carol PJ, Moore RY (1986): Neuropeptide Y localization in the rat amygdaloid complex. J Comp Neurol 251:349–362.

Hall E (1972): The amygdala of the cat: A Golgi study. Z Zellforsch, 134:439–458.

Heimer L, Alheid GF, Zaborszky L (1985): Basal ganglia. In Paxinos G (ed): "The Rat Nervous System." Orlando, FL: Academic Press, pp 37–86.

Herzog AG (1982): The relationship of dendritic branching complexity to ontogeny and cortical connectivity in the pyramidal cells of the monkey amygdala: A Golgi study. Dev Brain Res 4:73–77.

Humphrey T (1936): The telencephalon of the bat. I. The non-cortical nuclear masses and certain pertinent fiber connections. J Comp Neurol 65:603–711.

Johnston JB (1923): Further contributions to the study of the evolution of the forebrain. J Comp Neurol 35:337–481.

Ju G, Swanson LW (1989): Studies on the cellular architecture of the bed nuclei of the stria terminalis in the rat: I. Cytoarchitecture. J Comp Neurol 280:587–602.

Ju G, Swanson LW, Simerly RB (1989): Studies on the cellular architecture of the bed nuclei of the stria terminalis in the rat: II. Chemoarchitecture. J Comp Neurol 280:603–621.

Kamal AM, Tömböl T (1975): Golgi studies on the amygdaloid nuclei of the cat. J Hirnforsch 16:175–201.

Koikegami H (1963): Amygdala and other related limbic structures; experimental studies on the anatomy and function: I. Anatomical researches with some neurophysiological observations. Acta Med Biol (Niigata) 10:161–277.

Krettek JE, Price JL (1978a): Amygdaloid projections to subcortical structures within the basal forebrain and brainstem in the rat and cat. J Comp Neurol 178:225–254.

Krettek JE, Price JL (1978b): A description of the amygdaloid complex in the rat and cat with observations on intra-amygdaloid axonal connections. J Comp Neurol 178:255–280.

Lund JS (1984): Spiny stellate neurons. In Peters A, Jones EG (eds): "Cerebral Cortex." New York: Plenum Press, pp 255–308.

Luskin MB, Price JL (1983): The topographic organization of associational fibers of the olfactory system in the rat including centrifugal fibers to the olfactory bulb. J Comp Neurol 216:264–291.

McDonald AJ (1978): "The Cytoarchitecture and Projections of the Amygdala of the Opossum, *Didelphis virginiana*." Thesis, West Virginia University.

McDonald AJ (1982a): Cytoarchitecture of the central amygdaloid nucleus of the rat. J Comp Neurol 208:401–418.

McDonald AJ (1982b): Neurons of the lateral and basolateral amygdaloid nuclei: A Golgi study in the rat. J Comp Neurol 212:293–312.

McDonald AJ (1983a): Neurons of the bed nucleus of the stria terminalis: A Golgi study in the rat. Brain Res Bull 10:111–120.

McDonald AJ (1983b): Cytoarchitecture of the nucleus of the lateral olfactory tract: A Golgi study in the rat. Brain Res Bull 10:497–503.

McDonald AJ (1984): Neuronal organization of the lateral and basolateral amygdaloid nuclei in the rat. J Comp Neurol 222:586–606.

McDonald AJ (1985a): Morphology of peptide-containing neurons in the rat basolateral amygdaloid nucleus. Brain Res 338:186–191.

McDonald AJ (1985b): Immunohistochemical identification of gamma-aminobutyric acid-containing neurons in the rat basolateral amygdala. Neurosci Lett 53:203–207.

McDonald AJ (1986): Projections of amygdaloid neurons containing somatostatin, vasoactive intestinal peptide, or GABA. Soc Neurosci Abstr 12:1253.

McDonald AJ (1987): Organization of amygdaloid projections to the mediodorsal thalamus and prefrontal cortex: A fluorescence retrograde transport study in the rat. J Comp Neurol 262:46–58.

McDonald AJ (1989a): Coexistence of somatostatin with neuropeptide Y, but not with cholecystokinin or vasoactive intestinal peptide, in neurons of the rat amygdala. Brain Res 500:37–45.

McDonald AJ (1989b): Excitatory amino acid immunohistochemistry distinguishes basolateral amygdaloid neurons projecting to the prefrontal cortex versus mediodorsal thalamic nucleus. Soc Neurosci Abstr 15:1249.

McDonald AJ, Beitz AJ, Larson AA, Kuriyama R, Sellitto C, Madl JE (1989): Co-localization of glutamate and tubulin in putative excitatory neurons of the hippocampus and amygdala: An immunohistochemical study using monoclonal antibodies. Neuroscience 30:405–421.

McDonald AJ, Baimbridge KG (1990): Calcium binding protein containing neurons of the basolateral amygdala also exhibit GABA and cytochrome oxidase immunoreactivity. Soc Neurosci Abstr 16:431.

McDonald AJ, Culberson JL (1981): Neurons of the basolateral amygdala: A Golgi study in the opossum (*Didelphis virginiana*). Am J Anat 162:327–342.

McDonald AJ, Pearson JC (1989): Coexistence of GABA and peptide immunoreactivity in non-pyramidal neurons of the basolateral amygdala. Neurosci Lett 100:53–58.

Millhouse OE (1986): The intercalated cells of the amygdala. J Comp Neurol 247:246–271.

Millhouse OE, DeOlmos J (1981): Aspects of the neuronal organization of the amygdala. In Ben-Ari Y (ed): "The Amygdala Complex." Amsterdam: Elsevier/North-Holland Biomedical Press, pp 33–43.

Millhouse OE, DeOlmos J (1983): Neuronal configurations in lateral and basolateral amygdala. Neuroscience 10:1269–1300.

Millhouse OE, Uemura-Sumi M (1985): The structure of the nucleus of the lateral olfactory tract. J Comp Neurol 233:517–552.

Moga MM, Gray TS (1985): Evidence for corticotropin-releasing factor, neurotensin, and somatostatin in the neural pathway from the central nucleus of the amygdala to the parabrachial nucleus. J Comp Neurol 241:275–284.

Moga MM, Saper CB, Gray TS (1989): Bed nucleus of the stria terminalis: Cytoarchitecture, immunohistochemistry, and projection to the parabrachial nucleus in the rat. J Comp Neurol 283:315–332.

Mukhina YK, Leontovich TA (1970): Neuronal structure of some amygdaloid nuclei in dogs. Arkiv Anatomii Gistologii Embriologii (Moscow) 59:62–70.

Nitecka L, Amerski L, Narkiewicz O (1981a): The organization of intraamygdaloid connections: An HRP study. J Hirnforsch 22:3–7.

Nitecka L, Amerski L, Narkiewicz O (1981b): Interamygdaloid connections in the rat studied by the horseradish peroxidase method. Neurosci Lett 26:1–4.

Nitecka L, Ben-Ari Y (1987): Distribution of GABA-like immunoreactivity in the rat amygdaloid complex. J Comp Neurol 266:45–55.

Nitecka L, Frotscher M (1989): Organization and synaptic interconnections of GABAergic and cholinergic elements in the rat amygdaloid nuclei: Single- and double-immunolabeling studies. J Comp Neurol 279:470–488.

Ottersen OP (1980): Afferent connections to the amygdaloid complex of the rat and cat: II. Afferents from the hypothalamus and the basal telencephalon. J Comp Neurol 194:267–289.

Ottersen OP (1982): Connections of the amygdala of the rat: IV. Corticoamygdaloid and intraamygdaloid connections as studied with axonal transport of horseradish peroxidase. J Comp Neurol 205:30–48.

Ottersen OP, Fisher BO, Rinvik E, Storm-Mathisen J (1985): Putative amino acid transmitters in the amygdala. In Schwarz R, Ben-Ari Y (eds): "Excitatory Amino Acids and Epilepsy." New York: Plenum Press, pp 53–66.

Peters A (1984): Chandelier cells. In Peters A, Jones EG (eds): "Cerebral Cortex." New York: Plenum Press, pp 361–380.

Pitkänen A, Amaral DG (1990): Intrinsic connections of the monkey amygdala: A PHA-L analysis of projections originating in the lateral nucleus. Soc Neurosci Abstr 16:122.

Price JL, Russchen FT, Amaral DG (1987): The limbic region: II. The amygdaloid complex. In Björklund A, Hökfelt T, Swanson LW (eds): "Handbook of Chemical Neuroanatomy," Vol. 5. Amsterdam: Elsevier, pp 279–388.

Russchen FT (1982): Amygdalopetal projections in the cat: II. Subcortical afferent connections. A study with retrograde tracing techniques. J Comp Neurol 207:157–176.

Russchen FT (1986): Cortical and subcortical afferents of the amygdaloid complex. In Schwarz R, Ben-Ari Y (eds): "Excitatory Amino Acids and Epilepsy." New York: Plenum Press, pp 35–52.

Russchen FT, Amaral DG, Price JL (1987): The afferent input to the magnocellular division of the mediodorsal thalamic nucleus in the monkey, Macaca fascicularis. J Comp Neurol 256:175–210.

Saint Marie RL, Peters A (1985): The morphology and synaptic connections of spiny stellate neurons in monkey visual cortex (area 17): A Golgi-electron microscopic study. J Comp Neurol 233:213–235.

Shi C-J, Roberts L, Cassell MD (1990): A re-evaluation of neuronal configurations in the rat bed nucleus of the stria terminalis (BNST). Soc Neurosci Abstr 16:125.

Sripanidkulchai K, Sripanidkulchai B, Wyss JM (1984): The cortical projection of the basolateral amygdaloid nucleus in the rat: A retrograde fluorescent dye study. J Comp Neurol 229:419–431.

Tömböl T, Szafranska-Kosmal A (1972): A Golgi study of the amygdaloid complex in the cat. Acta Neurobiol Exp 32:835–848.

Turner BH, Zimmer J (1984): The architecture and some of the interconnections of the rat's amygdala and lateral periallocortex. J Comp Neurol 227:540–557.

Wakefield C (1979): The intrinsic connections of the basolateral amygdaloid nuclei as visualized with the HRP method. Neurosci Lett 12:17–21.

Yu HH (1969): "The Amygdaloid Complex in the Rat." Thesis, University of Ottawa.

The Amygdala: Neurobiological Aspects of Emotion,
Memory, and Mental Dysfunction, pages 97–114
© 1992 Wiley-Liss, Inc.

3
Distribution of Monoamines Within the Amygdala

JAMES H. FALLON AND PHILIPPE CIOFI
*Department of Anatomy and Neurobiology, University of California at
Irvine, Irvine, California*

INTRODUCTION

The amygdala is intimately involved in an impressive range of neuroendocrine, autonomic, limbic, and cognitive functions and has been implicated in a variety of human neural disorders from schizophrenia, dementia, and epilepsy to autonomic pathologies. The monoamines are neurotransmitters which have been shown to exert both subtle and profound influences on the functions of the amygdala. The monoamines include two groups of small cyclic compounds, the catecholamines and indolamines. The most prevalent catecholamines include dopamine, norepinephrine, and epinephrine, and the major indolamine is serotonin.

The study of monoamines in the central nervous system was greatly facilitated with the introduction of the fluorescence histochemical techniques (Falck et al., 1962; Lindvall and Björklund, 1974a). These techniques were used to reveal the location of monoamine cell bodies, fibers, and terminals throughout the central nervous system, including the amygdala (Fuxe, 1965; Anden et al., 1966; Ungerstedt, 1971; Lindvall and Björklund, 1974b; Fallon et al., 1978). The fluorescence data, combined with biochemical (Ben-Ari et al., 1975; Veersteg et al., 1976; Fallon et al., 1978) and connectional findings (Moore et al., 1978; Parent et al. 1981; Bobillier et al., 1979; Fallon and Moore, 1978; Pickel et al., 1974) demonstrated the rich monoamine innervation of the amygdala. By 1980, a significant body of information had been amassed on the general features of the monoamine innervation of the brain, including the amygdala. A series of reviews in the late seventies and eighties provided a comprehensive view of these neurotransmitter-defined neuronal systems in the rat (Moore and Bloom, 1978, 1979; Lindvall and Björklund, 1978, 1983; Steinbusch, 1981; Fallon, 1981; Moore and Card, 1984; Björklund and Lindvall, 1984; Hökfelt et al., 1984a,b; Fallon and Loughlin, 1985, 1987; Loughlin and Fallon, 1985). Unfortunately, there has been little work done on neuroanatomical distribution of the monoamine systems in the amygdala of

Address correspondence to James H. Fallon, Department of Anatomy and Neurobiology, University of California, Irvine, Irvine CA 92717.

the primate. Because of the wealth of information on the distribution of mono-amines in the rat amygdala, and the continued use of the rodent brain in bio-chemical, pharmacological, and behavioral analysis of the amygdala function, this chapter focuses on the rat amygdala. In this review, we have attempted to integrate the anatomical information from previous reports. In addition, we present new distributional maps of immunoreactivity for tyrosine hydroxylase (TH), dopamine-beta-hydroxylase (DBH) and phenylethanolamine-N-methyl-transferase (PNMT) in the amygdala of the rat. The immunoreactivities for these synthetic enzymes correspond closey to the respective distributions of their products dopamine, norepinephrine, and epinephrine using other anatomical and bio-chemial techniques. The distribution of serotonin in the amygdala is obtained using an antiserum directed against serotonin.

IMMUNOCYTOCHEMISTRY

Deeply anesthetized animals were transcardially perfused with 50 ml saline followed by 500 ml of ice-cold fixative (4% paraformaldehyde in 0.1 M phosphate-buffered saline, pH 7.4). Brains were dissected out, blocked, postfixed 4 h in the same fixative at 4°C and rinsed overnight at 4°C in phosphate-buffered saline containing 20% sucrose.

Four sets of adjacent 20 μm frozen coronal sections were cut on a sliding microtome and rinsed in phosphate-buffered saline before being processed free-floating for indirect immunoperoxidase reaction.

Primary rabbit antisera were applied for 20 h at room temperature, diluted in phosphate-buffered saline containing 0.25% Triton X-100. Anti-TH, anti-DBH, and anti-PNMT sera were diluted 1:1,000, 1:500, and 1:250, respectively, from crude commercial product, the antiserotonin was diluted 1:800. After rinsing in phosphate-buffered saline containing 0.05% Triton X-100, sections were then incubated for 90 min at room temperature in horseradish peroxidase-linked $F(ab')_2$ fragments of goat-antirabbit IgGs (Chemicon, Temecula, CA) diluted 1:100 in the same buffer. Peroxidase activity was revealed in 0.1 M TRIS buffer, pH 7.6, containing 0.02% H_2O_2 and 0.04% 3'3 diaminobenzidine-tetrahydrochloride (DAB) (Sigma, St. Louis, MO). After mounting sections on slides an air-drying over-night, the DAB immunostaining was enhanced by silver-intensification according to Gallyas et al. (1982). Sections ere observed under brightfield and/or darkfield illumination and photographed using Agfapan 25 film.

DISTRIBUTIONAL MAPS

The distributional maps in Figures 3–13 are photomicrographs or coronal sections of rat brain processed for immunocytochemistry using primary poly-clonal antibodies raised in rabbits against TH, DBH, PNMT, or serotonin. Anti-TH, DBH, and PNMT were purchased from Eugene Tech (Allendale, NJ) and the antiserotonin was obtained from Dr. Gérard Tramu (Bordeaux, France) (Tramu et al., 1983).

Although the distribution of TH, DBH, PNMT, and serotonin immunoreac-tivities correlate well with the respective distribution of dopamine, norepineph-rine, epinephrine, and serotonin using these techniques, it should be emphasized

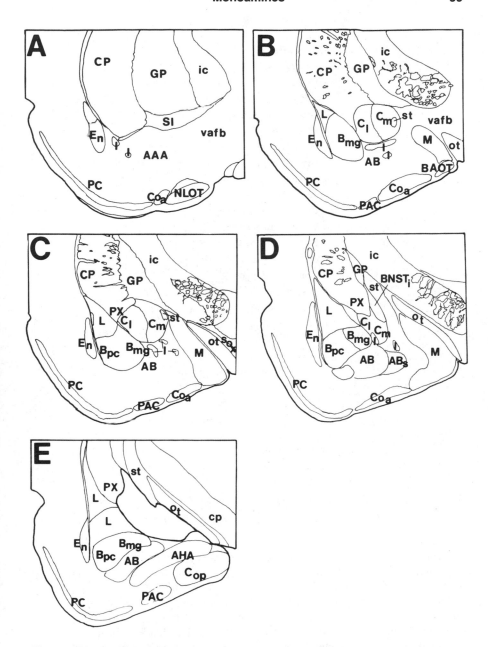

Fig. 1. Illustration of coronal sections of rat amygdala drawn from the A panels in Figures 3–7. Nomenclature is according to Price et al. (1987); see list of abbreviations.

ABBREVIATIONS IN LEGENDS

AAA	anterior amygdaloid area
AB	accessory basal nucleus
AB_s	accessory basal nucleus, superficial division
AHA	amygdalo-hippocampal area
BAOT	bed nucleus of accessory olfactory tract
B_{mg}	basal nucleus, magnocellular division
$BNST_i$	bed nucleus of the stria terminalis, interstitital part
B_{pc}	basal nucleus, parvicellular division
C_l	central nucleus, lateral division
C_m	central nucleus, medial division
Co_a	anterior cortical nucleus
Co_p	posterior cortical nucleus
cp	cerebral peduncle
CP	caudate/putamen
E_n	endopiriform nucleus
GP	globus pallidus
I	intercalated nuclei
ic	internal capsule
L	lateral nucleus
M	medial nucleus
NLOT	nucleus of the lateral olfactory tract
ot	optic tract
PAC	periamygdaloid cortex
PX	central nucleus, lateral capsular division
PC	pyriform cortex
SI	substantia innominata
sox	supraoptic nucleus
st	stria terminalis
vafb	ventral amygdalofugal bundle

that the distribution of the immunoreactivities for the catecholamine synthesizing enzymes (TH, DBH, PNMT) may reflect a mixture of these enzymes in different catecholaminergic fibers. For example, it is possible that TH, the first synthetic enzyme, could be present in fibers of not only dopamine neurons but also of norepinephrine and epinephrine neurons. Likewise, DBH could be present in some epinephrine fibers. However, the levels of the earlier enzymes in the sequence of catecholamine synthesis are thought to be quite low in catecholaminergic fibers and terminals. Therefore, we refer to dopamine, norepinephrine, and epinephrine distribution as revealed by TH, DBH and PNMT immunocytochemistry, respectively, although the aforementioned caveat should be considered.

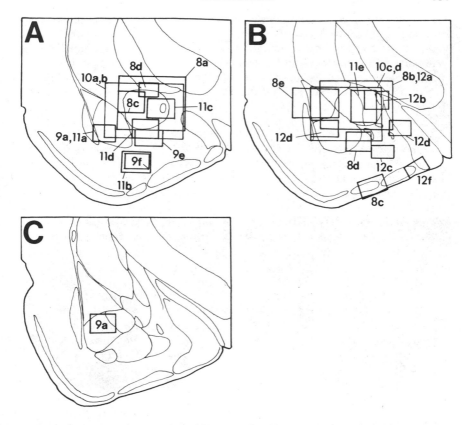

Fig. 2. Illustrations of coronal sections of rat amygdala drawn from the A panels of Figures 4–6. Numbers and correponding boxes denote approximate regions of amygdala from which photomicrographs of Figures 8–12 were taken.

The drawings in Figure 1 were generated from outline drawings for the sections of TH immunoreactivity in Figures 3A, 4A, 5A, 6A, and 7A. The drawings in Figure 1 may also be used to identify the coronal levels of the B (DBH), C (Serotonin), and D (PNMT) frames of Figures 3–7, but the illustrations in Figure 1 are only approximations of the location of nuclei in these figures. Figure 2 illustrates the approximate regions of the amygdala from which the high-power photomicrographs of Figures 8–12 were taken. As in Figure 1, the outline drawings in Figure 2 were from montages of TH immunoreactivity as seen in Figures 4A, 5A, and 6A. The nomenclature used for nuclei and areas of the amygdala is from Price et al. (1987).

Dopamine

The dopaminergic innervation of the amygdala arises from the continuum of dopamine-containing cell bodies in the subsantia nigra pars compacta (SN,

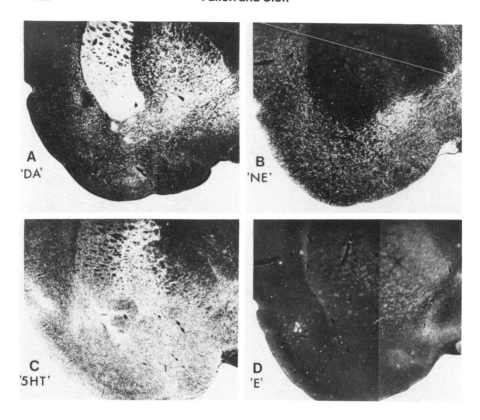

Fig. 3–7. Darkfield photomontages of coronal sections of five anterior to posterior levels of the rat amygdala. **A** panels in each figure are TH immunoreactivity (reflecting primarily dopamine, 'DA' fibers), **B** panels are DBH immunoreactivity (reflecting primarily norepinephrine fibers, 'NE'), **C** panels are serotonin immunoreactivity ('5HT') and **D** panels are PNMT immunoreactivity (reflecting primarily epinephrine fibers, 'E').

A9 cell group), ventral tegmental area (VTA, A10 cell group) and caudal extension of the SN (A8 cell groups) in the ventral midbrain. Two cell clusters provide the majority of the innervation, one located in the dorsal two-thirds of the VTA and the others in the lateral SN. Between these two cell clusters are scattered neurons in the dorsal tier of the SN and its caudal extension in the A8 cell group, which also project to the amygdala. Although the SN-VTA projection to the amygdala is known to be dopaminergic, many of the SN-VTA dopaminergic neurons innervating the amygdala also contain the peptide cholecystokinin (Seroogy et al., 1989). A small population of these neurons also provides a neurotensin-containing input to the amygdala (Seroogy et al., 1987). One feature of the dopaminergic innervation of the amygdala that is unique is the relative paucity of SN-VTA axon collaterals that also innervate other forebrain areas. Neu-

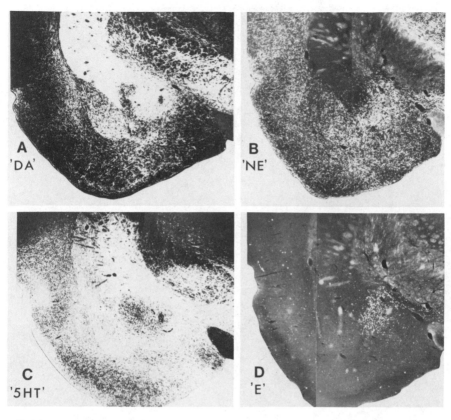

4

rons of the lateral VTA and medial SN give rise to axon collaterals hich innervate several cortical, striatal, and basal forebrain targets, but the amygdala does
not appear to share this highly collateralized input to the same degree as other
target areas of the SN-VTA (Fallon and Loughlin, 1982).

   The dopaminergic axons ascend in the ventral midbrain and enter the caudal hypothalamus in the medial forebrain bundle. The great majority of dopaminergic axons projecting to the amygdala enter at all levels of the ventral
amygdalofugal/ansa peduncularis pathway. At the anterior-posterior level of the
caudal and middle hypothalamus, fibers enter the amygdala by passing through
the supraoptic decussation between the optic tract and internal capsule to enter
the central and medial nuclei of the amygdala. Although a significant number of
TH immunoreactive fibers are present in the stria terminalis (Figs. 8F, 13), previous anterograde tracing techniques and combined lesion/biochemical studies
suggest that this is a minor dopaminergic pathway to the amygdala (Fallon et
al., 1978; Fallon and Moore, 1978).

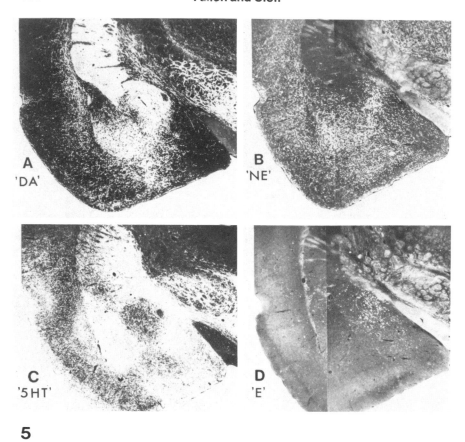

5

The distribution of dopaminergic axons and presumed terminals in the amygdala is heterogenous. The densest projections are to the medial division of the central nucleus, intercalated masses, and cell clusters at the borders of the basal and lateral nuclei (Figs. 8, 4A, 5A, 6A). A moderately dense innervation is present in both the parvicellular and magnocellular domains of the basal nucleus (Figs. 4A, 5A, 6A, 7A, 9A,D). Other areas containing moderate concentrations of dopaminergic fibers include the accessor basal nucleus, periamygdaloid cortex, the transition area between the accessory basal nucleus and periamygdaloid cortex (Figs. 4, 6A, 9F), lateral sector of the central nucleus (Figs. 4A, 5A, 6A, 8A–C), interstitial part of the bed nucleus of the stria terminalis (Fig. 9D), anterior (Fig. 8C), and posterior cortical nuclei, endopiriform nucleus (Figs. 4A, 5A, 6A, 9A), and anterior amygdaloid area (Fig. 1A). In addition, there are scattered fibers in the other amygdaloid nuclei and areas.

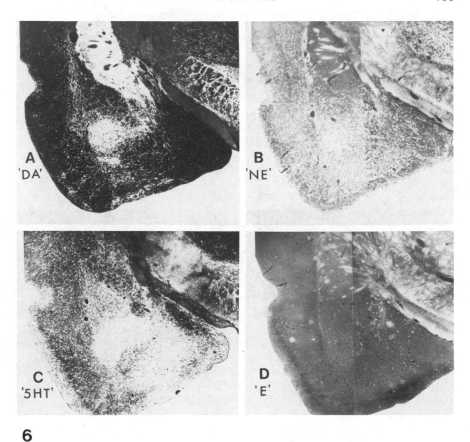

6

Norepinephrine

The noradrenergic innervation of the amygdala arises from the norepinephrine cell groups of the pons and medulla. Connectional (Pickel et al., 1974; Fallon
and Moore, 1978) and correlated lesion/biochemical studies (Fallon et al., 1978)
have shown that the majority of the innervation arises bilaterally from the locus
coeruleus (A6 cell group) and about 15% of the innervation arises from cell groups
caudal to the locus coeruleus (A1–5). Multiple labeling studies have demonstrated
that only a few "core" locus coeruleus neurons projecting to the amygdala also
project to other cortical and basal forebrain regions (Fallon and Loughlin, 1982).

The brain stem noradrenergic axons ascend in the dorsal and ventral noradrenergic bundles and enter the medial forebrain bundle in the hypothalamus.
Many fibers share the same ventral amygdalofugal pathway into the amygdala
as the dopaminergic fibers, and, in addition, approximately 25% of the noradrenergic input to the amygdala enters via the stria terminalis.

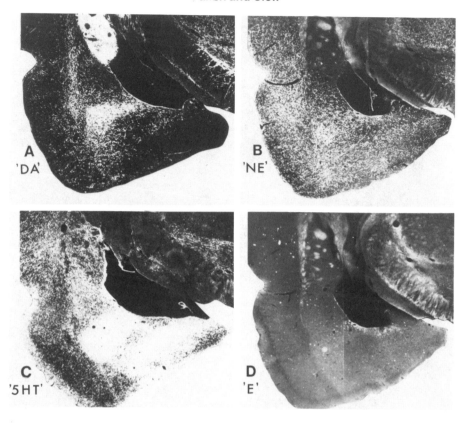

7

The distribution of noradrenergic axons and presumed terminals is more uniform than that of the dopaminergic input. Virtually every area of the amygdala contains at least a modest concentration of noradrenergic fibers (Figs. 4B, 5B, 6B, 7B). The densest concentrations of noradrenergic fibers are found in the medial part of the central nucleus (Figs. 10A,C, 11C). The basal nuclei are also well innervated (Figs. 5B, 6B, 7B, 11A,B). The other amygdaloid nuclei receive only a modest noradrenergic input. Noradrenergic fibers arising in the medulla concentrate in the anterior amygdaloid area, medial central nucleus, and basal nuclei (Fallon et al., 1978).

Serotonin

The serotonergic innervation of the amygdala arises from midbrain and pontine raphe nuclei. The major source of serotonin fibers is the dorsal raphe (B7 cell group), with additional input arising from the median raphe (B5 cell group) (Moore et al., 1978; Bobillier et al., 1979; Parent et al., 1981). The raphe projections to the forebrain, including the amygdala, arise from both ipsilateral and

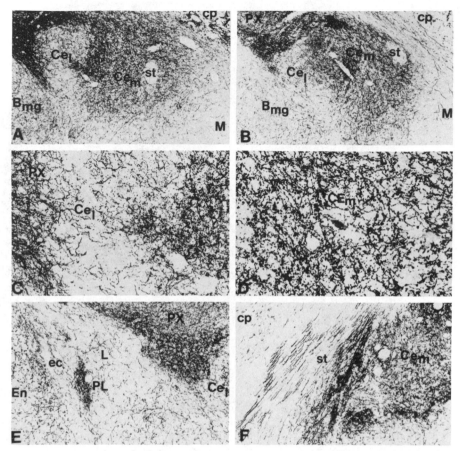

Fig. 8. Photomicrographs of TH-immunoreactive fibers ('dopaminergic') in the left amygdala: **A**: central nucleus; **B**: caudal central nucleus; **C**: high-power photomicrograph of border of medial (Ce$_m$) and lateral sectors (Ce$_l$ of central nucleus, as seen in panel A; **D**: high-power photomicrograph of medial sector of central nucleus, as seen in panel A; **E**: low-power photomicrograph of lateral (L) and paralaminar nuclei (PL) of amygdala just ventral to the caudoventral part of the putamen (PX); **F**: high-power photomicrograph of right amygdala at the level of the medial sector of the central nucleus, also demonstrating TH-positive fibers in the stria terminalis (st) and cerebral peduncle (cp).

contralateral raphe neurons, but the projection is unilateral (van der Kooy and Hattori, 1980). Some neurons in the central region of the dorsal raphe provide axon collaterals to the amygdala and other forebrain regions such as the septum, olfactory tubercle, nucleus accumbens, cortex, and caudate-putamen (Fallon and Loughlin, 1982).

The serotonin axons ascend in paramedian and periventricular bundles. Some fibers enter the medial forebrain bundle and enter the amygdala via the ventral

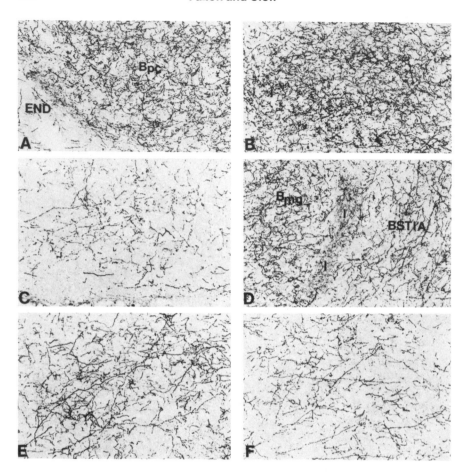

Fig. 9. High-power photomicrographs of TH-immunoreactive fibers ('dopaminergic') in the left amygdala; **A**: paricellular basal nucleus (B_{pc}) adjacent to the endopiriform nucleus (END); **B**: magnocellular basal nucleus; **C**: periamygdaloid cortex; **D**: interstitial part of the bed nucleus of the stria terminalis (BSTIA), intercalated masses (I), and magnocellular basal nucleus (B_{mg}); **E**: accessory basal nucleus; **F**: transition zone between accessory basal nucleus and periamygdaloid cortex.

amygdalofugal bundle. In addition, fibers can be seen entering the amygdala via the stria terminalis (Figs. 6C, 12B).

The distribution of serotonergic axons and presumed terminals in the amygdala is widespread and appears quite dense in most areas of the amygdala. Particularly dense innervation is present in the magnocellular and parvicellular parts of the basal nucleus (Figs. 4C, 5C, 6C, 7C, 12A,D), medial edge of the central nucleus (Figs. 12A,B), medial nucleus (Fig. 12C), and lateral nucleus (Figs. 4C, 5C, 6C, 7C). In comparison to these regions, there is a much lower density of fibers

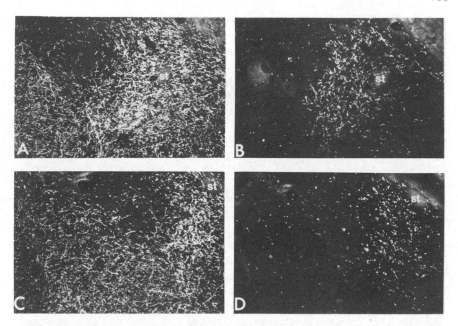

Fig. 10. Low-power darkfield photomicrographs of the central nucleus and stria terminalis (st) of the left amygdala at midrostral (**A,B**) and midcaudal (**C,D**) levels. In (A) and (C) note the dense DBH-immunoreactive nerve plexus ('norepinephrine') as compared to (B) and (D), where only a sparse to moderately dense number of PNMT-immunoreactive fibers ('epinephrine') are present.

in the bed nucleus of the accessory olfactory tract (Fig. 4C), lateral part of the central nucleus (Figs. 4C, 5C, 6C, 12D), and posterior cortical nucleus (Fig. 7C).

Epinephrine

In comparison to the dopamine, norepinephrine, and serotonin innervation of the amygdala, the details of the epinephrine input are less well known. The cells of origin of the ascending epinephrine projections are in the C1 region of the ventrolateral medulla and the C2 region of the dorsomedial medulla (Hökfelt et al., 1974, 1984a). The axons access the amygdala through the ventral amygdalofugal bundle.

The distribution of epinephrine in the amygdala is generally very sparse and localized in a few nuclei (Hökfelt et al., 1974, 1984a; Mezey, 1989). The densest projection is to the central nucleus, where fibers are prevalent in its medial sector (Figs. 4D, 5D, 6D, 10B,D, 11E,F). Sparse fibers are also present in the medial and basal nuclei.

SUMMARY

There is a rich heterogeneous monoamine innervation of the amygdala. The dopamine, norepinephrine, and serotonin inputs are moderately dense, while

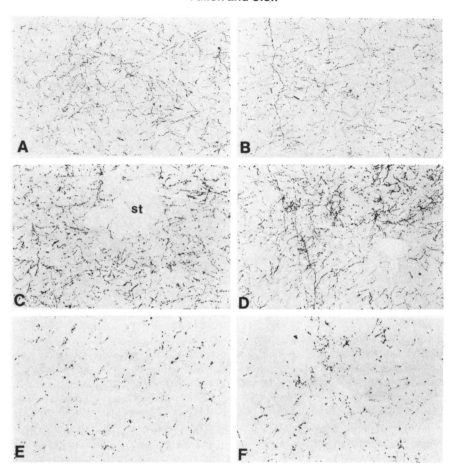

Fig. 11. High-power photomicrographs of DBH-immunoreactivity (**A–D** 'norepinephrine') and PNMT-immunoreactivity (**E,F** 'epinephrine') in the left amygdala; **A**: parvicellular basal nucleus; **B**: transition area between the accessory basal nucleus and periamygdaloid cortex; **C**: medial central nucleus in the region of the stria terminalis (st); **D**: ventral part of the central nucleus; **E**: PNMT fibers at the border of lateral and medial central nucleus.

Fig. 12. Photomicrographs of serotonin immunoreactivity in the left amygdala; **A**: low-power photomicrographs at the level of the medial (C_m) and lateral (C_l) central nucleus, magnocellular basal nucleus (B_{mg}), caudoventral putamen (PX), stria terminalis (st), and cerebral peduncle (cp); **B**: high-power photomicrograph of regions of stria terminalis as seen in panel A; **C**: high-power photomicrograph of accessory basal (AB) nucleus; **D**: high-power photomicrograph of border between magnocellular basal nucleus (B_{mg}) and endopiriform nucleus (E_n); **E**: high-power photomicrograph of medial (M) nucleus; **F**: high-power photomicrograph of anterior cortical (Co_a) nucleus.

Fig. 13. Darkfield contact photograph of TH immunoreactivity ('dopamine') through the rat brain at the level of the amygdala.

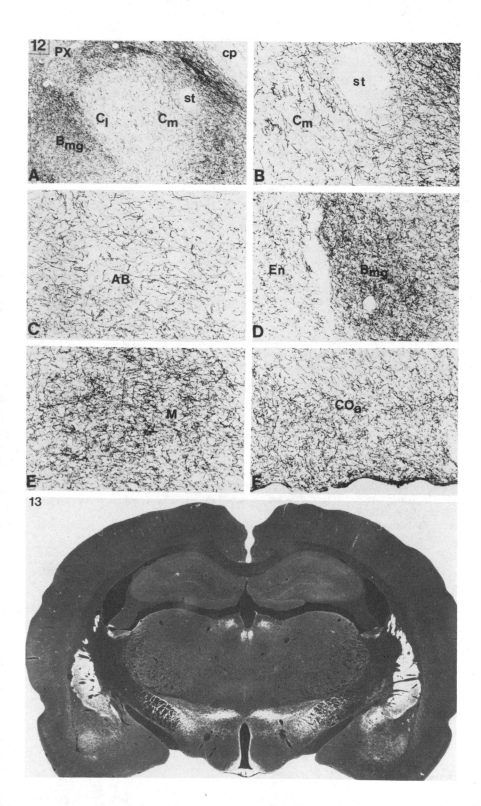

the epinephrine innervation is sparse. The densest monoamine inputs to the amygdala are in the medial sector of the central nucleus, where all four mono-amines are concentrated. The basal nuclei also receive moderately dense convergent inputs containing dopamine, norepinephrine, and serotonin. Other amygdaloid nuclei receive a variable concentration of input from monoaminergic neurons. The amygdala is different from other forebrain regions in that mono-aminergic neurons projecting to this region are not highly collateralized, sug-gesting a unique monoaminergic regulation of amygdala functions.

ACKNOWLEDGMENTS

This work was supported by the NIH grant 15321.

REFERENCES

Anden NE, Dahlstrom A, Fuxe K, Larsson K, Olson L, Ungerstedt U (1966): Ascending monoamine neurons to the telencephalon and diencephalon. Acta Physiol Scand 67:313–326.

Ben-Ari Y, Zigmond RE, Moore KI (1975): Regional distribution of tyrosine hydroxylase, norepinephrine and dopamine within the amygdaloid complex of the rat. Brain Res 87:91–101.

Björklund A, Lindvall O (1984): Dopamine-containing systems in the CNS. In Björklund A, Lindvall O (eds): "Handbook of Chemical Neuroanatomy," Vol 2, Part 1, "Classical Transmitters in the CNS." Amsterdam: Elsevier, pp 55–122.

Bobillier P, Seguin S, De Gueurce A, Lewis BD, Pujol JF (1979): The efferent connec-tions of the nucleus raphe centralis superior in the rat as revealed by radioautogra-phy. Brain Res 166:1–8.

Falck B, Hillarp NA, Thiene G, Torp A (1962): Fluorescence of catecholamines and related compounds condensed with formaldehyde. J Histochem Cytochem 10:348–354.

Fallon JH (1981): Histochemical characterization of dopaminergic, noradrenergic and serotonergic projections to the amygdala. In Ben-Ari Y (ed) "The Amygdaloid Com-plex." Amsterdam: Elsevier, pp 175–183.

Fallon JH, Koziell DA, Moore RY (1978): Catecholamine innervation of the basal fore-brain II. Amygdala, suprahinal cortex and entorhinal cortex. J Comp Neurol 180:509–531.

Fallon JH, Loughlin SE (1982): Monoamine innervation of the forebrain: Collateralization. Brain Res Bull 9:295–307.

Fallon JH, Loughlin SE (1985): Substantia nigra. In Paxinos G (ed): "The Rat Central Nervous System." Vol 1. Amsterdam: Elsevier, pp 353–374.

Fallon JH, Loughlin SE (1987): Monoamine innervation of cerebral cortex and a theory of the role of monoamines in cerebral cortex and basal ganglia. In Jones EG, Peters A (eds): "Cerebral Cortex," Vol 6. New York: Plenum pp 41–127.

Fallon JH, Moore RY (1978): Catecholamine innervation of the basal forebrain. IV Topog-raphy of dopamine cell projections to the basal forebrain and neostrintum. J Comp Neurol 180:545–580.

Fuxe K (1965): Evidence for the existence of monoamine neurons in the central nervous system IV. The distribution of monoamine terminals in the central nervous system. Acta Physiol Scand (Suppl 247) 64:37–84.

Gallyas F, Gorcs T, Merchenthaler I (1982): High-grade intensification of the end-product of the diaminobenzidine reaction for peroxidase histochemistry. J Histochem Cytochem 30:183–184.

Hökfelt T, Fuxe K, Goldstein M, Johansson O (1974): Immunohistochemical evidence for the existence of adrenaline neurons in the rat brain. Brain Res 66:235–251.

Hökfelt T, Johansson O, Goldstein M (1984a): Central catecholamine neurons as revealed by immunohistochemistry with special reference to adrenaline neurons. In Björklund A, Lindvall O (eds): "Handbook of Chemical Neuroanatomy." Vol 2, Part 1, "Classical Transmitters in the CNS." Amsterdam: Elsevier, pp 157–276.

Hökfelt T, Martensson R, Björklund A, Kleinau S, Goldstein M (1984b): Distributional maps of tyrosine-hydroxylase-immunoreactive neurons in the rat brain. In Björklund A, Lindvall O (eds): "Handbook of Chemical Neuroanatomy." Vol 2, Part 1, "Classical Transmitters in the CNS." Amsterdam: Elsevier, pp 277–386.

Lindvall O, Björklund A (1974a): The glyoxylic acid fluorescence method: A detailed account of the methodology for the visualization of central catecholamine neurons. Histochemistry 39:97–127.

Lindvall O, Björklund A (1974b): The organization of the ascending catecholamine neuron systems in the rat brain. Acta Physiol Scan (Suppl) 412:1–48.

Lindvall O, Björklund A (1978): Organization of catecholamine neurons in the rat central nervous systems. In Iversen LL, Iversen SD, Snyder SS (eds): "Handbook of Psychopharmacology," Vol 9. New York: Plenum Press, pp 139–231.

Lindvall O, Björklund A (1983): Dopamine and noradrenaline-containing neuron systems: Their anatomy in the rat brain. In Emson PC (ed): "Chemical Neuroanatomy." New York: Raven Press, pp 229–255.

Loughlin SE, Fallon JH (1985): Locus coeruleus. In Paxinos G (ed): "The Rat Nervous System," Vol 2. Sydney: Academic Press, pp 79–93.

Mezey E (1989): Phenylethanolamine-N-methyl-transferase-containing neurons in the limbic system of the young rat. Proc Natl Acad Sci USA 86:347–351.

Moore RY, Bloom FE (1978): Central catecholamine neurons systems: Anatomy and physiology of the dopamine systems. Ann Rev Neurosci 1:129–169.

Moore RY, Bloom FE (1979): Central catecholamine neurons systems: Anatomy and physiology of the norephinephrine and epinephrine systems. Ann Rev Neurosci 2:113–168.

Moore RY, Card P (1984): Noradrenaline-containing neuron systems. In Björklund A, Lindvall O (eds): "Handbook of Chemical Neuroanatomy." Vol 2, Part 1, "Classical Transmitters in the CNS." Amsterdam: Elsevier, pp 123–156.

Moore RY, Halaris AE, Jones BE (1978): Serotonin neurons of the midbrain raphe: Ascending projections. J Comp Neurol 180:417–438.

Parent A, Descarries C, Beaudet A (1981): Organization of ascending serotonin systems in the adult rat brain: A radioautographic study after intraventricular administration of ^{3}H hydroxytryptamine. Neuroscience 6:115–138.

Pickel VM, Segal M, Bloom FE (1974): A radioautographic study of the efferent pathways of the nucleus locus coeruleus. J Comp Neurol 155:15–42.

Price JL, Russchen FT, Amaral DG (1987): The limbic region II: The amygdaloid complex. In Björklund A, Hökfelt T, Swanson LW (eds): "Handbook of Chemical Neuroanatomy." Vol 5, Part 1, "Integrated Systems of the CNS." Amsterdam: Elsevier, pp 279–388.

Seroogy KB, Dangaran K, Lin S, Haycock J, Fallon JH (1989): Ventral mesencephalic neurons containing both cholecystokinin- and tyrosine hydroxylase-like immunoreactivities project to forebrain regions. J Comp Neurol 279:397–414.

Seroogy KB, Mehta A, Fallon JH (1987): Neurotensin and cholecystokinin coexistence within neurons of the ventral mesencephalon:Projections to forebrain. Exp Brain Res 68:277–289.

Steinbusch HWM (1981): Distribution of serotonin-immunoreactivity in the central nervous system of the rat: Cell bodies and terminals. Neuroscience 6:557–618.

Tramu G, Pillez A, Léonardelli J (1983): Serotonin axons of the ependyma and circumventricular organs in the forebrain of the guinea-pig. An immunohistochemical study. Cell Tissue Res 228:297–311.

Ungerstedt U (1971): Stereotaxic mapping of the monoamine pathways in the rat brain. Acta Physiol Scand (Suppl) 367:1–48.

van der Kooy D, Hattori T (1980): Bilaterally situated dorsal raphe cell bodies have only unilateral forebrain projections in the rat. Brain Res 192:550–554.

Veersteg DHG, van der Gugtan J, de Jong W, Palkovits M (1976): Regional concentrations of noradrenaline and dopamine in rat brain. Brain Res 113:563–574.

The Amygdala: Neurobiological Aspects of Emotion,
Memory, and Mental Dysfunction, pages 115–142
© 1992 Wiley-Liss, Inc.

4

Neuropeptides: Cellular Morphology, Major Pathways, and Functional Considerations

GARETH WYN ROBERTS

*Department of Anatomy and Cell Biology, St. Mary's Hospital
Medical School, London, UK*

INTRODUCTION

The amygdala has a variety of cells and fibres which contain one or some of virtually every neuropeptide found in the brain. The distribution patterns of neuropeptides within the amygdala reflect this diversity by displaying considerable complexity (see Roberts et al., 1982; Shiosaka et al., 1983; Price et al., 1987). Initial studies on the distribution patterns of peptides reported these patterns in some detail but commented on the mismatch between peptide distribution and the cytoarchitectonic boundaries of the amygdaloid nuclei derived from morphological studies (Roberts et al., 1982). These mismatches presumably have functional implications which are as yet largely unexplored.

The distribution of peptide-containing fibres in the amygdala shows both anteroposterior and mediolateral gradients and is best described pictorially (e.g., Fig. 1). The provision of an atlas detailing the distribution of every peptide in the amygdala is beyond the scope of the present chapter and the reader in need of such cartography is referred to the relevant literature outlined in several reviews (Roberts et al., 1982; Shiosaka et al., 1983; Price et al., 1987).

The aim of this chapter is to gather together recent studies which have described in detail some aspects of the cellular morphology of peptide systems in the amygdala and try to assess their functional implications. In a similar vein the coexistence of transmitters within amygdala neurons is reviewed and the main details of intra-amygdala peptide-containing pathways and the peptide pathways which link the amygdala with other brain regions and which underpin its functional capabilities will be re-examined.

CELLULAR MORPHOLOGY

Several detailed studies have attempted to correlate the morphological features of immunostained neurons in nuclei of the amygdala with the types of neurons characterized by Golgi stains (Fig. 2, Braak and Braak, 1983). Such attempts at correlation utilize a number of criteria to reconcile the features of neurons seen in the two types of preparations, including cell size and shape, dendritic mor-

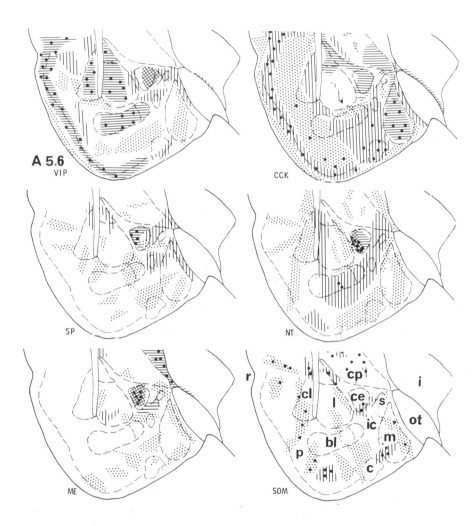

Fig. 1. Distribution of six neuropeptides in the rat amygdala at a level 5.6 mm anterior to the interaural zero plane. Note the enormous differences in distribution pattern of the various peptide-containing neurons (black circles) and fibres (stippled areas). bl: baso-lateral amygdaloid nucleus; bm: basomedial amygdaloid nucleus; c: cortical amygdaloid nucleus; ce: central amygdaloid nucleus; cl: claustrum; ic: intercalated amygdaloid nucleus; l: lateral amygdaloid nucleus; m: medial amygdaloid nucleus; ot: optic tract; p: piriform cortex; r: rhinal fissure; s: stria terminalis; v: ventral amygdalohypothalamic pathway. (Reproduced from Roberts et al., 1982 by kind permission of the editors and Pergamon Press.)

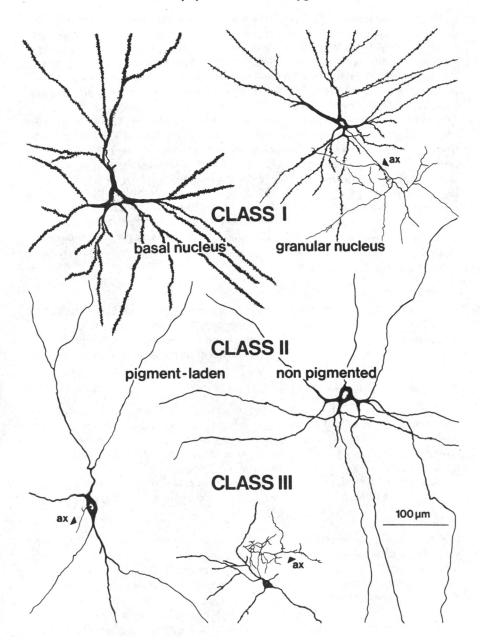

Fig. 2. Camera lucida drawings of cells in the human amygdala stained with the Golgi method. ax: axon. (Adapted from Price et al., 1987, courtesy of Dr. Haiko Braak.)

phology, orientation and branching pattern, and spine density. However, the degree to which the fine details of neuron morphology can be visualised differs considerably in Golgi and immunocytochemical techniques. A further relevant issue concerns the difference in the staining selectivity of the two techniques. It is well known that Golgi techniques are capricious and that the numbers and types of neurons stained are highly variable. In immunocytochemical studies (e.g., Cassell and Gray, 1989) between 5 and 30 times as many neurons per section were stained immunocytochemically as were visualised with the Golgi stain. Thus, given the large number of immunostained cells examined, it is unlikely that any but the scarcest cell types will have been overlooked. Therefore the few detailed studies which have been completed probably give a reasonably accurate picture of the morphology of peptide-containing neurons in some amygdaloid nuclei.

Central Nucleus

The details are taken largely from the study of Cassell and Gray (1989). The central nucleus can be divided into several subregions (see Chapter 2, McDonald, this volume, for details).

Substance P.

Substance P-immunoreactive (SP) cells have been identified only in the centromedial subdivision. Neurons were generally medium-sized with ovoid or pyramiform perikarya and with 3–4 long dendrites arising from the perikarya. Spines were rarely observed on the dendrites of SP neurons. Fusiform, bipolar SP neurons were not observed.

Vasoactive Intestinal Polypeptide (VIP)

Small numbers of VIP neurons were observed in the ventral subdivision and less commonly in lateral and medial divisions. The cells had ovoid perikarya, 10–15 μm long diameter, with thick primary dendrites. In some cases, a long, tapering secondary dendrite could be traced into the lateral subdivision. No spines were observed on these neurons. VIP neurons of a similar type were found scattered throughout ventral, medial, and lateral subdivisions, with spindle-shaped perikarya and a characteristic bipolar arrangement of primary dendrites.

Neurotensin

Neurotensin-immunoreactive (NT) neurons were identified in all subdivisions, with the greatest numbers in the lateral subdivision. In medial regions, NT neurons had medium-sized, pyramiform perikarya with 2–4 long, thick dendrites. In ventral regions the size (10–13 μm) of these neurons is within the diameter range of the medium, spine-sparse neuron, though a definite association could not be made with the minimal dendritic impregnation. Two forms of NT neurons were observed in the lateral subdivision. The most common form had round or ovoid perikarya (15–20 μm long diameter) with 3–5 primary dendrites possessing 2–4 secondary dendrites. These secondary dendrites, on which spines were occasionally seen, could be traced up to 200 μm from the body. These neurons closely resembled the medium spiny neuron in both perikaryal size and dendritic configuration. A small number of larger pyramiform NT neurons were observed in the lateral subdivision. NT neurons in the lateral capsular subdivision had perikaryal and dendritic configurations similar to medium spiny neurons, though no spines were observed on the dendrites of immunostained neurons.

Galanin

Galanin-immunoreactive (GAL) neurons were concentrated in the most medial subdivision, the GAL neurons being rare in ventral regions. Numerous GAL neurons were also located in the area between the central and medial amygdaloid nuclei. In contrast to SP neurons in medial regions, two forms of GAL neurons were identified. The most frequently observed type had irregular, pyramiform perikarya with 3–4 long dendrites arising from the cell body. Modest numbers of spines were observed on many of the dendrites of these neurons. The other, less common form of GAL neuron had a spindle-shaped perikaryon with two thick dendrites arising from the poles of the perikaryon. Dendritic spines were rarely observed on these neurons.

Somatostatin

Somatostain-immunoreactive (SOM) neurons were identified in all subdivisions (Fig. 3). Approximately 30% of SOM neurons in the lateral subdivision possessed 3–6 primary dendrites which arose from the perikarya (14–20 μm long axis) in configurations similar to those seen in the spiny neuron type. Many other neurons were observed possessing only two thick dendrites, though these were similar in size and orientation to the primary dendrites of medium spiny neurons. Secondary dendrites were observed on a number of neurons and in many cases these could be traced up to 150 μm from the cell body. The branching patterns of these dendrites were similar to the patterns observed in the medium spiny neurons described in Golgi preparations. In a few SOM neurons of this type, small numbers of dendritic spines could be seen on secondary dendrites. However, there was little evidence of the extensive and dense concentration of spines seen with Golgi-impregnated material. In the medial subdivision, small numbers of SOM neurons were observed resembling the pyramiform neurons found in Golgi preparations. However, the majority of SOM neurons in the medial subdivision had fusiform perikarya with long, thick dendrites arising from opposite poles of the perikaryon. These cells in general resembled the bipolar, fusiform cells seen in Golgi preparations. SOM neurons of this type were observed in ventral subdivision and less frequently in the lateral subdivision.

Corticotropin-Releasing Factor (CRF)

CRF neurons were observed in lateral, medial, and ventral subdivisions in that order of frequency. Neurons in the medial subdivision appeared to resemble the pyramiform, sparsely sinuous type, those in the lateral subdivision appeared similar to the medium spiny and pyramiform types (though spines were rarely observed). In the ventral subdivision, the few CRF neurons observed resembled the medium-sized, sparsely spinous neuron seen in Golgi preparations, and in several cases, dendrites could be followed into the lateral subdivision.

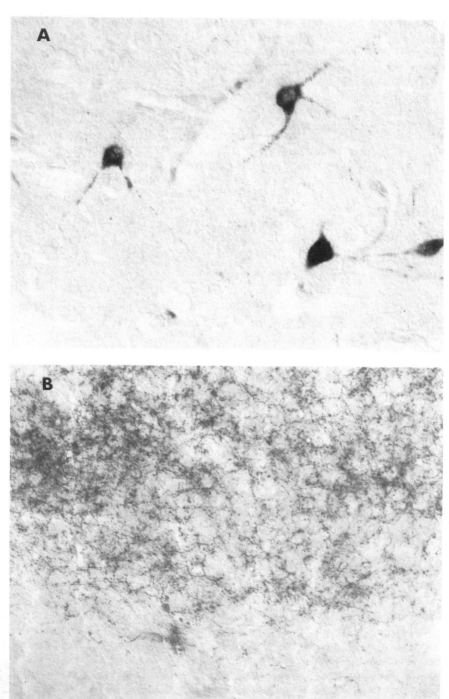

In a previous study (Cassell et al., 1986), NT and CRF neurons were observed to be concentrated in the rostral part of lateral subdivision corresponding to the location of the intermediate subdivision (CI) of the central nucleus as identified by McDonald (1982a). Neurons in this region reportedly resemble those in medial subdivision but possess greater numbers of dendritic spines (McDonald, 1982a). In the study of Gray et al. (1984) CRF and NT neurons in the CI retained the dendritic configurations and perikaryal size of the medium spiny neurons located more caudally.

Enkephalin

Leu-enkephalin can be derived from the pro-enkephalin and pro-dynorphin precursors, both of which are present in central nucleus neurons (Watson et al., 1982) and antisera often cross react with met-enkephalin. In view of this, the generic term enkephalin (ENK) has been applied to neurons immunoreactive to both leu- and met-enkephalin antibodies (Cassell et al., 1986; Gray and Magnusson, 1987).

Large numbers of ENK-immunostained neurons were observed in lateral and lateral capsular subdivisions. In the lateral region, ENK neurons resembled the medium spiny neuron type, though few spines were observed. In the lateral capsular regions, few ENK neurons were sufficiently stained to allow examination of their dendritic configuration. However, these cells had ovoid perikarya resembling in size and shape the characteristic medium spiny neuron.

Basolateral Complex

This data is derived largely from the study of McDonald (1985a).

VIP

The perikaryal size (11 μm) and dendritic branching pattern of VIP neurons in basolateral nucleus indicated that most, if not all, of these cells correspond to small class II neurons seen in Golgi preparations (McDonald, 1982b, 1984). Comparison of Nissl-stained cells with Golgi-impregnated neurons suggested that the great majority of large unlabeled neurons in Nissl-stained sections are class I neurons. VIP neurons in this nucleus are markedly smaller than large unlabeled neurons in counterstained sections. Examination of the dendritic arborization pattern of VIP cells suggests that these neurons correspond to the multipolar, bitufted, and bipolar class II neurons observed in Golgi preparations (McDonald, 1982b). It is possible that some of the VIP cells with small spherical perikary could be class III (neurogliaform) neurons (Fig. 2), but the latter cell type has a greater number of primary dendrites and dendritic branches than the VIP neurons observed.

SOM

The perikaryal size (15 μm) and dendritic branching pattern of SOM neurons suggests that these cells correspond to medium-sized multipolar, bitufted, and

---

Fig. 3. **(A)** Somatostatin immunoreactivity in Golgi type II cells in the central amygdaloid nucleus (× 475) and **(B)** neurotensin-immunoreactive fibres in the central amygdaloid nucleus (× 225).

bipolar class II neurons seen in Golgi preparations (Fig. 3A). Although a previous study (Gray, 1983) had suggested that SOM neurons in the basolateral complex corresponded not only to class II neurons but also to class I and class III cells, the cytoarchitecture in the lateral and basolateral nuclei is virtually identical, making it unlikely that the SOM cell types in these adjacent nuclei would differ. Size classification of immunohistochemically labeled neurons is more difficult in the lateral than in the basolateral nucleus because size variation among different classes of Golgi-impregnated neurons is less marked in the lateral nucleus. Although some large SOM neurons were seen in the lateral nucleus (McDonald, 1985), it has been suggested that the small number of primary and more distal dendrites of these cells, as well as the class I SOM cell illustrated by Gray (1983), means that these neurons correspond to large class II neurons rather than class I cells (McDonald, 1985a). On the other hand, it has been reported that secondary dendrites of large SOM neurons in the lateral nucleus exhibit dendritic spines. This finding suggests that more than one major cell class of neurons in the lateral nucleus contains SOM. However, in the basolateral nucleus, it appears that most SOM cells are class II neurons.

Cholecystokinin (CCK)

The large perikaryal size (10 μm) and pyramiform shape of CCK cells in the basolateral complex indicates that these cells are either class I neurons or large class II neurons (McDonald, 1985a). However, the small number of primary dendrites and dendritic branches, as well as the nonpyramidal shape of many of the cell bodies, suggests that most of the CCK neurons are actually large multipolar class II cells. In addition, the sparse distribution of CCK cells in the basolateral amygdala is also similar to that of large class II cells (Roberts et al., 1982; McDonald, 1982).

DISCUSSION

Few spines were identified on immunostained NT, SOM, or CRF neurons in the central nucleus. Dendritic spines were reported on GAL neurons (Cassell and Gray, 1989) and in morphological studies of immunostained neurons in other brain areas (e.g., Maley et al., 1983). The scarcity of spines on immunostained dendrites was most conspicuous in the lateral and lateral capsular subdivisions of the central nucleus (Cassell and Gray, 1989). Golgi stains indicate that the majority of neurons in these subdivisions have densely spinous secondary dendrites (McDonald, 1982a; Fig. 2). The association of somatostatin, neurotensin, CRF, and the enkephalins with the spiny neurons of the lateral and lateral capsular subdivisions is based on similarities in cell size, shape, and dendritic configuration. It is unlikely that these peptides are located in the medium-sized, sparsely spinous or small, aspinous neurons present in these subdivisions (McDonald, 1982a; Cassell and Gray, 1989) since there are few and they have different dendritic configurations from the medium spiny neurons. The ENK, NT, SOM, and CRF neurons in lateral and lateral capsular subdivisions of the central nucleus appear to be best classified as medium spiny neurons on the basis of the available perikaryal and dendritic morphology (Cassell and Gray, 1989).

Two general observations have been made regarding the morphology of peptide-immunoreactive neurons in the rat central amygdaloid nucleus (Cassell and Gray, 1989). First, the peptides neurotensin, somatostatin, VIP, galanin, met- and leu-enkephalin, and corticotrophin-releasing factor are each present within two or more morphologically distinct types of neuron, whereas thus far, substance P appears to be the only peptide in the central nucleus associated with a single cell type. Second, the major morphological classes of neurons identifiable with Golgi stains are each associated with more than one neuropeptide.

The mismatch between the distributions of peptide-containing neurons and the underlying cytoarchitecture of the central nucleus has been commented on frequently (Roberts et al., 1982; Wray and Hoffman, 1983; Veening et al., 1984; Cassell et al., 1986; Cassell and Gray, 1989). A chemoarchitectonic scheme of central nucleus organisation has been proposed to overcome this problem (Wray and Hoffman, 1983). Studies dealing with peptide distributions in the amygdala assume that the presence of peptide immunoreactivity implies a homogeneous cell type. This assumption is probably erroneous, as evidenced by the findings of the studies described, since they clearly indicate that peptides in the central nucleus are associated with several morphologically distinct classes of neuron rather than a single type with a variable size and shape.

The functional significance of the differences in spine density, dendritic branching, dendritic orientations, etc., that serve to distinguish central amygdala neurons remains unknown. The reported uniform electrical properties of medial central nucleus neurons, irrespective of their efferent target (Pascoe and Kapp, 1985), appears consistent with the relatively homogeneous morphologies of these neurons (McDonald, 1982a). However, the range of peptides contained within this type of neuron suggests that they have a variety of influences on target structures. Physiological studies have reported different effects from medial and lateral central nucleus stimulation but the degree to which these effects are attributable in any way to differences in cell morphology remains to be determined. Most likely, these differential effects are related to the differences in the efferent targets of neurons located in medial or lateral parts of the central nucleus (Veening et al., 1984; Moga and Gray, 1985a; Cassell et al., 1986). Whether morphologically different neurons have different connections, however, remains to be determined.

ANOVA of perikaryal sizes of peptide-containing neurons in basolateral amygdala also indicated that there was a size difference among peptide-containing cell types ($P < 0.001$, McDonald, 1985a). VIP-containing cells were significantly smaller than cells containing SOM and CCK. Most peptide-positive neurons, regardless of the peptide contained within the cell, had 2–4 processes that branched sparingly. Most, if not all, of the cells that contain VIP, SOM, or CCK correspond to the class II neurons described in Golgi studies (McDonald, 1982b, 1984).

These findings reveal several points of interest in regard to comparisons between the basolateral amygdala and the cerebral cortex. Golgi studies have demonstrated that the morphology of the basic cell types in both areas is very similar (McDonald, 1982b; Millhouse and DeOlmos, 1983; Carlsen and Heimer,

1988) although neuronal orientation in the basolateral amygdala is not as rigid as in the cortex. As in the basolateral amygdala, it is the spine-sparse nonpyramidal neurons in the cortex that contain VIP, SOM, and CCK (Emson and Hunt, 1981). In addition, both areas have spine-sparse nonpyramidal GABA-containing cells (Houser et al., 1983; McDonald, 1985b). The spine-sparse neurons in the basolateral amygdala and cerebral cortex are remarkably similar both morphologically and neurochemically; it seems possible that these cells are involved in similar types of circuits in both brain regions (McDonald and Pearson, 1989).

In previous Golgi studies of the basolateral amygdala, class II neurons had appeared to constitute a single population of spine-sparse neurons that exhibited a broad size range. However, it now appears that class II neurons consist of several discrete subpopulations of cells that differ both in size and in the neuropeptides that they contain (Roberts et al., 1982; McDonald, 1985a). In contrast, GABA-containing neurons in the basolateral amygdala, which also appear to be class II neurons, display a very broad size range (see also section on colocalisation below). Golgi studies have demonstrated that class II neurons often exhibit dense local axonal arborizations typical of local circuit neurons (interneurons). Since VIP, CCK, and perhaps SOM are thought to have excitatory actions, whereas GABA is inhibitory, it would appear that information processing in the basolateral amygdala involves complicated intrinsic circuits that require excitatory as well as inhibitory actions of class II neurons.

This cellular heterogeneity may reflect a complex interaction between the afferent and efferent wiring of amygdaloid neurons, since a widespread system of peptide-containing pathways linking the amygdala with more distant brain regions is well established (Roberts et al., 1982; Woodhams et al., 1983; Shiosaka et al., 1983; Price et al., 1987).

Multiple Transmitters in Peptide Neurons With:

GABA

Most GABA-immunoreactive cells do not exhibit peptide immunoreactivity, although there is extensive colocalization of peptides with GABA (McDonald and Pearson, 1989).

The following percentages of GABA-positive cells were also immunoreactive for the indicated peptide in the basolateral complex (data from McDonald and Pearson, 1989): SOM, 14.3%; neuropeptide Y (NPY), 14.9%; VIP, 17.4%; CCK, 7.9%. Double-labeled neurons, as well as single-labeled peptide-positive and GABA-positive neurons, appeared to be nonpyramidal cells.

The majority of SOM neurons in the basolateral amygdala also exhibited GABA immunoreactivity. Cell counts in rats indicated that approximately 80% of SOM cells in the lateral nucleus also contain GABA. Even greater percentages of GABA-SOM double-labeled cells were seen in the basolateral nucleus. There was also extensive colocalization of NPY and GABA but slightly greater percentages of double-labeled cells were seen in the lateral nucleus than in the basolateral nucleus (>85% and 80%, respectively).

Two populations of CCK-immunoreactive neurons were seen in the basolateral amygdala. Large CCK neurons (averaging 20 × 13 μm) predominate in the basolateral nucleus but are very rare in the lateral nucleus. Small CCK neurons (averaging 13×8 μm) predominate in the lateral nucleus but occasional cells are also seen in the basolateral nucleus. Virtually all large CCK neurons and a small percentage of small CCK neurons in the basolateral nucleus exhibited colocalization with GABA. About half of the small CCK neurons in the lateral nucleus were GABA-positive. More than half of the VIP-positive neurons in the lateral and basolateral nuclei were also GABA-positive. Previous studies (see above) show that SOM, VIP, and CCK-positive cells exhibited distinct perikaryal sizes, while the GABA-positive neurons demonstrated a wide range of perikaryal size. The variation in the size of GABA-positive cells is related, in part, to the finding that different GABA-positive cells contain different peptides (McDonald and Pearson, 1989).

At least 80% of the neurons in the lateral and basolateral amygdaloid nuclei that contain SOM or NPY immunoreactivity also contain GABA (McDonald and Pearson, 1989). Since there is also extensive coexistence of SOM and NPY in nonpyramidal neurons of the cerebral cortex, these findings support the idea that the basolateral amygdala shares many important features with the cortex. There also appears to be extensive coexistence of GABA, SOM, and NPY in nonpyramidal neurons of the cerebral cortex (Hendry et al., 1984a,b). There is considerable evidence that the nonpyramidal neurons in the cortex are local circuit neurons and that their principal synaptic targets are neighboring pyramidal neurons. A similar relationship appears to exist in the basolateral amygdala. Indeed, a light microscopic Golgi study of the basolateral amygdala found that axons of nonpyramidal neurons display dense local arborizations and frequently appear to contact pyramidal cells (McDonald, 1982b). Much of the GABA-mediated inhibition observed in the lateral amygdala (LeGal La Salle and Ben-Ari, 1981) could be accounted for by the possible GABA-ergic synaptic contacts of class II neurons on class I neuron. Thus, there is evidence that the pyramidal neurons in both the cerebral cortex and the basolateral amygdala are contacted by axons of nonpyramidal neurons that in some cases may contain the inhibitory neurotransmitter GABA and the neuropeptides SOM and NPY. The exact function of each of these peptides at these synapses has, however, yet to be determined.

Presumably the primary role of SOM-NPY neurons in the basolateral amygdala is to function as local circuit neurons. However, a subpopulation of these cells could be projection neurons. A small number of SOM neurons in the basolateral amygdala were retrogradely labeled by injections of horse radish peroxidase (HRP) into the rat striatum and cerebral cortex (McDonald, 1989). Preliminary experiments have also shown that striatal and cortical injections also retrogradely label NPY neurons and that the topography of the HRP-labeled NPY neurons in the basolateral amygdala is very similar to that of HRP-labeled SOM neurons in the same brain (McDonald, 1989). Whether SOM and NPY coexist in the same retrogradely labeled cells is not known.

Other Peptides

Previous studies have reported that the medial amygdaloid nucleus and the adjacent intra-amygdaloid portion of the bed nucleus of stria terminalis contain large numbers of SOM and NPY neurons, and that SOM and NPY coexist in many of these cells (McDonald and Pearson, 1989). There is evidence that some of the SOM neurons in these regions project through the stria terminalis to reach the bed nucleus of the stria terminalis proper (BST) and the medial preoptic-hypothalamic region (Roberts et al., 1982; Allen et al., 1984; McDonald, 1987). Since there is considerable colocalization of SOM and NPY, it is possible that some of the SOM neurons projecting through the stria also contain NPY. Although an NPY-containing efferent amygdaloid projection to the BST has been described, the exact origin of this projection has not been determined (Allen et al., 1984).

Since the striatum and lateral portions of the central amygdaloid nucleus share several cytoarchitectural and hodological features, it is of interest to compare the localization of SOM and NPY in these brain areas. There is 100% colocalization in the striatum (NPY immunoreactivity is equal to avian pancreatic polypeptide immunoreactivity) and these cells constitute a small subpopulation of medium-sized aspiny striatal cells that are found scattered throughout the striatum (Adrian et al., 1983). The majority of striatal neurons are medium-sized spiny neurons that do not exhibit SOM or NPY. The lateral capsular subdivision of the central nucleus, which merges with the laterally adjacent striatum, contains primarily medium-sized spiny neurons, although a few medium-sized aspiny cells are found. It may be inferred from the situation in the adjacent striatum that the small number of scattered SOM-NPY cells seen in lateral capsular division corresponds to the small population of medium-sized aspiny cells seen in Golgi preparations.

Golgi studies of the lateral subdivision of the central nucleus indicate that it consists almost entirely of medium-sized spiny neurons. Since there is a very high density of SOM cells in the lateral part of the central nucleus, most of the SOM cells must be medium-sized spiny neurons. These cells differ from the SOM neurons of lateral capsular division and the striatum in that they do not contain NPY. In support of this, NPY neurons have not been found in the lateral subdivision (Gustafson et al., 1986). Also, unlike the medium-sized aspiny striatal cells, which are thought to be local circuit neurons, some of the SOM cells in lateral subdivision are projection neurons that send efferents to the brain stem (see below).

Approximately 70% of SOM neurons in the medial nucleus were also NPY-immunoreactive and very few single-labeled NPY cells were observed (McDonald and Pearson, 1989). This scarcity of single-labeled NPY cells was seen in all portions of the amygdala. With the exception of the intercalated masses, all of the other amygdaloid nuclei contained scattered SOM-NPY neurons. The morphology of these neurons was similar to those seen in the medial nucleus. After the medial nucleus, the latereal nucleus and the intra-amygdaloid portion of the bed nucleus of the stria terminalis contained the greatest density of SOM-NPY neurons. There was a propensity for these neurons to be located along nuclear boundaries. In the basal and lateral amygdaloid nuclei all SOM-NPY neurons, as well as all single-labeled SOM and NPY cells, were nonpyramidal. Approximately 80% of SOM neurons in the lateral nucleus were SOM-NPY double-labeled cells. In the basolateral nucleus this figure was less than 40%. Virtually all NPY neurons in the latereal and basolateral nuclei also exhibited SOM.

CRF neurons are found throughout all subdivisions of the central amygdaloid nucleus (Shimada et al., 1989; Cassell and Gray, 1989). Numerous CRF cells were seen in the lateral subdivision of the nucleus, scattered CRF cells extended into its medial subdivision, and a few were found in the lateral capsular subdivision. Likewise, neurotensin cells were distributed predominantly in the lateral regions of the central nucleus and were scattered in the medial subdivision. They were sparse in the lateral capsular subdivision of the central nucleus. Investigation by the light microscopic mirror method revealed that about 90% of neurotensin cells werre immunoreactive to CRF in the lateral central nucleus (Shimada et al., 1989).

Unlike CRF and neurotensin neurons, SP neurons were concentrated in the medial subdivision of the central nucleus. A substantial number of SOM cells were distributed throughout the medial and lateral, but only a few were seen at scattered locations in the lateral capsular subdivision of the central nucleus. Immunofluorescent double staining showed that most of the somatostatin cells in the medial subdivision contained SP-like substances, while most of those in the lateral subdivision lacked evidence of SP-like immunoreactivity (Shimada et al., 1989). SP neurons in the dorsolateral part of the medial nucleus show colocalization with pro-dynorphin (Neal et al., 1989).

It has been suggested that regions of the bed nucleus of the stria terminalis resemble lateral and medial regions of the central nucleus. The distribution of peptides would support this view, since CRF/neurotensin neurons were found in lateral regions of the central nucleus and homologous areas of the bed nucleus and SP/somatostatin neurons were present in the medial subdivision and its homologous region of the bed nucleus (Shimada et al., 1989). However, there are substantial numbers of somatostatin cells in both regions which were not immunoreactive to SP.

It has been demonstrated that CRF, NT, SP, and SOM neurons in the central nucleus (and bed nucleus) project to parts of the lower brain stem such as the parabrachial nucleus and dorsal vagal complex (Gray and Magnusson, 1987; Moga and Gray, 1985a; Veening et al., 1984). After injections of tracer in these areas, retrogradely labeled CRF and neurotensin cells are seen in the lateral and medial parts of the central nucleus and the bed nucleus. Retrogradely labeled SP cells are found within the medial central nucleus and the ventral parts of the bed nucleus. The distribution pattern of the peptide-immunoreactive, projecting neurons overlaps that of CRF/neurotensin and SP/somatostatin neurons. Consequently, CRF/neurotensin and SP/somatostatin cells in the lateral central nucleus and bed nucleus contribute to the descending projections linking amygdala and brain stem.

The amygdala and bed nucleus are involved in autonomic function, and have reciprocal connections with brain stem autonomic regions (see Chapter 1, Amaral et al., this volume). It has been shown, for example, that electrical stimulation of the central nucleus results in increases in heart rate and blood pressure, changes in the inspiratory cycle, and gastric mucosal erosion (see Chapter 8, Kapp et al., and Chapter 11, Henke, this volume). CRF, neurotensin, SP, and somatostatin are also involved in these processes.

Intracerebroventricular injection of CRF increases mean arterial pressure and heart rate (Fisher et al., 1982), while microinjections of neurotensin into the central nucleus have an attenuating effect on cold-restraint gastric ulcers (Ray et al., 1987). Thus, the observed diversity of autonomic responses may correspond to a large variation in the pharmacological effects of these neuroactive substances in the central amygdaloid nucleus and the bed nucleus of the stria terminalis.

The functional significance of the coexistence of peptides in these areas is not clear, but it may be that CRF/neurotensin and SP/somatostatin neurons modulate autonomic responses by releasing these peptides simultaneously, causing a variety of effects in the central nucleus and BST, or via the efferent pathway, in the brain stem.

Intra-Amygdaloid Connections

Although some observations on intra-amygdaloid connectivity were made on the basis of axonal degeneration experiments in the rat, these fibre systems have been most extensively studied using modern anterograde and retrograde axonal transport techniques, especially in larger brained animals such as the cat and monkey (Price et al., 1987; see Chapter 2, McDonald, this volume) and the patterns of connections appear to be much the same in the different species.

There is general agreement that the major intra-amygdaloid connections arise in the lateral and basal nuclei and terminate in the more medial nuclei, particularly the accessory basal, central, medial, and anterior cortical nuclei, and the periamygdaloid cortex and amygdalohippocampal area (Fig. 4). The accessory basal nucleus also projects to the central, medial, and cortical nuclei and the amygdalohippocampal area. A consistent and striking feature of the intra-amygdaloid circuitry is that there are only weak projections from the medial, cortical, or central nuclei, or the amygdalohippocampal area back to the lateral and basal nuclei (see Chapter 2, Mcdonald, this volume). Other than these light and questionable projections it is clear that no other amygdaloid nucleus receives a heavy projection from the central nucleus. Thus, the flow of information through the amygdala is primarily unidirectional and in a lateral-to-medial direction. A very limited amount of data is available on the peptide compo-

---

Fig. 4. Organisation of Intra-amygdaloid peptide pathways. This summary figure links the data derived from axonal transport techniques (**A–E**) and from plotting the distribution of peptide immunoreactivity (**b–e**). Projections from the cortex enter into the lateral portion of the amygdala (**A**). Lateral nuclei send fibres toward the central nucleus and some VIP fibres follow this pattern (**B** and **b**). Basolateral nuclei connect with each other and with the central nucleus; a similar pattern is seen with SOM and NT immunoreactivity (**C** and **c**). Medial nuclei also show links with the central nucleus, as do CCK and SP (**D** and **d**). Finally the amygdaloid output leaves via the stria terminalis and ventral amygdalofugal pathway (**E**). Many peptide-containing systems also exit through the stria terminalis, and in addition this pathway carries peptide afferents which are then widely distributed through the amygdala. The enkephalin system (ME) is an example (**e**). For abbreviations, see Figure 1. (Derived from Price et al., 1987, and Roberts et al., 1982.)

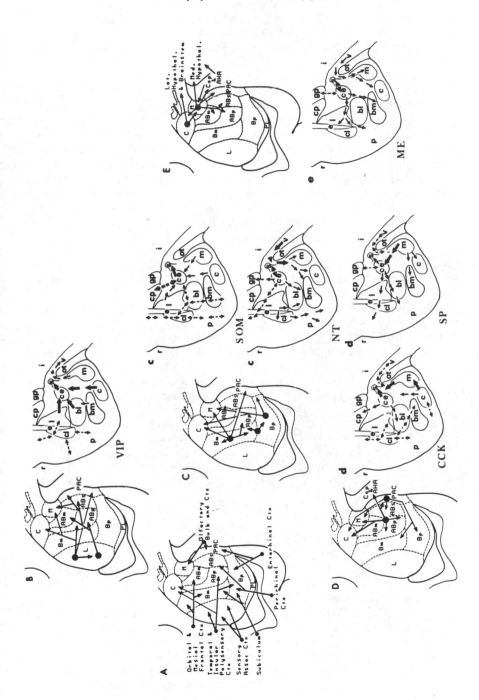

nents of intra-amygdaloid connections and this should be regarded as provisional until confirmed by dual labeling tracing techniques. The data is shown diagramatically (Fig. 4) with a corresponding diagram of known intra-amygdalised connections.

Catecholaminergic, peptidergic, and many other afferent terminal fields in the central nucleus are largely confined to individual cytoarchitectonic subdivisions (Price et al., 1987). Since these subdivisions principally reflect differences in cell morphology, afferents to the central nucleus may be directed toward specific types of neuron irrespective of their peptide content or efferent projections. However, specific interactions between peptide-containing terminals and both peptidergic and projection neurons have been demonstrated (Wray and Hoffman, 1983). Moreover, destruction of the noradrenergic input to the central nucleus markedly reduces the number of neurons expressing neurotensin immunoreactivity (Kawakami et al., 1984). Specific afferent inputs may therefore be important in the expression of individual peptides by both single and multiple classes of central nucleus neurons.

Major Peptide Pathways

The output of the amygdala is involved in modulating the activity of many different functional systems (see Chapter 1, Amaral et al., this volume). The pathways linking the amygdala with other brain regions are known to contain many peptides. These peptides originate in different regions of the amygdala, project in efferent amygdaloid pathways, and terminate in a topographic fashion in distant target areas (Roberts et al., 1981; Shiosaka et al., 1983; Price et al., 1987). The amygdala is connected to distant brain regions via a series of major and minor pathways, the most important pathways in terms of size being the stria terminalis and the pathways linking the amygdala and brain stem regions.

Stria Terminalis

The bed nucleus of the stria terminalis receives abundant peptidergic inputs of various kinds of peptides from the central nucleus (Roberts et al., 1982; Shiosaka et al., 1983; Woodhams et al., 1983; Fig. 5), suggesting that the amygdalofugal peptidergic system plays an important role in regulating the function of the BST (Fig. 6).

As data on the connections of specific cell types in the central nucleus are lacking, it appears premature to conclude that the presence of individual peptides in several neuron types indicates multifunctional roles for these peptides in the central nucleus. Nonetheless, those peptides (i.e., NT, SOM, and CRF) that are present in projections to the bed nucleus of the stria terminalis, dorsal medulla, central gray, and parbrachial complex (Roberts et al., 1982; Gray and Magnusson, 1987) are associated with at least four different types of neuron. In contrast, enkephalin, VIP, substance P, and galanin, which have only been identified in projections to either the bed nucleus of the stria terminalis (Roberts et al., 1982) or central gray (Gray, 1989), are contained within only one or two types of cell. The presence of NT, SOM, and CRF in multiple projections of the central nucleus may be based on the fact that they are contained within several neuron types. In support of this, all of the cell types associated here with NT,

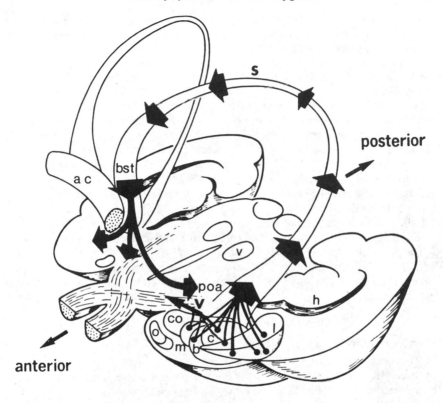

Fig. 5. The stria terminalis and ventral amygdalofugal pathways. These related systems carry the major peptidergic outflow from the amygdala. **s**: stria terminalis; **v**: ventral amygdalofugal pathway; ac: anterior commissure; bnst: bed nucleus stria terminalis; c, co, b, m, l: amygdaloid nuclei; h: hippocampus; poa: preoptic area; v: ventro-medial hypothalamas.

SOM, and CRF send axons toward the stria terminalis and ventral amygdalofugal pathway (McDonald, 1982a).

The major origin of VIP-containing fibres in the BST lies in the central amygdaloid nucleus and is supplied by two pathways; one from the stria terminalis which terminates diffusely in the BST, and the other from the ventral amygdalofugal pathway (Price et al., 1987), which terminates mainly in the ventral part of the BST. Such a topographic projection is very similar to that of L-ENK fibres, though L-ENK fibres projecting via the stria terminalis do not project diffusely to the BST but predominantly to the lateral subdivision of the BST. L-ENK and VIP may coexist in single cells of the central nucleus whose axons pass through the ventral amygdalofugal pathway, since distribution pattern of VIP fibres in the ventral subdivision of the BST and their fibre trajectories are similar to those of L-ENK.

Many L-ENK fibres in the lateral subdivision of the BST always remained after the destruction of the central nucleus or transection of both the stria terminalis and the ventral amygdalofugal pathway (Rao et al., 1987a). These fibres may be of intrinsic origin, because a small group of L-ENK neurons was detected in the lateral subdivision of the BST.

A dense plexus of substance P fibres was detected in the BST. This fibre plexus in the dorsal part of the BST is supplied by SP neurons in the central nucleus via the stria terminalis, and the remaining SP fibres in the BST originate in other parts (Roberts et al., 1982; Woodhams et al., 1983). The L-ENK fibre plexus is located in the lateral and ventral parts of the central nucleus and projects to the dorsal part of the BST (Inagaki and Parent, 1985; Rao et al., 1987b). Therefore, it is unlikely that L-ENK and SP coexist in same central nucleus neuron (Roberts et al., 1982; Woodhams et al., 1983). The descending SOM system from central amygdala to the hypothalamus and brain stem via the stria has been explored (Price et al., 1987). The destruction of the central amygdaloid nucleus failed to decrease the number of SOM fibres in the BST. Thus, the L-ENK and SOM amygdalofugal systems are different subpopulations.

Similarly, the descending CRF and NT neuron system from the central nucleus to the parabrachial nucleus has been described (Moga and Gray, 1985a). L-ENK and CRF or NT may not coexist in the same central nucleus neuron since destruction of the central nucleus failed to cause the reduction of L-ENK fibres in the parabrachial area.

Organization and Possible Function

Corticotropin-Releasing Factor

The central nucleus and BST contain a significant proportion of the forebrain population of CRF-immunoreactive neurons. It was estimated that a combined total of over 2,500 CRF-immunoreactive cells are located in these areas as compared to sightly over 2,000 cells within the paraventricular nucleus of the hypothalamus (Swanson et al., 1983). The majority are located in the dorsal part of the BST and the lateral part of the central nucleus (Veening et al., 1984; Cassell et al., 1986). The CRF-containing neurons of the BST and central nucleus also project to the parabrachial nucleus (Moga and Gray, 1985a), midbrain central gray (Gray, 1989), and the dorsal vagal complex (Veening et al., 1984). In fact, the BST and central nucleus contain the majority of forebrain CRF-immunoreactive neurons that project to these brain stem autonomic regions (Moga and Gray, 1985a; Gray, 1989). Both electrical stimulation of the central nucleus and central injections of CRF result in similar changes in centrally mediated cardiovascular responses. This includes increases in heart rate, blood pressure, and changes in visceral and somatic blood flow that are seen in "stresslike" or "defensive" behaviors. This suggests that CRF may be an important neurochemical mediator of cardiovascular changes seen following activation of the amygdala.

Neurotensin

Neurotensin-immunoreactive cells are especially numerous in the BST and the central nucleus. It is estimated that a combined total of over 3,000 NT-immunoreactive cells per side are present in these areas and, like the CRF-containing cells, they are located predominantly within the dorsal BST and lateral central nucleus. Neurotensin-immunoreactive cells in the same areas (like CRF) project to the parabrachial nucleus (Moga and Gray, 1985a), central gray (Gray, 1989), and the dorsal vagal complex (Veening et al., 1984). Injections of NT into the central nucleus and BST, as well as the midbrain central gray, have a strong antinocieptive action. Neurotensin-induced analgesia in the midbrain central gray is mediated via an excitatory pathway that activates the pain-suppressing regions of the nucleus raphe magnus. The reduced responsivity to painful stimuli induced by NT is unaffected by administration of naloxone. Studies using dopamine agonists and antagonists suggest that dopaminergic systems participate in neurotensin-induced analgesia (Hernandez et al., 1983).

In this regard it is interesting that the dopaminergic terminals are distributed most densely within the dorsal part of the BST and the lateral central nucleus where the majority of neurotensin-immunoreactive cells and fibres are located (see Chapter 3, Fallon and Ciofi, this volume). Thus, dopaminergic terminals that originate from the midbrain tegmentum are located in a position to influence directly amygdaloid neurotensin cells that in turn project to the brain stem. It has been suggested that NT may function in behavioral and affective responses to painful stimuli (Hernandez et al., 1983). In terms of amygdaloid-mediated functions, NT may integrate nonopioid analgesia associated with defensive reactions to stress-inducing or aversive stimuli.

Somatostatin

Somatostatin neurons represent another significant population of peptidergic neurons within the central nucleus. They are concentrated in the lateral central nucleus and dorsal BST in the regions with overlapping CRF, endorphin, and NT-immunoreactive neurons, but are also found scattered within the medial subdivision of the central nucleus and the ventral BST. The central nucleus and BST are the origin of somatostatin-containing pathways to the parabrachial nucleus (Moga and Gray, 1985a), central gray, and the dorsal vagal complex (Veening et al., 1984; Gray and Magnusson, 1987). This brain stem projection probably arises mainly from cells in the lateral central nucleus (Veening et al., 1984) and the dorsal BST (Moga and Gray, 1985a).

Enkephalin

Enkephalin-immunoreactive neurons are also prevalent with the BST and central nucleus, but are for the most part confined to their dorsal and lateral subdivisions, respectively. Enkephalin neurons in the lateral subdivision project heavily upon the BST and this projection is reciprocated. Enkephalin also coexists within individual glutamic acid decarboxylase-containing neurons of the central nucleus. Transection of the stria terminalis results in a reduction of GABA and enkephalin within the BST and central nucleus. Thus it may be that enkephalin/GABA neurons are interneurons that provide a functional link between the central nucleus and BST. This inhibition is thought to play a role in the susceptibility of the amygdala to experimentally induced epileptiform discharges (LeGal LaSalle and Ben-Ari, 1981). In this regard, it is interesting that cutting the stria terminalis facilitates the establishment of kindling (Itagaki

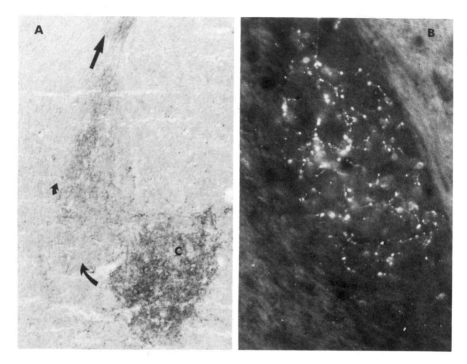

Fig. 6. The stria terminalis contains many peptidergic fibres. (**A**) SP fibres leave the central nucleus (**c**) and ascend into the stria terminalis (×35) and (**B**) NPY fibres are located within the arch of the stria terminalis. (×300).

et al., 1986; Loscher and Schwark, 1987). Enkephalin-containing cells in the central nucleus have been also implicated in opioid withdrawal and in learned cardiovascular responses to stressful stimuli.

Galanin

Like SP, galanin-immunoreactive neurons are sparsely distributed within the BST and central nucleus compared to the other peptidergic neuron types. However, unlike SP, no evidence was observed for the participation of galanin in the efferent pathway to the dorsal vagal complex. However, galanin cells in the BST and central amygdala do appear to project to the midbrain central gray and parabrachial nucleus (Skofitsch and Jacobowitz, 1985; Gray, 1989).

Dorsal Vagal Area

Peptidergic neurons within both the BST and the central nucleus innervate the dorsal vagal complex. The BST and central nucleus also send peptidergic efferents to the parabrachial nucleus (Moga and Gray, 1985a,b) and the central gray (Gray, 1989). These findings are not surprising in that the central nucleus and BST project to similar subregions of the parabrachial nucleus, central gray, and dorsal vagal complex (Fulwiler and Saper, 1984) from the same type of peptide-immunoreactive neurons. Thus, CRF, NT, SOM, and SP neurons within both the central nucleus and BST all contribute to the descending brain stem projections. It is estimated that over 20% of the central nucleus and 15% of the BST vagal efferent neurons are immunoreactive to these peptides (Gray, 1989). Retrogradely labeled CRF, NT, GAL, and SP-immunoreactive cells were also observed in the lateral hypothalamus-perifornical area and occasionally were present in the paraventricular nucleus.

The majority of vagally projecting neurons are located in the medial central nucleus and ventral part of the BST. The parabrachial nucleus of the pons receives projections from neurons located in all subdivisions of the central nucleus and BST (Moga and Gray, 1985a,b). Corticotropin-releasing factor, NT, and SOM projections to the parabrachial nucleus and dorsal vagal complex arise mainly from the ventral BST and lateral central nucleus (Moga and Gray, 1985a). SP projections to the dorsal vagal complex arise exclusively from the ventral BST and medial central nucleus. Also, Eiden et al. (1985) showed that some vasoactive intestinal polypeptide-immunoreactive terminals within the dorsal part of the BST and the lateral central nucleus have a common origin from cells in the brain stem, probably the dorsal raphe area. Thus, there is now substantial evidence indicating that the lateral and medial central nucleus are homologous to the dorsal and ventral BST with respect to their connections, morphology, and chemoarchitecture. Further studies are required to see if the dorsal BST has subdivisions that correspond to those of the lateral central nucleus (McDonald, 1982b; Cassell et al., 1986).

However, Higgins and Schwaber (1983) reported that the central nucleus projection to the dorsal vagal complex arises from SOM cells located in the medial central nucleus. The function of somatostatin in descending amygdaloid pathways is unclear. It has been demonstrated that the central administration of SOM acts to suppress vagal nerve activity and to a lesser degree sympathetic outflow to the stomach (Somiya and Tonoue, 1984). Also, SOM reduces adrenal nerve activity (Somiya and Tonoue, 1984) and adrenomedullary epinephrine secretion (Brown and Fisher, 1985).

Enkephalin neurons differ in that they do not appear to project to the parabrachial nucleus (Moga and Gray, 1985a), central gray, or the dorsal vagal complex (Veening et al., 1984). The substance P projection the dorsal vagal complex is relatively sparse on the basis of the low total number SP-immunoreactive neurons and low percentage of SP neurons that are also retrogradely labeled within the BST and central nucleus. This observation is consistent with evidence suggesting that most of the substance P terminals within the vagal complex originate from the periphery. The central nucleus also provides a sparse substance P input to the parabrachial nucleus.

Connections With the Parabrachial Nucleus

Previous studies have demonstrated that the central nucleus of the amygdala is innervated by neurons in the parabrachial nucleus (see Fulwiler and Saper, 1984, for review).

Recent studies which have combined retrograde transport techniques with immunohistochemistry have shown SOM and SP neurons in the central nucleus also accumulate retrograde tracers injected into the nucleus of the tractus solitarius (Higgins and Schwaber, 1983; Veening et al., 1984). Numerous SOM, NT, and CRF-containing central nucleus neurons project to the parabrachial nucleus (Moga and Gray, 1985a).

The double-label studies are of great functional interest. The fact that calcitonin gene-related peptide (CGRP) fibers in the central amygdaloid nucleus arise from neurons in the parabrachial nucleus suggests a role for this peptide in the ascending transmission of visceral sensory information (see Fulwiler and Saper, 1984, for review). The principal location of these CGRP-containing cells is in the ventral region of the parabrachial nucleus, which has been associated with cardiovascular regulation. Conversely, the recent findings of Cox et al. (1986) show that stimulation of the reciprocal pathway strongly influences neurons in the nucleus of the solitary tract and the dorsomedial nucleus of the hypothalamus involved in baroreflex regulation through descending projections of the central nucleus.

A large reciprocal connection from the parabrachial nucleus innervates the amygdala. Other peptide and neurotransmitter systems that terminate within the central nucleus also arborize selectively within the central nucleus subdivisions; for example, noradrenaline (NE), NPY, SOM, NT, ENK, SP, CRF, and VIP (Higgins and Schwaber, 1983; Wray and Hoffman, 1983; Cassell et al., 1986; Gustafson et al., 1986; Gray, 1989).

Those axons containing SP, ENK, NT, SS, VIP, and CRF exhibit differential distributions that overlap extensively with that of CGRP-containing axons (Schwaber et al., 1988). Within the lateral capsular subdivision of the central nucleus, CGRP is virtually coextensive with dense arborizations of SP, NT, and CRF-containing axons. In contrast, the heaviest overlap of VIP, ENK, and SOM-containing axons with the CGRP plexus occurs in the other regions of the central nucleus. Other systems, such as NPY and NE, also exhibit some overlap with the dense CGRP plexus, but the primary distribution of these fibre plexii is within the medial central nucleus. The origin of some of these peptidergic afferents is also located in the parabrachial nucleus—for example, NT and SP (Yamano et al., 1988a,b; Block and Hoffman, 1989). Other peptide systems do not form dense pericellular arbors analogous to those formed by the CGRP-immunoreactive axons. The dense overlap of these chemically distinct fibre systems within cytoarchitecturally distinct subdivisions suggests a functional interaction of these different systems in controlling the activity of the same neurons.

Sex Differences

The posterior medial amygdala and posterior medial BST are densely populated with neurons that contain estrogen and androgen receptors. Thus these regions contain estrogen neurons which may be direct targets of the organizational and/or activational effects of gonadal steroids (see also Chapter 8, Kapp et al., and Chapter 13, Kling and Brothers, this volume).

Other sexually dimorphic features of medial amygdala and the posterior medial BST have been described. Certain cell groups within the posterior medial BST are larger in male rats and guinea pigs (Del Abril et al., 1987). The cytoarchitecture of medial amygdala is also sexually dimorphic in that the volume of this region as a whole is approximately 20% larger in male than in female rats (Mizukami et al., 1983). This sex difference may be largely due to a difference in the volume of the posteriodorsal region, a region which receives a dense SP innervation (Malsbury and Mackay, 1989). Sex differences in synaptic organization within the medial amygdala have also been reported (Nishizuka and Ari, 1983).

The vomeronasal olfactory system provides one of the major afferents to the posterior medial amygdala. A number of features of the vomeronasal system, including the vomeronasal organ itself, show significantly greater development in male rats. For example, the accessory olfactory bulb is larger (Roos et al., 1988) and contains a greater number of mitral cells in males. Axons of these mitral cells form the accessory olfactory tract and terminate on dendrites of neurons in the posterior medial amygdala. Thus sex differences in the medial amygdala may be at least partly determined by sex differences in synaptic input to the medial amygdala. Furthermore, SP, vasopressin, and CCK-8 are known to have a sexually dimorphic distribution. Most of the vasopressin-immunoreactive cell bodies in the BST are present in the posterior part of the medial BST (Van Leeuwen et al., 1985) that is, in the same region which receives the most dense SP innervation.

Recently Micevych et al. (1988) described a dramatic sex difference in the number of CCK-8-immunoreactive perikarya in the posterior medial BST and posteriodorsal medial amygdala of the rat brain. In both areas the number of CCK-immunoreactive cells was several times greater in the male in the BST and medial amygdala innervate the regions which contain the sexually dimorphic populations of CCK-8-immunoreactive perikarya (Malsbury and Mackay, 1989). Thus it appears that these fields of SP fibers serve as a readily identifiable marker for sexually dimorphic cell groups within medial amygdala and BST.

Peptidergic neurons within these cell groups are clearly hormone-sensitive. For example, castration of adult male rats can reduce vasopressin staining in the BST (Van Leeuwen et al., 1985) and CCK staining in both the BST and posteriodorsal portion of the medial nucleus (Micevych et al., 1988). SP fibers in the medial amygdala and the posterior medial BST are responsive to both organizational and activational effects of testosterone. Injections of testoterone into newborn female rats can masculinize the SP innervation of the medial nucleus, while castration of adult males can reduce SP staining in the medial nucleus in rats and hamsters (see discussion in Malsbury and Mackay, 1989).

Although the functional significance of the SP innervation of the medial amygdala and BST is not known, these areas have been implicated in the regulation of a number of sexually differentiated brain functions in the rat. The evidence is particularly extensive for regulation of male sexual behavior and LH and prolactin release.

CONCLUSIONS

The amygdaloid complex receives sensory information from a variety of unimodal and polymodal association cortices. The apparent anatomical heterogeneity of the amygdala is reflected in the many shared afferent and efferent connections of its subdivisions and their extensive intra-amygdaloid interactions. The quantity and complexity of peptide systems, both within the amygdala and connecting the amygdala with other brain regions, makes them a linchpin in the control and regulation of the diversity of amygdaloid function. The basic concepts of amygdala organisation, that of an inhibitory lateral portion and a facilitatory medial portion, which can also be conceptualised as reflecting the external (lateral) and internal (medial) environments, are also reflected in the blueprint of peptide organisation. The peptide-containing neurons in the lateral basal complex show many similarities to the interneuron class of cortical neurons (mainly type II) both morphologically and in their transmitter (SOM, NPY, VIP) and cotransmitter (GABA) content, while the peptide-containing systems of the medial amygdala are closely connected with gender difference (SP, CCK) and by inference reproduction. The role of the amygdala in integrating external and internal environments and initiating behaviors which can modulate them is reflected in the gathering of amygdaloid output in the central nucleus (the most peptide-rich region in the brain outside the hypothalamus) and the funnelling of this output along peptide-containing fibres in the stria terminalis and the ventral amygdalofugal pathway. From the first the importance of the central nucleus and stria terminalis in the organisation of the amygdaloid peptide systems has been noted and it has been suggested that these inputs could act to gate amygdaloid output in the central nucleus (Roberts et al., 1982).

Several aspects of the role of peptides in the amygdala still need to be explored, such as the morphology of peptide neurons in the medial nuclei and the physiological mechanisms and significance of peptide and peptide-GABA cotransmitters. Further virgin territory is the role of peptides in brain development. The appearance of peptides during brain development and their subsequent levels vary significantly during the course of brain development (Shiosaka et al., 1983). In addition, a recent report indicates that tyrosine hydroxylase is also transiently expressed in SOM and SP neurons but not in CCK, NPY, or NE neurons in the central nucleus and BST during brain development (Verney et al., 1988). The transient expression of transmitters is thought to be related to synaptogenesis and the development of the stria terminalis. Peptide involvement in the development of the amygdala is assuredly of great functional importance; however, the extent of this involvement is only beginning to be realised.

The final profile of peptide distribution and function in the various amygdaloid nuclei is still some considerable way from completion. However, the gradual accretion of peptide cartography will ensure that a full understanding of the role of peptide transmitter systems in amygdaloid function and dysfunction systems will eventually emerge.

REFERENCES

Adrian TE, Allen JM, Bloom SR, Ghatei MA, Rosser MN, Roberts GW, Crow TJ, Tatemoto K, Polak JM (1983): Neuropeptide Y distribution in human brain. Nature, 306:584–588.

Allen YS, Roberts GW, Bloom SR, Crow TJ, Polak JM (1984): Neuropeptide Y in the stria terminalis: Evidence for an amygdalofugal projection. Brain Res 321:357–362.

Block CH, Hoffman G, Kapp BS (1989): Peptide-containing pathways from the parabrachial complex to the central nucleus of the amygdala. Peptides 10:465–471.

Braak H, Braak E (1983): Neuronal types in the basolateral amygdaloid nuclei of man. Brain Res Bull 11:349–365.

Brown, MR, Fisher LA (1985): Central nervous system actions of somatostatin related peptides. In YC Patel and GS Tannenbaum (eds): Somatostatin, Advances in Experimental Medicine and Biology. Proc Somatostatin Satellite Symposium, Montreal, Canada, pp 217–228.

Carlsen J (1988): Immunocytochemical localization of glutamate decarboxylase in the rat basolateral amygdaloid nucleus, with special reference to GABAergic innervation of amygdalostriatal projection neurons. J Comp Neurol 273:513–526.

Carlsen J, Heimer L (1988): The basolateral amygdaloid complex as a cortical-like structure. Brain Res 441:377–380.

Cassell MD, Gray TS, Kiss JZ (1986): Neuronal architecture in the rat central nucleus of the amygdala: A cytological, hodological, and immunocytochemical study. J Comp Neurol 246:478–499.

Cassell MD, Gray TS (1989): Morphology of peptide-immunoreactive neurons in the rat central nucleus of the amygdala. J Comp Neurol 281:320–333.

Cox, GE, Jordan D, Moruzzi P, Schwaber JS, Spyer KM, Turner SA (1986): Amygdaloid influences on brain-stem neurons in the rabbit. J Physiol (London) 381:135–148.

Del Abril A, Sogovia S, Guillamon A (1987): The bed nucleus of the stria terminalis in the rat: Regional sex differences controlled by gonadal steroids early after birth. Dev Brain Res 32:295–300.

Eiden LE, Hokfelt J, Brownstein MJ, Palkovits M (1985): Vasoactive intestinal polypeptide afferents to the bed nucleus of the stria terminalis in the rat: an immunohistorical and biochemical study. Neuroscience 15:999–1013.

Emson PC, Hunt SP (1981): Anatomical chemistry of the cerebral cortex. In Schmitt FO, Worden FG, Adelman G, Dennis SG (eds): "The Organization of the Cerebral Cortex." Cambridge, MA: MIT, pp 325–345.

Fisher LA, River J, River C, Spiess J, Vale W, Brown MR (1982): Corticotropin-releasing factor (CRF): Central effects on mean arterial pressure and heart rate in rats. Endocrinology 110:2222–2224.

Fulwiler CE, Saper CB (1984): Subnuclear organization of the efferents connections of the parabrachial nucleus in the rat. Brain Res Rev 7:229–259.

Gray TS (1983): The morphology of somatostatin-immunoreactive neurons in the lateral nucleus of the rat amygdala. Peptides 4:663–668.

Gray TS (1989): Autonomic neuropeptide connections of the amygdala. In Tache Y, Morley JE, Brown M (eds): "Neuropeptides and Stress: Symposia Hans Selye." New York: Springer Verlag, pp 92–106.

Gray TS, Cassell D, Kiss JZ (1984): The distribution of propiomelanocortin-derived peptides and enkephalins in the rat central nucleus of the amygdala. Brain Res 106:354–358.

Gray TS, Magnusson DJ (1987): Neuropeptide neuronal efferents from the bed nucleus of the stria terminalis and central amygdaloid nucleus to the dorsal vagal complex in the rat. J Comp Neurol 262:365–374.

Gustafson EL, Card PJ, Moore RY (1986): Neuropeptide Y localization in the rat amygdaloid complex. J Comp Neurol 251:349–362.

Hendry SHC, Jones EG, Defelipe J, Schmechel K, Brandon C, Emson PC (1984a): Neuropeptide-containing neurons of the cerebral cortex are also GABAergic. Proc Natl Acad Sci USA 81:6526–6530.

Hendry SHC, Jones EG, Emson PC (1984b): Morphology, distribution, and synaptic relations of somatostatin and neuropeptide Y-immunoreactive neurons in rat and monkey neocortex. J Neurosci 4:2497–2517.

Hernandez DE, Nemeroff CB, Orlando RC, Prange AJ Jr (1983): The effect of centrally administered neuropeptides on the development of stress-induced gastric ulcers in rats. J Neurosci Res 9:145–157.

Higgins GA, Schwaber JS (1983): Somatostatin: origin of projection from the central nucleus of the amygdala to the vagal nuclei. Peptides 4:657–662.

Houser CR, Hendry SHC, Jones EG, Vaughnn JE (1983): Morphological diversity of immunocytochemically identified GABA neurons in the monkey sensory-motor cortex. J Neurocytol 12:617–638.

Inagaki S, Parent A (1985): Distribution of enkephalin-immunoreactive neurons in the forebrain and upper brainstem of the squirrel monkey. Brain Res 359:267–280.

Itagaki S, Uemura S, Kimera H (1986): GABAergic system and amydaloid kindling studied by immunohistochemistry using antibody against GABA. Jpn J Psych Neurol 40:341–344.

Kawakami FK, Fukui H, Okamura N, Morimoto N, Yanaihara T, Nakajima, Ibata Y (1984): Influence of ascending noradrenergic fibers on the neurotensin-like immunoreactive perikarya and evidence of direct projection of ascending neurotensin-like immunoreactive fibers in the rat central nucleus of the amygdala. Neurosci Lett 51:225–230.

LeGal LaSalle G, Ben-Ari Y (1981): Unit activity in the amygdaloid complex: A review. In Ben-Ari Y (ed): "The Amygdaloid Complex." INSERM Symposium, No 20. Amsterdam: Elsevier, p 227.

Loscher W, Schwark WS (1987): Further evidence for abnormal GABAergic circuits in amygdala-kindled rats. Brain Res 420:385–390.

Maley B, Mullett T, Elde R (1983): The nucleus tractus solitarii of the cat: A comparison of Golgi impregnated neurons with methionine-enkephalin and substance P-immunoreactive neurons. J Comp Neurol 217:405–417.

Malsbury CW, Mackay K (1989): Sex difference in the substance P-immunoreactive innervation of the medial nucleus of the amygdala. Brain Res Bull 23:561–567.

McDonald AJ (1982a): Cytoarchitecture of the central amygdaloid nucleus of the rat. J Comp Neurol 208:401–418.

McDonald AJ (1982b): Neurons of the lateral and basolateral amygdaloid nuclei: A Golgi study in the rat. J Comp Neurol 212:293–312.

McDonald AJ (1984): Neuronal organization of the lateral and basolateral amygdaloid nuclei in the rat. J Comp Neurol 222:589–606.

McDonald AJ (1985a): Morphology of peptide-containing neurons in the rat basolateral amygdaloid nucleus. Brain Res 338:186–191.

McDonald AJ (1985b): Immunohistochemical identification of gamma-aminobutyric acid-containing neurons in the rat basolateral amygdala. Neurosci Lett 53:203–207.

McDonald AJ (1987): Somatostatinergic projections from the amygdala to the bed nucleus of the stria terminalis and medial preoptic-hypothalamic region. Neurosci Lett 75:271–277.

McDonald AJ (1989): Coexistence of somatostatin with neuropeptide Y, but not with cholecystokinin or vasoactive intestinal peptide in neurons of the rat amygdala. Brain Res 500:37–45.

McDonald AJ, Pearson JC (1989): Coexistence of GABA and peptide immunoreactivity in non-pyramidal neurons of the basolateral amygdala. Neurosci Lett 100:53–58.

Micevych P, Akesson T, Elde R (1988): Distribution of cholecystokinin-immunoreactive cell bodies in the male and female rat: II. Bed nucleus of the stria terminalis and amygdala. J Comp Neurol 269:381–391.

Millhouse OE, DeOlmos J (1983): Neuronal configurations in lateral and basolatereal amygdala. Neuroscience 10:1269–1300.

Mizukami S, Nishizuka M, Ari Y (1983): Sexual difference in nuclear volume and its ontogeny in the rat amygdala. Exp Neurol 70:569–575.

Moga MM, Gray TS (1985a): Evidence for corticotropin-releasing factor, neurotensin, and somatostatin in the neural pathway from the central nucleus of the amygdala to the parabrachial nucleus. J Comp Neurol 241:275–284.

Moga MM, Gray TS (1985b): Peptidergic efferents from the intercalated nuclei of the amygdala to the parabrachial nucleus in the rat. Neurosci Lett 61:13–18.

Neal CR Jr, Swann JM, Newman SW (1989): The co-localization of substance P and prodynorphin immunoreactivity in neurons of the medial preopic area, bed nucleus of the stria terminalis and medial nucleus of the amygdala of the Syrian hamster. Brain Res 496:1–13.

Nishizuka M, Ari Y (1983): Regional difference in sexually dimorphic synaptic organization of the medial amygdala. Exp Brain Res 49:462–465.

Pascoe JP, Kapp BS (1985): Electrophysiological characteristics of amygdaloid central nucleus neurons in the awake rabbit. Brain Res Bull 14:331–338.

Price JL, Ruschen FT, Amaral DG (1987): The amygdaloid complex. In Bjorklund A, Hokfelt T, Swanson LW (eds):, Vol 5. "Handbook of Chemical Neuroanatomy: Integrated systems of the CNS," Part 1. Amsterdam: Elsevier, pp 279–388.

Ray A, Henke PG, Sullivan RM (1987): The central amygdala and immobilization stress-induced gastric pathology in rats. Neurotensin and dopamine. Brain Res 409:398–402.

Rao ZR, Shiosaka S, Tohyama M (1987a): Origin of cholinergic fibers in the basolateral nucleus of the amygdaloid complex by using sensitive double-labeling technique of retrograde biotinized tracer and immunocytochemistry. J Hirnforsch 28:553–560.

Rao ZR, Yamano M, Shiosaka S, Shinohara A, Tohyama M (1987b): Origin of leucine-enkephalin fibers and their two main afferent pathways in the bed nucleus of the stria terminalis in the rat. Exp Brain Res 65:411–420.

Roberts GW, Woodhams PL, Polak JM, Crow TJ (1982): Distribution of neuropeptides in the limbic system of the rat: The amygdaloid complex. Neuroscience 7:99–131.

Roos J, Roos M, Schaeffer C, Aron C (1988): Sexual differences in the development of accessory olfactory bulbs in the rat. J Comp Neurol 270:121–131.

Schwaber JS, Sternini C, Brecha NC, Rogers WT, Card JP (1988): Neurons containing calcitonin gene-related peptide in the parabrachial nucleus project to the central nucleus of the amygdala. J Comp Neurol 270:416–426, 398–399.

Shimada S, Inagaki S, Kubota Y, Ogawa N, Shibasaki T, Takagi H (1989): Coexistence of peptides (corticotropin releasing factor/neurotensin and substance P/somatostatin) in the bed nucleus of the stria terminalis and central amygdaloid nucleus of the rat. Neuroscience 30:377–383.

Shiosaka SM, Sakanaka S, Inagaki E, Senba Y, Hare K, Takatsuki H, Takagi Y, Kawai, Tohyama M (1983): Putative neurotransmitters in the amygdaloid complex with special reference to peptidergic pathways. In Emson PC (ed): "Chemical Neuroanatomy." New York: Raven Press, pp 359–389.

Skofitsch G, Jacobowitz DM (1985): Immunohistochemical mapping of galanin-like neurons in the rat central nervous system. Peptides (Fayetteville) 6:509–546.

Somiya H, Tonoue T (1984): Neuropeptides as central integrators of autonomic nerve activity: Effects of TRH, SRIF, VIP and bombesin on gastric and adrenal nerves. Reg Pept: des 9:47–52.

Swanson LW, Sawchenko P (1983): Hypothalamic integration: Organization of the paraventricular and supraoptic nuclei. Ann Rev Neurosci 6:269–324.

Van Leeuwen FW, Caffe AR, De Vries GJ (1985): Vasopressin cells in the bed nucleus of the stria terminalis of the rat: Sex differences and the influence of androgens. Brain Res 325:391–394.

Veening JG, Swanson LW, Sawchenko PE (1984): The organization of projections from the central nucleus of the amygdala to brainstem sites involved in central autonomic regulation: A combined retrograde transport-immunohistochemical study. Brain Res 303:337–357.

Verney C, Gaspar P, Febvret A, Berger B (1988): Transient tyrosine hydroxylase-like immunoreactive neurons contain somatostatin and substance P in the developing amygdala and bed nucleus of the stria terminalis of the rat. Brain Res 470:45–58.

Watson SJ, Khachaturian H, Akil H, Coy D, Goldstein A (1982): Comparison of the distribution of dynorphin systems and enkephalin systems in brain. Science 218:1134–1136.

Woodhams PL, Roberts GW, Polak JM, Crow TJ (1983): Distribution of neuropeptides in the limbic system of the rat: The bed nucleus of the stria terminalis, septum and preoptic area. Neuroscience 8:677–703.

Wray S, Hoffman GE (1983): Organization and interrelationship of neuropeptides in the central amygdaloid nucleus of the rat. Peptides 4:525–541.

Yamano M, Hillyard CJ, Girgis S, MacIntyre I, Emson PC, Tohyama M (1988a): Presence of a substance P-like immunoreactive neuron system from the parabrachial area to the central amygdaloid nucleus of the rat with reference to coexistence with calcitonin gene-related peptide. Brain Res 451:179–188.

Yamano M, Hillyard CJ, Girgis S, Emson PC, MacIntyre I, Tohyama M (1988b): Projection of neurotensin-like immunoreactive neurons from the lateral parabrachial area to the central amygdaloid nucleus of the rat with reference to the coexistence with calcitonin gene-related peptide. Exp Brain Res 71:603–610.

The Amygdala: Neurobiological Aspects of Emotion,
Memory, and Mental Dysfunction, pages 143–165
© 1992 Wiley-Liss, Inc.

5
Neurophysiology and Functions of the Primate Amygdala

EDMUND T. ROLLS

Department of Experimental Psychology, University of Oxford, Oxford, UK

INTRODUCTION

It is the aim of this chapter to consider the functions of the primate amygdala in the light of the responsiveness of single neurons within the structure. This neuronal responsiveness is most informative when activity is recorded while the amygdala is functioning normally, and in situations in which the amygdala is required. The neurophysiology must thus proceed closely with lesion studies which help assess the functions of the amygdala. Because lesion studies are important in setting the context for neurophysiological studies of the amygdala, lesion studies which provide indications of the functions performed by the amygdala are considered first. The aim of the neurophysiology is then to show how the amygdala performs its functions. For this, it is important to analyse the information processing being performed by neurons in the amygdala, and for this reason some evidence on the input and output connections of the amygdala, and on the neuronal activity in these input and output regions, is considered. This helps to provide an understanding of how the amygdala operates at the systems level of brain function, and in particular how it transforms the inputs it receives, and what effects the results of its computations have on output regions. Particular attention is paid to research in nonhuman primates. Part of the reason for this is that the developments in primates in the structure and connections of neural systems associated with the amygdala (such as the temporal lobe cortical areas and the orbitofrontal cortex) make studies in primates particularly important for understanding amygdala function in humans, including its role in emotion and emotional disorders.

Systems Level Connections

The amygdala is a subcortical region in the anterior part of the temporal lobe. It receives massive projections in the primate from the overlying temporal

Address correspondence to Dr. E.T. Rolls, Department of Experimental Psychology, University of Oxford, South Parks Road, Oxford OX1 3UD, UK.

cortex (Herzog and Van Hoesen, 1976; Aggleton et al., 1980; Turner et al., 1980; Turner, 1981; Van Hoesen, 1981). These come in the monkey to overlapping but partly separate regions of the lateral and basal amygdala from the inferior temporal visual cortex, the superior temporal auditory cortex, the cortex of the temporal pole, and the cortex in the superior temporal sulcus. Thus the amygdala receives inputs from temporal lobe association cortex, but not from earlier stages of cortical visual information processing. It also receives projections from the posterior orbitofrontal cortex. Subcortical inputs to the amygdala include projections from the midline thalamic nuclei, the subiculum and CA1 parts of the hippocampal formattion, the hypothalamus and substantia innominata, the nucleus of the solitary tract (which receives gustatory and visceral inputs), and from olfactory structures (Ben-Ari, 1981). Although there are some inputs from early on in some sensory pathways, for example auditory inputs from the medial geniculate nucleus (LeDoux, 1987), this route is unlikely to be involved in most emotions, for which cortical analysis of the stimulus is likely to be required.

The outputs of the amygdala (Price, 1981; Ben-Ari, 1981) include the well-known projections to the hypothalamus, from the lateral amygdala via the ventral amygdalofugal pathway to the lateral hypothalamus, and from the medial amygdala, which is relatively small in the primate, via the stria terminalis to the medial hypothalamus. The ventral amygdalofugal pathway is now known to contain some long descending fibers that project to the autonomic centers in the medulla oblongata (Hopkins et al., 1981; Price, 1981; Schwaber et al., 1982), and provide a route for cortically processed signals to reach the brain stem. A further interesting output of the amygdala is to the ventral striatum (Heimer et al., 1982) including the nucleus accumbens, for via this route information processed in the amygdala could gain access to the basal ganglia and thus influence motor output. The amygdala also projects to the medial part of the mediodorsal nucleus of the thalamus (Nauta, 1961; Price, 1981), which projects to the orbitofrontal cortex and provides the amygdala with another output. In addition, the amygdala has direct projections back to many areas of the temporal, orbitofrontal, and insular cortices from which it receives inputs (Mufson et al., 1981; Porrino et al., 1981; Price, 1981; Amaral, 1986). It is suggested elsewhere (Rolls, 1989a) that the functions of these backprojections include the guidance of information representation and storage in the neocortex (when this is performed by reinforcing stimuli), and recall. Ways in which these functions of backprojections may be performed are discussed by Rolls (1989a). Another interesting set of output pathways of the amygdala projects to the entorhinal cortex, which provdes the major input to the hippocampus and dentate gyrus, and to the ventral subiculum, which provides a major output of the hippocampus (Price, 1981; Amaral, 1986).

These anatomical connections of the amygdala indicate that it is placed to receive highly processed information from the cortex and to influence motor systems, autonomic systems, some of the cortical areas from which it receives inputs, and other limbic areas. The functions mediated through these connections are now considered, using information available from the effects of damage to the amygdala and from the activity of neurons in the amygdala.

Effects of Lesions of the Amygdala

Bilateral removal of the amygdala in monkeys produces striking behavioral changes which include tameness, a lack of emotional responsiveness, excessive examination of objects, often with the mouth, and eating of previously rejected items such as meat (Weiskrantz, 1956). These behavioral changes comprise much of the Klüver-Bucy syndrome which is produced in monkeys by bilateral anterior temporal lobectomy (Klüver and Bucy, 1939). In analyses of the bases of these behavioral changes, it has been observed that there are deficits in some types of learning. For example, Weiskrantz (1956) found that bilateral ablation of the amygdala in the monkey produced a deficit on learning an active avoidance task. The monkeys failed to learn to make a response when a light signalled that shock would follow unless the response was made. He was perhaps the first to suggest that these monkeys had difficulty with forming associations between stimuli and reinforcement, when he suggested that "the effect of amygdalectomy is to make it difficult for reinforcing stimuli, whether positive or negative, to become established or to be recognized as such" (Weiskrantz, 1956). In this avoidance task, associations between a stimulus and negative reinforcement were impaired. Evidence soon became available that associations between stimuli and positive reinforcement (reward) were also impaired, in for example serial reversals of a visual discrimination made to obtain food (Jones and Mishkin, 1972). In this task the monkey must learn that food is under one of two objects, and after he has learned this, he must then relearn (reverse) the association as the food is then placed under the other object. Jones and Mishkin (1972) showed that the stages of this task which are particularly affected by damage to this region are those when the monkeys are responding at chance to the two visual stimuli or are starting to respond more to the currently rewarded stimuli, rather than the stage when the monkeys are continuing to make perserverative responses to the previously rewarded visual stimulus. They thus argued that the difficulty produced by this anterior temporal lobe damage is in learning to associate stimuli with reinforcement, in this case with food reward. More direct evidence for this is that amygdalectomized monkeys were impaired on a test in which they had to remember on the basis of a single presentation whether or not a trial-unique object had been paired with reward (Spiegler and Mishkin, 1981; Mishkin and Aggleton, 1981). In more recent experiments, Gaffan and Harrison (1987) and Gaffan et al. (1988) have shown that the tasks which are impaired by amygdala lesions in monkeys typically involve a cross-modal association from a previously neutral stimulus to a primary reinforcing stimulus (such as the taste of food), consistent with the hypothesis that the amygdala is involved in learning associations between stimuli and primary reinforcers (see also Gaffan et al., 1989). Further evidence linking the amygdala to reinforcement mechanisms is that monkeys will work in order to obtain electrical stimulation of the amygdala, and that single neurons in the amygdala are activated by brain-stimulation reward of a number of different sites (Rolls, 1975; Rolls et al., 1980).

Jones and Mishkin (1972) elaborated the hypothesis that many of the symptoms of the Klüver-Bucy syndrome, including the emotional changes, could be a result of this type of deficit in learning stimulus-reinforcement associations (see also Mishkin and Aggleton, 1981). For example, the tameness, the hypo-emotionality, the increased orality, and the altered responses to food would arise because of damage to the normal mechanism by which stimuli become associated with reward or punishment. Other evidence is also consistent with the hypothesis that there is a close relation between the learning deficit and the symptoms of the Klüver-Bucy syndrome. For example, in a study of subtotal lesions of the amygdala, Aggleton and Passingham (1981) found that in only those monkeys in which the lesions produced a serial reversal learning deficit was hypoemotionality present.

It may be noted here that the amygdala is well placed anatomically for such stimulus-reinforcement association learning, for not only does it receive highly processed visual and auditory inputs from the temporal lobe cortex, but it also receives inputs from the gustatory and somatosensory systems (via the insula in the primate; Mesulam and Mufson, 1982), and the olfactory and visceral systems (see Ben-Ari, 1981), so that a variety of well-processed stimuli and information about reinforcement should have access to the amygdala. This type of anatomical convergence is appropriate for a system implicated in stimulus-reinforcement association formation, in which it may be necessary to associate stimuli from different modalities. Thus in this function it may be necessary to "look up" (i.e., produce as output, or recall) for example a taste or a pleasant or painful somatosensory event using, for example, a visual or auditory "key" (or conditioned) stimulus which was previously associated with the taste or somatosensory event. Moreover, the outputs of the amygdala include connections to the autonomic centres of the brain stem and the hypothalamus through which the autonomic changes in emotion to learned stimuli could be elicited; to the ventral striatum and the central gray of the brain stem through which behaviour to learned reinforcing stimuli could be elicited; and to the basal forebrain magnocellular neurons and back to the cerebral cortex, through which effects of emotional state on memory could be produced. In line with this, LeDoux et al., (1988) were able to show that lesions of the lateral hypothalamus (which recieves from the central nucleus of the amygdala) blocked conditioned heart rate (autonomic) responses but not the conditioned behavioral emotional response of freezing to an aversive conditioned stimulus. In contrast, lesions of the central gray (which also receives from the central nucleus of the amygdala) blocked the conditioned freezing but not the conditioned autonomic response to the aversive conditioned stimulus. Further, Cador et al. (1989) obtained evidence consistent with the hypothesis that the learned incentive (conditioned reinforcing) effects of previously neutral stimuli paired with rewards are mediated by the amygdala acting through the ventral striatum, in that amphetamine injections into the ventral striatum enhanced the effects of a conditioned reinforcing stimulus only if the amygdala was intact (see Chapter 15, Everitt and Robbins, this volume).

Although much evidence is thus consistent with the hypothesis that the amygdala is involved in responses made to stimuli associated with reinforcement, there is evidence that it may also be involved to some extent in behavioral responses made to novel, as opposed to familiar, stimuli, in a different type of memory. It has been found, for example, that the alteration in responses to foods in rats with damage to the amygdala is due in part to decreased neophobia; that is, the rats more quickly accept new foods (E.T. Rolls and B.J. Rolls, 1973; see also Dunn and Everitt, 1988; and Wilson and Rolls, 1990b).

NEUROPHYSIOLOGY OF THE PRIMATE AMYGDALA
Multimodal Inputs to the Amygdala

Recordings from single neurons in the amygdala of the monkey have shown that some neurons do respond to visual stimuli, consistent with the inputs from the temporal lobe visual cortex (Sanghera et al., 1979). Other neurons responded to auditory, gustatory, olfactory, or somatosensory stimuli, or in relation to movements (see also Wilson and Rolls, 1991a,b).

Stimulus-Reinforcement Associations and the Responses of Amygdala Neurons in Primates

In tests of whether amygdala neurons in primates responded on the basis of the association of stimuli with reinforcement, Sanghera et al. (1979) showed that 19.5% of their sample of neurons with visual responses tended to respond on the basis of whether the stimuli were reinforcing in, for example, a visual discrimination task. Further examples of these amygdala neurons which respond more to reward-related than to punishment-related stimuli were analysed by Wilson and Rolls (1991a) (see Fig. 1). These neurons are found in the lateral, basal, and central nuclei of the amygdala (Sanghera et al., 1979; Wilson and Rolls, 1991a). However, although these neurons responded, for example, to the visual stimulus in the visual discrimination task, which indicated that reward was available, and responded to some other positively reinforcing stimuli such as some foods, they did not respond to all visual stimuli that were positively reinforcing, and they often responded to one or more stimuli that were not positively reinforcing (Sanghera et al., 1979; Rolls, 1981b). Thus these neurons tended to respond to reinforcing visual stimuli, but did not code uniquely for reinforcement. Moreover, eight of nine neurons tested in the reversal of a visual discrimination (in which the visual stimulus associated with food reward delivery becomes associated with aversive saline delivery and vice versa) did not reverse their responses (and for the remaining neuron the evidence was not clear). Thus these amygdaloid neurons did not respond whenever a reinforcing visual stimulus was shown, and did not alter their responses flexibly and rapidly when the reinforcement value of a visual stimulus was altered, although such neurons are found in the orbitofrontal cortex (Thorpe et al., 1983) and basal forebrain (Mora et al., 1976; Rolls et al., 1976; Rolls, 1985, 1986a,b; Wilson and Rolls, 1990a).

Neurons with responses which are probably similar to these have also been described by Ono and his coworkers (Ono et al., 1980; Nishijo, Ono, and Nishino, 1988; see also Chapter 6, Ono and Nishijo, this volume). Although the amygdaloid neurons studied by Sanghera et al. (1979) had a preference for reinforcing stimuli, they did not alter their responses flexibly and rapidly when the reinforcement value of a visual stimulus was altered during reversal. On the other hand,

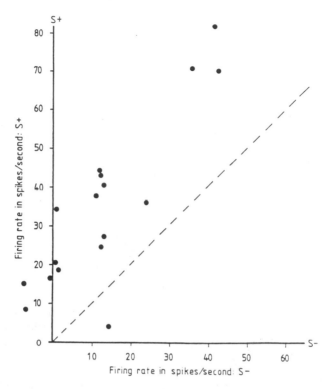

Fig. 1. Responses of amygdala neurons that responded more in a visual discrimination task to the reward-related visual stimulus (S +) than to the saline-related visual stimulus (S −). In the task, the macaque monkeys made lick responses to obtain fruit juice when the S + was the discriminandum, and had to withhold lick responses when the S − was the discriminandum in order to avoid the taste of saline. Each point shows the responses of one neuron to the S + and to the S − measured in a 0.5 sec period starting 100 msec after the visual stimulus was shown. Most of the points lie above the dashed line drawn at 45 degrees, showing that most of these neurons responded more to type S + than to the S −. (After Wilson and Rolls, 1991a).

Nishijo et al. (1988) have tested four amygdala neurons in a rather simpler relearning situation in which salt was added to a piece of food such as a watermelon, and the neurons' responses to the sight of the watermelon diminished. This was an extinction rather than a reversal test, and it was not clear whether in extinction with repeated trials the monkeys continued to fixate the piece of food once salt had been added to it. The advantage of the visual discrimination task (studied by Sanghera et al., 1979) is that the monkey must fixate the visual stimuli on every trial in the random trial sequence, to determine whether the visual stimulus currently associated with reward is being shown. It will be of interest in further studies to investigate whether in extinction evidence can be found for a rapid decrease in the responses to visual stimuli formerly associated with reward when reward is no longer given, even when fixation of the stimuli is adequate.

Comparison With Neuronal Responses to Reinforcing Stimuli in Other Brain Regions

The failure of this population of amygdala neurons to respond only to reinforcing stimuli, and the difficulty in reversing their responses, are in contrast to the responses of certain populations of neurons in the caudal orbitofrontal cortex and in a region to which it projects, the basal forebrain, which do show very rapid (in one or two trials) reversals of their responses in visual discrimination reversal tasks (Thorpe et al., 1983; Wilson and Rolls, 1990b; see below). On the basis of these findings, it is suggested that the obitofrontal cortex is more involved than the amygdala in the rapid readjustments of behavioral responses made to stimuli when their reinforcement value is repeatedly changing, as in discrimination reversal tasks (Thorpe et al., 1983; Rolls, 1986b, 1990b). The ability to flexibly alter responses to stimuli based on their changing reinforcement associations is important in motivated behavior (such as feeding) and in emotional behavior, and it is this flexibility which it is suggested the orbitofrontal cortex adds to a more basic capacity which the amygdala implements for stimulus-reinforcement learning (Rolls, 1986b, 1990b).

The basal forebrain neurons which respond to reinforcing stimuli provide a signal which more uniquely reflects the association of visual stimuli with previous primary reinforcers than do amygdala neurons. It is suggested that the basal forebrain neurons, which receive projections from the amygdala (Price and Amaral, 1981), sum inputs from many amygdala neurons so that the hypothalamic neurons come to reflect more generally than do individual amygdala neurons whether a visual stimulus has been previously paired with primary reinforcement. This population of basal forebrain neurons responds to real foods, comes to respond, as a result of stimulus-reinforcement association formation, to visual stimuli associated with food, and (in contrast to amygdala neurons; see Sanghera et al., 1979) only respond to these stimuli when the monkey is hungry (Rolls , 1975, 1981a,c, 1982, 1986c; Rolls et al., 1976; Burton et al., 1976; Mora et al., 1976; Wilson and Rolls, 1990a). Other neurons in the hypothalamus respond only to stimuli associated with punishment, that is, to aversive visual stimuli (Rolls et al., 1979). In that the responses of these neurons occurred to any visual stimuli associated with food reward, or in other cases to any aversive visual stimuli, the responses reflected the lookup by an associative memory mechanism to produce an output appropriate for a motivational or emotional response. This neuronal output would be appropriate for producing autonomic responses to emotional stimuli, via pathways which descend from the hypothalamus toward the brain stem autonomic motor nuclei (Saper et al., 1976; Schwaber et al., 1982). It is also possible that these outputs could influence emotional behavior, through, for example, the connections from the hypothalamus to the amygdala (Aggleton et al., 1980), to the substantia nigra (Nauta and Domesick, 1978), or even by the connections to the neocortex (Divac, 1975; Kievit and Kuypers, 1975). Indeed, it is suggested that the latter projection, by releasing acetylcholine in the cerebral cortex when emotional stimuli (including reinforcing and novel stimuli) are seen, provides one way in which emotion can influence the storage of memories in the cerebral cortex (Rolls, 1987; Wilson and Rolls, 1990a,c). In this case, the basal forebrain magnocellular neurons may act as a "strobe" which facilitates cortical plasticity for a short time.

Inputs to the hypothalamus that enable the neurons in it to respond in these ways reach the hypothalamus through both amygdala and orbitofrontal cortex connections. Thus the amygdala provides a route for highly processed visual information from the inferior temporal visual cortex to reach the hypothalamus (see further Fukuda et al., 1987). In the inferior temporal visual cortex, neurons have not been found which reflect the association of a visual stimulus with primary reinforcement, or which reverse their responses in the reversal of a visual discrimination task (Rolls et al., 1977). This adds to the evidence that it is the amygdala (and orbitofrontal cortex) which contain the learning mechanisms which enable representations of visual stimuli provided by the inferior temporal visual cortex to become associated with primary reinforcers such as the taste of food or touch, both of which are projected into the amygdala and orbitofrontal cortex (see above and Rolls, 1989b, 1990b).

Responses of Amygdala Neurons to Novel Stimuli That Are Reinforcing

Wilson and Rolls (1991a) confirmed the finding of Sanghera et al. (1979) that there is a population of neurons in the primate amygdala which discriminates between reward and punishment-associated visual stimuli in a visual discrimination task. These neurons also, in some cases, responded to some food-related visual stimuli, and two more neurons tested did not reverse their responses in the reversal of a visual discrimination task. They extended the previous results by recording from the same neurons in a recognition memory task. In this task the monkey used the rule that lick responses to novel stimuli were associated with the delivery of saline, and lick responses to the same stimulus when shown a second time (as familiar) were rewarded. Several trials separated the novel and familiar presentations of each stimulus, and each stimulus was shown only twice per day. In this running recognition memory task, the majority (12/14 analyzed) of these neurons responded equally well to novel and familiar stimuli even though these stimuli differentially signalled aversive saline or juice reward. Thus these amygdala neurons did not reflect the reinforcement value of visual stimuli when this was determined by a rule ("respond to familiar stimuli"), but did respond differentially when the reinforcement value of the visual stimuli was determined by a previous association with a primary reinforcer (the taste of food in the visual discrimination task). Expressed in another way, this shows that these amygdala neurons do not respond to all visual stimuli which signify reward, for example, when reward value is computed on the basis of a rule, but do respond to rewarding stimuli when this is based on a previous association between the visual stimulus and a primary reinforcer. As described above, the type of stimulus-reinforcement association learning implemented in the amygdala may not undergo very rapid reversal.

It was notable that these amygdaloid neurons responded to the S+ (the visual stimulus associated with fruit juice reward delivery) in the visual discrimination task and to the novel and familiar visual stimuli in the recognition memory task, but did not respond to the S − (the visual stimulus which indicated that the monkey should not lick or salt solution would be obtained) in the visual discrimination task. It is suggested that the lack of response to the S − was because it had been presented on many occasions without reinforcement, so that the monkey had no tendency to explore or approach it further. In contrast, the novel and familiar stimuli in the trial-unique recognition task had not been seen before on novel presentations, and for only 1.5 s on familiar presentations, and with this limited degree of exposure, the monkeys were likely to still be interested in the stimuli, and to wish to explore them further (Humphrey, 1972). The S + stimuli still elicited approach because of their previous association with primary reinforcement. The hypothesis proposed is that the responses of these amygdala neurons reflected the tendency of the monkeys to explore and/or approach the stimuli. According to this hypothesis, the deficit in visual discrimination learning produced in monkeys by amygdala lesions occurs in part because the normal habituation to a familiar and unrewarded object does not occur without the amygdala, so that the lesioned monkeys are more likely than normal monkeys to choose the S − .

Another way of formulating this hypothesis is that the amygdala is involved in determining whether on the basis of previous reinforcement history representations of visual stimuli should be made or retained, or attention should be paid to the stimuli. Amygdala neurons would signal that representations should be retained if a visual stimulus has been previously associated with a primary reinforcer; or for a relatively new visual stimulus for a period sufficiently long so that whether that stimulus is associated with a primary reinforcer can be determined. (It is suggested elsewhere and below that backprojections from the amygdala to the neocortex may influence whether a permanent representation of a stimulus is set up in the neocortex; see Rolls, 1989a, 1990b.) According to this formulation, in the visual discrimination task described above, the S − is never associated with juice reinforcement, and the amygdala therefore filters it out from further processing. In contrast, the S + , novel and familiar stimuli in the recognition memory task, and the two stimuli always used in the visual discrimination reversal task should have their representations retained as active, because they are sometimes *associated* with reinforcement or are reinforcing because they are relatively novel. Although these experiments (Wilson and Rolls, 1991a) were performed with positive reinforcers, it is suggested that an analogous function is performed by the amygdala in filtering out stimuli sometimes associated with punishment from those not associated with reinforcement. It is thus suggested that the amygdala neurons described operate as filters which provide an output if a stimulus is associated with a positive or negative reinforcer, or is reinforcing because of relative unfamiliarity, and which provide no output if a stimulus is familiar and has not been associated with a primary reinforcer. The functions of this output may be to influence the interest shown in a stimulus, whether it is approached or avoided, whether an affective response occurs to it, and whether a representation of the stimulus is made or maintained via an action mediated through either the basal forebrain nucleus of Meynert or the backprojections to the cerebral cortex (Rolls, 1987, 1989a, 1990b).

Responses of Amygdala Neurons to Novel Visual Stimuli

It has been suggested that the amygdala plays a role in recognition memory function, for lesions which damage the amygdala can potentiate the effects of damage to the hippocampus (Mishkin, 1978), and to the medial temporal cortex (Murray and Mishkin, 1986), on object recognition tasks in monkeys. However, the role of the amygdala in recognition memory is not yet fully understood, in that Zola-Morgan et al. (1989) showed that amygdala damage which avoided damage to the overlying entorhinal and perirhinal cortices did not impair performance on a delayed nonmatch to sample task, and did not potentiate the effects of hippocampal damage on that task (see Chapter 17, Murray, this volume). It is possible that if the memory task had been made more difficult, for example, by using intervening stimuli to make it a serial recognition task (Gaffan, 1974), or by using nontrial-unique stimuli, then a deficit would have been observed, but as it stands, the Zola-Morgan et al. (1989) study suggests that it is damage to the overlying cortex rather than to the amygdala itself which is implicated in memory. On the other hand, other evidence implicating the amygdala in recognition memory comes from a study by Bachevalier et al. (1985), in which major efferent pathways of the hippocampus and amygdala were damaged and cortical areas were not damaged. They showed that combined lesions of the fornix and the amygdalofugal pathways produced an impairment in an object recognition task that far exceeded the effects of a lesion restricted to one set of fibres alone.

In order to analyse further how the amygdala might contribute to recognition memory, Wilson and Rolls (1991b) recorded the responses of 659 amygdala neurons in monkeys performing recognition memory and visual discrimination tasks.

Three groups of neurons showed memory-like activity. One group (n = 10) responded maximally to novel stimuli and significantly less so to the same stimuli when they were familiar. The large differential response to novel and familiar presentation of the same stimuli occurred with an intertrial interval of 6 s between the two presentations of any given stimulus, indicating a memory for the stimulus that endured for at least 6 s. One limitation on the capacities of monkeys and people to accurately recognise a stimulus is the number of distractor stimuli presented between the first and second presentations of a stimulus; with increasing numbers of distractors, recognition accuracy declines. Thus Wilson and Rolls (1991b) examined how the differential neuronal responses were affected by intervening stimuli, each of which had to be remembered, in a running recognition memory task. It was found that, for each neuron, the magnitude of the differential response was attenuated by the intervening stimuli (see example in Fig. 2). The number of intervening trials over which the response to a familiar stimulus had increased to be similar to that to a novel stimulus was defined as the memory span. Of the five neurons for which this analysis was done, the average memory span was estimated to be five intervening trials (range = 2 to 10 intervening trials), a time period of approximately 80 s for the neuron with the most robust "memory span." Wilson and Rolls (1991b) ensured that the different reinforcement values of novel and familiar stimuli in the rec-

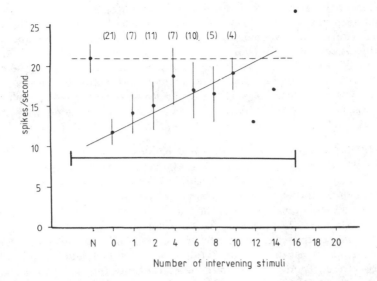

Fig. 2. Responses of an amygdala neuron to visual stimuli when they were novel (N), but not when they were familiar with no other stimuli intervening between the novel and familiar presentations of the visual stimuli (0 intervening stimuli). The neuronal responses gradually became like that to novel stimuli when a number of other stimuli intervened between the novel and familiar presentations of a stimulus. The neuronal responses shown are the mean ± the S.E.M. to different stimuli when novel (N) and when shown again as familiar after different numbers of intervening stimuli, recorded in a 500 msec period starting 100 msec after the visual stimuli were shown. The horizontal line shows the spontaneous firing rate ± the S.E.M. (After Wilson and Rolls, 1991b.)

ognition memory task (see above) were not responsible for the differential responses to the same stimulus when it was novel as compared with when it was familiar. This was done by recording the activity of these neurons during the performance of the visual discrimination task, in which the S + and the S − differed in their reinforcement value but were equally familiar. In almost all cases, the response to novel stimuli was significantly greater than to familiar stimuli, and to the S + and S − (Wilson and Rolls, 1991b). Thus the novelty of the stimuli, but not their differential reinforcement value, was the basis of the neuronal responses to novel stimuli. These neurons are found in part of the dorsal amygdala, and in part of the basal nucleus (see Wilson and Rolls, 1991b).

The two other groups of neurons responded to certain classes of visual stimuli, but included some neurons with memory-related activity in that their responses were greater to novel than to familiar visual stimuli. One such group of neurons (n = 6) with responses which occurred to some foods included four neurons that responded more to a food when it had not been seen recently, and three neurons which responded more to novel than to familiar nonfood visual stimuli. The third group of neurons (n = 10) responded to faces, and for two of these neurons the response to a novel face decreased as it became familiar.

These findings indicate that there is a small proportion of neurons in the primate amygdala which respond in recognition memory and similar tasks with information about the recency with which a visual stimulus has been seen. The memory spans of these neurons are up to 10 intervening stimuli. These neurons could contribute to the performance of recency memory tasks, and to the behavioral activation which is produced by novel stimuli, perhaps acting via ventral forebrain neurons (see Wilson and Rolls, 1990b). The activity of these neurons may also be related to the intrinsically rewarding properties of novel stimuli, and the behavioral tendency to approach such novel stimuli.

Neuronal Responses in the Primate Amygdala to Faces

Another interesting group of neurons in the amygdala responds primarily to faces (Rolls, 1981b; Leonard et al., 1985). Each of these neurons responds to some but not all of a set of faces, and thus across an ensemble could convey information about the identity of the face (see Figs. 3, 4). It will be of interest to investigate whether some of these amygdala face neurons respond on the basis of facial expression. It is probable that these neurons receive their inputs from a group of neurons in the cortex in the superior temporal sulcus which respond to faces, often on the basis of features present, such as eyes, hair, or mouth (Perrett et al., 1982), and consistent with this, the response latencies of the amygdala neurons tend to be longer than those of neurons in the cortex in the superior temporal sulcus (Rolls, 1984; Leonard et al., 1985). It has been suggested that this is part of a system which has evolved for the rapid and reliable identification of individuals from their faces, because of the importance of this in primate social behavior (Rolls, 1981b, 1984, 1985, 1991; Perrett and Rolls, 1982; Leonard et al., 1985). The part of this system in the amygdala may be particularly involved in emotional and social responses to faces. According to one possibility, such emotional and social responses would be "looked up" by a "key" stimulus, which consisted of the face of a particular individual (Rolls, 1984, 1987, 1991). Indeed, it is suggested that the tameness of the Klüver-Bucy syndrome, and the inability of amygdalectomized monkeys to interact normally in a social group (Kling and Steklis, 1976), arises because of damage to this system specialized for processing faces (Rolls, 1981a,b, 1984, 1985, 1991). The amygdala may allow neurons which reflect the social significance of faces to be formed using face representations received from the temporal cortical areas and information about primary reinforcers received from, for example, the somatosensory system (via the insula; Mesulam and Mufson, 1982), and the gustatory system (via, for example, the orbitofrontal cortex).

Fig. 3. The responses of four cells (**a–d**) in the amygdala to a variety of monkey and human face stimuli (A–E and K–P), and to nonface stimuli (F–J, objects, and foods). Each bar represents the mean response above baseline with the standard error calculated over 4 to 10 presentations. The F ratio for an analysis of variance calculated over the face sets indicates that the units shown range from very selective between faces (Y0809) to relatively nonselective (Z0264). Some stimuli for cells Y0801 and Y0809 produced inhibition below the spontaneous firing rate. (From Leonard et al., 1985.)

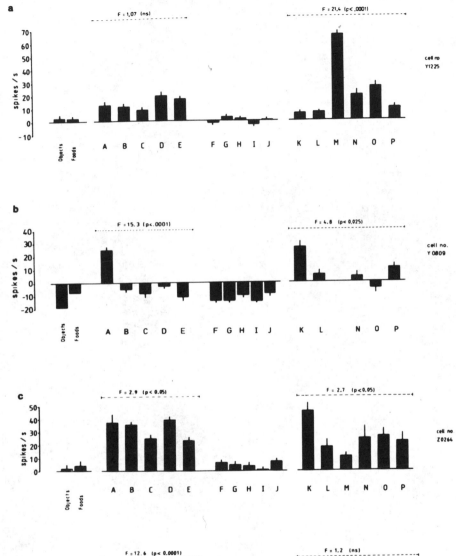

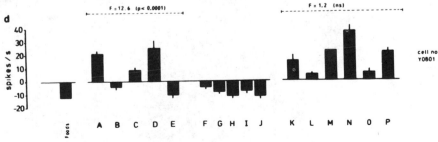

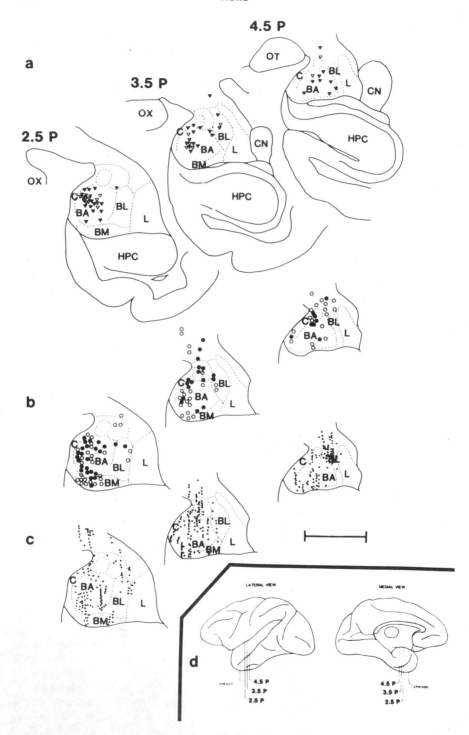

Cortical cells found in certain of the temporal lobe regions (e.g., TEa, TEm, and TPO; Baylis et al., 1987) which project into the amygdala have properties which would enable them to provide useful inputs for such an associative mechanism in the amygdala (see Rolls, 1987, 1989a, 1990c, 1991, 1992). These cortical neurons in many cases respond differently to the faces of different individuals, so that information about face identity which would be useful in recognition is represented by some of the neurons. However, the face of each individual is coded by the pattern of firing across a subpopulation of neurons (Baylis et al., 1985). That is, ensemble encoding rather than "grandmother cell" encoding is used. It is hypothesized that this type of tuning found is a delicate compromise between very fine tuning, which has the advantage of low interference in associative neuronal network operations but the disadvantage of losing the emergent properties of storage in such neuronal networks, and broad tuning, which has the advantage of allowing the emergent properties of neuronal networks to be realised but the disadvantage of leading to interference between the different memories stored in an associative network (Rolls, 1987, 1989a, 1990c; Rolls and Treves, 1990). Neurons in these areas are seen as filters, which as an ensemble give a unique representation of a particular stimulus in the environment. There is evidence that the responses of some of these neurons are altered by experience so that new stimuli become incorporated in the network (Rolls et al., 1989). Competition may play a role in the self-organization of such networks (Rolls, 1989a,c). The representation which is built in temporal cortical areas shows considerable size, contrast, spatial frequency, and translation invariance (Rolls and Baylis, 1986; Azzopardi and Rolls, 1989; Rolls, 1991, 1992). Thus the representation is in a form which is particularly useful for storage and as an output from the visual system. A further advantage for an input to such an associative system in the amygdala, where associations may be made to primary reinforcers, is that for some of the cortical neurons the representation which is built is object-based rather than viewer-centered (Hasselmo et al., 1989b). In addition to the population of neurons which code for face identity, there is a separate population in the cortex which conveys information about facial expression (Hasselmo et al., 1989a). These cortical neurons probably provide an input to the amygdaloid neurons which respond to faces, and one output from the amygdala for this information is probably via the ventral striatum, for a small population of neurons has been found in the ventral striatum with responses selective for faces (Rolls and Williams, 1987).

Fig. 4. (a) The distribution of neurons responsive to faces in the amygdala of four monkeys. The cells are plotted on three coronal sections at different distances (in mm) posterior (P) to the sphenoid (see **inset d**). Filled triangles: cells selective for faces; open triangles: cells responding to face and hands. (b) Other responsive neurons. Closed circles: cells with other visual responses; open circles: cells responding to cues, movement, or arousal. (c) The locations of nonresponsive cells. Abbreviations: BA, basal accessory nucleus of the amygdala; BL, basolateral nucleus of the amygdala; BM, basomedial nucleus of the amygdala; C, cortical nucleus of the amygdala; CN, tail of the caudate nucleus; HPC, hippocampus; L, lateral nucleus of the amygdala; OT, optic tract; OX, optic chiasm. (From Leonard et al., 1985.)

OUTPUT PATHWAYS

Amygdalectomy disrupts feeding and social behaviour (Kling and Steklis, 1976; Aggleton and Passingham, 1981, 1982), and it seems likely that the stimulus-selective neurons described in this chapter and elsewhere (Jacobs and McGinty, 1972; Sanghera et al., 1979; Rolls, 1981b; Leonard et al., 1985; Nishijo et al., 1988) participate in these types of behavior. The basis of this disruption appears to be at least partly related to a deficit in responding appropriately to stimuli that have great affective value, and it has been proposed that the amygdala participates in the establishment or recognition of the reinforcing or affective attributes of sensory stimuli (Weiskrantz, 1956; Jones and Mishkin, 1972; Rolls, 1985, 1986a, 1990b; see above). It may do this by containing modifiable synapses which enable associations to be formed between primary reinforcers such as taste, touch and visceral stimuli, and neutral stimuli such as visual and auditory stimuli, which by virtue of pairing with primary reinforcers become secondary reinforcers (Rolls, 1981, 1985, 1987, 1990b). Once formed, these associations may enable learned affective stimuli to influence behaviour by producing autonomic outputs (via the lateral hypothalamus) (see Rolls, 1990a; LeDoux, 1987; LeDoux et al., 1988); by influencing the striatum and orbitofrontal cortex (see Rolls, 1985, 1990b; Rolls and Williams, 1987; Rolls and Johnstone, 1991); by producing emotional arousal which could influence learning, perhaps via an action on the ventral forebrain cholinergic neurons which project to the cerebral cortex (see Rolls, 1987 and above); and by backprojections to the association areas of the cerebral cortex, as described more fully below.

Although our understanding of the functions of the amygdala is based largely on research in animals, the evidence that is available for the human is consistent with the evidence described above, suggesting that the amygdala is involved in emotion. Thus electrical stimulation of the human amygdala can give rise to emotional feelings such as fear, anxiety, or in some cases pleasure (see Halgren, 1981). Conversely, amygdalectomy in humans has been claimed to reduce emotional tension, to make fear and aggression harder to provoke, and to enhance emotional control, resulting in better concentration, a steadier mood, and more rewarding social interactions (see review by Halgren, 1981). However, the requirements for adequate controls, adequate and independent assessment of the behavioral changes, and long-term follow-up studies are difficult to meet in this type of work, and these claims must be regarded as being only tentative (see Halgren, 1981; Valenstein, 1973, 1980; Chapter 19, Aggleton, this volume). Robin and MacDonald (1975) and Valenstein (1973, 1980) have discussed many of the interpretive and major ethical problems endemic to this type of work and to psychosurgery in man.

THE ROLE OF THE AMYGDALA IN EMOTION

The evidence described above implicates the amygdala in the learning of associations between stimuli and reinforcement, and in social behaviour. This means that it must be important in learned emotional responses, which can be considered to be states elicited by reinforcing stimuli (Rolls, 1990b). Indeed, it is proposed that at least part of the importance of the amygdala in emotion is that it is involved in this type of emotional learning. This analysis provides a theoretical basis for understanding how the amygdala is involved in emotion.

The analyses above have been concerned primarily with how stimuli are decoded to produce emotional states, and with how these states can influence behavior. We have seen, for example, that the amygdala (and orbitofrontal cortex, see Rolls, 1991) are important in selecting out those stimuli which have been associated with primary reinforcers in the past, and in producing emotional responses to these stimuli. We have seen that the tuning of neurons in these structures, and in the structures which send projections to them, such as the inferior temporal cortex, can be understood as providing appropriate inputs to associative neuronal networks which perform the stimulus-reinforcement learning necessary for learned emotions. To finish this chapter, I wish to make a suggestion about how emotional states may influence cognitive processing.

Current mood state can affect the cognitive evaluation of events or memories (see Blaney, 1986). For example, happy memories are more likely to be recalled when happy. Why does this occur? It is suggested that whenever memories are stored, part of the context is stored with the memory. This is very likely to happen in associative neuronal networks such as those in the hippocampus (Rolls, 1987, 1989a, 1990a). In such networks, memories of particular events are stored by increasing the strengths of active synapses which make connections to strongly activated neurons. Consider the points that each neuron has many inputs (approximately 16,000 in the rat hippocampus), and that the networks in the CA3 part of the hippocampus appear to operate as an autoassociative memory capable of linking together almost arbitrary co-occurrences of inputs. It is therefore very likely that some of the input axons will be carrying information about the current emotional state, and that these synapses, as well as those conveying the particular event to be remembered, will be enhanced. Now recall of a memory occurs best in such networks when the input key to the memory is nearest to the original input pattern of activity which was stored. (Technically, optimal recall occurs when the key has a correlation of 1.0 with the original input to the memory; see Rolls, 1987, 1989a; Jordan, 1986.) It thus follows that a memory of, for example, a happy episode is recalled best when in a happy mood state, for then the key to the memory (the input pattern vector of axonal activity to each neuron) most closely resembles the pattern of modified synapses, so that the activation of those neurons with the matching synaptic pattern is optimal. This is a general theory of how context is stored with a memory, and of how context influences recall. (The "context" is simply part of what is stored, and it would be difficult in associative neural networks to arrange for no context to be stored, given that in principle the network should have considerable flexibility about what is connected to what.) The effect of emotional state on cognitive processing and memory is thus suggested to be a particular case of a more general way in which context can affect the storage and retrieval of memories, or can affect cognitive processing.

There are a number of sites in the brain where these effects of mood on storage and recall could be instantiated. One place is the hippocampus. The hippocampus receives projections (via the entorhinal cortex) from the amygdala, so that emotional states could easily gain access to the autoassociative network implemented by the CA3 recurrent collateral axons, and become linked into episodic memories (see Rolls, 1989a, 1990a). Another brain system where mood state could be stored with memories is in the backprojections from structures important in emotion, such as the amygdala and orbitofrontal cortex, to parts of the cerebral cortex important in the representation of objects, such as the inferior temporal visual cortex. It is suggested (Rolls, 1989a) that coactivity between forward inputs and backprojecting inputs to strongly activated cortical pyramidal cells would lead to both sets of synapses being modified (see Fig. 5). This may be part of a mechanism for allowing higher, often multimodal, stages of processing to influence the representations built in earlier cortical stages (see Rolls, 1989a). In the case of the amygdala backprojections, this could mean that the current emotion is stored by modification of the active backprojecting synapses onto cortical pyramidal cells activated via their forward inputs by, for example, a particular face or expression. Then later recognition of that stimulus by the forward activation of cortical pyramidal cells will be better when the mood-carrying backprojecting neurons are active with the pattern specifying the appropriate mood state, for then the amygdala backprojections will tend to make those cortical pyramidal cells with the matching modified synapses from backprojecting axons more easily activated by the forward input.

Thus emotional states may affect whether or how strongly memories are stored using the basal forebrain memory strobe (which may be activated via the amygdala, see above); be stored as part of many memories; and may influence both the recall of such memories, and the operation of cognitive processing, in the way described in the preceding paragraph.

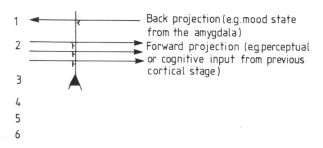

Fig. 5. Pyramidal cells in, for example, layers 2 and 3 of the temporal lobe association cortex receive forward inputs from preceding cortical stages of processing, and also backprojections from the amygdala. It is suggested that the backprojections from the amygdala make modifiable synapses on the apical dendrites of cortical pyramidal cells during learning, when amygdala neurons are active in relation to a mood state; and that the backprojections from the amygdala via these modified synapses allow mood state to influence later cognitive processing, for example, by facilitating some perceptual representations.

ACKNOWLEDGMENTS

The author has worked on some of the research described here with G.C. Baylis, M.J. Burton, M.E. Hasselmo, C.M. Leonard, F. Mora, D.I. Perrett, M.K. Sanghera, T.R. Scott, S.J. Thorpe, A. Treves, and F.A.W. Wilson, and their collaboration is sincerely acknowledged. Some of the research described was supported by the Medical Research Council.

REFERENCES

Aggleton JP, Burton MJ, Passingham RE (1980): Cortical and subcortical afferents to the amygdala in the rhesus monkey (Macaca mulatta). Brain Res 190:347–368.

Aggleton JP, Passingham RE (1981): Syndrome produced by lesions of the amygdala in monkeys (Macaca mulatta). J Comp Physiol 95:961–977.

Aggleton JP, Passingham RE (1982): An assessment of the reinforcing properties of foods after amygdaloid lesions in rhesus monkeys. J Comp Physiol Psychol 96:71–77.

Amaral DG (1986): Amygdalohippocampal and amygdalocortical projections in the primate brain. Schwarz R, Ben-Ari Y (eds): "Excitatory Amino Acids and Epilepsy." New York: Plenum Press, pp 3–17.

Azzopardi P, Rolls ET (1989): Translation invariance in the responses of neurons in the inferior temporal visual cortex of the macaque. Soc Neurosci Abstr 15:120.

Baylis GC, Rolls ET, Leonard CM (1985): Selectivity between faces in the responses of a population of neurons in the cortex in the superior temporal sulcus of the monkey. Brain Res 342:91–102.

Baylis GC, Rolls ET, Leonard CM (1987): Functional subdivisions of temporal lobe neocortex. J Neurosci 7:330–342.

Bachevalier J, Parkinson JK, Mishkin M (1985): Visual recognition in monkeys: Effects of separate versus combined transections of fornix and amygdalofugal pathways. Exp Brain Res 57:554–561.

Ben-Ari Y (ed) (1981): "The Amygdaloid Complex." Amsterdam: Elsevier.

Blaney PH (1986): Affect and memory: A review. Psych Bull 99:229–246.

Burton MJ, Rolls ET, Mora F (1976): Visual responses of hypothalamic neurones. Brain Res 107:215–216.

Cador M, Robbins TW, Everitt BJ (1989): Involvement of the amygdala in stimulus-reward associations: Interaction with the ventral striatum. Neuroscience 30:77–86.

Divac I (1975): Magnocellular nuclei of the basal forebrain project to neocortex, brain stem, and olfactory bulb. Review of some functional correlates. Brain Res 93:385–398.

Dunn LT, Everitt BJ (1988): Double dissociations of the effects of amygdala and insular cortex lesions on conditioned taste aversion, passive avoidance, and neophobia in the rat using the excitotoxin ibotenic acid. Behav Neurosci 102:3–23.

Fukuda M, Ono T, Nakamura K (1987): Functional relations among inferotemporal cortex, amygdala, and lateral hypothalamus in monkey operant feeding behavior. J Neurophys 57:1060–1077.

Gaffan D (1974): Recognition impaired and association intact in the memory of monkeys after transection of the fornix. J Comp Physiol Psychol 86:1100–1109.

Gaffan D, Harrison S (1987): Amygdalectomy and disconnection in visual learning for auditory secondary reinforcement by monkeys. J Neurosci 7:2285–2292.

Gaffan EA, Gaffan D, Harrison S (1988): Disconnection of the amygdala from visual association cortex impairs visual reward-association learning in monkeys. J Neurosci 8:3144–3150.

Gaffan D, Gaffan EA, Harrison S (1989): Visual-visual associative learning and reward-association learning in monkeys: The role for the amygdala. J Neurosci 9:558–564.

Halgren E (1981): The amygdala contribution to emotion and memory: Current studies in humans. In Ben Ari Y (ed): "The Amygdaloid Complex." Amsterdam: Elsevier, pp 395–408.

Hasselmo ME, Rolls ET, Baylis GC (1989a): The role of expression and identity in the face-selective responses of neurons in the temporal visual cortex of the monkey. Behav Brain Res 32:203–218.

Hasselmo ME, Rolls ET, Baylis GC, Nalwa V (1989b): Object-centered encoding by face-selective neurons in the cortex in the superior temporal sulcus of the monkey. Exp Brain Res 75:417–429.

Heimer L, Switzer RD, Van Hoesen GW (1982): Ventral striatum and ventral pallidum. Components of the motor system? Trends in Neurosci 5:83–87.

Herzog AG, Van Hoesen GW (1976): Temporal neocortical afferent connections to the amygdala in the rhesus monkey. Brain Res 115:57–69.

Hopkins DA, McLean JH, Takeuchi Y (1981): Amygdalotegmental projections: Light and electron microscopic studies utilizing anterograde degeneration and the anterograde and retrograde transport of horseradish peroxidase (HRP). In Ben-Ari Y (ed): "The Amygdaloid Complex." Amsterdam: Elsevier, pp 133–147.

Humphrey NK (1972): "Interest" and "pleasure": Two determinants of a monkey's visual preferences. Perception 3:105–114.

Jacobs BL, McGinty DJ (1972): Participation of the amygdala in complex stimulus recognition and behavioural inhibition: Evidence from single unit studies. Brain Res 36:431–436.

Jones B, Mishkin M (1972): Limbic lesions and the problem of stimulus-reinforcement associations. Exp Neurol 36:362–377.

Jordan MI (1986): An introduction to linear algebra in parallel distributed processing. In Rumelhart DE, McClelland JL (eds): "Parallel Distributed Processing," Vol 1, Ch 9. Cambridge, MA: MIT Press, pp 365–442.

Kling A, Steklis HD (1976): A neural substrate for affiliative behavior in nonhuman primates. Brain Behav Evol 13:216–238.

Kievit J, Kuypers HGJM (1975): Subcortical afferents to the frontal lobe in the rhesus monkey studied by means of retrograde horseradish peroxidase transport. Brain Res 85:261–266.

Klüver H, Bucy PC (1939): Preliminary analysis of functions of the temporal lobes in monkeys. Arch Neurol Psychiatr 42:979–1000.

LeDoux JE (1987): Emotion. In Plum F, Mouncastle VB (eds): "Handbook of Physiology, The Nervous System. V. Higher Function." Washington, DC: American Physiological Society, pp 419–459.

LeDoux JE, Iwata J, Cicchetti P, Reis DJ (1988): Different projections of the central amygdaloid nucleus mediate autonomic and behavioral correlates of conditioned fear. J Neurosci 8:2517–2229.

Leonard CM, Rolls ET, Wilson FAW, Baylis GC (1985): Neurons in the amygdala of the monkey with responses selective for faces. Behav Brain Res 15:159–176.

Mesulam M-M, Mufson EJ (1982): Insula of the old world monkey. III. Efferent cortical output and comments on function. J Comp Neurol 212:38–52.

Mishkin M (1978): Memory in monkeys severely impaired by combined but not separate removal of amygdala and hippocampus. Nature 273:297–299.

Mishkin M, Aggleton J (1981): Multiple functional contributions of the amygdala in the monkey. In Ben-Ari Y (ed): "The Amygdaloid Complex." Amsterdam: Elsevier, pp 409–420.

Mora F, Rolls ET, Burton MJ (1976): Modulation during learning of the responses of neurones in the lateral hypothalamus to the sight of food. Exp Neurol 53:508–519.

Mufson EJ, Mesulam M-M, Pandya DN (1981): Insular interconnections with the amygdala in the rhesus monkey. Neuroscience 6:1231–1248.

Murray EA, Mishkin M (1986): Visual recognition in monkeys following rhinal cortical ablations combined with either amygdalectomy or hippocampectomy. J Neurosci 6:1991–2003.

Nauta WJH (1961): Fiber degeneration following lesions of the amygdaloid complex in the monkey. J Anat 95:515–531.

Nauta WJH, Domesick VB (1978): Crossroads of limbic and striatal circuitry: Hypothalamonigral connections. In Livingston KE, Hornykiewicz O (eds): "Limbic Mechanisms." New York: Plenum Press, pp 75–93.

Nishijo H, Ono T, Nishino H (1988): Single neuron responses in amygdala of alert monkey during complex sensory stimulation with affective significance. J Neurosci 8:3570–3583.

Ono T, Nishino H, Sasaki K, Fukuda M, Muramoto K (1980): Role of the lateral hypothalamus and amygdala in feeding behavior. Brain Res Bull 5 (Suppl 4):143–149.

Perrett DI, Rolls ET (1982): Neural mechanisms underlying the visual analysis of faces. In Evert J-P, Capranica RR, Ingle DJ (eds): "Advances in Vertebrate Neuroethology." New York: Plenum Press.

Perrett DI, Rolls ET, Caan W (1982): Visual neurons responsive to faces in the monkey temporal cortex. Exp Brain Res 47:329–342.

Porrino LJ, Crane AM, Goldman-Rakic PS (1981): Direct and indirect pathways from the amygdala to the frontal lobe in rhesus monkeys. J Comp Neurol 198:121–136.

Price JL (1981): The efferent projections of the amygdaloid complex in the rat, cat and monkey. In Ben-Ari Y (ed): "The Amygdaloid Complex." Amsterdam: Elsevier, pp 121–132.

Price JL, Amaral DG (1981): An autoradiographic study of the projections of the central nucleus of the monkey amygdala. J Neurosci 1:1242–1259.

Robin A, MacDonald D (1975): "Lessons of Leucotomy." London: Kimpton.

Rolls ET (1975): "The Brain and Reward." Oxford: Pergamon.

Rolls ET (1981a): Processing beyond the inferior temporal visual cortex related to feeding, memory, and striatal function. In Katsuki Y, Norgren R, Sato M (eds): "Brain Mechanisms of Sensation." New York: Wiley, pp 241–269.

Rolls ET (1981b): Responses of amygdaloid neurons in the primate. In Ben-Ari Y (ed): "The Amygdaloid Complex." Amsterdam: Elsevier, pp 383–393.

Rolls ET (1981c): Central nervous mechanisms related to feeding and appetite. Brit Med Bull 37:131–134.

Rolls ET (1982): Feeding and reward. In Novin D, Hoebel BG (eds): "The Neural Basis of Feeding and Reward." Brunswick, ME: Haer Institute for Electrophysiological Research.

Rolls ET (1984): Neurons in the cortex of the temporal lobe and in the amygdala of the monkey with responses selective for faces. Human Neurobiol 3:209–222.

Rolls ET (1985): Connections, functions and dysfunctions of limbic structures, the prefrontal cortex, and hypothalamus. In Swash M, Kennard C (eds): "The Scientific Basis of Clinical Neurology." London: Churchill Livingstone, pp 201–213.

Rolls ET (1986a): A theory of emotion, and its application to understanding the neural basis of emotion. In Oomura Y (ed): "Emotions: Neural and Chemical Control." Tokyo: Japan Scientific Societies Press and Basel: Karger, pp 325–344.

Rolls ET (1986b): Neural systems involved in emotion in primates. In Plutchik R, Kellerman H (eds): "Emotion: Theory, Research, and Experience." New York: Academic Press, pp 125–143.

Rolls ET (1986c): Neuronal activity related to the control of feeding. In Ritter RC, Ritter S, Barnes CD (eds): "Feeding Behavior: Neural and Humoral Controls." New York: Academic Press, pp 163–190.

Rolls ET (1987): Information representation, processing and storage in the brain: Analysis at the single neuron level. In Changeux J-P, Konishi M (eds): "The Neural and Molecular Bases of Learning. Chichester: Wiley, pp 503–540.

Rolls ET (1989a): The representation and storage of information in neuronal networks in the primate cerebral cortex and hippocampus. In Durbin R, Miall C, Mitchison G (eds): "The Computing Neuron." Wokingham, UK: Addison-Wesley, pp 125–159.

Rolls ET (1989b): Information processing in the taste system of primates. J Exp Biol 146:141–164.

Rolls ET (1989c): Functions of neuronal networks in the hippocampus and cerebral cortex in memory. In Cotterill RMJ (ed): "Models of Brain Function." Cambridge: Cambridge University Press, pp 15–33.

Rolls ET (1990a): Functions of the primate hippocampus in spatial processing and memory. In Olton DS, Kesner RP (eds): "Neurobiology of Comparative Cognition." Hillsdale, NJ: L. Erlbaum, pp 339–362.

Rolls ET (1990b): A theory of emotion, and its application to understanding the neural basis of emotion. Cognition and Emotion 4:161–190.

Rolls ET (1990c): The representation of information in the temporal lobe visual cortical areas of macaques. In Eckmiller R (ed): "Advanced Neural Computers." Amsterdam: North-Holland, pp 69–78.

Rolls ET (1991): The processing of face information in the primate temporal lobe. In Bruce V, Burton M (eds): "Processing Images of Faces." Norwood, NJ: Ablex.

Rolls ET (1992): Neuropsychological mechanisms underlying face processing within and beyond the temporal cortical visual areas. Phil Trans Roy Soc (in press).

Rolls ET, Rolls BJ (1973): Altered food preferences after lesions in the basolateral region of the amygdala in the rat. J Comp Physiol Psychol 83:248–259.

Rolls ET, Burton MJ, Mora F (1976): Hypothalamic neuronal responses associated with the sight of food. Brain Res 111:53–66.

Rolls ET, Judge SJ, Sanghera M (1977): Activity of neurones in the inferotemporal cortex of the alert monkey. Brain Res 130:229–238.

Rolls ET, Sanghera MK, Roper-Hall A (1979): The latency of activation of neurons in the lateral hypothalamus and substantia innominata during feeding in the monkey. Brain Res 164:121–135.

Rolls ET, Burton MJ, Mora F (1980): Neurophysiological analysis of brain-stimulation reward in the monkey. Brain Res 194:339–357.

Rolls ET, Baylis GC (1986): Size and contrast have only small effects on the responses to faces of neurons in the cortex of the superior temporal sulcus of the monkey. Exp Brain Res 65:38–48.

Rolls ET, Williams GV (1987): Sensory and movement-related neuronal activity in different regions of the primate striatum. In Schneider JS, Lidsky TI (eds): "Basal Ganglia and Behavior: Sensory Aspects and Motor Functioning. Bern: Hans Huber, pp 37–59.

Rolls ET, Baylis GC, Hasselmo ME, Nalwa V (1989): The effect of learning on the face-selective responses of neurons in the cortex in the superior temporal sulcus of the monkey. Exp Brain Res 76:153–164.

Rolls ET, Johnstone S (1991): Neurophysiological analysis of striatal function. In Wallesch C, Vallar G (eds): "Neuropsychological Disorders Associated with Subcortical Lesions." Oxford: Oxford University Press.

Rolls ET, Treves A (1990): The relative advantages of sparse versus distributed encoding for associative neuronal networks in the brain. Network 1:407–421.

Sanghera MK, Rolls ET, Roper-Hall A (1979): Visual responses of neurons in the dorsolateral amygdala of the alert monkey. Exp Neurol 63:610–26.

Saper CB, Loewy AD, Swanson LW, Cowan WM (1976): Direct hypothalamo-autonomic connections. Brain Res 117:305–312.

Schwaber JS, Kapp BS, Higgins GA, Rapp PR (1982): Amygdaloid and basal forebrain direct connections with the nucleus of the solitary tract and the dorsal motor nucleus. J Neurosci 2:1424–1438.

Spiegler BJ, Mishkin M (1981): Evidence for the sequential participation of inferior temporal cortex and amygdala in the acquisition of stimulus-reward associations. Behav Brain Res 3:303–317.

Thorpe SJ, Rolls ET, Maddison S (1983): Neuronal activity in the orbitofrontal cortex of the behaving monkey. Exp Brain Res 49:93–115.

Turner BH (1981): The cortical sequence and terminal distribution of sensory related afferents to the amygdaloid complex of the rat and monkey. In Ben-Ari Y (ed): "The Amygdaloid Complex." Amsterdam: Elsevier, pp 51–62.

Turner BH, Mishkin M, Knapp M (1980): Organization of the amygdalopetal modality-specific cortical association areas in the monkey. J Comp Neurol 191:515–543.

Valenstein ES (1973): "Brain Control: A Critical Examination of Brain Stimulation and Psychosurgery." New York: Wiley.

Valenstein ES (ed) (1980): "The Psychosurgery Debate: Scientific, Legal, and Ethical Perspectives." San Francisco: Freeman.

Van Hoesen GW (1981): The differential distribution, diversity and sprouting of cortical projections to the amygdala in the rhesus monkey. In Ben-Ari Y (ed): "The Amygdaloid Complex." Amsterdam: Elsevier, pp 77–90.

Weiskrantz L (1956): Behavioral changes associated with ablation of the amygdaloid complex in monkeys. J Comp Physiol Psychol 49:381–391.

Wilson FAW, Rolls ET (1990a): Neuronal responses related to reinforcement in the primate basal forebrain. Brain Res 502:213–231.

Wilson FAW, Rolls ET (1990b): Neuronal responses related to the novelty and familiarity of visual stimuli in the substantia innominata, diagonal band of Broca and periventricular region of the primate. Exp Brain Res 80:104–120.

Wilson FAW, Rolls FT (1990c): Learning and memory are reflected in the responses of reinforcement-related neurons in the primate basal forebrain. J Neurosci 10:1254–1267.

Wilson FAW, Rolls ET (1991a): The primate amygdala and reinforcement: A dissociation between rule-based and associatively-mediated memory revealed in amygdala neuronal activity.

Wilson FAW, Rolls ET (1991b): The effects of stimulus novelty and familiarity on neuronal activity in the amygdala of monkeys performing recognition memory tasks.

Zola-Morgan S, Squire LR, Amaral DG (1989): Lesions of the amygdala that spare adjacent cortical regions do not impair memory or exacerbate the impairment following lesions of the hippocampal formation. J Neurosci 9:1922–1936.

The Amygdala: Neurobiological Aspects of Emotion,
Memory, and Mental Dysfunction, pages 167–190
© 1992 Wiley-Liss, Inc.

6

Neurophysiological Basis of the Klüver-Bucy Syndrome: Responses of Monkey Amygdaloid Neurons to Biologically Significant Objects

TAKETOSHI ONO AND HISAO NISHIJO

Department of Physiology, Faculty of Medicine, Toyama Medical and Pharmaceutical University, Toyama, Japan

INTRODUCTION

Bilateral lesions of the temporal cortex that include the amygdala produce the Klüver-Bucy syndrome in monkeys (Klüver and Bucy, 1939; Weiskrantz, 1956; Gloor, 1960). This syndrome consists of a complex set of several affective disorders: tameness coupled with a willingness to approach normally fear-inducing stimuli such as humans, gloves, or animal models (loss of fear); increased and inappropriate sexual behavior (hypersexuality); and a tendency to investigate the environment orally and put inedible objects into the mouth (oral tendency). The habits of approaching aversive stimuli and failing to discriminate food from nonfood have been referred to as "psychic blindness," an overall deficit in the ability to identify the biological significance of stimuli. Lesion studies have indicated that the amygdala is a focal point of causes contributing to the Klüver-Bucy syndrome (Gloor, 1960; Goddard, 1964), while electrical stimulation and unit recording studies have further helped demonstrate the crucial role of this structure in emotional behavior (Kaada, 1972; Sanghera et al., 1979; Ono et al., 1980, 1983).

The Klüver-Bucy syndrome might be interpreted in terms of a deficit in sensory processing. It has been proposed that sequential processing of sensory information takes place in the neocortex (Turner et al., 1980; Pons et al., 1987) and that the amygdala receives highly integrated sensory information from all modalities in a late stage of this sequential cortical processing (Gloor, 1960; Aggleton et al., 1980; Turner et al., 1980; Iwai and Yukie, 1987). In turn, the amygdala projects to the hypothalamus (Oomura et al., 1970; Krettek and Price, 1978; Amaral et al., 1982; Ono et al., 1985), and lower brain stem areas (Hopkins et al., 1978; Krettek et al., 1978; Price and Amaral, 1981; Schwaber et al., 1982;

Address correspondence to: Dr. Taketoshi Ono, Department of Physiology, Faculty of Medicine, Toyama Medical and Pharmaceutical University, Toyama 930-01, Japan.

Veening et al., 1984). It has been suggested that the Klüver-Bucy syndrome may be produced by lesions that interrupt this pathway (Horel et al., 1975), such as lesions of the entire temporal neocortex or inferotemporal cortex (Horel et al., 1975; Gaffan et al., 1988), lesions of the amygdala (Horel et al., 1975), or lesions of the pathway from the amygdala to the hypothalamus or brain stem (Hilton and Zbrozyna, 1963).

In this information flow (see a hypothetical schema in Fig. 11), the amygdala might be involved in the process through which sensory stimuli gain motivational and emotional significance as a result of the interaction between the higher sensory cortex and the limbic system, i.e., stimulus-affective association (Weiskrantz, 1956; Jones and Mishkin, 1972; Spiegler and Mishkin, 1981). Thus, bilateral lesions of the monkey amygdala or temporal cortex produce visual-limbic disconnections (Geschwind, 1956) or sensory-affective dissociations (Jones and Mishkin, 1972), which are suggested to be underlying defects responsible for the Klüver-Bucy syndrome. These assumptions imply that amygdala neurons will respond to the affective significance of sensory stimuli (Mishkin and Aggleton, 1981).

In an attempt to examine this proprosal, we have studied the arousal and aversive reactions of the monkey amygdala (Ono et al., 1980, 1983; Fukuda et al., 1987; Nishijo et al., 1986, 1988a,b) to stimuli that were considered to be biologically significant (Weiskrantz, 1956; Horel et al., 1975; Perrett et al., 1982). Animals were tested on a variety of behavioral tasks which involved the discrimination of different rewarding and aversive stimuli. At the same time we examined the discharge patterns of single amygdala neurons. Some neurons were also tested by changing the affective significance of the stimuli presented (Nishijo et al., 1988a,b). Another objective of these studies was to investigate the changes in neural responses following reversible disconnection of the inferotemporal cortex from the amygdala (by cooling the inferotemporal cortex) and the amygdala from the lateral hypothalamus (by cooling the amygdala) (Fukuda et al., 1987).

The experiments described here were performed on eight monkeys (*Macaca fuscata*, 4–6 kg). A common feature of these experiments was the painless restraint of the monkeys in a stereotaxis apparatus by a previously prepared, surgically fixed head holder designed in our laboratory (Ono et al., 1980, 1981a, 1983, 1988). A monkey sat on a chair facing a panel containing shutters and an operant responding bar (Fig. 1A). Juice, water, and saline were made available through a small spout with an electromagnetic valve. Weak electric shock could be applied between the two ear lobes to produce an aversive stimulation. The tasks included feeding, drinking, active avoidance, and auditory discrimination.

In one feeding task (Fig. 1B), an opaque shutter (W1) was opened at random intervals so the monkey could see an object, either food or nonfood, on a turntable through a transparent shutter (W2). The animal had to then press the bar a prefixed number of times (fixed ration, FR 10–30) to obtain the food. The transparent shutter was opened at the last bar press and the animal could extend its arm, take the available food, and ingest it. In another modified feeding task, a one-way mirror (S1) in front of the turntable was used in place of the W1 and

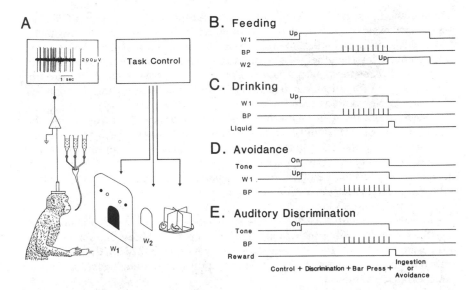

Fig. 1. Experimental setup and protocol of monkey discrimination task. **A:** Monkey sits in a chair facing a panel which has a bar and a window covered by two shutters (W1 and W2). Liquid is provided from a small spout while a weak electric shock can be applied between ear lobes. **B,C,D,E:** Time sequences of feeding, drinking, avoidance, and auditory discrimination tasks. W1: Opaque shutter in front of turntable, opens at Up (B,C,D). BP: Indications of individual bar presses and time during which they occur (B–E). Liquid: dispensed from spout after the last bar press (C). Tone: warns of imminent application of shock if avoidance criterion is not met (D), and indicates availability of reward in auditory discrimination test (**E**). Reward: drop of juice is dispensed from spout after the last bar press, or cookie or raisin on turntable is made available by simultaneous opening of W1 and W2 after the last bar press.

W2 shutters, and another shutter (S2) temporarily prevented access to the bar. When the light behind S1 was turned on, the monkey could see an object on the turntable. After a delay of at least 2 sec, S2 was opened automatically, and the animal could obtain the object by pressing the bar. The monkey's behavior and neural responses were basically similar in both original and modified tasks. Each feeding task was divided into four phases: control, visual (discrimination), bar press (operant responding), and ingestion (reward) or avoidance (aversion). Comparably, when the FR criterion was met in a drinking trial (Fig. 1C) a drop of palatable or unpalatable liquid (juice, water, or saline), signaled by some symbolic object (cylinder, cube, etc.), could be licked from a small spout. Usually white and red cylinders were associated with juice and water, respectively. In active avoidance (Fig. 1D) one of two objects, either a brown cylinder associated with electric shock or a roll of tape that was not associated with electric shock, was presented with a 1200 Hz tone. The brown cylinder plus 1200 Hz tone meant that the monkey had to complete a FR schedule within a predetermined period (4–6 sec) to avoid shock. In an auditory discrimination (Fig. 1E) task, a buzzer noise was associated with food (cookie or raisin) and an 800 Hz tone with a drop of juice. Two other pure tones (2800 and 4300 Hz) had no significance with any other part of the task. Upon hearing the buzzer or the 800 Hz tone, a FR response was needed to obtain, respectively, food or a drop of juice. The rest of the design matched that in the visual feeding task except that the food was not visible behind W1.

To test the effects of disconnection, cooling probes were chronically implanted bilaterally over the dura of the anterior inferotemporal cortex in one monkey, and bilaterally in the amygdala in two monkeys. The temperature in the cortex ranged from 18 to 23°C, while the temperature around the cooling probes in the amygdala was below 20°C. These temperature ranges are sufficient to depress synaptic transmission (Jasper et al., 1970).

AMYGDALA NEURAL RESPONSES DURING VISUAL DISCRIMINATION

Of 585 amygdala neurons tested, 312 (53.3%) responded to at least one stimulus. Based on their responsiveness to sensory modalities, 238 of these 312 neurons fell into five categories: vision related, audition related, ingestion related, multimodal, and selective.

Vision-Related Type

Of the 585 neurons tested, 40 (6.8%) responded (all excited) to visual stimuli, but not to auditory, oral sensory, or somesthetic stimuli. These neurons responded strongly to the sight of unfamiliar objects regardless of whether they were food or nonfood, and to the sight of some familiar nonfood objects.

Of these 40 vision-related neurons, 26 responded consistently to both rewarding objects, such as familiar food and the red or white cylinders associated with water or juice, and to certain nonfood objects such as the brown cylinder that was associated with electric shock, a syringe, a glove, etc., but not to neutral nonfood stimuli (tape) (Vis-I-type). Figure 2 illustrates an example of a vision-related neuron. This neuron responded strongly to both familiar positive (a, orange) and negative (b, brown cylinder) objects, and to unfamiliar objects (c, dried yam; d, small bottle). In contrast to its responses to visual stimuli, this

---

Fig. 2. Responses of a Vis-I neuron. **A:** Activity increases at the sight of positive (**a**) and negative (**b**) affectively related objects, and unfamiliar objects (**c,d**), but not to auditory (**e**) or somesthetic (**f**) stimuli. Note absence of neural response after animal had put orange into mouth (Aa, arrow). Bar presses are shown by histograms on time scales. W1 opened at time 0. Ordinates: summed responses for N trials, calibration at the right of each histogram indicates the number of spikes in each bin. **B:** Comparison of responses to various visual stimuli. Solid circles connected by heavy lines indicate mean firing rate (spikes/sec) of each of four sequential trials lasting 5 sec after W1 was opened. The histograms show the overall mean of each set of four trials, the broken line indicates the spontaneous firing rate. The order of stimulus presentation is shown by the number at the bottom of each bar, the food and nonfood objects being separated for clarity. A total of 27 stimuli were tested, 12 of which are shown here.

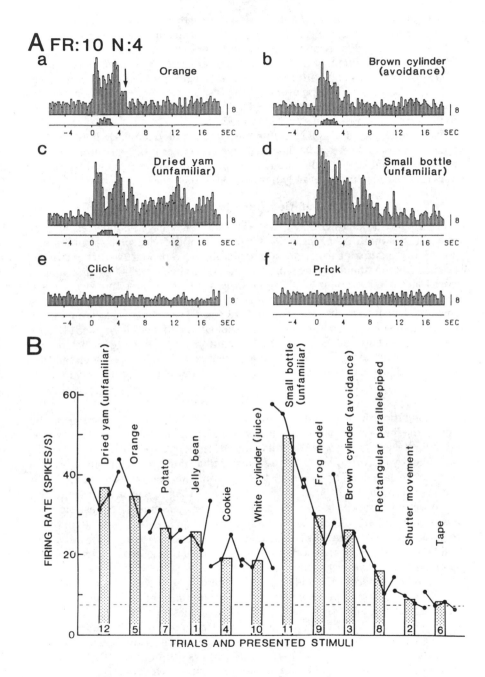

neuron did not respond to auditory (e) or somesthetic (f) stimuli. These stimuli did, however, elicit various overt reactions (but not bar pressing). Figure 2Aa shows the lack of response after putting orange into the mouth (indicated by arrow), suggesting that this neuron did not respond to oral sensory stimuli. The responses of this neuron to various food and nonfood objects are compared in Figure 2B. It can be seen that the response magnitude differed significantly between the various objects and that the neuron responded more strongly to preferred rather than less preferred food.

The remaining 14 vision-related neurons responded similarly both to unfamiliar objects and certain familiar negative objects. But these neurons did not respond to familiar reward-related objects, such as food or red and white cylinders associated with water and juice (Vis-II type).

Audition-Related Neurons

There were 26 neurons among the 585 tested (4.4%) that responded exclusively to auditory stimuli. All of these 26 neurons responded vigorously to unfamiliar sounds and habituated to certain auditory stimuli in repeated trials if the monkey learned that the stimuli had no biological meaning; none responded to the familiar pure tones used as controls. These neurons were subdivided into two groups: those that responded to familiar cue tones associated with a cookie or juice reward, as well as to unfamiliar sounds (8 aud-I); and those that responded to unfamiliar sounds but not to cue tones associated with cookie or juice (18 aud-II). Figure 3 shows an example of aud-I neurons. Although the associated rewards were the same, this neuron did not respond to visual cues associated with feeding and drinking (a,b), but did respond to auditory cues (c,d).

Ingestion-Related Neurons

Among the 585 neurons tested there were 41 (7%) that responded primarily during the ingestion phase of the tasks. Depending on responsiveness to other stimuli, these neurons were subdivided into three groups: 27 oral sensory, 11 oral sensory plus vision, and 3 oral sensory plus audition. Figure 4 shows representative data of an oral sensory-type neuron. This neuron responded only in the ingestion phases of food (Aa,b,e,f), juice (Ac), and saline (Ad) trials, but there were differences in its responses to the various stimuli. The responses to a watermelon (Ae) and the cucumber (Af) were apparently greater than those to cookies (Aa) or to raisins (Ab), and this tendency was evident for other palatable food (not shown). Another characteristic of this neuron was its responsiveness to negative oral sensory stimuli (Ad).

Some oral sensory neurons tended to habituate to certain kinds of food. Of the 27 oral sensory type neurons, five habituated in repeated trials (Fig. 4B). Although bar pressing and mouth movement did not change, neural responses to both cabbage (trails 1–5) and mushroom (trials 6–10) habituated over successive trials. The previous response levels did, however, reappear when the mushroom was salted (trials 11 and 12). These results imply that the activity of this neuron was not dependent on the motor actions of feeding.

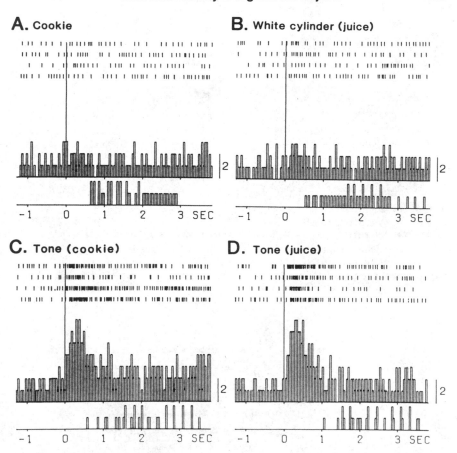

Fig. 3. Responses of aud-I neurons shown as raster displays and summed histograms (40 msec bins, 5.12 sec) for four trials. Although associated rewards were the same, the neuron responded only to auditory (**C,D**), and not to visual (**A,B**), stimuli. Other descriptions as for Figure 2.

Multimodal Neurons

The responses of 117 of the 585 neurons (20.0%) were multimodal. Of these, 40 (6.8%) responded phasically and nonspecifically to various sensory stimuli. These responses were independent of the nature of the stimuli. The multimodal phasic neuron shown in Figure 5A responded to rewarding stimuli (cookie, a), to known aversive or potentially aversive stimuli (punishment-associated brown cylinder, b; experimenter's hand approaching, c), and to neutral stimuli (shutter opening, d), as well as to a light flash (e). This particular neuron was also sensitive to auditory (g,h) and somesthetic (f) stimuli.

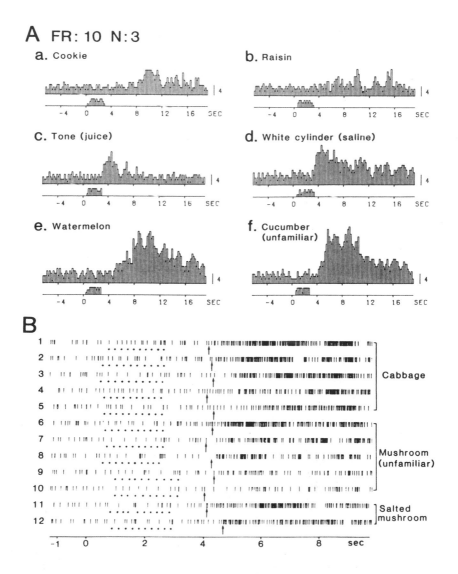

Fig. 4. Responses of oral sensory type neurons displayed as peristimulus time histograms (200 msec bins, 25.6 sec). **A:** Neuronal activity increases only in the ingestion phase (**a–f**). Note response to saline (**d**), and prominent responses to watermelon (**e**) and unfamiliar food (**f**). Other descriptions as for Figure 2. **B:** Raster display of neural responses in sequential food trials. Note habituation of responses to cabbage (trials 1–5), mushroom (trials 6–10), and reinstatement of response to mushroom after salting (trials 11–12). Other descriptions as for Figure 3.

In contrast with these phasic-type neurons, 77 (13.2%) amygdala neurons responded tonically to biologically significant stimuli but not to neutral stimuli. Typical results from one neuron of this type are shown in Figure 5B. This neuron responded to both visual and auditory cues during ingestion (a,b), as well as to somesthetic stimuli (gentle pricking the back with a pencil) (c). This neuron also responded strongly to an unfamiliar object (e, glass pyramid), but not to a familiar, neutral nonfood object (d, tape).

Selective Neurons

Responses of 14 of the 585 neurons (2.4%) were highly selective for only particular familiar objects or sounds (selective): six (1.0%) were selective for one specific food item or for a cylinder associated with a palatable liquid; five (0.9%) were selective for one specific nonfood item, and three (0.5%) were selective for one specific sound. Examples of responses that indicated selectivity for one specific food item are shown in Figure 6A. The neuron was tested with 16 objects and seven somesthetic and auditory stimuli (not all shown), and the magnitude of its response to the sight and ingestion of watermelon was much greater than its responses to any other stimulus (A). An example of a neuron that responded to a specific nonfood item is shown in Figure 6B. This neuron was tested with 16 objects and eight somesthetic and auditory stimuli (only four stimuli shown in Fig. 6B), and responded only to the sight of a spider model (a).

Effects of Reversal on Amygdala Neural Activity

Although vis-I neurons responded similarly to both positive and negative stimuli, the change in response that occurred when the affective significance of a stimulus was altered indicates that this factor was more important than the physical characteristics of the stimulus. For example, the neuron characterised in Figure 2 was also studied in a modified situation (Fig. 7). It was found that responses to an unfamiliar object (dried yam) habituated gradually over successive trials (1 to 14) as the object became familiar and the monkey learned that it was biologically unimportant. Later when the dried yam was presented with the same 1200 Hz tone that had been paired with the brown cylinder in the avoidance task but without the accompanying electric shock (trial 15), the initial response increased slightly but quickly habituated over subsequent trials (15 to 18) as the monkey learned that the dried yam was still unimportant. Finally the dried yam was presented with the tone and followed by an electric shock (broad line below raster display in trials 19 and 20). Under this condition, bar pressing and neural responses were quickly reinstated (trials 19 to 22). In trial 20, neural responses were elicited without bar pressing for avoidance, and in trials 20 to 22 the neural responses were time-locked to presentation of dried yam. These observations reveal that the neural responses were not related directly to the avoidance situation, but to the dried yam associated with electric shock. Thus, the response of the neuron to visual stimulation was modified when it was associated with other stimuli (1200 Hz tone and electric shock). Of seven other vis-I neurons tested with other nonfood objects in the same way, all showed a reinstatement of responses when the stimulus was associated with electric shock.

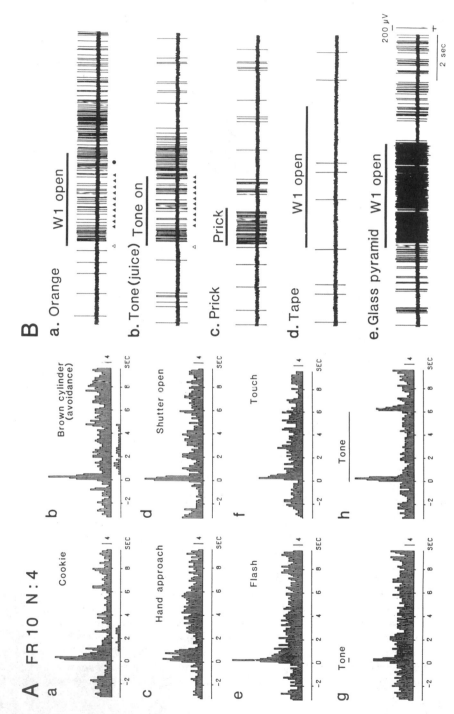

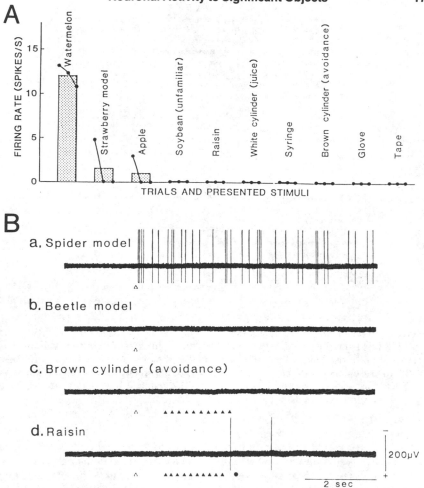

Fig. 6. Responses of two selective neurons. **A:** Responses of neuron selective to watermelon. Solid circles connected by heavy lines indicate mean firing rate in each of three successive trials lasting 5 sec after the opaque shutter was opened. Other descriptions as for Figure 2B. **B:** Responses of neuron selective to spider model (**a**) shown as raw records. The neuron did not respond at the sight of any other objects presented [examples shown: beetle model (**b**), brown cylinder used in avoidance task (**c**), raisin (**d**)]. Other descriptions as for Figure 5B.

Fig. 5. Responses of multimodal type neurons (two examples). **A:** Responses of phasic type neuron displayed as peristimulus time histograms (100 msec bins, 12.8 sec). Activity increased in response to presentation of positive (**a**) and negative (**b**) affectively related objects, approach of experimenter's hand (**c**), shutter open (**d**), flash (**e**), touching monkey's back (**f**), and turning tone on and off (**g,h**). Other description as for Figure 2A. **B:** Responses of tonic type neuron. Neuron responded at sight and ingestion of orange (**a**), to tone associated with juice and ingestion of juice (**b**), and to pricking of animal's back with pencil (**c**). Neuron did not respond at sight of neutral nonfood (**d**) but responded strongly at sight of unfamiliar object (**e**). Open triangles, times W1 opened; filled triangles, bar presses; filled circle, food put into mouth.

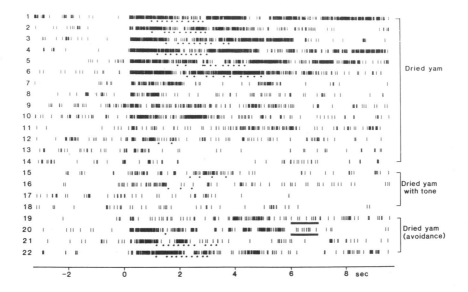

Fig. 7. Raster display of other responses of neuron depicted in Figure 2. The dried yam, which was handled and smelled but never tasted, was not accepted by the monkey as food. In trials 1–14, the response gradually habituated. In trials 15–18, the dried yam was presented with the 1200 Hz tone that was used in the active avoidance task. In trials 19–22, the response appeared again after association with electric shock (underbars in 19, 20). Shock was avoided in trials 21 and 22. W1 opened at time 0. Each dot below a raster display indicates one bar press.

Eight neurons that responded to the sight of food-related objects (four oral sensory plus vision and four selective neurons) were also challenged by altering the affective significance of the stimulus object. It was found that not only visual but also ingestion responses of all eight neurons were attenuated by salting the food. Figure 8A illustrates the modulation of responses of one of the oral sensory plus vision neurons. In trials 1 and 2 the neuron may have responded slightly in the late ingestion phase to a white cylinder associated with juice and to a cookie. In contrast, responding in both the visual and ingestion phases was found for apple, potato, raisin, and orange (trials 3–5, 9, and 13–15). As in our feeding paradigm, mouth movement is slight or absent during the discrimination and bar press phases, it is likely that the neural responses preceding ingestion were not preparatory to mouth movement. Similarly, bar-pressing behavior did not correlate with neural activity (see trials 6, 13, and 14), but visual presentation of a normally ingested food did elicit activity in trials 9 and 15. In addition, the neuron represented in Figure 8A did not respond to any known aversive or neutral objects such as the brown cylinder that was associated with electric shock, a syringe, or tape (trials 6–8, and others, not shown).

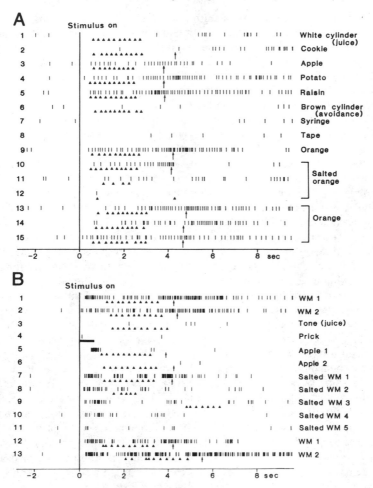

Fig. 8. Modulation of neural responses by reversal tests. *A:* Raster display of responses of an oral sensory plus vision neuron. The neuron responded slightly to the ingestion of juice and cookie in trials 1 and 2. Activity increased primarily in and immediately preceding ingestion phase in trials 3–5. Note no neural response in bar-press phase in avoidance task (trial 6). Trials 9–15 show reversal associated with salted food. Note that neural responses disappeared at the moment when animal put a salted orange into its mouth (arrow in trial 10). Other details as in Figure 7. *B:* Raster display of responses of neuron selective to watermelon. The neuron responds to the sight and ingestion of normal watermelon in trials 1 and 2 but not to a tone associated with juice in trial 3, or somesthetic stimulation (prick) in trial 4. In trials 5 and 6, responses to apple habituated in only one trial. Note that neural responses decreased the moment the animal put salted watermelon into its mouth (arrow in trial 7). In trials 8–11, the neural and bar-pressing responses gradually decreased and finally disappeared. Activity levels were then reinstated with normal watermelon (trials 12 and 13). Triangle under raster indicates one bar press, arrow shows when food is in the mouth.

Trials 9–15 show the effects of salting food. The response attentuation was apparent during both the visual inspection and ingestion phases of the task. In the first salted food trial (trial 10), the response disappeared immediately after putting salted orange into the animal's mouth. Salting of food was always done in such a way that the salt could not be seen, so it was first detected by the animal upon ingestion. The response to the sight of orange then diminished on subsequent salted food trials (trials 11 and 12), as well as on the first two unsalted food trials that followed (trials 13 and 14). After the experimenter had given a piece of unsalted orange to the animal by hand, bar pressing to obtain orange began again in trials 13 to 15, and neuronal responses to the sight and ingestion of orange quickly recovered.

Figure 8B shows the modulation of activity of a neuron that selectively responded to watermelon. The neuron responded consistently at the sight and ingestion of watermelon in trials 1 and 2, but did not respond to the rewarding cue tone associated with juice and its ingestion in trial 3, nor to a presumably aversive somesthetic stimulus (prick) in trial 4. The neuron responded slightly at the sight of an apple, but only in the first trial with this stimulus (trial 5). In trials 7–11 it was found that salted watermelon, which was visually indistinguishable from unsalted watermelon, reversibly modified the neuronal activity that occurred during both the sight and ingestion of that stimulus. In trial 7 the neuron responded as previously until the salted watermelon was ingested (indicated by arrow), at which point the neuronal activity suddenly decreased. In trials 8–11, responses to the sight of watermelon gradually decreased and finally disappeared. After the experimenter gave a piece of unsalted watermelon to the animal, neuronal and bar pressing responses resumed in trials 12 and 13. The suppression of neuronal activity associated with salted food could not be ascribed to diverted attention. We monitored adjunctive behavior in three different ways: by recording the animal's gaze with two TV cameras, by electrooculogram (EOG), or by both methods and the experimenter's observations (Nishijo et al., 1988a,b). All observations indicated that the animal continued to watch the object during reversal trials. In fact, two monkeys continued to press the bar even after experiencing the salty taste of the food, but they struck the food off the turntable instead of eating it. In these cases, neuronal activity remained suppressed.

Location of Each Neuron Type

The distribution of the various neuron types is illustrated in Figure 9. We adopted the atlas of Kusama and Mabuchi (1970) for *Macaca fuscata* based on Johnston's classification (1923). The corticomedial (CM) group includes the central, medial, and periamygdaloid nuclei and the anterior amygdaloid area. The lateral, basolateral, and basomedial nuclei in the atlas correspond, respectively, to the lateral, basal, and basal accessory nuclei in the terminology adopted by Price (1981).

Vis-II neurons tended to be located in the anterior laterodorsal part of the amygdala and were concentrated in the lateral nucleus (Fig. 9A, open triangles, 14 vis-II/57 tested). (The denominators of this and all of the other fractions

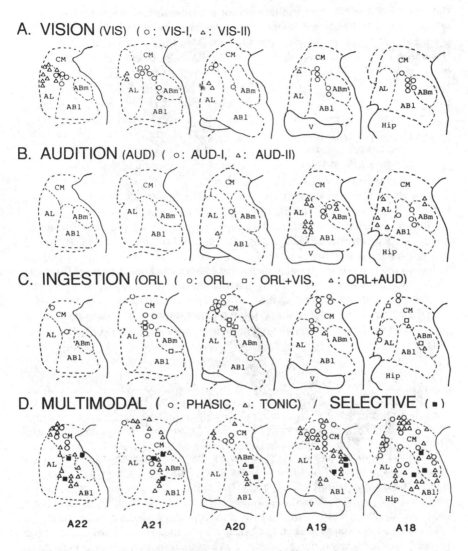

Fig. 9. Recording sites of five major neuron types. **A:** Vision related; open circles, vis-I; open triangles, vis-II. **B:** Audition related; open circles, aud-I; open triangles, aud-II. **C:** Ingestion related; open circles, oral sensory (ORL); open squares, oral sensory plus vision (ORL + VIS); open triangles, oral sensory plus audition (ORL + AUD). **D:** Multimodal or selective; open circles, multimodal phasic; open triangles, multimodal tonic; filled squares, selective. CM, corticomedial group of amygdala; AL, lateral nucleus; ABl, basolateral nucleus; ABm, basomedial nucleus. Numbers below each section indicate distance (mm) anterior from interaural line.

that follow represent the total number of neurons tested in the region within which the vis-II, or other respective neuron types, were found.) Vis-I neurons were located more medially than vis-II, that is, in the border area between the basolateral nucleus and the other nuclei (Fig. 9A, open circles, 26/72). The aud-II neurons were located in the posterolateral part of the amygdala (mainly in the lateral nucleus and its border with the basolateral nuclei) and in the border zone between the basomedial nucleus and the corticomedial group (Fig. 9B, open triangles, 18/69). The aud-I neurons were located in the posterior basolateral nucleus (Fig. 9C, open circles, 8/51). Most of the oral sensory plus vision type neurons were found along the dorsal edge of the basolateral nucleus, and one was in the border area between the putamen and the corticomedial group (Fig. 9C, open squares, 11/62). The oral sensory plus audition type neurons were located on the posterior dorsal surface of the basolateral nucleus (Fig. 9C, open triangles, 3/44). The multimodal tonic type neurons were widely distributed across the amygdala except for the lateral nucleus (Fig. 9D, open triangles, 77/585). A similar distribution was found for the multimodal phasic type neurons (Fig. D, open circles, 40/516). Lastly, the selective type neurons were located in the basolateral and basomedial nuclei (D, filled squares, 14/312).

DISCONNECTION EXPERIMENT BY REVERSIBLE COOLING OF INFEROTEMPORAL CORTEX OR THE AMYGDALA

Of 43 amygdala neurons tested, the spontaneous firing rate of 13 neurons decreased and that of two increased when the inferotemporal cortex was cooled. Of these 43 amygdala neurons, 38 responded to visual stimulation before cooling the inferotemporal cortex. According to the patterns of responses to the sight of food and nonfood, the amygdaloid responsive neurons were classified into three groups: food predominant type (n = 6), nonfood predominant type (n = 11), and arousal (nondifferential) type (n = 21).

Cooling the inferotemporal cortex suppressed visual responses in 2 of 6 food predominant neurons. Figure 10A shows an example of this modulatory effect of inferotemporal cooling. Before cooling it was found that neuron activity increased at the sight of food and during ingestion in all trials (Fig. 10Aa), but about 3 min after the start of inferotemporal cooling, visual responses to the sight of the food disappeared in each of the four trials (Fig. 10Ab). Cooling the inferotemporal cortex did not, however, change the responses of this particular neuron during ingestion of the food (Fig. 10Ab). Of 11 nonfood predominant neurons, inferotemporal cooling was found to nondiscriminately enhance visual responses in two, and suppress visual responses in another four. Of 17 neurons that responded differentially to the sight of food or nonfood, eight became nondiscriminative during inferotemporal cooling.

Of 55 lateral hypothalamic neurons tested, 44 responded in the visual discrimination phase, 8 during bar press, and 12 during ingestion. It was found that amygdala cooling changed the spontaneous firing rates of 38% (12 increased,

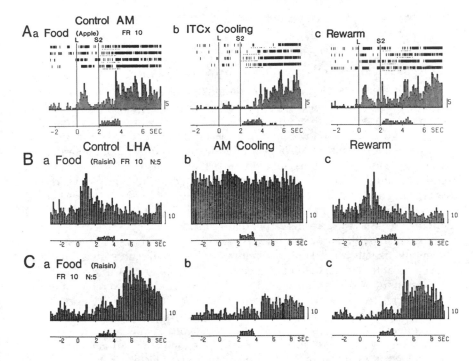

Fig. 10. Effects of inferotemporal cortex (ITCx) and amygdala (AM) cooling during a feeding task. **A:** Effects of ITCx cooling on food predominant neurons in amygdala. Raster displays and histograms (80 msec bins, 10.24 sec) show neural responses to sight of food (apple) before (**a**), during ITCx cooling (**b**), and after rewarming (**c**), and bar presses (lower histogram of each set) for four trials. Time L (0), light on; S2, shutter in front of bar opened. Note no visual responses to sight of food during ITCx cooling (**b**). **B:** Effects of amygdala cooling on lateral hypothalamic (LHA) food predominant neurons. Histograms (100 msec bins, 12.8 sec) show responses for five trials during control (**a**), amygdala cooled (**b**), and rewarmed (**c**) states. No significant visual responses to sight of food during amygdala cooling, although spontaneous firing rate increased remarkably (**b**). **C:** Effects of amygdala cooling on responses of ingestion-related LHA neurons. Neuron responded substantially before (**a**) and after (**c**), but less during AM cooling (**b**). Histograms: accumulated in five trials (100 msec bins, 12.8 sec). Other descriptions as in A.

9 decreased) of these neurons. Of 22 neurons that responded both to food and nonfood, two were depressed by amygdala cooling. Of 22 neurons that responded preferentially to the sight of food (food responsive), the responses of 9 were weakened or depressed by amygdala cooling (Fig. 10B). As the spontaneous firing rate was greatly increased by bilateral amygdala cooling (Fig. 10Bb), none of the excitatory visual responses were significantly greater than the background activity. In contrast to the effects of cooling the inferotemporal cortex on amygdala responses during the ingestion phase, amygdala cooling depressed the

responses of 3 of 12 lateral hypothalamic neurons that responded during the ingestion phase (Fig. 10C).

FUNCTIONAL RELATIONS
Amygdala Neural Activity, Sensory Stimuli, and Operant Responding

There was not always a direct correlation between bar pressing and neural activity, while a direct link between neural activity in the amygdala and individual bar presses (i.e., direct one-to-one motor coupled response) was never observed. Although spontaneous bar pressing during intertrial intervals was rare, when such spontaneous pressing did occur no concomitant neural activity change was ever observed. In high FR (FR 30) trials the responses of vis-I, aud-I, and multimodal tonic type neurons returned to the control level during bar pressing and then reappeared after the transparent shutter (W2) was opened following the last bar press. Even when there was no bar pressing, vis-I and multimodal tonic type neurons responded to visual stimuli. Both of these results are consistent with a previous study (Ono et al., 1980). In the bar-press phase, the animal usually looked at the window, and vis-I and multimodal tonic type neuron responses depended on the nature of the stimulus. During this phase the responses of some neurons to the most preferred food were significantly stronger than the responses of the same neurons to less preferred food. Nevertheless, differences in the duration of the bar-press phase, which directly reflected the frequency of bar pressing, were not statistically significant, except in the reversal tests when some confusion might be expected. Vis-II and aud-II neurons seldom responded to familiar positive stimuli even though the animal responded behaviorally. There were, however, some indications of an indirect relationship between neural and behavioral responses. For instance, stronger neural responses accompanied normal bar pressing, but the same neurons responded less vigorously when bar pressing was delayed or absent (Figs. 7, 8A,B) as in reversal or extinction trials. Similar relations have been reported in the lateral hypothalamic area (Fukuda et al., 1986).

Our results imply that neural activity in the amygdala is not directly related to either sensory inputs or to overt acts of the individual. Neuronal activity may, however, reflect motivational aspects of an animal's behavioral responses. This conclusion is not new. Other investigators, using different paradigms, have made similar inferences (Sanghera et al., 1979; Ono et al., 1980; Nishijo et al., 1986; Nakano et al., 1987; Gaffan et al., 1988).

Amygdala Neural Responsiveness and Affective Significance

The activity of eight neurons that responded to food-related stimuli (four oral sensory plus vision and four selective neurons), along with related behavioral responses, were suppressed by reversal tests (Fig. 8). During these tests the neural and behavioral responses (not individual bar presses) were well correlated. Initial ingestion of the salted food brought about a suppression of the responses of both types of neurons. This was followed by a suppression of the visual responses to the food, even though the visual appearance of the food had not altered. In preliminary experiments, we have also observed the suppression of gustatory responses by quinine in a very similar manner to that brought about by salt.

In general, the reward value (palatability) of food can be estimated through its ingestion (Norgren et al., 1989), the gustation phase being an important factor in the evaluation of food palatability (Bartoshuk, 1989). This in turn suggests that the suppression of neuronal activity described above is related to an aversion to salted food. This is a reasonable speculation since behavioral responses were also suppressed after the first of a series of salted food trials. Thus, the discovery based on ingestion that the salted food was aversive led to the decision that the visual appearance of the same food was also aversive (suppression of visually dependent neural responses). This dependence of visual responses on ingestion-related sensations suggests that these neurons are involved in visual-oral sensory (possibly gustatory) associations (Nishijo et al., 1988a,b). Geschwind (1965) also suggested a role for the limbic system in visual-gustatory association, a process which is essential for normal stimulus-reinforcement association.

Nondifferential vision-related, audition-related, and multimodal tonic neurons responded equally to rewarding and aversive stimuli, but did not respond to neutral stimuli. The responses of these neurons were easily modulated by extinction or by changing the affective significance of the stimulus (Fig. 7). One function of these neurons might be to help differentiate stimuli that are biologically significant from those that are nonsignificant. This rapid and flexible neuronal change could in turn form the neurophysiological basis, depending on the affective significance of the stimulus, for the role of the basolateral amygdala in the acquisition of fear-potentiated startle (Miserendino et al., 1990). These response changes might also be part of an attentional mechanism, reflected by the animal's concentration on one biologically significant stimulus among various exteroceptive stimuli (Nishijo et al., 1988a,b).

Neural Mechanisms for Discrimination of Food and Nonfood

Although monkeys with amygdala lesions cannot distinguish food from nonfood immediately after surgery, they are eventually able to make this discrimination (Iwai et al., 1986). Furthermore, animals with amygdala lesions can learn visual discriminations (Pribram and Bagshan, 1953; Schwartzbaum, 1965; Horel et al., 1975; Zola-Morgan et al., 1982), but this occurs gradually (Spiegler and Mishkin, 1981; Zola-Morgan and Squire, 1984). Discrimination of food from nonfood can be regarded as a simple visual discrimination (Zola-Morgan and Squire, 1984) and it has been suggested that the temporal stem (Zola-Morgan and Squire, 1984) or direct visual projections from the visual cortex to the striatum (Mishkin et al., 1984) are responsible for such simple discriminations. Mishkin and his colleagues (Spiegler and Mishkin, 1981; Mishkin et al., 1984) have proposed that this inferotemporal-striatal system corresponds to a neural counterpart of habit or procedural memory (Cohen and Squire, 1980), while the inferotemporal-amygdala system is responsible for associative memory by which animals discriminate positive and negative affective objects. Animals with amygdala lesions may learn to substitute the inferotemporal-striatal system for the inferotemporal-amygdala system. Previously, we reported food-responsive neurons in the rostroventral putamen (Nishijo et al., 1986), an area which receives afferents from both the inferotemporal cortex and the amygdala (Selemon and Goldman-Rakic, 1985; Russchen et al., 1985). In contrast to the amygdala food-responsive neurons, the responses of the putamen neurons were highly task-dependent, and not multimodal (i.e., did not respond during the ingestion phase). These characteristics are seen as consistent with a relationship to procedural memory (Nishijo et al., 1986).

Effects of Inferotemporal Cooling on Amygdala Activity and Amygdala Cooling on Lateral Hypothalamic Activity

Of 17 amygdala neurons that responded differentially to the sight of food or nonfood in the cooling experiment, eight became nondiscriminative during cooling of the inferotemporal cortex. Thus the main amygdala response to inferotemporal cooling was a depression of both vision-related neural responses and spontaneous firing rates. Previous recording studies have indicated that some inferotemporal neurons will respond to only one pattern regardless of size or color (Gross et al., 1969; Sato et al., 1980; Desimone et al., 1984; Miyashita, 1988; Miyashita and Chang, 1988) while other studies have found units that respond to specific colors (Fuster and Jervey, 1982; Desimone et al., 1984). Furthermore, a lesion study provided evidence that the inferotemporal cortex is critical for storing "prototypes" of visual objects (Weiskrantz and Saunders, 1984). These findings, along with those of the present study, strongly suggest that the inferotemporal cortex is in one of the paths (Fig. 11) by which object-related information passes from the visual cortex to the amygdala (Fukuda et al., 1987).

It is interesting that cooling of the inferotemporal cortex did not suppress neural responses during ingestion in spite of its effect on visual responses (Fig. 10A). It is presumed that in this condition visual information normally reaching the amygdala is disconnected by cooling the inferotemporal cortex, while estimation of the reward value of food is apparently possible through oral sensory information. Similar observations were reported previously: Animals with visual

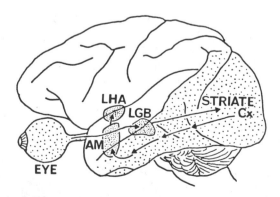

Fig. 11. Simplified diagrammatic schema for sequential visual processing. Abbreviations: AM, amygdala; LGB, lateral geniculate body; LHA, lateral hypothalamic area.

disconnection of the amygdala tried to check objects through other available sensory modalities such as gustatory (oral tendency?) or somesthetic information (Horel and Keating, 1969). Similarly, animals in which the amygdala was visually disconnected did not respond to visually presented stimuli with biological significance, but did show fear responses to somesthetic stimuli (Downer, 1961).

Amygdala cooling mainly depressed excitatory or inhibitory lateral hypothalamic responses related to visual or ingestion signals, and decreased or increased the spontaneous firing rates of lateral hypothalamic neurons. This is consistent with our previous studies, in which the effects of amygdala stimulation on lateral hypothalamic neurons were generally caused by either inhibition or disinhibition (Oomura et al., 1970; Ono et al., 1981b; Oomura and Ono, 1982). Taken together, our analysis of the neural relationships between the inferotemporal cortex, amygdala, and lateral hypothalamus indicates that the amygdala mediates sensory integration and permits links between the inferotemporal cortex and the lateral hypothalamus. These views, which are similar to a suggestion proposed by Rolls (1981), based on the finding that the latency of neurons to respond to visual stimuli increased as one went from the inferotemporal cortex to the lateral hypothalamic area, are summarized in Figure 11.

ACKNOWLEDGMENTS

We thank Dr. A. Simpson, Showa University, for advice and help with the manuscript and Ms. A. Tabuchi and Ms. Yamazaki for typing. Parts of this work were supported partly by Japanese Ministry of Education, Science and Culture Grants-in-Aid for Scientific Research 02255106 and 382350018577, and by Uehara Memorial Foundation.

REFERENCES

Amaral DG, Veazey RB, Cowan WM (1982): Some observations on hypothalamo-amygdaloid connections in the monkey. Brain Res 252:13–27.

Aggleton JP, Burton MJ, Passingham RE (1980): Cortical and subcortical afferents to the amygdala of the rhesus monkey (*Macaca mulatta*). Brain Res 190:347–368.

Bartoshuk LM (1989): The functions of taste and olfaction. In Schneider LH, Cooper SJ, Halmi KA (eds): "The Psychology of Human Eating Disorders" (Ann NY Acad Sci vol 575). New York: New York Academy of Science, pp 353–362.

Cohen NJ, Squire LR (1980): Preserved learning and retention of pattern analyzing skill in amnesia: Dissociation of knowing how and knowing that. Science 210:207–209.

Desimone R, Albright TD, Gross CG, Bruce C (1984): Stimulus-selective properties of inferior temporal neurons in the macaque. J Neurosci 4:2051–2062.

Downer JDeC (1961): Changes in visual gnostic functions and emotional behavior following unilateral temporal lobe damage in 'split-brain' monkey. Nature (Lond) 191:50–51.

Fukuda M, Ono T, Nishino H, Sasaki K (1986): Visual responses related to food discrimination in monkey lateral hypothalamus during operant feeding behavior. Brain Res 374:249–259.

Fukuda M, Ono T, Nakamura K (1987): Functional relations among inferotemporal cortex, amygdala, and lateral hypothalamus in monkey operant feeding behavior. J Neurophysiol 57:1060–1077.

Fuster JM, Jervey JP (1982): Neuronal firing in the inferotemporal cortex of the monkey in a visual memory task. J Neurosci 2:361–375.

Gaffan EA, Gaffan D, Harrison S (1988): Disconnection of the amygdala from visual association cortex impairs visual reward association learning in monkeys. J Neurosci 8:3144–3150.

Geschwind N (1965): Disconnection syndromes in animals and man. Brain 88:237–294.

Gloor P (1960): Amygdala. In Field J (ed): "Handbook of Physiology, Neurophysiology," Vol 2. Washington, DC: American Physiological Society, pp 1395–1420.

Goddard GV (1964): Functions of the amygdala. Psych Bull 62:89–109.

Gross CG, Bender DB, Rocha-Miranda CF (1969): Visual receptive fields of neurons in inferotemporal cortex of the monkey. Science 116:1303–1306.

Hilton SM, Zbrozyna AW (1963): Amygdaloid region for defence reactions and its afferent pathways to the brain stem. J Physiol (Lond) 165:160–173.

Hopkins DA, Holstege G (1978): Amygdaloid projections to the mesencephalon, pons and medulla oblongata in the cat. Exp Brain Res 32:529–547.

Horel JA, Keating EG (1969): Partial Klüver-Bucy syndrome produced by cortical disconnection. Brain Res 16:281–284.

Horel JA, Keating EG, Misantone LJ (1975): Partial Klüver-Bucy syndrome produced by destroying temporal neocortex or amygdala. Brain Res 94:347–359.

Iwai E, Nishino T, Yamaguchi K (1986): Neuropsychological basis of a K-B sign in Klüver-Bucy syndrome produced following total removal of inferotemporal cortex of macaque monkeys. In Oomura Y (ed): "Emotions: Neural and Chemical Control." Tokyo: Japan Scientific Societies Press, pp 299–321.

Iwai E, Yukie M (1987): Amygdalofugal and amygdalopetal connections with modality-specific visual cortical areas in Macaques (Macaca fuscata, M. mulatta, and M. fascicularis). J Comp Neurol 261:362–387.

Jasper H, Shacter DG, Montplaisir J (1970): The effects of local cooling upon spontaneous and evoked electrical activity of cerebral cortex. Can J Physiol Pharmacol 48:640–652.

Johnston JB (1923): Further contributions to the study of the evolution of the forebrain. J Comp Neurol 35:337–481.

Jones B, Mishkin M (1972): Limbic lesions and the problem of stimulus-reinforcement associations. Exp Neurol 36:362–377.

Kaada BR (1972): Stimulation and regional ablation of the amygdaloid complex with reference to functional representations. In Eleftheriou BE (ed): "The Neurobiology of the Amygdala." New York: Plenum Press, pp 205–281.

Klüver H, Bucy PC (1939): Preliminary analysis of functions of the temporal lobes in monkeys. Arch Neurol Psychiatr 42:979–1000.

Krettek JE, Price JL (1978): Amygdaloid projections to subcortical structures within the basal forebrain and brainstem in the rat and cat. J Comp Neurol 178:225–254.

Kusama T, Mabuchi M (1970): "Stereotaxic Atlas of the Brain of Macaca fuscata." Tokyo: Tokyo University Press.

Miserendino MDJ, Sananes CB, Melia KR, Davis M (1990): Blocking of acquisition but not expression of conditioned fear-potentiated startle by NMDA antagonists in the amygdala. Nature 345:716–718.

Mishkin M, Aggleton J (1981): Multiple functional contributions of the amygdala in the monkey. In Ben-Ari Y (ed): "The Amygdaloid Complex." Amsterdam: Elsevier/North-Holland Biomedical, pp 409–420.

Mishkin M, Malamut B, Bachevalier J (1984): Memories and habits: Two neural systems. In Lynch G, McGaugh JL, Weinberger NM (eds): "Neurobiology of Learning and Memory." New York: Guilford, pp 65–77.

Miyashita Y (1988): Neuronal correlate of visual associate long-term memory in the primate temporal cortex. Nature 335:817–820.

Miyashita Y, Chang HS (1988): Neuronal correlate of pictorial short-term memory in the primate temporal cortex. Nature 331:68–70.

Nakano Y, Lenard L, Oomura Y, Nishino H, Aou S, Yamamoto T (1987): Functional involvement of catecholamines in reward related neuronal activity of the monkey amygdala. J Neurophysiol 57:72–91.

Nishijo H, Ono T, Nakamura K, Kawabata M, Yamatani K (1986): Neuron activity in and adjacent to the dorsal amygdala of monkey during operant feeding behavior. Brain Res Bull 17:847–854.

Nishijo H, Ono T, Nishino H (1988a): Single neuron responses in amygdala of alert monkey during complex sensory stimulation with affective significance. J Neurosci 8:3570–3583.

Nishijo H, Ono T, Nishino H (1988b): Topographic distribution of modality-specific amygdalar neurons in alert monkey. J Neurosci 8:3556–3569.

Norgren R, Nishijo H, Travers SP (1989): Taste responses from the entire gustatory apparatus. In Schneider LH, Cooper SJ, Halmi KA (eds): "The Psychology of Human Disorders" (Ann NY Acad Sci, vol 575). New York: New York Academy of Science, pp 246–264.

Ono T, Fukuda M, Nishino H, Sasaki K, Muramoto K (1983): Amygdaloid neuronal responses to complex visual stimuli in an operant feeding situation in the monkey. Brain Res Bull 11:515–518.

Ono T, Luiten PGM, Nishijo H, Fukuda M, Nishino H (1985): Topographic organization of projections from the amygdala to the hypothalamus of the rat. Neurosci Res 21:221–239.

Ono T, Nishijo H, Nakamura K, Tamura R, Tabuchi E (1988): Role of amygdala and hypothalamic neurons in emotion and behavior. In Takagi H, Oomura Y, Ito M, Otsuka M (eds): "Biowarning System in the Brain." Tokyo: University of Tokyo Press, pp 309–331.

Ono T, Nishino H, Sasaki K, Fukuda M, Muramoto K (1980): Role of the lateral hypothalamus and the amygdala in feeding behavior. Brain Res Bull (Suppl 4) 5:143–149.

Ono T, Nishino H, Sasaki K, Fukuda M, Muramoto K (1981a): Monkey lateral hypothalamic neuron response to sight of food, and during bar press and ingestion. Neurosci Lett 21:99–104.

Ono T, Oomura Y, Nishino H, Sasaki K, Fukuda M, Muramoto K (1981b): Neural mechanisms of feeding behavior. In Katsuki Y, Norgren R, Sato M (eds): "Brain Mechanisms of Sensation." New York: John Wiley & Sons, pp 271–286.

Oomura Y, Ono T (1982): Mechanism of inhibition by the amygdala in the lateral hypothalamic area of rats. Brain Res Bull 8:653–666.

Oomura Y, Ono T, Ooyama H (1970): Inhibitory action of the amygdala on the lateral hypothalamic area in rats. Nature 228:1108–1110.

Perrett DI, Rolls ET, Caan W (1982): Visual neurons responsive to faces in the monkey temporal cortex. Exp Brain Res 47:329–342.

Pons TP, Garraghty PE, Friedman DP, Mishkin M (1987): Physiological evidence for serial processing in somatosensory cortex. Science 237:417–420.

Pons TP, Garraghty PE, Friedman DP, Mishkin M (1987): Physiological evidence for serial processing in somatosensory cortex. Science 237:417–420.

Pribram KH, Bagshaw M (1953): Further analysis of the temporal lobe syndrome utilizing frontotemporal ablations. J Comp Neurol 99:347–357.

Price JL (1981): Toward a consistent terminology for the amygdaloid complex. In Ben-Ari Y (ed): "The Amygdaloid Complex." Amsterdam: Elsevier/North Holland Biomedical, pp 13–18.

Price JL, Amaral DG (1981): An autoradiographic study of the projections of the central nucleus of the monkey amygdala. J Neurosci 1:1242–1259.

Rolls ET (1981): Processing beyond the inferior temporal visual cortex related to feeding, memory, and striatal function. In Katsuki Y, Norgren R, Soto M (eds): "Brain Mechanisms of Sensation." New York: John Wiley and Sons.

Russchen FT, Bakst I, Amaral DG, Price JL (1985): The amygdalostriatal projections in the monkey. An anterograde tracing study. Brain Res 329:241–257.

Sanghera MK, Rolls ET, Roper-Hall A (1979): Visual responses of neurons in the dorsolateral amygdala of the alert monkey. Exp Neurol 63:610–626.

Sato T, Kawamura T, Iwai E (1980): Responsiveness of inferotemporal single units to visual pattern stimuli in monkeys performing discrimination. Exp Brain Res 38:313–319.

Schwaber JS, Kapp BS, Higgins GA, Rapp PR (1982): Amygdaloid and basal forebrain direct connections with the nucleus of the solitary tract and the dorsal motor nucleus. J Neurosci 2:1424–1438.

Schwartzbaum JS (1965): Discrimination behavior after amygdalectomy in monkeys: Visual and somesthetic learning and perceptual capacity. J Comp Physiol Psychol 60:314–319.

Selemon LD, Goldman-Rakic PS (1985): Longitudinal topography and interdigitation of corticostriatal projections in the rhesus monkey. J Neurosci 5:776–794.

Spiegler BJ, Mishkin M (1981): Evidence for the sequential participation of inferior temporal cortex and amygdala in the acquisition of stimulus-reward associations. Behav Brain Res 3:307–317.

Turner BH, Mishkin M, Knapp M (1980): Organization of the amygdalopetal projections from modality-specific cortical association areas in the monkey. J Comp Neurol 191:515–543.

Veening JG, Swanson LW, Sawchenko PE (1984): The organization of projections from the central nucleus of the amygdala to brainstem sites involved in central autonomic regulation: A combined retrograde transport-immunohistochemical study. Brain Res 303:337–357.

Weiskrantz L (1956): Behavioral changes associated with ablation of the amygdaloid complex in monkeys. J Comp Physiol Psychol 49:381–391.

Weiskrantz L, Saunders RC (1984): Impairments of visual object transforms in monkeys. Brain 107:1033–1072.

Zola-Morgan S, Squire LR (1984): Preserved learning in monkeys with medial temporal lesions: Sparing of motor and cognitive skills. J Neurosci 4:1072–1085.

Zola-Morgan S, Squire LR, Mishkin M (1982): The neuroanatomy of amnesia: Amygdala-hippocampus versus temporal stem. Science 218:1337–1339.

The Amygdala: Neurobiological Aspects of Emotion,
Memory, and Mental Dysfunction, pages 191–228

7

Emotional Neurophysiology of the Amygdala Within the Context of Human Cognition

ERIC HALGREN

Regional Epilepsy Center, Wadsworth Veterans Affairs Medical Center; the Department of Psychiatry and Brain Research Institute, University of California, Los Angeles, California; and INSERM, Clinique Neurologique, Hôpital Pontchaillou, Rennes, France

INTRODUCTION

The amygdala has all of the right connections with the cognitive neocortex and visceral brain stem to provide the link between them that is central to emotion. This role has been confirmed by the dramatic effects on emotional behavior of amygdala lesions in animals. In humans, the case reports of Klüver-Bucy syndromes after lesions that include the amygdala (Terzian and Ore, 1955), or of uncontrolled rage after electrical stimulation of the amygdala (Mark et al., 1975), seem to imply that it plays the same critical role in our species.

However, explaining the phenomena of emotion by reference to neural mechanisms in the amygdala still requires the use of enigmas to explain mysteries. Conflated with emotion are centuries of religious and philosophical speculations as to why we act and feel (Jaynes, 1982). These echoes and reflections of emotion are lost when emotion is experimentally studied, especially in animals. Conversely, animal experiments frequently provoke overt manifestations of fear and aggression—e.g., defecating from fear, or physically attacking to kill—that few of us will ever experience firsthand.

Since its birth, psychology has been centrally concerned with the mechanism of emotion. Specifically at issue has been the necessity and order of Conscious versus preConscious versus Unconscious evaluations, and the temporal/epistemological primacy of Conscious versus bodily events in emotion (for reviews, see Plutchik, 1980; Panksepp, 1982; Ohman, 1987). Classically, the controversy begins with the assertion by James (1884) that physiological responses are necessary antecedents to emotional feelings (Fig. 1A). Stimuli are thought to directly activate bodily responses and these responses are then introspectively noted. With the resulting cognitive inferences, these introspections constitute the emotion. This theory was countered by Cannon (1939; Fig. 1B), who demonstrated that visceral responses were neither necessary nor sufficient for emotion, and that the range and rate of autonomic changes did not correspond to

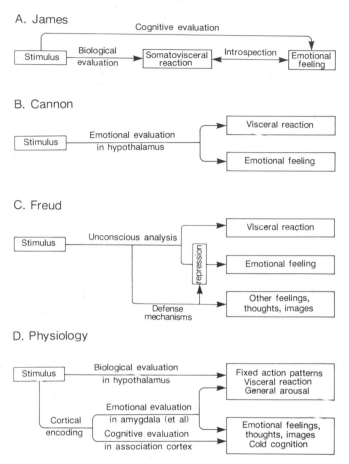

Fig. 1. Four different views of the order and necessity of preConscious, Unconscious, ·or Conscious processing, and of Bodily or Cognitive events, in the genesis of emotional experience.

changes in emotion. Based upon his finding that rage could easily by evoked in cats after transection above but not below the hypothalamus, Cannon proposed that stimuli directly activate the hypothalamus, which then evoke both somatic and subjective aspects of emotion through its descending and ascending projections, respectively.

This model bears some functional resemblance to that earlier proposed by Freud (1949; Fig. 1C). However, psychoanalytic models incorporate much more complex processing (by the Unconscious) prior to entry of the emotion into Consciousness. This processing can lead to defense mechanisms (repression, denial, undoing, projection, displacement, etc.) that may distort or eliminate the Conscious experience of the emotion (Rado, 1969; Brenner, 1974).

These disparate models continue to animate experimental investigation. Although Cannon's claim that the visceral concomitants of various emotions are essentially identical has continued to be supported, claims of differential responses persist (Ohman, 1987; Levenson, 1988; Levenson et al., 1990). In addition, cognition has received an increasingly important role in assigning emotional specificity based upon the psychosocial context in which the autonomic arousal occurs (Lazarus et al., 1970; Mandler, 1975; Schachter, 1975; but see Plutchik and Ax, 1967; Plutchik, 1980). It should also be noted that James included somatomotor as well as visceromotor reactions as direct responses to an arousing stimulus. Specifically, facial expressions are rapid and emotion-specific (Izard and Buechler, 1979), consistent across widely isolated cultural groups (Ekman, 1982), and even similar across species (Darwin, 1872). Thus facial expressions are to some degree innate, and could provide a biologically reliable system for intrapersonal as well as interpersonal communication of emotional state (Levenson et al., 1990).

While these studies show that visceral and facial responses have a role in emotion, they do not demonstrate that they are necessary precursors for the Conscious appreciation of emotional significance. The alternative view, dating from Cannon, that emotional significance is immediately appreciated, without visceral or cognitive mediation, has found experimental support in the work of Zajonc (1980). He showed that nonsense figures, presented so rapidly that they are not consciously perceived, may later be preferred to figures that have never been presented. As important as this finding is, it is not clear that one can make a general conclusion regarding the genesis of emotion from a slight aesthetic preference which may be due to greater ease of processing, rather than to any primary affective evaluation.

Thus, these important issues regarding the temporal and causal relationship of cognition versus visceral activation in emotion, raised and defined by psychological analysis, remain unresolved by psychological experiments. The apparent evolutionary continuity of emotions suggests that brain research in animals may provide a solution. Cannon's hypothalamic theory survives, but surrounded and elaborated by various intermediary limbic structures (Papez, 1937; Pribram and Kruger, 1954; Arnold, 1960; Maclean, 1972). In these theories, the amygdala plays a prominent role, but only in situations that are complex because the affective stimulus is either complex, or must be learned, or the required response runs counter to those already prepotent (e.g., type B rather than type A behaviors in Fig. 2; Goddard, 1964).

This poses the question: Does the additional complexity of human motivational structure (Fig. 2C) make the amygdala relatively even more important than in mammals, or does it make the amygdala superfluous? I argue here that the effects of lesioning or stimulating the human amygdala suggests that it has a less crucial role in behavior than in lower animals. However, this decreased necessity for the amygdala is not due to a role confined to reflexive actions that are unimportant in humans. Rather, recording as well as stimulation and lesion evidence clearly indicates that the human amygdala receives both high-level cognitive as well as visceral inputs, and that it influences the contents

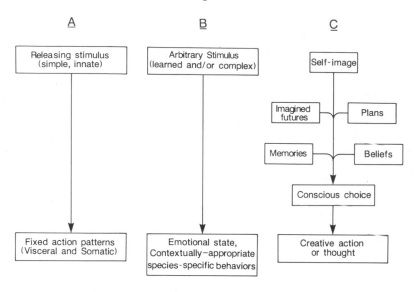

Fig. 2. Three levels of complexity in the evolution of motivated behavior. The first level (**A**) is hypothesized to be mediated by the hypothalamic/brain stem axis. The second level (**B**) is mediated by the amygdala in concert with the hypothalamus. Complex perceptions and memories are integrated in the amygdala with the autonomic state, resulting in the assignment of emotional valence to stimuli by evoking appropriate visceromotor accompaniments. The highest level (**C**) is something of a caricature of the "higher-level" motivational mechanisms that nonetheless must be considered in explaining such prominent aspects of human behavior as voluntary fasts during Ramadan.

and quality of awareness as well as the autonomic state. While the human amygdala may thus play a key role in relating biologically motivated emotions to cognition, its role in humans is limited by the development of alternate pathways (involving especially the prefrontal cortex), and possibly of motivations that are not biological in origin. Finally, the evidence reviewed below clearly indicates that the amygdala is involved in the evaluation of complex stimuli long before they are completely analyzed cognitively, and probably long before they enter awareness. However, this amygdala processing appears to be integrated with the neocortical cognitive processing that leads to conscious awareness, resulting in a model for the genesis of emotion that is distinct from the James, Cannon, and Freud models (see Fig. 1D).

LESIONS

The effects of unilateral or bilateral amygdala lesions on memory were exhaustively reviewed 10 years ago (Halgren, 1981). No convincing evidence for a decrement in verbal or nonverbal, primary, recent or remote memory had been reported, and subsequent studies only confirm this conclusion. For example, no deficit in cross-modal learning was found in one patient after bilateral amygdala lesions (Lee et al., 1988). One patient with bilateral amygdala lesions was reported to have a deficit in nonverbal recent memory (Tranel and Hyman, 1990) but this patient also had probable complex partial seizures, which are often accompanied by hippocampal dysfunction (Halgren et al., 1991b). Furthermore, additional cases of amnesia with hippocampal but no amygdala damage have been reported (e.g., Zola-Morgan et al., 1986). It cannot, however, be definitively concluded that human amygdala lesions have no effect on memory because most studies have been of stereotaxically induced lesions, which may destroy less than half of the amygdala (Adams and Rutkin, 1969). Furthermore, the amygdala may be specialized for learning to associate visceral states with complex cognitions (see below and Fig. 9), and such high-level emotional learning has apparently not been tested after amygdala lesions.

The overall finding reported previously (Halgren, 1981), that amygdala lesions produce a general decrease in emotional tension, continues to be reported, albeit based upon clinical evaluations that are neither done blindly nor incorporate a control group of any kind (see Chapter 19, Aggleton, this volume). For example, Ramamurthi (1988) reports that of a large series (603 total, 481 bilateral amygdalotomies, some with epilepsy, many children) operated on for extreme restlessness and unprovoked aggression due to presumed brain damage, 70–76% showed a moderate or excellent improvement. A case study of the well-known subject H.M., who had received bilateral surgical removal of the hippocampal formation, uncus, temporal pole, and amygdala, reported that he lacks the ability to introspect into his state of hunger, thirst, or pain (Hebben et al., 1985).

The classical evidence for the involvement of the amygdala in emotion is the Klüver-Bucy syndrome, first observed in monkeys after bilateral anterior temporal lobectomy (Klüver and Bucy, 1939). In humans, the full syndrome consisting of psychic blindness, hyperorality, extreme distractability, and altered sexual behavior, is extremely rare (Rossitch et al., 1989). This rarity suggests that other damage may be necessary for its appearance. For example, H.M. displays none of the classic symptoms (Corkin, 1984), and as noted earlier, amygdalotomy is commonly performed as elective surgery to decrease restlessness. Even the original highly cited case of Terzian and Ore (1955) was suicidal and had rage attacks before receiving bilateral anterior temporal lobectomy, strongly suggesting the possibility of extratemporal brain abnormalities. At a minimum, lesions causing the Klüver-Bucy syndrome have been noted to damage, in addition to the amygdala and uncus, the hippocampal formation and cingulate gyrus, and the orbitofrontal, insular, and temporal cortices (Guard et al., 1982).

Consistent with this view is the finding of Klüver-Bucy-like symptoms in more diffuse diseases that include the amygdala. For example, in Alzheimer's disease, amygdala pathology is common, and appears to be correlated with Klüver-Bucy symptoms (Herzog and Kemper, 1980; see Chapter 23, Mann, this volume). These symptoms are also characteristic of Pick's disease, a presenile dementia that preferentially attacks the temporal lobes (Cummings and Duchen, 1981). Lastly, there is growing evidence of an amygdaloid involvement in schizophrenia, and the serotonin metabolite 5HIAA is increased in the amygdala of people who have committed suicide (Cheetham et al., 1989; Kirkpatrick and Buchanan, 1990; Roberts and Burton, 1990; Chapter 22, Reynolds, this volume).

One may conclude that by itself, amygdala damage seems to have little effect, although controlled and blinded pre/postoperative studies with large patient groups still have not been performed. Nonetheless, current evidence suggests the possibility that major psychological abnormalities could result from amygdala damage in the presence of pre-existing or concomitant diffuse brain abnormalities. If true, this would be consistent with a role for the amygdala in emotion that is crucial, but which can be compensated for by other structures if amygdala damage occurs in the otherwise normal brain. This view is supported by the results of stimulating, or recording from, the human amygdala, to which we now turn.

STIMULATION

Extensive reviews of the effects of amygdala stimulation have been published (see Halgren et al., 1978a; Halgren, 1981, 1982; Gloor, 1991; Wieser, 1991). Such stimulation can result in a broad variety of phenomena, including hallucinations (dreamlike, memorylike, or thoughtlike), emotions (almost always fear), *déjà vu*, visceral sensations (usually epigastric, but also referred to the heart or chest), autonomic changes, hormonal secretions, oroalimentary movements, and loss of contact. Even within a group of patients who were all implanted in the same multiple locations in the medial temporal lobe (including amygdala), which of these phenomena occurred was not related to electrode position, but rather to factors specific to the person stimulated, and in particular to his or her personality (Fig. 3). Within a given patient, the category of mental phenomenon evoked tends to be constant across sites within a given session, but may be different on another day (e.g., Halgren et al., 1978a). Furthermore, the content of the auditory, visual, or olfactory hallucination may be related to the patient's personality and ongoing concerns, and to the psychodynamic context of the stimulation session (Mahl et al., 1964; Horowitz, 1967; Horowitz et al., 1968; Ferguson et al., 1969; Horowitz and Adams, 1970; Rayport and Ferguson, 1974).

A variety of viscerosensory phenomena have been reported, referred to the head, heart, chest, or stomach. Gustatory sensations may also be evoked, most likely when the discharge spreads to the insular cortex (Hausser-Hauw and Bancaud, 1987), as well as thirst (Remillard et al., 1981). Sexual feelings (Bancaud et al.,1970; Stoffels et al., 1980) have also occasionally been reported, especially in women (Remillard et al., 1983). By far the most common evoked visceral feeling is the epigastric sensation, which typically rises from the stomach up the chest to the throat and head (Herpin, 1867; Gowers, 1907). Interestingly, patients may describe this sensation physically (like "being about to belch," or like nausea), or like an emotion (usually fear, sometimes guilt, or nervousness, or even anger) (Van Buren, 1963; Halgren et al., 1978a). Intragastric recordings during these sensations indicate that they are true hallucinations, rather than indirectly due to evoked gastric movements (Van Buren, 1963). Again, Bancaud (1981) has suggested that epigastric sensations are evoked by amygdala stimulation when the discharge spreads to the insular cortex. The possibility that the cortical representation of visceral sensations is located in the insula is difficult to evaluate because the large number of blood vessels traversing this region has generally prevented its exploration with depth electrodes. However, Penfield

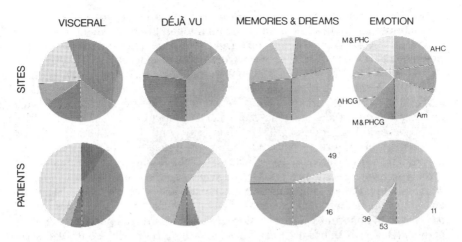

Fig. 3. Distribution of different categories of stimulation-evoked mental phenomena, according to the site (**above**), or to the person (**below**), that was stimulated. Note that each of the different categories of mental phenomena tended to be evoked from all of the medial temporal lobe sites (M&PHC: middle and posterior hippocampus; AHC: anterior hippocampus; Am: amygdala; M&PHCG: middle and posterior parahippocampal gyrus; AHCG: anterior parahippocampal gyrus). In contrast, most of the stimulations evoking a given category were obtained from only two or three of the 36 patients studied (different patients are indicated by their patient numbers: 11, 16, 36, 49, and 53. Data from Halgren et al., 1978a.

and Faulk (1955) found that in contrast to the amygdala, stimulation of the insular cortex only evokes epigastric sensations in conjunction with clear changes in gastric motility, and that gastric movements may be evoked by insular stimulation without any conscious sensation. It thus seems possible that amygdala stimulation evokes epigastric sensations directly through activation of learned associations with previous events that had more actively involved the insula (see below and Fig. 9).

In contrast to epigastric sensations, sexual feelings evoked by amygdala stimulation are usually accompanied by appropriate autonomic and visceral output, and other visceromotor phenomena are also commonly observed; bradypnea or polynea (Bancaud, 1981), transient increases in heart rate (Chapman et al., 1954), mydriasis (Bancaud et al., 1965; Wieser, 1983; Swartz et al., 1990), and a decrease in skin resistance (Van Buren, 1963). Interestingly, these phenomena are seldom reported by the patients themselves, even though their awareness is still intact. At somewhat higher levels of activation, but still without necessarily any loss of contact, characteristic chewing and lip-smacking movements (termed "oro-alimentary automatisms") may occur (Munari et al., 1979; Bancaud, 1981). Amygdala stimulation that provokes a high-frequency afterdischarge results in an increased secretion of prolactin and ACTH (Parra et al., 1980; Sperling and Wilson, 1986; Gallagher et al., 1987).

It is interesting to note that sexual automatisms are not evoked from amygdala stimulation, but rather from the frontal lobe, and especially the anterior cingulate gyrus (Spencer et al., 1983; Delgado-Escueta et al., 1987). Similarly, rage has occasionally been reported (Heath and Mickle, 1960; Hitchcock and Cairns, 1973; Mark et al., 1975), but not in the larger series of patients (Chapman, 1958; Halgren et al., 1978a; Gloor et al., 1982; Wieser, 1991). Reports of aggression during seizures involving the amygdala are rare, and appear usually or always to reflect a confusional state due to postictal depression of the forebrain (Delgado-Escueta et al., 1981). Attempts to control the patient in this state can evoke poorly directed attacks that seem defensive, rather than a well-coordinated attack intended to inflict harm. Thus this "aggression" resembles the "hypothalamic sham rage," which has a clearly dissociated anatomical substrate from predatory killing in other mammals (Albert and Walsh, 1984). Similarly, the often-quoted "temporal lobe" personality characteristics, hypothesized to arise from abnormal affective coloring due to amygdala epileptiform hyperactivity (Bear, 1979), has not been possible to confirm in well-controlled studies (Rodin, 1969; Stevens, 1991).

At higher stimulus intensities, when the afterdischarge appears to spread to the diencephalon, the patient becomes unresponsive with a fixed motionless stare ("arrest reaction": Munari et al., 1980; Gloor et al., 1980). The mechanism of this loss of contact is unknown. However, it is interesting to note that it is accompanied by widespread electroencephalogram (EEG) changes (Delgado-Escueta et al.,1977), that amygdala stimulation may also have diffuse EEG effects (Laitinen and Toivakka, 1980), and that the amygdala is one of the principal sources of afferents to the nucleus basalis of Meynert (Price et al., 1981; Russchen et al., 1985; Irle and Markowitsch, 1986; Alheid and Heimer, 1988), whose cholinergic cells may control neocortical EEG (Riekkinen et al., 1991).

One may conclude that amygdala stimulation can evoke the various subjective mental phenomena of emotion (feelings, dreamlike or memorylike images, and visceral sensations), as well as the bodily signs of emotion (visceromotor activation, general arousal, hormal secretion, and facial movements). It is somewhat disturbing that although all of these modalities of emotional experience and expression are evoked, the categories of emotion within a given modality are somewhat limited. That is, different aspects of fear may be represented as the feeling itself, or as associated visceral sensations, autonomic phenomena, formed hallucinations, or general arousal, alone or in combination. Sexual feelings, and thirst, while they occur, are much less common, as are their associated visceral phenomena, and anger, elation, and hunger are nearly absent. While this may suggest that the amygdala has a special role in the integration of fear, it is also possible that this apparent focus is an artifact of the psychosocial context of the stimulation, and/or of the fact that stimulation does not provoke normal activity but a hypersynchronous activation/inhibition whose relation to normal activity is problematical, but certainly involves some degree of disruption. This disrupted amygdala firing would presumably be part of the neural network that encodes the emotion, and might bias the label of the emotion toward fear (cf. Fischer, 1970).

Within a few synapses, every part of the brain is connected with every other part. What then is the real significance of this overwhelming richness of mental and behavioral phenomena? Do they simply represent the spread of activation to other structures, or do they confirm that the amygdala is a central integrative structure normally capable of evoking all of the various aspects of emotion? The fact that most amygdala stimulations evoke no mental phenomenon even when they are strong enough to provoke an afterdischarge supports the importance of spread to distant structures (Halgren et al., 1978a). Indeed, behaviorally effective stimulation of the amygdala nearly always evokes either afterdischarges or evoked potentials in the neighboring hippocampal formation, and vice versa. Thus, localization of sites that when stimulated evoke different mental phenomena within the medial temporal lobe seems fruitless. However, similar phenomena have also been evoked by stimulation of distant sites where the amygdala is known to project. For example, memorylike and dreamlike hallucinations have been reported after stimulation of lateral temporal sites (Penfield and Perot, 1963; Brunet-Bourgin, 1984), fear can be evoked in various limbic sites (Halgren, 1982), and horror with sympathetic arousal in the hypothalamus (Laitinen, 1988; Sano and Mayanagi, 1988). However, the full constellation of phenomena observed after medial temporal lobe stimulation has not been observed elsewhere. Furthermore, it is much more difficult to evoke memory- or dreamlike hallucinations from temporal neocortex than from the amygdala, and when they are evoked they seem to involve a spread of activation from neocortex to amygdala (Gloor et al., 1982; Gloor, 1990; Wieser, 1991). It seems reasonable in fact to suppose that a phenomenon as complex as a formed mental image reflects the activity of quite widespread and integrated neural networks, and this is why their occurrence and content is so dependent on personal and contextual variables (Chauvel et al., 1989).

RECORDING
Emotional Correlates

Narabayashi et al. (1963) and Andy and Jurko (1977) have reported that the amygdala of aggressive nonepileptic patients seems more prone to generate EEG spikes, EEG spindles, and injury discharges than that of nonaggressive patients. Several different groups of researchers, in rather large numbers of psychotic patients, have reported spikes in the amygdala or surrounding structures during psychotic behavior or psychological stress (Sem-Jacobsen et al., 1955, 1956; Stevens et al., 1969; Hanley et al., 1970). During the recall of emotional memories, Heath and coworkers (Heath, 1958, 1964; Less et al., 1965) reported that 14 of 51 psychotic patients displayed 18–35 Hz spindles in the amygdala and anterior hippocampus. Similar spindles have found to be evoked in the amygdala by sniffing (see below), which was not controlled for in Heath's study.

We examined amygdala EEG and unit activity in seven nonpsychotic patients during the recall and discussion of emotional memories. Electrodes were implanted in order to localize the onset of medically uncontrolled complex partial seizures so that the focus could be surgically removed (Walter, 1973). Fifty amygdala units were discriminated from 19 fine-wire electrodes. Three units

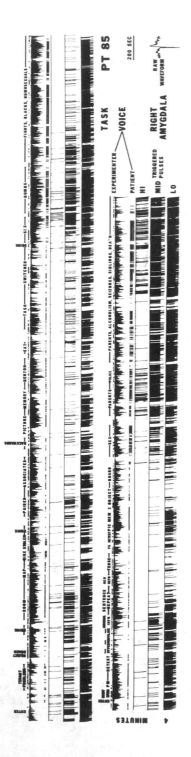

Fig. 4. Activity of three units from a right amygdala electrode during a 2 3/4 hour interview showing large increases in firing when the patient is speaking about emotional topics. Periods when the patient is speaking are indicated by the lines below the voice track. A single line underscores unemotional speech (e.g, digit span), two lines denote mildly emotional topics (e.g., theft of a bicycle), three lines indicate still more emotive content (e.g., sex), while four lines indicate when the patient's speech was interrupted by sobs. The units also respond, but less strongly, when the patient hyperventilates. Speech from the experimenter is indicated by lines above the voice track. Procedures used in the indicated tasks are described in Halgren et al. (1978b) and Halgren (1991a).

on one electrode showed a delayed but powerful and prolonged increase in firing that seemed to be related to the emotionality of the discussion (Fig. 4). No EEG changes were noted. However, these units also responded after hyperventilation. Subsequent studies have shown that this is a response by the neurons to cardiovascular changes (see below). Since discussion of the emotional memories caused the patient to breathe heavily, and at times to sob, the unit response in Figure 4 may be associated with cardiovascular rather than emotional changes. Thus, the above findings provide some support for activation of the amygdala during highly charged emotional episodes, but also permit alternative interpretations. In any case, the studies are too crude to reveal the cause or significance of this activation.

Sensory Stimuli

Amygdala stimulation evokes various mental and somatic aspects of emotion. Any role of the amygdala in evoking these phenomena will be limited to the information that the amygdala receives. Originally, the amygdala was thought to be closely involved in the reception of olfactory input (Pribram and Kruger, 1954). Modern neuroanatomy has revealed paths whereby information from unimodal and polymodal visual, auditory, and somatosensory association cortices may cascade down into the amygdala (see Chapter 1, Amaral, this volume). An alternate pathway carrying less processed sensory information directly from the thalamus also exists, especially in rodents (Turner et al., 1980; LeDoux, 1986, 1987). In contrast to lower mammals, the human amygdala shows little if any responsiveness to sensory inputs unless they have specific cognitive relevance.

Olfactory

Direct projections of the lateral olfactory tract are limited to nuclei in the corticomedial group, which is relatively small in humans. Although olfactory hallucinations can occur with amygdala stimulation, they are rare and are thought to reflect spread of activation to the uncus (Jackson and Stewart, 1899; Penfield and Jasper, 1954). Most studies have revealed little or no effect of amygdala lesions upon human olfactory function (Eslinger et al., 1982; but see Andy et al., 1975). Eskenazi et al. (1986) recently examined the effect of unilateral removal of the amygdala and hippocampal formation, together with overlying cortex of the temporal pole, uncus, as well as rhinal cortex on olfaction. They found a small decrease in odor identification accuracy, and a larger decrease in odor recognition memory with monorhinic stimulation ipsilateral to the lesion. The specific contribution of the amygdala to this deficit remains problematic.

Fully 40% of rat amygdala units are responsive to odors (Cain and Bindra, 1972). However, the size and distribution of potentials evoked in the amygdala by olfactory bulb stimulation show a clear phylogenetic decrease (Cragg, 1960). We examined the responses of 116 human amygdala units to sniffing from an odorant-filled beaker (Halgren et al., 1977a). No response was found with a latency of less than 8 seconds. When an odorant was introduced into a continuous stream of air passing over the olfactory mucoa, the method used by Cain and Bindra (1972), no response at all was observed, signaling a clear phylogenetic decrease in the importance of smell for the human amygdala.

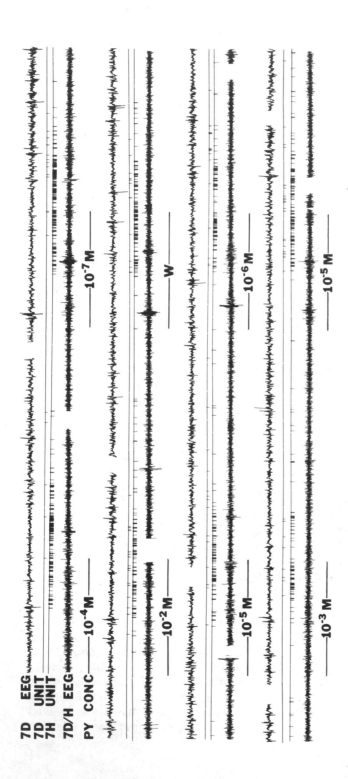

Fig. 5. Odorants evoke in the human amygdala a high-frequency EEG rhythm (to sniffing) and powerful unit-responses (to cere-brovascular changes), but no olfactory responses per se. The patient sniffed from a flask during the underlined 20 second periods. Fast activity is not seen in the amygdala fine-wire 7D when it is referred to the vertex (7D EEG) but is visible in differential recordings 7H (7D/7H EEG). The fast rhythm is strongest with subthreshold odors (10^{-6}M, 10^{-5}M and 10^{-4}M) and weaker with suprathreshold odors (10^{-3}M, 10^{-2}M, and 10^{-1}M), presumably because the patient sniffed more vigorously to identify the weaker odors.

In contrast to the lack of a unit response, respiration-linking spindles (20–30 Hz, 30–50 microV, 1–3 sec duration) have frequently been observed (Angeleri et al., 1964; Pagni and Marrossero, 1965). The spindle is larger medially (Narabayashi, 1980). Monorhinal sniffing produces only ipsilateral spindles (Ganzha, 1986). Some evidence in animals suggests that this spindle is dependent on trigeminal input from the nasal mucosa (Ueki and Domino, 1961), and it is enhanced by more vigorous sniffing (trigeminal input), rather than stronger odorants (olfactory) (Fig. 5). Nonetheless, Hughes and Andy (1979a,b) claim that the frequency of the spindles encodes the type of odor, but this has not been confirmed by Ganzha (1986).

Auditory and Visual

Essentially no responses can be observed in human amygdala unit-firing to simple, moderately bright flashes (none of 166 units) or moderately loud clicks (one of 157 units), which are attended but not responded to (Wilson et al., 1984). Again, this may represent a true phylogenetic decrease in responsiveness to sensory stimuli. Nishijo et al. (1988) found in the macaque that 6.8% of basolateral neurons were responsive to visual stimuli, 4% to auditory, and 20% to both visual and auditory. A similar proportion of visually responsive cells was found in monkeys by Sanghera et al. (1979) and in cats by O'Keefe and Bouma (1968). It seems unlikely that the lack of visually or auditorily responsive cells in humans was due to electrode location—both monkey and human recordings were from the basolateral nuclear complex. The lack of a behavioral task might have decreased the number of responsive units in humans. However, Halgren et al. (1978c) and Heit et al. (1990) recorded from a total of 66 amygdala units during a variety of tasks presented on slides. Only two units responded to all slides, suggesting a visual response.

Interoceptive

A strikingly greater proportion of cells in the cat amygdala are responsive to input from the carotid body (46%) than from exteroceptors (17%: Schutze et al., 1987; Avatisian et al., 1988). Substantial convergence was found between interoceptive and exteroceptive inputs. This led us to reevaluate our previous finding that about 25% of 116 human amygdala units have clear firing-rate changes to hyperventilation (Halgren et al., 1977b). Hyperventilation decreases arterial CO_2 concentration, raising blood pH and evoking cerebral vasoconstriction. When the patients hyperventilated 93% O_2/7% CO_2, the units that were inhibited after hyperventilation of room air were now excited, and vice versa, confirming that it is the cardiovascular rather than sensory or motor effects of hyperventilation that influence amygdala firing. Recently, Frysinger and Harper (1989) extended these results, showing that not only did 11% of human amygdala units have a tonic firing rate related to tonic respiratory period, but 19% had a tonic rate correlated with the tonic heart rate, and 26% were related to the cardiac cycle. Neither our data nor that of Frysinger and Harper (1989) eliminate a possible role of local input (for example, a change in the local partial pressure of oxygen) in modulating cell firing (Halgren et al., 1977b). However, the entrainment of the amygdala firing by the cardiac cycle is similar to that which is characteristic of brain stem neurons involved in the sympathetic system (Gebber and Barman, 1988). Given that a path from carotid body receptors to the amygdala has been demonstrated electrophysiologically and anatomically in cats (Cechetto and Calaresu, 1985; Volz et al., 1990), it seems likely that these responses by human amygdala neurons reflect a strong viscerosensory input.

Cognitive Tasks

Orienting Response

In contrast to the lack of responses to simple auditory and visual stimuli in the human amygdala, very large and consistent responses are seen to stimuli with cognitive significance, regardless of their sensory qualities (Fig. 6). Cognitive brain activity has been studied in the human, mainly using scalp-recording event-related potentials (Hillyard and Picton, 1988; Halgren, 1990a). Typically,

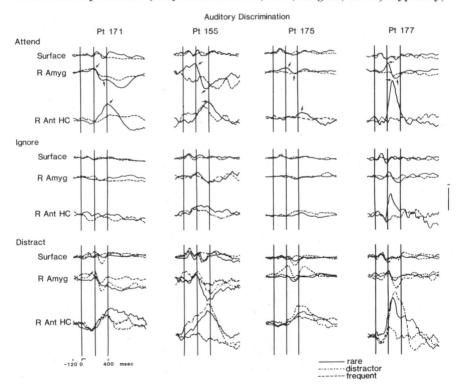

Fig. 6. Potentials evoked in the human medial temporal lobe during auditory discrimination tasks in four patients. Arrows indicate the N2 (at about 200 msec) and P3 in the amygdala and hippocampus (at about 360 msec). The N2/P3 are evoked by task-relevant stimuli in any modality, and are correlated with the Orienting Reflex. The surface site is Cz except for patient 155, for whom it is Fz. The tasks are: Attend, count rare (20%) high tones; Ignore, read a book while the same stimuli are presented; Distract, count rare (15%) high tones in the context of 70% frequent and 15% unique, distracting tones. Calibration = 100 microV, negativity up. From Stapleton and Halgren (1987) with permission.

the EEG is averaged at different delays with respect to the repeated brief presentation of sensory stimuli that must be discriminated, recognized, or otherwise evaluated. Cognitive components are identified as those that change with the cognitive significance of the stimuli, while controlling across trials for sensory characteristics. Across hundreds of such studies using a wide variety of tasks, a series of cognitive evoked potential components labeled N2/P3/SW (also known as N200/P300 or late positive complex/Slow Wave) are observed to follow the sensory components in the auditory, visual, and somatosensory modalities. These components, especially the N2, are prominent within the amygdala (Halgren et al., 1980; Stapleton and Halgren, 1987; McCarthy et al., 1989).

Like the scalp N2/P3 complex, the N2/P3 intracranially recorded from the amygdala is evoked by both visual and auditory stimuli, is much larger to attended than ignored stimuli, and is large to rare attended events in a series, especially if they are behavioral targets or are somehow bizarre (Squire et al., 1983; Stapleton and Halgren, 1987). These potentials are even evoked following the absence of an expected stimulus that is missing from a regular train of stimuli (Stapleton and Halgren, 1987). Within the amygdala, the N2 is generally negative, with an onset latency of 110 msec and a peak latency to simple auditory stimuli of 200 msec (about 40 msec before the scalp). The P3 is positive within the amygdala, but much smaller than in the nearby anterior hippocampus, suggesting that the P3 might be passively volume-conducted from the hippocampus to the amygdala recording electrode. In contrast, the N2 is usually larger in the amygdala than in the hippocampal formation, and thus it is more likely to be locally generated.

One may summarize the cognitive conditions that evoke the N2/P3 as being the presentation of stimuli that are novel or that are signals for behavioral tasks, and thus need to be attended to, and processed. These evoking conditions and functional consequences are identical to these that have been found for the orienting reflex (Sokolov, 1963; Ohman, 1979).

In contrast to the N2/P3, the orienting reflex is usually measured not with the EEG but autonomically (as increased skin conductance, heart rate, and/or blood pressure), in tasks that present fewer trials at longer interstimulus intervals, and that use stimuli that are novel rather than task-relevant. However, when recorded simultaneously, it is found that the visceromotor responses and the N2/P3 are well correlated, even across individual trials (Dykman, 1987), or after startling loud noises (Putnam and Roth, 1987), but can be dissociated on the basis of details of their reaction to repetition or to changes in the task relevance of the stimuli (Naatanen and Gaillard, 1983; Roth et al., 1984; Rosler et al., 1987). An interesting possibility is that there are separable components both of the autonomic orienting reflex and of the N2/P3, one component of each being evoked by task-relevant signals (showing little or no habituation), and the other by surprising, novel but irrelevant stimuli (showing rapid habituation: Maltzman and Pendery, 1991). The signals would evoke a more parietal P3b, and the novel stimuli a more frontal P3a (Verbaten, 1983). Both task-relevant targets and task-irrelevant novel stimuli evoke the amygdala N2/P3 (Stapleton and Halgren, 1987).

In conclusion, the N2/P3 and the autonomic orienting reflex may be considered as constituting different parts of an overall organismic reaction complex evoked by stimuli that merit further evaluation (Roth, 1983; Donchin et al., 1984). This overall reaction is termed in the following discussion the Orienting Complex. Given that the human amygdala not only displays a large N2/P3 but also projects to visceromotor areas, it is clear that the amygdala is crucially situated so as to link the autonomic and cognitive aspects of the Orienting Complex. However, it must be noted that other limbic areas with efferents to visceromotor areas, notably the anterior cingulate gyrus and posterior orbitofrontal cortex, also generate fairly robust N2/P3/SW potentials (Smith et al., 1990). Thus, like the lesion and stimulation evidence reviewed above, recording studies also suggest pathways paralleling the amygdala for cortical-brain stem interaction.

Since the Orienting Complex functions to reorient behavior and cognition toward significant stimuli, it embodies the essence of emotion, as defined by those theories that consider emotion to be a generalized arousal that disrupts ongoing behavior (e.g., Young, 1943; Tolman, 1923). However, for other theorists (e.g., (Panksepp, 1982), the Orienting Complex is too brief and nonspecific to be considered as more than a larval, or preemotion, constituting the primary emotional appraisal that may then lead to secondary appraisal and true emotion. This position has been developed by Ohman (1979; 1987), who suggests that the orienting reflex is associated with "controlled processing." Controlled processing is effortful, slow, at the center of awareness, sequential, single-channel, and creative, as opposed to "automatic," which is effortless, fast, unavailable to awareness, parallel, multiple-channel, and routinized (Shiffrin and Schneider, 1977).

It may seem paradoxical to include the orienting reflex within awareness. However, many studies have found that the orienting reflex is only learned when the subject becomes conscious of the contingency between the conditioned and unconditioned stimuli (Ohman, 1988). Lazarus and McCleary (1951) have found that the orienting reflex may still be expressed to stimuli that have been presented too briefly to be verbally reported. However, even in these studies the interpretation may be made that, at very short stimulus duration, perception occurs but is indirectly and imperfectly linked to either verbal report or autonomic response (Eriksen, 1960). This interpretation receives indirect support from the finding of Dawson and Schell (1982) in a dichotic listening shadowing task that skin conductance responses in the absence of a verbal report are only evoked by stimuli given to the left ear. In any case, it is clear that with some very few and controversial exceptions, the orienting reflex requires awareness for both learning and expression.

The N2/P3 has also been associated with controlled or conscious processing (Posner, 1975; Donchin et al., 1983; Naatanen and Picton, 1986; Hillyard and Picton, 1988; Hoffman, 1990). For example, the P3 is present if, and only if, independent behavioral data show that the stimulus has captured the subject's attention and reached his or her awareness. (Although more controversial, it is possible that, among stimuli that are perceived but otherwise equated, the P3 is larger to stimuli with greater affective valence: Sutton and Ruchkin, 1984; Johnston et al., 1987; but see Vanderploeg et al., 1987.)

The exact point in time within the N2/P3 sequence when the stimulus enters awareness remains unclear. Libet (1973) found that it is difficult to evoke a conscious perception by electrical stimulation of the postcentral gyrus with a single pulse. Interestingly, such stimulation evokes early but not late evoked potential components. Trains of stimulation evoke conscious percepts at much lower current levels than single pulses, with the threshold level decreasing with increasingly long trains, reaching a minimum level at train durations of about 500 to 600 msec. Furthermore, application of direct cortical stimulation up to about 150 msec after a peripheral stimulus can block conscious perception of that stimulus. This time is consistent with studies of "backwards-masking," where a peripheral stimulus blocks the perception of a previously presented peripheral stimulus (although in such experiments the level of the neuraxis where the interference takes place is often unclear: Turvey, 1973). By examining the time-course of the interference by a primary task upon the reaction time to a secondary probe, Posner and Klein (1973) concluded that the "limited capacity mechanism" associated with consciousness begins to be engaged about 150 to 500 msec following the presentation of a letter.

The time from stimulus onset to P3 onset is also about 200 to 400 msec, suggesting that the P3 follows the entry of the stimulus to awareness. Comparison of P3 to reaction time latencies across single trials, or across task conditions, tends to support this conclusion. The peak of the P3 occurs at about the same latency as the subject's response, indicating that the stimulus has been accurately classified (Kutas et al., 1977; McCarthy and Donchin, 1981). Since the time from P3 onset to P3 peak is about equal to the time from motor command to behavioral response, this suggests that the P3 begins when the stimulus has been sufficiently processed to be accurately perceived (Desmedt, 1981). The N2 (and the N4, see below) occur before the P3, and thus could embody processing that is prior to conscious awareness, but that is within the "single-channel" to consciousness. To the extent, then, that amygdala processing evaluates emotional significance, the large amygdala N2 implies that emotional evaluation occurs in parallel with cognitive evaluation, perhaps prior to, but in any case on the path to, consciousness.

Semantic and Contextual Integration

This conclusion can be drawn more strongly after considering the response of the human amygdala to stimuli that are intrinsically meaningful within a complex semantic system: spoken, written, or signed words; faces; and objects. Such stimuli, when presented within a task that invokes their meaning, evokes an N4 (or N400) at the scalp, following the N2 and prior to the P3 (Rugg et al., 1986; Halgren and Smith, 1987; Kutas and Van Petten, 1988). The N4 has been studied, mainly with respect to words, in many cognitive tasks, leading to refined concepts of its antecedent conditions (determining whether the N4 occurs), and modulatory conditions (given the N4 occurs, determining its amplitude and duration) (Halgren, 1990b). Since a complete N4 occurs to pronounceable nonwords as well as to genuine words, lexical access cannot be completed before the N4 starts (Smith and Halgren, 1987b). Conversely, since nonpronounceable nonwords evoke no N4, phonemic lexical encoding sufficient to determine that the letter-string is potentially meaningful appears to be an adequate antecedent condition for the N4. Once the N4 is evoked, its amplitude and duration is decreased according to how easy it is to integrate the word into the current cognitive context. Thus, for example, a smaller N4 will be evoked by a target word if it is preceded by a semantically related word, or by a sentence that establishes a contextual expectation for the target word (Kutas and Hillyard, 1980). Similarly, common words evoke smaller N4s than uncommon words, and words that have been processed recently in the same task context evoke smaller N4s than words that have not (Smith and Halgren, 1987b, 1989; Rugg and Nagy, 1989; Van Petten and Kutas, 1990). Thus, the N4 appears to embody the integration of a potentially meaningful stimulus with the current cognitive context in order to extract its meaning (Halgren, 1990b).

A large N4 is recorded in the human amygdala (Fig. 7: McCarthy and Wood, 1984, 1985; Smith et al., 1986). It is difficult to know for certain if this N4 is locally generated, inasmuch as a large polarity-inverting N4 is also recorded in the hippocampal formation inferior to the amygdala. However, local generation seems likely, in that the amygdala N4 is usually larger in the amygdala than in the hippocampal formation, the N4 decreases very rapidly in amplitude immediately upon passing to recording sites just medial to the amygdala, and the amygdala N4 is maintained even when the adjacent hippocampus appears to be too damaged by epileptiform activity to generate cognitive potentials (Fig. 8). In any case, the N4 is larger in the amygdala than in any other brain site yet sampled, and conversely, the largest evoked potentials so far observed in the human amygdala have been to words and faces.

Across a variety of tasks, including recognition memory, lexical decision, and sentence reading, the amygdala N4 to words has what appears to be the same cognitive correlates as the N4 recorded at the scalp. The N4 to words is about threefold larger in the dominant than in the nondominant hemisphere. Furthermore, four of six amygdala units recorded during the N4 showed increased firing specifically ($P < .005$) to one out of the 10 repeated words in a recognition task (Heit et al., 1988). Thus the N4 appears to participate in some aspect of semantic contextual integration during the N4.

Preceding the N4 at the scalp are the N2 and other processing negativities (Pritchard et al., 1988). These potentials are also evoked by letter-matching tasks, where they appear to represent lexical encoding/template-matching processes (Ritter et al., 1984; Lovrich et al., 1986). These components are largest over the posterior temporal lobe, and they are unilaterally diminished by removal of this cortex in anterior temporal lobectomy (Smith and Halgren, 1988), consistent with a progression of processing from inferotemporal visual association cortex to the amygdala (Mishkin, 1982; Marrocco, 1986).

This progression is supported by observations of the potentials evoked by faces, again culminating in an amygdala N4 (Fig. 8). In monkeys, unit responses specific to faces have been recorded at a latency of 90–140 msec in the superior temporal sulcus (Hasselmo et al., 1989) and 110–200 msec in the amygdala

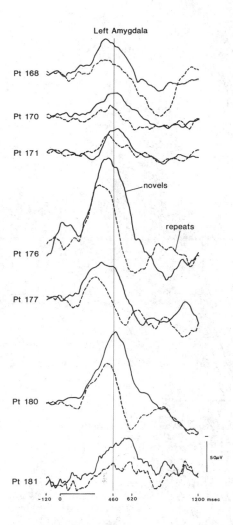

Fig. 7. Average wave forms recorded from the left amygdala of seven patients during word recognition memory testing. A large N4 (or N400), with average latency-to-peak of 460 ms that declines in amplitude with word repetition is observed. In some patients the repeated words also evoke a P3 (or P300) with average latency-to-peak of 620 ms. The N4 is only evoked by "semantic" stimuli such as words or faces, and its size is determined by the ease with which the word or face can be integrated with the current cognitive context. Negativity is up. From Smith et al. (1986) with permission.

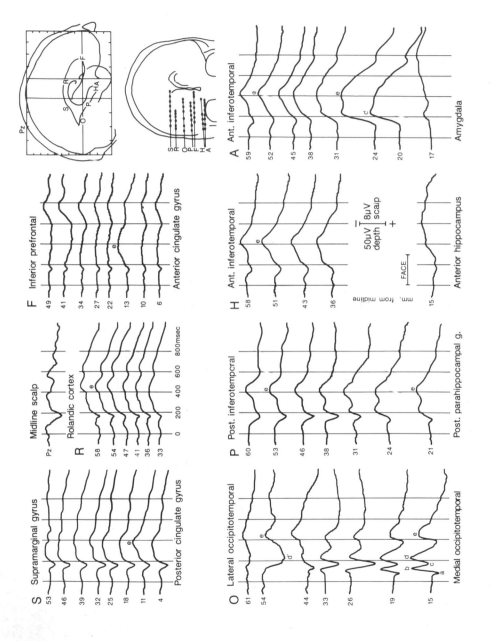

(Leonard et al., 1985). The reduced visual responses in the amygdala after cooling of the monkey inferotemporal cortex supports this path of information flow (Fukuda et al., 1987). In humans, preceding the N4 are what may be face-specific evoked potential components at latencies of 150 and 225 msec, with a scalp distribution suggestive of posterior temporal cortex origin (Srebo, 1985; Smith and Halgren, 1987a; Barrett et al., 1988; Botzel and Grusser, 1989). In depth recordings, the earliest potentials evoked by faces, peaking at 70 and 110 msec, are recorded medially at the occipitotemporal junction near the primary visual cortex, where they are thought to be generated by excitation-inhibition in the thalamorecipient laminae (Darcey et al., 1980; Streletz et al., 1981; Kraut et al., 1985; Mitzdorf, 1986; Ducati et al., 1988). Somewhat lateral and anterior is a peak at 150 ms, followed by a widespread negativity at 225 msec that polarity-inverts in the posterior inferotemporal cortex (Fig. 8). This apparent N2, as well as the following N4 at 420 msec, attain maximal amplitude in the amygdala, but are also present in multiple medial and lateral inferotemporal cortex locations. The N4 is also seen in frontal and posterior supramodal association neocortex, as well as limbic neocortex.

This distribution suggests that a medial as well as lateral route functions to transmit information from primary visual cortex to the amygdala. A medial route is also supported by the visually responsive units we have recorded in the human posterior parahippocampal gyrus (Wilson et al., 1983, 1984), as well as the fact that prosopagnosia is generally associated with bilateral lesions in the medial occipitotemporal cortex (Damasio, 1989). Apparently, the lateral route is sufficient to support the preserved ability to cognitively process faces (de Haan et al., 1987), as well as preserved skin conductance response to familiar faces (Bauer, 1984; Tranel and Damasio, 1988) in prosopagnosics.

Fig. 8. Potentials evoked by slides of unfamiliar human faces (exposure 300 ms). A series of peaks from 70 to 460 msec are seen, with an anatomical distribution consistent with known pathways beginning in the primary visual cortex, passing to visual association cortex, then to supramodal limbic association cortex, and ending in the amygdala. The late cognitive potential in the amygdala is simultaneous with (but larger than) similar potentials observed at several association cortex sites. Thus, amygdala information processing appears to be integrated within the cognitive cortext, rather than following it, or independent from it. The earliest potentials are observed in the medial occipitotemporal cortex (electrode O), near area 19. The P70 (a) is thought to be generated by depolarization of layer IV cells in primary visual cortex by geniculocortical afferents and the N110 (b) by the following hyperpolarization. This is followed by a P160 with a somewhat more anterior and lateral distribution (c), and then a large, widespread N210 (d). This evoked potential component polarity inverts in posterior inferotemporal cortex (d'), and reaches maximal amplitude in the amygdala. The final component, an N460 (e), has a very widespread distribution, including sites in posterior cingulate gyrus (**S**), rolandic (**R**), inferior prefrontal cortex (**F**), inferotemporal cortex at four anteroposterior levels (**O,P,H,A**), and posterior parahippocampal gyrus. Again, it is largest in the basolateral amygdala complex. Trials with epileptiform spikes in the remaining channels, or with eye movements, were rejected from analysis. From Marinkovic, Baudena, Halgren, Heit, Devaux, Broglin, and Chauvel, in preparation.

IMPLICATIONS
Amygdala Processing for Emotional Significance Is Simultaneous and Interactive With Neocortical Processing for Cognitive Integration

We noted above that psychological theories of emotion differ as to whether they consider the emotional evaluation of events to be automatic, preceding conscious evaluation (Fig. 1B), or whether conscious evaluation is a necessary antecedent of emotion (Fig. 1A). Experiments have attempted to support the first model by demonstrating that stimuli can evoke emotional responses even though they are not perceived. However, the unconscious emotional evaluation models do not require that there be no conscious processing of the event, only that such processing does not *precede* the emotional evaluation. The large N2 and N4 generated in the amygdala strongly imply that amygdala processing of events (and thus presumably their emotional evaluation) occurs synchronously with their cognitive evaluation, and thus prior to any conclusion being obtained from that processing. That is, by comparing the time-course of processing in the amygdala versus the neocortex, these studies obviate the need to determine if there are emotional responses to unconscious events—the amygdala potentials indicate preConscious emotional processing of events that are on the route to Consciousness.

This argument against the necessary priority of conscious processing is in some respects similar to that made by LeDoux (1986, 1987). However, LeDoux bases his argument on the important role that the direct thalamo-amygdala pathway plays in the conditioned emotional response in rats. The studies reviewed above suggest that this early simple sensory input is very weak or nonexistent in humans. Rather, cognitive inputs reflected in the N2 and N4 dominate human amygdala activity. When evoked by words or faces, this activity appears to arrive in the amygdala from visual association cortex in the medial and lateral inferotemporal cortex, and is correlated with N2s and N4s recorded simultaneously in multiple supramodal association cortical areas.

These correlated potentials, as well as the cognitive-semantic correlates of the N2 and N4, strongly suggest that the amygdala functions within the cognitive processing system. Certainly, from the onset of the amygdala N2 at 120 msec poststimulus onset to the completion of the N4 about 500 msec later, there is ample time for many iterations of cortico-amygdala communication. That such communication occurs is confirmed by the apparent high frequency of word-specific cells within the amygdala. Furthermore, the complex memory- and dreamlike images evoked by amygdala stimulation must reflect a cortical output, especially given their eloquence in representing psychosocial concerns.

Thus, while presumably the amygdala performs emotional evaluation, it does so within the cognitive system. This could explain why it has been so difficult to dissociate emotional from cognitive processing in humans. Words and faces evoke components in visual association cortex correlated with stimulus preprocessing/encoding. These components and sites appear to be necessary prerequisites for later components in the polymodal association neocortal areas that support cognitive processing, as well as for the amygdala components. Thus, degradation of the signal will tend to eliminate both cognitive and emotional processing.

Finally, it should be noted that the present data allow no conclusion regarding whether amygdala neurons participate in the networks that embody Consciousness. However, they are certainly well qualified: Some of the cognitive evoked potential components most closely associated with conscious processing are maximal in the amygdala, and the variety, intensity, complexity, and number of mental phenomena evoked by amygdala stimulation exceeds anything observed after cortical stimulation.

In summary, the results of human amygdala lesions, stimulation, and recordings suggest the model for emotional interaction presented in Figure 1D. This model is more consistent with that of Cannon than that of James in suggesting that emotional evaluation precedes conscious appreciation. Perhaps it is most similar to the psychoanalytic viewpoint (Fig. 1C), in that preConscious emotional processing is complicated and has multiple possible consequences that are highly dependent on the person and the context.

Emotional Learning in a Cognitive and Visceral Context

Animal studies have shown that the amygdala is necessary for the conditioned emotional response, and presumably is the site where synapses from neurons activated by the conditioned stimulus (a tone) have attained the ability to fire neurons that produce the conditioned response (a change in heart rate), after pairing with the unconditioned stimulus (a shock) (see Davis, Gallagher, LeDoux, this volume, Chapters 9, 10, 12, and Fig. 9A). The human amygdala also appears to receive viscerosensory inputs, and stimulation of the human amygdala produces visceromotor responses. However, in place of simple sensory inputs, the human amygdala receives highly processed cognitive information. Thus, the human equivalent of the conditioned emotional response may consist of learning to produce visceral responses to faces, words, thoughts, or other meaningful stimuli that have previously been associated with visceral upset (Fig. 9B).

However, human amygdala stimulation not only produces visceromotor and hormonal responses (which could be innate unconditioned responses), it also can evoke images, thoughts, and feelings (which are learned, idiosyncratic, and context-determined, not innate unconditioned responses). Furthermore, the neural substrate for these mental phenomena is undoubtedly a complex widespread pattern of neural activation in the neocortex. Thus, any model for learning by the human amygdala must specify how a complex input pattern could be associated with an equally complex output pattern. Recurrent excitatory synapses between amygala neurons with Hebbian plasticity properties would allow it to function as such an associative network (e.g., Fig. 9C; Hinton and Anderson, 1981). While the periamygdaloid cortex has such properties (Lynch, 1986), the physiology of the intrinsic amygdala connections is as yet insufficiently specified to precisely define a theory for associative learning within the amygdala.

Nonetheless, the reciprocal connections of the amygdala with brain stem viscerosensory and visceromotor nuclei as well as with association cortex, together with the lesion, recording, and stimulation studies reviewed above, suggest that in contrast to other brain structures, learning in the amygdala is likely to be a hybrid of simple visceral conditioning with complex pattern asso-

A. Conditioned Emotional Response

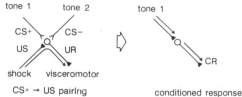

CS+ → US pairing   conditioned response

B. Human Equivalent of CER?

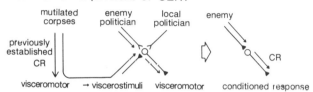

C. Associative Learning

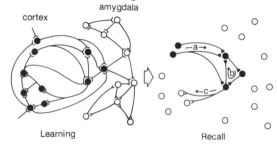

Learning   Recall

D. Hybrid of Conditioning and Associative Learning

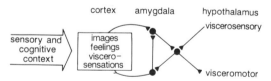

Fig. 9. Possible mechanisms of memory mediated by the amygdala, in animals (**A**) and humans (**B–D**). **A**: One neuron with three inputs and one output is sufficient to model the conditioned emotional response, where pairing of the positive conditioned stimulus (CS+) with the unconditioned stimulus (US) eventually permits it to evoke the conditioned response (CR) by itself. **B**: The same mechanism could be used to learn discriminative visceral reactions in humans. **C**: However, the complexity of human amygdala outputs (implied by the formed images and other mental phenomena evoked by stimulation) suggests that it may learn to associate patterns of neural activity. In a typical such model, a cortical network embodies current feelings, images, thoughts, and viscerosensations. Amygdala circuits are activated by input from these cortical networks, plus intra-amygdaloid recurrent excitation, and long-loop recurrent cortex ↔ amygdala excitation. During the learning phase, convergent excitation above a threshold (in this Figure set to

ciation (Fig. 9D). In one such model, visceral stimulation or other brain stem activation (the unconditioned stimulus) would prime the amygdala to potentiate the currently activated amygala synapses, and these synapses would reflect the current activity patterns in the various cortices associated with amygdala, for example, an image encoded by inferotemporal cortex and a visceral sensation by insular cortex. This neocortical activity would project to the amygdala during the N2/N4, and after multiple neocortical amygdala feedback cycles, the pattern of activated cells in the amygdala would come to reflect those that participate in the distributed neural networks that include both neocortex and amygdala, and that specifically encode the currently experienced event. That is, the emotional unconditioned stimulus would enhance those amygdala synapses currently participating in the neocortical amygdala positive feedback loop. Recall would be triggered by either a visceral input, or by a pattern in one of the associated cortical areas. Recall would consist not only of a visceral output but also of the associated patterns in several cortical structures. The amygdala output to these cortices would only be one of several influences upon their activity, as evidenced by the contextual and personality influences on the mental phenomena evoked by amygdala stimulation.

In this formulation, the importance for emotion of visceral sensations is maintained, but with the additional possibility that the "gut feelings" may actually be hallucinations induced by previous association of the presented image, thought or word. These viscero-hallucinations would neither be as slow nor as unspecific as sensations resulting from actual visceromotor activation, and thus they could play a greater role in secondary cognitive appraisal (cf. Mandler, 1975, who proposed a similar mechanism for overcoming Cannon's telling criticisms of James's theory).

Even if associative learning in the amygdala is not adequate by itself to interrelate complex novel patterns of cortical activation, the amygdala could presumably access such traces through the hippocampus. By virtue of its reciprocal connections with association cortex, as well as its intrinsic anatomy and plasticity, the hippocampus has been proposed to function as an autoassociative memory for recent events (Marr, 1971; Halgren, 1984; Teyler and DiScenna, 1986; Rolls, 1989). The human amygdala is so densely interconnected with the hippocampal formation that it is virtually impossible to distinguish between the subjective effects of stimulating the two structures (Halgren et al., 1978a). Furthermore, the N2/N4/P3 cycle is also prominent in the hippocampal formation and thus may form an envelope uniting its information processing with that in the amygdala (Smith et al., 1986; Stapleton and Halgren, 1987). Indeed, hippocampal formation neurons also fire specifically to individual words and faces during the same

---

3) results in potentiation of the synapses that are activated both pre- and postsynaptically. During retrieval, partial activation of the original cortical circuit (a) is projected to the amygdala, where the amygdala curcuit is reconstructed (b), and this in turn aids or influences the cortical reconstruction (c). **D:** The human amygdala is likely to function as a hybrid of B and C.

time period, as do amygdala neurons (Heit et al., 1988). Thus, it is likely that the amygdala and hippocampal formation function together as a unit in interrelating the complex patterns embodying mental phenomena with viscerosensory and visceromotor activity.

Cognitive Integration in the Amygdala: An Evolutionary Link From Primate Social Communication to Human Language

Primates typically use a rich repertoire of vocalizations, gestures, and facial expressions to communicate a variety of information, suggesting that human language may have evolved from primate social communication (Seyfarth, 1987). A corollary proposal would suggest that human general cognitive abilities evolved from the primate cognitive abilities that are more focused on social interactions (Cheney et al., 1986; Essock-Vitale and Seyfarth, 1987). Clearly, an analogy may be drawn between sentence structure in human language (where auditory or visual words are sequentially integrated within an internally constructed cognitive context) and social exchanges in primates (where gestures, cries, and especially facial expressions are sequentially integrated within an internally constructed social context). However, other authors have challenged this position, noting that compared to human language, primate social communication seems far more innate, involuntary, and linked to the animal's immediate emotional state (Lancaster, 1975; Ploog, 1981; Terrace, 1985).

This challenge has been supported by the apparent lack of homology between brain structures supporting human language versus those supporting primate social communication. Whereas lesions of the left temporo-parieto-occipital junction are well known to render humans aphasic, they do not disrupt social communication in primates (Heffner and Heffner, 1989). Conversely, lesions of the human amygdala do not disrupt language (Halgren, 1981), whereas lesions of the primate amygdala do render their social communication abnormal and contextually innappropriate (see Chapter 13, Kling, this volume; Klüver and Bucy, 1939; Steklis and Kling, 1985). Furthermore, stimulation of the primate amygdala evokes the species-specific vocalizations essential for primate social communication (Jurgens, 1982). Finally, recording studies in primates have found amygdala neurons that respond specifically to faces of a particular individual, or to faces that express a particular social communication (see Chapter 5, Rolls, this volume; Leonard et al., 1985).

Thus, the lesions that disrupt language in humans do not disrupt social communication in primates, and the lesions that disrupt social communication in primates do not disrupt language in humans. This double dissociation would appear to argue against the evolution of human language from primate social communication. It remains theoretically possible, however, that human language and primate social communication share very similar neural substrates, but that the areas within this substrate that are essential for language versus social communication are distinct. Since the effects of lesions only show what areas are *essential* for a function, and not those that are involved in its production, the effects of lesions would then give a false impression that language and social communication have distinct neural substrates.

The areas involved in the production of a cognitive function are revealed by their differential physiological activation when this function is differentially invoked by a task. The only evoked potential component specifically evoked by semantic stimuli is the N4. As reviewed above, the N4 is closely linked to language processing, in that an antecedent condition for the triggering of the N4 to words is lexical encoding, and N4 amplitude is modulated by the ease of integration of the word with the current semantic context. Although the N4 appears to have widespread generators in both cerebral hemispheres, including polymodal and supramodal association cortices, as well as in limbic areas, it is largest in the amygdala. Since the N4 appears to be generated in both the language cortex and the amygdala, in response to both words and to faces, it is an excellent candidate for a neurocognitive process common to human language and to primate social communication.

If true, this formulation would provide a natural explanation for the dissociative effects of lesions on language and social communication referred to above. In this view, both language understanding and social integration are conceived of as having very widespread neural substrates in polymodal and supramodal cortex as well as the limbic system of both hemispheres. Although it has not been specifically tested, there is little doubt that complete ablation of all cortical and limbic areas where the N4 is recorded would abolish both language and social communication. However, it is postulated that in Wernicke's area there exists an essential entry point for words into the cognitive system (Halgren, 1990b). Conversely, it is postulated that the amygdala is an essential point for contact between cognitive representations and emotional significance. Since Wernicke's area is not necessary for the relation of cognitive representations to emotional significance, and the amygdala is not necessary for lexicophonemic encoding, lesions of these respective areas have dissociated effects on language and social communication. Nonetheless, following the entry of a word or a social signal (carried, for example, by a face), their contextual integration is postulated to be embodied by a common process, the N4.

FROM MYTH AND METAPHOR TO MECHANISM

An axiom of our experience is the separate realities of our minds and bodies. The amygdala lies, functionally and anatomically, between these two poles, between the enormous thinking mantle that creates an objective model of external reality, and the subjective inner reality of pain and fear, of surviving to mate and ensuring that our offspring do also. The amygdala fits so well this paradoxical axis of human existence from biology to spirit that it has a tendency to achieve an almost mythical status that goes beyond its true significance. One suspects that if the amygdala did not exist, it would have been invented as a metaphor for the connection of mind and body.

It must be borne in mind that despite the drama of the Klüver-Bucy syndrome, even massive amygdala damage in an otherwise intact brain is consistent with a grossly normal personality; that despite the rich complexity and intensity of mental phenomena that can be evoked from the human amygdala by electrical stimulation, most such stimulations evoke no subjective response even when they evoke an afterdischarge; that despite their greater size in the amygdala, the cognitive potentials associated with orienting and semantic integration can also be recorded in many other sites. The amygdala probably has little to do with voluntary planned actions, especially if they are based upon faith, hope, love, insight, curiosity, or integrity. Even for relating the visceral and the cognitive realms, parallel paths exist in posterior orbitofrontal cortex, temporal pole, insula, and anterior cingulate gyrus.

Nonetheless, the stimulation and recording studies reviewed above indicate that the human amygdala plays a very important role in the integration of cognition with biological motivations: In the presence of collateral damage eliminating parallel cognitive and/or limbic pathways for behavioral modulation, amygdala damage can have devastating effects on the subject's emotional life; electrical activation of the amygdala can evoke all aspects of emotion, including affects, visceral sensations, thoughts, memories, and autonomic output; human amygdala neurons are very sensitive to both visceral and cognitive inputs, and very probably participate with the cognitive brain from the onset to the completion of event evaluation. Hopefully, these studies will help lead to concrete mechanistic models for the contribution of the amygdala to human emotion.

ACKNOWLEDGMENTS

I thank Michael Smith, Gary Heit, Ksenija Marinkovic, June Stapleton, and Patrick Baudena for contributing to the research results reported here, and Ksenija Marinkovic, Bertrand Deputte, Robert Frysinger, and Patrick Chauvel for discussions contributing to the ideas proposed in this chapter.

REFERENCES

Adams JR, Rutkin BB (1969): Treatment of temporal lobe epilepsy by stereotactic surgery. Confin Neurol 21:80–85.

Albert DJ, Walsh ML (1984): Neural systems and the inhibitory modulation of agonistic behavior: A comparison of mammalian species. Neurosci Biobehav Rev 8:5–24.

Alheid GF, Heimer L (1988): New perspectives in basal forebrain organization of special relevance for neuropsychiatric disorders: The striatopallidal, amygdaloid, and corticopetal components of substantia innominata. Neuroscience 27:1–39.

Andy OJ, Jurko MF, Hughes JR (1975): Amygdalotomy for bilateral temporal lobe seizures. South Med J 68:743–748.

Andy OJ, Jurko M (1977): The human amygdala: Excitability state and aggression. In Sweet WH, Obrador S, Martin-Rodriguez JG (eds): "Neurosurgical Treatment in Psychiatry, Pain and Epilepsy." Baltimore: University Park Press, pp 417–427.

Angeleri F, Ferro-Milone F, Parigi S (1964): Electrical activity and reactivity of the rhinencephalic, pararhinencephalic and thalamic structures: Prolonged implantation of electrodes in man. Electroencephalogr Clin Neurophysiol 16:100–129.

Arnold MB (1960): "Emotion and Personality." New York: Columbia University Press.

Avatisian EA, Baklavadzhian OS, Mikaelian RN (1988): Unit responses of the amygdaloid corticomedial nuclei to stimulation of the vagal, splanchnic and sciatic nerves. Fiziol Z 74:41–48.

Bancaud J, Talairach J, Bonis A, Schaub C, Szikla G, Morel P, Bordas Ferrer M (1965): "La Stereoelectroencephalographie dans l'epilepsie." Paris: Masson et Cie.

Bancaud J, Favel P, Bonis A, Bordas-Ferrer M, Miravet J, Talairach J (1970): Manifestations sexuelles paroxystiques et epilepsie temporale. Etude clinique, EEG et SEEG d'une epilepsie d'origine temporale. Rev Neurol (Paris) 123:217–230.

Bancaud J (1981): Epileptic attacks of temporal lobe origin in man. Jap J EEG EMG 61–71.

Barrett SE, Rugg MD, Perrett DI (1988): Event-related potentials and the matching of familiar and unfamiliar faces. Neuropsychologia 26:105–117.

Bauer RM (1984): Autonomic recognition of names and faces in prosopagnosia: A neuropsychological application of the Guilty Knowledge Test. Neuropsychologia 22:457–469.

Bear DM (1979): Temporal lobe epilepsy: A syndrome of sensory-limbic hyperconnection. Cortex 15:357–384.

Botzel K, Grusser OJ (1989): Electric brain potentials evoked by pictures of faces and non-faces: A search for "face-specific" EEG-potentials. Exp Brain Res 77:349–360.

Brenner C (1974): On the nature and development of affects: A unified theory. Psychoanal Q 43:532–556.

Brunet-Bourgin F (1984): "Semiologie et Pathophysiologie du Dreamystate." Rennes: Universite de Rennes I (Medical Thesis).

Cain DP, Bindra D (1972): Responses of amygdala single units to odors in the rat. Exp Neurol 35:98–110.

Cannon WB (1939): "The Wisdom of the Body." New York: Norton.

Cechetto DF, Calaresu FR (1985): Central pathways relaying cardiovascular afferent information to amygdala. Am J Physiol 248:R38–R45.

Chapman WP, Schroeder HR, Geyer G, Brazier MAB, Eager C, Poppen JL, Solomon HC, Yakovlev P (1954): Physiological evidence concerning importance of the amygdaloid nuclear region in the intergration of circulatory function and emotion in man. Science 120:849–950.

Chapman WP (1958): Studies of the periamygdaloid area in relation to human behavior. Publ Assoc Res Nerv Ment Dis 36:258–277.

Chauvel P, Brunet-Bourgin F, Halgren E (1989): L'etat de reve. Neuro-Psy 4:443–450.

Cheetham SC, Crompton MR, Czudek C, Horton RW, Katona CL, Reynolds GP (1989): Serotonin concentrations and turnover in brains of depressed suicides. Brain Res 502:332–340.

Cheney D, Seyfarth R, Smuts B (1986): Social relationships and social cognition in non-human primates. Science 234:1361–1366.

Corkin S (1984): Lasting consequences of bilateral medial temporal lobectomy: Clinical course and experimental findings in H.M. Sem Neurol 4:249–259.

Cragg BG (1960): Responses of the hippocampus to stimulation of the olfactory bulb and various afferent nerves in five mammals. Exp Neurol 2:547–572.

Cummings JL, Duchen LW (1981): Klüver-Bucy syndrome in Pick disease: Clinical and pathologic correlations. Neurology 31:1415–1422.

Damasio AR (1989): Neural mechanisms. In Young AW, Ellis HD (eds): "Handbook of Research on Face Processing." Amsterdam: Elsevier, pp 405–425.

Darcey TM, Wieser HG, Meles HP, Skrandies W, Lehmann D (1980): Intracerebral and scalp fields evoked by visual stimulation. Electroencephalogr Clin Neurophysiol 49:111.

Darwin C (1872): "The Expression of the Emotions in Man and Animals." London: Murray.

Dawson ME, Schell AM (1982): Electrodermal responses to attended and nonattended significant stimuli during dichotic listening. J Exp Psychol [Hum Percept] 8:315–324.

de Haan EHF, Young A, Newcombe F (1987): Face recognition without awareness. Cogn Neuropsychol 4:385–415.

Delgado-Escueta AV, Kunze U, Waddell G, Boxley J, Nadel A (1977): Lapse of consciousness and automatisms in temporal lobe epilepsy: A video tape analysis. Neurology 27: 144–155.

Delgado-Escueta AV, Mattson RH, King L, Goldensohn ES, Spiegel H, Madsen J, Crandall P, Dreifuss F, Porter RJ (1981): The nature of aggression during epileptic seizures. N Engl J Med 305:711–716.

Delgado-Escueta AV, Swartz BE, Maldonado HM, Walsh GO, Rand RW, Halgren E (1987): Complex partial seizures of frontal lobe origin. In Wieser HG, Elger CE (eds): "Presurgical Evaluation of Epileptics." Berlin, Heidelberg: Springer-Verlag, pp 268–299.

Desmedt JE (1981): Scalp-recorded cerebral event-related potentials in man as point of entry into the analysis of cognitive processing. In Schmitt FO, Worden FG, Edelmann G, Dennis SD (eds): "The Organization of the Cerebral Cortex." Cambridge: MIT Press, pp 441–473.

Donchin E, McCarthy G, Kutas M, Ritter W (1983): Event-related potentials in the study of consciousness. In Davidson RJ, Schwartz GE, Shapiro D (eds): "Consciousness and Self-Regulation. Advances in Research and Theory," Vol 3. New York: Plenum Press, pp 81–122.

Donchin E, Heffley E, Hillyard SA, Loveless N, Maltzman I, Ohman A, Rosler F, Ruchkin D, Siddle D (1984): Cognition and event-related potentials II. The orienting reflex and P300. In Karrer R, Cohen J, Tueting P (eds): "Brain and Information: Event-Related Potentials." New York: New York Academy of Sciences, pp 39–57.

Ducati A, Fava E, Motti ED (1988): Neuronal generators of the visual evoked potentials: Intracerebral recording in awake humans. Electroencephalogr Clin Neurophysiol 71:89–99.

Dykman RA (1987): Commentary: Event-related potentials (ERPs) in simple conditioning paradigms. In Johnson R, Rohrbaugh JW, Parasuraman R (eds): "Current trends in event-related potential research" (EEG Suppl 40). Amsterdam: Elsevier, pp 311–315.

Ekman P (1982): "Emotion in the Human Face." Cambridge: Cambridge University Press.

Eriksen CW (1960): Discrimination and learning without awareness: A methodological survey and evaluation. Psychol Rev 67:279–300.

Eskenazi B, Cain WS, Novelly RA, Mattson R (1986): Odor perception in temporal lobe epilepsy patients with and without temporal lobectomy. Neuropsychologia 24:553–562.

Eslinger PJ, Damasio AR, Van Hoesen GW (1982): Olfactory dysfunction in man: Anatomical and behavioral aspects. Brain Cogn 1:259–285.

Essock-Vitale S, Seyfarth RM (1987): Intelligence and social cognition. In Smuts BB, Cheney DL, Seyfarth RM, Wrangham RW, Struhsaker TT (eds): "Primate Societies." Chicago: University of Chicago Press, pp 452–461.

Ferguson SM, Rayport M, Gardner R, Kass W, Weiner H, Reisner MF (1969): Similarities in mental content of psychotic states, spontaneous seizures, dreams, and responses to electrical brain stimulation in patients. Psychosom Med 31:478–498.

Fischer WF (1970): "Theories of Anxiety." New York: Harper and Row.

Freud S (1949): "Collected Papers," Vol IV. London: Hogarth Press.

Frysinger RC, Harper RM (1989): Cardiac and respiratory correlations with unit discharge in human amygdala and hippocampus. Electroencephalogr Clin Neurophysiol 72:463–470.

Fukuda M, Ono T, Nakamura K (1987): Functional relations among inferotemporal cortex, amygdala, and lateral hypothalamus in monkey. J Neurophysiol 57:1060–1077.

Gallagher BB, Flanigin HF, King DW, Littleton WH (1987): The effect of electrical stimulation of medial temporal lobe structures in epileptic patients upon ACTH, prolactin, and growth hormone. Neurology 37:299–303.

Ganzha BL (1986): Olfactory rhythm in the electrical activity of the amygdaloid nucleus of the human brain. Neirofiziologiia 18:61–69.

Gebber GL, Barman SB (1988): Studies on the origin and generation of sympathetic nerve activity. Clin Exp Hypertens [A] A10(Suppl 1):33–44.

Gloor P, Olivier A, Ives J (1980): Loss of consciousness in temporal lobe seizures: Observations obtained with stereotaxis depth electrode recordings and stimulations. In Canger R, Angeleri F, Penry JK (eds): "Advances in Epileptology: XIth Epilepsy International Symposium." New York: Raven Press, pp 349–353.

Gloor P, Olivier A, Quesney LF, Andermann F, Horowitz S (1982): The role of the limbic system in experiential phenomena of temporal lobe epilepsy. Ann Neurol 12:129–144.

Gloor P (1990): Experiential phenomena of temporal lobe epilepsy: Facts and hypotheses. Brain 113:1673–1694.

Gloor P (1991): Neurobiological substrates of ictal behavioral changes. In Smith DB, Treiman DM, Trimble MR (eds): "Neurobehavioral Problems in Epilepsy (Advances in Neurology, Vol 55)." New York: Raven Press, pp 1–34.

Goddard GV (1964): Functions of the amygdala. Psychol Bull 62:89–109.

Gowers WR (1907): "Borderland of Epilepsy; Faints, Vagal Attacks, Vertigo, Migraine, Sleep Symptoms, and Their Treatment." London: Churchill.

Guard O, Couailler J-F, Graule A, Dumas R (1982): Le sydrome de Klüver et Bucy chez l'homme: Presentation d'un cas et revue de la litterature. In Sizaret P (ed): "Comptes Rendu du Congres de Psychiatrie et de Neurologie de langue Francaise." Paris: Masson, pp 276–293.

Halgren E, Babb TL, Rausch R, Crandall PH (1977a): Neurons in the human basolateral amygdala and hippocampal formation do not respond to odors. Neurosci Lett 4:331–335.

Halgren E, Babb TL, Crandall PH (1977b): Responses of human limbic neurons to induced changes in blood gases. Brain Res 132:43–63.

Halgren E, Walter RD, Cherlow DG, Crandall PH (1978a): Mental phenomena evoked by electrical stimulation of the human hippocampal formation and amygdala. Brain 101:83–117.

Halgren E, Babb TL, Crandall PH (1978b): Activity of human hippocampal formation and amygdala neurons during memory testing. Electroencephalogr Clin Neurophysiol 45:585–601.

Halgren E, Babb TL, Crandall PH (1978c): Human hippocampal formation EEG desynchronizes during attentiveness and movement. Electroencephalogr Clin Neurophysiol 44:778–781.

Halgren E, Squires NK, Wilson CL, Rohrbaugh JW, Babb TL (1980): Endogenous potentials generated in the human hippocampal formation and amygdala by infrequent events. Science 210:803–805.

Halgren E (1981): The amygdala contribution to memory and emotion: Current studies in humans. In Ben-Ari Y (ed): "The Amygdaloid Complex." Amsterdam: Elsevier, pp 395–408.

Halgren E (1982): Mental phenomena induced by stimulation in the limbic system. Hum Neurobiol 1:251–260.

Halgren E (1984): Human hippocampal and amygdala recording and stimulation: Evidence for a neural model of recent memory. In Butters N, Squire L (eds): "The Neuropsychology of Memory." New York: Guilford, pp 165–181.

Halgren E (1990a): Evoked potentials. In Boulton AA, Baker G, Vanderwolf C (eds): "Neuromethods, Vol. 15: Neurophysiological Techniques—Applications to Neural Systems." Clifton, NJ: Humana, pp 147–275.

Halgren E (1990b): Insights from evoked potentials into the neuropsychological mechanisms of reading. In Scheibel A, Weschsler A (eds): "Neurobiology of Cognition." New York: Guilford, pp 103–150.

Halgren E, Smith ME (1987): Cognitive evoked potentials as modulatory processes in human memory formation and retrieval. Hum Neurobiol 6:129–139.

Halgren E (1991a): Firing of human hippocampal units in relation to voluntary movements. Hippocampus 1:153–161.

Halgren E, Stapleton J, Domalski P, Swartz BE, Delgado-Escueta A, Treiman D, Walsh GO, Mandelkern M, Blahd W, Ropchan J (1991b): Memory dysfunction in epileptics as a derangement of normal physiology. In Smith D, Treiman DM, Trimble M (eds): "Advances in Neurology, Vol 55: Neurobehavioral Problems in Epilepsy." New York: Raven Press, pp 385–410.

Hanley J, Berkhout J, Crandall P, Rickles WR, Walter RD (1970): Spectral characteristics of EEG activity accompanying deep spiking in a patient with schizophrenia. Electroencephalogr Clin Neurophysiol 28:90.

Hasselmo ME, Rolls ET, Baylis GC (1989): The role of expression and identity in the face-selective responses of neurons in the temporal visual cortex of the monkey. Behav Brain Res 32:203–218.

Hausser-Hauw C, Bancaud J (1987): Gustatory hallucinations in epileptic seizures: Electrophysiological, clinical and anatomical correlates. Brain 110:339–359.

Heath RG (1958): Correlation of electrical recordings from cortical and subcortical regions of the brain with abnormal behavior in human subjects. Confin Neurol 18:305–313.

Heath RG, Mickle WA (1960): Evaluation of seven years' experience with depth electrode studies in human patients. In Ramey ER, O'Doherty D (eds): "Electrical Studies of the Unanesthetized Brain." New York: Paul B. Hoeber, pp 214–247.

Heath RG (1964): Activity of the human brain during emotional thought. In Heath RG (ed): "The Role of Pleasure in Behavior." New York: Hoebe, Harper and Row, pp 83–106.

Hebben N, Corkin S, Eichenbaum H, Shedlack K (1985): Diminished ability to interpret and report internal states after bilateral medial temporal resection: Case H.M. Behav Neurosci 99:1031–1039.

Heffner HE, Heffner RS (1989): Effect of restricted cortical lesions on absolute thresholds and aphasia-like deficits in Japanese macaques. Behav Neurosci 103:158–169.

Heit G, Smith ME, Halgren E (1988): Neural encoding of individual words and faces by the human hippocampus and amygdala. Nature 333:773–775.

Heit G, Smith ME, Halgren E (1990): Neuronal activity in the human medial temporal lobe during recognition memory. Brain 113:1093–1112.

Herpin TH (1867): "Des Acces Incomplets d'Epilepsie." Paris.

Herzog AG, Kemper TL (1980): Amygdaloid changes in aging and dementia. Arch Neurol 37:625–629.

Hillyard SA, Picton TW (1988): Electrophysiology of cognition. In Mountcastle V, Plum F (eds): "Handbook of Physiology—The Nervous System V." Bethesda: American Physiological Society, pp 519–584.

Hinton GE, Anderson JA (eds) (1981): "Parallel Models of Associative Memory." Hillsdale, NJ: Lawrence Erlbaum Associates.

Hitchcock E, Cairns V (1973): Amygdalotomy. Postgrad Med 49:894–904.

Hoffman JE (1990): Event-related potentials and automatic and controlled processes. In Rohrbaugh JW, Parasuraman R, Johnson R Jr (eds): "Event-related Brain Potentials: Basic Issues and Applications." New York: Oxford, pp 145–157.

Horowitz MJ (1967): Visual imagery and cognitive organization. Am J Psychiatry 123:938–946.

Horowitz MJ, Adams JE, Rutkin BB (1968): Visual imagery on brain stimulation. Arch Gen Psychiat 19:469–486.

Horowitz MJ, Adams JE (1970): Hallucinations on brain stimulation: Evidence for revision of the Penfield hypothesis. In Keup W (ed): "Origin and Mechanism of Hallucinations." New York: Plenum Press, pp 13–23.

Hughes JR, Andy OJ (1979a): The human amygdala. I. Electrophysiological responses to odorants. Electroencephalogr Clin Neurophysiol 46:428–443.

Hughes JR, Andy OJ (1979b): The human amygdala. II. Neurophysiological correlates of olfactory perception before and after amygdalotomy. Electroencephalogr Clin Neurophysiol 46:444–451.

Irle E, Markowitsch HJ (1986): Afferent connections of the substantia innominata/basal nucleus of Meynert in carnivores and primates. J Hirnforsch 27:343–367.

Izard CE, Buechler S (1979): Aspects of consciousness and personality in terms of differential emotions theory. In Plutchik R, Kellerman H (eds): "Emotion: Theory, Research and Experience." New York: Academic Press.

Jackson JH, Stewart P (1899): Epileptic attacks with warning sensations of smell and with intellectual aura (dreamy state) in a patient who had symptoms pointing to gross organic disease of the right temporo-sphenoidal lobe. Brain 22:534–549.

James W (1884): What is an emotion? Mind 9:188–205.

Jaynes J (1982): A two-tiered theory of emotions: Affect and feeling. Behav Brain Sci 5:434–435.

Johnston VS, Burleson MH, Miller DR (1987): Emotional value and late positive components of ERPs. In Johnson R, Rohrbaugh JW, Parasuraman R (eds): "Current Trends in Event-Related Potential Research (EEG Suppl 40)." Amsterdam: Elsevier/North-Holland Biomedical Press, pp 198–203.

Jurgens U (1982): Amygdalar vocalization pathways in the squirrel monkey. Brain Res 241:189–196.

Kirkpatrick B, Buchanan RW (1990): The neural basis of the deficit syndrome of schizophrenia. J Nerv Men Dis 178:545–555.

Klüver H, Bucy PC (1939): Preliminary analysis of the temporal lobe in monkeys. Arch Neurol Psychiat 42:979–1000.

Kraut MA, Arezzo JC, Vaughan HG (1985): Intracortical generators of the flash VEP in monkeys. Electroencephalogr Clin Neurophysiol 62:300–312.

Kutas M, Hillyard SA (1980): Reading senseless sentences: Brain potentials reflect semantic incongruity. Science 207:203–205.

Kutas M, McCarthy G, Donchin E (1977): Augmenting mental chronometry: The P300 as a measure of stimulus evaluation time. Science 197:792–795.

Kutas M, Van Petten C (1988): Event-related brain potential studies of language. In Ackles PK, Jennings JR, Coles MGH (eds): "Advances in Psychophysiology." Greenwich, CT: JAI Press, pp 139–187.

Laitinen L, Toivakka E (1980): Slowing of scalp EEG after electrical stimulation of amygdala in man. Acta Neurochir [Suppl] (WIEN) 30:177–181.

Laitinen LV (1988): Psychosurgery today. Acta Neurochir [Suppl] (WIEN) 44:158–162.

Lancaster J (1975): "Primate Behavior and the Emergence of Human Culture." New York: Holt, Rinehart and Winston.

Lazarus RS, Averill JR, Opton EMJr (1970): Towards a cognitive theory of emotion. In Arnold M (ed): "Feelings and Emotions." New York: Academic Press.

Lazarus RS, McCleary RA (1951): Autonomic discrimination without awareness: A study of subception. Psychol Rev 8:113–122.

LeDoux JE (1986): Sensory systems and emotion: A model of affective processing. Integr Psychiat 4:237–248.

LeDoux JE (1987): Emotion. In Mountcastle VB, Plum F (eds): "Handbook of Physiology: The Nervous System V." Bethesda: American Physiological Society, pp 419–459.

Lee GP, Meador KJ, Smith JR, Loring DW, Flanigin HF (1988): Preserved crossmodal association following bilateral amygdalotomy in man. Int J Neurosci 40:47–55.

Leonard CM, Rolls ET, Wilson FA, Baylis GC (1985): Neurons in the amygdala of the monkey with responses selective for faces. Behav Brain Res 15:159–176.

Less H, Heath RG, Mickle WA (1965): Rhinencephalic activity during thought. Electroencephalogr Clin Neurophysiol 18:260–271.

Levenson RW (1988): Emotion and the autonomic nervous system: A prospectus for research on autonomic specificity. In Wagner HL (ed): "Social Psychophysiology and Emotion: Theory and Clinical Application." New York: John Wiley & Sons, pp 17–42.

Levenson RW, Ekman P, Friesen WV (1990): Voluntary facial action generates emotion-specific autonomic nervous system activity. Psychophysiology 27:363–383.

Libet B (1973): Electrical stimulation of cortex in human subjects, and conscious sensory aspects. In Iggo A (ed): "Handbook of Sensory Physiology," Vol 2. New York: Springer, pp 743–790.

Lovrich D, Simson R, Vaughan HGJr, Ritter W (1986): Topography of visual event-related potentials during geometric and phonetic discriminations. Electroencephalogr Clin Neurophysiol 65:1–12.

Lynch G (1986): "Synapses, Circuits, and the Beginnings of Memory." Cambridge: MIT Press.

Maclean PD (1972): Cerebral evolution and emotional processes: new findings on the striatal complex. Ann NY Acad Sci 193:137–149.

Mahl GF, Rothenberg A, Delgado GMR, Hamlin H (1964): Psychological responses in the human to intracerebral electrical stimulation. Psychosom Med 26:337–368.

Maltzman I, Pendery M (1991): An interpretation of human classical conditioning of electrodermal activity. In Galbraith GC, Kietzman ML, Donchin E (eds): "Neurophysiology and Psychophysiology: Experimental and Clinical Applications." Hillsdale, NJ: Lawrence Erlbaum Associates.

Mandler G (1975): "Mind and Emotion." New York: Wiley.

Mark VH, Sweet W, Ervin FR (1975): Deep temporal lobe stimulation and destructive lesions in episodically violent temporal lobe epileptics. In Fields WS, Sweet WH (eds): "Neural Bases of Violence and Aggression." St. Louis: Waren H. Green, pp 379–391.

Marr D (1971): A theory of archicortex. Philos Trans R Soc Lond [Biol] 262:23–81.

Marrocco RT (1986): The neurobiology of perception. In LeDoux JE, Hirst W (eds): "Mind and Brain, Dialogues in Cognitive Neuroscience." Cambridge: Cambridge University Press, pp 33–79.

McCarthy G, Donchin E (1981): A metric for thought: A comparison of P300 latency and reaction time. Science 211:77–80.

McCarthy G, Wood CC (1984): Intracranially recorded event-related potentials during sentence processing. Soc Neurosci Abstr 10:847 (Abstract).

McCarthy G, Wood CC (1985): Human intracranial ERPs during lexical decision. Soc Neurosci Abstr 11:880–880.

McCarthy G, Wood CC, Williamson PD, Spencer DD (1989): Task-dependent field potentials in human hippocampal formation. J Neurosci 9:4253–4268.

Mishkin M (1982): A memory system in the monkey. Philos Trans R Soc Lond [Biol] 298:83–95.

Mitzdorf U (1986): The physiological causes of VEP: Current source density analysis of electrically and visually evoked potentials. In Cracco R, Bodis-Wollner I (eds): "Evoked Potentials." New York: Alan R. Liss, pp 141–154.

Munari C, Bancaud J, Bonis A, Buser P, Talairach J, Szikla G, Philippe A (1979): Role du noyau amygdalien dans la survenue de manifestations oro-alimentaires au cours des crises epileptiques chez l'homme. Electroencephalogr Clin Neurophysiol 3:236–240.

Munari C, Bancaud J, Bonis A, Stoffels C, Szikla G, Talairach J (1980): Impairment of consciousness in temporal lobe seizure: A stereoelectroencephalographic study. In Canger R, Angeleri F, Penry JK (eds): "Advances in Epileptology: XIth Epilepsy International Symposium." New York: Raven Press, pp 111–113.

Naatanen R, Gaillard AWK (1983): The orienting reflex and the N2 deflection of the ERP. In Gaillard AWK, Ritter W (eds): "Tutorials in Event Related Potential Research: Endogenous Components." Amsterdam: Elsevier, pp 119–141.

Naatanen R, Picton TW (1986): N2 and automatic versus controlled processes. In McCallum WC, Zappoli R, Denoth F (eds): "Cerebral Psychophysiology Studies in Event-Related Potentials" (Electroencephalogr Clin Neurophysiol Suppl 38). Amsterdam: Elsevier, pp 169–186.

Narabayashi H, Nagao T, Saito Y, Yoshida M, Nagahata M (1963): Stereotaxic amygdalotomy for behaviour disorders. Arch Neurol 9:1–16.

Narabayashi H (1980): From experiences of medial amygdalotomy on epileptics. Acta Neurochir [Suppl] (WIEN) 30:75–81.

Nishijo H, Ono T, Nishino H (1988): Topographic distribution of modality-specific amygdalar neurons in alert monkey. J Neurosci 8:3556–3569.

O'Keefe J, Bouma H (1968): Complex sensory properties of certain amygdala units in the freely moving cat. Exp Neurol 23:384–396.

Ohman A (1979): The orienting response, attention, and learning: An information-processing perspective. In Kimmel HD, Van Olst EH, Orlebeke JF (eds): "The Orienting Reflex in Humans." Hillsdale, NJ: Erlbaum, pp 443–467.

Ohman A (1987): The psychophysiology of emotion: An evolutionary-cognitive perspective. In Ackles PK, Jennings JR, Coles MGH (eds): "Advances in Psychophysiology: A Research Annual," Vol 2. Greenwich, CT: JAI Press, pp 79–127.

Ohman A (1988): Nonconscious control of autonomic responses: A role for Pavlovian conditioning? Biol Psychol 27:113–135.

Pagni CA, Marrossero F (1965): Some observations on the human rhinencephalon—A rheo-electroencephalographic study. Electroencephalogr Clin Neurophysiol 18:260–271.

Panksepp J (1982): Toward a general psychobiological theory of emotion. Behav Brain Sci 5:407–422.

Papez JW (1937): A proposed mechanism of emotion. Archneurol Psychiat 38:725–743.

Parra A, Velasco M, Cervantes C, Munoz H, Cerbon MA, Velasco F (1980): Plasma prolactin increase following electric stimulation of the amygdala in humans. Neuroendocrinology 31:60–65.

Penfield W, Jasper H (1954): "Epilepsy and the Function Anatomy of the Human Brain." Boston: Little, Brown.

Penfield WP, Faulk ME (1955): The insula: Further observations on its function. Brain 78:445–470.

Penfield WP, Perot P (1963): The brain's record of auditory and visual experience: A final summary annd discussion. Brain 86:595–696.

Ploog D (1981): Neurobiology of primate audio-vocal behavior. Brain Res 228:35–61.

Plutchik R, Ax AF (1967): A critique of "Determinants of Emotional State" by Schacter and Singer. Psychophysiol 4:79–82.

Plutchik R (1980): "Emotion: A Psychoevolutionary Synthesis." New York: Harper and Row.

Posner MI (1975): Psychobiology of attention. In Gazzaniga M, Balkemore C (eds): "Handbook of Psychobiology." New York: Academic Press, pp 441–480.

Posner MI, Klein RM (1973): On the functions of consciousness. In Kornblum S (ed): "Attention and Performance," Vol IV. New York: Academic Press, pp 21–35.

Pribram KH, Kruger L (1954): Functions of the "olfactory brain." Ann NY Acad Sci 58:109–138.

Price JL, Russchen FT, Amaral DG (1981): An autoradiographic study of the projections of the central nucleus of the monkey amygdala. J Neurosci 11:1242–1259.

Pritchard WS, Shappell SA, Brandt ME (1988): Psychophysiology of N200/N400: A review and classification scheme. In Ackles PK, Jennings JR, Coles MGH (eds): "Advances in Psychophysiology." Greenwich, CT: JAI Press (in press).

Putnam EL, Roth WT (1987): Automatic elicitation of cognitive components by startling stimuli. In Johnson R Jr, Rohrbaugh JW, Parasuraman R (eds): "Current Trends in Event-Related Potential Research," (EEG Suppl 40). Amsterdam: Elsevier, pp 256–307.

Rado S (1969): "Adaptational Psychodynamics: Motivation and Control." New York: Science House.

Ramamurthi B (1988): Stereotactic operation in behaviour disorders. Amygdalotomy and hypothalamotomy. Acta Neurochir [Suppl] (WIEN) 44:152–157.

Rayport M, Ferguson SM (1974): Qualitative modification of sensory responses to amygdaloid stimulation in man by interview content and context. Electroencephalogr Clin Neurophysiol 34:714.

Remillard GM, Andermann F, Gloor P, Olivier A, Martin JB (1981): Water-drinking as ictal behavior in complex partial seizures. Neurology 31:117–124.

Remillard G, Andermann F, Testa GF, Gloor P, Aube M, Martin JB, Feindel W (1983): Sexual ictal manifestations in women with temporal lobe epilepsy: A finding suggesting sexual dimorphism in the human brain. Neurology 33:323–330.

Riekkinen P, Buzsaki G, Riekkinen P Jr, Soininen H, Partanen J (1991): The cholinergic system and EEG slow waves. Electroencephalogr Clin Neurophysiol 78:89–96.

Ritter W, Ford JM, Gaillard AW, Harter MR, Kutas M, Naatanen R, Polich J, Renault B, Rohrbaugh J (1984): Cognition and event-related potentials. I. The relation of negative potentials and cognitive processes. Ann NY Acad Sci 425:24–38.

Roberts GW, Bruton CJ (1990): Notes from the graveyard: Neuropathology and schizophrenia. Neuropathol Appl Neurobiol 16:3–16.

Rodin E (1969): Psychomotor epilepsy and aggressive behavior. Arch Gen Psychiat 28:210–213.

Rolls ET (1989): Functions of neuronal networks in the hippocampus and neocortex in memory. In Byrne JH, Berry WO (eds): "Neural Models of Plasticity." San Diego: Academic Press, pp 240–265.

Rosler F, Hasselmann D, Sojka B (1987): Central and peripheral correlates of orienting and habituation. In Johnson R Jr, Rohrbaugh JW, Parasuraman R (eds): "Current Trends in Event-Related Potential Research" (EEG Suppl 40). Amsterdam: Elsevier Science, pp 366–372.

Rossitch E Jr, Carrazana EJ, Ellenbogen R, Alexander Eben III (1989): Klüver-Bucy syndrome following recovery from transtentorial herniation. Br J Neurosurg 3:503–506.

Roth WT (1983): A comparison of P300 and skin conductance response. In Gaillard AWK, Ritter W (eds): "Tutorials in ERP Research: Endogenous Components." Amsterdam: North-Holland, pp 177–199.

Roth WT, Dorato KH, Kopell BS (1984): Intensity and task effects on evoked physiological responses to noise bursts. Psychophysiology 21:466–481.

Rugg MD, Kok A, Barrett G, Fischler I (1986): ERPs associated with language and hemispheric specialization. A review. Electroencephalogr Clin Neurophysiol [Suppl] 38:273–300.

Rugg MD, Nagy ME (1989): Event-related potentials and recognition memory for words. Electroencephalogr Clin Neurophysiol 72:395–406.

Russchen FT, Amaral DG, Price JL (1985): The afferent connections of the substantia innominata in the monkey, Macaca fascicularis. J Comp Neurol 242:1–27.

Sanghera MK, Rolls ET, Roper-Hall A (1979): Visual responses of neurons in the dorsolateral amygdala of the alert monkey. Exp Neurol 63:610–626.

Sano K, Mayanagi Y (1988): Posteromedial hypothalamotomy in the treatment of violent, aggressive behaviour. Acta Neurochir (Wien) 44:145–151.

Schachter S (1975): Cognition and peripheralist-centralist controversies in motivation and emotion. In Gazzaniga MS, Blakemore C (eds): "Handbook of Psychobiology." New York: Academic Press.

Schutze I, Knuspfer MM, Eismann A, Stumpf H, Stock G (1987): Sensory input to single neurons in the amygdala of the cat. Exp Neurol 97:499–515.

Sem-Jacobsen CW, Peterson MC, Lazarte JA, Dodge HW Jr, Holman CB (1955): Intracerebral electrographic recordings from psychotic patients during hallucinations and agitation. Am J Psychiat 112:278–288.

Sem-Jacobsen CW, Peterson MC, Lazarte JA, Dodge HW Jr, Holman CB (1956): Electroencephalographic rhythms from the depths of the parietal, occipital and temporal lobes in man. Electroencephalogr Clin Neurophysiol 8:263–278.

Seyfarth RM (1987): Vocal communication and its relation to language. In Smuts BB,

Cheney DL, Seyfarth RM, Wrangham RW, Struhsaker TT (eds): "Primate Societies." Chicago: University of Chicago Press, pp 440–451.

Shiffrin RM, Schneider W (1977): Controlled and automatic human information processing: II. Perceptual learning, automatic attention and a general theory. Psychol Rev 84:127–190.

Smith ME, Halgren E (1987a): Event-related potentials elicited by familiar and unfamiliar faces. Electroencephalogr Clin Neurophysiol [Suppl] 40:422–426.

Smith ME, Halgren E (1987b): Event-related potentials during lexical decision: Effects of repetition, word frequency, pronounceability, and concreteness. Electroencephalogr Clin Neurophysiol [Suppl] 40:417–421.

Smith ME, Stapleton JM, Halgren E (1986): Human medial temporal lobe potentials evoked in memory and language tasks. Electroencephalogr Clin Neurophysiol 63:145–159.

Smith ME, Halgren E (1988): Attenuation of a sustained visual processing negativity after lesions that includes the inferotemporal cortex. Electroencephalogr Clin Neurophysiol 70:366–370.

Smith ME, Halgren E (1989): Dissociation of recognition memory components following temporal lobe lesions. J Exp Psychol [Learn Mem Cogn] 15:50–60.

Smith ME, Halgren E, Sokolik M, Baudena P, Mussolino A, Liegeois-Chauvel C, Chauvel P (1990): The intracranial voltage distribution of endogenous potentials elicited during auditory discrimination. Electroencephalogr Clin Neurophysiol 76:235–248.

Sokolov EN (1963): Higher nervous functions: The orienting reflex. Annu Rev Physiol 25:545–580.

Spencer SS, Spencer DD, Williamson PD, Mattson RH (1983): Sexual automatisms in complex partial seizures. Neurology 33:527–533.

Sperling MR, Wilson CL (1986): The effect of limbic and extralimbic electrical stimulations upon prolactin secretion in humans. Brain Res 371:293–297.

Squires NK, Halgren E, Wilson CL, Crandall PH (1983): Human endogenous limbic potentials: Cross-modality and depth/surface comparisons in epileptic subjects. In Gaillard AWK, Ritter W (eds): "Tutorials in ERP Research: Endogenous Components." Amsterdam: North Holland, pp 217–232.

Srebo R (1985): Localization of cortical activity associated with visual recognition in humans. J Physiol 360:247–259.

Stapleton JM, Halgren E (1987): Endogenous potentials evoked in simple cognitive tasks: Depth components and task correlates. Electroencephalogr Clin Neurophysiol 67:44–52.

Steklis HD, Kling A (1985): Neurobiology of affiliative behavior in non-human primates. In Reite M, Field T (eds): "The Biology of Social Attachment." New York: Academic Press.

Stevens JR, Mark VH, Ervin F, Pacheco P, Suematsu K (1969): Deep temporal lobe stimulation in man: Long-latency, long-lasting psychological changes. Arch Neurol 21:157–169.

Stevens JR (1991): Psychosis and the temporal lobe. In Smith DB, Treiman DM, Trimble MR (eds): "Advances in Neurology (Vol 55): Neurobehavioral Problems in Epilepsy." New York: Raven Press, pp 79–96.

Stoffels C, Munari C, Bonis A, Bancaud J, Talairach J (1980): Manifestations genitales et "sexuelles" lors des crises epileptiques partielles chez l'homme. Rev Electroencephalogr Neurophysiol Clin 10:386–392.

Streletz LJ, Bae SH, Roeshman RM, Schatz NJ, Savino PJ (1981): Visual evoked potentials in occipital lobe lesions. Arch Neurol 38:80–85.

Sutton S, Ruchkin D (1984): The late positive complex: Advances and new problems. In Karrer R, Cohen J, Tueting P (eds): "Brain and Information: Event-Related Potentials (Annals of the New York Academy of Sciences, Vol 425)." New York: NY Academy of Sciences, pp 1–23.

Swartz BE, Delgado-Escueta AV, Maldonado HM (1990): A stereoencephalographic study of ictal propagation producing anisocoria, auras of fear, and complex partial seizures of temporal lobe origin. J Epilepsy 3:149–156.

Terrace HS (1985): Animal cognition: Thinking about language. Philos Trans R Soc Lond [Biol] 308:113–128.

Terzian J, Ore GD (1955): Syndrome of Klüver and Bucy. Neurology 5:373–380.

Teyler TJ, DiScenna P (1986): The hippocampal memory indexing theory. Behav Neurosci 100:147–154.

Tolman EC (1923): A behavioristic account of the emotions. Psychol Rev 30:217–227.

Tranel D, Damasio AR (1988): Non-conscious face recognition in patients with face agnosia. Behav Brain Res 30(3):235–249.

Tranel D, Hyman BT (1990): Neuropsychological correlates of bilateral amygdala damage. Arch Neurol 47:349–355.

Turner BH, Mishkin M, Knapp M (1980): Organization of the amygdalopetal projections from modality-specific cortical association areas in the monkey. J Comp Neurol 191:515–543.

Turvey MT (1973): On peripheral and central processes in vision: Inferences from an information-processing analysis of masking with patterned stimuli. Psychol Rev 80:1–52.

Ueki S, Domino EF (1961): Some evidence for a mechanical receptor in olfactory function. J Neurophysiol 24:12–25.

Van Buren JM (1963): The abdominal aura: A study of abdominal sensation occurring in epilepsy and produced by depth stimulation. Electroencephalogr Clin Neurophysiol 15:1–19.

Vanderploeg RD, Brown WS, Marsh FT (1987): Judgements of emotion in words and face: ERP correlates. Int J Psychophysiol 5:193–205.

VanPetten C, Kutas M (1990): Interactions between sentence context and word frequency in event-related brain potentials. Mem Cogn 18:380–393.

Verbaten MN (1983): The influence of information on habituation of cortical, autonomic and behavioral components of the orienting response (or). In Gaillard AWK, Ritter W (eds): "Tutorials in ERP Research: Endogenous Components." Amsterdam: North-Holland, pp 201–218.

Volz HP, Rehbein G, Triepel J, Knuepfer MM, Stumpf H, Stock G (1990): Afferent connections of the nucleus centralis amygdalae. A horseradish peroxidase study and literature survey. Anat Embryol 181:177–194.

Walter RD (1973): Tactical considerations leading to surgical treatment of limbic epilepsy. In Brazier MAB (ed): "Epilepsy: Its Phenomena in Man." New York: Academic Press, pp 99–119.

Wieser HG (1983): "Electroclinical Features of the Psychomotor Seizure." London: Butterworths.

Wieser H (1991): Ictal manifestations of temporal lobe seizures. In Smith DB, Treiman DM, Trimble MR (eds): "Advances in Neurology (Vol 55): Neurobehavioral Problems in Epilepsy." New York: Raven Press, pp 301–315.

Wilson CL, Babb TL, Halgren E, Crandall PH (1983): Visual receptive fields and response properties of neurons in human temporal lobe and visual pathways. Brain 106:473–502.

Wilson CL, Babb TL, Halgren E, Wang ML, Crandall PH (1984): Habituation of human limbic neuronal response to sensory stimulation. Exp Neurol 84:74–97.

Young PT (1943): "Emotion in Man and Animals." New York: Wiley.

Zajonc RB (1980): Feeling and thinking. Preferences need no inferences. Am Psychol 35:151–175.

Zola-Morgan S, Squire LR, Amaral DG (1986): Human amnesia and the medial temporal region: Enduring memory impairment following a bilateral lesion limited to field CA1 of the hippocampus. J Neurosci 6:2950–2967.

The Amygdala: Neurobiological Aspects of Emotion,
Memory, and Mental Dysfunction, pages 229–254
© 1992 Wiley-Liss, Inc.

8

Amygdaloid Contributions to Conditioned Arousal and Sensory Information Processing

BRUCE S. KAPP, PAUL J. WHALEN, WILLIAM F. SUPPLE, AND
JEFFREY P. PASCOE
Department of Psychology, University of Vermont, Burlington, Vermont

INTRODUCTION

As is apparent from the chapters in this volume concerning the behavioral functions of the amygdala, much research of late has been devoted to amygdaloid contributions to learning and memory processes. Indeed, as is summarized in the following sections, our research has been concerned with delineating a specific neural circuit by which the amygdala contributes to the acquisition and expression of a well-defined conditioned response (CR): conditioned heart rate deceleration (i.e., bradycardia) in the rabbit during Pavlovian fear conditioning. This CR has long served as a model response for analyses designed to elucidate neural circuits which contribute to associative learning (Schneiderman, 1972). In addition, it has served as a model to investigate the neural substrates by which emotional arousal affects autonomic responding, as well as the conditions and neural substrates by which emotional arousal elicits cardiopathology (Markgraf and Kapp, 1988). As detailed below, our own research and that of others prompted our initial hypothesis that the central nucleus of the amygdala is a component of a circuit essential to the expression of this CR (Kapp et al., 1981). However, more recent research, also to be reviewed below, suggests that the central nucleus possesses the appropriate characteristics for the plasticity required for the acquisition of this CR.

While in a restricted sense the central nucleus and anatomically associated structures appear to function in the acquisition and expression of the bradycardiac CR, emerging anatomical, physiological, and behavioral research dictates that it possesses a more general function, necessitating an expansion of our original hypothesis. In this chapter, therefore, we review evidence which supports the hypothesis that the central nucleus and associated structures contribute to the rapid acquisition of an increased level of nonspecific attention or arousal,

Address correspondence to Bruce S. Kapp, Department of Psychology, University of Vermont, Burlington, VT 05405.

as manifested in a variety of rapidly acquired CRs (e.g., bradycardia, EEG desynchronization, pupillary dilation) which emerge during Pavlovian conditioning; CRs which function to enhance sensory information processing. These CRs are expressed by the extensive projections of the central nucleus to, for example, (1) the basal forebrain, including magnocellular cholinergic neurons, (2) the brain stem, including the lateral tegmental fields, and (3) the dorsal medulla, including autonomic regulatory nuclei. They provide optimal conditions for sensory processing by lowering detection thresholds for environmental stimuli and by enhancing neuronal responsiveness of central structures to such stimuli. In essence, the nucleus enhances sensory information processing.

While the validity of this hypothesis has yet to be vigorously tested, it is consistent with earlier formulations suggesting the contribution of the amygdala to arousal or attentional processes (Kaada, 1972). Furthermore, it aids in the unification of a large amount of anatomical, electrophysiological, and behavioral data concerning amygdaloid contributions to behavior. We now turn to the evidence which led to our initial and expanded hypotheses.

THE RABBIT BRADYCARDIAC CONDITIONED RESPONSE AND THE CENTRAL NUCLEUS OF THE AMYGDALA: A RESEARCH FOCUS

For a variety of reasons which we have detailed previously (Kapp et al., 1984a), the rabbit bradycardiac CR was chosen for our analysis of amygdaloid contributions to learning and memory processes. This CR rapidly develops in response to an auditory conditioned stimulus (CS) during Pavlovian fear conditioning trials in which the offset of a 5.0 second tone CS is coincident with the onset of a 0.5 second electric shock unconditioned stimulus (US). It can be considered a primary response not secondary to increased blood pressure and is accompanied by a slight depressor response (Powell and Kazis, 1976). In addition, it results primarily from activation of the vagus nerves (Fredericks et al., 1974). Since preganglionic, vagal cardioinhibitory neurons in the rabbit were reported to be located in the vagal dorsal motor nucleus and nucleus ambiguous (Schwaber and Schneiderman, 1975; Jordan et al., 1982), these combined findings would prove advantageous for identifying a descending pathway(s) which might activate these cardioinhibitory neurons and which might serve as a potential CR pathway(s).

Given the heterogeneous nature of the amygdaloid complex, we adopted a neuroanatomical systems approach by concentrating our efforts on one nucleus, the central nucleus, in an initial attempt to elucidate amygdaloid function in associative learning (Fig. 1). We postulated that an attempt to determine if this nucleus contributed to the acquisition and/or expression of the bradycardiac CR, followed by an analysis of the information carried by the afferents and efferents of this nucleus, would lead us closer to understanding its role and perhaps the role of other components of the amygdala in learning. Our initial focus on the central nucleus was guided by several factors which have been described previously (Kapp et al., 1981). Hence, we will not elaborate upon them here.

CONTRIBUTIONS OF THE CENTRAL NUCLEUS TO THE EXPRESSION OF THE BRADYCARDIAC CONDITIONED RESPONSE

Our earlier research, as well as that of others, suggested that the central nucleus was critical to the expression of the bradycardiac CR. First, lesions

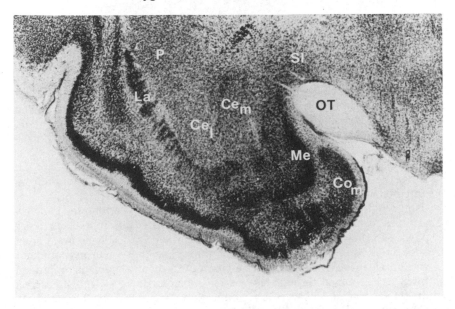

Fig. 1. The amygdaloid complex of the rabbit shown in coronal section. Abbreviations: Ce_m, medial component of the central nucleus; Ce_l, lateral component of the central nucleus; Co_m, posteromedial cortical nucleus of the amygdala; La, lateral nucleus of the amygdala; Me, medial nucleus of the amygdala; OT, optic tract; P, putamen; SI, sublenticular substantia innominata.

(Kapp et al., 1979) or pharmacological manipulations (Gallagher et al., 1980, 1981, 1982) of the nucleus prior to conditioning markedly attenuated or augmented the magnitude of the bradycardiac CR. The effects appeared to be selective to an effect on a mechanism involving the elaboration of the CR since the results could not be readily attributed to a decreased sensitivity to the CS and US intensities used, nor to an interference with resting heart rate. Second, as we have demonstrated in the rabbit (Schwaber et al., 1980, 1982), and as others have demonstrated in other species (Hopkins and Holstege, 1978; Price and Amaral, 1981; Higgins and Schwaber, 1983), the central nucleus projects directly, and most probably indirectly, to cardioregulatory nuclei of the dorsal medulla; the nucleus of the solitary tract (NTS), nucleus ambiguous, and the vagal dorsal motor nucleus. As stated above, the latter two nuclei contain vagal preganglionic cardioinhibitory neurons in the rabbit, and this projection offered an anatomical substrate for the activation of these neurons by the central nucleus. Third, we and others have subsequently demonstrated that electrical stimulation of the central nucleus in the rabbit elicits profound, short-latency bradycardia and depressor responses (Kapp et al.,1982; Applegate et al.,1983; Cox et al., 1987), a response pattern similar to that observed in response to a CS during Pavlovian aversive conditioning (Powell and Kazis, 1976). Such stimulation also has been shown to produce short-latency activation of NTS neurons and of cardioinhibitory neurons within the vagal dorsal motor nucleus of the rabbit (Cox et al., 1986). Fourth, we have observed changes in short-latency multiple unit activity which rapidly develop in the central nucleus to the presentation of the CS when paired with an aversive US (Applegate et al., 1982) (Fig. 2). In subsequent single unit analyses we used a differential conditioning procedure in which a tone of one frequency, the CS +, was always followed by the US, but that of another frequency, the CS −, was never paired with the US (Pascoe and Kapp, 1985a). We found that the majority of central nucleus neurons demonstrated differential responses to these CSs, as did the heart rate (Fig. 3). Importantly, for some neurons the magnitude of the neuronal response to the CS + was correlated significantly with the magnitude of the bradycardiac CR to the CS +. Hence, one could predict the magnitude of heart rate deceleration from the rate of neuronal firing in response to the CS +.

Using antidromic activation and collision techniques, we attempted to determine if these central nucleus neurons which demonstrated differential excitatory responses to the two CSs were projection neurons to the lower brain stem (Pascoe and Kapp, 1985a). Somewhat to our surprise, these neurons could not be antidromically activated from stimulation of the central nucleus projection pathway as it coursed through the mesencephalon. However, other neurons within the central nucleus were antidromically activated from such simulation. The latter were characterized by very slow spontaneous rates (0.01–0.4 Hz) and decreased their activity more to the CS + than to the CS −. This suggested that during the presentation of the CS, influences normally exerted by these neurons on the brain stem were reduced. The observation that neurons demonstrating differential excitatory responses to the CSs did not appear to project to the lower brain stem raises the possibility that any influence that they exert on medullary cardioinhibitory neurons may be via an oligosynaptic pathway(s). In this context we have observed in rabbit a projection from the central nucleus to an area of the periaqueductal gray from which arise projections to the NTS/vagal dorsal motor nucleus complex (Kapp et al., 1986; Wilson and Kapp, 1990a). However, while chemical stimulation at sites within this region of the periaqueductal gray elicited bradycardia and depressor responses, lesions of this region did not affect the expression of the bradycardiac CR (Wilson and Kapp, 1990b). This suggests that a central nucleus-periaqueductal gray-dorsal medullary oligosynaptic pathway is not essential for the expression of conditioned bradycardia. An obvious second oligosynaptic pathway by which the central nucleus may drive the vagus nerve in the expression of the bradycardiac CR is via its projection to the hypothalamus, which in turn projects directly to the NTS/vagal dorsal motor nucleus complex. The contribution of this pathway to the expression of this CR has not been adequately investigated in the rabbit. However, recent work by LeDoux and colleagues (LeDoux et al., 1988) has demonstrated its possible importance in the expression of a blood pressure CR in the rat in response to a fear-arousing auditory CS (see Chapter 12, LeDoux, this volume). In summary, our earlier results suggested that auditory CS information influences the central nucleus, which in turn, via both direct and indirect pathways, leads to an activation of medullary cardioinhibitory neurons which slow the heart.

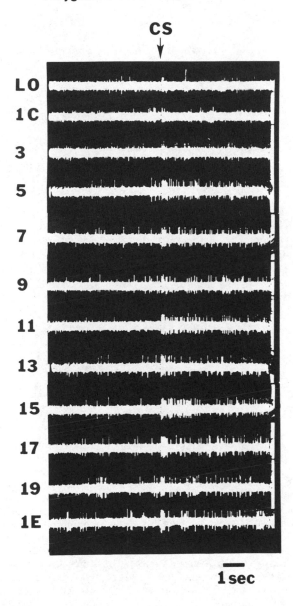

Fig. 2. Oscilloscope traces of multiple unit activity recorded from the amygdala central nucleus over Pavlovian conditioning trials. Arrow at top center marks the onset of the 5.0 second tone CS for each trial. The last of 20 tone alone orienting trials (LO) followed by alternate CS-US paired conditioning trials (1C–19) for the 20 trial conditioning phase are shown. Note the early emergence of increased unit activity to the CS over the course of conditioning. The first extinction trial following the 20 conditioning trials is depicted in 1E.

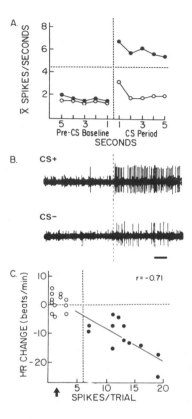

Fig. 3. Characteristics of central nucleus neurons which demonstrate an increase in activity in response to CS + and CS − presentations during the expression of conditioned bradycardia. **A:** Cumulative records of the activity of 13 neurons during the course of 114 presentations each of the CS + (●) and CS − (○). The dashed horizontal line indicates the point at which unit activity is significantly elevated over pre-CS baseline rates ($P < .05$). **B:** Oscilloscope traces showing the response of one such neuron to the presentation of the CS + and CS −. Dashed vertical line depicts onset of the 5.0 second CS. Calibration bar = 1.0 second. **C:** The relationship between heart rate change and the activity of the neuron depicted in B during the course of 12 presentations each of the CS + (●) and CS − (○). The correlation coefficient and regression line are based only upon those trials during which the CS + was presented. The arrow depicts spontaneous rate and the dashed vertical line indicates the point above which the activity of this neuron is significantly increased over baseline rates ($P < .05$). [Adapted with permission from Elsevier Science Publishers, from Pascoe and Kapp (1985a). We thank Dr. A.D. Loewy for the adaptation.]

Research consistent with this hypothesis has been offered by others. First, Gentile et al. (1986a) have reported that selective neuronal cell body destruction within the central nucleus with ibotenic acid prior to Pavlovian fear conditioning in the rabbit attenuated the magnitude of the bradycardiac CR. Gentile et al. (1986b) also reported that electrolytic lesions administered following acquisition of this CR attenuated its magnitude during subsequent CS presentations. Second, lesions of the central nucleus block the acquisition of conditioned heart rate responding during Pavlovian conditioning in neonatal rats (Sananes and Campbell, 1989). Third, lesions made in the region of the central nucleus prior to Pavlovian fear conditioning trials in rats attenuated the magnitude of conditioned blood pressure and freezing responses to auditory CS presentations during subsequent retention testing (Iwata et al., 1986). Electrical or chemical stimulation of the central nucleus in the awake rat elicits blood pressure responses of a pattern similar to that observed in response to a CS (Iwata et al., 1987). Fourth, a potentiated acoustic startle response elicited in the rat by an auditory startle stimulus during a fear-arousing CS is markedly attenuated by lesions located in the region of the central nucleus (Hitchcock and Davis, 1986). Conversely, electrical stimulation within this region immediately prior to the presentation of the auditory startle stimulus potentiates the startle response (Rosen and Davis, 1988). Finally, cooling of the central nucleus in cat during presentation of a fear-arousing CS has been demonstrated to attenuate the blood pressure CR to that stimulus (Zhang et al., 1986). The importance of these observations lies in the fact that the central nucleus may contribute to the acquisition and expression of a variety of CRs across several species. This suggests that this nucleus possesses a more general function(s) during Pavlovian conditioning than the expression of cardiovascular responses, a function to which we return below.

THE CENTRAL NUCLEUS OF THE AMYGDALA: WIDESPREAD INFLUENCES ON FOREBRAIN AND BRAIN STEM

While our earlier anatomical studies focused upon the projections of the central nucleus to cardioregulatory nuclei of the dorsal medulla and their contribution to conditioned cardiovascular responding, it must be emphasized that this nucleus sends extensive projections to a variety of brain stem sensory, motor, and sensorimotor-related regions, suggesting its potential for widespread influences on the brain stem. For example, it has been reported to project to the parabrachial nuclear complex (Hopkins and Holstege, 1978), mesencephalic trigeminal nucleus (Ruggiero et al., 1982), the ventral aspects of the periaqueductal gray (Hopkins and Holstege, 1978), the lateral tegmental field (Hopkins and Holstege, 1978), and the medial and ventral regions of the cervical spinal cord (Sandrew et al., 1986). A particularly heavy projection innervates the entirety of the lateral tegmental field, a continuous region extending from the caudal medulla to rostral pons (Holstege et al., 1977). This field is characterized by populations of interneurons which project upon a variety of cranial nerve motor nuclei (Holstege et al., 1977), including motorneurons of the trigeminal, facial, hypoglossal, and abducens nuclei, as well as to autonomic and somatic motor neurons of the spinal cord. These projections suggest that these interneurons are important components of a variety of brain stem reflex pathways (Holstege et al.,

1977; Ruggiero et al., 1982). In this sense, the lateral tegmental field is postulated to be homologous to the dorsolateral part of the spinal cord intermediate zone, which contains interneurons that innervate spinal motorneuron pools.

The central nucleus possesses the potential for widespread influences not only on the brain stem but also, indirectly, on the cortex. Given its projections to the region of cholinergic neurons located within the sublenticular substantia innominata (Price and Amaral, 1981; Grove, 1988; Russchen et al., 1985), the central nucleus has the potential for widespread influences on the cortex via modulation of the activity of cholinergic neurons which in turn project upon cortex. In summary, the efferent projection system of the central nucleus is extensive and suggests a function(s) for the nucleus during Pavlovian conditioning that exceeds the expression of cardiovascular conditioned CRs.

Before proceeding with a discussion of this function(s), it should be noted that based upon a variety of anatomical observations (Schwaber et al., 1982; DeOlmos et al., 1985; Holstege et al., 1985; Grove, 1988), the suggestion has been offered that the central nucleus may be a component of a more extensive forebrain continuum which includes neighboring portions of the sublenticular substantia innominata, bed nucleus of the stria terminalis, and nucleus accumbens (see DeOlmos et al., 1985). These observations suggest the anatomical unity of this continuum as a single entity, perhaps with a defined function. From a functional perspective, therefore, any functions attributed to the central nucleus may best be understood in the context of the functions of the other components of this continuum as knowledge of their functions emerges.

THE CENTRAL NUCLEUS: A SUBSTRATE FOR CONDITIONED AROUSAL RESPONSES

We adopted the rabbit bradycardiac CR as a model to identify brain circuits which contribute to learning. However, the rapid emergence of this CR during aversive Pavlovian conditioning procedures in a variety of species (Fitzgerald et al., 1966; Hein, 1969), including the human (Obrist et al., 1965) suggests that it serves an important, adaptive function. Given that the central nucleus contributes to its expression, an understanding of the function of this response should lead to an understanding of a more general function(s) of the central nucleus, particularly with respect to its extensive projection system.

A perusal of the conditions under which conditioned bradycardia occurs in the rabbit demonstrates that during Pavlovian conditioning procedures it not only occurs to a CS that predicts negative reinforcement but also to one that predicts positive reinforcement (Sideroff et al., 1972; Gibbs, personal communication). Further, it has been documented repeatedly in humans that bradycardia occurs in response to a variety of motivationally significant stimuli, and not exclusively to those that predict an aversive event (Lacey and Lacey, 1974; Obrist, 1981). It must be concluded from these results that bradycardia is not simply a manifestation of an emotional state of fear but of a more general central process.

Insight into the functional significance of the bradycardiac response comes from human studies showing that vagus-mediated bradycardia occurs to anticipatory, attention-commanding stimuli (Bohlin and Graham, 1977; Lacey and

Lacey, 1970, 1974, 1978), for example, during the signaled preparatory interval of reaction time tasks during which the subject awaits in anticipation for a stimulus to respond. Lacey and Lacey (1974) have proposed that this bradycardia is a component of an attentional or arousal mechanism which functions to enhance the receptivity of the organism to sensory input, as well as its response to such input. They suggest that bradycardia decreases baroreceptor feedback, an inhibitory feedback which has been shown, for example, to (1) produce increased EEG slow-wave activity, an index of decreased arousal, (2) increase the threshold for the elicitation of reflexes, and (3) depress sensory and motor neuron activity (see Lacey and Lacey, 1970, 1974, 1978). The extent to which bradycardia is causally related to enhanced sensory input and the facilitation of motor output has not received extensive investigation and remains a subject of debate (Hahn, 1973).

Nevertheless, the hypothesis of Lacey and Lacey (1974) receives support from others. For example, Schell and Catania (1975) have reported a significant relationship between the degree of bradycardia and visual acuity during an anticipatory auditory stimulus of a reaction time task; greater visual acuity was associated with greater degrees of bradycardia during the auditory stimulus. Furthermore, Bohlin and Graham (1977) reported that the bradycardiac response in humans to the presentation of an attention-commanding stimulus was associated with an enhancement (e.g., increased amplitude, decreased latency) of an eyeblink reflex in response to an auditory startle stimulus. Similar results were reported by Papakostopolous and Cooper (1973), who reported that an increase in the excitability of a spinal monosynaptic reflex was associated with bradycardia during the signaled preparatory interval of a reaction time task. Although Bohlin and Graham (1977) do not address the causal relationship between bradycardia and eyeblink reflex facilitation, they suggest that an attentional-orienting process enhances sensory input, that the reflex facilitation may be simply a secondary consequence of this enhancement, and that their results are compatible with Lacey and Lacey's (1974) hypothesis. Finally, it is a common observation in humans that stimuli which elicit bradycardia also elicit EEG desynchronization reflected in low voltage fast activity (Lansing et al., 1959). A general enhancement of somatic reflexes and the occurrence of low voltage fast activity in the human has been interpreted as a reflection of heightened arousal (Lindsley, 1960; Brunia et al., 1982).

These human observations are relevant to any attempt to understand the more general functions of the central nucleus, for not only does the nucleus appear to function in anticipatory bradycardia as described above, but also in reflex modulation and in the elicitation of EEG low voltage fast activity. Two lines of evidence suggest its contribution to reflex modulation. First, from a physiological perspective, electrical stimulation of the nucleus has been reported to modulate the gain of a variety of reflexes, including the baroreceptor reflex in cat (Schlor et al., 1984) and rabbit (Pascoe et al., 1989), the jaw closure (masseteric) reflex in cat (Gary Bobo and Bonvallet, 1975), and the acoustic startle reflex in rat (Rosen and Davis, 1988). More recently, we have found that stimulation at sites within the nucleus which elicit bradycardia also enhance the amplitude of the nictitating membrane *unconditioned* reflex (a third eyelid reflex which is a component of a coordinated blink reflex) in the rabbit when electrical stimulation of the nucleus immediately precedes the elicitation of the reflex by an eyelid stimulus (Whalen and Kapp, 1991; Figs. 4, 5). The anatomy of the central nucleus and of the nictitating membrane unconditioned reflex pathway in rabbit is consistent with this finding; a multisynaptic component of the reflex circuit is believed to synapse in the medullary lateral tegmental field (Harvey et al., 1984), in an area recipient of substantial projections from the central nucleus (Whalen and Kapp, 1991). Since facilitation of the reflex occurred with current levels which did not cause movement of the nictitating membrane, the data are also consistent with the hypothesis that the enhancement could be due, at least in part, to an effect on the sensory side of the reflex, leading to enhanced motor output. As described above, the eyeblink unconditioned reflex facilitation during an anticipatory stimulus in humans has been interpreted in this context (Bohlin and Graham, 1977).

Second, from a behavioral perspective, during conditioning of the nictitating membrane response in rabbit, the nictitating membrane unconditioned response is enhanced in amplitude when the CS immediately precedes the US compared to elicitation of the reflex by the US in the absence of the CS (Weisz and LoTurco, 1988). This enhancement appears to be learned (Weisz and McInerney, 1990), and similar to the bradycardiac CR, it emerges within few conditioning trials, at a time when the CS has yet to elicit a nictitating membrane CR. The relationships between (1) bradycardia and reflex facilitation (including eyeblink reflex) during attention-commanding, anticipatory stimuli in humans and (2) bradycardia and facilitation of the nictitating membrane unconditioned response during an anticipatory CS in rabbit are intriguing. This is particularly so in light of (a) our findings that sites within the central nucleus which, when stimulated, elicit both bradycardia and facilitation of the nictitating membrane unconditioned response (Whalen and Kapp, 1991), (b) the recent report that lesions of the central nucleus block the conditioned enhancement of the nictitating membrane unconditioned reflex in rabbit (Harden et al., 1990) in

---

Fig. 4. A: Data from an individual rabbit in which facilitation of the amplitude of the nictitating membrane (NM) reflex was obtained from stimulation at a site located within the central nucleus. The abscissa represents the percent change in NM reflex amplitude when stimulation (100 µA, 100 msec) of the central nucleus preceded (by 100 msec) the elicitation of the NM reflex compared to the temporally adjacent baseline trial, in which stimulation did not precede the elicitation of the reflex. A 0% change indicates no effect of stimulation on the amplitude of the NM reflex. Eight baseline and eight stimulation trials were presented with a 90 second variable intertrial interval. **B:** A thionin-stained coronal section illustrating the electrode placement which when stimulated produced the facilitation of the reflex as shown in A. The arrow denotes the placement of the ventral tip of the electrode where stimulation was applied, located in the dorsal region of the central nucleus. **C:** The bradycardiac response produced by a 3 second stimulus train (100 µA, 100Hz) applied to the site depicted in B. The bar represents the 3 second stimulus period. Abbreviations as in Figure 1. (Reprinted by permission of the American Psychological Association, from Whalen and Kapp, 1991.)

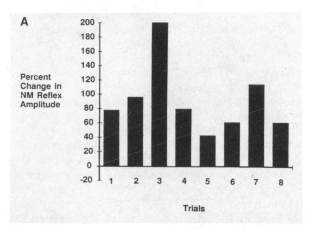

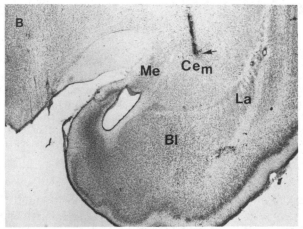

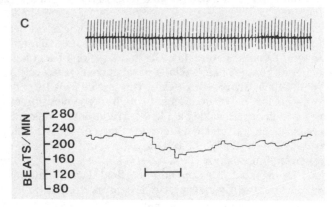

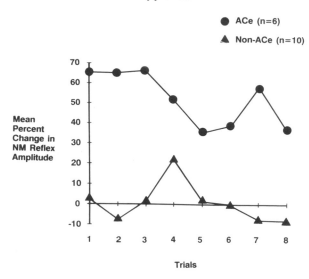

Fig. 5. Mean percent change in NM reflex amplitude following stimulation at electrode placements lying within the central nucleus (ACe, n = 6) versus stimulation of placements lying outside of the nucleus (non-ACe, n = 10). Sites lying outside the nucleus were located in the internal capsule, globus pollidus, optic tract, stria terminalis, and the lateral amygdala nucleus. A 100 uA, 100Hz, 400 msec stimulus train was applied to all sites 400 msec prior to elicitation of the reflex on stimulation trials. See Figure 4A for further details. (Reprinted by permission of the American Psychological Association from Whalen and Kapp, 1991.)

addition to the bradycardiac CR, and (c) the suggestion that reflex facilitation during an anticipatory stimulus in human may be secondary to enhanced sensory input (Bohlin and Graham, 1977) and reflect a general increase in arousal (Brunia et al., 1982).

As stated above, evidence also suggests a contribution for the central nucleus in the generation of neocortical EEG low voltage fast activity. First, extensive projections exist from the central nucleus to the region of acetylcholine (ACh)-containing neurons of the magnocellular basal nucleus (Price and Amaral, 1981; Russchen et al., 1985; Grove, 1988). The latter nucleus, via its widespread projections to neocortex, plays an essential role in the generation of neocortical low voltage fast activity (Busaki et al., 1988). Traditionally, this desynchronized EEG pattern has been considered a function of neocortical ACh release (Celesia and Jasper, 1966; Szerb, 1967), and reflective of a state of cortical readiness for processing sensory information (Steriade and McCarley, 1990). Consistent with this view are findings that ACh applied to cortical sensory neurons produces a striking enhancement of their response to sensory stimuli (Sillito and Kemp, 1983; Metherate et al., 1987, 1988a,b). Conversely, lesions of the magnocellular basal nucleus which deplete the neocortex of ACh reduce the responsiveness of neurons to visual stimuli (Sato et al., 1987). The projections from the central nucleus to the region of the magnocellular basal nucleus suggest that it may contribute directly to cortical ACh release via modulation of the activity of the magnocellular basal nucleus, resulting in neocortical low voltage fast activity. Second, and consistent with this suggestion, are the observations that electrical stimulation of the central nucleus in cat elicits low voltage fast activity (Ursin and Kaada, 1960; Kreindler and Steriade, 1964), and in recent work we have found that stimulation at sites within the central nucleus which elicit bradycardia also elicit atropine-sensitive low voltage fast activity in the rabbit (Kapp et al., 1990a) (Fig. 6). Third, central nucleus neuronal activity increases immediately preceding episodes of neocortical low voltage fast activity in the cat (Langhorst et al., 1987). Fourth, much data demonstrate that a generalized neocortical low voltage fast activity can be rapidly conditioned using Pavlovian conditioning procedures (see Morrell, 1961), and *in rabbit this EEG pattern is acquired during Pavlovian aversive conditioning concurrently with, and at a rate similar to, the conditioning of the bradycardiac CR* (Yehle et al., 1967) (Fig. 7). The concurrent conditioning of low voltage fast activity and bradycardia also has been demonstrated in cat (Hein, 1969). It follows that the central nucleus may function in the acquisition/expression of conditioned low voltage fast activity via its activation of ACh neurons within the magnocellular basal nucleus. This would enhance the readiness of cortical neurons to respond to sensory input, thereby facilitating sensory processing, a function similar to the enhancement of sensory input via central nucleus projections to the brain stem as theorized previously in our discussion of the functional significance of bradycardia and reflex facilitation.

Many of these observations led us to revise our hypothesis of central nucleus function during Pavlovian conditioning (Kapp et al., 1990b). *This revision states that the nucleus and its associated structures function, at least in part, in the acquisition of an increased state of nonspecific attention or arousal manifested in a variety of CRs which function to enhance sensory processing. This mechanism is rapidly acquired, perhaps via an inherent plasticity within the nucleus and associated structures in situations of uncertainty but of potential import; for example, when a neural stimulus (CS) precedes either a positive or negative reinforcing, unexpected event (US).* This rapid acquisition is manifested in (1) conditioned bradycardia, (2) conditioned facilitation of the nictitating membrane unconditioned reflex, and (3) conditioned, cholinergically mediated neocortical low voltage fast activity, as well as in a variety of additional CRs indicative of arousal and mediated by the nucleus. For example, in mapping the nucleus for cardioreactive sites (Applegate et al., 1983), we found that low-level stimulation produced a variety of responses in addition to bradycardia, which may function to enhance sensory input. One potent response was pupillodilation, which (a) also has been observed upon stimulation of the central nucleus in the cat (Ursin and Kaada, 1960), (b) like bradycardia, is rapidly conditioned in the cat (Weinberger, 1982), (c) is considered to be a correlate of conditioned arousal in the cat (Weinberger, 1982), and (d) occurs in association with bradycardia in the human during attention (Lacey and Lacey, 1974). The possibility exists that either the direct (Sandrew et al., 1986) or indirect

A

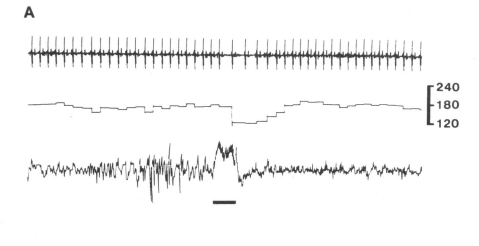

B
20 min POST — ATROPINE (5.0 mg/kg)

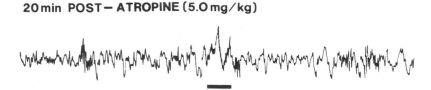

Fig. 6. Elicitation of bradycardia and neocortical low voltage fast activity upon electrical stimulation of the central nucleus in the conscious rabbit. **A:** The upper two traces depict the bradycardiac response as reflected in the electrocardiogram and cardiotachograph (beats per min) to a 1 second stimulus train (100 μA; 100 Hz). The lower trace depicts the production of low voltage fast activity in the electroencephalogram recorded from the frontal cortex in response to the stimulus. **B:** The effects of stimulation on the electroencephalogram 20 minutes following an injection of atropine sulfate (5.0 mg/kg, i.v.). Note that atropine blocks the elicitation of low voltage fast activity.

projections of the central nucleus to the intermediolateral cell columns of the cervical spinal cord, where motor neurons which contribute to pupillary dilation are located (Budge and Waller, 1851), may mediate this response. Further, we observed pinna orientation upon stimulation of the nucleus, a response which presumably functions to enhance sensitivity to auditory stimuli. Pinna orientation may be mediated by the projections of the nucleus to the region of the lateral tegmental field, which in turn projects to motor neurons of the dorsomedial facial subnucleus (Holstege et al., 1977, 1984). The latter innervates the muscles of the ear which contribute to pinna movement.

Finally, stimulation of the central nucleus in the rabbit (Kapp et al., 1982; Applegate et al , 1983) and in the cat (Ursin and Kaada, 1960) elicits a decreased tidal volume and increased frequency of respiration, as well as an arrest of ongoing somatomotor behavior. The functional significance of this respiratory pat-

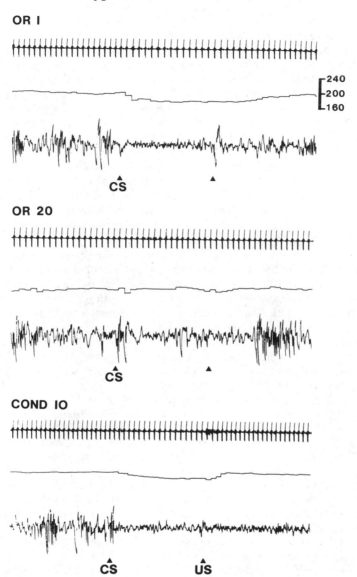

Fig. 7. Conditioning of frontal cortex low voltage fast activity and bradycardia in the rabbit. **OR1:** The upper two traces depict the bradycardiac orienting response to a novel 5.0 second tone stimulus (CS). The lower trace demonstrates the elicitation of low voltage fast activity to that same stimulus. Cursors represent the onset and offset of the 5.0 sec CS. **OR20:** These traces depict the heart rate and frontal cortex response to the twentieth presentation of the tone CS. Note the habituation of the bradycardiac and electroencephalographic response. **COND10:** These traces depict the presence of the conditioned bradycardiac and low voltage fast activity responses to the tenth presentation of the CS during conditioning trials in which the offset of the CS was coincident with the onset of the aversive US.

tern in terms of arousal is not readily apparent. Nevertheless, a respiratory CR of a similar pattern emerges with a time course similar to that of the bradycardiac CR during Pavlovian conditioning in the rabbit (Yehle et al., 1967) and cat (Hein, 1969). Demonstrated projections from the central nucleus to the regions of respiratory regulatory neurons located within the parabrachial nucleus, NTS, nucleus ambiguous, and/or cervical spinal cord (Hopkins and Holstege, 1978; Price and Amaral, 1981; Schwaber et al., 1982; Sandrew et al., 1986; Ellenberger et al., 1990) may contribute to this respiratory pattern. The arrest of ongoing motor behavior observed in response to the CS during Pavlovian conditioning in rabbit (Schneiderman, 1972) may well serve to increase the animal's ability to detect environmental auditory stimuli. The central nucleus projections by which this response is elicited by a CS or by electrical stimulation of the nucleus have yet to be identified in the rabbit. Recent research by LeDoux et al. (1988), however, suggests that the projections from the nucleus to the periaqueductal gray may represent a component of the descending pathway(s) which mediates CS-induced immobility or freezing behavior in the rat.

From our discussion it is apparent that the efferent projections of the central nucleus may contribute to a coordinated pattern of responses which can best be interpreted within an arousal or nonspecific attentional framework. This interpretation is consistent with the classic description of responses elicited by electrical stimulation of the nucleus in cat provided by Ursin and Kaada (1960) and others (Magnus and Lammers, 1956; Shealy and Peele, 1957). They described the "attention or orienting" response in unanesthetized cats, the most common response elicited upon stimulation. It was characterized by a nearly immediate arrest of all spontaneous activities, alterations in respiration, and an attitude change of the animal to one of attention or alertness as if it were bewildered, surprised, or expectant of an impending event. In this sense it closely resembled the "investigatory" or orienting reflex described by Pavlov (1927) and was indistinguishable from the orienting response induced by activation of the brain stem reticular formation. This initial response was soon followed by orienting-like responses, in which the animal would raise its head and look around with quick and anxious glancing or searching movements. The eyes opened and the pupils dilated, at times accompanied by directional movements of the ears, similar to that observed in the rabbit as described above. While stimulation at sites within the central nucleus elicits an orienting response, it is important to note that it is not the only nucleus which when stimulated elicits this reaction in cat. For example, stimulation of points within the anterior amygdaloid area and the lateral and basolateral nuclei were also reported to elicit the response (Ursin and Kaada, 1960). The extent of involvement of these nuclei and/or their projections of the central nucleus in this response pattern is deserving of further research. Nevertheless, given the extensive brain stem projections to the central nucleus in comparison to these other amygdaloid nuclei, it would appear that the former plays a pivotal role in the expression of various components of the orienting response. Consistent with this functional interpretation is the recent research by Gallagher et al. (1990) demonstrating that neurotoxic lesions of the nucleus abolish conditioned orienting responses in the rat (see Chapter 10, Gallagher, this volume).

THE CENTRAL NUCLEUS: A SITE OF PLASTICITY FOR THE ACQUISITION OF CONDITIONED AROUSAL?

While the central nucleus appears to contribute to the expression of a variety of CRs which serve to enhance sensory processing, the question arises concerning the extent to which it may be a site for the plasticity required for their acquisition. Such a function implies that information about the CS and US must converge upon central nucleus neurons if training-induced plasticity in neuronal activity is to occur within the nucleus per se. While the convergence of the auditory CS and somatosensory US on central nucleus neurons has not been systematically investigated over the course of conditioning, we have observed individual neurons within the nucleus which responded in an excitatory manner to visual, auditory, and somatosensory stimuli (Pascoe and Kapp, 1985b). In addition, some neurons which showed differential excitatory activity to the two auditory CSs during differential conditioning also demonstrated excitatory responses to the somatosensory US (Pascoe and Kapp, 1985a). Given these findings, we directed our efforts to an identification of the major pathways by which auditory CS and somatosensory US information is carried to the nucleus (Kapp et al., 1984b, 1985, 1989).

Our research in rabbit, as well as research in other species, have demonstrated that a variety of structures project to the nucleus. Two areas, the insular cortex and magnocellular medial geniculate nucleus, were of particular interest with respect to transmitting auditory CS information. The insular cortex was of interest for two reasons. First, consistent with findings in other species (Mufson et al., 1981; Saper, 1982), we observed in the rabbit a prominent projection from this cortex to all major components of the forebrain continuum: the central nucleus, sublenticular substantia innominata, and bed nucleus of the stria terminalis (Kapp et al., 1985). This projection overlapped the source of origin of descending projections of these components to the dorsomedial medulla. Second, sensory cortex, including auditory, projects to insular cortex (Mesulam and Mufson, 1982). These combined observations suggested that the insular cortex may relay auditory information to the central nucleus, thereby representing the pathway by which the auditory CS accesses the central nucleus.

In initial investigations of the insular cortex, we found that short-latency responses in central nucleus brain stem projection neurons were evoked by electrical stimulation of the insular cortex (Pascoe and Kapp, 1987a). In addition, lesions of the insular cortex produced a small but significant attenuation of the magnitude of the bradycardiac CR (Markgraf, 1984), a finding similar to that reported in rabbit by Powell et al. (1985). However, in an initial electrophysiological investigation, none of 21 insular cortical neurons which were antidromically identified to project to the central nucleus were CS-responsive (Pascoe and Kapp, 1987b). This result is not consistent with the hypothesis that auditory CS information accesses the central nucleus via a projection from the insular cortex. However, our initial analysis of the CS responsiveness of insular neurons was directed toward the rostral insula, and we have not yet explored the more posterior regions. Thus, any final conclusions concerning the CS responsiveness of insular neurons which project to the central nucleus cannot be made at this time.

Several observations suggest that the magnocellular medial geniculate nucleus (MGm) may convey CS information to the amygdala. First, LeDoux and colleagues have implicated on MGm-amygdala projection in the mediation of conditioned blood pressure and freezing responses to an auditory CS in the rat (Iwata et al., 1986; Chapter 12, LeDoux, this volume). Second, the MGm projects to the amygdala. Unlike the projections from the insular cortex, the bulk of the MGm-amygdala projection surrounds the dorsal and lateral aspects of the central nucleus in both rat (LeDoux et al., 1990a) and rabbit (Kapp et al., 1984b) and enters the lateral amygdala nucleus, which in turn projects to the central nucleus (Krettek and Price, 1978). Third, Ryugo and Weinberger (1978) demonstrated that associative changes in MGm neuronal activity develop to an auditory CS during the Pavlovian conditioning of pupillary dilation in the cat, and this development paralleled the development of the pupillary CR. A similar development in MGm neuronal responsiveness was observed in the rabbit during the early conditioning trials of a differential avoidance conditioning procedure (Gabriel et al., 1976). Fourth, lesions of the MGm block the acquisition of conditioned bradycardia in the rabbit using an auditory CS (Schneiderman et al., 1988).

These combined observations prompted us to record from single neurons in the MGm during the differential expression of conditioned bradycardia in the rabbit (Supple and Kapp, 1989). The results demonstrated that neurons located in the region of the MGm responded differentially to the CS + versus CS − , just as did those in the central nucleus (Pascoe and Kapp, 1985a). Of particular interest was the finding that MGm neurons responded to the CS with latencies which were in some instances 10–20 msec shorter than latencies recorded from neurons within the central nucleus (Pascoe and Kapp, 1985a). Furthermore, responses from neurons in naive rabbits did not demonstrate differential responsiveness to the CS + and CS − , suggesting the associative nature of the response observed in trained rabbits. These data are consistent with the hypothesis of LeDoux and colleagues (Iwata et al., 1986) that the critical projection for the conditioning of blood pressure and freezing responses to an auditory CS during Pavlovian aversive conditioning in the rat involves a projection from the MGm to the amygdala, particularly to the lateral amygdala nucleus (Chapter 12, LeDoux, this volume). Lesions of the latter significantly reduce these CRs in rats to such a CS (LeDoux et al., 1990). Presumably, intrinsic direct and/or indirect amygdala projections from the lateral nucleus to the central nucleus (Krettek and Price, 1978) conveys CS information to the latter.

While considerable progress has been made in identifying the structures which send CS information to the central nucleus, less is known concerning the structures by which US information is transmitted. There are several likely candidates: the locus coeruleus, MGm, and parabrachial nucleus. Both the locus coeruleus and parabrachial nucleus send projections directly to the central nucleus, while the MGm projects to anatomically associated amygdala nuclei as discussed previously. Neurons of the locus coeruleus respond to somatosensory stimuli (Aston-Jones and Bloom, 1981), and evidence has been presented suggesting that it provides a pathway for US input to the pigeon lateral geniculate homologue (Gibbs et al., 1983, 1986). The neurons of the latter demonstrate conditioning-induced modification of activity to a visual CS over repeated Pavlovian conditioning trials. Since neuronal activity within the central nucleus of the cat is affected by stimulation of the locus coeruleus (Schutze et al., 1987), this structure may convey US information to the central nucleus, information which is necessary if the central nucleus is a site of neuronal plasticity.

A second candidate for a source of US input to the central nucleus is the parabrachial nucleus. This nucleus receives significant projections from neurons in lamina I of the spinal cord (Light et al., 1987) and from neurons in the caudal trigeminal nucleus (Cechetto et al., 1985), and both structures are recipient of nociceptive stimuli. In addition, neurons within the rat parabrachial nucleus which respond to nociceptive stimuli have been demonstrated to project directly to the central nucleus using antidromic identification techniques (Bernard and Besson, 1990). Further, we have observed that a prominent projection from the parabrachial nucleus to the central nucleus exists in the rabbit (Kapp et al., 1989), as it does in other species (Fulwiler and Saper, 1984). A putative pathway for transmission of the eyelid US, therefore, may originate in the caudal trigeminal nucleus and terminate in the central nucleus via a relay within the parabrachial nucleus. The extent to which this is indeed the case is currently a focus of our research (Pascoe and Kapp, 1989, 1990).

Finally, that the MGm may serve as a source of origin for the transmission of US information to the amygdala, and eventually to the central nucleus, is based upon the findings that MGm neurons respond to somatosensory stimuli (Love and Scott, 1969; Wepsic, 1966), and as described above, may transmit their response to the amygdala via projections to the lateral amygdala nucleus. Consistent with this notion is the recent research by Hitchcock and Davis (1987), which suggests that the MGm may relay US information from the spinal cord to the amygdala during fear conditioning to a visual CS in the rat.

As is apparent from the above discussion, several parallel pathways may serve as candidates for the transmission of information about the CS and US to the central nucleus (see Fig. 8). In the final analysis no single pathway may exlusively transmit information about each of these stimuli. Furthermore, in addition to the central nucleus, there may exist several sites of plasticity within the circuit, including the MGm, and the basolateral and lateral nuclei of the amygdala. Consistent with this notion are the findings that (1) as described previously, conditioning-induced modifications in neuronal activity occur in both the central nucleus and the MGm (Ryugo and Weinberger, 1978; Pascoe and Kapp, 1985a), (2) conditioning-induced modifications occur in the basolateral nucleus in rabbit during the early stages of avoidance conditioning (Maren et al., 1989), and (3) synaptic plasticity in the form of long-term potentiation is induced in the lateral nucleus of the amygdala in the rat from stimulation of the MGm (Clugnet and LeDoux, 1990).

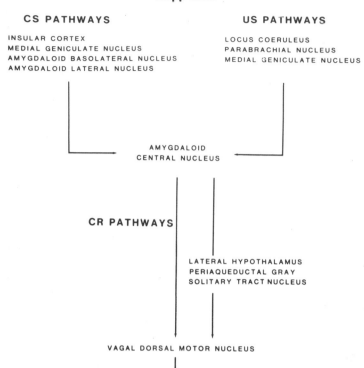

Fig. 8. Possible pathways by which CS and US information may access the amygdala central nucleus and thereby contribute to the plasticity which forms the substrate for the conditioned bradycardiac response. Alternate CR pathways are proposed to contribute to the expression of other conditioned responses indicative of arousal.

CONCLUSIONS

The research reviewed above suggests that the amygdala central nucleus contributes importantly to the expression of a variety of CRs which are indicative of heightened arousal and which serve to enhance sensory information processing. The widespread efferent projections of the nucleus form the substrate(s) for the expression of these CRs. In addition, the nucleus possesses characteristics which make it a candidate for the site of plasticity required for the acquisition of these CRs. Additional research will be necessary to test the validity of these hypotheses, and the extent to which the nucleus contributes to other behavioral functions, which to date have been less intensely investigated.

REFERENCES

Applegate CD, Frysinger RC, Kapp BS, Gallagher M (1982): Multiple unit activity recorded from the amygdala central nucleus during Pavlovian heart rate conditioning in the rabbit. Brain Res 238:457–462.

Applegate CD, Kapp BS, Underwood M, McNall CL (1983): Autonomic and somatomotor effects of amygdala central n. stimulation in awake rabbits. Physiol Behav 31:353–360.

Aston-Jones G, Bloom FE (1981): Norepinephrine-containing locus coeruleus neurons in behaving rats exhibit pronounced responses to non-noxious environmental stimuli. J Neurosci 1:887–900.

Bernard JF, Besson JM (1990): The Spino (Trigemino) pontoamygdaloid Pathway: Electrophysiological evidence for an involvement in pain processes. J Neurophysiol 63:473–490.

Bohlin G, Graham FK (1977): Cardiac deceleration and reflex blink facilitation. Psychophysiology 14:423–430.

Brunia CHM, Scheirs JGM, Haagh AVM (1982): Changes of achilles tendon reflex amplitudes during a fixed foreperiod of four seconds. Psychophysiology 19:63–70.

Budge JL, Waller AV (1851): Action de la partie cervicale du nerf grand sympathique et d'une portion de la moelle epiniere sur la dilatation de la pupille. CR Acad Sci (Paris) 33:370–374.

Busaki G, Bickford RG, Ponomareff G, Thal LJ, Mandel R, Gage FH (1988): Nucleus basalis and thalamic control of neocortical activity in the freely moving rat. J Neurosci 8:4007–4026.

Cechetto DF, Standaert DG, Saper CB (1985): Spinal and trigeminal dorsal horn projections to the parabrachial nucleus in the rat. J Comp Neurol 240:153–160.

Celesia GG, Jasper HH (1966): Acetylcholine released from cerebral cortex in relation to state of activation. Neurology 16:1053–1064.

Clugnet MC, LeDoux JE (1990): Synaptic plasticity in fear conditioning circuits: Induction of LTP in the lateral nucleus of the amygdala by stimulation of the medial geniculate body. J Neurosci 10:2818–2824.

Cox GE, Jordan D, Moruzzi P, Schwaber JS, Spyer KM, Turner SA (1986): Amygdaloid influences on brain-stem neurons in the rabbit. J Physiol (Lond) 381:135–148.

Cox GE, Jordan D, Paton JFR, Spyer KM, Wood LM (1987): Cardiovascular and phrenic nerve responses to stimulation of the amygdala central nucleus in the anesthetized rabbit. J Physiol (Lond) 389:341–356.

deOlmos J, Alheid GF, Beltramino CA (1985): Amygdala. In Paxinos G (ed): "The Rat Nervous System." Sydney: Academic Press, pp 223–334.

Ellenberger HH, Vera PL, Haselton JR, Haselton CL, Schneiderman N (1990): Brainstem projections to the phrenic nucleus. An anterograde and retrograde HRP study in the rabbit. Brain Res Bull 24:4007–4026.

Fitzgerald RD, Vardaris RM, Brown JS (1966): Classical conditioning of heart-rate deceleration in the rat with continuous and partial reinforcement. Psychonom Sci 6:437–438.

Fredericks A, Moore JW, Metcalf FV, Schwaber JS, Schneiderman N (1974): Selective autonomic blockade of conditioned and unconditioned heart rate changes in rabbit. Pharmacol Biochem Behav 2:493–501.

Fulwiler CE, Saper CB (1984): The subnuclear organization of the efferent connections of the parabrachial nucleus in the rat. Brain Res Rev 7:229–259.

Gabriel M, Miller JD, Saltwick SE (1976): Multiple unit activity of the rabbit medial geniculate nucleus in conditioning, extinction and reversal. Physiol Psychol 4:124–134.

Gallagher M, Kapp BS, Frysinger RC, Rapp PR (1980): B-adrenergic manipulation in amygdala central n. alters rabbit heart rate conditioning. Pharmacol Biochem Behav 12:419–426.

Gallagher M, Kapp BS, McNall CL, Pascoe JP (1981): Opiate effects in the amygdala central n. alters rabbit heart rate conditioning. Pharmacol Biochem Behav 14:497–505.

Gallagher M, Kapp BS, Pascoe JP (1982): Enkaphalin analogue effects in the amygdala central nucleus on conditioned heart rate. Pharmacol Biochem Behav 17:217–222.

Gallagher M, Graham PW, Holland PC (1990): The amygdala central nucleus and appetitive Pavlovian conditioning: Lesions impact one class of conditioned behavior. J Neurosci 10:1906–1911.

Gary Bobo E, Bonvallet M (1975): Amygdala and masseteric reflex. I. Facilitation, inhibition and diphasic modifications of the reflex induced by localized amygdaloid stimulation. EEG Clin Neurophysiol 39:329–339.

Gentile CG, Romanski LM, Jarrell TW, McCabe PM, Schneiderman N (1986a): Ibotenic acid lesions in amygdaloid central nucleus prevent the acquisition of differentially conditioned bradycardiac responses in rabbits. Soc Neurosci Abstr 12:755.

Gentile CG, Jarrell TW, Teich AH, McCabe PM, Schneiderman N (1986b): The role of amygdaloid central nucleus in differential Pavlovian conditioning of bradycardia in rabbits. Behav Brain Res 20:263–276.

Gibbs CM, Broyles JL, Cohen DH (1983): Further studies of the involvement of locus coeruleus in plasticity of avian lateral geniculate neurons during learning. Soc Neurosci Abstr 9:641.

Gibbs CM, Cohen DH, Broyles JL (1986): Modification of the discharge of lateral geniculate neurons during visual learning. J Neurosci 6:627–636.

Grove EA (1988): Efferent connections of the substantia innominata in the rat. J Comp Neurol 277:347–364.

Hahn WW (1973): Attention and heart rate: A critical appraisal of the hypothesis of Lacey and Lacey. Psych Bull 79:59–70.

Harden DG, Xiang Z, David J, Weisz DJ (1990): Lesions of the amygdala disrupt reflex facilitation of the nictitating membrane (NM) response in rabbit. Neurosci Abstr 16:269.

Harvey JA, Land T, McMaster SE (1984): Anatomical study of the rabbits' corneal-VIth nerve reflex: Connections between cornea, trigeminal sensory complex, and the abducens and accessory abducens nuclei. Brain Res 301:307–321.

Hein PL (1969): Heart rate conditioning in the cat and its relationship to other physiological responses. Psychophysiology 5:455–464.

Higgins GA, Schwaber JS (1983): Somatostatinergic projections from the central nucleus of the amygdala to the vagal nuclei. Peptides 4:1–6.

Hitchcock JM, Davis M (1986): Lesions of the amygdala, but not of the cerebellum or red nucleus, block conditioned fear as measured with the potentiated startle paradigm. Behav Neurosci 100:11–22.

Hitchcock JM, Davis M (1987): Proposed neural pathways for conditioned and unconditioned stimuli in the fear-potentiated startle paradigm. Neurosci Abstr 13:643.

Holstege G, Kuypers HGJM, Dekker JJ (1977): The organization of the bulbar fibre connections to the trigeminal, facial and hypoglossal motor nuclei. Brain 100:265–286.

Holstege G, Tan J, van Ham J, Bos A (1984): Mesencephalic projections to the facial nucleus in the cat. An autoradiographic study. Brain Res 311:7–22.

Holstege G, Meiners L, Tan K (1985): Projections of the bed nucleus of the stria terminalis to the mesencephalon, pons and medulla in the cat. Exp Brain Res 58:379–391.

Hopkins DA, Holstege D (1978): Amygdaloid projections to the mesencephalon, pons, and medulla oblongata in the cat. Exp Brain Res 32:529–547.

Iwata J, LeDoux JE, Meeley MP, Americ S, Reis DJ (1986): Intrinsic neurons in the amygdaloid field projected to by the medial geniculate body mediate emotional responses conditioned to acoustic stimuli. Brain Res 383:195–214.

Iwata JK, Chida K, LeDoux JE (1987): Cardiovascular responses elicited by stimulation of neurons in the central amygdaloid nucleus in awake but not anesthetized rats resemble conditioned emotional responses. Brain Res 418:183–188.

Jordan D, Khalid MEM, Schneiderman N, Spyer KM (1982): The location and properties of preganglionic vagal cardiomotor neurons in the rabbit. Pflugers Arch 395:244–250.

Kaada BR (1972): Stimulation and regional ablation of the amygdaloid complex with reference to functional representations. In BF Eleftherlou (ed): "The Neurobiology of the Amygdala." New York: Plenum Press, pp 205–292.

Kapp BS, Frysinger RC, Gallagher M, Haselton J (1979): Amygdala central nucleus lesions: Effects on heart rate conditioning in the rabbit. Physiol Behav 23:1109–1117.

Kapp BS, Gallagher M, Frysinger RC, Applegate CD (1981): The amygdala, emotion and cardiovascular conditioning. In Ben-Ari Y (ed): "The Amygdaloid Complex," INSERIM symposium no. 20. Amsterdam: Elsevier/North Holland Biomedical Press, pp 355–367.

Kapp BS, Gallagher M, Underwood MD, McNall CL, Whitehorn D (1982): Cardiovascular responses elicited by electrical stimulation of the amygdala central nucleus in the rabbit. Brain Res 234:251–262.

Kapp BS, Pascoe JP, Bixler MA (1984a): The amygdala: A neuroanatomical systems approach to its contribution to aversive conditioning. In Butters N, Squire LR (eds): "The Neuropsychology of Memory." New York: Guilford Press, pp 473–488.

Kapp BS, Schwaber JS, Driscoll PA (1984b): Subcortical projections to the amygdaloid central nucleus in the rabbit. Soc Neurosci Abstr 10:831.

Kapp BS, Schwaber JS, Driscoll PA (1985): Frontal cortex projections to the amygdaloid central nucleus in the rabbit. Neuroscience 15:327–346.

Kapp BS, Wilson A, Schwaber JS, Bilyk-Spafford T (1986): The organization of amygdaloid central nucleus projections to the midbrain periaqueductal gray and dorsomedial medulla in rabbit. Neurosci Abstr 12:55.

Kapp BS, Markgraf CG, Schwaber JS, Bilyk-Spafford T (1989): The organization of dorsal medullary projections to the central amygdaloid and parabrachial nuclei in the rabbit. Neuroscience 3:717–732.

Kapp BS, Supple WF, Doherty JL (1990a): Effects of stimulation of the amygdaloid central nucleus (ACe) on cortical electroencephalographic (EEG) activity in the rabbit. Neurosci Abstr 16:606.

Kapp BS, Wilson A, Pascoe JP, Supple W, Whalen PJ (1990b): A neuroanatomical systems analysis of bradycardia in the rabbit. In Gabriel M, Moore J (eds): "Neurocomputation and Learning: Foundations of Adaptive Networks." Bradford Books, MIT Press, pp 53–90.

Kreindler A, Steriade M (1964): EEG patterns of arousal and sleep induced by stimulating various amygdaloid levels in the cat. Arch Ital Biol 102:576–586.

Krettek JE, Price JL (1978): A description of the amygdaloid complex in the rat and cat with observations on intra-amygdaloid axonal connections. J Comp Neurol 178:255–280.

Lacey JL, Lacey BC (1970): Some autonomic-central nervous system interrelationships. In Black P (ed): "Physiological Correlates of Emotion." New York: Academic Press, pp 205–227.

Lacey BC, Lacey JI (1974): Studies of heart rate and other bodily processes in sensorimotor behavior. In Obrist PA, Black AH, Brener J, DiCara LV (eds): "Cardiovascular Psychophysiology: Current Issues in Response Mechanisms, Biofeedback and Methodology." Chicago: Aldine, pp 538–564.

Lacey BC, Lacey JI (1978): Two-way communication between the heart and brain. Significance of time within the cardiac cycle. Am Psychol 99:99–114.

Langhorst P, Lambertz M, Schulz G, Stock G (1987): Role played by amygdala complex and common brainstem system in integration of somatomotor and autonomic components of behavior. In Ciriello J, Calaresu FR, Renaud LP, Polosa C (eds): "Organization of the Autonomic Nervous System: Central and Peripheral Mechanisms." New York: Alan R. Liss, pp 347–361.

Lansing RW, Schwartz E, Lindsley DB (1959): Reaction time and EEG activation under alerted and non-alerted conditions. J Exp Psychol 58:1–7.

LeDoux JE, Iwata J, Cicchetti P, Reis DJ (1988): Different projections of the central amygdaloid nucleus mediate autonomic and behavioral correlates of conditioned fear. J Neurosci 8:2517–2529.

LeDoux JE, Cichetti P, Xagoraris A, Romanski L (1990a): The lateral amygdaloid nucleus: Sensory interface of the amygdala in fear conditioning. J Neurosci 10:1062–1069.

LeDoux JE, Farb C, Ruggiero DA (1990b): Topographic organization of neurons in the acoustic thalamus that project to the amygdala. J Neurosci 10:1043–1054.

Light AR, Casale E, Sedivec M (1987): The physiology and anatomy of spinal laminae I and II neurons antidromically activated by stimulation in the parabrachial region of the midbrain and pons. In Schmidt RF, Schaible HG, Vahle-Hinz C, (eds): "Fine Afferent Nerve Fibers and Pain." Weinheim, FRG: VCH, pp 347–356.

Lindsley DB (1960): Attention, consciousness, sleep and arousal. In Field J, Magoun HW, Hall VE (eds): "Handbook of Physiology: Section I: Neurophysiology," 3:1553–1593. Washington, DC: American Physiological Society.

Love JA, Scott JW (1969): Some response characteristics of cells of the magnocellular division of the medial geniculate body of the cat. Can J Physiol Pharmacol 47:881–888.

Magnus O, Lammers HJ (1956): The amygdaloid nuclear complex: Part I. "Folia Psychiatrica, Neurologica et Neurochirurgia Neerlandica." 59:555–581.

Markgraf CG (1984): Contributions of the insular cortex to cardiovascular regulation during aversive Pavlovian conditioning in the rabbit. Unpublished master's thesis, University of Vermont.

Markgraf CG, Kapp BS (1988): Neurobehavioral contributions to cardiac arrhythmias during aversive Pavlovian conditioning in the rabbit receiving digitalis. J Auto Nerv Syst 23:35–46.

Maren S, Cox A, Gabriel M (1989): Unit activity in the amygdaloid basolateral nucleus during acquisition and overtraining of discriminative avoidance behavior in rabbits. Neurosci Abstr 15:82.

Mesulam MM, Mufson EJ (1982): The insula of the old world monkey. III: Efferent cortical output and comments on function. J Comp Neurol 212:38–52.

Metherate R, Tremblay N, Dykes W (1987): Acetylcholine permits long-term enhancement of neuronal responsiveness in cat primary somatosensory cortex. Neuroscience 22:75–81.

Metherate R, Tremblay N, Dykes RW (1988a): The effects of acetylcholine on response properties of cat somatosensory cortical neurons. J Neurophysiol 59:1231–1252.

Metherate R, Tremblay N, Dykes RW (1988b): Transient and prolonged effects of acetylcholine on responsiveness of cat somatosensory cortical neurons. J Neurophysiol 59:1253–1276.

Morrell F (1961): Electrophysiological contributions to the neural basis of learning. Physiol Rev 41:443–494.

Mufson EJ, Mesulam MM, Pandya DN (1981): Insular connections with the amygdala in the rhesus monkey. Neuroscience 7:1231–1248.

Obrist PA, Wood DM, Perez-Reyes M (1965): Heart rate during conditioning in humans: Effects of UCS intensity, vagal blockade and adrenergic block of vasomotor activity. J Exp Psychol 70:32–42.

Obrist PA (1981): "Cardiovascular Psychophysiology: A Perspective." New York: Plenum Press.

Papakostopoulos D, Cooper R (1973): The contingent negative variation and the excitability of the spinal monosynaptic reflex. J Neurol Neurosurg Psych 36:1003–1010.

Pascoe JP, Kapp BS (1985a): Electrophysiological characteristics of amygdaloid central nucleus neurons during Pavlovian fear conditioning in the rabbit. Behav Brain Res 16:117–133.

Pascoe JP, Kapp BS (1985b): Electrophysiological characteristics of amygdaloid central nucleus neurons in the awake rabbit. Brain Res Bull 14:331–338.

Pascoe JP, Kapp BS (1987a): Some electrophysiological characteristics of insular cortex efferents to the amygdaloid central nucleus in awake rabbits. Neurosci Lett 78:288–294.

Pascoe JP, Kapp BS (1987b): Responses of amygdaloid central nucleus neurons to stimulation of the insular cortex in awake rabbits. Neuroscience 21:471–485.

Pascoe JP, Bradley DJ, Spyer KM (1989): Interactive responses to stimulation of the amygdaloid central nucleus and baroreceptor afferents in the rabbit. J Auto Nerv Syst 26:157–167.

Pascoe JP, Kapp BS (1989): Responses of amygdaloid central nucleus (ACE) neurons to stimulation of the parabrachial nucleus (PBN) in rabbits. Neurosci Abstr 15:1246.

Pascoe JP, Kapp BS (1990): Single unit activity in the parabrachial region (PB) during stimulation of the amygdaloid central nucleus (ACE) and Pavlovian conditioning in rabbits. Neurosci Abstr 16:1234.

Pavlov IP (1927): "Conditioned Reflexes. An Investigation of the Physiological Activity of the Cerebral Cortex." Oxford: Oxford University Press.

Powell DA, Kazis E (1976): Blood pressure and heart rate changes accompanying classical eyeblink conditioning in the rabbit (*Oryctolagus cuniculis*). Psychophysiology 13:441–447.

Powell DA, Buchanan S, Hernandez L (1985): Electrical stimulation of insular cortex elicits cardiac inhibition but insular lesions do not abolish conditioned bradycardia in rabbits. Behav Brain Res 17:125–144.

Price JL, Amaral DG (1981): An autoradiographic study of the projections of the central nucleus of the monkey amygdala. J Neurosci 1:1242–1259.

Rosen JB, Davis M (1988): Enhancement of acoustic startle by electric stimulation of the amygdala. Behav Neurosci 102:195–202.

Ruggiero DA, Ross CA, Kumada M, Reis DJ (1982): Reevaluation of projections from the mesencephalic trigeminal nucleus to the medulla and spinal cord: New projections. A combined retrograde and anterograde horseradish peroxidase study. J Comp Neurol 206:278–292.

Russchen FT, Amaral DG, Price JL (1985): The afferent connections of the substantia innominata in the monkey, *Macaca fasicularis*. J Comp Neurol 242:1–27.

Ryugo DK, Weinberger NM (1978): Differential plasticity of morphologically distinct neuron populations in the medial geniculate body of the cat during classical conditioning. Behav Biol 22:275–301.

Sananes CB, Campbell BA (1989): Role of the central nucleus in olfactory heart rate conditioning. Behav Neurosci 103:519–525.

Sandrew BB, Edwards DL, Poletti CE, Foote WE (1986): Amygdalospinal projections in the cat. Brain Res 373:235–239.

Saper CB (1982): Convergence of autonomic and limbic connections in the insular cortex of the rat. J Comp Neurol 210:163–173.

Sato H, Hata Y, Hagihara K, Tsumoto T (1987): Effects of cholinergic depletion on neuron activities in the cat visual cortex. J Neurophysiol 58:781–793.

Schell AM, Catania J (1975): The relationship between cardiac activity and sensory acuity. Psychophysiology 12:147–151.

Schlor KH, Stumpf H, Stock G (1984): Baroreceptor reflex during arousal induced by electrical stimulation of the amygdala or by natural stimuli. J Auto Nerv Syst 10:157–165.

Schneiderman N (1972): Response system divergencies in aversive classical conditioning. In Black AH, Prokasy WF (eds): "Classical Conditioning Vol. III: Current Research and Theory." New York: Appleton-Century-Crofts, pp 341–378.

Schneiderman N, Markgraf CG, McCabe PM, Liskowsky DR, Winters RW (1988): Ibotenic acid lesions in the magnocellular medial geniculate nucleus prevent the acquisition of classically conditioned bradycardia to single tones in rabbits. Neurosci Abstr 14:784.

Schutze I, Knuepfer MM, Eismann A, Stumpf H, Stock G (1987): Sensory input to single neurons in the amygdala of the cat. Exp Neurol 97:499–515.

Schwaber JS, Schneiderman N (1975): Aortic nerve activated cardioinhibitory neurons and interneurons. Am J Physiol 299:783–790.

Schwaber JS, Kapp BS, Higgins G (1980): The origin and extent of direct amygdala projections to the region of the dorsal motor nucleus of the vagus and the nucleus of the solitary tract. Neurosci Lett 20:15–20.

Schwaber JS, Kapp BS, Higgins GA, Rapp PR (1982): Amygdaloid and basal forebrain direct connections with the nucleus of the solitary tract and the dorsal motor nucleus. J Neurosci 2:1424–1438.

Shealy CN, Peele TL (1957): Studies on amygdaloid nucleus of the cat. J Neurophysiol 20:125–139.

Sideroff S, Elster AJ, Schneiderman N (1972): Cardiovascular conditioning in rabbits using appetitive or aversive hypothalamic stimulation as the US. J Comp Physiol Psych 81:501–508.

Sillito AM, Kemp JA (1983): Cholinergic modulation of the functional organization of the cat visual cortex. Brain Res 289:143–155.

Steriade M, McCarley RW (1990): "Brainstem Control of Wakefullness and Sleep." New York: Plenum Press.

Supple WF, Kapp BS (1989): Response characteristics of neurons in the medial component of the medial geniculate nucleus during Pavlovian differential fear conditioning in rabbits. Behav Neurosci 103:1276–1286.

Szerb JC (1967): Cortical acetylcholine release and electroencephalographic arousal. J Physiol (Lond) 192:329–343.

Ursin H, Kaada BR (1960): Functional localization within the amygdaloid complex in the cat. EEG Clin Neurophysiol 12:109–122.

Weinberger NM (1982): Effects of conditioned arousal on the auditory system. In Beckman AL (ed): "The Neural Basis of Behavior." Jamaica, NY: Spectrum Publications, pp 63–91.

Weisz DJ, LoTurco JJ (1988): Reflex facilitation of the nictitating membrane response remains after cerebellar lesions. Behav Neurosci 102:203–209.

Weisz DJ, McInerney J (1990): As associative process maintains reflex facilitation of the unconditioned nictitating membrane response during the early stages of training. Behav Neurosci 104:21–27.

Wepsic JG (1966): Multimodal sensory activation of cells in the magnocellular medial geniculate nucleus. Exp Neurol 15:299–318.

Whalen PJ, Kapp BS (1991): Contributions of the amygdaloid central nucleus to the modulation of the nictitating membrane reflex in the rabbit. Behav Neurosci 105:141–153.

Wilson A, Kapp BS (1990a): Midbrain periaqueductal gray projections to the dorsomedial medulla in the rabbit. Brain Res Bull (In press).

Wilson A, Kapp BS (1990b): The effects of stimulation and lesions of the ventrolateral periaqueductal gray on cardiovascular responses in the rabbit. Brain Res Bull (submitted).

Yehle A, Dauth G, Schneiderman N (1967): Correlates of heart rate classical conditioning in curarized rabbits. J Comp Physiol Psychol 64:98–104.

Zhang JX, Harper RM, Ni H (1986): Cryogenic blockade of the central nucleus of the amygdala attenuates aversively conditioned blood pressure and respiratory responses. Brain Res 386:136–145.

The Amygdala: Neurobiological Aspects of Emotion,
Memory, and Mental Dysfunction, pages 255–305
© 1992 Wiley-Liss, Inc.

9

The Role of the Amygdala in Conditioned Fear

MICHAEL DAVIS

*Ribicoff Research Facilities of the Connecticut Mental Health Center,
Department of Psychiatry, Yale University School of Medicine, New Haven,
Connecticut*

INTRODUCTION

Converging evidence now indicates that the amygdala plays a crucial role in the development and expression of conditioned fear. Conditioned fear is a hypothetical construct that is used to explain the cluster of behavioral effects that are produced when an initially neutral stimulus is consistently paired with an aversive stimulus. For example, when a light, which initially has no behavioral effect, is paired with an aversive stimulus such as a footshock, the light alone can now elicit a constellation of behaviors that are typically used to define a state of fear in animals. To explain these findings it is generally assumed (cf. McAllister and McAllister, 1971) that during light-shock pairings (training session) the shock elicits a variety of behaviors that can be used to infer a central state of fear (unconditioned responses, Fig. 1). After pairing, the light can now produce the same central fear state and thus the same set of behaviors formerly produced by the shock. Moreover, the behavioral effects that are produced in animals by this formerly neutral stimulus (now called a conditioned stimulus, CS) are similar in many respects to the constellation of behaviors that are used to diagnose generalized anxiety in humans (Table I).

The purpose of this chapter is to describe one example of conditioned fear, namely the elevation in the amplitude of the startle reflex elicited in the presence of a cue previously paired with shock. Using this paradigm, we have found that the amygdala is critically involved in the expression of conditioned fear through its direct projection to the brain steam nuclei involved in mediating the startle reflex. The amygdala may also be a site where neural activity produced by conditioned and unconditioned stimuli converge. In fact, local infusion of N-methyl-D-aspartate antagonists into the amygdala block the acquisition but not the expression of conditioned fear. In addition, central administration of the peptide, corticotropin-releasing factor produces a constellation of behavioral effects similar to conditioned fear, including increased startle, and this effect can also be blocked by lesions of the amygdala. Hence, the amygdala,

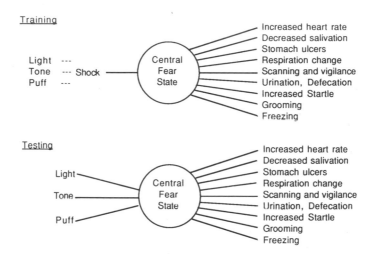

Fig. 1. General scheme believed to occur during classical conditioning using an aversive unconditioned stimulus. During training, the aversive stimulus (e.g., shock) activates a central fear system which produces a constellation of behaviors generally associated with aversive stimuli (unconditioned responses). After consistent pairings of some neutral stimulus such as a light or tone or puff of air with shock during the training phase, the neutral stimulus is now capable of producing a similar fear state and hence the same set of behaviors (conditioned responses) formerly only produced by the shock.

and its many efferent projections, may represent a central fear system involved in both the expression and acquisition of conditioned fear. Studies supporting this conclusion are reviewed at the end of the chapter.

THE FEAR-POTENTIATED STARTLE PARADIGM
A Central State of Fear Inferred From Increased Startle in the Presence of a Cue Previously Paired With Shock

Brown et al. (1951) demonstrated that the amplitude of the acoustic startle reflex in the rat can be augmented by presenting the eliciting auditory startle stimulus in the presence of a cue (e.g., a light) that has previously been paired with a shock. This phenomenon has been termed the "fear-potentiated startle effect" and has been replicated using either an auditory or visual conditioned stimulus and when startle has been elicited by either a loud sound or an airpuff (cf. Davis, 1986).

In this paradigm a central state of fear is considered to be the conditioned response (cf. McAllister and McAllister, 1971). Conditioned fear is operationally defined by elevated startle amplitude in the presence of a cue previously paired with a shock (see Fig. 2). Thus, the conditioned stimulus does not elicit startle. Furthermore, the startle-eliciting stimulus is never paired with a shock.

TABLE I. Comparison of Measures in Animals Typically Used to Index Fear and Those in the DSM-III Manual to Index Generalized Anxiety in People

Measures of Fear in Animal Models	DSM-III Criteria: Generalized Anxiety
Increased heart rate	Heart pounding
Decreased salivation	Dry mouth
Stomach ulcers	Upset stomach
Respiration change	Increased respiration
Scanning and vigilance	Scanning and vigilance
Increased startle	Jumpiness, easy startle
Urination	Frequent urination
Defecation	Diarrhea
Grooming	Fidgeting
Freezing	Apprehensive expectation— something bad is going to happen

Instead, the conditioned stimulus is paired with a shock and startle is elicited by another stimulus either in the presence or absence of the conditioned stimulus. Fear-potentiated startle is said to occur if startle is greater when elicited in the presence of the conditioned stimulus. Potentiated startle only occurs following paired versus unpaired or "random" presentations of the conditioned stimulus and the shock, which indicates that it is a valid measure of classical conditioning (Davis and Astrachan, 1978). Discriminations between visual and auditory conditioned stimuli (Davis et al., 1987) or between auditory cues or visual cues that differ in duration (Siegel, 1967; Davis et al., 1989) have also been demonstrated with potentiated startle. Increased startle in the presence of the conditioned stimulus still occurs very reliably at least one month after original training, making it appropriate for the study of long-term memory as well (Cassella and Davis, 1985; Campeau et al., 1990).

It has been suggested, however, that potentiated startle may not reflect increased fear in the presence of a conditioned stimulus, but instead results from the animal making a postural adjustment (e.g., crouching) in anticipation of the impending footshock that is especially conducive to startle (Kurtz and Siegel, 1966). We have found, however, that in spinally transected rats rigidly held in a modified stereotaxic instrument, which prevented obvious postural adjustments, the pinna component of startle was enhanced in the presence of a cue previously paired with a footshock (Cassella and Davis, 1986). Potentiation of startle measured electromyographically in neck muscles also occurs in the absence of any obvious postural adjustment (Cassella et al., 1986a). In addition, the magnitude of potentiated startle correlates highly with the degree of freezing, a very common measure of fear (Leaton and Borszcz, 1985). Taken together, therefore, the data indicate that potentiated startle is a valid measure of classical fear conditioning.

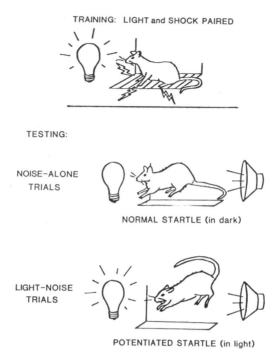

TRAINING: LIGHT and SHOCK PAIRED

TESTING:

NOISE–ALONE
TRIALS

NORMAL STARTLE (in dark)

LIGHT–NOISE
TRIALS

POTENTIATED STARTLE (in light)

Fig. 2. Cartoon depicting the fear-potentiated startle paradigm. During training, a neutral stimulus (conditioned stimulus) such as a light is consistently paired with a footshock. In training, a 3,700 msec light is typically paired with a 500 msec, 0.6 mA shock presented 3,200 msec after the light onset. During testing, startle is elicited by an auditory stimulus (e.g., a 100-dB burst of white noise) in the presence (Light-Noise trial type) or absence (Noise-Alone trial type) of the conditioned stimulus. In testing, the noise burst is typically presented 3,200 msec after light onset (i.e., at the same time as the shock was presented in training). It is important to note that the rat does not startle to light onset, but only to the noise burst presented alone or 3,200 msec after light onset. The positions and postures that are pictured may not exactly mimic the actual behavior of the animals.

Fear-Potentiated Startle as a Model of Anticipatory Anxiety

Recently, we have found that fear-potentiated startle in rats shows considerable temporal specificity, because the magnitude of fear-potentiated startle in testing is maximal at the time after light onset in which the shock would have occurred in training (Davis et al., 1989). This suggests that fear-potentiated startle may be a sensitive measure of anticipatory anxiety. To evaluate this, three different groups of rats were used. In training, two groups received 30 light-shock pairings, using a 200-msec light-shock interval in one group and a 51,200-msec interval in the other group. The third group had lights and shocks presented in a random relationship to each other. Several days later, all groups

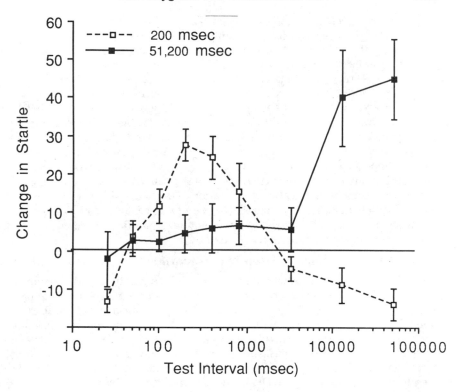

Fig. 3. A possible measure of anticipatory fear in rats. Mean change in startle amplitude at various intervals after light onset in testing following either 200 or 51,200 msec
light-shock intervals in training.

were tested identically by presenting startle stimuli at different intervals after
light onset. Figure 3 shows the change in startle of the two paired groups, relative to the random group, at various times after light onset. The group trained
with a 200-msec light-shock interval had maximum potentiation 200-msec after
light onset with no potentiation at much longer intervals. In contrast, the group
trained with the 51,200-msec light-shock interval had maximum potentiation
51,200 msec after light onset, with little or no potentiation at much shorter intervals. These data suggest, therefore, that fear-potentiated startle was maximal
at the time when the animal was anticipating receipt of shock, making it a sensitive measure of anticipatory fear or anxiety.

Fear-Potentiated Startle in Humans

Early studies indicated that the eyeblink component of airpuff-elicited startle in humans could be potentiated when elicited at various intervals after presentation of a visual stimulus previously paired with shock (Spence and Runquist,
1958; Ross, 1961). The human eyeblink component of startle can also be ele-

vated when subjects view unpleasant slides and reduced when they view pleasant ones (cf. Lang et al., 1990). Recently, we have been using the eyeblink component of startle in humans to measure anticipatory anxiety (Grillon et al., in press). Subjects were fitted with an electrode on the wrist through which they were told they might get a painful shock. During alternate blocks of stimuli, the acoustic startle reflex was elicited either during a period in which the subjects were told they might get a shock or a period when they were told they definitely would not get a shock. In each of the nine subjects tested so far, the eyeblink component of the startle reflex has been larger during periods in which subjects anticipated shock (Anxiety) than in periods when they did not (Safe) (Fig. 4). Importantly, this effect occurred in each of the periods when they were anticipating shock, before the actual shock was given. Potentiation during shock anticipation then persisted after presentation of the single shock, which, in fact, was not very painful. These data indicate, therefore, that anticipation of a shock is sufficient to elevate the eyeblink component of startle in humans, making it a sensitive measure of anticipatory anxiety.

Effects of Different Drugs on Fear-Potentiated Startle in Animals

Table II shows that a variety of drugs that reduce fear or anxiety in humans decrease potentiated startle in rats. Drugs like clonidine, morphine, diazepam, and buspirone, which differ considerably in their mechanism of action, all block potentiated startle. In most cases, these treatments do not depress baseline levels of startle, although drugs like clonidine do have marked depressant effects on baseline levels. In most cases there has been good agreement in the literature regarding drug effects on potentiated startle, although some inconsistencies do exist (e.g., ipsapirone, 8-OH-DPAT). Drugs like yohimbine and piperoxane, which induce anxiety in normal people and exaggerate it in anxious people (Goldenberd et al., 1947; Soffer, 1954; Holmberg and Gershon, 1961; Charney et al., 1984), actually increase potentiated startle in rats. Thus, at very low doses, these drugs increase startle amplitude in the presence of the light without having any effect on startle in the absence of the light and this only occurs in rats conditioned to fear the light (Davis et al., 1979).

NEURAL SYSTEMS INVOLVED IN FEAR-POTENTIATED STARTLE

A major advantage of the potentiated startle paradigm is that fear is measured by a change in a simple reflex. Hence, with potentiated startle, fear is expressed through some neural circuit that is activated by the conditioned stimulus and ultimately impinges on the startle circuit. Figure 5 shows a schematic summary diagram of the neural pathways which we believe are required for fear-potentiated startle. These pathways involve convergence of the conditioned visual stimulus and the unconditioned shock stimulus at the lateral and basal amygdala nuclei, which then project to the central nucleus of the amygdala, which then projects directly to a particular nucleus in the acoustic startle pathway.

The Acoustic Startle Pathway

In the rat, the latency of acoustic startle is 6 msec recorded electromyographically in the foreleg and 8 msec in the hindleg (Ison et al., 1973). This very short

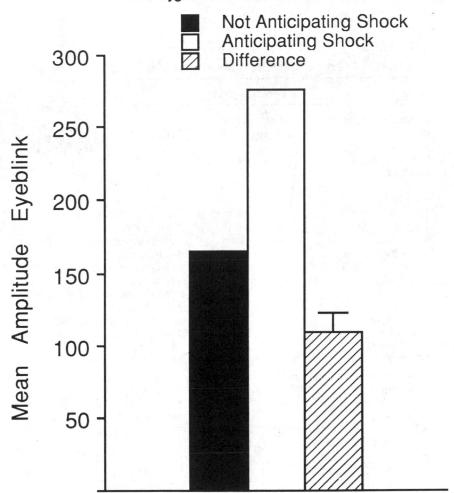

Fig. 4. Anticipatory anxiety in humans produces potentiation of the eyeblink. Mean amplitude of the eyeblink during periods in which subjects were told either they would not get a shock (black bar) or that they might get a shock (white bar) and the difference between those two trial types (+ standard error of the mean).

latency indicates that only a few synapses could be involved in mediating acoustic startle. Using a variety of techniques (Davis et al., 1982; Cassella and Davis, 1986b), we have proposed that the acoustic startle reflex is mediated by the ventral cochlear nucleus (VCN), an area just medial to the ventral nucleus of the lateral lemniscus (VLL) (the paralemniscal zone or the central nucleus of the acoustic tract), an area just dorsal to the superior olives in the nucleus reticularis pontis caudalis, and motor neurons in the spinal cord. Bilateral lesions using ibotenic

TABLE II. Effects of Different Drugs on Fear-Potentiated Startle

Drug	Dose Range (mg/kg)	Reference
Drugs that block potentiated startle		
Alcohol	10% solution	Williams, 1960
		(cited in Miller and Barry, 1960)
Sodium amytal	10–40	Chi, 1965
Diazepam	0.3–2.5	Davis, 1979a;
		Berg and Davis, 1984
Flurazepam	2.5–20	Davis, 1979a
Midazolam	0.5–2.0	Hijzen and Slangen, 1989
Morphine	2.5–10	Davis, 1979b
Nicotine[a]	0.4	Sorenson and Wilkinson, 1983
Buspirone	0.6–10	Kehne et al., 1988;
		Mansbach and Geyer, 1988
Gepirone	0.6–10	Kehne et al., 1988;
		Mansbach and Geyer, 1988
Clonidine	0.01–0.04	Davis et al., 1979
Methysergide[a]	0.3–10	Mansbach and Geyer, 1988
Ipsapirone[a]	0.3–10	Mansbach and Geyer, 1988
8-OH-DPAT	0.12–0.5	Mansbach and Geyer, 1988
Propranolol[a]	20	Davis et al., 1979
Drugs that don't block potentiated startle		
Cinanserin	10	Davis et al., 1988a
Cyproheptadine	5	Davis et al., 1988a
Ipsapirone	5–20	Davis et al., 1988a
8-OH-DPAT	2.5–10	Davis et al., 1988a
p-chloroamphetamine	5	Davis et al., 1988a
Naloxone	2.0	Davis et al., 1988a
Ro-15-1788	1.0	Davis et al., 1988a
WB-4101	1.0	Davis et al., 1979
1-PP	0.5–40	Kehne et al., 1988
(buspirone metabolite)		
Imipramine	5–10	Cassella and Davis, 1985
(chronic or acute)		
WB-4101	1.0	Davis et al., 1979
Drugs that increase potentiated startle		
Piperoxane	0.25–1.0	Davis et al., 1979
Yohimbine	0.125–.25	Davis et al., 1979
Lindane	7.5–30	Hijzen and Slangen, 1989
DMCM	0.1–0.4	Hijzen and Slangen, 1989
p-Chlorophenylalanine	400 × 2	Davis et al., 1988a

[a]Partial blockade.

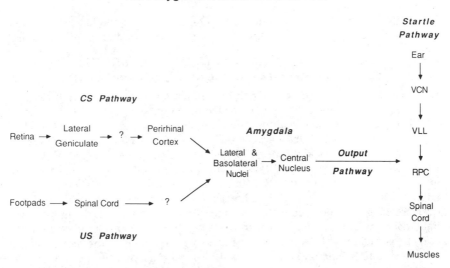

Fig. 5. Proposed neural pathways involved in fear-potentiated startle using a visual conditioned stimulus. Inputs from both the retina, via a projection involving the ventral lateral geniculate nucleus and the perirhinal cortex, and pain afferents in the spinal cord may converge at the lateral and basal nuclei of the amygdala. After being paired with a shock, the light may activate the lateral and basal amygdaloid nuclei, which in turn project to the central amygdaloid nucleus. Activation of the central nucleus of the amygdala may be both necessary and sufficient to facilitate startle through a direct connection to the nucleus reticularis pontis caudalis (RPC), an obligatory part of the acoustic startle pathway. VCN = ventral cochlear nucleus. VLL = ventral nucleus of the lateral lemniscus.

acid in each of these nuclei eliminate startle, whereas lesions in a variety of other auditory or motor areas do not. Startlelike responses can be elicited electrically from each of these nuclei, with progressively shorter latencies as the electrode is moved down the pathway.

Determining the Point Within the Startle Pathway Where Fear Alters Neural Transmission so as to Elevate Startle

Having delineated the startle reflex circuit involved in fear-potentiated startle, we have attempted to determine the point within the startle circuit where the visual conditioned stimulus ultimately modulates transmission following conditioning. To do this, startlelike responses were elicited electrically from various points along the startle pathway before and after presentation of a light that was either paired or not paired with a shock in different groups of rats (Berg and Davis, 1985). These experiments showed that startle elicited electrically from either the ventral cochlear nucleus or from the paralemniscal zone was potentiated by a conditioned fear stimulus, whereas elicitation of startle in the nucleus reticularis pontis caudalis or beyond was not. Potentiation of electrically elicited startle could be blocked by diazepam at doses that had no effect whatsoever on baseline levels of electrically elicited startle (Berg and

Davis, 1984). Based on these and other data (see below), we have concluded that fear ultimately alters transmission at the nucleus reticularis pontis caudalis.

SENSITIZATION OF STARTLE BY FOOTSHOCKS
Effects of Footshock on Acoustically Elicited Startle

Fear-potentiated startle is defined by an increase in startle in the presence of a cue previously paired with shock. One might expect, therefore, that shock itself would increase startle amplitude. Curiously, however, Brown et al. (1951) reported that acoustic startle was actually depressed when elicited from 15 to 60 sec after a footshock, although longer intervals were not tested. However, Blanchard and Blanchard (1969) and Fanselow and colleagues (e.g., Fanselow and Bolles, 1979; Fanselow, 1981, 1982, 1984) have shown that shock leads to an increase in freezing, a traditional measure of fear in rats. Interestingly, however, freezing does not occur immediately after the shock, but develops gradually over several minutes. Because the magnitude of fear-potentiated startle correlates highly with the amount of freezing measured in the same experimental situation (Leaton and Borszcz, 1985), we reasoned that startle should increase for several minutes following footshock with a time course similar to that of freezing.

To test this, rats were presented with 40 105-dB noise bursts once every 30 sec before and after a train of 10 shocks (0.6 mA, 0.5 sec in duration) presented at a rate of 1 shock per sec (Davis, 1989). Another group was treated identically except that no shocks were given. Footshocks led to a progressive increase in startle amplitude that peaked in about 10 min, leading to a significant difference in startle amplitude in the shocked and nonshocked group during the postshock series of startle stimuli. Other studies showed that the magnitude of startle facilitation was directly related to the number or intensity of intervening shocks. Moreover, shocks given prior to presenting any startle stimuli also led to an elevation of startle, indicating that enhanced startle results from sensitization rather than simply from dishabituation (e.g., Groves and Thompson, 1970).

Effects of Footshock on Electrically Elicited Startle

Using the electrically elicited startle technique described earlier, we found that shock sensitization, like conditioned fear, appears to ultimately modulate startle at the level of the nucleus reticularis pontis caudalis (Boulis and Davis, 1989). Thus, startle elicited electrically from either the ventral cochlear nucleus or the paralemniscal zone was elevated following footshock, whereas startle elicited from the reticulospinal tract connecting the nucleus reticularis pontis caudalis to the spinal cord was not.

THE ROLE OF THE AMYGDALA IN FEAR-POTENTIATED STARTLE
The Role of the Central Nucleus of the Amygdala
Effects of Lesions of the Central Nucleus of the Amygdala on Fear-Potentiated Startle

Several studies have indicated that lesions of the cerebellum or lesions of efferents from the cerebellum to the red nucleus eliminate classically conditioned motor responses, such as the nictitating membrane response and conditioned leg flexion (cf. Thompson et al., 1987). Interestingly, however, these lesions did not block heart rate conditioning (Lavond et al., 1984), suggesting that the cerrebellum may not be required for fear conditioning. On the other hand, lesions of the central nucleus of the amygdala block heart rate conditioning (Cohen, 1975; Kapp et al., 1979; Gentile et al., 1986) as well as other measures of conditioned fear in several other experimental paradigms (see Chapter 8, Kapp, this volume). Because of these results, we hypothesized that lesions of the amygdala should block potentiated startle, whereas lesions of the cerebellum or red nucleus might not.

To test this, rats were given 10 light-shock pairings on two successive days (Hitchcock and Davis, 1986). At 24–48 hr following training, groups of rats received either bilateral transection of the cerebellar penducles, bilateral lesions of the red nucleus (which receives most of the cerebellar efferents), or bilateral lesions of the central nucleus of the amygdala. Control animals were sham operated. Three to four days after surgery, the rats were tested for potentiated startle. Fear-potentiated startle was completely blocked by lesions of the central nucleus of the amygdala. In this same experiment, transection of the cerebellar peduncles or lesions of the red nucleus did not block potentiated startle. A visual prepulse test indicated that the blockade of potentiated startle observed in animals with lesions of the amygdala could not be attributed to visual impairment. In fact, blockade of fear-potentiated startle by amygdala lesions is not specific to the visual modality, because lesions of the central nucleus of the amygdala also blocked fear-potentiated startle when an auditory rather than a visual conditioned stimulus was used (Hitchcock and Davis, 1987). This is consistent with other investigators who have shown that lesions of the central nucleus of the amygdala block the increased blood pressure or freezing in the presence of an auditory cue previously paired with footshock (Iwata et al., 1986). Finally, the absence of potentiation in the animals with amygdala lesions did not simply result from a lowered startle level ceiling, because animals with amygdala lesions could show increased startle with increased stimulus intensity or following administration of strychnine (Hitchcock and Davis, 1986), a drug that reliably increases startle at subconvulsant doses (Kehne et al., 1981). Taken together, the results of these experiments support the hypothesis that the amygdala is involved in the expression of conditioned fear. Moreover, the cerebellum does not seem to play a role in fear-potentiated startle, even though more recent data now indicate that the cerebellar vermis is apparently very important for other measures of fear (cf. Supple and Leaton, 1990).

Effects of Electrical Stimulation of the Amygdala on Acoustic Startle

Electrical stimulation of the amygdala has been reported to produce fearlike behaviors in many animals, including humans (see Chapter 20, Gloor, this volume). We have found that startle is an extremely sensitive index of amygdala stimulation because low-level electrical stimulation of the amygdala (e.g., 40–400 μA, 25 ms trains of 0.1 ms square wave cathodal pulses) markedly increases acoustic startle amplitude (Rosen and Davis, 1988a) with no obvious signs of behavioral activation during stimulation at these stimulation currents and durations.

Moreover, the duration of stimulation is well below that used to produce kindling in rats (Handforth, 1984), so that the effects on startle are not associated with convulsions. This excitatory effect has occurred in every rat that we have tested in which electrodes were found to be placed in the central, intercalated, or medial nucleus of the amygdala or in the area just medial to the amygdaloid complex. In fact, stimulation of this area had the lowest threshold for increasing acoustic startle, consistent with the effects of electrical stimulation on heart rate in rabbits (e.g., Kapp et al., 1982; Applegate et al., 1983). This area coincides with the initial part of the ventral amygdalofugal pathway as it begins its projection to the lower brain stem (Krettek and Price, 1978a; Post and Mai, 1980; Schwaber et al., 1982). Low-level electrical stimulation at this site would be expected to activate a large number of fibers projecting down to the brain stem because they are highly concentrated at this part of the pathway. In contrast, stimulation of the amygdaloid nuclei themselves, where the neurons of these fibers originate, would require higher currents (i.e., more current spread) to activate the same number of brain stem projections because the neurons are dispersed throughout the nuclei. Further studies involving stimulation of the area just medial to the amygdala where the ventral amygdalofugal pathway begins, in combination with lesions of cell bodies (e.g., ibotenic acid lesions) in the central, medial, intercalated, or basal nucleus, would help clarify whether enhancement of startle by stimulation in this pathway actually results from activation of the axons originating from these amygdaloid nuclei.

With electrical stimulation of the amygdala, the excitatory effect on startle appears to develop very rapidly. By eliciting startle at various times before and after electrical stimulation of the amygdala, we estimate a transit time of about 5 msec from the amygdala to the startle pathway (Rosen and Davis, 1988b), comparable to the very short latency (2–5 msec) of facilitation of trigeminal motoneurons following amygdala stimulation reported by Ohta (1984). The rapidity of action means that the increase in startle is not secondary to autonomic or hormonal changes that might be produced by amygdala stimulation, because these would have a much longer latency. In addition, electrical stimulation of the amygdala alone does not elicit startle at these currents. Moreover, electrical stimulation of several other nearby brain areas such as the endopiriform nucleus, fundus striati, internal capsule, or some sites in the basal nucleus of the amygdala does not increase startle. Finally, using electrically elicited startle, electrical stimulation of the amygdala appears to modulate startle at the level of the nucleus reticularis pontis caudalis (Rosen and Davis, 1990), like conditioned fear and shock sensitization.

A paired pulse technique (Rosen and Davis, 1988a) indicated that the population of stimulated axons of the amygdala which is responsible for enhancing startle is quite homogeneous. Most neurons recovered from refractoriness between 0.8 and 1.0 ms, and enhancement was not increased with longer conditioning-test intervals. The refractory periods of the axons of the amygdala neurons which enhance acoustic startle are in the same range as those which subserve self-stimulation in the medial forebrain bundle in the rat (Yeomans, 1975) and callosal axons of the rabbit visual system (Swadlow and Waxman, 1976). The medial forebrain bundle and visual callosal axons are considered small and myelinated with conduction velocities estimated to be 1 to 8 m/s (Swadlow and Waxman, 1976; Shizgal et al., 1980). This suggests that the axons subserving the enhancement of startle are also small and myelinated with similar conduction velocities and these values are consistent with the estimated 4–5 msec transit time from the amygdala to the startle pathway, which in the rat are about 8–9 mm apart. At the present time it is not clear how the amygdala participates in fear-potentiated startle. It is possible that the light, after being paired with shock, activates the amygdala, which would then increase startle.

The Role of Various Amygdala Projection Areas in Fear-Potentiated Startle

As discussed previously, lesions of the central nucleus of the amygdala block fear-potentiated startle. The central nucleus of the amygdala projects to a variety of brain regions via two major efferent pathways, the stria terminalis and the ventral amygdalofugal pathway. The caudal part of the ventral amygdalofugal pathway is known to project directly to many parts of the pons, medulla, and spinal cord (Krettek and Price, 1978a; Post and Mai, 1980; Price and Amaral, 1981; Schwaber et al., 1982; Mizuno et al., 1985; Sandrew et al., 1986). Inagaki et al. (1983) reported direct connections between the central nucleus of the amygdala and the exact part of the nucleus reticularis pontis caudalis that is critical for startle (an area just dorsal to the superior olives). We have confirmed this direct connection using anterograde [*Phaseolus vulgaris*-leucoagglutinin (PHA-L)] and retrograde (Fluro-Gold) tracing techniques (Rosen et al., 1991) and have been systematically lesioning various points along the output pathways of the amygdala to evaluate the role of these projections in fear-potentiated startle (Hitchcock and Davis, 1991).

A diagram of the output pathways of the central nucleus of the amygdala and the effects of lesions at various points along this pathway is summarized in Figure 6. Lesions of the stria terminalis itself, or the bed nucleus of the stria terminalis, a major projection area of this pathway, do not block potentiated startle. Knife cuts of the rostral part of the ventral amygdalofugal pathway, which would interrupt its projections to the rostral lateral hypothalamus and substantia innominata, also fail to block potentiated startle. On the other hand, lesions of the caudal part of the ventral amygdalofugal pathway, at the point where it passes through the subthalamic area and cerebral peduncles, completely block potentiated startle. Interestingly, Jarrell et al. (1986) found that lesions of this area also block heart rate conditioning. Lesions of the substantia nigra, which receives central amygdaloid nucleus projections as well as fibers of passage from the central nucleus of the amygdala to more caudal brain stem regions, also block potentiated startle. This blockade does not seem to involve dopamine cells in the zona compacta because infusion of the dopamine neurotoxin 6-OHDA into the substantia nigra did not block potentiated startle despite over a 90% depletion of dopamine in the caudate nucleus. Finally, lesions of the lateral tegmental field, caudal to the substantia nigra, also block fear-potentiated startle.

The projection from the central nucleus of the amygdala to the startle pathway is completely ipsilateral (Rosen et al., 1991). Consistent with this, lesions of one central nucleus of the amygdala and the contralateral subtha-

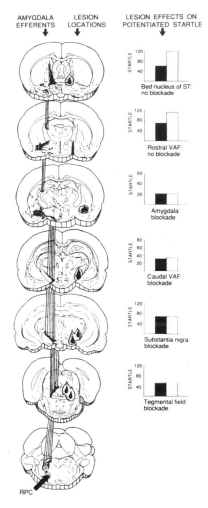

AMYGDALA   LESION   LESION EFFECTS ON
EFFERENTS   LOCATIONS   POTENTIATED STARTLE

Bed nucleus of ST:
no blockade

Rostral VAF:
no blockade

Amygdala:
blockade

Caudal VAF:
blockade

Substantia nigra:
blockade

Tegmental field:
blockade

RPC

Fig. 6. Lesions interrupting the pathway from the central nucleus of the amygdala to the RPC, but not lesions interrupting other central nucleus efferent pathways, block fear-potentiated startle. **Left panel:** A series of coronal rat brain sections, with the top section being the most rostral. The left sides of the sections show a schematic representation, based on PHA-L tracing studies, of the efferent pathways of the central nucleus of the amygdala. The right sides of the sections show representative lesions that interrupted the central nucleus efferent pathways at various levels. The black areas represent the cavities produced by the lesions and the stippled areas represent the surrounding gliosis. **Right panel:** Graphs showing the effects of bilateral lesions in each area on fear-potentiated startle. The graphs show the mean amplitude startle response on Noise-Alone trials (black bars) and Light-Noise trials (white bars) in rats given bilateral lesions in the locations shown in the corresponding brain section to the left of the graph. (Adapted from Hitchcock and Davis, 1991.)

lamic area also completely block fear-potentiated startle (Hitchcock and Davis, 1991). Fluro-Gold deposited in the nucleus reticularis pontis caudalis confirmed labeled cells primarily in the anterior and medial division of the central nucleus of the amygdala. Consistent with this, lesions of the central nucleus were only effective in blocking potentiated startle if they destroyed the anterior medial division of the central nucleus. Even a small amount of sparing of this area was sufficient to allow potentiated startle to occur.

Effects of Lesions of the Central Nucleus or the Ventral Amygdalofugal Pathway on Shock Sensitization

Because footshock is both aversive and fear-producing, it is quite possible that footshock activates the amygdala, which then leads to an elevation of startle via connections between the amygdala and the startle pathway. In fact, lesions of the central nucleus of the amygdala (Fig. 7), or of the ventral amygdalofugal pathway at the subthalamic level, prevent footshocks from sensitizing startle (Hitchcock et al., 1989).

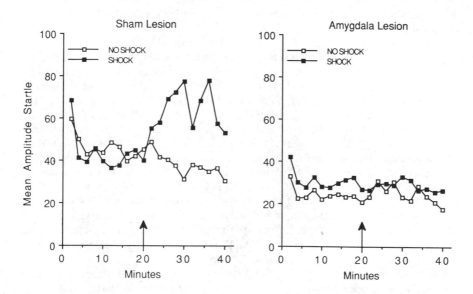

Fig. 7. Effect of lesions of the central nucleus of the amygdala on the enhancement of startle by footshock. The graphs show the mean amplitude startle response of animals given sham lesions **(left panel)** or central nucleus lesions **(right panel)** prior to and following a series of 10 0.6 mA, 500 msec footshocks (indicated by the arrow) presented once per second (solid) or no intervening shock (open). Forty noise bursts were presented at a 30 sec interval both before and after the shocks. Adapted from Hitchcock et al., 1989.

The Role of the Lateral and Basal Nuclei of the Amygdala

Effects of Lesions of the Lateral and Basal Nuclei of the Amygdala on Fear-Potentiated Startle

Most sensory information enters the amygdala through its lateral and basal nuclei (Ottersen, 1980; Turner, 1981; Van Hoesen, 1981; Amaral, 1987; LeDoux et al., 1990a). In turn, these nuclei project to the central nucleus (Krettek and Price, 1978b; Nitecka et al., 1981; Ottersen, 1982; Roberts et al., 1982; Russchen, 1982; Millhouse and DeOlmos, 1983; Aggleton, 1985; Smith and Millhouse, 1985; Amaral, 1987; Nitecka and Frotscher, 1989), which, as discussed above, then projects directly to the acoustic startle pathway. Recent evidence indicates that the lateral nucleus of the amygdala provides a critical link for relaying auditory information to the central nucleus of the amygdala involved in fear conditioning using an auditory conditioned stimulus (LeDoux et al., 1990a). Hence, we wondered how lesions of the lateral and basal nuclei would affect both fear-potentiated startle and shock sensitization (Sananes and Davis, 1992). Selective destruction of the lateral and basal nuclei was accomplished by local infusion of N-methyl-D-aspartate (NMDA) into the basal nucleus (Lewis et al., 1989; Crooks et al., 1989), based on extensive work with this technique in Dr. Michela Gallagher's laboratory, who generously supplied us with the details of the methodology.

Figure 8 shows that NMDA lesions of the lateral and basal nuclei caused a complete blockade of fear-potentiated startle when the lesions were made before training. Histological examination of the nine animals used in this study indicated that six rats were judged to have complete, bilateral lesions of the lateral and basal nucleus. In addition, in most animals there was also damage to the dorsal endopiriform nucleus. Partial damage of the amygdalastriatal transition zone, medial aspects of the perirhinal cortex, and the ventral endopiriform nucleus was seen in some animals, although this was typically only unilateral. Most animals had sparing of the accessory basal nucleus and ventral basal nucleus and all animals had sparing of the central nucleus. In the remaining three animals, a similar pattern of damage was seen except for obvious sparing of the most anterior regions of at least one basal nucleus. Figure 9 shows photomicrographs of animals judged to have a normal basal nucleus (A), complete destruction following NMDA (B), or sparing of ventral and anterior aspects of the basal nucleus (C). Importantly, NMDA lesions of the basal nucleus did not destroy cells in the central nucleus of the amygdala.

In these studies, the NMDA lesions were performed before training, so that the blockade of potentiated startle could have resulted from a blockade of acquisition or a blockade of the expression of potentiated startle, or both. In a subsequent study, NMDA lesions of the lateral and basal nuclei were also found to block the expression of fear-potentiated startle, because they caused a complete blockade of fear-potentiated startle when surgeries were performed after training. Hence, these lesions clearly block the expression of fear-potentiated startle, probably because they prevent visual information from activating the amygdala. However, these animals can clearly see, because they still demonstrate visual prepulse inhibition comparable to that shown by normal rats.

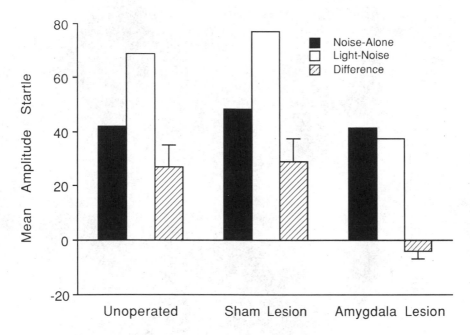

Fig. 8. Mean amplitude startle response on Noise-Alone trials (black bars) and Light-Noise trials (white bars), and the difference between these two trial types (+ standard error of the mean), in rats given bilateral NMDA lesions of the lateral and basal nuclei of the amygdala. (From Sananes and Davis, in press).

Effects of Lesions of the Lateral and Basal Nuclei of the Amygdala on Shock Sensitization

Figure 10 shows the effects of NMDA lesions on shock sensitization, comparing the unoperated and sham animals with the six NMDA lesioned animals judged to have complete basal lesions and the three judged to have basal sparing. Animals with complete lateral and basal NMDA lesions had a complete blockade of shock sensitization. In contrast, shock sensitization was within normal limits in the three animals with partial lesions of the basal nucleus. These differences did not seem attributable to a decrease in the reception of footshock, at least based on the degree to which the animals reacted during presentation of the footshocks, which was measured and found not to differ in the various groups. These data indicate, therefore, that sparing of the most anterior part of the basal nucleus was sufficient to allow normal shock sensitization. As mentioned earlier, lesions of the central nucleus of the amygdala or of the ventral amygdalofugal pathway also blocked shock sensitization (Hitchcock et al., 1989). In contrast, electrolytic lesions of the lateral nucleus of the amygdala did not (Hitchcock et al., 1989), consistent with a lack of blockade of shock sensitization in the three rats which had sparing of the anterior part of the basal nucleus, but extensive damage to the lateral nucleus. Hence, at least for shock sensitiza-

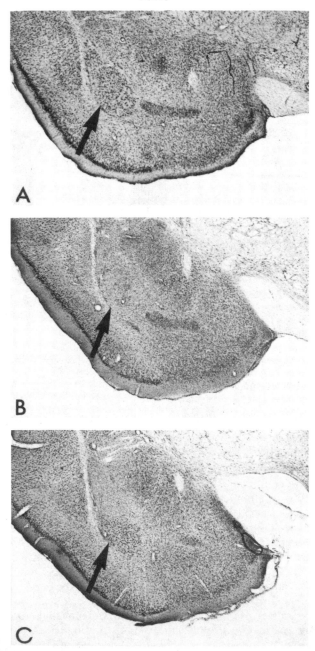

Fig. 9. Photomicrograph of a rat with a normal amygdala (**A**), cell loss in the lateral and basal nuclei but not in the central (**B**), or with sparing of cells in the ventral aspect of the anterior part of the basal nucleus (**C**). Arrow points to basal nucleus. (From Sananes and Davis, in press).

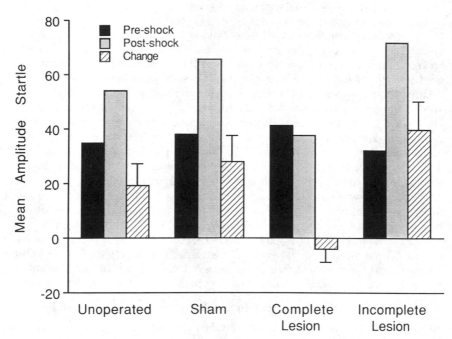

Fig. 10. Mean amplitude startle response during the last 10 min before and the first 20 min after a series of 10 0.6 mA footshocks in unoperated rats or in rats with sham lesions, complete NMDA-induced lesions of the lateral and basal nuclei of the amygdala, or in rats with sparing in the most anterior part of the basal nucleus. (From Sananes and Davis, in press).

tion, these two sets of data point to an involvement of the basal nucleus, including its most anterior aspect, and not the lateral nucleus, in shock sensitization.

Using Golgi techniques, McDonald (1984) has made a distinction between anterior and posterior divisions of the basal nucleus, noting that "the organization of class I and class II neurons in the posterior basolateral nucleus suggests that this subnucleus may process information differently from other portions of the basolateral amygdala" (p. 602). Consistent with this, the present results suggest that the anterior basal nucleus may be especially important for shock sensitization. Hence, selective inputs to this part of the basal nucleus may be part of the shock pathway involved in shock sensitization. Moreover, because shock sensitization may provide a kind of readout of activation of the amygdala by shock important for aversive conditioning (Davis, 1989), this anterior part of the basal nucleus may also be critical for acquisition of aversive conditioning.

The Visual Pathway Involved in Fear-Potentiated Startle Using a Visual Conditioned Stimulus

These data suggest, therefore, that visual input critical for the acquisition, as well as the expression of fear-potentiated startle using a visual conditioned stimulus, may enter the amygdala through the lateral and/or basal nuclei. At the present time, however, the visual pathway(s) critical for fear-potentiated startle using a visual conditioned stimulus linking the retina to these basal nuclei are still unclear. Recently, we have found that complete removal of all primary and secondary visual cortices does not block the expression of fear-potentiated startle using a visual conditioned stimulus (Rosen et al., submitted). In contrast, relatively small lesions of the perirhinal cortex completely block fear-potentiated startle, provided the lesion included an area of perirhinal cortex just dorsal and ventral to the rhinal sulcus (Rosen et al., submitted). Animals with dorsal but not ventral damage did not have a blockade of potentiated startle. This is especially interesting because McDonald and Jackson (1987) find heavy retrograde and anterograde labeling in the basal, accessory basal, and especially the lateral nucleus of the amygdala after deposits in the perirhinal cortex. Most of the connections between the lateral nucleus and the perirhinal cortex involve the area of the perirhinal cortex dorsal to the rhinal sulcus, whereas the connections between the basal and accessory basal nucleus and the perirhinal cortex involve the area below the rhinal sulcus. Thus, it is possible that visual information is relayed from the area of the perirhinal cortex just below the rhinal sulcus to the basal nucleus. Currently, we are using retrograde tracing techniques to evaluate how subcortical visual information might get to this area of the perirhinal cortex.

The Role of NMDA Receptors in the Amygdala in Conditioned Fear

Effects of NMDA Antagonists on the Acquisition of Fear-Potentiated Startle

One of the most promising models of learning in vertebrates is long-term potentiation (LTP). The finding that NMDA receptor antagonists, such as 2-amino-5-phosphonovalerate (AP5), block the induction or acquisition of LTP in certain hippocampal synapses, but not the expression of LTP, has lead to very powerful biochemical models of learning in vertebrates (Collingridge and Bliss, 1987; cf. Brown et al., 1988; Nicoll et al., 1988). Moreover, a number of behavioral studies have now shown that competitive as well as noncompetitive NMDA antagonists attenuate or block various measures of learning (Kesner et al., 1983; Tang and Franklin, 1983; Morris et al., 1986; Handelmann et al., 1987; Benvenga and Spaulding, 1988; Butelman, 1989, 1990; Tang and Ho, 1988; Tonkiss et al., 1988; Danysz and Wroblewski, 1989; Hauber and Schmidt, 1989; Laroche et al., 1989; Mondadori et al., 1989; Morris, 1989; Morris et al., 1989; Robinson et al., 1989; Staubli et al., 1989; Tan et al., 1989; Whishaw and Auer, 1989; Chiamulera et al., 1990; Gandolfi et al., 1990; Heale and Harley, 1990; Jones et al., 1990; McLamb et al., 1990; Myhall and Fleming, 1990; Paoli et al., 1990; Shapiro and Caramanos, 1990; Welzl et al., 1990; Kim et al., 1991). However, at the present time, very little is known about the anatomical substrates of these behavioral actions of NMDA antagonists. Recent studies have shown that LTP can occur in amygdala brain slices (Chapman et al., 1990) or in vivo following tetanic stimulation of the part of the medial geniculate nucleus that projects to the lateral nucleus of the amygdala (Clugnet and LeDoux, 1990). In some cases its induction can be blocked by AP5 (T.H. Brown, personal communication). If convergence between the light and shock occurs at the amygdala, and an NMDA-dependent process is involved in the acquisition of conditioned fear, then local infusion of NMDA antagonists into the amygdala should block the acquisition of conditioned fear measured with the fear-potentiated startle effect.

To test this (Miserendino et al., 1990), 132 rats were implanted with bilateral cannulae aimed for the basal nucleus of the amygdala, which is known to have high levels of NMDA receptors (Monaghan and Cotman, 1985). One week later, rats were infused with either artificial cerebrospinal fluid (CSF), or 6, 12, 25 or 50 nmol/side of the selective NMDA antagonist AP5. Five minutes later they were presented with the first of 10 light-shock pairings presented at an average intertrial interval of 4 min, creating a 45-min training session. The infusions and training procedures were then repeated 24 h later, because we have found that this 2-day training procedure results in potentiated startle in virtually every control animal. One week later, all animals were tested for fear-potentiated startle without any drug infusions. AP5 caused a dose-related attenuation of fear-potentiated startle retention, with a total blockade at the higher doses. Observation of the animals during training found no evidence of catalepsy or ataxia (e.g., Leung and Desborough, 1988). The effect did not seem to result from a decrease in sensitivity to footshock, because local infusion of AP5 into the amygdala did not alter either overall reactivity to footshock or the slope of reactivity as a function of different footshock intensities. In contrast to the blockade of retention, AP5 did not block the expression of fear-potentiated startle because infusion of AP5 immediately before testing did not block potentiated startle in animals previously trained in the absence of the drug. We also found that either 25 or 50 nmol of the more selective NMDA antagonist, 3-(2-carboxy-piperazin-4-yl)-propyl-1-phosphonic acid (CPP), blocked retention of fear-potentiated startle.

Other studies showed that 40 nmol/side of propanolol, which has local anesthetic effects (Weiner, 1985) and alters one-trial inhibitory avoidance conditioning (Liang et al., 1986), did not block or even attenuate fear conditioning after local infusion into the amygdala prior to training. In addition, AP5 given after training but one week before testing did not block potentiated startle, ruling out any permanent damage to the amygdala or blockade caused by residual drug during testing. Local infusion of AP5 did not affect visual prepulse inhibition, a sensitive measure of vision in rats (Wecker and Ison, 1986). Finally, infusion of AP5 into deep cerebellar nuclei did not block retention, even at a dose eight times that required to block retention after local infusion into the amygdala. These data indicate, therefore, that AP5's blockade of conditioning probably did not result from local anesthetic effects, permanent damage to the amygdala, or blockade of visual transmission, and did not occur if placed into a different part of the brain.

To reduce the time period in which the drugs would have to act and hence the dose required to block retention, we have used a shorter training paradigm in which a total of five light-shock pairings are given over a single 8-min training session, compared to the 45-min training session used previously (Campeau et al., 1990). Using this paradigm we find an eightfold reduction in the dose of AP5 required to significantly attenuate fear conditioning and a four-

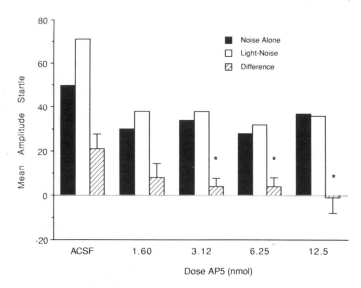

Fig. 11. Mean amplitude startle response during the test session on Noise-Alone trials (black bars) and Light-Noise trials (white bars), and the difference between these two trial types (+ standard error of the mean), following bilateral infusion of various doses of the NMDA antagonist AP5 into the amygdala during the training session which occurred one week before the test session.

fold reduction in the dose required to completely block retention (Fig. 11). Finally, recent studies indicate that local infusion of NMDA antagonists in the amygdala can block other measures of fear conditioning such as freezing (M.S. Fanselow, personal communication) or inhibitory avoidance (Kim and McGaugh, 1990; Liang and Davis, 1990).

Effects of NMDA Antagonists on the Extinction of Fear-Potentiated Startle

Clinically, the inability to eliminate fear and anxiety ranks as one of the major problems in psychiatry. Although a good deal is known about neural systems involved in the acquisition of fear, much less is known about the neural systems that might be involved in extinction of conditioned fear (cf. LeDoux et al., 1990b). To begin to approach this problem, we measured whether blockade of NMDA receptors at the level of the amygdala would alter the process of experimental extinction (Falls et al., 1992). Rats were implanted with bilateral cannulae in the basal nucleus of the amygdala and trained for potentiated startle in the usual way. One week later, all animals were given a short test session and, based on their levels of fear-potentiated startle during this session, matched into four groups of 10 rats each which had equivalent levels of fear-potentiated startle. The next day half the animals were presented with

30 lights at 1-min intervals without any shocks. Five minutes before this extinction session, one group was infused with 50 nmol/side of the selective NMDA receptor antagonist APS and one group with its vehicle, artificial CSF. The two other groups were treated identically, except no lights were presented. They were simply placed into the test cages and given either artificial CSF or APS. Twenty-four hours later, all rats were again tested for fear-potentiated startle. Animals infused with artificial CSF or APS, but not exposed to lights, had levels of fear-potentiated startle that did not differ from their first test session or from each other. Animals infused with artificial CSF during the extinction day in which lights were presented had very little potentiated startle on their second test day, indicating that extinction had occurred. In contrast, animals infused with APS during extinction had levels of potentiated startle that did not differ from their pretest level or from the groups not exposed to lights and significantly higher than those of rats infused with artificial CSF and exposed to lights. These data indicate, therefore, that APS infused into the amygdala blocked the normal process of extinction. Taken together, these data suggest that the amygdala may be importantly involved in both the retention and extinction of conditioned fear and that an NMDA-dependent process may be critical for both of these forms of learning.

Lesions of the Central Nucleus of the Amygdala Block the Excitatory Effect of Corticotropin-Releasing Factor on Startle

Corticotropin-releasing factor (CRF), a 41-amino acid peptide which regulates the release of adrenocorticotropin (Vale et al., 1981), has been implicated in many neural and behavioral functions in addition to its hypophysiotropic effect (Koob and Bloom, 1985). Intracerebroventricular injection of CRF produces a constellation of behavioral and physiological responses similar to those seen during periods of stress or fear (cf. Dunn and Berridge, 1990). These findings led to the suggestion that release of CRF may mediate many of the behavioral effects observed during stress or fear (Koob and Bloom, 1985). This suggestion is further supported by the finding that many of the behavioral effects of stress can be blocked by intraventricular infusion of the CRF antagonist, α-helical CRF(9-41) (cf. Dunn and Berridge, 1990). Swerdlow et al. (1986) reported that intraventricular infusion of CRF causes a dose-dependent increase in the amplitude of the acoustic startle reflex which can be blocked by intraventricular infusion of the CRF antagonist, α-helical CRF(9-41) (Swerdlow et al., 1989). Because CRF immunoreactivity and binding sites are present in the amygdala (DeSouza et al., 1985; Sakanaka et al.,1987) as well as in the spinal cord (Merchenthaler et al., 1983; Skofitsch et al., 1985), and CRF containing neurons in the amygdala may be critical for some of the autonomic effects seen during a state of fear (cf. Gray, 1990), we evaluated the role of the amygdala in the excitatory effect of CRF on startle (Liang et al., 1989).

The left panel of Figure 12 shows that intraventricular infusion of CRF produced a pronounced, dose-dependent and long-lasting enhancement of the acoustic startle reflex. The right panel shows that intrathecal infusion of CRF also elevated startle, but the magnitude of this effect was much lower than that

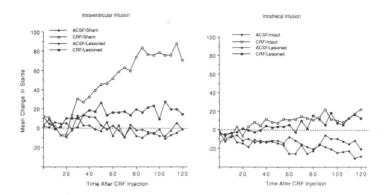

Fig. 12. Left panel shows the mean change in startle (relative to a 15 min preinfusion baseline) after intraventricular infusion of 1 μg corticotropin-releasing factor (CRF) or artificial cerebrospinal fluid (ACSF) in sham lesioned animals or animals with bilateral lesions of the central nucleus of the amygdala. **Right panel** shows comparable data when 1 μg of CRF was infused into the subarachnoid space of the spinal cord (intrathecal infusion).

produced by intraventricular administration. Bilateral lesions of the amygdala caused a marked attenuation of the excitatory effect of CRF on startle given intraventricularly but no blockade of the much weaker excitatory effect of CRF given intrathecally. These data suggest that CRF given intraventricularly elevates startle by both spinal and supraspinal sites of action. The major excitatory effect results from a supraspinal site of action which is completely blocked by lesions of the central nucleus of the amygdala.

The simplest interpretation of these data would be that CRF given intraventricularly diffuses to the amygdala and elevates startle by binding to CRF receptors in the amygdala. While we cannot rule out this interpretation, we have only found very weak excitatory effects of CRF after direct infusion into the brain in the 55 animals we have tested thus far (Liang et al., 1989). In contrast, local infusion of CRF into the parabrachial nucleus of the brain stem produces a marked facilitation of startle (Liang et al., 1989). Because the parabrachial nucleus sends heavy projections to the central nucleus of the amygdala (Otterson and Ben-Ari, 1978; Saper and Loewy, 1980; Otterson, 1981; Voshart and Vander-Kooy, 1981; Takeuchi et al., 1982; Block and Schwartzbaum, 1983; Fulwiler and Saper, 1984; Ma and Peschanski, 1988) it is possible that this is a critical site of action for CRF which then elevates startle via activation of the amygdala. However, it remains unclear as to how CRF given intraventricularly could activate cells in the parabrachial nucleus, and whether lesions of the amygdala would also block the excitatory effects on startle of CRF given locally into the parabrachial nucleus. Nonetheless, it is striking that lesions of the amygdala appear to interact importantly with a peptide which produces a constellation of behaviors similar to fear and anxiety.

ANXIETY AND THE AMYGDALA

A variety of animal models have been used to infer a central state of fear or anxiety. In some models fear is inferred when an animal freezes, thus interrupting some ongoing behavior such as pressing a bar or interacting socially with other animals. In other models, fear is measured by changes in autonomic activity, such as heart rate, blood pressure, or respiration. Fear can also be measured by a change in simple reflexes or a change in facial expressions and mouth movements. Thus fear appears to produce a complex pattern of behaviors that are highly correlated with each other.

Anatomical Connections Between the Amygdala and Brain Areas Involved in Fear and Anxiety

Similar to suggestions of several previous reviews (Gloor, 1960; Kapp et al., 1984, 1990; Sarter and Markowitsch, 1985; Kapp and Pascoe, 1986; LeDoux, 1987; Gray, 1989), Figure 13 summarizes work done in many different laboratories indicating that the central nucleus of the amygdala has direct projections to hypothalamic and brain stem areas that might be expected to be involved in many of the symptoms of fear or anxiety. Direct projections from the central nucleus of the amygdala to the lateral hypothalamus (Krettek and Price, 1978a, Shiosaka et al., 1980; Price and Amaral, 1981) appear to be involved in activation of the sympathetic autonomic nervous system seen during fear and anxiety (cf. LeDoux et al., 1988). Direct projections to the dorsal motor nucleus of the vagus (Hopkins and Holstege, 1978; Schwaber et al., 1982; Takeuchi et al., 1983; Veening et al., 1984) may be involved in several autonomic measures of fear or anxiety, since the vagus is involved in many different autonomic functions. Projections of the central nucleus of the amygdala to the parabrachial nucleus (Hopkins and Holstege, 1978; Krettek and Price, 1978a; Price and Amaral, 1981; Takeuchi et al., 1982) may be involved in respiratory changes during fear, since electrical stimulation (Cohen, 1971, 1979; Berstrand and Hugelin, 1971; Mraovitch et al., 1982) or lesions (Von Euler et al., 1976; Baker et al., 1981) of the parabrachial nucleus are known to alter various measures of respiration.

Projections from the amygdala to the ventral tegmental area (Beckstead et al., 1979; Phillipson, 1979; Simon et al., 1979; Wallace et al., 1989) may mediate stress-induced increases in dopamine metabolites in the prefrontal cortex (Thierry et al., 1976). Direct amygdala projections to the locus coeruleus (e.g., Cedarbaum and Aghajanian, 1978; Wallace et al., 1989), or indirect projections via the paragigantocellularis nucleus (Aston-Jones et al., 1986), or perhaps via the ventral tegmental area (e.g., Deutch et al., 1986), may mediate the response of cells in the locus coeruleus to conditioned fear stimuli (Rasmussen and Jacobs, 1986), as well as being involved in other actions of the locus coeruleus linked to fear and anxiety (cf. Redmond, 1977). Direct projections of the amygdala to the lateral dorsal tegmental nucleus (e.g., Hopkins and Holstege, 1978) and parabrachial nuclei (see above), which have cholinergic neurons that project to the thalamus (cf. Pare et al., 1990), may mediate increases in synaptic transmission in thalamic sensory relay neurons (Pare et al., 1990; Steriade et al., 1990)

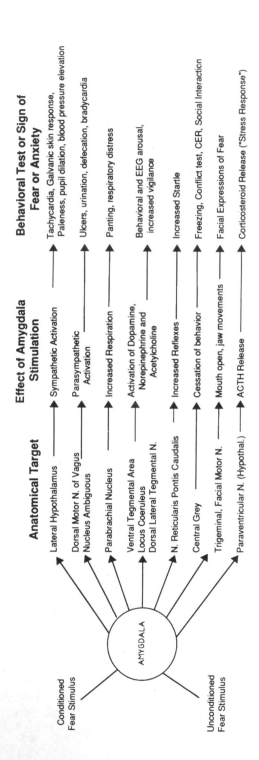

Fig. 13. Schematic diagram showing direct connections between the central nucleus of the amygdala and a variety of hypothalamic and brain stem target areas that may be involved in different animal tests of fear and anxiety.

during states of fear. This cholinergic activation, along with increases in thalamic transmission accompanying activation of the locus coeruleus (Rogawski and Aghajanian, 1980), may thus lead to increased vigilance and superior signal detection in a state of fear or anxiety. In addition, release of norepinephrine onto motor neurons via amygdala activation of the locus coeruleus, or via amygdala projections to serotonin containing raphe neurons (Magnuson and Gray, 1990), could lead to enhanced motor performance during a state of fear, because both norepinephine and serotonin facilitate excitation of motor neurons (e.g., McCall and Aghajanian, 1979; White and Neuman, 1980).

As outlined earlier, projections of the amygdala to the nucleus reticularis pontis caudalis (Inagaki et al., 1983; Rosen et al., 1991) probably are involved in fear-potentiation of the startle reflex (Hitchcock and Davis, 1991). The central nucleus of the amygdala projects to a region of the central grey (Gloor, 1978; Hopkins and Holstege, 1978; Krettek and Price, 1978a; Post and Mai, 1980; Beitz, 1982) that has been implicated in conditioned fear in a number of behavioral tests (Liebman et al., 1970; Hammer and Kapp, 1986; LeDoux et al., 1988; Borszcz et al., 1989), as well as a critical part of a general defense system (cf. Adams, 1979; Blanchard et al., 1981; Bandler and Depaulis, 1988; Graeff, 1988; LeDoux et al., 1988; Zhang et al., 1990; Fanselow, 1991). Direct projections to the trigeminal and facial motor nuclei (Holstege et al., 1977; Post and Mai, 1980; Ruggiero et al., 1982) may mediate some of the facial expressions of fear. Finally, direct projections of the central nucleus of the amygdala to the paraventricular nucleus of the hypothalamus (Silverman et al., 1981; Tribollet and Dreifuss, 1981; Gray, 1989), or indirect projections by way of the bed nucleus of the stria terminalis and preoptic area, which receive inputs from the amygdala (Krettek and Price, 1978a; Weller and Smith, 1982; DeOlmos et al., 1985) and project to the paraventricular nucleus of the hypothalamus (Sawchenko and Swanson, 1983; Swanson et al., 1983), may mediate the prominent neuroendocrine responses to fearful or stressful stimuli.

At the present time, the identity of the transmitters released onto these target sites by amygdaloid neurons is just beginning to emerge. Gray (1989) estimates that 25% of the neurons in the central nucleus of the amygdala and bed nucleus of the stria terminalis contain known neuropeptides. The main output neurons of the amygdala contain corticotropin-releasing factor, somatostatin, and neurotensin, with smaller contributions from substance P and galanin-containing cells.

Elicitation of Fear by Electrical Stimulation of the Amygdala

Importantly, it has also been shown that electrical stimulation of the amygdala can produce a complex pattern of behavioral and autonomic changes that, taken together, highly resembles a state of fear. Thus, stimulation of the amygdala can also alter heart rate and blood pressure, both measures used to study cardiovascular changes during fear conditioning (Kaada, 1951; Anand and Dua, 1956; Koikegami et al., 1957; Hilton and Zbrozyna, 1963; Reis and Oliphant, 1964; Bonvallet and Gary Bobo, 1972; Heinemann et al., 1973; Morgenson and Calaresu, 1973; Faiers et al., 1975; Stock et al., 1978, 1981; Timms, 1981; Kapp et al., 1982; Applegate et al., 1983; Galeno and Brody, 1983; Frysinger et al., 1984; Harper et al., 1984; Schlor et al.,1984; Cox et al., 1987; Gelsema et al., 1987; Iwata et al., 1987; Pascoe et al., 1989). In many cases, these effects are critically dependent on the state of the animal and level of anesthesia (e.g., Stock et al., 1978; Timms, 1981; Galeno and Brody, 1983; Frysinger et al., 1984; Harper et al., 1984; Iwata et al., 1987), and in some instances these effects may result from stimulation of fibers of passage rather than cell bodies (cf. Lewis et al., 1989). Amygdala stimulation can also produce gastric ulceration (Sen and Anand, 1957; Henke, 1980b, 1982; Innes and Tansy, 1980), which may result from chronic fear or anxiety.

Electrical stimulation of the amygdala also alters respiration (Anand and Dua, 1956; Bonvallet and Gary Bobo, 1972; Applegate et al., 1983; Harper et al., 1984), a prominent symptom of fear, especially in panic disorders. Electrical stimulation of the central nucleus of the amygdala produces a cessation of ongoing behavior (Gloor, 1960; Applegate et al., 1983; Kaada, 1972; Ursin and Kaada, 1960). In fact, cessation of ongoing behavior is the critical measure of fear or anxiety in several animal models such as freezing (Blanchard and Blanchard, 1969; Bolles and Collier, 1976; Fanselow and Bolles, 1979), the operant conflict test (Geller and Seifter, 1960), the conditioned emotional response (Estes and Skinner, 1941) which correlates with freezing (e.g., Bouton and Bolles, 1980; Mast et al., 1982), and the social interaction test (File, 1980). Electrical stimulation of the amygdala also elicits jaw movements (Gloor, 1960; Applegate et al.,1983; Kaku, 1984; Ohta, 1984) and activation of facial motoneurons (Fanardjian and Manvelyan, 1987), which probably mediate some of the facial expressions seen during the fear reaction. These motor effects may be indicative of a more general effect of amygdala stimulation, namely that of modulating brain stem reflexes such as the massenteric (Bonvallet and Gary Bobo, 1975; Gary Bobo and Bonvallet, 1975), baroreceptor (Schlor et al., 1984; Lewis et al., 1989; Pascoe et al., 1989), nictitating membrane (Whalen and Kapp, 1990), and startle reflex (Rosen and Davis, 1988a,b). In most cases stimulation of the amygdala facilitates these reflexes, although that may depend on the exact amygdala sites being stimulated [see Whalen and Kapp (1991) for a discussion of this point]. Electrical stimulation of the amygdala elicits feelings of fear or anxiety as well as autonomic reactions indicative of fear (Chapman et al.,1954; Gloor et al., 1981). In fact, it has been proposed that some of the emotional content of dreams may result from activation of the amygdala, stimulation of which increases ponto-geniculo-occipital activity, which occurs during paradoxical (dream) sleep (cf. Calvo et al., 1987).

Finally, electrical stimulation of the amygdala has been shown to increase plasma levels of corticosterone, indicating an excitatory effect of the amygdala on the hypothalamo-pituitary-adrenal axis (HPA) (Mason, 1959; Setekliev et al., 1961; Matheson et al.,1971; Redgate and Fahringer, 1973; Yates and Maran,1974; Smelik and Vermes, 1980; Feldman et al., 1982; Dunn and Whitener, 1986). As mentioned above, some of these excitatory effects may be mediated through the pre-optic area and bed nucleus of the stria terminalis, which receive input from the amygdala (Krettek and Price, 1978a; Weller and Smith, 1982; DeOlmos et al., 1985) and project to the paraventricular nucleus of the hypothalamus (Sawchenko and Swanson, 1983; Swanson et al., 1983). Electrical stimulation of these nuclei increases plasma corticosterone levels (Saphier and Feldman, 1986; Dunn, 1987), and elevated plasma levels of corticosterone produced by amygdala stimulation can be attenuated by bilateral lesions of the stria terminalis, medial preoptic area, and the bed nucleus of the stria terminalis (Feldman et al., 1990). In addition, direct projections from the medial nucleus of the amygdala to the hypothalamus exist as well (Silverman et al., 1981; Tribollet and Dreifuss, 1981; Gray et al., 1989), and these projections may also mediate some of the excitatory effects of the amygdala on the HPA axis.

Viewed in this way, the highly correlated set of behaviors seen during fear may result from activation of a single area of the brain (the amygdala, especially its central nucleus), which then projects to a variety of target areas which themselves are critical for each of the specific symptoms of fear, as well as the perception of anxiety. Moreover, it must be assumed that all of these connections are already formed in an adult organism, because electrical stimulation produces these effects in the absence of prior explicit fear conditioning. Thus, much of the complex behavioral pattern seen during fear conditioning has already been "hard wired" during evolution. In order for a formerly neutral stimulus to produce the constellation of behavioral effects used to define a state of fear or anxiety, it is only necessary for that stimulus to now activate the amygdala, which in turn will produce the complex pattern of behavioral changes by virtue of its innate connections to different brain target sites. Viewed in this way, plasticity during fear conditioning probably results from a change in synaptic inputs prior to or in the amygdala, rather than from a change in its efferent target areas. The ability to produce long-term potentiation (Chapman et al., 1990; Clugnet and LeDoux, 1990) in the amygdala and the finding that local infusion of NMDA antagonists into the amygdala blocks the retention of fear conditioning (Miserendino et al., 1990) is consistent with this hypothesis.

The Role of the Amygdala in Fear Elicited by a Conditioned Stimulus

If fear conditioning results from an activation of the amygdala, one would expect that a conditioned stimulus would activate units in the amygdala and that lesions of the amygdala would prevent a conditioned stimulus from producing fear. Thus far, it has been difficult to record single-unit activity in the amygdala because many of the cells are small and have very low spontaneous rates of firing. Nonetheless, several studies have shown that a neutral stimulus paired with aversive stimulation will now alter neural firing in the amygdala (Umemoto and Olds, 1975; Applegate et al., 1982; Henke, 1983; Pascoe and Kapp, 1985b) as well as an induction of increased neural activity. In addition, many studies indicate that lesions of the amygdala block the effects of a conditioned stimulus in a variety of behavioral test situations. Lesions of the amygdala eliminate or attenuate conditioned freezing normally seen in response to a stimulus formerly paired with shock (Blanchard and Blanchard, 1972; LeDoux et al., 1988, 1990) or a dominant male rat (Bolhuis et al., 1984; Luiten et al., 1985) or in a continuous passive avoidance test (Slotnick, 1973). Lesions of the amygdala counteract the normal reduction of bar pressing in the operant conflict test (Shibata et al., 1986) or the conditioned emotional response paradigm (Kellicut and Schwartzbaum, 1963; Spevack et al., 1975). In birds, lesions of the archistriatum, believed to be homologous with the mammalian amygdala, block the development of a conditioned emotional response (Dafters, 1976) or heart rate acceleration in response to a cue paired with a shock (Cohen, 1975). In both adult (Gentile et al., 1986; Kapp et al.,1979) and infant mammals (Sananes and Campbell, 1989), lesions of the central nucleus block conditioned changes in heart rate. Ibotenic acid lesions of the central nucleus of the amygdala (Iwata et al., 1986) or localized cooling of this nucleus (Zhang et al., 1986) also block conditioned changes in blood pressure. Lesions of the lateral amygdala (basal, lateral, and accessory basal nuclei) attenuate, and lesions of the medial amygdala (corticomedial and central nucleus) eliminate, negative contrast following sucrose reduction (Becker et al., 1984), a measure of emotionality sensitive to anxiolytic drugs (cf. Flaherty, 1990). Perhaps similarly, lesions of the amygdala block the effects of positive behavioral contrast (Henke, 1972; Henke et al., 1972); decreasing the responsiveness to shifts in reward magnitude in monkeys (Schwartzbaum, 1960) and rats (Kemble and Beckman, 1970), and the effects of frustrative nonreward (e.g., Henke, 1973, 1977). Data outlined earlier indicate that lesions of the central nucleus or of the lateral and basal nuclei of the amygdala block fear-potentiated startle (Hitchcock and Davis, 1986, 1987; Sananes and Davis, 1992). This, along with a large literature implicating the amygdala in many other measures of fear such as active and passive avoidance (for reviews see Kaada, 1972; Sarter and Markowitsch, 1985; Ursin et al., 1981) and evaluation and memory of emotionally significant sensory stimuli (Bennett et al., 1985; Bresnahan and Routtenberg, 1972; Ellis and Kesner, 1983; Gallagher et al., 1980; Gallagher and Kapp, 1981; 1978; Gold et al., 1975; Handwerker et al., 1974; Kesner, 1982; Liang et al., 1985; Liang et al., 1986; McGaugh et al., 1990; Mishkin and Aggleton, 1981) provide strong evidence for a crucial role of the amygdala in fear.

The Role of the Amygdala in Unconditioned Fear

Lesions of the amygdala are known to block several measures of innate fear in different species (cf., Blanchard and Blanchard, 1972; Ursin et al., 1981). Lesions of the cortical amygdaloid nucleus and perhaps the central nucleus markedly reduce emotionality in wild rats measured in terms of flight and defensive behaviors (Kemble et al., 1984; Kemble et al., 1990). Large amygdala lesions or those which damaged the cortical, medial, and in several cases the central nucleus, dramatically increase the number of contacts a rat will make with a sedated cat (Blanchard and Blanchard, 1972). In fact, some of these lesioned animals crawl all over the cat and even nibble its ear, a behavior never shown by the non-lesioned animals. Following lesions of the archistriatum, believed to be homologous with the mammalian amygdala, birds become docile and show little tendency to escape from humans (Phillips, 1964; 1968), consistent with a general taming effect of amygdala lesions reported in many species (cf. Goddard, 1964). Finally, lesions of the amygdaloid complex inhibit adrenocortical responses following olfactory or sciatic nerve stimulation (Feldman and Conforti, 1981) and attenuate the compensatory hypersecretion of ACTH that normally occurs following adrenalectomy (Allen and Allen, 1974). Lesions of the central nucleus have been found to significantly attenuate ulceration (Henke, 1980) or elevated levels of plasma corticosterone produced by restraint

stress (Beaulieu et al., 1986, 1987) and lesions of the medially projecting component of the ventroamygdalofugal pathway, which carries the fibers connecting
the central nucleus of the amygdala to the hypothalamus, attenuate the increase
in ACTH secretion following adrenalectomy, lesions of the stria terminalis do
not (Allen and Allen, 1974). Finally, lesions of the amygdala have been reported
to block the ability of high levels of noise, which may be an unconditioned fear
stimulus (cf. Leaton and Cranney, 1990), to produce hypertension (Galeno et
al., 1984) or activation of tryptophan hydroxylase (Singh et al., 1990).

It should be pointed out, however, that other measures that have been used
to index innate fear have produced less consistent data concerning amygdala
lesions. Large electrolytic lesions of the amygdaloid complex (Schwarzbaum
and Gay, 1966; Corman et al., 1967; Jonason and Enloe, 1971; Bresnahan et al.,
1976; Eclancher and Karli, 1979; Greidanus et al., 1979) or electrolytic or ibotenic
acid lesions of the central nucleus of the amygdala (e.g., Werka et al., 1978;
Jellestad et al., 1986; Grijalva et al., 1990) or of the lateral and basal nuclei
(Jellestad and Cabrera, 1986) produce an increase in exploratory behavior in
the open field test. However, this does not seem to occur when open field testing
is preceded by other tests on the same animals (Grossman et al., 1975), when
test conditions are especially familiar (e.g., McIntyre and Stein, 1973), when
testing occurs after considerable handling and a long time after surgery (Kemble
et al., 1979), when the lesions are very small (Riolobos and Garcia, 1987) and
may depend on the age of the animal when the lesions are performed (Eclancher
and Karli, 1979). However, because increased exploratory behavior is not always
associated with changes in corticosterone (Jellestad and Cabrera, 1986; Jellestad
et al., 1986) or other measures usually associated with a loss of fear of the open
field, these authors have concluded that increased locomotor activity cannot
easily be explained by a general loss of fear after amygdala lesions. Moreover,
other measures of neophobia, such as the time to begin eating in a novel environment, do not show consistent changes with lesions of the amygdala as one
might expect from a lesion that reduced fear (cf. Aggleton et al., 1989). However, the exact way in which neophobia is measured may determine whether it
is a valid measure of fear, at least based on the measurement of corticosterone
(e.g., Misslin and Cigrang, 1986).

Other data indicate that the amygdala appears to be involved in some types
of aversive conditioning, but this depends on the exact unconditioned aversive
stimulus that is used. For example, electrolytic lesions of the basal nucleus
(Pellegrino, 1968), or fiber sparing chemical lesions of most of the amygdaloid
complex (Cahill and McGaugh, 1990), attenuate avoidance of thirsty rats to
approach an electrified water spout through which they were previously accus-
tomed to receiving water. Importantly, however, these same lesioned animals
did not differ from controls in the rate at which they found the water spout
over successive test days or their avoidance of the water spout when quinine
was added to the water (Cahill and McGaugh, 1990), prompting Cahill and
McGaugh to suggest that "the degree of arousal produced by the unconditioned
stimulus, and not the aversive nature per se, determined the level of amygdala
involvement" (p. 541). It is especially interesting in this regard that although

many studies have shown that electrolytic lesions of the amygdala can interfere with taste aversion learning, an elegant series of experiments have now shown that these effects result from an interruption of gustatory fibers passing through the amygdala on route to the insular cortex (Dunn and Everitt, 1988). In these studies, ibotenic acid lesions of the amygdala fail to block taste aversion learning, whereas ibotenic acid lesions of the gustatory insular cortex do. Once again, the amygdala does not seem critical for all types of aversive conditioning, but instead conditioning that involves an obvious fear component such as that produced by aversive shocks.

Finally, it should be acknowledged that the amygdala may also be importantly involved in stimulus-response associations that do not obviously involve aversive conditioning (e.g., Murray and Mishkin, 1985; Aggleton and Mishkin, 1986; Cador et al., 1989; Everitt et al., 1989; Kesner et al., 1989; Murray, 1990; Peinado-Manzano, 1990; but see Zola-Morgan et al., 1989). Hence, some of the deficits in aversive conditioning following alterations of amygdala function may be part of a more general deficit in attention (Gallagher et al., 1990; Kapp et al., 1990).

Conditioned Fear Versus Anxiety

Clinically, fear is regarded to be more stimulus-specific than anxiety, despite very similar symptoms. Figure 13 suggests that spontaneous activation of the central nucleus of the amygdala would produce a state resembling fear in the absence of any obvious eliciting stimulus. In fact, fear and anxiety often precede temporal lobe epileptic seizures (Gloor et al., 1981), which are usually associated with abnormal electrical activity of the amygdala (Crandall et al., 1971). An important implication of this distinction is that treatments that block conditioned fear might not necessarily block anxiety. For example, if a drug decreased transmission along a sensory pathway required for a conditioned stimulus to activate the amygdala, then that drug might be especially effective in blocking conditioned fear. However, if anxiety resulted from activation of the amygdala not involving that sensory pathway, then that drug might not be especially effective in reducing anxiety. On the other hand, drugs that act specifically in the amygdala should affect both conditioned fear and anxiety. Moreover, drugs that act at various target areas might be expected to provide selective actions on some but not all of the somatic symptoms associated with anxiety.

It is noteworthy in this regard that the central nucleus of the amygdala is known to have high densities of opiate receptors (Goodman et al., 1980), whereas the basal nucleus, which projects to the central nucleus (Krettek and Price, 1978b; Nitecka et al., 1981; Ottersen, 1982; Russchen, 1982; Millhouse and DeOlmos, 1983; Aggleton, 1985; Smith and Millhouse, 1985) has high densities of benzodiazepine receptors (Niehoff and Kuhar, 1983). In fact, local infusion of the opiate agonists into the central nucleus of the amygdala blocks the acquisition of conditioned bradycardia in rabbits (Gallagher et al., 1981, 1982), and has anxiolytic effects in the social interaction test (File and Rodgers, 1979). Furthermore, local infusion of benzodiazepines into the amygdala has anxiolytic effects in the operant conflict test (Nagy et al., 1979; Petersen and Scheel-Kruger, 1982; Scheel-Kruger and Petersen, 1982; Shibata et al., 1982; Petersen et al., 1985;

Thomas et al., 1985; Hodges et al., 1987), the light-dark box measure in mice (Costall et al., 1989) and antagonizes the discriminative stimulus properties of pentylenetetrazol (Benjamin et al., 1987). The anticonflict effect can be reversed by systemic administration of the benzodiazepine antagonist flumazenil (Petersen et al., 1985; Hodges et al., 1987; Shibata et al., 1989) or coadministration into the amygdala of the GABA antagonist bicuculline (Scheel-Kruger and Petersen, 1982) and mimicked by local infusion into the amygdala of GABA (Hodges et al., 1987) or the GABA agonist muscimol (Scheel-Kruger and Petersen, 1982). In general, anticonflict effects of benzodiazepines occur after local infusion into the lateral and basal nuclei (Petersen and Scheel-Kruger, 1982; Scheel-Kruger and Petersen, 1982; Petersen et al., 1985; Thomas et al., 1985), those nuclei of the amygdala that have high densities of benzodiazepine receptors, and not after local infusion into the central nucleus (Petersen and Scheel-Kruger, 1982; Scheel-Kruger and Petersen, 1982). However, Shibata et al. (1982) found just the opposite effect, perhaps because of local anesthetic effects, which can occur when high doses of these compounds are infused into the central nucleus (e.g., Heule et al., 1983). More recently it has been shown that the anterior part of the basal and central nucleus are especially important for conflict performance based on both lesion and local infusion of benzodiazepines (Shibata et al., 1989). Taken together, therefore, these results suggest that drug actions in the amygdala may be sufficient to explain both fear-reducing and anxiety-reducing effects of various drugs given systemically. In fact, local infusion into the amygdala of the benzodiazepine antagonist flumazenil significantly attenuated the anticonflict effect of the benzodiazepine agonist chlordiazepoxide given systemically (Hodges et al., 1987). This is a very powerful experimental design and strongly implicates the amygdala in mediating the anxiolytic effects of benzodiazepines. However, in a very important recent study, the benzodiazepine chlordiazepoxide still had a marked anticonflict effect after amygdala lesions (Yadin et al., 1991), so more work clearly needs to be done on this issue.

Recently, a new class of anxiolytic compounds acting as $5-HT_3$ receptor subtype antagonists have been shown to produce anxiolytic effects after local infusion into the amygdala (Costsall et al., 1989). Such infusions also can block some of the signs of withdrawal following subchronic administration of diazepam, ethanol, nicotine, or cocaine (Costall et al., 1990) or increases in levels of dopamine or the serotonin metabolite 5-HIAA in the amygdala after activation of dopamine neurons in the ventral tegmental area (Hagan et al., 1990). These later effects, which may relate to the way in which sensory information is gated in the amygdala (Maeda and Maki, 1986), were more pronounced in the right amygdala vs. the left (Hagen et al., 1990), consistent with other lateralized effects reported previously (Costall et al., 1987). It is interesting in this regard that measures of emotionality, including fear-potentiated startle in humans, also show lateralization (cf. Lang et al., 1990), consistent with a greater participation of the right versus the left hemisphere and hence perhaps the right amygdala. Future studies employing local infusion of benzodiazepine or opiate antagonists into the amygdala, coupled with systemic administration of various agonists, may be able to determine if local binding to receptors in the amygdala is necessary to explain their anxiolytic effects. Eventually, local infusion of various drugs into specific target areas may be used to evaluate whether highly specific anxiolytic actions are produced. These results could then serve as a guide for eventually producing more selective anxiolytic compounds.

CONCLUSIONS

An impressive amount of evidence from many different laboratories using a variety of experimental techniques indicates that the amygdala plays a crucial role in conditioned fear and probably anxiety. Many of the amygdaloid projection areas are critically involved in specific signs that are used to measure fear and anxiety. Electrical stimulation of the amygdala elicits a pattern of behaviors that mimic natural or conditioned states of fear. Lesions of the amygdala block innate or conditioned fear and local infusion of drugs into the amygdala have anxiolytic effects in several behavioral tests. Finally, the amygdala may be a critical site of plasticity that mediates both the acquisition and extinction of conditioned fear. A better understanding of brain systems that inhibit the amydala, as well as the role of its very high levels of peptides (cf. Gray, 1989), may eventually lead to the development of more effective pharmacological strategies for treating clinical anxiety disorders.

ACKNOWLEDGMENTS

Research reported in this chapter was supported by NIMH grant MH-25642, MH-47840, NINCDS grant NS-18033, Research Scientist Development Award MH-00004, a grant from the Air Force Office of Scientific Research, and the State of Connecticut. Our sincere thanks are extended to Lee Schlesinger, who tested many of the animals used for these studies, to Bruce Kapp for helpful discussions about the brain stem projections of the amygdala, and to Leslie Fields for help in typing the paper.

REFERENCES

Adams DB (1979): Brain mechanisms for offense, defense and submission. Behav Brain Sci 2:201–241.

Aggleton JP (1985): A description of intra-amygdaloid connections in the old world monkeys. Exp Brain Res 57:390–399.

Aggleton JP, Blindt HS, Rawlins JNP (1989): Effect of amygdaloid and amygdaloid-hippocampal lesions on object recognition and spatial working memory in rats. Behav Neurosci 103:962–974.

Aggleton JP, Mishkin M (1986): The amygdala, sensory gateway to the emotions. In Plutchik R, Kellerman H (eds): "Emotion: Theory, Research and Experience." New York: Academic Press, pp 281–299.

Allen JP, Allen CF (1974): Role of the amygdaloid complexes in the stress-induced release of ACTH in the rat. Neuroendocrinology 15:220–230.

Amaral D (1987): Memory: Anatomical organization of candidate brain regions. In Plum F (ed): "Handbook of Physiology, Sec. 1: Neurophysiology, Vol. 5: Higher Functions of the Brain." Bethesda, MD: American Physiological Society, pp 211–294.

Anand BK, Dua S (1956): Circulatory and respiratory changes induced by electrical stimulation of limbic system (visceral brain). J Neurophysiol 19:393–400.

Applegate CD, Frysinger RC, Kapp BS, Gallagher M (1982): Multiple unit activity recorded from amygdala central nucleus during Pavlovian heart rate conditioning in rabbit. Brain Res 237:457–462.

Applegate CD, Kapp BS, Underwood MD, McNall CL (1983): Autonomic and somatomotor effects of amygdala central n. stimulation in awake rabbits. Physiol Behav 31:353–360.

Aston-Jones G, Ennis M, Pieribone VA, Nickell WT, Shipley MT (1986): The brain nucleus locus coeruleus: Restricted afferent control of a broad efferent network. Science 234:734–737.

Baker T, Netick A, Dement WC (1981): Sleep-related apneic and apneustic breathing following pneumotaxic lesion and vagotomy. Resp Physiol 46:271–294.

Bandler R, Depaulis A (1988): Elicitation of intraspecific defence reactions in the rat from midbrain periaqueductal grey by microinjection of kainic acid, without neurotoxic effects. Neurosci Lett 88:291–296.

Beaulieu S, DiPaolo T, Barden N (1986): Control of ACTH secretion by central nucleus of the amygdala: Implication of the serotonergic system and its relevance to the glucocorticoid delayed negative feed-back mechanism. Neuroendocrinology 44:247–254.

Beaulieu S, DiPaolo T, Cote J, Barden N (1987): Participation of the central amygdaloid nucleus in the response of adrenocorticotropin secretion to immobilization stress: Opposing roles of the noradrenergic and dopaminergic systems. Neuroendocrinology 45:37–46.

Becker HC, Jarvis MF, Wagner GC, Flaherty CF (1984): Medial and lateral amygdalectomy differentially influences consummatory negative contrast. Physiol Behav 33:707–712.

Beckstead RM, Domesick VB, Nauta WJH (1979): Efferent connections of the substantia nigra and ventral tegmental area in the rat. Brain Res 175:191–217.

Beitz AJ (1982): The organization of afferent projections to the midbrain periaqueductal gray of the rat. Neuroscience 7:133–159.

Benjamin D, Emmett-Oglesby MW, Lal H (1987): Modulation of the discriminative stimulus produced by pentylenetetrazol by centrally administered drugs. Neuropharmacology 26:1727–1731.

Bennett C, Liang KC, McGaugh JL (1985): Depletion of adrenal catecholamines alters the amnestic effect of amygdala stimulation. Behav Brain Res 15:83–91.

Benvenga MJ, Spaulding TC (1988): Amnesic effect of the novel anticonvulsant MK-801. Pharmacol Biochem Behav 30:205–207.

Berg WK, Davis M (1984): Diazepam blocks fear-enhanced startle elicited electrically from the brainstem. Physiol Behav 32:333–336.

Berg WK, Davis M (1985): Associative learning modifies startle reflexes at the lateral lemniscus. Behav Neurosci 99:191–199.

Bertrand S, Hugelin A (1971): Respiratory synchronizing function of the nucleus parabrachialis medialis: Pneumotaxic mechanisms. J Neurophysiol 34:180–207.

Blanchard DC, Blanchard RJ (1969): Crouching as an index of fear. J Comp Physiol Psychol 67:370–375.

Blanchard DC, Blanchard RJ (1972): Innate and conditioned reactions to threat in rats with amygdaloid lesions. J Comp Physiol Psychol 81:281–290.

Blanchard DC, Williams G, Lee EMC, Blanchard RJ (1981): Taming of wild *Rattus norvegicus* by lesions of the mesencephalic central gray. Physiol Psychol 9:157–163.

Block CH, Schwartzbaum JS (1983): Ascending efferent projections of the gustatory parabrachial nuclei in the rabbit. Brain Res 259:1–9.

Boluis JJ, Fitzgerald RE, Dijk DJ, Koolhaas JM (1984): The corticomedial amygdala and learning in an agonistic situation in the rat. Physiol Behav 32:575–579.

Bolles RC, Collier AC (1976): Effects of predictive cues on freezing in rats. Animal Learn Behav 4:6–8.

Bonvallet M, Gary Bobo E (1972): Changes in phrenic activity and heart rate elicited by localized stimulation of the amygdala and adjacent structures. Electroencephalogr Clin Neurophysiol 32:1–16.

Bonvallet M, Gary Bobo E (1975): Amygdala and masseteric reflex. II. Mechanism of the diphasic modifications of the reflex elicited from the "Defence Reaction Area." Role of the spinal trigeminal nucleus (pars oralis). Electroencephalogr Clin Neurophysiol 39:341–352.

Borszcz GS, Cranney J, Leaton RN (1989) Influence of long-term sensitization on long-term habituation of the acoustic startle response in rats: Central gray lesions, preexposure, and extinction. J Exp Psychol: Animal Behav Process 15:54–64.

Boulis N, Davis M (1989): Footshock-induced sensitization of electrically elicited startle reflexes. Behav Neurosci 103:504–508.

Bouton ME, Bolles RC (1980): Conditioned fear assessed by freezing and by the suppression of three different baselines. Animal Learn Behav 8:429–434.

Bresnahan E, Routtenberg A (1972): Memory disruption by unilateral low level, sub-seizure stimulation of the medial amygdaloid nucleus. Physiol Behav 9:513–525.

Bresnahan JC, Meyer PM, Baldwin RB, Meyer DR (1976): Avoidance behavior in rats with amygdala lesions in the septum, fornix longus, and amygdala. Physiol Psychol 4:333–340.

Brown JS, Kalish HI, Farber IE (1951): Conditioned fear as revealed by magnitude of startle response to an auditory stimulus. J Exp Psychol 41:317–328.

Brown TH, Chapman PF, Kairiss EW, Keenan CL (1988): Long-term synaptic potentiation. Science 242:724–728.

Butelman ER (1989): A novel NMDA antagonist, MK-801, impairs performance in a hippocampal-dependent spatial learning task. Pharmacol Biochem Behav 34:13–16.

Butelman ER (1990): The effect of NMDA antagonists in the radial arm maze task with an interposed delay. Pharmacol Biochem Behav 35:533–536.

Cador M, Robbins TW, Everitt BJ (1989): Involvement of the amygdala in stimulus-reward associations: Interaction with the ventral striatum. Neuroscience 30:77–86.

Cahill L, McGaugh JL (1990): Amygdaloid complex lesions differentially affect retention of tasks using appetitive and aversive reinforcement. Behav Neurosci 104:532–543.

Calvo JM, Badillo S, Morales-Ramirez M, Palacios-Salas P (1987): The role of the temporal lobe amygdala in ponto-geniculo-occipital activity and sleep organization in cats. Brain Res 403:22–30.

Campeau S, Liang KC, Davis M (1990): Long-term retention of fear-potentiated startle following a short training session. Animal Learn Behav 18:462–468.

Campeau S, Hayward MD, Hope BT, Rosen JB, Nestler EJ, Davis M (1991): Induction of c-Fos proto-oncogene in rat amygdala during unconditioned fear. Brain Res (in press).

Cassella JV, Davis M (1985): Fear-enhanced acoustic startle is not attenuated by acute or chronic imipramine treatment in rats. Psychopharmacology (Berlin) 87:278–282.

Cassella JV, Davis M (1986a): Habituation, prepulse inhibition, fear conditioning, and drug modulation of the acoustically elicited pinna reflex in rats. Behav Neurosci 100:39–44.

Cassella JV, Davis M (1986b): Neural structures mediating acoustic and tactile startle reflexes and the acoustically-elicited pinna response in rats: Electrolytic and ibotenic acid studies. Soc Neurosci Abstr 12:1273.

Cassella JV, Harty PT, Davis M (1986): Fear conditioning, pre-pulse inhibition and drug modulation of a short latency startle response measure electromyographically from neck muscles in the rat. Physiol Behav 36:1187–1191.

Cedarbaum JM, Aghajanian GK (1978): Afferent projections to the rat locus coeruleus as determined by a retrograde tracing technique. J Comp Neurol 178:1–16.

Chapman PF, Kairiss EW, Keenan CL, Brown TH (1990): Long-term synaptic potentiation in the amygdala. Synapse 6:271–278.

Chapman WP, Schroeder HR,Guyer G, Brazier MAB, Fager C, Poppen JL, Solomon HC, Yakolev PI (1954): Physiological evidence concerning the importance of the amygdaloid nuclear region in the integration of circulating function and emotion in man. Science 129:949–950.

Charney DS, Heninger GR, Breier A (1984): Noradrenergic function in panic anxiety. Arch Gen Psychiat 41:751–763.

Chi CC (1965): The effect of amobarbital sodium on conditioned fear as measured by the potentiated startle response in rats. Psychopharmacology 7:115–122.

Chiamulera C, Costa S, Reggiani A (1990): Effect of NMDA- and strychnine-insensitive glycine site antagonists on NMDA-mediated convulsions and learning. Psychopharmacology 102:551–552.

Clugnet MC, LeDoux JE (1990): Synaptic plasticity in fear conditioning circuits: Induction of LTP in the lateral nucleus of the amygdala by stimulation of the medial geniculate body. J Neurosci 10:2818–2824.

Cohen DH (1975): Involvement of the avian amygdala homologue (archistriatum posterior and mediale) in defensively conditioned heart rate change. J Comp Neurol 160:13–36.

Cohen MI (1971): Switching of the respiratory phases and evoked phrenic responses produced by rostral pontine electrical stimulation. J Physiol (London) 217:133–158.

Cohen MI (1979): Neurogenesis of respiratory rhythm in the mammal. Physiol Rev 59:1105.

Collingridge GL, Bliss TVP (1987): NMDA receptors—their role in long-term potentiation. Trends Neurosci 10:288–293.

Corman CD, Meyer PM, Meyer DR (1967): Open-field activity and exploration in rats with septal and amygdaloid lesions. Brain Res 5:469–476.

Costall B, Domeney AM, Naylor RJ, Tyers MB (1987): Effects of the 5-HT-3 receptor antagonist, GR38032F, on raised dopaminergic activity in the mesolimbic system of the rat and marmoset brain. Br J Pharmacol 92:881–894.

Costall B, Jones BJ, Kelly ME, Naylor RJ, Onaivi ES, Tyers MB (1990): Sites of action of ondasetron to inhibit withdrawal from drugs of abuse. Pharmacol Biochem Behav 36:97–104.

Costall B, Kelly ME, Naylor RJ, Onaivi ES, Tyers MB (1989): Neuroanatomical sites of action of 5-HT-3 receptor agonist and antagonists for alteration of aversive behaviour in the mouse. Br J Pharmacol 96:325–332.

Cox GE, Jordan D, Paton JFR, Spyer KM, Wood LM (1987): Cardiovascular and phrenic nerve responses to stimulation of the amygdala central nucleus in the anaesthetized rabbit. J Physiol (Lond) 389:541–556.

Crandall PH, Walter RD, Dymond A (1971): The ictal electroencephalographic signal identifying limbic system seizure foci. Proc Am Assoc Neurol Surg 1:1.

Crooks GB Jr, Robinson GS, Hatfield TJ, Graham PW, Gallagher M (1989): Intraventricular administration of the NMDA antagonist APV disrupts learning of an odor aversion that is potentiated by taste. Soc Neurosci Abstr 15:464.

Dafters RI (1976): Effect of medial archistriatal lesions on the conditioned emotional response and on auditory discrimination performance of the pigeon. Physiol Behav 17:659–665.

Danysz W, Wroblewski JT (1989): Amnesic properties of glutamate receptor antagonists. Neurosci Res Commun 5:10–18.

Davis M (1979a): Diazepam and flurazepam: Effects on conditioned fear as measured with the potentiated startle paradigm. Psychopharmacology 62:1–7.

Davis M (1979b): Morphine and naloxone: Effects on conditioned fear as measured with the potentiated startle paradigm. Eur J Pharmacol 54:341–347.

Davis M (1986): Pharmacological and anatomical analysis of fear conditioning using the fear-potentiated startle paradigm. Behav Neurosci 100:814–824.

Davis M (1989): Sensitization of the acoustic startle reflex by footshock. Behav Neurosci 103:495–503.

Davis M, Astrachan DI (1978): Conditioned fear and startle magnitude: Effects of different footshock or backshock intensities used in training. J Exp Psychol: Animal Behav Process 4:95–103.

Davis M, Cassella JV, Kehne JH (1988): Serotonin does not mediate anxiolytic effects of buspirone in the fear-potentiated startle paradigm: Comparison with 8-OH-DPAT and ipsapirone. Psychopharmacology 94:14–20.

Davis M, Gendelman DS, Tischler MD, Gendelman PM (1982): A primary acoustic startle circuit: Lesion and stimulation studies. J Neurosci 6:791–805.

Davis M, Hitchcock JM, Rosen JB (1987): Anxiety and the amygdala: Pharmacological and anatomical analysis of the fear-potentiated startle paradigm. In Bowen GH (ed): "The Psychology of Learning and Motivation," Vol. 21. New York: Academic Press, pp 263–305.

Davis M, Redmond DE Jr, Baraban JM (1979): Noradrenergic agonists and antagonists: Effects on conditioned fear as measured by the potentiated startle paradigm. Psychopharmacology 65:111–118.

Davis M, Schlesinger LS, Sorenson CA (1989): Temporal specificity of fear-conditioning: Effects of different conditioned stimulus-unconditioned stimulus intervals on the fear-potentiated startle effect. J Exp Psychol: Animal Behav Process 15:295–310.

DeOlmos J, Alheid GF, Beltramino CA (1985): Amygdala. In Paxinos G (ed): "The Rat Nervous System," Vol 1. Orlando, FL. Academic Press, pp 223–334.

DeSouza EB, Insel TR, Perrin MH, Rivier J, Vale WW, Kuhar MJ (1985): Corticotropin-releasing factor receptors are widely distributed within the rat central nervous system: An autoradiographic study. J Neurosci 5:3189–3203.

Deutch AY, Goldstein M, Roth RH (1986): Activation of the locus coeruleus induced by selective stimulation of the ventral tegmental area. Brain Res 363:307–314.

Dunn AJ, Berridge CW (1990): Physiological and behavioral responses to corticotropin-releasing factor administration: Is CRF a mediator of anxiety or stress response? Brain Res Revs (in press).

Dunn JD (1987): Plasma corticosterone responses to electrical stimulation of the bed nucleus of the stria terminalis. Brain Res 407:327–331.

Dunn JD, Whitener J (1986): Plasma corticosterone responses to electrical stimulation of the amygdaloid complex: Cytoarchitectural specificity. Neuroendocrinology 42:211–217.

Dunn LT, Everitt BJ (1988): Double dissociations of the effects of amygdala and insular cortex lesions on conditioned taste aversion, passive avoidance, and neophobia in the rat using the excitotoxin ibotenic acid. Behav Neurosci 102:3–23.

Eclancher F, Karli P (1979): Effects of early amygdaloid lesions on the development of reactivity in the rat. Physiol Behav 22:1123–1134.

Ellis ME, Kesner RP (1983): The noradrenergic system of the amygdala and aversive information processing. Behav Neurosci 97:399–415.

Estes WK, Skinner BF (1941): Some quantitative properties of anxiety. J Exp Psychol 29:390–400.

Everitt BJ, Cador M, Robbins TW (1989): Interactions between the amygdala and ventral striatum in stimulus-reward associations: Studies using a second-order schedule of sexual reinforcement. Neuroscience 30:63–75.

Faiers AA, Calaresu FR, Mogenson GJ (1975): Pathway mediating hypotension elicited by stimulation of the amygdala in the rat. Am J Physiol 288:1358–1366.

Falls WA, Miserendino MJD, Davis M (1992): Extinction of fear-potentiated startle: blockade by infusion of an NMDA antagonist into the amygdala. J Neurosci (in press).

Fanardjian VVG, Manvelyan LR (1987): Mechanisms regulating the activity of facial nucleus motoneurons. III. Synaptic influences from the cerebral cortex and subcortical structures. Neuroscience 20:835–843.

Fanselow MS (1981): Naloxone and pavlovian fear conditioning. Learn Motiv 12:398–419.

Fanselow MS (1982): The postshock activity burst. Animal Learn Behav 10:448–454.

Fanselow MS (1984): Shock-induced analgesia on the formalin test: Effect of shock severity, naloxone, hypophysectomy, and associative variables. Behav Neurosci 98:79–95.

Fanselow MS (1991): The midbrain periaqueductal gray as a coordinator of action in response to fear and anxiety. In Depaulis A, Bandler R (eds): "The Midbrain Periaqueductal Grey Matter: Functional, Anatomical and Immunohistochemical Organization." New York: Plenum Press (in press).

Fanselow MS, Bolles RC (1979): Naloxone and shock-elicited freezing in the rat. J Comp Physiol Psychol 93:736–744.

Feldman S, Conforti N (1981): Amygdalectomy inhibits adrenocortical responses to somatosensory and olfactory stimulation. Neuroendocrinology 32:330–334.

Feldman S, Conforti N, Saphier D (1990): The preoptic area and bed nucleus of the stria terminalis are involved in the effects of the amygdala on adrenocortical secretion. Neuroscience 37:775–779.

Feldman S, Conforti N, Siegal RA (1982): Adrenocortical responses following limbic stimulation in rats with hypothalamic deafferentations. Neuroendocrinology 35:205–211.

File SE (1980): The use of social interaction as a method for detecting anxiolytic activity of chlordiazepoxide-like drugs. J Neurosci Meth 2:219–238.

File SE, Rodgers RJ (1979): Partial anxiolytic actions of morphine sulphate following microinjection into the central nucleus of the amygdala in rats. Pharmacol Biochem Behav 11:313–318.

Flaherty CF (1990): Effect of anxiolytics and antidepressants on extinction and negative contrast. Pharmac Ther 46:308–320.

Frysinger RC, Marks JD, Trelease RB, Schechtman VL, Harper RM (1984): Sleep states attenuate the pressor response to central amygdala stimulation. Exp Neurol 83:604–617.

Fulwiler CE, Saper CB (1984): Subnuclear organization of the efferent connections of the parabrachial nucleus in the rat. Brain Res Rev 7:229–259.

Galeno TM, Brody MJ (1983): Hemodynamic responses to amygdaloid stimulation in spontaneously hypertensive rats. Am J Physiol 245:281–286.

Galeno TM, VanHoesen GW, Brody MJ (1984): Central amygdaloid nucleus lesion attenuates exaggerated hemodynamic responses to noise stress in the spontaneously hypertensive rat. Brain Res 291:249–259.

Gallagher M, Graham PW, Holland PC (1990): The amygdala central nucleus and appetitive pavlovian conditioning: Lesions impair one class of conditioned behavior. J Neurosci 10:1906–1911.

Gallagher M, Kapp BS (1978): Manipulation of opiate activity in the amygdala alters memory processes. Life Sci 23:1973–1978.

Gallagher M, Kapp BS (1981): Effect of phentolamine administration into the amygdala complex of rats on time-dependent memory processes. Behav Neural Biol 31:90–95.

Gallagher M, Kapp BS, Frysinger RC, Rapp PR (1980): β-Adrenergic manipulation in amygdala central n. alters rabbit heart rate conditioning. Pharmacol Biochem Behav 12:419–426.

Gallagher M, Kapp BS, McNall CL, Pascoe JP (1981): Opiate effects in the amygdala central nucleus on heart rate conditioning in rabbits. Pharmacol Biochem Behav 14:497–505.

Gallagher M, Kapp BS, Pascoe JP (1982): Enkephalin analogue effects in the amygdala central nucleus on conditioned heart rate. Pharmacol Biochem Behav 17:217–222.

Gandolfi O, Dall'Olio R, Roncada P, Montanaro N (1990): NMDA antagonists interact with 5-HT-stimulated phosphatidylinositol metabolism and impair passive avoidance retention in the rat. Neurosci Lett 113:304–308.

Gary Bobo E, Bonvallet M (1975): Amygdala and masseteric reflex. I. Facilitation, inhibition and diphasic modifications of the reflex, induced by localized amygdaloid stimulation. Electroencephalogr Clin Neurophysiol 39:329–339.

Geller, I, Seifter J (1960): The effects of memprobamate, barbiturates, d-amphetamine and promazine on experimentally induced conflict in the rat. Psychopharmacologia 1:482–492.

Gelsema AJ, McKitrick DJ, Calaresu FR (1987): Cardiovascular responses to chemical and electrical stimulation of amygdala in rats. Am J Physiol 253:R712–R718.

Gentile CG, Jarrel TW, Teich A, McCabe PM, Schneiderman N (1986): The role of amygdaloid central nucleus in the retention of differential pavlovian conditioning of bradycardia in rabbits. Behav Brain Res 20:263–273.

Gloor P (1960): Amygdala. In Field J (ed): "Handbook of Physiology: Sec. I. Neurophysiology." Washington, DC: American Physiological Society, pp 1395–1420.

Gloor P (1978): Inputs and outputs of the amygdala: What the amygdala is trying to tell the rest of the brain. In Livingston K, Hornykiewicz K (eds): "Limbic Mechanisms: The Continuing Evolution of the Limbic System Concept." New York: Plenum Press, pp. 189–209.

Gloor P, Olivier A, Quesney LF (1981): The role of the amygdala in the expression of psychic phenomena in temporal lobe seizures. In Ben-Ari Y (ed): "The Amygdaloid Complex." New York, Elsevier/North-Holland, pp 489–507.

Goddard GV (1964): Functions of the amygdala. Psychol Bull 62:89–109.

Gold PE, Hankins L, Edwards RM, Chester J, McGaugh JL (1975): Memory interference and facilitation with posttrial amygdala stimulation: Effect varies with footshock level. Brain Res 86:509–513.

Goldenberg M, Snyder CH, Aranow H Jr (1947): New test for hypertension due to circulating epinephrine. JAMA 135:971–976.

Goodman RR, Snyder SH, Kuhar MJ, Young WS III (1980): Differential delta and mu opiate receptor localizations by light microscopic autoradiography. Proc Natl Acad Sci USA 77:2167–2174.

Graeff FG (1988): Animal models of aversion. In Simon P, Soubrie P, Wildlocher D (eds): "Selected Models of Anxiety, Depression and Psychosis." Basel: Karger, pp 115–142.

Gray TS (1989): Autonomic neuropeptide connections of the amygdala. In Tache Y, Morley JE, Brown MR (eds): Vol. 1: "Neuropeptides and Stress." New York: Springer Verlag, pp 92–106.

Gray TS (1990): The organization and possible function of amygdaloid corticotropin-releasing factor pathways. In DeSouza EB, Nemeroff CB (eds): "Corticotropin-Releasing Factor: Basic and Clinical Studies of a Neuropeptide." Boca Raton: CRC Press, pp 53–68.

Gray TS, Carney ME, Magnuson DJ (1989): Direct projections from the central amygdaloid nucleus to the hypothalamic paraventricular nucleus: Possible role in stress-induced adrenocorticotropin release. Neuroendocrinology 50:433–446.

Greidanus TBVW, Croiset G, Bakker E, Bouman H (1979): Amygdaloid lesions block the effect of neuropeptides (vasopressin, ACHT) on avoidance behavior. Physiol Behav 22:291–295.

Grijalva CV, Levin ED, Morgan M, Roland B, Martin FC (1990): Contrasting effects of centromedial and basolateral amygdaloid lesions on stress-related responses in the rat. Physiol Behav 48:495–500.

Grillon C, Ameli R, Woods SW, Merikangas K, Davis M (1990): Fear-potentiated startle in humans: Effect of anticipatory anxiety on the acoustic blink reflex. Psychophysiology (in press).

Grossman SP, Grossman L, Walsh L (1975): Functional organization of the rat amygdala with respect to avoidance behavior. J Comp Physiol Psychol 88:829–850.

Groves PM, Thompson RF (1970): Habituation: A dual process theory. Psychol Rev 77:419–450.

Hagan RM, Jones BJ, Jordan CC, Tyers MB (1990): Effect of 5-HT-$_3$ receptor antagonists on responses to selective activation of mesolimbic dopaminergic pathways in the rat. Br J Pharmacol 99:227–232.

Hammer GD, Kapp BS (1986): The effects of naloxone administered into the periaqueductal gray on shock-elicited freezing behavior in the rat. Behav Neural Biol 46:189–195.

Handelmann GE, Contreras PC, O'Donohue TL (1987): Selective memory impairment by phencyclidine in rats. Eur J Pharmacol 140:69–73.

Handforth A (1984): Implications of stimulus factors governing kindled seizure threshold. Exp Neurol 86:33–39.

Handwerker MJ, Gold PE, McGaugh JL (1974): Impairment of active avoidance learning with posttraining amygdala stimulation. Brain Res 75:324–327.

Harper RM, Frysinger RC, Trelease RB, Marks JD (1984): State-dependent alteration of respiratory cycle timing by stimulation of the central nucleus of the amygdala. Brain Res 306:1–8.

Hauber W, Schmidt WJ (1989): Effects of intrastriatal blockade of glutamatergic transmission on the acquisition of T-maze and radial maze tasks. J Neural Trans 78:29–41.

Heale V, Harley C (1990): MK-801 and AP5 impair acquisition, but not retention, of the morris milk maze. Pharmacol Biochem Behav 36:145–149.

Heinemann W, Stock G, Schaeffer H (1973): Temporal correlation of responses in blood pressure and motor reaction under electrical stimulation of limbic structures in the unanesthetized unrestrained cat. Pflugers Arch Gen Physiol 343:27–40.

Henke PG (1972): Amygdalectomy and mixed reinforcement schedule contrast effects. Psychon Sci 28:301–302.

Henke PG (1973): Effects of reinforcement omission on rats with lesions in the amygdala. J Comp Physiol Psychol 84:187–193.

Henke PG (1977): Dissociation of the frustration effect and the partial reinforcement extinction effect after limbic lesions in rats. J Comp Physiol Psychol 91:1032–1038.

Henke PG (1980a): The amygdala and restraint ulcers in rats. J Comp Physiol Psychol 94:313–323.

Henke PG (1980b): The centromedial amygdala and gastric pathology in rats. Physiol Behav 25:107–112.

Henke PG (1982): The telencephalic limbic system and experimental gastric pathology: A review. Neurosci Biobehav Rev 6:381–390.

Henke PG (1983): Unit-activity in the central amygdalar nucleus of rats in response to immobilization-stress. Brain Res Rev 10:833–837.

Henke PG, Allen JD, Davison C (1972): Effect of lesions in the amygdala on behavioral contrast. Physiol Behav 8:173–176.

Heule F, Lorez H, Cumin R, Haefely W (1983): Studies on the anticonflict effect of midazolam injected into the amygdala. Neurosci Lett 14:S164.

Hijzen TH, Slangen JL (1989): Effects of midazolam, DMCM and lindane on potentiated startle in the rat. Psychopharmacology 99:362–365.

Hilton SM, Zbrozyna AW (1963): Amygdaloid region for defense reactions and its efferent pathway to the brainstem. J Physiol (Lond) 165:160–173.

Hitchcock JM, Davis M (1986c): Lesions of the amygdala, but not of the cerebellum or red nucleus, block conditioned fear as measured with the potentiated startle paradigm. Behav Neurosci 100:11–22.

Hitchcock JM, Davis M (1987): Fear-potentiated startle using an auditory conditioned stimulus: Effect of lesions of the amygdala. Physiol Behav 39:403–408.

Hitchcock JM, Davis M (1991): Efferent pathway of the amygdala involved in conditioned fear as measured with the fear-potentiated startle paradigm. Beh Neurosci 105:826–842.

Hitchcock JM, Sananes CB, Davis M (1989): Sensitization of the startle reflex by footshock: Blockade by lesions of the central nucleus of the amygdala or its efferent pathway to the brainstem. Behav Neurosci 103:509–518.

Hodges H, Green S, Glenn B (1987): Evidence that the amygdala is involved in benzodiazepine and serotonergic effects on punished responding but not on discrimination. Psychopharmacology 92:491–504.

Holmberg G, Gershon S (1961): Autonomic and psychic effects of yohimbine hydrochloride. Psychopharmacologia (Berlin) 2:93–106.

Holstedge G, Kuypers HGJM, Dekker JJ (1977): The organization of the bulbar fibre connections to the trigeminal, facial and hypoglossal motor nuclei. II. An autoradiographic tracing study in cat. Brain 100:265–286.

Hopkins DA, Holstege G (1978): Amygdaloid projections to the mesencephalon, pons and medulla oblongata in the cat. Exp Brain Res 32:529–547.

Inagaki S, Kawai Y, Matsuzak T, Shiosaka S, Tohyama M (1983): Precise terminal fields of the descending somatostatinergic neuron system from the amygdala complex of the rat. J Hirnforsch 24:345–365.

Innes DL, Tansy MF (1980): Gastric mucosal ulceration associated with electrochemical stimulation of the limbic system. Brain Res Bull 5:33–36.

Ison JR, McAdam DW, Hammond GR (1973): Latency and amplitude changes in the acoustic startle reflex of the rat produced by variation in auditory prestimulation. Physiol Behav 10:1035–1039.

Iwata J, Chida K, LeDoux JE (1987): Cardiovascular responses elicited by stimulation of neurons in the central amygdaloid nucleus in awake but not anesthetized rats resemble conditioned emotional responses. Brain Res 418:183–188.

Iwata J, LeDoux JE, Meeley MP, Arneric S, Reis DJ (1986): Intrinsic neurons in the amygdala field projected to by the medial geniculate body mediate emotional responses conditioned to acoustic stimuli. Brain Res 383:195–214.

Jarrell TW, McCabe PM, Teich A, Gentile CG, VanDercar DH, Schneiderman N (1986): Lateral subthalamic area as mediator of classically conditioned bradycardia in rabbits. Behav Neurosci 100:3–10.

Jellestad FK, Cabrera IG (1986): Exploration and avoidance learning after ibotenic acid and radio frequency lesions in the rat amygdala. Behav Neural Biol 46:196–215.

Jellestad FK, Markowska A, Bakke HK, Walther B (1986): Behavioral effects after ibotenic acid, 6-OHDA and electrolytic lesions in the central amygdala nucleus of the rat. Physiol Behav 37:855–862.

Jonason KR, Enloe LJ (1971): Alterations in social behavior following septal and amygdaloid lesions in the rat. J Comp Physiol Psychol 75:286–301.

Jones KW, Bauerle LM, DeNoble VJ (1990): Differential effects of σ and phencyclidine receptor ligands on learning. Eur J Pharmacol 179:97–102.

Kaada BR (1951): Somatomotor, autonomic and electrophysiological responses to electrical stimulation of "rhinencephalic" and other structures in primates, cat, and dog. Acta Physiol Scand (Suppl 83) 24:1–285.

Kaada BR (1972): Stimulation and regional ablation of the amygdaloid complex with reference to functional representations. In Eleftheriou BE (ed): "The Neurobiology of the Amygdala." New York: Plenum Press, pp 205–281.

Kaku T (1984): Functional differentiation of hypoglossal motoneurons during the amygdaloid or cortically induced rhythmical jaw and tongue movements in the rat. Brain Res Bull 13:147–154.

Kapp BS, Frysinger RC, Gallagher M, Haselton JR (1979): Amygdala central nucleus lesions: Effects on heart rate conditioning in the rabbit. Physiol Behav 23:1109–1117.

Kapp BS, Gallagher M, Underwood MD, McNall CL, Whitehorn D (1982): Cardiovascular responses elicited by electrical stimulation of the amygdala central nucleus in the rabbit. Brain Res 234:251–262.

Kapp BS, Pascoe JP (1986): Correlation aspects of learning and memory: Vertebrate model systems. In Martinez JL, Kesner RP (eds): "Learning and Memory: A Biological View." New York: Academic Press, pp 399–440.

Kapp BS, Pascoe JP, Bixler MA (1984): The amygdala: A neuroanatomical systems approach to its contribution to aversive conditioning. In Butters N, Squire LS (eds): "The Neuropsychology of Memory." New York: Guilford Press, pp 473–488.

Kapp BS, Wilson A, Pascoe JP, Supple WF, Whalen PJ (1990): A neuroanatomical systems analysis of conditioned bradycardia in the rabbit. In Gabriel M, Moore J (eds): "Neurocomputation and Learning: Foundations of Adaptive Networks." New York: Bradford Books.

Kehne JH, Cassella JV, Davis M (1988): Anxiolytic effects of buspirone and gepirone in the fear-potentiated startle paradigm. Psychopharmacology 94:8–13.

Kehne JH, Gallager DW, Davis M (1981): Strychnine: Brainstem and spinal mediation of excitatory effects on acoustic startle. Eur J Pharmacol 76:177–186.

Kellicut MH, Schwartzbaum JS (1963): Formation of a conditioned emotional response (CER) following lesions of the amygdaloid complex in rats. Psychol Rev 12:351–358.

Kemble ED, Beckman GJ (1970): Runway performance of rats following amygdaloid lesions. Physiol Behav 5:45–47.

Kemble ED, Blanchard DC, Blanchard RJ (1990): Effects of regional amygdaloid lesions on flight and defensive behaviors of wild black rats (*Rattus rattus*). Physiol Behav 48:1–5.

Kemble ED, Blanchard DC, Blanchard RJ, Takushi R (1984): Taming in wild rats following medial amygdaloid lesions. Physiol Behav 32:131–134.

Kemble ED, Studelska DR, Schmidt MK (1979): Effects of central amygdaloid nucleus lesions on ingestation, taste reactivity, exploration and taste aversion. Physiol Behav 22:789–793.

Kesner RP (1982): Brain stimulation: Effects on memory. Behav Neural Biol 36:315–367.

Kesner RP, Hardy JD, Novak JM (1983): Phencyclidine and behavior: II. Active avoidance learning and radial arm maze performance. Pharmacol Biochem Behav 18:351–356.

Kesner RP, Walser RD, Winzenried G (1989): Central but not basolateral amygdala mediates memory for positive affective experiences. Behav Brain Res 33:189–195.

Kim M, McGaugh JL (1990): Microinfusion of an N-methyl-D-aspartate antagonist into the amygdala impairs avoidance learning in rats. Soc Neurosci Abstr 16:767.

Kim JJ, DeCola JP, Landeira-Fernandez J, Fanselow MS (1991): N-methyl-d-aspasate receptor antagonist APV blocks acquisition but not expression of fear conditioning. Behav Neurosci 105:126–133.

Koikegami H, Dudo T, Mochida Y, Takahashi H (1957): Stimulation experiments on the amygdaloid nuclear complex and related structures: Effects upon the renal volume, urinary secretion, movements of the urinary bladder, blood pressure and respiratory movements. Folia Psychiat Neurol Japan 11:157–207.

Koob GF, Bloom FE (1985a): Corticotropin-releasing factor and behavior. Fed Proc 44:259–263.

Krettek JE, Price JL (1978a): Amygdaloid projections to subcortical structures within the basal forebrain and brainstem in the rat and cat. J Comp Neurol 178:225–254.

Krettek JE, Price JL (1978b): A description of the amygdaloid complex in the rat and cat with observations on intraamygdaloid axonal connections. J Comp Neurol 178:255–280.

Kurtz KH, Siegel A (1966): Conditioned fear and magnitude of startle response: A replication and extension. J Comp Physiol Psychol 62:8–14.

Lang PJ, Bradley MM, Cuthbert BN (1990): Emotion, attention, and the startle reflex. Psychol Rev 97:377–395.

Laroche S, Doyere V, Bloch V (1989): Linear relation between the magnitude of long-term potentiation in the dentate gyrus and associative learning in the rat. A demonstration using commissural inhibition and local infusion of an N-methyl-D-aspartate receptor antagonist. Neuroscience 28:375–386.

Lavond DG, Lincoln JS, McCormick DA, Thompson RF (1984): Effect of bilateral lesions of the lateral cerebellar nuclei on conditioning of the heart-rate and nictitating membrane/eyelid responses in rabbit. Brain Res 305:323–330.

Leaton RN, Borszcz GS (1985): Potentiated startle: Its relation to freezing and shock intensity in rats. J Exp Psychol: Animal Behav Process 11:421–428.

Leaton RN, Cranney J (1990): Potentiation of the acoustic startle response by a conditioned stimulus paired with acoustic startle stimulus in rats. J Exp Psychol: Animal Behav Process 16:279–287.

LeDoux JE (1987): Emotion. In Plum F (ed): "Handbook of physiology: nervous system V." Washington, DC: American Physiological Society, pp 419–459.

LeDoux JE, Cicchetti P, Xagoraris A, Romanski LM (1990a): The lateral amygdaloid nucleus: Sensory interface of the amygdala in fear conditioning. J Neurosci 10:1062–1069.

LeDoux JE, Iwata J, Cicchetti P, Reis DJ (1988): Different projections of the central amygdaloid nucleus mediate autonomic and behavioral correlates of conditioned fear. J Neurosci 8:2517–2529.

LeDoux JE, Romanski L, Xagoraris A (1990b): Indelibility of subcortical emotional memories. J Cogn Sci 1:238–243.

Leung LWS, Desborough KA (1988): APV, an N-methyl-D-aspartate receptor antagonist, blocks the hippocampal theta rhythm in behaving rats. Brain Res 463:148–152.

Lewis SJ, Verberne AJM, Robinson TG, Jarrott B, Louis WJ, Beart PM (1989): Excitotoxin-induced lesions of the central but not basolateral nucleus of the amygdala modulate the baroreceptor heart rate reflex in conscious rats. Brain Res 494:232–240.

Liang KC, Bennett C, McGaugh JL (1985): Peripheral epinephrine modulates the effects of post-training amygdala stimulation on memory. Behav Brain Res 15:93–100.

Liang KC, Juler RG, McGaugh JL (1986): Modulating effects of posttraining epinephrine on memory: Involvement of the amygdala noradrenergic systems. Brain Res 368:125–133.

Liang KC, Davis M (1990): Intra-amygdala injection of N-methyl-D-aspartate receptor antagonists impairs memory in an inhibitory avoidance task. Soc Neurosci Abstr 16:767.

Liang KC, Miserendino MJD, Melia KR, Davis M (1989): Corticotropin releasing factor enhances the acoustic startle reflex: Involvement of the amygdala and the spinal cord. Soc Neurosci Abstr 15, p. 1069.

Liebman JM, Mayer DJ, Liebeskind JC (1970): Mesencephalic central gray lesions and fear-motivated behavior in rats. Brain Res 23:353–370.

Luiten PGM, Koolhaas JM, deBoer S, Koopmans SJ (1985): The cortico-medial amygdala in the central nervous system organization of agonistic behavior. Brain Res 332:283–297.

Ma W, Peschanski M (1988): Spinal and trigeminal projections to the parabrachial nucleus in the rat: Electron-microscopic evidence of a spino-ponto-amygdalian somatosensory pathway. Somatosensory Res 5:247–257.

Maeda H, Maki S (1986): Dopaminergic facilitation of recovery from amygdaloid lesions which affect hypothalamic defensive attack in cats. Brain Res 363:135–140.

Magnuson DJ, Gray TS (1990): Central nucleus of amygdala and bed nucleus of stria terminalis projections to serotonin or tyrosine hydroxylase immunoreactive cells in the dorsal and median raphe nucleus in the rat. Soc Neurosci Abstr 16:121.

Mansbach RS, Geyer MA (1988): Blockade of potentiated startle responding in rats by 5-hydroxytryptame1A receptor ligands. Eur J Pharmacol 156:375–383.

Mason JW (1959): Plasma 17-hydroxycorticosteroid levels during electrical stimulation of the amygdaloid complex in conscious monkeys. Am J Physiol 196:44–48.

Mast M, Blanchard RJ, Blanchard DC (1982): The relationship of freezing and response suppression in a CER situation. Psychol Rec 32:151–167.

Matheson BK, Branch BJ, Taylor AN (1971): Effects of amygdaloid stimulation on pituitary-adrenal activity in conscious cats. Brain Res 32:151–167.

McAllister WR, McAllister DE (1971): Behavioral measurement of conditioned fear. In Brush FR (ed): "Aversive Conditioning and Learning." New York: Academic Press, pp 105–179.

McCall RB, Aghajanian GK (1979): Serotonergic facilitation of facial motoneuron excitation. Brain Res 169:11–27.

McDonald AJ (1984): Neuronal organization of the lateral and basolateral amygdaloid nuclei in the rat. J Comp Neurol 222:589–606.

McDonald AJ, Jackson TR (1987): Amygdaloid connections with posterior insular and temporal cortical areas in the rat. J Comp Neurol 262:59–77.

McGaugh JL, Introinicollision IB, Nagahara AH, Cahill L, Brioni JD, Castellano C (1990): Involvement of the amygdaloid complex in neuromodulatory influences on memory storage. Neurosci Biobehav Rev 14:425–432.

McIntyre M, Stein DG (1973): Differential effects of one- vs. two-stage amygdaloid lesions on activity, exploration, and avoidance behavior in the albino rat. Behav Biol 9:451–465.

McLamb RL, Williams LR, Nanry KP, Wilson WA, Tilson HA (1990): MK-801 impedes the acquisition of a spatial memory task in rats. Pharmacol Biochem Behav 37:41–45.

Merchenthaler I, Hynes MA, Vigh S, Shally AV, Petrusz P (1983): Immunocytochemical localization of corticotropin releasing factor (CRF) in the rat spinal cord. Brain Res 275:373–377.

Miller NE, Barry H III (1960): Motivational effects of drugs: Methods which illustrate some general problems in psychopharmacology. Psychopharmacologia 1:169–199.

Millhouse OE, DeOlmos J (1983): Neuronal configuration in lateral and basolateral amygdala. Neuroscience 10:1269–1300.

Miserendino MJD, Sananes CB, Melia KR, Davis M (1990): Blocking of acquisition but not expression of conditioned fear-potentiated startle by NMDA antagonists in the amygdala. Nature 345:716–718.

Mishkin M, Aggleton J (1981): Multiple functional contributions of the amygdala in the monkey. In Ben-Ari Y (ed): "The Amygdaloid Complex." New York: Elsevier/North-Holland, pp 409–420.

Misslin R, Cigrang M (1986): Does neophobia necessarily imply fear or anxiety? Behav Process 12:45–50.

Mizuno N, Takahashi O, Satoda T, Matsushima R (1985): Amygdalospinal projections in the macaque monkey. Neurosci Lett 53:327–330.

Monaghan DT, Cotman CW (1985): Distribution of N-methyl-D-aspartate-sensitive L-[3H]glutamate-binding sites in rat brain. J Neurosci 5:2909–2919.

Mondadori C, Weiskrantz L, Buerki H, Petschke F, Fagg GE (1989): NMDA receptor antagonists can enhance or impair learning performance in animals. Exp Brain Res 75:449–456.

Morgenson GJ, Calaresu FR (1973): Cardiovascular responses to electrical stimulation of the amygdala in the rat. Exp Neurol 39:166–180.

Morris RGM, Anderson E, Lynch GS, Baudry M (1986): Selective impairment of learning and blockade of long-term potentiation by an N-methyl-D-asparate receptor antagonist, AP5. Nature 319:774–776.

Morris RGM, Halliwell R, Bowery N (1989): Synaptic plasticity and learning: II. Do different kinds of plasticity underlie different kinds of learning? Neuropsychologia 27:41–59.

Morris RGM (1989): Synaptic plasticity and learning: Selective impairment of learning in rats and blockade of long-term potentiation in vivo by the N-methyl-aspartate receptor antagonist AP5. J Neurosci 9:3040–3057.

Mraovitch S, Kumada M, Reis DJ (1982): Role of the nucleus parabrachialis in cardiovascular regulation in cat. Brain Res 232:57–75.

Murray EA (1990): Representational memory in nonhuman primates. In Kesner RT, Olton DS (eds): "Neurobiology of Comparative Cognition." Hillsdale, NJ: Erlbaum, pp 127–155.

Murray EA, Mishkin M (1985): Amygdalectomy impairs crossmodal association in monkeys. Science 228:604–606.

Myhal N, Fleming AS (1990): MK-801 effects on a learned food preference depends on dosage: Is it disruption of learning or a conditioned aversion? Psychobiology 18:428–434.

Nagy J, Zambo K, Decsi L (1979): Anti-anxiety action of diazepam after intra-amygdaloid application in the rat. Neuropharmacology 18:573–576.

Nicoll RA, Kauer JA, Malenka RC (1988): The current excitement in long-term potentiation. Neuron 1:97–103.

Niehoff DL, Kuhar MJ (1983): Benzodiazepine receptors: Localization in rat amygdala. J Neurosci 3:2091–2097.

Nitecka L, Amerski L, Narkiewicz O (1981): The organization of intraamygdaloid connections: an HRP study. J Hirnforsch 22:3–7.

Nitecka L, Frotscher M (1989): Organization and synaptic interconnections of GABAergic and cholinergic elements in the rat amygdaloid nuclei: Single- and double-immunolabeling studies. J Comp Neurol 279:470–488.

Ohta M (1984): Amygdaloid and cortical facilitation or inhibition of trigeminal motoneurons in the rat. Brain Res 291:39–48.

Ottersen OP (1980): Afferent connections to the amygdaloid complex of the rat and cat. II. Afferents from the hypothalamus and the basal telencephalon. J Comp Neurol 194:267–289.

Ottersen OP (1981): Afferent connections to the amygdaloid complex of the rat with some observations in the cat. III. Afferents from the lower brain stem. J Comp Neurol 202:335–356.

Ottersen OP (1982): Connections of the amygdala of the rat. IV. Corticoamygdaloid and intraamygdaloid connections as studied with axonal transport of horseradish peroxidase. J Comp Neurol 205:30–48.

Ottersen OP, Ben-Ari Y (1978): Pontine and mesencephalic afferents to the central nucleus of the amygdala of the rat. Neurosci Lett 8:329–334.

Paoli F, Spignoli G, Pepeu G (1990): Oxiracetam and D-pyroglutamic acid antagonize a disruption of passive avoidance behaviour induced by the N-methyl-D-aspartate receptor antagonist 2-amino-5-phosphonovalerate. Psychopharmacology 100:130–131.

Pare D, Steriade M, Deschenes M, Bouhassiri D (1990): Prolonged enhancement of anterior thalamic synaptic responsiveness by stimulation of a brain-stem cholinergic group. J Neurosci 10:20–33.

Pascoe JP, Bradley DJ, Spyer KM (1989): Interactive responses to stimulation of the amygdaloid central nucleus and baroreceptor afferents in the rabbit. J Auton Nerv Sys 26:157–167.

Pascoe JP, Kapp BS (1985a): Electrophysiological characteristics of amygdaloid central nucleus neurons in the awake rabbit. Brain Res Bull 14:331–338.

Pascoe JP, Kapp BS (1985b): Electrophysiological characteristics of amygdaloid central nucleus neurons during Pavlovian fear conditioning in the rabbit. Behav Brain Res 16:117–133.

Peinado-Manzano MA (1990): The role of the amygdala and the hippocampus in working memory for spatial and non-spatial information. Behav Brain Res 38:117–134.

Pellegrino L (1968): Amygdaloid lesions and behavioral inhibition in the rat. J Comp Physiol Psychol 65:483–491.

Petersen EN, Braestrup C, Scheel-Kruger J (1985): Evidence that the anticonflict effect of midazolam in amygdala is mediated by the specific benzodiazepine receptors. Neurosci Lett 53:285–288.

Petersen EN, Scheel-Kruger J (1982): The GABAergic anticonflict effect of intraamygdaloid benzodiazepines demonstrated by a new water lick conflict paradigm. In Spiegelstein MY, Levy A (eds): "Behavioral Models and the Analysis of Drug Action." Amsterdam: Elsevier Scientific.

Phillips RE (1964): "Wildness" in the Mallard duck; effects of brain lesions and stimulation on "escape behavior" and reproduction. J Comp Neurol 122:139–156.

Phillips RE (1968): Approach-withdrawal behavior of peach-faced lovebirds, *Agapornis roseicolis*, and its modification by brain lesions. Behavior 31:163–184.

Phillipson OT (1979): Afferent projections to the ventral tegmental area of Tsai and intrafascicular nucleus. A horseradish peroxidase study in the rat. J Comp Neurol 187:117–143.

Post S, Mai JK (1980): Contribution to the amygdaloid projection field in the rat: A quantitative autoradiographic study. J Hirnforsch 21:199–225.

Price JL, Amaral DG (1981): An autoradiographic study of the projections of the central nucleus of the monkey amygdala. J Neurosci 1:1242–1259.

Rasmussen K, Jacobs BL (1986): Single unit activity of locus coeruleus in the freely moving cat: II. Conditioning and pharmacologic studies. Brain Res 371:335–344.

Redgate ES, Fahringer EE (1973): A comparison of the pituitary-adrenal activity elicited by electrical stimulation of preoptic, amygdaloid and hypothalamic sites in the rat brain. Neuroendocrinology 12:334–343.

Redmond DE Jr (1977): Alteration in the function of the nucleus locus coeruleus: A possible model for studies on anxiety. In Hanin IE, Usdin E (eds): "Animal Models in Psychiatry and Neurology." Oxford: Pergamon Press, pp 293–304.

Reis DJ, Oliphant MC (1964): Bradycardia and tachycardia following electrical stimulation of the amygdaloid region in the monkey. J Neurophysiol 27:893–912.

Riolobos AS, Garcia AIM (1987): Open field activity and passive avoidance responses in rats after lesion of the central amygdaloid nucleus by electrocaogulation and ibotenic acid. Physiol Behav 39:715–720.

Roberts GW, Woodhams PL, Polak JM, Crow TJ (1982): Distribution of neuropeptides in the limbic system of the rat: The amygdaloid complex. Neuroscience 7:99–131.

Robinson GS, Jr, Crooks GB Jr, Shinkman PG, Gallagher M (1989): Behavior effects of MK-801 mimic deficits associated with hippocampal damage. Psychobiology 17: 156–164.

Rogawski MA, Aghajanian GK (1980): Modulation of lateral geniculate neuron excitability by noradrenaline microiontophoresis or locus coeruleus stimulation. Nature 287:731–734.

Rosen JB, Davis M (1988a): Enhancement of acoustic startle by electrical stimulation of the amygdala. Behav Neurosci 102:195–202.

Rosen JB, Davis M (1988b): Temporal characteristics of enhancement of startle by stimulation of the amygdala. Physiol Behav 44:117–123.

Rosen JB, Davis M (1990): Enhancement of electrically elicited startle by amygdaloid stimulation. Physiol Behav 48:343–349.

Rosen JB, Hitchcock JM, Miserendino MJD, Davis M (1990a): Lesions of the perirhinal cortex, but not of the frontal, visual or insular cortex block fear-potentiated startle using a visual conditioned stimulus (Submitted).

Rosen JB, Hitchcock JM, Sananes CB, Miserendino MJD, Davis M (1991): A direct projection from the central nucleus of the amygdala to the acoustic startle pathway: Anterograde and retrograde tracing studies. Behav Neurosci 105:817–825.

Ross LE (1961): Conditioned fear as a function of CS-UCS and probe stimulus intervals. J Exp Psychol 61:265–273.

Ruggiero DA, Ross CA, Kumada M, Reis DJ (1982): Reevaluation of projections from the mesencephalic trigeminal nucleus to the medulla and spinal cord: New projections. A combined retrograde and anterograde horseradish peroxidase study. J Comp Neurol 206:278–292.

Russchen FT (1982): Amygdalopetal projections in the cat. II. Subcortical afferent connections. A study with retrograde tracing techniques. J Comp Neurol 207:157–176.

Sakanaka M. Shibasaki T, Lederis K (1987): Corticotropin releasing factor-like immunoreactivity in the rat brain as revealed by a modified cobalt-glucose oxidase-diaminobenzidine method. J Comp Neurol 260:256–298.

Sananes CB, Campbell BA (1989): Role of the central nucleus of the amygdala in olfactory heart rate conditioning. Behav Neurosci 103:519–525.

Sananes CB, Davis M (1992): N-M-D-A lesions of the lateral and basolateral nuclei of the amygdala block and shock of sensitization of fear-potentiated startle. Behav Neurosci (in press).

Sandrew BB, Edwards DL, Poletti CE, Foote WE (1986): Amygdalospinal projections in the cat. Brain Res 373:235–239.

Saper CB, Loewy AD (1980): Efferent connections of the parabrachial nucleus in the rat. Brain Res 197:291–317.

Saphier D, Feldman S (1986): Effects of stimulation of the preoptic area on hypothalamic paraventricular nucleus unit activity and corticosterone secretion in freely moving rats. Neuroendocrinology 42:167–173.

Sarter M, Markowitsch HJ (1985): Involvement of the amygdala in learning and memory: A critical review, with emphasis on anatomical relations. Behav Neurosci 99:342–380.

Sawchenko PE, Swanson LW (1983): The organization of forebrain afferents to the paraventricular and supraoptic nucleus of the rat. J Comp Neurol 218:121–144.

Scheel-Kruger J, Petersen EN (1982): Anticonflict effect of the benzodiazepines mediated by a GABAergic mechanism in the amygdala. Eur J Pharmacol 82:115–116.

Schlor KH, Stumpf H, Stock G (1984): Baroreceptor reflex during arousal induced by electrical stimulation of the amygdala or by natural stimuli. J Auton Nerv Sys 10:157–165.

Schwaber JS, Kapp BS, Higgins GA, Rapp PR (1982): Amygdaloid and basal forebrain direct connections with the nucleus of the solitary tract and the dorsal motor nucleus. J Neurosci 2:1424–1438.

Schwartzbaum JS (1960): Changes in reinforcing properties of stimuli following ablation of the amygdaloid complex in monkeys. J Comp Physiol Psychol 53:388–395.

Schwartzbaum JS, Gay PE (1966): Interacting behavioral effects of septal and amygdaloid lesions in the rat. J Comp Physiol Psychol 61:59–65.

Sen RN, Anand BK (1957): Effect of electrical stimulation of the limbic system of brain ("visceral brain") on gastric secretory activity and ulceration. Ind J Med Res 45:515–521.

Setekleiv J, Skaug OE, Kaada BR (1961): Increase of plasma 17-hydroxy-corticosteroids by cerebral cortical and amygdaloid stimulation in the cat. J Endocrinol 22:119–126.

Shapiro ML, Caramanos Z (1990): NMDA antagonist MK-801 impairs acquisition but not performance of spatial working and reference memory. Psychobiology 18:231–243.

Shibata K, Kataoka Y, Gomita Y, Ueki S (1982): Localization of the site of the anticonflict action of benzodiazepines in the amygdaloid nucleus of rats. Brain Res 234:442–446.

Shibata K, Kataoka Y, Yamashita K, Ueki S (1986): An important role of the central amygdaloid nucleus and mammillary body in the mediation of conflict behavior in rats. Brain Res 372:159–162.

Shibata S, Yamashita K, Yamamoto E, Ozaki T, Ueki S (1989): Effect of benzodiazepine and GABA antagonists on anticonflict effects of antianxiety drugs injected into the rat amygdala in a water-lick suppression test. Psychopharmacol 98:38–44.

Shiosaka S, Tokyama M, Takagi H, Takahashi Y, Saitoh T, Sakumoto H, Nakagawa H, Shimizu N (1980): Ascending and descending components of the medial forebrain bundle in the rat as demonstrated by the horseradish peroxidase-blue reaction. I. Forebrain and upper brainstem. Exp Brain Res 39:377–388.

Shizgal P, Bielajew C, Corbett D, Skelton R, Yeomans J (1980): Behavioral methods for inferring anatomical linkage between rewarding brain stimulation sites. J Comp Physiol Psychol 94:227–237.

Siegel A (1967): Stimulus generalization of a classically conditioned response along a temporal dimension. J Comp Physiol Psychol 64:461–466.

Silverman AJ, Hoffman DL, Zimmerman EA (1981). The descending afferent connections of the paraventricular nucleus of the hypothalamus (PVN). Brain Res Bull 6:47–61.

Simon H, LeMoal M, Calas A (1979): Efferents and afferents of the ventral tegmental-A10 region studies after local injection of [3H]leucine and horseradish peroxidase. Brain Res 178:17–40.

Singh VB, Onaivi ES, Phan TH, Boadle-Biber MC (1990): The increases in rat cortical and midbrain tryptophan hydroxylase activity in response to acute or repeated sound stress are blocked by bilateral lesions to the central nucleus of the amygdala. Brain Res 530:49–53.

Skofitsch G, Insel TR, Jacobowitz DM (1985): Binding sites for corticotropin releasing factor in sensory areas of the rat and hindbrain and spinal cord. Physiol Behav 35:519–522.

Slotnick BM (1973): Fear behavior and passive avoidance deficits in mice with amygdala lesions. Physiol Behav 11:717–720.

Smelik PG, Vermes I (1980): The regulation of the pituitary-adrenal system in mammals. In Jones IC, Henderson IW (eds): "General Comparative and Clinical Endocrinology of the Adrenal Cortex." London: Academic Press, pp 1–55.

Smith BS, Millhouse OE (1985): The connections between basolateral and central amygdaloid nuclei. Neurosci Lett 56:307–309.

Soffer A (1954): Regitine and benodaine in the diagnosis of pheochromocytoma. Med Clin N Am 38:375–384.

Sorenson CA, Wilkinson LO (1983): Behavioral evidence that nicotine administration has anxiolytic actions in rats. Soc Neurosci Abstr 9:137.

Spence KW, Runquist WN (1958): Temporal effects of conditioned fear on the eyelid reflex. J Exp Psychol 55:613–616.

Spevack AA, Campbell CT, Drake L (1975): Effect of amygdalectomy on habituation and CER in rats. Physiol Behav 15:199–207.

Staubli U, Thibault O, DiLorenzo M, Lynch G (1989): Antagonism of NMDA receptors impairs acquisition but not retention of olfactory memory. Behav Neurosci 103:54–60.

Steriade M, Datta S, Pare D, Oakson G, Dossi RC (1990): Neuronal activities in brainstem cholinergic nuclei related to tonic activation processes in thalamocortical systems. J Neurosci 10:2541–2559.

Stock G, Schlor KH, Heidt H, Buss J (1978): Psychomotor behaviour and cardiovascular patterns during stimulation of the amygdala. Pflugers Arch Ges Physiol 376:177–184.

Stock G, Rupprecht U, Stumpf H, Schlor KH (1981): Cardiovascular changes during arousal elicited by stimulation of amygdala, hypothalamus and locus coeruleus. J Auton Nerv Syst 3:503–510.

Supple WF Jr, Leaton RN (1990): Lesions of the cerebellar hemispheres: Effects on heart rate conditioning in rats. Behav Neurosci 104:934–947.

Swadlow HA, Waxman SG (1976): Variations in conduction velocity and excitability following single and multiple impulses of visual callosal axons in the rabbit. Exp Neurol 53:128–150.

Swanson LW, Sawchenko PE, Rivier J, Vale W (1983): Organization of ovine corticotropin-releasing factor immunoreactive cells and fibers in the rat brain: An immunohistochemical study. Neuroendocrinology 36:165–186.

Swerdlow NR, Britton KT, Koob GF (1989): Potentiation of acoustic startle by corticotropin-releasing factor (CRF) and by fear are both reversed by alpha-helical CRF (9-41). Neuropsychopharmacology 2:285–292.

Swerdlow NR, Geyer MA, Vale WW, Koob GF (1986): Corticotropin-releasing factor potentiates acoustic startle in rats: Blockade by chlordiazepoxide. Psychopharmacology 88:147–152.

Takeuchi Y, Matsushima S, Matsushima R, Hopkins DA (1983): Direct amygdaloid projections to the dorsal motor nucleus of the vagus nerve: A light and electron microscopic study in the rat. Brain Res 280:143–147.

Takeuchi Y, McLean JH, Hopkins DA (1982): Reciprocal connections between the amygdala and parabrachial nuclei: Ultrastructural demonstration by degeneration and axonal transport of horseradish peroxidase in the cat. Brain Res 239:538–588.

Tan S, Kirk RC, Abraham WC, McNaughton N (1989): Effects of the NMDA antagonists CPP and MK-801 on delayed conditional discrimination. Psychopharmacology 98:556–560.

Tang AH, Franklin SR (1983): Acquisition of brightness discrimination in the rat is impaired by opiates with psychotomimetic properties. Pharmacol Biochem Behav 18:873–877.

Tang AH, Ho PM (1988): Both competitive and non-competitive antagonists of N-methyl-D-aspartic acid disrupt brightness discrimination in rats. Eur J Pharmacol 151:143–146.

Thierry AM, Tassin JP, Blanc G, Glowinski J (1976): Selective activation of the mesocortical DA system by stress. Nature 263:242–243.

Thomas SR, Lewis ME, Iversen SD (1985): Correlation of [3H]diazepam binding density with anxiolytic locus in the amygdaloid complex of the rat. Brain Res 342:85–90.

Thompson RF, Donegan NH, Clark GA, Lavond DG, Lincoln JS, Madden J IV, Mamounas LA, Mauk MD, McCormick DA (1987): Neuronal substrates of discrete, defensive conditioned reflexes, conditioned fear states, and their interactions in the rabbit. In Gormezano I, Prokasy WF, Thompson RF (eds): "Classical Conditioning III: Behavioral, Neurophysiological, and Neurochemical Studies in the Rabbit." Hillsdale, NJ: Lawrence Erlbaum, pp 371–400.

Timms RJ (1981): A study of the amygdaloid defence reaction showing the value of althesin anesthesia in studies of the functions of the forebrain in cats. Pflugers Arch 391:49–56.

Tonkiss J, Morris RGM, Rawlins JNP (1988): Intraventricular infusion of the NMDA antagonist AP5 impairs DRL performance in the rat. Exp Brain Res 73:188.

Tribollet E, Dreifuss JJ (1981): Localization of neurones projecting to the hypothalamic paraventricular nucleus of the rat: A horseradish peroxidase study. Neurosci 7:1215–1328.

Turner BJ (1981): The cortical sequence and terminal distribution of sensory related afferents to the amygdaloid complex of the rat and monkey. In Ben-Ari Y (ed): "The Amygdaloid Complex." Amsterdam: Elsevier, North-Holland Biomedical Press, pp 51–62.

Umemoto M, Olds ME (1975): Effects of chlordiazepoxide, diazepam and chlorpromazine on conditioned emotional behaviour and conditioned neuronal activity in limbic, hypothalamic and geniculate regions. Neuropharmacology 14:413–425.

Ursin H, Jellestad F, Cabrera IG (1981): The amygdala, exploration and fear. In Ben-Ari Y (ed): "The Amygdaloid Complex." Amsterdam: Elsevier, pp 317–329.

Ursin H, Kaada BR (1960): Functional localization within the amygdaloid complex in the cat. Electroencephalogr Clin Neurophysiol 12:1–20.

Vale W, Spiess J, Rivier C, Rivier J (1981): Characterization of a 41-residue ovine hypothalamic peptide that stimulates secretion of corticotropin and beta-endorphin. Science 213:1394–1397.

Van Hoesen GW (1981): The differential distribution, diversity and sprouting of cortical projections to the amygdala in the Rhesus monkey. In Ben-Ari Y (ed): "The Amygdaloid Complex." Amsterdam: Elsevier/North Holland, pp 77–90.

Veening JG, Swanson LW, Sawchenko PE (1984): The organization of projections from the central nucleus of the amygdala to brain stem sites involved in central autonomic regulation: A combined retrograde transport-immunohistochemical study. Brain Res 303:337–357.

Von Euler C, Martila I, Remmers JE, Trippenbach J (1976): Effects of lesions in the parabrachial nucleus on the mechanisms for central and reflex termination of inspiration in the cat. Acta Physiol Scand 96:324–337.

Voshart K, VanderKooy D (1981): The organization of the efferent projections of the parabrachial nucleus to the forebrain in the rat: A retrograde fluorescent double-labeling study. Brain Res 212:271–286.

Wallace DM, Magnuson DJ, Gray TS (1989): The amygdalo-brainstem pathway: dopaminergic, noradrenergic and adrenergic cells in the rat. Neurosci Lett 97:252–258.

Wecker JR, Ison JR (1986): Visual function measured by reflex modification in rats with inherited retinal dystrophy. Behav Neurosci 100:679–684.

Weiner N (1985): Drugs that inhibit adrenergic nerves and block adrenergic receptors. In Gilman A, Goodman LS, Rall TW, Murad F (eds): "The Pharmacological Basis of Therapeutic." New York: Macmillan, p 181.

Weller KL, Smith DA (1982): Afferent connections to the bed nucleus of the stria terminalis. Brain Res 232:255–270.

Welzl H, Alessandri B, Battig K (1990): The formation of a new gustatory memory trace in rats is prevented by the noncompetitive NMDA antagonist ketamine. Psychobiology 18:43–47.

Werka T, Skar J, Ursin H (1978): Exploration and avoidance in rats with lesions in amygdala and piriform cortex. J Comp Physiol Psychol 92:672–681.

Whalen PJ, Kapp BS (1991): Contributions of the amygdaloid central nucleus to the modulation of the nictitating membrane reflex in the rabbit. Behav Neurosci 105:141–153.

Whishaw IQ, Auer RN (1989): Immediate and long-lasting effects of MK-801 on motor activity, spatial navigation in a swimming pool and EEG in the rat. Psychopharmacology 98:500–507.

White SR, Neuman RS (1980): Facilitation of spinal motoneuron excitability by 5-hydroxytryptamine and noradrenaline. Brain Res 185:1–9.

Yadin E, Thomas E, Strickland CE, Grishkat HL (1991): Anxiolytic effects of benzodiazepines in amygdala-lesioned rats. Psychopharmacol 103:473–479.

Yates EF, Maran JW (1974): Stimulation and inhibition of adrenocorticotropin release. In Knobil E, Sawyer WH (eds): "Handbook of Physiology, Sec 7, Endocrinology, the Pituitary Gland and Its Neuroendocrine Control." Am J Physiol IV:367–404.

Yeomans JS (1975): Quantitative measurement of neural post-stimulation excitability with behavioral methods. Physiol Behav 15:593–602.

Zhang JX, Harper RM, Ni H (1986): Cryogenic blockade of the central nucleus of the amgydala attenuates aversively conditioned blood pressure and respiratory responses. Brain Res 386:136–145.

Zhang SP, Bandler R, Carrive P (1990): Flight and immobility evoked by excitatory amino acid microinjection within distinct parts of the subtentorial midbrain periaqueductal gray of the cat. Brain Res 520:73–82.

Zola-Morgan S, Squire LR, Amaral DG (1989): Lesions of the amygdala that spare adjacent cortical regions do not impair memory or exacerbate the impairment following lesions of the hippocampal formation. J Neurosci 9:1922–1930.

The Amygdala: Neurobiological Aspects of Emotion,
Memory, and Mental Dysfunction, pages 307–321
© 1992 Wiley-Liss, Inc.

10
Understanding the Function of the Central Nucleus: Is Simple Conditioning Enough?

MICHELA GALLAGHER AND PETER C. HOLLAND

*Department of Psychology, University of North Carolina at Chapel Hill
(M.G.); and Department of Psychology, Duke University, Durham, North
Carolina (P.C.H.)*

INTRODUCTION

Research on the neural basis of associative learning has profited greatly from the use of a simple model system approach, a strategy used to describe a discrete chain of events between stimulus input and response output. As implemented in neurobiological studies, the strategy consists of mapping discrete events, conditioned responses, and sites where learning occurs onto specific neural circuits. As a result of this strategy, there is now little doubt that the central nucleus of the amygdala is a critical component of a forebrain system for associative learning. Anatomical studies link the central nucleus to inputs for events that serve as a basis for learning and to output systems for the expression of relevant learned behavior, electrophysiological studies show that the activity of neurons in the central nucleus during conditioning is consistent with an associative function, and the acquisition of learning in a number of tasks is dramatically impaired by central nucleus damage (see Chapters 8, 9, and 12, by Kapp, Davis, and LeDoux, this volume). Still, much more work will be needed to establish whether this nucleus is a locus where associative learning actually occurs. Yet another question that needs to be answered concerns the nature of the learning process served by this system. What is learned, or in the case of an animal with central nucleus damage, what is the nature of the learning defect? This question is the main focus of this chapter.

One view of the learning function served by the central nucleus has enjoyed remarkable consensus over the past decade, such that some might wonder whether further inquiry is really necessary. The psychological explanation of the learning deficit in animals with central nucleus damage has flowed naturally from the behavioral paradigms used to study it. Thus, the proposal that this system is a

Address correspondence to: Dr. Michela Gallagher, Department of Psychology, CB# 3270,
Davie Hall, University of North Carolina, Chapel Hill, NC 27599.

substrate for the acquisition of conditioned fear became widely accepted, because deficits after central nucleus damage are found in a variety of fear conditioning tasks (Kapp et al., 1984; Davis, 1986). By this view, the function of this nucleus, or the neural system of which it is a part, is to associate the emotional significance of aversive events with the relevant cues for those events. Animals with central nucleus damage are seen as deficient in the ability to acquire conditioned fear, i.e., a conditioned stimulus (CS) that predicts an aversive event fails to elicit the negative effect appropriate to the impending unconditioned stimulus (US). This interpretation of the role of the central nucleus in associative learning is also compatible with more global views of amygdala function, such as those ascribing a key role for the amygdala in the regulation of innate and acquired motivational states, and in mediating the reinforcing impact of stimuli on learning (e.g., Klüver and Bucy, 1939; Weizkrantz, 1956).

Recent studies we conducted have yielded data that do not support such views of central nucleus function. We have found that rats with damage in this nucleus have deficits in appetitive classical conditioning that are not only incompatible with the specific interpretation of impaired fear conditioning, but also are not amenable to the broader view of a deficit in acquired motivational states. It is not our intent to use these data to challenge the view that the central nucleus of the amygdala is critical for these learning functions. At the very least, however, our results indicate that another learning function is intermingled in this system, and perhaps some of the data previously found compatible with a fear conditioning interpretation (by virtue of its collection in aversive conditioning tasks) could be usefully re-examined in the new context provided by our studies.

EFFECTS OF CENTRAL NUCLEUS LESIONS ON APPETITIVE CLASSICAL CONDITIONING

Our recent examination of central nucleus function used a conditioning preparation employed extensively by one of us to study behavioral aspects of Pavlovian conditioning to CSs paired with food (Holland, 1977). As shown in prior behavioral studies, both visual and auditory CSs paired with food delivery come to elicit behaviors that resemble those produced by food delivery iself: Rats stand relatively motionless with their heads inserted into the recessed area where food is delivered and/or make short rapid movements of the head directed toward the food cup during the CS. The form of these conditioned responses (CR) depends critically on the event used as the US, and they do not occur in response to the auditory and visual cues prior to conditioning. Thus,we refer to this class of behavior as *US-generated behavior*.

In addition to the above class of CR, however, CSs acquire high levels of another type of CR that resembles the behavior elicited by cues prior to conditioning: Food-reinforced visual cues come to elicit *rearing* on the hind legs and orientation toward the light source, whereas auditory cues provoke a *startle* response. Each of these CRs is observed prior to conditioning when rats orient to novel visual or auditory cues, and during conditioning the re-emergence of these behaviors is dependent on the CS/US contingency. Thus, some would refer to the latter class of CRs as examples of alpha conditioning. We prefer to describe these learned responses as *CS-generated CRs*. As illustrated in our car-

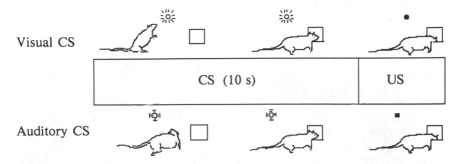

Fig. 1. Illustration of the types of behaviors observed during appetitive Pavlovian conditioning. After pairing the visual CS with food, a *rear* response is elicited by the light. This behavior resembles the orienting response to this visual cue. The auditory CS, in contrast, elicits a *startle* behavior which resembles the orienting response evoked by this cue prior to conditioning. Both visual and auditory CSs also elicit behavior that is directed toward the food cup prior to the delivery of the US (food). Unlike rear and startle CRs, food-cup behavior is not elicited by the CSs prior to conditioning but depends on the event used as the US.

toon (Fig. 1), both types of CR can be observed as a consequence of simple CS/US pairings. However, considerable evidence indicates that these two classes of CRs involve different behavioral mechanisms, a point to which we return in our later discussion.

We recently examined the effects of discrete neurotoxic lesions of the central nucleus on the development of US- and CS-generated CRs in appetitive Pavlovian conditioning. Throughout these studies, we reliably observed that such lesions severely impaired the acquisition of CS-generated CRs while sparing the acquisition of the US-generated type of learning. Thus, unlike normal rats, animals with central nucleus damage show little evidence of behavior directed toward the CS during conditioning. However, rats with such damage do resemble control subjects in learning behavior that is evoked by, and/or directed toward, the food US. Another important aspect of our findings is that orienting responses to the CSs monitored prior to conditioning remain intact in rats with central nucleus lesions, in spite of the fact that the CRs with a similar topography are virtually abolished.

The data shown in Figure 2 illustrate the effect of such damage on the two types of CR. Before turning to those data, we provide a brief account of the experiment which is described in detail elsewhere (Gallagher et al., 1990). Experimental subjects (CN) received stereotaxic surgery in which 0.2 μl of ibotenic acid (10 mg/ml) was injected bilaterally into the central nucleus of the amygdala. Control subjects (VE) received injections of the nontoxic buffered vehicle. Following postoperative recovery, rats were adapted to a restricted feeding regimen at 80% of their free-feeding weights. After a session in which rats were adapted to delivery of food pellets in the test chamber, rats received two sessions in which CS-generated orienting and habituation were monitored to

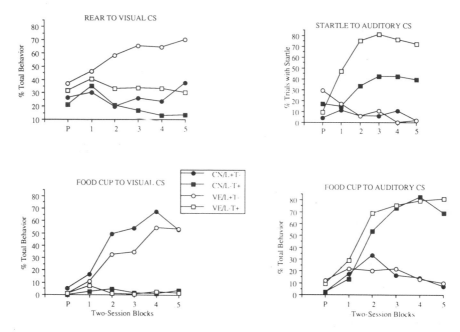

Fig. 2. CS-generated (**top panels**) and US-generated (**bottom panels**) behaviors in the Conditioning phase. The points labeled "P" refer to mean responding during the last session of the Pretraining phase, when rats were habituated to nonreinforced presentations of the visual and auditory cues. Group CN had bilateral central nucleus lesions; group VE received only injections of vehicle into the central nucleus during surgery. In the L + T − training condition, the visual cue was reinforced but the auditory cue was nonreinforced. In the L − T + condition, animals received reinforced auditory and nonreinforced visual cue presentations. The measure of startle behavior, which invariably occurred during the first 1.25 s after onset of the auditory S, was the percentage of trials on which that response occurred. The index of each of the other behaviors was *percentage total behavior*, obtained by dividing the frequency of the target behavior by the total number of observations made. Note that because the number of observations was constant within each observation interval, this measure is an absolute frequency measure rather than a relative one. See text for description of results and statistical analyses.

presentations of a light (L) and a tone (T). Rats were then assigned to one of four groups for differential conditioning. Two of these groups (CN/L + T − and VE/L + T −) received reinforced presentations of a visual cue and nonreinforced presentation of the auditory cue (L + T −). The other groups (CN/T + L − and VE/T + L −) received reinforced auditory and nonreinforced visual cue presentations (T + L −). The three categories of behavior described above were monitored from videotapes by an observer who was unaware of the rats' lesion condition.

The CN lesions had no significant effect on the initial elicitation of unconditioned orienting responses (*rear* to L or *startle* to T) or on the habituation of those behaviors (data not shown, see Gallagher et al., 1990). The emergence of these same behaviors during conditioning, however, was severely impaired (top panels in Fig. 2). Acquisition of rear behavior in the vehicle control group (group VE/L + T −) was substantial, but failed to develop in the corresponding CN group (group CN/L + T −). Significant differential conditioning was also evident in the vehicle control rats (rear in group VE/L + T − vs. VE/L −T +), but this was not the case for the CN rats (group CN/L + T − vs. CN/L − T +). A similar pattern of results was evident for *startle* behavior during conditioning. Although both the VE and CN rats acquired startle behavior to the tone paired with food (upper right panel of Fig. 2), that CR was significantly more frequent in the control rats. The effect of the lesions on the startle response was confined to conditioning, however, as startle responding elicited by nonreinforced tones was similar in VE and CN rats (groups VE/L + T − and CN/L + T −). In contrast to the deficits in the acquisition of these CS-generated CRs, central nucleus lesions had no reliable effect on the acquisition of US-generated CRs by either visual or auditory cues (lower panels of Fig. 2).

These results are supported by the results of another experiment (Gallagher et al., 1989) that was designed to investigate the effects of small central nucleus lesions on complex discrimination learning. That experiment involved nonreinforced pretraining and conditioning with a visual cue and several auditory cues. Eight rats with lesions and eight control rats received nonreinforced pretraining with a visual stimulus and three auditory stimuli, followed by reinforced training of one of the auditory cues and of a serial-trace compound CS, which comprised a visual cue followed by an empty trace interval and another auditory cue. As in the first experiment, central nucleus lesions spared US-generated CRs, but prevented acquisition of the CS-generated CRs. In addition, there was no detectable difference between the groups in unconditioned orienting behavior, including initial level of orienting, habituation, or spontaneous recovery.

These effects of central nucleus damage in our appetitive conditioning experiments were highly selective. Novel stimuli elicited comparable orienting in control and CN-lesioned rats. Only conditioned behaviors that topographically resembled orienting were impaired. Contrary to the frequent claim that amygdala damage impairs the ability to evaluate and associate the motivational significance of USs, the CSs in our experiment appear to have acquired the appropriate motivational significance, as indicated by normal acquisition of US-generated CRs in rats with central nucleus lesions. Further evidence that the food USs in these experiments were processed similarly by experimental and control rats was provided by the results of a potentiated eating experiment, conducted with a sample of subjects from an experiment that is described in detail in a later section of this chapter. This test is based on the observation by Weingarten (1983) that food-sated rats will consume substantial amounts of food if presented with a CS previously paired with food. As described below, we found that CS-potentiated eating was unaffected by lesions of the central nucleus.

CENTRAL NUCLEUS LESIONS DO NOT ALTER CS-POTENTIATED FEEDING

At the conclusion of an experiment in which animals received paired presentations of CSs (panel light and tone) and food USs, 16 animals with central

TABLE I. Unblocking Experiment

Group	Phase 1	Phase 2	Test
HI-CON (high US control)	—	LT $\to$ US$_H$	T
HI (High US)	L $\to$ US$_H$	LT $\to$ US$_H$	T
LO (low US)	L $\to$ US$_L$	LT $\to$ US$_L$	T
UP (upshift)	L $\to$ US$_L$	LT $\to$ US$_H$	T
DN (downshift)	L $\to$ US$_H$	LT $\to$ US$_L$	T

Conditioned stimuli consisted of a light (L) and a tone (T). The subscripts H and L refer to high- and low-value reinforcers, respectively.

nucleus lesions and 16 control subjects were randomly selected from all prior treatment conditions (shown in Table I), and were given free access to their usual chow in their home cages for one week. Two tests of consumption of the 450 mg pellets used as the USs during prior training were then given on successive days. One of the tests included CS presentations ("signaled" condition) and one did not ("unsignaled"); the order of the tests was counterbalanced across subjects. Thirty minutes before each test, a standard procedure of exposure to food pellets was used to eliminate almost all tendency to eat the food pellets in the test chambers (Holland, 1988). Then in the "signaled" test condition, the rats were placed in the test chamber for 10 min, during which 10 10-s presentations of the panel light + tone compound were followed immediately by the delivery of two pellets (20 pellets total). In the "unsignaled" test condition, 20 food pellets were placed in the food cup immediately prior to the 10-min session, during which no other events were delivered. Thus, in both test conditions, the rats had a 10-min opportunity to consume 20 pellets, but in the signaled test condition, each two-pellet delivery was preceded by a previously conditioned CS. At the end of the 10-min period in both conditions, the rats were removed, and the numbers of pellets remaining in the food cups and/or spilled were counted.

The control rats consumed a mean of 15.2 of the 20 pellets in the signaled test, and 0.2 in the unsignaled test. Similarly, the rats with lesions ate a mean of 16.9 pellets in the signaled condition and 3.8 in the unsignaled condition. All 32 subjects consumed more pellets in the signaled than in the unsignaled test condition, indicating a substantial CS-induced facilitation of eating. Furthermore, this effect did not differ between lesion and control subjects: Difference scores constructed by subtracting each rat's consumption in the unsignaled condition from that in the signaled condition did not distinguish the two groups, U(16,16) = 121. Thus, the central nucleus lesions had no effect on the CS's ability to potentiate normal consummatory behavior, providing additional evidence that CN damage did not measurably affect the rat's response to the food USs or the ability of the CS to acquire motivational significance appropriate to an appetitive US. In the next section we turn to a consideration of the nature of the deficit in acquisition of CS-generated CRs that is produced by central nucleus damage in appetitive conditioning.

A ROLE FOR CENTRAL NUCLEUS IN THE MODULATION OF CS PROCESSING?

Perhaps the simplest account of the effects of central nucleus lesions in our experiments is that there is a deficit in conditioned orienting only at the level of response production. This would account for the selective effect of such damage on CS-generated CRs while, at the same time, sparing the acquisition of US-generated CRs. Alternately, the deficits produced by central nucleus damage may reflect a change in CS processing. By this view, the increase in frequency of conditioned orienting behavior in intact rats might reflect an increase in attention to the CS over the course of conditioning. Thus, rats with central nucleus damage might be deficient in allocating attention to the CS. In agreement with this concept, a recent experiment from our labs suggests that the effects of central nucleus damage go beyond a simple deficit in the production of conditioned orienting responses. A description of this experiment requires a brief digression to explain the behavioral paradigm.

Use of an Unblocking Paradigm to Study CS Processing

The phenomenon of blocking, first described by Kamin (1968), is relatively well known. Conditioning to one element (X) of a compound CS (AX) may be prevented (blocked) by prior conditioning to the other element (A) with the same US. The question of why pretraining of A should block subsequent conditioning of X has caused considerable debate. Two broad classes of solutions have been proposed by learning theorists (Rescorla and Holland, 1982).

One account of blocking suggests that training of A affects the extent to which the added X cue is processed ("attended to") on AX compound trials. For example, Pearce and Hall (1980; described more fully later) proposed that a CS engages attentional processing only to the extent that its consequences are not predicted. In a blocking procedure, because prior training of A alone ensures that the US is well predicted on compound trials, X will lose attention over the course of AX compound training. Because little attention is directed toward X during compound training, there is relatively little opportunity for learning about the X-US relation.

In the context of this type of account for blocking, many investigators have examined the effects of lesions of various brain systems on blocking as a means of addressing the neural substrates of attention (e.g., Solomon, 1977; Rickert et al., 1978; Lorden et al., 1980). The results of such studies, however, are not exclusively interpretable in terms of attentional processes. A second account for blocking suggests that the reinforcing power of a US varies to the extent that it is already well-signaled. Rescorla and Wagner (1972) suggested that the effective reinforcing power of a US is a function of the difference between its intrinsic reinforcing power and the conditioning strength of the CSs that predict it. Thus, prior training of A blocks conditioning of X because the US that is contiguous with X on compound trials is rendered ineffective by A's conditioning strength. The "US-processing" approach has been extremely successful in accounting for a variety of learning phenomenon (including blocking) without reference to attentional processes.

Although various theoretical accounts of classical conditioning predict blocking, other related experimental procedures more effectively isolate the effects of modulating CS- and US-processing on learning. One such procedure is that of "unblocking," in which the reinforcer is changed in number or magnitude when compound AX trials are introduced (e.g., Dickinson et al., 1976). Under many circumstances the normal blocking of conditioning to X by prior training of A is disrupted by these changes; that is, X acquires substantial conditioning. For example, Holland (1984, 1988) paired one cue, A, with either a single pellet US or a multiple pellet US that comprised one pellet followed 5 s later by two more pellets. Then in a second phase, an AX compound was paired with either the same US or the other US. No conditioning of X was observed if the same US was used in both phases (i.e., blocking occurred), but X acquired substantial conditioning if the US was changed (i.e., unblocking occurred).

The occurrence of unblocking when the US was changed from the single pellet to the multiple pellet is consistent with US processing accounts such as the Rescorla-Wagner model—the added effectiveness of the US caused by the shift to an increased (multiple pellet) magnitude would support additional conditioning to both elements of the compound. In contrast, the occurrence of unblocking when the US was shifted from the multiple to the single pellet US is not anticipated by the Rescorla-Wagner model. Indeed, the Rescorla-Wagner model predicts that X should acquire conditioned inhibitory, rather than excitatory, tendencies as a consequence of a downward shift in US magnitude (e.g., Wagner et al., 1980): The previously established strength of A would exceed the reinforcing power of the smaller US. Contrary to these different outcomes for upshifts and downshifts predicted by US-processing theories, according to CS-processing theories like Pearce and Hall's (1980), any detectable variation in the US would maintain processing of the added X cue. This maintained attention to X would permit the acquisition of excitatory associations between X and the new US after either upshifts or downshifts in US value. Thus the occurrence of unblocking with downshifts in US value may uniquely reflect modulation of CS-attentional processes (e.g., Dickinson et al., 1976; Holland, 1988).

In order to examine the role of the central nucleus in attentional processes, we examined the effects of lesions in this nucleus on the occurrence of unblocking (conditioning) with US downshifts. If central nucleus damage produces deficits in attentional processing beyond mere reduction of conditioned orienting, such lesions might interfere with the enhanced CS processing thought to cause unblocking under downshift conditions. Conversely, if central nucleus damage affects only potentiation of specific response production mechanisms, then unblocking might be unaffected, even while conditioned orienting is substantially reduced.

Effects of Central Nucleus Lesions on Blocking and Unblocking

Although the main purpose of this experiment was to examine the effect of central nucleus lesions on unblocking (conditioning) with downshifts in the value of the US, we also examined the effects of those lesions on unblocking after upshifts in US value, and on the occurrence of blocking itself. The design of this experiment is shown in Table I.

In the first phase, most rats received trials in which a 10-s panel light CS (L) was paired with either a low- or high-value food US. In the low-value condition (+), a single 45-mg food pellet was delivered at the termination of the light; in the high-value condition (+ +), a single pellet was delivered immediately, followed 5 s later by the delivery of two more food pellets. Other rats (group HI-CON) received only the high-value US, in the absence of the panel light CS in this phase. This last group of rats served as a control for identifying the occurrence of blocking in the other groups. Phase 1 comprised eight sessions, each containing eight trials.

In each of the five sessions in the second phase, all rats received eight pairings of a 10-s compound of the panel light and a 1,500 Hz tone (TL) with one of the food USs. Group HI received the high-value US in both phases; group LO, the low-value US in both phases. Rats in group UP were shifted up from the low-value US in phase 1 to the high-value US in phase 2, and rats in group DN were shifted down from the high-value US to the low-value CS. Finally, subjects in group HI-CON received pairings of TL with the high-value US in phase 2.

In the test session, responding was assessed in the presence of the 10-s tone (T) alone. There were eight nonreinforced presentations of the tone in this single session.

Both rats with lesions and rats with vehicle control injections were re-presented in each of the five training conditions described above, and are identified by the respective suffixes -LES and -VEH. Lesions were made by the same methods used in our previous studies and the same criteria were used to evaluate histological material obtained at the completion of the behavioral study (Gallagher et al., 1990).

Although both CS-generated and US-generated behaviors were monitored in this experiment, it is important to note that the critical effects of central nucleus lesions were assessed with US-generated behaviors, those behaviors that are *spared* by such damage. The question of interest is whether central nucleus damage impairs more general attentional mechanisms implicated in the acquisition of all classes of conditioned behavior in blocking/unblocking procedures.

Consistent with our previous results, during the initial training with the panel light, subjects with central nucleus lesion (CN) were impaired in their acquisition of CS-generated (rear) responses (left side of Fig. 3), but not of US-generated behavior (right side of Fig. 3). Over all training sessions, the frequency of rear behavior was greater in control subjects than in subjects with lesions, with both the low- and high-valued USs [Us (27, 17) $\leq$ 48], but the frequency of magazine behavior did not differ [Us (27, 17) $\geq$ 211]. Although Figure 3 suggests that the high-value US supported more behavior than the low-value US, this difference was not reliable.

The data of main interest came from tests with the tone element alone, conducted after LT compound training in all groups. Figure 4 shows the US-generated behavior during this test session. There were three major findings. First, there were no detectable effects of central nucleus damage (-LES) on blocking: Conditioning to the added tone was blocked by prior training of the light in both lesion and control subjects. The rats in the groups that received the same US in both phases of the experiment (groups HI-LES, HI-VEH, LO-LES, and LO-VEH)

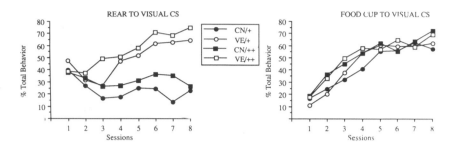

Fig. 3. CS-generated (**left panel**) and US-generated (**right panel**) behaviors in the initial conditioning phase of the unblocking experiment. During this phase, the panel light was paired with either low or high reinforcement. Groups CN had bilateral central nucleus lesions; group VE received injections of vehicle during surgery. See text for description of results and statistical analyses.

responded considerably less than rats in group HI/CON-LES and HI/CON-VEH (Us ≤ 15.5), which received LT-food pairings, but no prior training with L. Furthermore, responding of CN rats in the blocking groups did not differ from that in the corresponding control subjects: Responding in group HI-LES did not differ significantly from that in group HI-VEH [U (13, 8) = 45], nor did responding in group LO-LES differ from that in group LO-VEH [U (15, 9) = 62.5].

Second, there were no reliable effects of central nucleus damage on unblocking when the US was shifted upward: Unblocking (conditioning to the added tone) occurred in both rats with lesions (group UP-LES) and control (group UP-VEH) rats. Among the rats with lesions, responding was significantly greater in group UP-LES, which received upshifts, than in group HI-LES, which received the higher-value US in both phases, U (13, 12) = 40. A similar pattern was apparent

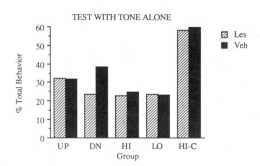

Fig. 4. US-generated behavior during the final test phase of the unblocking experiment. This phase, which followed training with the compound CS (panel light and tone), consisted of presentation of the tone alone. Group treatments were as indicated in Table I. See text for description of results and statistical analyses.

for control subjects (groups UP-VEH and HI-VEH), but the corresponding difference was unreliable, U $(8, 8) = 21.5, P > .10$. Furthermore, the responding of rats with lesions in the upshift condition (group UP-LES) did not differ from that of similar control subjects (group UP-VEH), U $(12, 8) = 47$.

Third, and perhaps most important, central nucleus lesions eliminated unblocking with downshifts in US value, thought to reflect variations in CS processing. Downshifts in US value engendered conditioning to the added tone only in control subjects. Rats in group DN-VEH, who were shifted from the high-value to the low-value US when the tone was added in phase 2, showed reliably more responding to the tone in testing than rats in group LO-VEH, which received the low-value US in both stages of the experiment [U$(9, 9) = 9$]. There was, however, no difference in responding between the corresponding groups of rats with lesions, groups DN-LES and LO-LES [U $(15, 14) = 100$]. Furthermore, responding was reliably greater in group DN-VEH than in group DN-LES [U $(14, 9) = 30.5$].

A ROLE FOR THE CENTRAL NUCLEUS OF THE AMYGDALA IN A CS-PROCESSING (ATTENTIONAL) SYSTEM

These data suggest that the central nucleus of the amygdala regulates a process responsible for the enhancement of conditioning to an added CS when US value is shifted downward in an unblocking design, but is not necessary for those processes responsible for the occurrence of blocking itself, or unblocking when US value is shifted upward. Recall that the latter phenomena may be attributable in many circumstances to US-processing mechanisms like those specified by the Rescorla-Wagner model, but that the enhancement of conditioning that occurs with downshifts in US value has been attributed to changes in CS processing (e.g., Dickinson et al., 1976; Holland, 1988). Thus, the present data support the concept that the central nucleus is involved in the modulation of attentional processing of CSs, specifically, in the maintenance or enhancement of attention to a stimulus that heralds a change in the reinforcer.

Our results are compatible with a popular conditioning theory proposed by Pearce and Hall (1980). They distinguished between an "automatic" processing of CSs, which determines the performance of unconditioned responses and responses already conditioned to a CS, and a "controlled" processing, which determines a CS's ability to enter into new associations, i.e., its "associability."

Pearce and Hall suggest that automatic processing is essentially unaltered by conditioning, but that controlled processing varies as a function of learning. Specifically, controlled processing of a CS occurs only to the extent that its consequences were not well predicted: CSs that reliably predict their consequences are less able to enter into new associations than those that are less valid predictors. Only unpredicted consequences engage mechanisms that maintain or enhance attention to a CS. In other words, it is reasoned that there is not much point wasting scarce resources attending to cues whose predictive relations are already well known; organisms must attend most closely to those events whose significance has not yet been discovered.

Thus, for example, a CS consistently followed by no US, or one consistently followed by the same US, will be less readily associated with new consequences than a CS that is unpredictably followed by the US on some occasions but not on others. Experiments that examine the effects of shifting the reinforcer on new learning to a cue after either consistently nonreinforced, consistently reinforced, or partially reinforced training support this claim: New learning is most rapid after partial reinforcement (e.g., Pearce and Collins, 1985). Similarly, in a blocking experiment in which the US is the same in both phases, the added cue rapidly loses associability because its consequences are already predicted by the pretrained stimulus. But if the US is altered when the second cue is added, that cue's associability is maintained (thus making possible learning about the added cue) until the new US is well predicted.

If the engagement of Pearce and Hall's (1980) mechanism for maintaining or enhancing attention to cues with low predictive validity is mediated by the central nucleus of the amygdala, then lesions in this nucleus would be anticipated to interfere with unblocking, as observed. We are currently conducting experiments to examine the effects of central nucleus damage on learning in other experimental paradigms in which associability of CSs is presumably maintained by their low predictive validity (e.g., Pearce and Collins, 1985). If this attentional mechanism is mediated by the central nucleus, then rats with damage to this nucleus should not show any of these examples of maintained associability when the CS is a relatively poor predictor of the US; indeed, rats with central nucleus lesions should perform essentially as predicted by US-processing theories like the Rescorla-Wagner model.

Other accounts for the present data are worth considering. Some investigators have suggested that amygdala damage reduces rats' sensitivity to differences in US magnitude (e.g., Kemble and Beckman, 1970). It is possible that in the present experiment, subjects with central nucleus damage were simply insensitive to the change from the high-value, multiple-pellet US to the low-value, single-pellet US. By this account, the behavior of rats in the downshifted group DN-LES was indistinguishable from that of the rats with lesions in the unshifted groups, not because of a failure of the shift to engage attentional processing of the CS, but simply because the shift was undetected.

Two aspects of the data argue against this account. First, although rats with lesions in groups DN-LES and HI-LES showed the same high level of US-related behavior during the CS in phase 1, when they both received the high-value US, group DN-LES showed less of that behavior (67%) than group HI-LES (87%) during the CS in phase 2, when the former group received the low-value US and the latter received the high-value US. Second, the lack of lesion effects on the consequences of upshifts in US value indicates that the individual lesioned rats were unimpaired in their ability to distinguish between the low- and high-value USs.

Another possibility is that central nucleus damage affected unblocking after downshifts in US value by interfering with some process of frustration that normally engenders unblocking in these circumstances. From this perspective, downshifts in US value produce a frustration response which is conditioned to the added tone, and which is capable of motivating other behaviors as well. Consequently, when the tone was presented in testing, the conditioned frustration response served to enhance the otherwise low levels of US-related behaviors controlled by that cue. If, as suggested by several investigators (e.g., Henke and Maxwell, 1973), the amygdala is crucial to the display of frustrative behaviors, then downshifts might not generate frustration in central nucleus damaged subjects, and those subjects would then fail to show unblocking under downshift conditions.

Data from the present experiment do not directly address this possibility. However, the frustration account for unblocking in intact rats is not well supported. First, similar blocking and unblocking effects occur with shock USs (e.g., Dickinson et al., 1976), the omission of which is unlikely to engender frustration. Second, Holland (1985) showed that unblocking with downshifts in the value of food USs can be prevented if the compound is paired with the high-value US prior to the downshift. Within the frustration account, the downshift should still induce frustration, despite prior exposure to the compound without a change in reinforcement conditions. In contrast, accounts like Pearce and Hall's (1980) anticipate Holland's (1985) results: Because the added cue did not initially signal any change in the US, attention to that cue would be decremented. So, by the time the US was downshifted, attention to the added cue would already have been driven very low, minimizing the conditioning that could accrue to that cue after the downshift. We are currently examining the effects of central nucleus damage on unblocking using these procedures.

A Note on the Connectivity of the Central Nucleus of the Amygdala as Part of a CS-Processing (Attentional) System

The neural connectivity of the central nucleus is interesting to consider in the light of its function as suggested by the results of our behavioral work. The central nucleus occupies a strategic position with efferent projections that gain access to brain stem circuity-including systems where orienting reflexes may be largely organized (Price and Amaral, 1981; DeOlmos et al, 1985). Other projections gain direct access to corticopetal systems, e.g., direct projections onto magnocellular basal forebrain neurons (for review, see Alheid and Heimer, 1988). The descending targets of central nucleus efferents include both somatomotor systems in the reticular formation and brain stem nuclei for regulation of autonomic functions. These projections have been frequently discussed as possible pathways for the expression of simple conditioned responses that are impaired by central nucleus damage, e.g., autonomic CRs, conditioned potentiation of startle, and conditioned immobility (Pascoe and Kapp, 1985; Hitchcock and Davis,1986; Chapter 12, LeDoux, this volume). By comparison, the role of central nucleus outputs in the regulation of forebrain function has received less attention. There are reports that "alerting" behavior, elicited by direct microstimulation of this nucleus, occurs in conjunction with desynchronization of the cortical EEG (Stock et al., 1981; Kapp et al., 1990 and Chapter 8, this volume) Perhaps these general manifestations of "alerting" reflect a role for the central nucleus in a controlled processing function that maintains or enhances the associability of cues. Thus, the central nucleus may be part of a forebrain system by which attentional mechanisms engage and/or regulate associative functions.

A FINAL NOTE ABOUT SIMPLE SYSTEMS AND SIMPLE CONDITIONING

The use of simple classical conditioning procedures has done much to draw attention to the study of the central nucleus of the amygdala in associative learning. In this chapter we have described some new and interesting findings about the function of this nucleus in experiments using procedures that extend beyond the study of simple acquisition of a conditioned response. Firm conclusions about the significance of the results generated in our recent experiments will require further work, much of which will depend on the use of a behavioral analysis that has come from the development and study of specific theoretical models of classical conditioning. Our understanding of the neurobiological basis of learning may profit substantially from this approach. Despite impressive strides made with a simple model system approach, there is still little contact between the study of simple Pavlovian conditioning and the complex associative processes that characterize mammalian adaptive behavior. The study of complex processes in Pavlovian conditioning may be used to bridge this gap, while still providing an analysis of learning based on the strides made with reduced/simplified models. In the process, a more accurate view of the complexity of learning systems in the mammalian forebrain may be achieved.

ACKNOWLEDGMENTS

This work was supported by a Research Scientist Development Award (NIMH KO2-MH00406) to M.G., NIMH research grant MH35554 to M.G., and NSF research grant BNS8513603 to P.C.H. We are grateful to Vicki Fowler for her assistance in preparation of the figures for this chapter.

REFERENCES

Alheid GF, Heimer L (1988): New perspectives in basal forebrain organization of special relevance for neuropsychiatrc disorders: The striopallidal, amygdaloid, and corticopetal components of substantia innominata. Neuroscience 27:1–39.

Davis M (1986): Pharmacological and anatomical analysis of fear conditioning using the fear-potentiated startle paradigm. BehavNeurosci 100:814–824.

DeOlmos J, Alheid GF, Beltramino CA (1985): Amygdala. In Paxinos G (ed): "The Rat Nervous System." Sydney: Academic Press, pp 223–234.

Dickinson A, Hall G, Mackintosh NJ (1976): Surprise and the attenuation of blocking. J Exp Psychol: Animal Behav Proc 2:313–322.

Gallagher M, Graham PW, Holland PC (1989): The amygdala central nucleus and appetitive Pavlovian conditioning: Lesions impair one class of conditioned behavior. Soc Neurosci Abstr 15:891.

Gallagher M, Graham PW, Holland PC (1990): The amygdala central nucleus and appetitive Pavlovian conditioning: Lesions impair one class of conditioned behavior. J Neurosci 10:1906–1911.

Henke PG, Maxwell D (1973): Lesions in the amygdala and the frustration effect. Physiol Behav 10:647–650.

Hitchcock J, Davis M (1986): Lesions of the amygdala, but not the cerebellum or red nucleus, block conditioned fear as measured with the potentiated startle paradigm. Behav Neurosci 100:12–22.

Holland PC (1977): Conditioned stimulus as a determinant of the form of the Pavlovian conditioned response. J Exp Psychol 3:77–104.

Holland PC (1984): Unblocking in Pavlovian appetitive conditioning. J Exp Psychol: Animal Behav Proc 10:476–497.

Holland PC (1985): Pretraining a compound conditioned stimulus reduces unblocking. Bull Psychonom Soc 23:237–240.

Holland PC (1988): Excitation and inhibition in unblocking. J Exp Psychol: Animal Behav Proc 14:261–279.

Kamin LJ (1968): Attention-like processes in classical conditioning. In Jones MR (ed): "Miami Symposium on the Prediction of Behavior: Aversive Stimulation." Coral Gables, FL: University of Miami Press, pp 9–32.

Kapp BS, Pascoe JP, Bixler MA (1984): The amygdala: A neuroanatomical systems approach to its contribution to aversive conditioning. In Squire L, Butters N (eds): "The Neuropsychology of Memory." New York: Guilford Press, pp 473–488.

Kapp BS, Supple WP, Doherty JL (1990): Effects of stimulation of the amygdaloid central nucleus (ACe) on cortical electroencephlographic (EEG) activity in the rabbit. Soc Neurosci Abstr 16:606.

Kemble ED, Beckman GJ (1970): Runway performance of rats following amygdaloid lesions. Physiol Behav 5:45–47.

Klüver H, Bucy PC (1939): Preliminary analysis of the temporal lobes in monkeys. Arch Neurol Psychiat 42:979–1000.

Lorden JF, Rickert EJ, Dawson R Jr, Pelleymounter MA (1980): Forebrain norepinephrine and selective processing of information. Brain Res 190:369–373.

Pascoe JP, Kapp BS (1985): Electrophysiological characteristics of amygdaloid central nucleus neurons during Pavlovian fear conditioning in the rabbit. Behav Brain Res 16:117–133.

Pearce JM, Collins L (1985): Predictive accuracy and the effects of partial reinforcement on serial autoshaping. J Exp Psychol: Animal Behav Proc 11:548–564.

Pearce JM, Hall G (1980): A model for Pavlovian learning: Variations in the effectiveness of conditioned but not of unconditioned stimuli. Psychol Rev 106:532–552.

Price JL, Amaral DG (1981): An autoradiographic study of the projections of the central nucleus of the monkey amygdala. J Neurosci 11:1242–1259.

Rescorla RA, Holland PC (1982): Behavioral studies of associative learning in animals. Ann Rev Psychol 33:265–308.

Rescorla RA, Wagner AR (1972): A theory of Pavlovian conditioning: Variations in the effectiveness of reinforcement and nonreinforcement. In Black AH, Prokasy WF (eds): "Classical conditioning II." New York: Appleton-Century-Crofts, pp 64–99.

Rickert EJ, Bennett TL, Lane P, French J (1978): Hippocampectomy and the attenuation of blocking. Behav Biol 22:147–160.

Solomon PR (1977): Role of the hippocampus in blocking and conditioned inhibition of the rabbit's nictitating membrane response. J Comp Physiol Psychol 91:407–417.

Stock G, Rupprecht U, Stumpf H, Schlor KH (1981): Cardiovascular changes during arousal elicited by stimulation of the amygdala, hypothalamus and locus coeruleus. J Autonom Nerv Sys 3:503–510.

Wagner AR, Mazur JE, Donegan NH, Pfautz PL (1980): Evaluation of blocking and conditioned inhibition to a CS signaling a decrease in US intensity. J Exp Psychol: Animal Behav Proc 6:376–385.

Weingarten HP (1983): Conditioned cues elicit feeding in sated rats: A role for learning in meal initiation. Science 220:431–433.

Weiskrantz L (1956): Behavioral changes associated with ablations of the amygdaloid complex in monkeys. J Comp Physiol Psychol 9:381–391.

The Amygdala: Neurobiological Aspects of Emotion,
Memory, and Mental Dysfunction, pages 323–338
© 1992 Wiley-Liss, Inc.

11

Stomach Pathology and the Amygdala

PETER G. HENKE

St. Francis Xavier University, Antigonish, Nova Scotia, Canada

INTRODUCTION

The amygdala has had a long history of being associated with responses to threatening conditions, on the one hand, and gut reactions on the other. During the past decade, evidence has accumulated indicating that this limbic structure plays an important role in gastric stress ulcer modulation; that is, individual differences, which are reflected in degrees of severity of the pathology, may be coded in this area. Several studies have shown that the amygdala is a nodal point in a series of temporal lobe circuits (which also include hippocampus and entorhinal cortex) that modify gastric stress pathologies, possibly based on what the organism has experienced in the past in similar circumstances. In fact, it seems that specific changes in the neurophysiology of these temporal lobe circuits, as well as the behaviors shown by the animal, are frequently better predictors of the severity of stress ulceration than the imposition of the specific stress procedure.

GASTROINTESTINAL FUNCTIONS OF THE
AMYGDALA AND STRESS ULCERS

Electrical stimulation in widespread regions of the amygdala produces changes in gut activity. Increases in acid secretions have been obtained by stimulating the anteromedial area of the amygdala, as well as the central and medial nuclei (Sen and Anand, 1957; Shealy and Peele, 1957; Zawoiski, 1967). Stimulation of the latter nuclei also produced increased gastric motility (Sen and Anand, 1957). A reduction in mucosal blood flow has also been reported after stimulation of the central amygdala (Stock et al., 1981; Timms, 1981). These factors (acid, motility, and blood flow) have been prominently mentioned as possible peripheral mechanisms for ulcer development (Guth et al., 1975; Weiner, 1977; Guth and Leung, 1987; Garrick et al., 1989; Garrick, 1990).

Inhibitions of gastric secretions and motility have been found after electrical stimulations of more posterior, lateral, and basal regions of the amygdala

Address correspondence to: Dr. Peter G. Henke, Department of Psychology, St. Francis Xavier University, Antigonish, Nova Scotia, Canada, B2G 1CO.

(Koikegami et al., 1953; Koikegami, 1964). Vagotomy abolished both these excit-atory and inhibitory effects (Eliasson, 1952; Fennegan and Puiggari, 1966).

Stimulation of the anteromedial (Sen and Anand, 1957; Innes and Tansy, 1980) or central (Henke, 1980b, 1985) areas of the amygdala also produced gastric erosions (Fig. 1). These pathological effects of stimulation, however, could be prevented by peripheral vagotomy (Innes and Tansy, 1980), or by lesions of the ventral amygdalofugal pathway (Henke, 1980b).

Histologically, these stimulation-induced erosions are indistinguishable from so-called stress ulcers. Usually, these stress ulcers are fairly shallow erosions of the gastric mucosa (Fig. 2). They rarely penetrate the muscularis layer of the stomach, and they heal relatively fast (usually within 72 h). Various techniques have been used to produce this type of stomach pathology in a large variety of species (Ader, 1971; Henke, 1979; Glavin, 1980; Paré and Glavin, 1986). Studies on the role of the amygdala, however, have mostly used physical restraint, some-times in combination with cold temperatures, to produce stress ulcers. Restraint

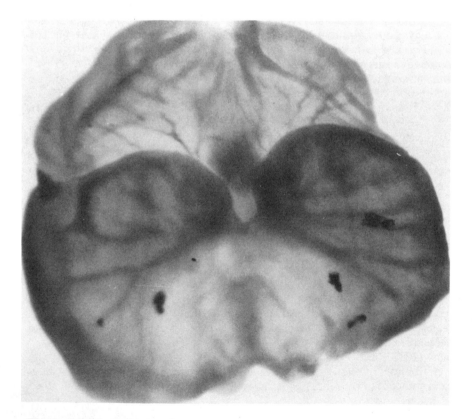

Fig. 1. Gastric erosions produced in the acid-secreting part of the rat stomach by stim-ulation of the central nucleus of the amygdala (Reprinted with permission from Henke, 1980b, Pergamon Press).

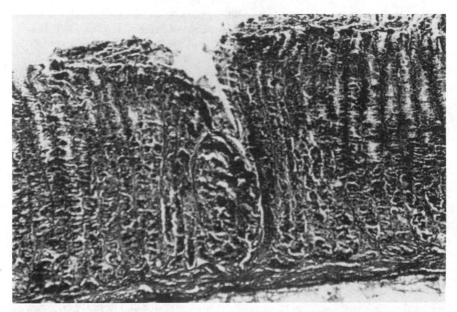

Fig. 2. Photomicrograph of restraint-induced mucosal erosion; eosin and hematoxylin stain (From Henke, 1988a. Copyright 1988 by the American Psychological Association. Reprinted by permission of the publisher).

is one of the most commonly used methods and, as a consequence, many of the variables and parameters influencing this type of stress ulcer are known. For example, prior food deprivation enhances the severity of ulceration, and species differences exist (rats and mice being particularly susceptible). Other relevant variables include age, sex, genetic selection, activity cycles, developmental history, and seasonal variations (Ader, 1971; Glavin, 1980; Henke, 1982; Paré and Glavin, 1986).

An examination of the behavior of neurons in the amygdala during restraint showed that this stress treatment affected the mutiple-unit activity recorded from the medial, central, and lateral nuclei (Henke, 1985). Similar changes were also noted from units in the bed nucleus of the stria terminalis (BNST) (Henke, 1984). However, stomach erosions were only produced when the areas of the units found in the central nucleus were stimulated electrically (Henke, 1985, 1988a). Previous data had also shown that units found in the central nucleus and BNST responded when an auditory stimulus was presented which had been present while the rat was restrained. These animals also escaped from that stimulus in behavioral tests, indicating that it had acquired aversive properties (Henke, 1983, 1984).

Bilateral lesions in the centromedial amygdala have been reported to attenuate the effects of stress conditions on gastric functions. Centromedial lesions reduced restraint- and shock-induced ulcers and also eliminated the ulcer-aggravating effects of posterolateral lesions in the amygdala (Henke, 1980a,c,

1981). Similar lesions in the centromedial region also attenuated the gastric damage usually seen after lateral hypothalamic lesions in rats (Grijalva et al., 1986).

Kindling of the amygdala, on the other hand, made rats more susceptible to subsequently induced restraint ulcers (Henke and Sullivan, 1985), whereas long-term potentiation of the amygdala by stimulating the ventral CA1 regions of the hippocampus produced opposite effects (Henke, 1990c). The reasons for these differences are unclear, at this point, but the afterdischarges elicited by the kindling procedure presumably reflected an abnormal functional state of neurons in the amygdala.

Cells in the central nucleus have been found which behave differently in ulcer-susceptible as compared to ulcer-resistant rats. Multiple-unit recordings could distinguish several activity profiles obtained during the restraint session. One type of unit, found in stress-susceptible animals, showed increased activity which was followed by a suppression in rate (type 1). The other profile, however, showed baseline responding after the initial increase during restraint (type 2). These latter neurons were mostly seen in ulcer-resistant rats (Henke, 1988a).

The results indicate that distinct neural "signatures" correlated with the animal's resistance to the effects of restraint-stress on gastric functions. In agreement with these findings, an examination of unit profiles in the central nucleus of rats which had been bred for extreme differences in avoidance performance, the so-called Roman High- (RHA) and Roman Low- (RLA) Avoidance strains, showed similar differences (Henke, 1988a). The RLA rats, which also "freeze" more, defecate more, and ambulate less in an open field (Driscoll and Bättig, 1982), displayed mostly type 1 activity; the opposite was the case for RHA rats. Data obtained on Wistar rats which had been divided into high- and low-emotional categories (based on the criterion of defecation in an open-field area before five rearing responses had occurred) also support these findings. High-emotional rats showed predominantly type 1 activity in the central nucleus, but low-emotional animals displayed the type 2 pattern under stress conditions. Low-level electrical stimulation of either type of units, however, produced stomach erosions in all cases (Henke, 1988a). These data may be interpreted to indicate that (1) distinct neural signatures in the central nucleus reflect emotionality differences in rats, (2) these unit profiles also differentiate ulcer-susceptible from ulcer-resistant animals under stress conditions, and (3) electrical stimulation of type 1 and type 2 units can override any such differences and lead to the development of stomach ulcers.

NEUROPHARMACOLOGY OF THE CENTRAL NUCLEUS AND STOMACH PATHOLOGY

The central nucleus is rich in aminergic transmitters and neuropeptides (Ben-Ari, 1981; Gray, 1989). Several studies (Taché and Ishikawa, 1989; Hernandez, 1990) have implicated these transmitters/modulators in the central control of gastric stress ulcer development (Table I). Consequently, a series of experiments examined the effects of applications of putative transmitters within the central nucleus on stress ulcers produced by cold-restraint in rats.

A number of previous studies have shown that catecholamines are protective (Lauterbach and Mattes, 1977; Nemeroff et al., 1983; Glavin, 1985b; Glavin et

TABLE I. Intraventricular Injections of Peptides and Stomach Ulcers

Protective	Ulcerogenic	No Effect
Bombesin	TRH[a]	Somatostatin
Calcitonin	NPY	Bradykinin
Opioids	VIP	Substance P
Neurotensin	PP	Gastrin
		CCK-8

[a]TRH, thyrotropin-releasing hormone; NPY, neuropeptide Y; VIP, vasoactive-intestinal peptide; PP, pancreatic polypeptide; CCK, cholecystokinin.

al., 1986; Sikiric et al., 1986; Ray et al., 1987b; Szabo and Moriga, 1989). The protection afforded by norepinephrine in the central nucleus seems to be a beta-adrenoceptor effect (Ray et al., 1990b), whereas the dopamine (DA)-mediated actions (Table II), probably from cells originating in the ventral tegmental area (Ray et al., 1988a), occur in interaction with a number of neuropeptides (Table III) in this nucleus of the amygdala (Henke, 1988b).

Several studies have suggested that DA and neurotensin are closely associated in the brain (Bissette and Nemeroff, 1988; Davis and Kilts, 1988; Phillips et al.,

TABLE II. Injections Into the Central Nucleus of the
Amygdala and Stress Ulcers

Injections	Stomach Pathology
Adrenergic	
Norepinephrine	Decrease
Propranolol	Increase
Dopaminergic	
Dopamine	Decrease
Apomorphine	Decrease
Haloperidol	Increase
Clozapine	Increase
GABAergic	
GABA	Decrease
Chlorodiazepoxide	Decrease
RO 15-1788	Increase
Peptidergic	
Neurotensin	Decrease
Beta-endorphin	Decrease
Met-enkephalin	Decrease
Leu-enkephalin	Decrease
Naloxone	Increase
Thyrotropin-releasing hormone	Increase
Bombesin	No effect
Vasoactive-intestinal peptide	No effect

TABLE III. Dopamine-Peptide Interactions in the Central Nucleus
of the Amygdala and Gastric Ulcers

Treatment	Pathology
DA + TRH[a]	Decrease
Cloz + DA + TRH	Increase
Cloz + DAMEA	Increase
Hal + NT	Control Level

[a]DA, dopamine; TRH, thyrotropin-releasing hormone; Cloz, clozapine; DAMEA, [D-Ala^2]
Met-enkephalinamide; Hal, haloperidol; NT, neurotensin.

1988; Tassin et al., 1988). Intraventricular injections of neurotensin have been
reported to attenuate stress ulcers in rats (Nemeroff et al., 1982; Hernandez et al.,
1985, 1986). A similar decrease in stress ulcer severity occurs following injections
of DA and neurotensin into the central nucleus. This attenuation of neurotensin
is reversed by prior treatment in the central nucleus with 6-hydroxydopamine
(6-OHDA) or intraperitoneal injections of dopamine antagonists (Ray et al. 1987a;
Ray and Henke, 1989; Henke et al., 1988b). It was also found, however, that
6-OHDA lesions of the central nucleus produced only weak and inconsistent effects on stress erosions (Ray et al., 1987a). The reasons for these latter findings
are unknown, but could be related to data showing that this damage in the
amygdala frequently produces compensatory increases in DA activity in the
nucleus accumbens (Simon and LeMoal, 1988). This area has also been implicated
in stress ulcer development (Kauffman, 1989). In fact, recent measurements
of stress-induced changes in glucose-utilization rates in various brain regions
indicate that the protective effects of intraventricular applications of neurotensin
may be mediated by the amygdala and nucleus accumbens (Xing et al., 1989).

The central nucleus has been reported to contain endorphinergic and enke-
phalinergic terminals, as well as opioid receptors (Hökfelt et al., 1977; Roberts
et al., 1982; Gray, 1989). Peripheral and central injections of opioid drugs have
been shown to influence stress ulcer severity in rats (Morley et al., 1982; Dai and
Chan, 1983; Ferri et al., 1983; Hernandez et al., 1983; Glavin, 1985a). An effective
central site for these effects seems to be the central nucleus and this action on
gastric functions occurs in conjunction with altered DA transmission. For example, injections of beta-endorphin, met-enkephalin, and leu-enkephalin into the
central nucleus reduced the stomach pathology seen after cold-restraint. These
effects were reversible with Naloxone or Naltrexone. Further data showed that
Naloxone also produced an intrinsic aggravation of the stress ulcer severity,
implicating endogenous mechanisms (Ray et al., 1988c; Ray and Henke, 1990a).

Tests of DA-enkephalin interactions in the central nucleus revealed that intraperitoneal injections of the DA antagonist clozapine or applications of the DA
neurotoxin 6-OHDA within the nucleus reversed the protective effects of met-
enkephalin injections into the central nucleus (Ray et al., 1988c). These results
suggest, perhaps, that endogenous opioids modulate DA transmission in this area
during stressful treatments. In general, the data showed that beta-endorphin

(which is potent at both delta and mu receptors) seemed a more effective inhibitor of the stress pathology than leu-enkephalin (which is mostly a delta agonist). One conclusion from these findings may be that both delta and mu receptors in the central nucleus are involved (Henke, 1988b).

A potent ulcerogenic peptide is thyrotropin-releasing hormone (TRH). This tripeptide is widely distributed in brain and gut (Morley et al., 1977; Jackson and Lechan, 1983). In the CNS, most TRH-positive fibers originate in the caudal raphe nuclei, and they project from there to the dorsal vagal complex, hypothalamus, and limbic system (Eskay et al., 1983; Kubek et al., 1983; Sharif and Burt, 1985; Palkovits et al., 1986).

Peripheral factors by which TRH damages the gastric mucosa include an increase in acid secretions and gastric contractility (Taché et al., 1985; Garrick, 1990). Both of these effects are prevented by vagotomy or atropine injections (Henke et al., 1988; Garrick, 1990; Hernandez et al., 1990a). Intraventricular infusions of TRH antiserum have been reported to reduce stress-induced erosions in the stomach. These data support the idea that endogenous TRH may mediate some aspects of the ulcerogenic response to stress conditions (Hernandez et al., 1990b).

Microinjections of TRH into the dorsal vagal complex also produce similar changes in the gut (Hernandez and Emerick, 1988; Garrick, 1990). Electrophysiological studies have also found that TRH stimulates a large number of cells in the dorsal motor nucleus of the vagus (Rogers et al., 1988), further supporting a role of this peptide in the central regulation of gastric functions.

Similar results are seen following microinjections of TRH into the central nucleus of the amygdala. These injections induced gastric ulcers and stimulated acid secretions in nonstressed rats, and truncal vagotomy or intraperitoneal injections of methyl atropine prevented these pathological effects. Under cold-restraint conditions, injections of TRH within the central nucleus aggravated stress ulcers, dose-dependently (Henke et al., 1988; Hernandez et al., 1990a).

As shown in Table III, TRH interacts with DA and neurotensin in the central nucleus (Henke et al., 1988), similar to the effects seen in other physiological conditions (Prange and Nemeroff, 1982; Maeda-Hagiwara and Watanabe, 1983). The increase in stomach pathology produced by TRH was prevented when neurotensin was also injected into the central nucleus. The attenuation produced by injections of DA into the central nucleus, however, was not affected by TRH. But furthermore, the DA antagonist clozapine (given intraperitoneally) severely aggravated the pathology produced by application of TRH within the central nucleus (Henke et al., 1988). These findings suggest that DA also interacts with TRH in the central nucleus during stressful circumstances; that is, DA release inhibits the effects of TRH on gastric ulcer formation.

In addition to DA-peptide interactions in the central nucleus, recent studies also reported that GABA (gamma aminobutyric acid) transmission in this area is affected by benzodiazepines during stress treatments (Table II). Previous data had shown that these antianxiety drugs, when given intraperitoneally in rats, reduced the gastric erosions produced by restraint (File and Pearce, 1981; Henke, 1987). Benzodiazepine treatment also influenced the multiple-unit activity in the central nucleus during stressful experiences. Low-level electrical stimulation of these units, however, produced stomach erosions in the rats (Henke, 1985). Receptors for these antianxiety drugs are thought to interact with GABA receptors, as part of a supramolecular complex, and enhance GABAergic activity (Costa et al., 1983). Both GABA and benzodiazepine receptors exist in the central nucleus (Young and Kuhar, 1980; Ben-Ari, 1981).

Microinjections into the central nucleus of either GABA or the benzodiazepine chlorodiazepoxide attenuated the stress ulcer formation in rats. Both of these effects, however, were blocked by prior injections of the benzodiazepine antagonist RO 15-1788. Maybe even more importantly, it was also found that RO 15-1788 produced an intrinsic aggravation of stress ulcers (Sullivan et al.,1989).

Taken together, these neuropharmacological data implicate the central nucleus as being an important site in which stressful experiences influence gastric functions. Several "classical" transmitters, as well as a number of so-called brain-gut peptides, apparently modulate the severity of the gastric ulcers which are known to occur in response to such aversive conditions. This modulaton may depend on inputs from temporal lobe circuits, which also include the hippocampus and entorhinal cortex.

TEMPORAL LOBE PATHWAYS AND ULCER SUSCEPTIBILITY

Some time ago, data were reported that showed that bilateral lesions in the posterolateral amygdala aggravated stress ulcers, lesions in the centromedial regions attenuated ulcers, and combined lesions in these two areas also attenuated the pathology. The interpretation, at that time, was that posterolateral structures directly influenced the development of stress ulcers through the centromedial amygdala (Henke, 1980c). Recent data, however, suggest that the circuitry involved in these effects may be more extensive than was originally thought. Indications are now that the defensive capabilities of a number of temporal lobe structures are recruited when the organism is faced with threatening circumstances.

In a preliminary study, the evoked potentials in the dentate gyrus of the hippocampus were recorded following electrical stimulation of the perforant path prior to as well as after restraining the rats. The finding was that stress-resistant animals, as shown by little stomach pathology, also developed increased granule cell potentials. On the other hand, stress-vulnerable rats displayed suppressed potentials, relative to prestress baselines. A similar suppression was seen in the dentate gyrus when the animal showed impaired coping responses, the so-called learned-helplessness effect, following uncontrollable shock stimulation. Taken together, these results were interpreted to indicate that suppressed hippocampal activity might be associated with a reduced coping ability under stressful conditions (Henke, 1990a). In general agreement with this hypothesis, data also showed that an enhancement of transmission at these dentate granule cells, by inducing long-term potentiation (LTP), also made the animal more resistant to stress ulcer development (Henke, 1989b). On the other hand, when LTP was prevented at these synapses, by intraventricular infusions of the selective N-methyl-D-aspartate receptor blocker aminophosphonovaleric acid (AP5), it increased the stress ulcer severity in the rats and, additionally, aggravated the behavioral helplessness of the animal (Henke, 1989a). It has been reported that LTP of dentate granule cells can also be induced by high-frequency electrical stimulation of the amygdala (Racine et al., 1983). Presumably, a pathway originating in the lateral amygdala, through the entorhinal cortex, may be involved in this effect (Price 1981; Thomas et al., 1984; Finch et al., 1986). In an additional study, when so-called stress units (multiple units that had been found to respond during restraint) in the posterolateral amygdala were stimulated at high frequencies, LTP was also seen in the dentate gyrus. Furthermore, this treatment reduced the severity of stress ulcers produced by restraint. Intraventricular injections of AP5, however, reversed this attenuation of the pathology and prevented LTP. Dentate LTP, elicited by stimulation of the posterolateral amygdala, also reduced the behavioral "struggling" activity of rats during the last half of a one-hour session of supine restraint. The data from this series of studies were interpreted to indicate that an augmented efficacy of transmission in this temporal lobe pathway, linking the posterolateral amygdala to dentate gyrus, facilitates the habituation to uncontrollable stressors, presumably an adaptive reaction, conserving bodily resources (Henke, 1990d).

There are other data implicating the hippocampal formation in habituation, a simple form of learning. Large lesions as well as granule cell destructions interfere with habituation responses (Coover and Levine, 1972; Douglas, 1967; Mickley and Ferguson, 1989). Suppression of the electrophysiological activity also seems to be associated with behavioral helplessness and increased stomach pathology following stressful experiences (Henke, 1990a). Lesions in the hippocampus produce similar effects (Elmes et al., 1975; Henke, 1990c).

If, as the data suggest, potentiations or suppressions in this temporal lobe pathway reflect the animal's resiliency or vulnerability under stress conditions, the question still remains how outputs from the hippocampal formation might influence stress ulcers in the stomach. Bilateral large lesions or ventral lesions in the hippocampus aggravated stress ulcers in rats. However, dorsal hippocampal lesions or fimbria-fornix cuts produced no differential effects (Henke et al., 1981; Henke, 1990c). There are a numer of anatomical and functional investigations that indicate that nonfornical connections include caudally directed fibers which reach the amygdala from the ventral CA1 hippocampal region (Morrison and Poletti, 1980; Adamec and Stark-Adamec, 1984; Poletti et al., 1984; DeOlmos et al., 1985). Recent results showed that high-frequency stimulation near the pyramidal cells of the ventral CA1 area induced LTP recorded from the lateral edge of the central nucleus of the amygdala. This LTP also attenuated stress-induced stomach erosions (Henke, 1990c). In other words, these findings implicate output fibers from the ventral hippocampus to the central amygdala in the modulation of stress ulcer severity.

CONCLUSIONS

A number of studies have been reported that show that individual differences exist in the ways in which organisms react to stressful conditions (Brush et al., 1988; Natelson et al., 1988; Dess and Chapman, 1990). The amygdala and its temporal lobe connections, apparently, modulates the degree to which aversive experiences can produce pathological changes in the gastrointestinal system—in other words, a kind of resiliency or vulnerability the animal brings into the stressful situation. These differences, indexed in the central nucleus of the amygdala by distinct neural signatures, correlate with the emotional reactions to threat shown by the animal (Henke, 1988a). Furthermore, cells in the central nucleus not only respond to the initial stress experience, but they also respond to external stimuli that had been present while the animal experienced the stressful situation (Henke, 1983, 1984).

Transmission in a pathway connecting the posterolateral amygdala to the dentate gyrus seemingly links coping styles and the degree to which gastric pathology develops. An increased efficacy of transmission produced faster behavioral habituation and less ulceration; suppressed activity led to greater behavioral

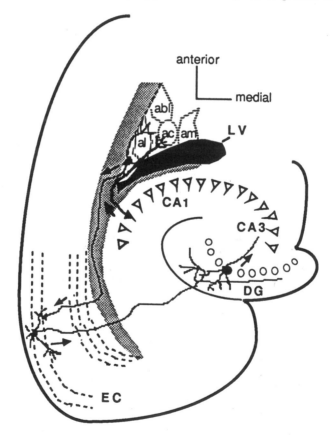

Fig. 3. Diagram of horizontal section through the temporal lobe. It shows the pathways proposed to modulate stress ulcer severity. Abbreviations: abl, basolateral n. amygdala; am, medial n. amygdala; ac, central n. amygdala; al, lateral n. amygdala; LV, lateral ventricle; EC, entorhinal cortex; DG, dentate gyrus; CA1-CA3, hippocampal fields.

helplessness and more ulceration. Fibers from the ventral CA1 area of the hippocampus to the lateral edge of the central amygdala may transmit this information, modulating the severity of the gastric pathology (Henke, 1989a,b, 1990a,c,d). This neural loop in the temporal region (Fig. 3) may, therefore, represent some aspects of the "visceral brain" described by MacLean in 1949, in which threatening experiences can influence gastrointestinal functions (Henke, 1990b, 1991).

ACKNOWLEDGMENTS

Funding was provided by the Natural Sciences and Engineering Research Council of Canada.

REFERENCES

Adamec RE, Stark-Adamec C (1984): The contribution of limbic connectivity to stable behavioural characteristics of aggressive and defensive cats. In Bandler R (ed): "Modulation of Sensorymotor Activity During Alterations in Behavioral States." New York: Alan R. Liss, pp 325–339.

Ader R (1971): Experimentally induced gastric lesions. Adv Psychosom Med 6:1–39.

Ben-Ari Y (1981): Transmitters and modulators in the amygdaloid complex: A review. In Ben-Ari Y (ed): "The Amygdaloid Complex." Amsterdam: Elsevier/North-Holland Biomedical Press, pp 163–174.

Bissette G, Nemeroff CB (1988): Neurotensin and mesocorticolimbic dopamine system. Ann NY Acad Sci 537:397–404.

Brush FR, Del Paine SN, Pellegrino LJ, Rykaszewski IM, Dess NK, Collins PY (1988): CER suppression, passive avoidance learning, and stress-induced suppression of drinking in the Syracuse high- and low-avoidance strains of rats (Rattus norvegicus). J Comp Psychol 102:337–349.

Coover GD, Levine S (1972): Auditory startle response of hippocampectomized rats. Physiol Behav 9:75–77.

Costa E, Corda MG, Epstein B, Forchetti C, Guidotti A (1983): GABA-benzodiazepine interactions. In Costa E (ed): "The Benzodiazepines: From Molecular Biology to Clinical Practice." New York: Raven Press, pp 117–136.

Dai S, Chan M (1983): Effects of naloxone on serum corticosterone and gastric lesions in stressed rats. Pharmacology 27:180–184.

Davis MD, Kilts CD (1988): Influence of neurotensin on endogenous dopamine release from explanted mesoaccumbens neurons in Vitro: Selective activation of somatodentritic receptor sites. Ann NY Acad Sci 537:493–495.

DeOlmos J, Alheid GF, Beltramine GA (1985): Amygdala. In Paxinos G (ed): "The Rat Nervous System. Vol 1. Forebrain and Midbrain" Sydney: Academic Press, pp 223–334.

Dess NK, Chapman CD (1990): Individual differences in taste, body weight, and depression in the "helplessness" rat model and in humans. Brain Res Bull 24:669–676.

Douglas RJ (1967): The hippocampus and behavior. Psychol Bull 67:416–442.

Driscoll P, Bättig K (1982): Behavioral, emotional and neurochemical profiles of rats selected for extreme differences in active, two-way avoidance performance. In Lieblich I (ed): "Genetics of the Brain." Amsterdam: Elsevier, pp 95–123.

Eliasson S (1952): Cerebral influence on gastric motility in the cat. Acta Physiol Scand (Suppl 95) 26:1–70.

Elmes DG, Jarrard LE, Swart PD (1975): Helplessness in hippocampectomized rats: Response perseveration? Physiol Psychol 3:51–5.

Eskay RL, Long RT, Palkovits M (1983): Localization of immunoreactive thyrotropin-releasing hormone in the lower brain stem in the rat. Brain Res 277:159–162.

Fennegan RM, Puiggari MJ (1966): Hypothalamic and amygdaloid influences on gastric motility in dogs. J Neurosurg 24:497–504.

Ferri S, Arrigo-Reina R, Candeletti S, Costa G, Murari G, Speroni E, Scot G (1983): Central and peripheral sites of action for the protective effects of opioids on the rat stomach. Pharmacol Res Commun 15:409–418.

File SA, Pearce JB (1981): Benzodiazepines reduce gastric ulcers induced in rats by stress. Br J Pharmacol 74:593–599.

Finch DM, Wong EE, Derian EL, Chen XH, Nowlin-Finch NL, Brothers LE (1986): Neurophysiology of limbic system pathways in the rat: Projections from the amygdala to the entorhinal cortex. Brain Res 370:273–284.

Garrick T (1990): The role of gastric contractility and brain thyrotropin-releasing hormone in cold restraint-induced gastric mucosal injury. Ann NY Acad Sci 597:51–70.

Garrick T, Weiner H, Bass T (1989): Cold restraint and tail shock stimulate gastric contractility in the rat. In Buéno L, Collins S, Junien JL (eds): "Stress and Digestive Motility." London: John Libbey, pp 175–177.

Glavin GB (1980): Restraint ulcer: History, current research and future implications. Brain Res Bull (Suppl 1) 5:51–58.

Glavin GB (1985a): Effects of morphine and naloxone on restraint stress ulcers in rats. Pharmacology 31:57–60.

Glavin GB (1985b): Stress and brain noradrenalin. Neurosci Biobehav Rev 9:233–243.

Glavin GB, Dugani AM, Pinsky C (1986): L-Deprenyl attenuates stress ulcer formation in rats. Neurosci Lett 70:379–381.

Gray TS (1989): Autonomic neuropeptide connections of the amygdala. In Taché Y, Morley JE, Brown MR (eds): "Neuropeptides and Stress." New York: Springer-Verlag, pp 92–106.

Grijalva CV, Taché Y, Gunion MW, Walsh JM, Geiselman PJ (1986): Amygdaloid lesions attenuate neurogenic gastric mucosal erosions but do not alter gastric secretory changes induced by intracisternal bombesin. Brain Res Bull 16:55–61.

Guth PH, Paulsen G, Foroozan P (1975): Experimental chronic gastric ulcer due to ischemia in rats. Am J Digest Dis 20:824–834.

Guth PH, Leung FW (1987): Physiology of the gastric circulation. In Johnson LR (ed): "Physiology of the Gastrointestinal Tract." New York: Raven Press, pp 1031–1053.

Henke PG (1979): The hypothalamus-amygdala axis and experimental gastric ulcers. Neurosci Biobehav Rev 3:75–82.

Henke PG (1980a): The amygdala and restraint ulcers in rats. J Comp Physiol Psychol 94:313–323.

Henke PG (1980b): The centromedial amygdala and gastric pathology in rats. Physiol Behav 25:107–112.

Henke PG (1980c): Facilitation and inhibition of gastric pathology after lesions in the amygdala of rats. Physiol Behav 25:575–579.

Henke PG (1981): Attenuation of shock-induced ulcers after lesions in the medial amygdala. Physiol Behav 27:143–146.

Henke PG (1982): The telencephalic limbic system and experimental gastric pathology: A review. Neurosci Biobehav Rev 6:381–390.

Henke PG (1983): Unit-activity in the central amygdalar nucleus of rats in response to immobilization-stress. Brain Res Bull 10:833–837.

Henke PG (1984): The bed nucleus of the stria terminalis and immobilization-stress: Unit activity, escape behaviour, and gastric pathology in rats. Behav Brain Res 11:35–45.

Henke PG (1985): The amygdala and forced immobilization of rats. Behav Brain Res 16:19–24.

Henke PG (1987): Chlorodiazepoxide and stress tolerance in rats. Pharmacol Biochem Behav 26:561–563.

Henke PG (1988a): Electrophysiological activity in the central nucleus of the amygdala: Emotionality and stress ulcers in rats. Behav Neurosci 102:77–83.

Henke PG (1988b): Recent studies of the central nucleus of the amygdala and stress ulcers. Neurosci Biobehav Rev 12:143–150.

Henke PG (1989a): N-methyl-D-aspartate receptors and stress ulcers in rats: gastric ulcers, hippocampal long-term potentiation, and coping. In Buéno L, Collins S, Junien JL (eds): "Stress and Digestive Motility." London: John Libbey, pp 247–249.

Henke PG (1989b): Synaptic efficacy in the entorhinal-dentate pathway and stress ulcers in rats. Neurosci Lett 107:110–113.

Henke PG (1990a): Granule cell potentials in the dentate gyrus of the hippocampus: Coping behavior and stress ulcers in rats. Behav Brain Res 36:97–103.

Henke PG (1990b): Limbic system modulation of stress ulcer development. Ann NY Acad Sci 597:201–206.

Henke PG (1990c): Hippocampal pathway to the amygdala and stress ulcer development. Brain Res Bull 25:691–695.

Henke PG (1990d): Potentiation of inputs from the posterolateral amygdala to the dentate gyrus and resistance to stress ulcer formation in rats. Physiol Behav 48:659–664.

Henke PG (1991): The limbic system and stress ulcers. In Szabo S (ed): "Neuroendocrinology of Gastrointestinal Ulceration." New York: Springer (in press).

Henke PG, Savoie RJ, Callahan BM (1981): Hippocampal deafferentation and deefferentation and gastric pathology in rats. Brain Res Bull 7:395–398.

Henke PG, Sullivan RM (1985): Kindling in the amygdala and susceptibility to stress ulcers. Brain Res Bull 14:5–8.

Henke PG, Sullivan RM, Ray A (1988): Interactions of thyrotropin-releasing hormone with neurotensin and dopamine in the central nucleus of the amygdala during stress ulcer formation in rats. Neurosci Lett 91:95–100.

Hernandez DE (1989): Neurobiology of brain-gut interactions: Implications for ulcer disease. Digest Dis Sci 34:1809–1816.

Hernandez DE (1990): The role of brain peptides in the pathogenesis of experimental stress gastric ulcers. Ann NY Acad Sci 597:28–35.

Hernandez DE, Nemeroff CB, Orlando RC, Prange AJ Jr (1983): The effect of centrally administered neuropeptides on the development of stress-induced gastric ulcers in rats. J Neurosci Res 9:143–157.

Hernandez DE, Stanley DA, Allen JA, Prange AJ Jr (1985): Role of brain neurotransmitters in neurotensin induced cytoprotection. Parmacol Biochem Behav 22:509–513.

Hernandez DE, Stanley DA, Melvin JA, Prange AJ Jr (1986): Involvement of brain dopamine systems in neurotensin-induced protection against stress gastric lesions. Brain Res 381:159–163.

Hernandez DE, Emerick SG (1988): Thyrotropin-releasing hormone: Medullary site of action to induce gastric ulcers and stimulate acid secretions. Brain Res 459:148–152.

Hernandez DE, Salaiz AB, Morin P, Moreira MA (1990a): Administration of thyrotropin-releasing hormone into the central nucleus of the amygdala induces gastric lesions in rats. Brain Res Bull 24:697–699.

Hernandez DE, Arredondo ME, Xue BG, Jennes L (1990b): Evidence for a role of brain thyrotropin-releasing hormone (TRH) on stress gastric lesion formation in rats. Brain Res Bull 24:693–695.

Hökfelt T, Elde R, Johansson O, Terenius L, Stein L (1977): The distribution of enkephalin-immunoreactive cell bodies in rat central nervous system. Neurosci Lett 5:25–31.

Hopkins DA (1975): Amygdalotegmental projections in the rat, cat and rhesus monkey. Neurosci Lett 1:262–270.

Innes DL, Tansy MF (1980): Gastric mucosal ulceration associated with electrochemical stimulation of the limbic brain. Brain Res Bull (Suppl 1) 5:33–36.

Jackson IMD, Lechan RM (1983): Thyrotropin releasing hormone. In Krieger DT, Brownstein MJ, Martin JB (eds): "Brain Peptides." New York: Wiley-Interscience, pp 661–685.

Kauffman GL (1989): The effect of central neurotensin-monamine interactions during stress on gastric mucosal function. Digest Dis Sci 34:1316.

Koikegami H (1964): Amygdala and other related limbic structures: Experimental studies in the anatomy and function. II. Functional experiments. Acta Med Biol 12:73–266.

Koikegami HA, Komoto A, Kido C (1953): Studies on the amygdaloid nuclei and peri-amygdaloid complex: Experiments on the influence of their stimulation upon motility of small intestine and blood pressure. Folia Psychiat Neurol Jap 7:86–108.

Kubek MJ, Rea MA, Hades ZI, Apriban MH (1983): Quantitation and characterization of thyrotropin-releasing hormone in vagal nuclei and other regions of the medulla oblongata of the rat. J Neurochem 40:1307–1313.

Lauterbach HH, Mattes DB (1977): Effect of dopamine in stress ulcers in rats. Eur Surg Res 9:258–263.

MacLean PD (1949): Psychosomatic disease and the "visceral brain": Recent developments bearing on the Papez theory of emotion. Psychosom Med 11:338–353.

Maeda-Hagiwara M, Watanabe K (1983): Influence of dopamine agonists on gastric acid secretion induced by intraventricular administration of thyrotropin-releasing hormone in the perfused stomach of anesthetized rat. Br J Pharmacol 79:297–303.

Mickley GA, Ferguson JL (1989): Enhanced acoustic startle responding in rats with radiation-induced hippocampal granule cell hypoplasia. Exp Brain Res 75:28–34.

Morley JE, Garvin TJ, Pekary HE, Hershman JM (1977): Thyrotropin-releasing hormone in the gastrointestinal tract. Biochem Biophys Res Commun 79:314–318.

Morley JE, Levine AS, Silvis SE (1982): Endogeneous opiates and stress ulceration. Life Sci 31:693–699.

Morrison F, Poletti CE (1980): Hippocampal influence on amygdala unit activity in awake squirrel monkeys. Brain Res 192:353–369.

Natelson BH, Ottenweller JE, Cook JA, Pitman D, McCarty R, Tapp WN (1988): Effect of stressor intensity on habituation of the adenocortical stress response. Physiol Behav 43:41–46.

Nemeroff CE, Hernandez DE, Orlando RC, Prange AJ Jr (1982): Cytoprotective effect of centrally administered neurotensin on stress induced gastric ulcers. Am J Physiol 242:G342–G346.

Nemeroff CB, Luttinger D, Hernandez DE, Mailman RB, Mason GA, Davis SD, Widerlov E, Fry GD, Kilts CA, Beaumont K, Breese GR, Prange AJ Jr (1983): Interactions of neurotensin with brain dopamine systems: Biochemical and behavioral studies. Pharmacol Exp Ther 225:337–345.

Palkovits M, Mezey E, Eskay RL, Brownstein NJ (1986): Innervation of the tractus solitarius and the dorsal vagal nucleus by thyrotropin-releasing hormone-containing raphe neurons. Brain Res 373:246–251.

Paré WP, Glavin GB (1986): Restraint stress in biomedical research: A review. Neurosci Biobehav Rev 10:339–370.

Phillips AG, Blaha CD, Fibiger HC, Lane RF (1988): Interactions between mesolimbic dopamine neurons, cholecystokinin, and neurotensin: Evidence using *in vivo* voltammetry. Ann NY Acad Sci 537:347–361.

Poletti Ce, Kliot M, Boytin G (1984): Metabolic influences of the hippocampus on hypothalamus, preoptic and basal forebrain is exerted through amygdalofugal pathways. Neurosci Lett 45:211–216.

Prange AJ, Nemeroff CB (1982): The manifold actions of neurotensin: A first synthesis. Ann NY Acad Sci 400:368–375.

Price JL (1981): The efferent projections of the amygdaloid complex in the rat, cat and monkey. In Ben-Ari Y (ed): "The Amygdaloid Complex." Amsterdam: Elsevier/North-Holland Biomedical Press, pp 121–132.

Racine RJ, Milgram NW, Hafner S (1983): Long-term potentiation phenomena in the rat limbic forebrain. Brain Res 260:217–231.

Ray A, Henke PG, Sullivan RM (1987a): The central amygdala and immobilization stress induced gastric pathology in rats: Neurotensin and dopamine. Brain Res 409:398–402.

Ray A, Sullivan RM, Henke PG (1987b): Adrenergic modulation of gastric stress pathology in rats: A cholinergic link. J Autonom Nerv Sys 20:265–268.

Ray A, Henke PG, Sullivan RM (1988a): Central dopamine systems and gastric stress pathology in rats. Physiol Behav 42:359–364.

Ray A, Henke PG, Sullivan RM (1988b): Effects of intra-amygdalar dopamine agonists and antagonists on gastric stress lesions in rats. Neurosci Lett 84:302–306.

Ray A, Henke PG, Sullivan RM (1988c): Opiate mechanisms in the central amygdala and gastric stress pathology in rats. Brain Res 442:195–198.

Ray A, Henke PG (1989): Role of dopaminergic mechanisms in the central amygdalar nucleus in the regulation of stress-induced gastric ulcer formation in rats. Ind J Med Res 90:224–228.

Ray A, Henke PG (1990a): Enkephalin-dopamine interactions in the central amygdalar nucleus during gastric stress ulcer formation in rats. Behav Brain Res 36:179–183.

Ray A, Henke PG (1990b): Noradrenergic mechanisms in the central amygdalar nucleus and gastric stress ulcer formation in rats. Neurosci Lett 110:331–336.

Roberts GW, Woodham PL, Polak JM, Crow JJ (1982): Distribution of neuropeptides in the limbic system of the rat: The amygdaloid complex. Neuroscience 7:99–131.

Rogers RC, McCann MJ, Hermann GE (1988): TRH effects on physiologically-identified neurons in the dorsal vagal complex: *In vivo* and *in vitro* studies. Soc Neurosci Abstr 14:538.

Sen RN, Anand BK (1957): Effect of electrical stimulation of the limbic system of brain ("visceral brain") on gastric secretory activity and ulceration. Ind J Med Res 45:515–521.

Sharif N, Burt D (1985): Limbic, hypothalamic, cortical and spinal regions are enriched with receptors of thyrotropin-releasing hormone: Evidence from [^{3}H] ultrafilm autoradiography and correlation with cerebral effects of the tripeptide in rat brain. Neurosci Lett 60:337–342.

Shealy CN, Peele TL (1957): Studies on amygdaloid nucleus in the cat. J Neurophysiol 20:125–139.

Sikiric P, Geber J, Ivanovic D, Suckanek E, Gjuris V, Tucan-Foretic M, Mise R, Cvitanovic B, Rotkovic I (1986): Dopamine antagonists induce gastric lesions in rats. Eur J Pharmacol 131:105–109.

Simon H, LeMoal M (1988): Mesencephalic dopaminergic neurons: Role in the general economy of the brain. Ann NY Acad Sci 537:235–253.

Stock G, Rupprecht U, Stumpf H, Schlör K (1981): Cardiovascular changes during arousal elicited by stimulation of amygdala, hypothalamus and locus coeruleus. J Autonom Nerv Sys 3:503–510.

Sullivan RM, Henke PG, Ray A, Hebert MA, Trimper JM (1989): The GABA/benzodiazepine receptor complex in the central amygdalar nucleus and stress ulcers in rats. Behav Neurol Biol 51:262–269.

Szabo S, Moriga M (1989): Neuropeptides and duodenal ulcer: The cysteamine story. In Taché Y, Morley JE, Brown MR (eds): "Neuropeptides and Stress." New York: Springer-Verlag, pp 158–174.

Taché Y, Lesiege D, Vale W, Collu R (1985): Gastric hypersecretion by intracisternal TRH: Dissociation from hypophysiotropic activity and role of central catecholamine. Eur J Pharmacol 107:149–155.

Taché Y, Ishikawa T (1989): Role of brain peptides in the ulcerogenic response to stress. In Taché Y, Morley JE, Brown MR (eds): "Neuropeptides and Stress." New York: Springer-Verlag, pp 146–157.

Tassin JP, Kitabgi P, Tramu G, Studler JM, Hervé D, Trovero F, Glowinski J (1988): Rat mesocortical dopaminergic neurons are mixed neurotensin/dopamine neurons: Immunohistochemical and biochemical evidence. Ann NY Acad Sci 537:531–533.

Thomas SR, Assaf SY, Iversen SD (1984): Amygdaloid complex modulates neurotransmission from the entorhinal cortex to the dentate gyrus of the rat. Brain Res 307:363–365.

Timms RJ (1981): A study of the amygdaloid defense reaction showing the value of Althesin anesthesia in studies of the function of the fore-brain in cats. Pflügers Arch 391:49–56.

Weiner H (1977): "Psychobiology and Human Disease." New York: Elsevier/North Holland, pp 29–101.

Xing L, King J, Bryan R, Kauffman G (1989): Effect of neurotensin on regional cerebral glucose utilization during restraint-induced gastric mucosal injury. Digest Dis Sci 34:1321.

Young WS, Kuhar MJ (1980): Radiohistochemical localization of benzodiazepine receptors in rat brain. J Pharmacol Exp Therapeut 12:337–346.

Zawoiski EJ (1967): Gastric secretory response of the unrestrained cat following electrical stimulation of the hypothalamus, amygdala and basal ganglia. Exp Neurol 17:128–139.

The Amygdala: Neurobiological Aspects of Emotion,
Memory, and Mental Dysfunction, pages 339–351
© 1992 Wiley-Liss, Inc.

12
Emotion and the Amygdala

JOSEPH E. LEDOUX
Center for Neural Science, New York University, New York, New York

INTRODUCTION

Although the amygdala is now believed to be a key structure in the brain's emotional system, it has not always been held in such esteem. Early influential theories of brain and emotion either ignored or diminished the importance of the amygdala relative to other structures. In the Cannon-Bard hypothesis, for example, the hypothalamus and cerebral cortex played the key integrative roles in emotional processes (Bard, 1929; Cannon, 1931). Along similar but more detailed anatomical lines, Papez (1937) proposed a circuit of emotion involving the hypothalamus, anterior thalamus, cignulate cortex, and hippocampus. The amygdala was not included. Maclean's (1949, 1952) limbic system hypothesis expanded the emotional system to include much of the subcortical forebrain and several additional cortical structures as well. While the amygdala was one of the subcortical nuclei of Maclean's limbic system, it was clearly a lesser companion of the hippocampus, which was the centerpiece of the limbic system theory of emotion. Today, the hippocampus and other limbic areas with which it is connected are generally viewed as more involved in cognitive than emotional processes, with the amygdala standing out as the brain region most often implicated in emotional processes.

The importance of the amygdala to emotional processes was not really appreciated until it was determined that the dramatic emotional changes characteristic of the Klüver-Bucy syndrome (Klüver and Bucy, 1937), produced by damage to the temporal lobe, are attributable to damage to the amygdala (Weiskrantz, 1956). Subsequently, a wealth of findings implicating the amygdala in a variety of emotional processes were reported. In the following, the aim is to survey some of this literature. The chapter is organized around various emotional processes in which the amygdala has been implicated. We begin, appropriately enough, with the Klüver-Bucy syndrome.

THE KLÜVER-BUCY SYNDROME

More than 100 years ago, Brown and Schafer (1888) observed that large lesions of the temporal lobe transformed normaly wild and fierce monkeys into tame, indifferent creatures. Prior to surgery, the animals would assault anyone who teased or tried to handle them. Following surgery, however, they could be handled and teased without consequence. Later, Klüver and Bucy (1937, 1939) reported similar findings. They noted that temporal lobe lesions, in addition to producing tameness or hypoemotionality, also resulted in "psychic blindness" (visual agnosia) and changes in dietary and sexual behavior. Subsequent studies demonstrated that the critical site of temporal lobe damage producing these behavioral disturbances is the amygdala (Weiskrantz, 1956; Downer, 1961; Horel et al., 1975; Aggleton and Passingham, 1981). The collection of behavioral changes produced by lesions of the amygdala in primates has come to be referred to as the "Klüver-Bucy syndrome."

Downer (1961), studying the Klüver-Bucy syndrome, helped to identify specific pathways involved in emotional information processing by the amygdala. He placed a unilateral lesion in one amygdala. In addition, he sectioned the optic chiasm and forebrain commissures. This preparation left each eye connected to only the ipsilateral hemisphere and prevented interhemispheric communication. Thus, visual input restricted to one eye remained in the ipsilateral hemisphere. When the monkeys viewed the world through the eye connected to the amygdalectomized hemisphere, they exhibited tameness to visual stimuli. If the animal viewed the world through the other eye, which was connected to a hemisphere with an intact amygdala, it reacted in the normal wild fashion to threatening visual stimuli. Interestingly, regardless of which hemisphere was viewing the world, touch stimuli evoked defensive behavior. Downer's lesions thus produced a tameness restricted to visual stimuli.

Downer's work suggested that unless visual information processed in cortical areas reaches the amygdala, its affective significance will not be registered. Anatomical studies have shown that each primary sensory receiving area of the cortex is linked with the amygdala through a series of corticocortical projections (e.g., Whitlock and Nauta, 1956; Jones and Powell, 1970; Turner et al., 1980). In the visual system, these involve transmission through striate cortex, prestriate cortex, and temporal neocortex, which then projects to amygdala. It should, therefore, be possible to reproduce the effects of amygdala lesions by cortical lesions which interrupt this processing sequence. This view is in fact supported by studies showing that partial or complete Klüver-Bucy symptoms can be produced by lesions of the temporal neocortex (Akert et al., 1961; Horel et al., 1975) or by destruction of the input or output pathways of the temporal lobe (Horel and Misantone, 1976).

Studies of the Klüver-Bucy syndrome have contributed significantly to the view that the amygdala is a focal structure in the processing of emotion. Specifically, this work has led to the view that the sensory stimuli are endowed with emotional and motivational significance by transmission of sensory input to the amygdala (Weiskrantz, 1956; Geschwind, 1965; Jones and Mishkin, 1972; Horel et al., 1975; Aggleton and Mishkin, 1986; Rolls, 1986; LeDoux, 1987). Thus, when the amygdala is damaged, monkeys act tame in the presence of humans because the sight of a human is no longer coded as a threatening stimulus. Smilarly, dietary and sexual preferences change since environmental stimuli no longer elicit their normal affective responses. Stimuli are still perceived as objects when the amygdala is damaged, but they are no longer perceived as emotionally significant objects.

Recently it has been proposed that amygdala lesions interfere with the formation of cross-model (intersensory) associations and that the Klüver-Bucy syndrome may result in part from an inability to associate stimuli across different modalities, as well as deficits in affective processing (Murray and Mishkin, 1985). This conclusion is based on studies involving lesions of the amygdala and adjacent cortical areas. While amygdala lesions alone produce the emotional changes of the Klüver-Bucy syndrome (Zola Morgan et al., in press), it remains to be determined whether amygdala lesions alone result in cross-modal association deficits.

STIMULUS-REWARD ASSOCIATION LEARNING

Studies of the Klüver-Bucy syndrome clearly implicate the amygdala in emotional processing. This syndrome has been useful as a functional marker in studies of the underlying anatomy of emotion. However, the Klüver-Bucy syndrome is based on cinical observation and is not well suited for addressing questions about the nature of the underlying emotional process that is disturbed.

Experimental tasks have been designed to directly test the hypothesis, suggested by the Klüver-Bucy syndrome, that the amgdala processes the affective significance of visual stimuli (Jones and Mishkin, 1972; Sunshine and Mishkin, 1975; Spiegler and Mishkin, 1981; Gaffan and Harrison, 1987; Gaffan et al., 1988). These tasks are typically designed to determine whether an animal is able to associate sensory stimuli with rewards and are thus often viewed as measures of stimulus-reward association learning. For example, the task used by Jones and Mishkin involved the rapid switching of the reward value of two stimuli. The animals were fist trained to obtain a peanut under stimulus A but not B. Once they were able to reliably retrieve the peanut, the task was changed so that the peanut was located under stimulus B. Following reliable performance, the peanut was switched back to A, and so forth. While all animals learned the initial task, animals with amygdala lesions performed poorly when the relationship between stimuls and reward was reversed. These data suggest that the amygdala is necessary for learning to modify the associations between visual stimuli and rewards. Similar findings have been reported with one-trial object reversal learning (Spiegler and Mishkin, 1981), with the use of secondary rather than primary reinforcers (Gaffan and Harrison, 1987), and following surgical disconnection of the amygdala and the visual association cortex (Gaffan et al., 1988).

Nevertheless, not all studies support a role for the amygdala in the formation of stimulus-reward associations. For example, while lesion studies have long implicated the amygdala in taste aversion learning (for review, see Sarter and Markowitsch, 1985), recent work questions this view. When lesions are made using neurotoxic agents that destroy cell bodies but not fibers of passage fibers passing through the amygdala en route to the insular cortex appear to be more important than fibers terminating within the amygdala (Dunn and Everitt, 1988).

Other studies using neurotoxic lesions also question the generality of the amygdala's involvement in stimulus-reward association learning, suggesting that the amygdala is more involved in aversively motivated than appetitively motivated tasks (Cahill and McGaugh, 1990). Nevertheless, other studies using neurotoxic agents to lesion the amygdala indicate a key role for the amygdala in appetitively motivated tasks (Gallagher et al., 1990; Cador et al., 1989; Itiori and White, 1991).

Much work needs to be done in order to resolve the contradictory conclusions that exist in the literature. Important variables that need to be controlled include the size and location of lesions, the method of lesion production, and the tasks used to assess the lesion effects. It might also be useful to reconsider just what stimulus-reward association learning is, whether the tasks used to measure it are really sensitive to it, and the extent to which stimulus-reward association learning is relevant to the issue of emotional processing.

CHANGES IN NEURAL ACTIVITY DURING EXPOSURE TO EMOTIONAL STIMULI

The notion that the amygdala contributes to the processing of the emotional significance of sensory stimuli is also supported by findings from studies where neural activity has been recorded in the amygdala during exposure to emotional stimuli. Early studies using simple sensory stimuli, such as flashing lights, clicks, and sciatic nerve stimulation, revealed that amygdala neurons are responsive to sensory stimuli of various modalities (Machne and Segundo, 1956; Creutzfeldt et al., 1963). Later studies emphasized that amygdala neurons were more sensitive to complex sensory events with biological significance than to simple, meaningless stimuli (O'Keefe and Bouma, 1969; Jacobs and McGinty, 1972). Amygdala units responsive to faces, complex visual stimuli with clear emotional signal value, have been reported (Rolls, 1986). Further, amygdala units have been found to be selectively sensitve to rewarding and aversive stimulus properties (Fuster and Uyeda, 1971; Sanghera et al., 1979; Ono et al., 1983; Nishijo et al. 1986, 1988). Interestingly, the discharge properties of amygdala units change as a result of emotional conditioning, as described below.

While the discharge properties of amygdala units are consistent with the conclusion that amygdala neurons are involved in the processing of the emotional significance of stimuli, it appears that amygdala units are not capable of rapidly modifying their responsivity to changing stimulus-reward relations (Rolls, 1986). This suggests that the amygdala has a tendency to maintain the emotional status quo over the short run, a conclusion that fits with the results of lesion studies suggesting that emotional memories established through the amygdala are indelible (see below). Rapid modifications of emotional responsivity may require other structures. A likely candidate is the orbitofrontal cortex, which contains neurons that do undergo rapid modifications in stimulus-reward relations (Rolls, 1986). However, given that following removal of the amygdala animals perform poorly on tasks requiring rapid switching of stimulus-reward relations (see above), it would seem that the neural changes occurring in regions such as frontal cotex nevertheless depend upon the amygdala as either an input or output in the regulation of emotionally guided behavior.

FEAR CONDITIONING

It is well established that emotionally neutral stimuli can acquire the capacity to evoke striking emotional reaction following temporal pairing with an aversive event. Conditioning does not create new emotional responses but instead simply allow new stimuli to serve as triggers capable of activating existing, often hard-wired, species-specific emotional reactions. In the rat, for example, a pure tone previously paired with footshock evokes a conditioned fear reaction consisting of freezing behavior accompanied by a host of autonomic adjustments, including increases in arterial pressure and heart rate (Blanchard and Blanchard, 1972; Bouton and Bolles, 1980; LeDoux et al., 1984). Similar responses are expressed when laboratory rats are exposed to a cat for the first time, but following amygdala lesions such responses are no longer present (Blanchard and Blanchard, 1972), suggesting that the responses are genetically specified (since they appear when the rat sees a cat, a natural predator, for the first time) and involve the amygdala. The fact that electrical stimulation of the amygdala is capable of eliciting the similar response patterns (e.g., Kapp et al., 1984; Iwata et al., 1987) further supports the notion that the responses are hard wired.

Recent studies have identified neural circuits which are essential for the conditioning of these autonomic and behavioral fear responses. The pathway involves the relay of the auditory stimulus through the primary acoustic structures of the brain stem to the inferior colliculus and then to the medial geniculate body (LeDoux et al., 1984; LeDoux, 1986a,b). From there, the auditory signal is transmitted directly to the amygdala (LeDoux et al., 1985; LeDoux, 1986a,b; Iwata et al., 1986). In the amygdala, the input sructure appears to be the lateral nucleus (LeDoux et al., 1990a,b), while the central nucleus functions as the amygdala output relay (Iwata et al., 1987; LeDoux et al., 1988). The pathway then separates into two components after the amygdala, with changes in autonomic activity and emotional behavior evoked by the acoustic conditioned stimulus taking different routes. Projections from the central amygdala to the lateral hypothalamic area, which, in turn, is connected with brain stem and spinal premotor neurons of the autonomic nervous system, are critically involved in the control of the autonomic changes, whereas, behavioral fear responses depend upon projections to the midbrain central gray region from the central amygdala (LeDoux et al., 1988). Descending connections from the central amygdala to other motor control systems have been shown to mediate the potentiation of startle responses by conditioned fear stimuli (Davis et al., 1987). Findings from studies of other species are consistent with the observations in the rat implicating the central amygdaloid nucleus as a key output to motor control areas (Kapp et al., 1979, 1984; Gentile et al., 1986).

The pathways mediating fear conditioning involve a direct thalamo-amygdala projection and thus bypass the neocortical auditory system (LeDoux, 1986). This observation indicates that fear conditioning does not require the auditory cortex when a simple acostic event serves as the conditioned stimulus. Presumably, however, if the conditioned stimulus information is increased in complexity, such that cortical analysis is required, the pathway would indeed involve the auditory cortex and cortico-amygdala projections. It is thus important to point out that the lateral amygdala also receives acoustic input from the auditory cortex. The lateral amygdala is thus a site of convergence of acoustic pathways originating in the thalamus and neocortex (LeDoux et al., 1987). While the thalamic pathway provides the amygdala with a rapid but crude representation, the auditory cortex transmits a slower but refined message. Interactions between thalamic and cortical sensory information in the amygdala may play an important role in emotional processing (LeDoux, 1986).

Recent studies suggest that emotional memories established through the amygdala are impervious to extinction and forgetting processes (LeDoux et al., 1989). This effect was unmasked by examing the consequences of visual cortex lesions on the acquisition and extinction of fear responses conditioned to visual stimuli. As expected from the auditory conditioning studies, visual cortex lesions did not interfere with acquisition. And when the animals were subsequently given unreinforced presentations of the conditioned stimulus, it was found that they failed to extinguish over the period of time tested (about one month). This suggested that emotional memories established through subcortical inputs to the amygdala are highly resistant to extinction. It is unlikely that the sensory cortex itself plays a significant role in extinction but may instead provide the essential connection to other cortical areas, such as the orbitofrontal cortex or hippocampus, both of which have been implicated in extinction regulation. These observations are consistent with the results of the physiological studies described above, suggesting that the amygdala does not easily switch the emotional valence it assigns to a stimulus and that for such switching to take place, other structures, such as orbitofrontal cortex, may have to intervene.

ANXIETY

The concepts of fear and anxiety are closely related. It is thus of interest that Gray (1982) has developed a model of anxiety built around the function of the hippocampus and septum (septo-hippocampal system). Gray's model is based on the fact that the effects of antianxiety drugs (alcohol, barbituates, benzodiazepines) on behavioral tasks mirror the effects of lesions of the septo-hippocampal system.

A shortcoming of Gray's model is that lesions of the septo-hippocampal system do not interfere with one of the standard procedures for studying experimental anxiety, namely, fear conditioning. Gray dismisses fear conditioning studies as not being directly relevant to the problem of anxiety. Thus, the amygdala is only peripherally involved in Gray's model. This is curious for several reasons. First, lesions of the amygdala are generally believed to reduce experimental fear and anxiety. Second, receptors for benzodiazepines, the major class of anxiolytic drugs in therapeutic use, are heavily concentrated in the amygdala, as well as the hippocampus. Third, microinjection of benzodiazepines into the amygdala, but not the hippocampus, reduces experimental fear and anxiety. Gray deals with this latter observation by arguing that benzodiazepines act on hippocampal activity indirectly, by way of the locus coeruleus. However, the locus coeruleus also innervates the amygdala and other forebrain areas, as well as the hippocampus. Even if the locus coeruleus system is a site of benzodiazepine action relevant to anxiety, the amygdala is not ruled out. And given the known action of benzodiazepines in the amygdala in reducing anxiety, it it likely that any role of the locus coeruleus sysem is to complement the action in the amygdala.

Any model of fear and anxiety, it would seem, will have to account for the contribution of the amygdala. However, in spite of the problems with Gray's model, the hippocampus may also be involved in anxiety. One hypothesis is suggested here, based on the traditional distinction between fear and anxiety. Fear is generally thought to be tied to a specific stimulus, whereas anxiety is not. As we have seen, the pathways of fear involve interactions between sensory processing areas and the amygdala. These pathways pesumably transmit emotionally neutral sensory signals to the amygdala, where the affective implications are assessed. The amygdala also receives inputs from the hippocampal formation, which is believed to be involved in higher cognitive functions (e.g., Squire, 1987). Interestingly, the same region of the amygdala (i.e., the lateral nucleus) which receives convergent inputs from thalamic and cortical sensory processing areas also receives inputs from the hippocampus. Thoughts and memories processed in the hippocampus might, therefore, receive emotional coloration by way of information transmission to the amygdala. By this account, the distinction between fear and anxiety is based on whether the emotional processing mechanisms of the amygdala are activated directly by sensory information originating in thalamic and cortical areas or by cognitive processes organized in the hippocampus. The hippocampus (and other areas of the limbic system with which it is connected), then, would contribute to anxiety as a cognitive rather than as an affective processing structure. It would constitute the third and most complex tier in the cascade of inputs of increasing complexity to the amygdala, with sensory transmission from the thalamus and perceptual transmission from modality-specific cortex constituting the first two.

DEFENSE RESPONSES EVOKED BY BRAIN STIMULATION

One of the classic methods for mapping the pathways of emotion involves the application of electrical or chemical stimuli to discrete brain regions. It has been known for some time that stimulation of the hypothalamus in anesthetized animals evokes widespread activation of the sympathetic nervous system (Karplus and Kreidel, 1927; Ranson and Magoun, 1939). Studies by Hess and Brugger (1943) demonstrated that hypothalamic stimulation in the awake animal produced a coordinated pattern of emotional behavior which began as an alerting response, progressed to include piloerection, hissing, and exposure of the claws, and culminated in attack or flight responses. They termed this behavior pattern the "defense response." Later studies demonstrated that hypothalamic sites from which sympathetic activation can be elicited in anesthetized animals are the same sites from which defensive behavior can be evoked in awake animals (Abrahams et al., 1960).

Autonomic and behavioral defense responses can also be evoked by amygdala stimulation (Hilton and Zbrozyna, 1963; Reis and Gunne, 1965; Fernandez de Molina and Hunsperger, 1959, 1962; Kapp et al., 1984; Iwata et al., 1987). Lesions of the hypothalamus or of pathways connecting the amygdala with the hypothalamus prevent the evocation of defense responses by amygdala stimulation (Hilton and Zbrozyna, 1963; Fernandez de Molina and Hunsperger, 1962), suggesting that projections from the amygdala to the hypothalamus play a critical role in the expression of autonomic and behavioral defense responses. However, recent work using chemical rather than electrical stimuli suggests that the hypothalamus may not be a synaptic link in the pathway mediating behavioral defense responses. Thus, microinjection of excitatory amino acids into the hypothalamus fails to evoke defensive behaviors, whereas injections in the central gray region does (Bandler, 1982). Since excitatory amino acids activate local neurons but not fibers of passage (Goodchild et al., 1982), the behaviors evoked by electrical stimulation of the hypothalamus may be due to activation of fibers connecting the amygdala with the central gray and running through the hypothalamus. The hypothalamus does, however, appear to be a synaptic station in the sympathoexcitatory pathway, as excitatory amino acids do evoke autonomic changes when injected there (Sun ad Guyenet, 1986). These findings are consistent with the results of studies of conditioned fear responses described above, which suggest that amygdalo-hypothalamic connections mediate the learned autonomic changes and that amygdalo-central gray projections mediate the behavioral fear responses.

While stimulation of other limbic areas generally does not evoke defensive or aggressive behaviors, when certain limbic area are stimulated concurrently with hypothalamic stimulation, hypothalamically evoked attack responses can be inhibited or facilitated (Siegel and Edinger, 1981). For example, stimulation of the dorsal hippocampus suppresses hypothalamic attack, while stimulation of the vental hippocampus enhances hypothalamic attack. Further, stimulation of the orbitofrontal or anterior cingulate cortex inhibits hypothalamic attack. These data suggest that information processed in several limbic areas can modulate the activity of the primary attack pathway involving the amygdala and its projections to hypothalamus.

EMOTIONAL CONSEQUENCES OF BRAIN STIMULATION IN MAN

One of the major gaps in our understanding of the brain mechanisms of emotion is the relationship between human and animal emotional systems. Most of the techniques available for studying emotion in animals have focused on problems concerning how the brain processes the emotional significance of stimuli and produces emotional responses. These are important problems but they only relate indirectly to the question of how the brain generates the variety of subjective emotional states that we refer to as "emotions." We have no neurobiology of love or jealousy and it is unlikely that animal research will shed much light on these human conditions. Fortunately, one technique has been available for studying emotional states in man. It involves electrical stimulation of brain areas.

It has been known for over 100 years that epileptic seizure activity of the temporal lobe can give rise to "psychic" or experiential states (Jackson, 1880). Later studies by Penfield and associates confirmed and extended these observations by delivering electrical impulses to the temporal lobe in the course of surgical procedures aimed at relieving the epileptic condition (Penfield and Jasper, 1954; Penfield and Perot, 1963; Penfield, 1975). Such stimulations were found to produce hallucinations, illusions, memory flashbacks, "*déjà vu*" experiences, and fear and other emotions (Gloor et al., 1982). Penfield attributed these phenomena to activation of neocortical memory networks. However, more recent work has suggested that the effects are due mainly to activation of limbic areas, such as amygdala and hippocampus (Halgren, 1981; Gloor et al., 1982). For example, Gloor et al., (1982) found that experiential phenomena did not occur unless spontaneous seizure discharges or electrical stimulation involved limbic structures. Further, activation of temporal neocortex by the seizure discharge or stimulus was not necessary for the occurrence of experiential phenomena. Given the role of the amygdala in emotion and the hippocampus in declarative memory, that is, conscious recollection of facts and experiences (Squire, 1987), it is possible that together these structures and their connections are involved in the affective coloration of conscious experiences. Needless to say, much remains unknown about the mechanisms of subjective emotional experience. However, the information available suggests that the amygdala, which has been consistently implicated in emotion in animals, is also important for the mediation of subjective emotional states in man.

BRAIN SYSTEMS AND EMOTION: CONCLUSIONS

While the contribution of the amygdala is undeniable, this should not imply that the problem of relating brain mechanisms to emotion has been solved. The amygdala and its connections almost certainly do not constitute the only brain system involve in emotional processes. Moreover, emotion is surely not the only function of the amygdala. And while we are on fairly safe ground in extrapolating from animal to human emotion for relatively primitive emotional processes (i.e., fear, anger, pleasure), we know almost nothing about the neurobiology of complex human emotions (love, jealousy, a sense of personal fulfillment) and it is unlikely that animal work will tell us very much about these. What is clear is that much more work needs to be done, that existing techniques need to be improved, and/or that new techniques need to be developed before the important questions concerning the relation between human and animal emotion will be better understood. It seems likely, given what we now know, that the amygdala will play a central role in the emotional system of the human brain, once we understand it. However, that day is not yet here. In the meantime, we should continue to pursue the neurobiology of emotion in animals in the hope that most of what we learn will apply to man and will help in not only understanding how emotion is normally processed but also will shed some light on what goes wrong in emotional disorders.

REFERENCES

Abrahams VC, Hilton SM, Zbrozyna A (1960): Active muscle vasodilation produced by stimulation of the brain stem: Its significance in the defence reaction. J Physiol 154:491–513.

Aggleton JP, Mishkin M (1986): The amygdala: Sensory gateway to the emotions. In Plutchik

R, Kellerman H (eds): "Emotion: Theory, Research and Experience," Vol 3, Orlando: Academic Press, pp 281–299.

Aggleton JP, Passingham RE (1981): Syndrome produced by lesions of the amygdala in monkeys (*Macaca mulatta*). J Comp Physiol Psychol 95:961–977.

Akert K, Gruesen RA, Woolsey CN, Meyer DR (1961): Klüver-Bucy syndrome in monkeys with neocortical ablations of temporal lobe. Brain 84:480–497.

Bandler, RJ (1982): Induction of "rage" following microinjection of glutamate into midbrain but not hypothalamus of cats. Neurosci Lett 30:183–188.

Bard P (1929): The central representation of the sympathetic system: As indicated by certain physiological observations. Arch Neurol Psychiat 22:230–246.

Blanchard DC, Blanchard RJ (1972): Innate and conditioned reactions to threat in rats with amygdaloid lesions. J Comp Physiol Psychol 81:281–290.

Bouton ME, Bolles RC (1980): Conditioned fear assessed by freezing and by the suppression of three different baselines. Anim Learn Behav 8:429–434.

Brown S, Schafer A (1888): An investigation into the functions of the occipital and temporal lobes of the monkey's brain. Philos Trans R Soc Lond [Biol] 179:303–327.

Cador M, Robbins TW, and Everitt BJ (1989): Involvement of the amygdala in stimulus-reward associations: interaction with the ventral striatum. Neuroscience 30:77–86.

Cahill L, McGaugh JL (1990): Amygdaloid complex lesions differentially affect retention of tasks using appetitive and aversive reinforcement. Behav Neurosci 104:532–543.

Cannon WB (1931): Again the James-Lange and the thalamic theories of emotion. Psychol Rev 38:281–295.

Creutzfeldt OD, Bell FR, Ross Adey W (1963): The activity of neurons in the amygdala of the cat following afferent stimulation. Prog Brain Res 3:31–49.

Davis M, Hitchcock JM, Rosen JB (1987): Anxiety and the amygdala: Pharmacological and anatomical analysis of the fear-potentiated startle paradigm. In Bower GH (ed): "The Psychology of Learning and Motivation," San Diego: Academic Press, pp 263–305.

Downer JDC (1961): Changes in visual gnostic function and emotional behavior following unilateral temporal lobe damage in the "split-brain" monkey. Nature 191:50–51.

Dunn LT, Everitt BJ (1988): Double dissociations of the effects of amygdala and insular cortex lesions on conditioned taste aversion, passive avoidance, and neophobia in the rat using the excitotoxin ibotenic acid. Behav Neurosci 102:3–23.

Fernandez de Molina A, Hunsperger RW (1959): Central representation of affective reactions in forebrain and brain stem: Electrial stimulation of amygdala, stria terminalis, and adjacent structures. J Physiol 145:251–265.

Fuster JM and Uyeda AA (1971): Reactivity of limbic neurons of the monkey to appetitive and aversive signals. Electroencephalogr Clin Neurophysiol (In Press).

Fernandez de Molina A, Hunsperger RW (1962): Organization of the subcortical system governing defense and flight reactions in the cat. J Physiol 160:200–213.

Gaffan D, Harrison S (1987): Amygdalectomy and disconnection in visual learning for auditory secondary reinforcement by monkeys. J Neurosci 7:2285–2292.

Gaffan EA, Gaffan D, Harrison S (1988): Disconnection of the amygdala from visual association cortex impairs visual reward-association learning in monkeys. J Neurosci 8(9):3144–3150.

Gallagher M, Graham PW, Holland PC (1990): The amygdala central nucleus and appetitive pavlovian conditioning: Lesions impair one class of conditioned behavior. Behav Neurosci 10:1906–1911.

Gentile CG, Jarrel TW, Teich A, McCabe PM, Schneiderman N (1986): The role of amygdaloid central nucleus in the retention of differential Pavlovian conditioning of bradycardia in rabbits. Behav Brain Res 20:263–273.

Geschwind N (1965): The disconnexion syndromes in animals and man. Part I. Brain 88:237–294.

Gloor P, Olivier A, Quesney LF, Andermann F, Horowitz S (1982): The role of the limbic system in experiential phenomena of temporal lobe epilepsy. Ann Neurol 12:129–144.

Goodchild AK, Dampney RAL, Bandler RJ (1982): A method for evoking physiological responses by stimulation of cell bodies, but not axons of passage within localized regions of the central nervous system. J Neurosci Meth 6:351–363.

Gray JA (1982) Precis of "The Neuropsychology of Anxiety: An Enquiry into the Functions of the Septo-Hippocampal System." Behav Brain Sci 5:469–534.

Halgren E (1981): The amygdala contribution to emotion and memory: Current studies in humans. In Ben-Ari Y (ed): "The Amygdaloid Complex." Amsterdam: Elsevier, pp 395–408.

Hess WR, Brugger M (1943): Das subkortikale Zentrum der affektiven Abwehrreaktion. Helv Physiol Pharmacol Acta 1:35–52.

Hilton SM, Zbrozyna AW (1963): Amygdaloid region for defense reactions and its efferent pathway to the brainstem. J Physiol 165:60–173.

Hiroi N and White N M (1991): The lateral nucleus of the amygdala mediates expression of the amphetamine conditioned place preference.

Horel JA, Keating EG, Misantone LJ (1975): Partial Klüver-Bucy syndrome produced by destroying temporal neocortex or amygdala. Brain Res 94:347–359.

Horel JA, Misantone LJ (1976): Visual discrimination impaired by cutting temporal lobe connections. Science 193:336–338.

Iwata J, LeDoux JE, Meeley MP, Arneric S, Reis DJ (1986): Intrinsic neurons in the amygdaloid field projected to by the medial geniculate body mediate emotional responses conditioned to acoustic stimuli. Brain Res 383:195–214.

Iwata J, Chida K, LeDoux JE (1987): Cardiovascular responses elicited by stimulation of neurons in the central amygdaloid nucleus in awake but not anesthetized rats resemble conditioned emotional responses. Brain Res 418:183–188.

Jackson JH (1880): On right or left sided spasm at the onset of epileptic paroxysms, and on crude sensation warnings and elaborate mental states. Brain 3:192–306.

Jacobs BL, McGinty DJ (1972): Participation of the amygdala in complex stimulus recognition and behavioral inhibition: Evidence from unit studies. Brain Res 36:431–436.

Jones B, Mishkin M (1972): Limbic lesions and the problem of stimulus-reinforcement associations. Exp Neurol 36:362–377.

Jones EG, Powell TPS (1970): An anatomical study of converging sensory pathways within the cerebral cortex of the monkey. Brain 93:793–820.

Kapp BS, Frysinger RC, Gallagher M, Haselton J (1979): Amygdala central nucleus lesions: Effect on heart rate conditioning in the rabbit. Physiol Behav 23:1109–1117.

Kapp BS, Pascoe JP, Bixler MA (1984): The amygdala: A neuroanatomical systems approach to its contributions to aversive conditioning. In Buttlers N, Squire LR (eds): "Neuropsychology of Memory." New York: Guilford.

Karplus JP, Kreidl A (1927): Gehirn und Sympathicus. VII. Uber beziehungen der hypothalamuszentren zu blutdruck und innerer sekretion. Pfluegers Arch Gesamte Physiol Menschen Tiere 215:667–670.

Klüver H, Bucy PC (1937): "Psychic blindness" and other symptoms following bilateral temporal lobectomy in rhesus monkeys. Am J Physiol 119:352–353.

Klüver H, Bucy PC (1939): Preliminary analysis of functions of the temporal lobes in monkeys. Arch Neurol Psychiat 42:979–1000.

LeDoux JE, Sakaguchi A, Reis DJ (1984): Subcortical efferent projections of the medial geniculate nucleus mediate emotional responses conditioned to acoustic stimuli. J Neurosci 4:683–698.

LeDoux JE, Ruggiero DA, Reis DJ (1985): Projections to the subcortical forebrain from anatomically defined regions of the medial geniculate body in the rat. J Comp Neurol 242:182–313.

LeDoux JE (1986a): Sensory systems and emotion. Integ Psychiat 4:237–248.

LeDoux JE (1986b): Neurobiology of emotion. In LeDoux JE, Hirst W (eds): "Mind and Brain." New York: Cambridge University Press, pp 301–354.

LeDoux JE, Sakaguchi J, Iwata J, Reis D (1986): Destruction of intrinsic neurons in the lateral hypothalamus disrupts the associative conditioning of autonomic but not behavioral emotional responses in the rat. Brain Res 368:161–166.

LeDoux JE, Farb C, Ruggiero DA, Reis DJ (1987a): Thalamic and cortical auditory pathways converge in the rat amygdala. Soc Neurosci Abstr 13:1467–1467.

LeDoux JE (1987): Emotion. In Plum F (ed): "Handbook of Physiology. 1: The Nervous System. Vol V, Higher Functions of the Brain" Bethesda: American Physiological Society, pp 419–460.

LeDoux JE, Iwata J, Cicchetti P, Reis DJ (1988): Different projections of the central amygdaloid nucleus mediate autonomic and behavioral correlates of conditioned fear. J Neurosci 8:2517–2529.

LeDoux JE, Cicchetti P, Xagoraris A, Romanski LR (1990a): The lateral amygdaloid nucleus: Sensory interface of the amygdala in ear conditioning. J Neurosci 10:1062–1069.

LeDoux JE, Romanski LM, Xagoraris AE (1989): Indelibility of subcortical emotional memories. J Cog Neurosci 1:238–243.

LeDoux JE, Farb CF, Ruggiero DA (1990b): Topographic organization of neurons in the acoustic thalamus that project to the amygdala. J Neurosci 10:1043–1054.

Machne X, Segundo JP (1956): Unitary responses to afferent volleys in amygdaloid complex. J Neurophysiol 19:232–240.

Maclean PD (1949): Psychosomatic disease and the "viseral brain": Recent developments bearing on the Papez theory of emotion. Psychosom Med 11:338–353.

Maclean PD (1952): Some psychiatric implications of physiological studies on frontotemporal portion of limbic system (visceral brain). Electroencephalogr Clin Neurophysiol 4:407–418.

Murray EA, Mishkin M (1985): Amygdalectomy impairs crossmodal association in monkeys. Science 228:604–606.

Nishijo H, Ono T, Nakamura K, Kawabata M, Yamatani K (1986): Neuron activity in and adjacent to the dorsal amygdala of monkey during operant feeding behavior. Brain Res Bull 17:847–854.

Nishijo H, Ono T, Nishino H (1988): Topographic distribution of modality-specific amygdalar neurons in alert monkey. J Neurosci 8:3556–3569.

O'Keefe J and Bouma H (1969): Complex sensory properties of certain amygdala units in the freely moving cat. Exp Neurol 23:384–398.

Ono T, Fukuda M, Nishino H, Sasaki K, Muramoto K-I (1983): Amygdaloid neuronal responses to complex visual stimuli in an operant feeding situation in the monkey. Brain Res Bull 11:515–518.

Papez JW (1937): A proposed mechanism of emotion. Arch Neurol Psychiat 79:217–224.

Penfield W, Jasper H (1954): "Epilepsy and the Functional Anatomy of the Human Brain." Boston: Little, Brown.

Penfield W, Perot P (1963): The brain's record of auditory and visual experience. A final summary and discussion. Brain 86:595–596.

Penfield W (1975): "The Mystery of the Mind. A Critical Study of Consciousness and the Human Brain." Princeton: Princeton University Press.

Ranson SW, Magoun HW (1939): The hypothalamus. Ergebn Physiol 41:56–163.

Reis DJ, Gunne L-M (1965): Brain catecholamines: Relation to defense reaction evoked by brain stimulation in cat. Science 149:450–451.

Rolls ET (1986): A theory of emotion, and its application to understanding the neural basis of emotion. In Oomur Y (ed): "Emotions: Neural and Chemical Control." Tokyo: Japan Scientific Societies Press, pp 325–344.

Sanghera MK, Rolls ET, Roper-Hall A (1979): Visual responses of neurons in the dorso-lateral amygdala of the alert monkey. Exp Neurol 63:610–626.

Sarter M, Markowitsch IIJ (1985): Involvement of the amygdala in learning and memory: A critical review, with emphasis on anatomical relations. Behav Neurosci 99:342–380.

Siegel A, Edinger H (1981): Neural control of aggression and rage behavior. In Morgane PJ, Panksepp J (eds): "Handbook of the Hypothalamus, Vol 3, Behavioral Studies of the Hypothalamus." New York: Marcel Dekker, pp 203–240.

Spiegler BJ, Mishkin M (1981): Evidence for the sequential participation of inferior temporal cortex and amygdala in the acquisition of stimulus-reward associations. Behav Brain Res 3:303–317.

Squire LR (1987): Memory: Neural organization and behavior. In Plum F (ed): "Handbook of Physiology, Section 1: The Nervous System. Vol V. Higher Functions of the Brain." Bethesda: American Physiological Society, pp 295–371.

Sun MK, Guyenet PG (1986): Hypothalamic glutamatergic input to medullary sympatho-excitatory neurons in the rat. Am J Physiol 251:R798–R810.

Sunshine J, Mishkin M (1975): A visual-limbic pathway serving visual associative functions in rhesus monkey. Fed Proc 34:440.

Turner BH, Mishkin M, Knapp M (1980): Organization of the amygdalopetal projections from modality-specific cortical association areas in the monkey. J Comp Neurol 191:515–543.

Weiskrantz L (1956): Behavioral changes associated with ablation of the amygdaloid complex in monkeys. J Comp Physiol Psychol 4:381–391.

Whitlock DG, Nauta WJH (1956): Subcortical projections from the temporal neocortex in *Macaca mulatta*. J Comp Neurol 106:183–212.

Zola-Morgan S, Squire LR, Alvarez-Royo P, Clower RP (1991): Independence of memory functions and emotional behavior: Separate contributions of the hippocampal formation and the amygdala. Hippocampus (in press).

The Amygdala: Neurobiological Aspects of Emotion,
Memory, and Mental Dysfunction, pages 353–377
© 1992 Wiley-Liss, Inc.

13
The Amygdala and Social Behavior

ARTHUR S. KLING AND LESLIE A. BROTHERS
*Psychiatry Service, Sepulveda Veterans Affairs Medical Center and
Department of Psychiatry and Biobehavioral Sciences, University of
California School of Medicine, Los Angeles, California*

INTRODUCTION

This chapter reviews and comments on the role of the amygdala in the social behavior of animals, from reptiles to primates. We do not consider human data in any detail, as they are reviewed in other chapters in this volume. In the discussion that follows, we include under the larger heading "social behavior" any socially relevant communicative behaviors: that is, we consider elicited behavioral elements in the light of the social contexts in which they would have occurred under natural conditions. Our rationale is that the evolutionary history of affective displays, including aggression and defense, is best understood as the development of a signaling system useful for intraspecific communication. Thus, we view the stereotyped motor and autonomic effects of amygdala stimulation as components of social routines which have both internal physiologic and external signaling aspects. Similarly, we focus on amygdala neural responses to stimuli which normally would have social significance, even when these have been deployed under artificial laboratory studies of isolation. Evidence from lesion studies for the role of the amygdala in social behavior is examined from this perspective as well.

Since the early reports on the behavioral consequences of temporal lobectomy by Klüver and Bucy in the monkey (1939), there has been an increasing interest in understanding the mechanisms by which this syndrome is produced. Klüver originally held the view that damage to the entire temporal lobe, including the cortical and more mesial structures, was responsible for this syndrome. However, he could not reproduce the syndrome by ablation of temporal cortex or interruption of frontal-temporal connections. Subsequent studies showed that the syndrome could be produced by ablation of the amygdala alone (Schreiner and Kling, 1953). Nevertheless, I (A.K.) remember vividly a conversation with Dr. Klüver which took place in 1968 shortly before my departure for Zambia to

Address correspondence to: Dr. Arthur Kling, Chief, Psychiatry Service (116A), Veterans Affairs Medical Center, Sepulveda, CA 91343.

study the effects of amygdalectomy in free-ranging monkeys. He admonished me to be sure to remove the whole temporal lobe and not to restrict the lesion to the amygdala, as he believed that the cortical structures were important to the syndrome.

While Klüver's principal interest was the psychic blindness which occurs after bitemporal lobectomy, his remarkable ability to foresee the implications of his observations is revealed in the following excerpt from his 1939 paper: "We may consider the outstanding characteristic of the behavioral changes following bilateral temporal lobectomy to be that they affect the relation between animal and environment so deeply. A monkey which approaches every enemy to examine it orally will conceivably not survive longer than a few hours if turned loose in a region with a plentiful supply of enemies. We doubt that a monkey would be seriously impaired under natural conditions, in the wild, by a loss of its prefrontal region, its parietal lobes or its occipital lobes, as long as small portions of the striate cortex remained intact" (Klüver and Bucy, 1939).

While subsequently our studies showed that amygdalectomized subjects in the wild do not display the characteristic hyperorality seen in confinement and instead become social isolates, it remained true that the eventual consequence of the lesion was inability to survive longer than several weeks (Kling et al., 1970). It was also the case, as we learned in other studies, that lesions of dorsolateral frontal cortex were compatible with survival, as they did not impair the subjects' social bonds with their group (Kling and Steklis, 1976). It is entirely possible, had we followed Klüver's advice and removed the entire temporal lobes, that the operates would have exhibited the complete syndrome irrespective of the setting. These experiments have yet to be accomplished.

Since Klüver and Bucy's seminal experiments, the amygdaloid nuclei have been found to have a regulatory influence on autonomic, endocrine, somatosensory and motor function, reproduction, memory, sleep and wakefulness, and orientation (Eleftheriou, 1972; Ben-Ari, 1981). Over the past two decades, we have focused on the role of the amygdala and related structures (temporal pole; posterior medial orbital cortex) in affective and social behavior in monkeys, and particularly on the processing of emotionally significant sensory stimuli in a social context.

The results of these investigations support the following general framework for understanding amygdala function. While the importance of social bonding for the survival of any individual varies with the specific adaptational mechanisms of its species, it is true for any animal that uses displays, defends territory, and reproduces and cares for young that effective communication with conspecifics is essential. Such communication depends upon the attachment of appropriate significance to sensory information, such that an appropriate response may be generated. It is the attachment of significance which appears to be the critical process lost following amygdalectomy: With that failure, the capacity to respond to important external cues is lost, unless extensive processing through alternate routes is undertaken. In intact animals, once appropriate significance is attached to sensory stimuli, a response is effected (e.g., flight, defense) along with associated autonomic, endocrine, and somatomotor activity. With the expansion and increasing specialization of cerebral cortex seen in primate evolution, the amygdala continues to expand as well (Stephan et al., 1984), presumably to receive increasingly discrete and more highly processed sensory information. The accurate analysis of complex social information made possible by such an arrangement appears to be critical for survival and reproductive success in primates and other highly social animals. It is within this conceptual framework that we review and discuss the role of the amygdala in the regulation of social and affective behavior.

ANATOMICAL CONSIDERATIONS

The pattern of afferent and efferent connections of the amygdala suggests that it is strategically situated for generating rapid, specific autonomic and endocrine patterns in response to complex social signals. The following outline, which highlights some of these connections, draws primarily on the authoritative anatomical review of Price et al. (1987), and on the results of other investigations cited below.

In primates, the amygdala receives inputs primarily from higher order sensory cortices, both unimodal and polysensory (e.g., Herzog and Van Hoesen, 1976; Iwai and Yukie, 1987). In the case of auditory, visual, gustatory, and somesthetic modalities, regions with the most elaborated processing of sensory input have the heaviest projections to the amygdala (Turner et al. 1980). Olfactory input is distinctive, however, for the olfactory bulb projects directly onto the anterior cortical nucleus and periamygdaloid cortex, without intervening processing (Price, 1973). The amygdala's intimate tie with olfaction is even more pronounced in nonprimates because of input from the accessory olfactory bulb as well (Scalia and Winans, 1975). The persisting tie with olfaction in relatively nonolfactory primates may be residual from the archaic predominance of olfaction over vision in ancestral primates (Allman, 1982).

Amygdala outputs can be conceptualized under two major headings. The first is the reciprocal of the sensory input just described: The amygdala has widespread outputs to sensory association cortex. Indeed, there is evidence in primates for amygdala projections to visual areas which handle sensory information in relatively early stages of processing (Tigges et al., 1983; Iwai and Yukie, 1987). Here we wish to emphasize the second category of major amygdala efferents, those directed to the hypothalamus, which is critical for orchestrating endocrine and autonomic activity. These projections appear to arise from all except the lateral nucleus of the amygdala. In addition, the central nucleus of the amygdala innervates specific brain stem centers which control heart rate and respiratory rate (Kapp et al., 1981; Harper et al., 1984).

The amygdala, then, receives highly processed sensory information in all modalities, and projects directly to subcortical structures which effect changes in physiological state. The value of such a system for a socially living animal may be understood as follows: The perception of another individual's approach should give rise to a specific pattern of autonomic and endocrine activity, tailored to whether the approaching individual's intent is to threaten, to initiate a friendly grooming session, or to copulate. Indeed, exposure of animals in laboratory settings to particular types of social interactions with other animals gives rise to highly specific endocrine and autonomic changes (Weiner, 1977). The finely tuned links between the meanings of social stimuli on the one hand, and the patterns of physiologic activity set into play on the other, presumably are embodied in the network of intrinsic connections in the amygdala. Below, we shall see that the results of amygdala activity are not restricted to changes in internal physiological parameters, but are expressed in complex, patterned behavioral sequences as well.

Reciprocal connections between the amygdala and mesial and orbital frontal cortices are of particular interest in light of the selective deficit in interpreting social stimuli described in patients with lesions in this area (Eslinger and Damasio, 1985; Damasio and Tranel, 1988). Also of significance is a substantial reciprocal pathway between cingulate cortex and the amygdala: The cingulate appears to play a role in the production of vocalizations in monkeys (Robinson, 1967; Jürgens and Ploog, 1970), and in the initiation of speech in humans (Barris and Schuman, 1953; Jürgens and von Cramon, 1982), behavior which is preeminently social.

Finally, reciprocal connections between amygdaloid nuclei and the hippocampal formation may serve to link affective response patterns with the encoding of perceptions in memory, thus providing rapid access to appropriate motivational states when complex social situations or particular individuals are re-encountered.

LESION STUDIES
Aggression, Defense, and Flight Behavior

There have been a number of studies of the effects of complete and partial lesions of the amygdala (or, in reptiles, of homologous structures) on aggression toward conspecifics and toward humans. Studies of reptiles, inbred and wild rats, domestic and wild cats, and New and Old World nonhuman primates have all shown a decrease of aggressive behavior and an increase in tameness (see Table Ia–d). An exception to this was reported by Wood (1958), who found an increase in aggression in half of his cats following discrete lesions of central and basal nuclei. Other studies of cats have also shown occasional increases in aggression toward human experimenters, particularly in females. In studies involving partial or selective lesions of amygdaloid nuclei, which have been carried out mainly in rats, the lateral, basal, and medial nuclei have all been implicated in reduced aggression. Lesions of central nucleus had no effect on aggressive behavior directed at conspecifics but reduced aggressive responses to nociceptive stimuli.

Distinct zones for fear and flight behavior were described by Kaada (1967), who suggested that these two behavioral patterns have separate neural mechanisms, at least in the cat, although not corresponding exactly to anatomically defined nuclei within the amygdala. However, the "defense zone" was found by these authors to be located mainly within the basal nucleus, and its activity conducted to the hypothalamus mainly by the ventral amygdalofugal pathway, as opposed to the stria terminalis. Interruption of the latter, conversely, affected

TABLE Ia. Effects of Amygdala Lesions on Social Behavior in Reptiles

Species	Age	Sex	Group Composition	Observational Setting	Behavior	Reference
Caiman *C. sklerops*	18–24 inches	M & F	Solitary-response	Aquaria	Decreased aggression	Keating et al. (1970)
Fence lizard *S. occidentalis*	Adult	M & F	Groups of 6–8 subjects	Laboratory enclosure	Decreased attention and responsiveness, loss of display behavior for dominance or submission; loss of fear and response to visual social signals	Tarr (1977)

TABLE Ib. Effects of Amygdala Lesions on Social Behavior in Rodents

Species	Age at Lesion	Sex	Group Composition	Observational Setting	Behavior	Reference
D. agouti	Adult	M & F	Solitary and with other species	Large cage and room enclosure	Decreased aggression, tameness, hyperorality, hypersexuality	Schreiner and Kling (1956)
Rat Sprague-Dawley	Adult and pre-weaning	M & F	Conspecific M/F dyads	Cage	Aphagia and adipsia; males would not copulate, females normally receptive	Schwartz and Kling (1964)
Deermouse *P. manculabs bairdii*	Adult	F	Lesioned female paired with normal male	Cage	Lesions of medial n.; no mating in females but they cycled; lesions of basal and lateral n. resulted in hypersexuality	Eleftheriou and Zolovick (1966)
Golden hamster *M. aurtus* LAK-LVG	90–120 days	M & F	Dyads as well as groups of 6	Large hexagonal enclosure with 6 cages in perimeter	Lesions of basal lateral nuclei in dominant subject decreased total social activity; only small loss in submissive subjects; reduced aggression in both groups, no change in rank	Bunnell et al. (1970)
Rat Long-Evans	90–120 days	M & F	Dyads	Circular open-field diam = 4 ft	Reduced contact and social responsiveness with amygdala lesion; septal lesion had reverse effect	Jonason and Enloe (1971)
Golden hamster *M. aurtus* LAK-LVG	90–120 day ovariectomized hormone replacement	F	Lesioned females with normal males	Sound attenuated glass aquaria	Cortical and medial n. lesions resulted in reduced lordosis and ultrasound calls	Kirn and Floody (1985)
Rat Wistar	Adult	F	Lesioned female with pups and male intruder	Large enclosure	Injection of bicuculline results in reduced aggression to males	Hansen and Ferreira (1986)

Rat Tryonmaze dull 53	6 mo	M	Male dyads, intruder vs. resident	Cage	Lesions of medial n. results in reduced offensive behavior, especially in experienced rats	Vochteloo and Koolhaas (1987)
Golden hamster *M. auratus*	Adult virgin and with sex exper. males	M & F	M & F dyads	Plexiglass enclosure with door separating compartments	Lesion of medial n. results in reduced pre- and postcopulatory attack and reduced vaginal scent marking; increase in duration of copulation	Takahashi and Gladstone (1988)
Rat Wistar naive	Adult	M	Normal males with castrated, lesioned males	Cage	Lesions of cortical medial n. suppresses lordosis; lateral n. lesions are without effect; lesions of posterior lateral n. resulted in increased lordosis; anterior lateral lesion decreased lordosis	Chateau and Aron (1988)
Rat Wistar naive	Adult	M	Normal males with castrated, lesioned males	Cage	Lesions of posterior cortical medial n. result in decreased lordosis; anterior cortical medial lesions increased lordosis	Chateau and Aron (1989)
Rat Long-Evans	Sexually experienced adults	F	Lesioned males paired with receptive females	Cage	Males with basolateral lesions show normal or slight increase in copulation; those with cortical medial lesions show severe deficits in copulation and ejaculation	Harris and Sachs (1975)
Albino rat	Adult ovariectomized with hormone replacement	F	M & F dyads	Cage	Lesions of anterior cortical and medial n. result in decreased frequency of lordosis; lesions in posterior lateral n. result in increased receptivity; opposite results with electrical stimulation	Masco and Carrer (1980)

(continued)

TABLE Ib. Effects of Amygdala Lesions on Social Behavior in Rodents (continued)

Species	Age at Lesion	Sex	Group Composition	Observational Setting	Behavior	Reference
Golden hamster *M. aurtus* LAK-LVG	Adult	M	M & F dyads	Cage	Lesions of cortical and medial n. eliminate mating behavior in males; also reduced sniffing and licking	Lehman and Winans (1980)
Rat Wistar	60–90 day	F virgin	Lesioned ovariectomized with 4–10 day old rat pups	Cage: pups placed adjacent to female daily for 11 days	Females with lesion of amygdala or cortex became maternal more rapidly than controls, possibly reduced avoidance; MPOA lesions inhibited maternal behavior	Fleming et al. (1983)
Rat *R. norvegicus* and *R. rattus*	Adult	M & F	Solitary-man	Enclosure	Lesions of medial n. reduced defensiveness; lesion in region of cortical n. reduced flight behavior	Kemble et al. (1984)
Rat Sprague-Dawley albino	Adult	M	Dyads	Plexiglass tube with compartments for confrontations	Lesions of central or lateral n. did not affect aggression or rank; lesions of cortical n. did affect attack and threat; pyriform cortex lesions abolished aggressive behavior as did lesions of BNST and accumbens	Miczek et al. (1974)
Rat Sprague-Dawley albino	Adult	M	Pain induced aggression between conspecifics	Plexiglass tube with compartments for confrontations	Decreased aggression from central or lateral n. but not cortical pyriform or BNST	Miczek et al. (1974)

TABLE Ic. Effects of Amygdala Lesions on Social Behavior in Carnivora

Species	Age at Lesion	Sex	Group Composition	Observational Setting	Behavior	Reference
Domestic cat	Adult	M & F	Pairs and small groups of conspecifics and other species	Cages and free associations in large room	Tameness, decreased fear and aggression, hyperorality; hypersexuality with conspecifics and other species	Schreiner and Kling (1953)
Domestic cat	2–75 days	M & F	Small groups of conspecifics	Room enclosure	Sparing of above syndrome when lesioned prior to 75 days of age	Kling (1962)
Canada lynx L. rufus	Adult	M	With other species	Cage and room enclosure	Tameness, hypersexuality	Schreiner and Kling (1956)
Domestic cat, tame and wild strays	Adult	M & F	Solitary	Laboratory cages	Stereotaxic lesions of flight region results in reduction of flight behavior, less so for defense region	Ursin (1965)
Domestic cat	Adult	M & F	Small groups	Laboratory	Stereotaxic lesions of lateral n. resulted in hypersexuality, lesion of central and basal nuclei in increased aggression, lesions of central and medial nuclei in hyperphagia and hyperorality	Wood (1958)
Domestic cat	Adult	M	Paired with estrous female or with rabbits or with toys	Laboratory enclosure	Lesions of lateral and basal n. resulted in inappropriate mounting and decreased latency to mount	Aronson and Cooper (1979)
Domestic dog spanish beagle terrier	Adult	M & F	Pairs	Enclosure	Loss of preoperative social rank, decrease in aggression, hyperphagia; maternal behavior intact	Fuller et al. (1957)
Domestic dog	Adult	NS	Solitary	Cage	Tame, less fearful	Fonberg, (1968)

TABLE Id. Effects of Bilateral Amygdala Lesions on Social Behavior in Nonhuman Primates

Species	Age at Lesion	Sex	Group Composition	Observational Setting	Behavior	Reference
M. arctoides M. mulatta M. radiata	2–5 days	F	Mother-infant dyads or alone	Laboratory cage	Normal infant behavior; no effect of lesion on maternal deprivation syndrome	Kling and Green (1967)
M. mulatta	2.5 mos	F	Dyads	Laboratory enclosure	Operates show more social fear; decreased social interaction, grooming, and proximity; same deficits at 3.5 and 6 yrs of age when tested with normals	Thompson et al. (1969)
M. mulatta	Juv	M	Dyads	Laboratory enclosure	Hypersexuality, increased grooming and play	Kling (1968)
M. arctoides	Juv	F	Dyads	Laboratory	Decreased grooming, increased mounting; received more aggression from normals	Miller (1968)
M. mulatta	Juv	M	Artificial group	Laboratory enclosure	Fall in rank, decreased aggression in group; in individual cage increase in fear and aggression	Rosvold et al. (1954)
M. arctoides	Adult, juv	M & F	Artificial heterosexual group	Large enclosure	Decreased aggression, grooming, and huddling; fall in rank, hyperorality, hyperphagia	Kling and Cornell (1971)
C. aethiops	Adult, juv	M & F	Artificial heterosexual group	Laboratory cage	Decreased aggression, fall in rank receives more aggression from normals, hyperoral; diminished vocal and postural threat behavior	Kling et al. (1968)

Species	Age	Group	Location	Effects	Reference
S. sciureus	Adult	M	Homosexual group	Laboratory group cage	Fall in rank, hyperorality, decreased fear of snakes, social proximity and aggression	Kling et al. (unpublished observation)
S. sciureus	Adult	M	Homosexual group	Laboratory group cage	Fall in rank, decreased aggression	Plotnik (1968)
M. arctoides	Adult	M & F	Normal heterosexual group with operates	Fenced enclosure and 1/2 acre enclosure LaParaguerra, P.R.	In laboratory: decreased affiliation, hypersexuality fall in rank; in enclosure: social isolation, social indifference, attack by normals	Kling and Dunne (1976)
M. mulatta	Adult, juv	M & F	Natural semi-free-ranging group	Cayo-Santiago, P.R.	Social indifference, decreased aggression, adults expelled from group and died; juvenile operates rejoined group	Dicks et al. (1969)
C. aethiops	Adult, juv	M & F	Natural free-ranging group	Central Africa Savannah, natural habitat	In captivity, decreased aggression, fear, grooming; hyperoral in field; social withdrawal, isolation, and death; juveniles less affected but did not rejoin group	Kling et al. (1970)

flight behavior. A decrease in flight behavior has also been observed following amygdala lesions in the lizard, lesions of the cortical and medial nuclei in the rat, and large amygdala ablations in Old and New World primates (see Table I).

It deserves emphasis that aggressive, fear, and flight behavior are all elements of social interaction. In socially living aimals they will occur predominantly in social encounters, and only occasionally in situations involving predators or other danger. Finally, the ability to signal a disposition to fight or to flee, by producing some elements of the behavior pattern, may be more important in successfully negotiating a social situation than the fully executed behavior.

Social Rank

Studies of the effects of amygdala lesions on social rank in appropriate species have consistently found a decrease in rank in lesioned subjects when confronted with conspecifics. Such effects have been described in the hamster following lesions of the lateral nucleus, while in lizards, dogs, and monkeys, large lesions which included both medial and lateral areas were used (see Table I). However, we have observed alterations in rank in monkeys following lesions which spared portions of the cortical and medial nuclei (Kling and Cornell, 1971).

Social Affiliation

In nonhuman primates, one of the most consistent effects of amygdalectomy is a decrease of affiliative behavior, a decrease which may be expressed as frank social isolation when the subject is placed in a sufficiently complex environment. These findings have been reviewed in several publications (Kling and Steklis, 1976; Steklis and Kling, 1985). A generalized decrease in social interaction has also been noted in the lizard following lesions of structures homologous to the amygdala, and in hamster and rats following lesions of the lateral nucleus (see Table I). No studies specifically addressing this issue have been reported in dogs or cats. The effects of amygdala lesions on the complex social behavior characteristic of canine packs, which includes patterns of affiliative bonding between individuals, have not been studied but would be of considerable interest. The social isolation observed in nonhuman primates does not ameliorate over time. In fact, our observations suggest this symptom intensifies over time.

Reproductive Behavior

Effects of amygdalectomy on copulation and related reproductive behaviors show great variability across species, while remaining consistent across studies carried out within a species. The variability is presumably owing to differences in neural organization which underlie diverse reproductive behavioral strategies. As an example, the hypersexuality observed in *Macaca arctoides* after amygdala lesions is characterized by a broad spectrum of sexual behavior-bizarre forms of homosexual activity, fellatio, and mutual masturbation-which interestingly extended to nonlesioned animals housed with lesioned subjects (Kling and Dunn, 1976). Hypersexuality has not been observed after amygdalectomy in *Cercopithicus aethiops* or *Saimiri sciureus*. It is tempting to speculate that in general, animals whose copulatory activities normally are cued by a variety of stimuli, as opposed to being strictly confined to intervals of hormone-dependent receptivity and triggered by a few stereotyped olfactory or simple visual signals, are likely to display a wider range of aberrant behaviors when amygdalectomized. In fact, however, the striking behavior seen in lesioned *M. arctoides* remains in need of explanation.

The expression of hypersexuality in lesioned monkeys is sensitive to a number of factors, for example, the social environment and age at lesion. The hypersexuality observed in *M. mulatta* is not restricted to conspecifics or to other animals, but is directed toward inanimate objects as well, as first described by Klüver and Bucy (1939).

Turning to other mammals, hypersexuality has also been observed in domestic cat, dog, and lynx (see Table Ic). As in primates, damage to the lateral and basal nuclei have been identified as critical to its expression in carnivores. Also analogous to findings in primates is the observation that hypersexuality in carnivores does not occur if the lesions were originally sustained in the neonatal period (Kling, 1962). In both primates and carnivores, complete ablation of the amygdala, including the medial nuclei, is consistent with the appearance of hypersexuality. Thus, it does not appear that the integrity of the medial group of nuclei is essential for the expression of hypersexuality in these species. It remains unknown to what extent the expression of hypersexuality in cats might be modified if operates were studied under more natural, free-ranging conditions, as has been done in monkeys. This reflects the more general fact that study of the interaction of amygdala lesions with environments of varying complexity has been largely ignored in nonprimates.

In male rodents, lesions of the medial and cortical nucleus abolish copulatory behavior, while basolateral lesions may cause it to increase (see Table Ib). In an early study, Schwartz and Kling (1964) found that large amygdala lesions including medial nuleus did not impair receptivity in female albino rats. Lesioned males, however, failed to copulate. This dichotomy is similar to effects on copulatory behavior after large cortical ablations in rats (Beach, 1940).

In female monkeys, amygdalectomy has devastating effects on maternal behavior, resulting in death for the infants unless they are removed and artificially reared (Steklis and Kling, 1985). The impact of amygdala lesions on maternal behavior has not been studied in cats or dogs. In rodents, virgin females with amygdala lesions appear less fearful of newborn pups and are more maternal than unoperated virgin females (Takahashi and Gladstone, 1988). This effect has been interpreted as a decrease in fear of strange pups. This contrast between the effects of amygdala lesions on maternal behavior in monkey and rat may reflect the more complex functions of the amygdala with evolution.

In summary, review of the literature on amygdala lesions in animals reveals effects on aggression, defense, rank, affiliation, and reproductive behavior. Except in primates, there has been little examination of the impact of the social complexity of the environment on behavioral alteration caused by amygdalectomy.

RECORDING STUDIES

Studies of electrical activity from the amygdaloid nuclei in response to social communications have been carried out mostly in primate species (Table II). In multiunit recordings analyzed by power spectral analysis, it was found that a hierarchy of responses was recorded which correlated with the emotional significance of the stimulus. This was the case for both auditory stimuli (broadcasting of conspecific calls) and projection of visual stimuli. It is of interest that in the squirrel monkey, "isolation peeps" were the most potent stimuli as measured by the power of the delta band (Kling et al., 1987). This is the most primitive of vocalizations and is essential for localization of infants or juveniles separated from their mother or group. Other calls which were very potent were "snake calls" and "alarm peeps." In the case of visual stimuli, primate "threat face" and human faces were consistently more potent than pictures of food or conspecifics.

In a social group, using radiotelemetry, amygdaloid electrical activity also showed a hierarchy of power: The highest power was recorded when the subjects were given ambiguous social communications which could have resulted in a number of different outcomes (e.g., genital inspection, threat face). Other potent stimuli included being chased and aggressed upon. The lowest power outputs were recorded during the tension-reducing behaviors of grooming and huddling.

In squirrel monkeys, ablation of cortical areas projecting to the amygdala had differential effects on electrical activity and social behavior. For example, ablation of the temporal pole resulted in a deficit in social behavior similar to amygdalectomy with a concomitant profound decrease in power from both lateral and medial nuclei. In contrast, ablation of inferior temporal cortex did not impair affiliative behavior and caused reduced power in only the lateral and basal nuclei, leaving the medial nuclei as responsive as before the cortical lesion. This experiment led us (A.K. and R.L., 1987) to conclude that the integrity of the medial nucleus was essential for the maintenance of social bondings, at least in primate species.

Environmental factors also play a role in electrical activity of the amygdala. We found that broadcasting the same conspecific calls when the subject was freely moving in a group cage produced greater power output than to the same stimulus when the subject was seated in a restraining chair and separated from its conspecifics. Thus, the context in which the stimulus is presented modifies amygdala activity.

STIMULATION STUDIES

As Table III shows, behavior produced by amygdala stimulation in animals includes expressions of fearfulness and components of escape, instances of rage and attack behavior, components of copulation sequences such as penile erection (in monkeys), and lordosis (in rats), and vocalization.

In general, the effects of amygdala stimulation are the opposite of those produced by lesions and are accompanied by overt expressions of autonomic discharge. As seen in Table III, nearly all studies of electrical stimulation have

TABLE II. Recording Studies

Species	Age	Sex	Location in the Amygdala	Composition	Setting	Results	Reference
Cat	Adult	NS	Throughout	Solitary	Cage	Single-unit recording; meowing the most effective sensory stimulus	Sawa and Delgado (1963)
Monkey (C. aethiops)	Adult	M & F	NS	Mixed group of 14	Cage	Multiunit recording; highest power outputs in some frequencies occurred in response to ambiguous approaches	Kling et al. (1979)
Monkey (S. sciureus)	Adult	M & F	Throughout	Group of 4	Restraining chair; group	Multiunit recording; medial nucleus critical for social bonding, based on responses to vocalizations	Kling et al. (1987)
Monkey (M. mulatta)	NS	NS	NS	Solitary	Restraining chair	Single-unit recording; 10% of visually responsive neurons responded to faces	Rolls (1981)
Monkey (M. mulatta)	NS	NS	Basal accessory n	Solitary	Restraining chair	Single-unit recording; neurons were selective for faces as opposed to other objects; some were selective for individuals	Leonard et al. (1985)
Monkey (C. aethiops, M. mulatta)	Adult	M & F	Basal n	Small social group	Cage	Multiunit recording; lesions of temporal pole caused decreased amplitude in all frequencies in amygdala, and behavioral effects similar to amygdala lesions	Kling (1981)
Monkey (M. arctoides)	Adult	F	NS	Solitary	Restraining chair	Single-unit recording; responses to components of expressive behavior and social interactions	Brothers et al. (1990)

TABLE III. Stimulation Studies

Species	Age	Sex	Location in Amygdala	Group Composition	Observational Setting	Results	Reference
Rat	Adult	F	Anterior cortical and lateral n.	With 1 male	Observation cage	Increased lordosis to anterior cortical n. stimulation; decreased lordosis to posterior lateral n. stimulation	Masco and Carrer (1980)
Cat	Adult	NS	Medial and central n.	Solitary	NS	Rage	Shealy and Peele (1957)
Cat	Adult	NS	Rostral lateral and central n.; posterior lateral and basal n.	Solitary	NS	Rostral lateral and central n. produced fear; posterior lateral and basal n. stimulation produced anger	Ursin and Kaada (1960)
Cat	Adult	NS	Basolateral n.	Solitary	NS	Defense reaction (pupil dilatation, piloerection, restlessness, growling)	Hilton and Zbrozyna (1963)
Cat	3 wks	M & F	Throughout	Solitary	Cage	Only after 3 weeks of age could affective behavior, including autonomic components, be elicited	Kling and Coustan (1964)

Species	Age	Sex	Brain region	Social condition	Restraint condition	Results	Reference
Dog	NS	NS	Central lateral and basal n.	NS	NS	Defensive behavior resulted from stimulation of dorsomedial part; basolateral stimulation produced fear	Fonberg (1968)
Monkey, cat, dog (*M. mulatta, C. aethiops*)	NS	NS	"Anterior limbic cortex"	Solitary	Under anesthesia	Vocalizations with facial movements seen in monkeys but not in cats or dogs; vocalization occurred in absence of precentral motor cortex	Kaada (1951)
Monkey *M. mulatta*	Adult	M	Basolateral and cortico-medial n.	Solitary	NS	"Krr" and rhythmic grunts accompanied by piloerection	Robinson (1967)
Monkey *M. mulatta*	Adult	M	Cortical	Solitary	Restraining chair	Penile erection	Robinson and Mishkin (1968)
Monkey (*S. sciureus*)	Adult	M & F	Central and basal n.	Solitary	Restraining chair	Growling and cackling elicited; attributed to effects on "inner state"	Jürgens and Ploog (1970)
Monkey *M. mulatta*	NS	NS	Throughout	Solitary	Restraining chair	Rostral and lateral stimulation produced fear responses; caudal and medial zone stimulation produced defense behavior	Ursin (1972)

been carried out in a solitary condition. It would be of interest to know how social and environmental factors would affect responses elicited in a social milieu, as has been done for other structures by Delgado (1967), who found major differences in the effects of stimulation in the same site depending on the social rank of the experimental subject.

THE ROLE OF THE AMYGDALA IN SOCIAL SIGNALING SYSTEMS

It is of note that the amygdala appears to participate both in encoding social events and in producing patterned motor-autonomic behavioral sequences pertinent to social interactions.

As outlined in Table II, single neurons in the amygdala take part in encoding social events. In 1963, Sawa and Delgado demonstrated that the most effective sensory stimulus for driving amygdala units in cats was a miaowing sound. Later, in macaque monkey, Rolls (1981) and then Leonard et al. (1985) demonstrated that some amygdala units were selective for faces from among a wide array of visual objects. While such units did not respond exclusively to faces, responses to this category greatly exceeded response to any other objects, as well as to nonface stimuli which were known to be arousing and aversive. Furthermore, some of these neurons responded selectively to pictures of particular individuals. These responsive neurons were found primarily in the region of the basal accessory nucleus.

Recent observations in our laboratory, using short moving sequences containing a variety of body views and movements as stimuli, extend these findings (Brothers et al., 1990). For example, we have recorded unit activity in central and medial regions of the macaque amygdala which is selectively responsive to views of swinging limb movements in monkeys typical of walking or trotting; we have detected responses to movements of the head and of facial features; and we have described a neuron which appears tuned to various depictions of an interaction taking place between two other individuals (Brothers et al., in preparation). Such findings suggest that the amygdala is an integral part of a neural system, highly developed in group living primates, that has undergone considerable selection pressure favoring the accurate encoding of social events. This hypothesized system presumably also includes regions of the superior temporal sulcus and inferotemporal cortex (Perrett et al., 1982; Desimone et al., 1984; Baylis et al., 1985; Yamane et al. 1988) as well as other areas with direct amygdala connections.

AFFECTIVE BEHAVIOR

One of the pervasive changes observed after amygdalectomy in monkeys is affective blunting. This symptom was noted by Klüver and Bucy (1939) and has been described in virtually all studies since. The absence of affective responses to normally arousing or exciting stimuli occurs in all environments and is not restricted to either field or confined conditions. This deficit (affect) may be responsible for the failure of social affiliation in amygdalectomized monkeys. That is, without affect, social affiliations are meaningless and would appear to the observer as social indifference. Since carnivores exhibit a diminished repertoire of affective social expression compared with primates, blunting is less demonstrable; it has, however, been noted in wild species.

Corollary neurophysiological findings in the monkey amygdala shed interesting light on the neural basis of emotion. In multiunit recording studies, a stable hierarchy of power in the delta frequency range is produced in various sites in the amygdala in response to a set of emotionally significant visual and auditory stimuli (Kling et al., 1987). Ablation of inferior temporal cortex which projects to the amygdala, fails to produce either alterations of affective expression in response to the stimulus set or alterations of social behavior. Such lesions do, however, cause reduction in delta power elicited by the stimuli, but only in the lateral group of nuclei, not the medial. In contrast, ablation of temporal pole causes behavioral deficits similar to those following amygdalectomy, and also causes marked reduction in delta power in the medial amygdala (Kling, 1981). From this one can conclude that, at least in primates, the medial but not the lateral nuclei are essential for the response to emotionally arousing stimuli, that is, for affective expression. Whether medial nuclei possess a similar role in carnivores and rodents has not been studied. In light of its evolutionary history, however, this group of nuclei would seem likely to have preserved a consistent functional relationship to affective and social behavior through phylogeny.

As pointed out above, the amygdala is known to receive highly processed sensory input from all modalities, and from polymodal cortex. The relative roles of the lateral and medial groups in the processing sequence are still being worked out. What emerges, however, is that there are multiple opportunities for sensory convergence, at the level of cortical inputs and at the level of single neurons. This anatomical arrangement, together with the behavioral and physiological observations described above, leads us to propose the following: Affect is no more and no less than the confluence and integration of sensory information in several modalities, combined with immediate coactivation of somatic effector systems (motor, autonomic, and endocrine). In support of this assertion, we note that brain regions which possess both the connectivity necessary for polymodal sensory convergence and direct access to effector structures are capable of generating emotional experience upon stimulation.

We may here touch on a few points regarding this proposal. One, it is consistent with the peripheralism of William James, but it requires an important addition to the effector aspect, namely, concomitant sensory integration. For our purposes, integrated sensory experience need not, however, be tied to current stimulation: While primary sensory cortical activation may occur and ultimately give rise to emotional experience, such experience could also be generated by the activation of mnemonic traces at polymodal or high-order sensory levels alone (provided several modalities are involved and they activate structures such as the amygdala which are linked to effectors). Thus, this proposal is consistent with the well-known tie between memory and emotion. Finally, it encompasses both the display (effector) aspects of emotion dear to ethologists and behaviorists, and the subjective (sensory) aspects dear to psychoanalysts and artists, without resorting to nonneural terms of explanation.

It deserves to be noted that amygdala lesions do not necessarily result in a total inability to generate emotional responses or appropriate reactions: In the presence of a strong-enough stimulus or threat, the offended subjects are seen to be capable of retreating or defending themselves. It appears that the affective response can still be elicited, but with a higher threshold. It is possible that anatomically related structures such as orbital frontal cortex, temporal pole, or cingulate are recruited, or that cortical projections directly to hypothalamus are capable of effecting the responses.

DISCUSSION

From this review we can safely infer that a perceptual apparatus and an effector apparatus are colocalized in the amygdala. This suggests that, for social stimuli, perception and reaction are intimately entwined. And, indeed, when an animal subject views a display (or is mounted, or groomed, or hears a call), a behavioral sequence is called forth ("released"). For example, an animal which is confronted by the threat expression of another grimaces and crouches quickly and automatically without prolonged evaluation and assessment. Such automatic, patterned reactions to social displays are ubiquitous, occurring in all mobile animals which mate and which defend territory. Apparently, automatic social responses not mediated by neocortical processing have worked well in non-mammals, and are the substrate of social behavior in mammals as well. There is no reason to postulate an elaborate evaluative process occurring prior to the released behavior. Instead, as is implied in our discussion of affects above, we believe that the internal and external states which constitute the response to the stimulus are identical with the "evaluation" of the stimulus. This understanding sheds light on what otherwise appears to be a dual aspect of amygdala function, namely, that responses to social sensory stimuli may be elicited in amygdala recordings, while amygdala stimulation produces patterned social displays.

An animal whose pupils are dilated, whose fur is erect, and which is hissing or growling also may be presumed to be feeling something. In consequence, not only overt behavior but also subjective sensations are integral to acts of social response. While it is well known that electrical stimulation of the amygdala in humans may elicit subjective emotional states, of which fear is the most frequent, the findings of Gloor with respect to elicited mnemonic fragments in patients undergoing amygdala stimulation have been insufficiently appreciated in respect to their implications for the mechanisms of social perception (Gloor, 1986). Often such fragments contain representations of other individuals directing an action toward the subject (speaking to him, threatening him physically, having sexual intercourse with him), and these scenes are accompanied by subjective feelings such as fear or pleasure. Such feelings, we suggest, would under normal circumstances be part of the automatically released responses to significant acts of others. As such, they would constitute the cognitive core of the evaluations of others' intentions ("displays") (Brothers, 1990). From the foregoing, it would appear likely that in human beings, the neural representations of the dispositions and intentions of others are mediated at least in part by amygdala activity.

One of us (L.B.) has speculated that a trend seen in primates toward increasingly complex group life has created the conditions for an expansion of the array of innate affects which the central nervous system can generate (Brothers, 1990). Such affects would constitute critical inner signals to their possessor, immediately differentiating the playful intentions of an ally from those of a foe, or the solicitations of a dominant from those of a subordinate, etc. Far from some idealized "primary emotions" or blends of these, social affects form a vast but discriminable palette of feeling, for example, "as if you are demanding," and "as if I am guilty," or "as if I did not belong here (like being at a party and not being welcome)" (Gloor, 1986). Such feelings, elicited in these examples by electrical stimulation, could under normal circumstances be thought of as the "readouts" of others' displays.

Hypotheses regarding the effects of amygdalectomy on social behavior have been largely species-specific. For example, it has been tacitly assumed that in primates it is the failure to correctly evaluate visual information which accounts for the behavioral effects. Split-brain experiments, however, which produce unusually docile behavior only when visual information is presented to the amygdalectomized hemisphere (Downer, 1962), have been carried out in species which rely heavily on visual signaling. Studies of multiunit electrical activity in species which rely heavily on auditory signaling, however, suggest that an emotional evaluation of auditory signals takes place in the amygdala as well (Lloyd and Kling, 1987). What remains to be studied is how, in species with differing predominance of sensory modalities, amygdala activity is affected by activation in the various modalities. For example, does the amygdala favor auditory input in anosmic animals such as cetacea and chiroptera? It also remains to be understood at what level integration of different modalities occurs; that is, whether single neurons in the amygdala might respond to combinations of auditory, visual, olfactory, or somesthetic aspects of complex social stimuli. Perhaps some answers to these questions will be presented in the next volume.

ACKNOWLEDGMENTS

This work was supported by the Department of Veterans Affairs.

REFERENCES

Allman J (1982): Reconstructing the evolution of the brain in primates through the use of comparative neurophysiological and neuroanatomical data. In Armstrong E, Falk D (eds): "Primate Brain Evolution: Methods and Concepts." New York: Plenum Press.

Aronson LR, Cooper ML (1979): Amygdaloid hypersexuality in male cats re-examined. Physiol Behav 22:257–265.

Barris RW, Schuman HR (1953): Bilateral anterior cingulate gyrus lesions. Neurology 3:44–52.

Baylis GC, Rolls ET, Leonard CM (1985): Selectivity between faces in the responses of a population of neurons in the cortex in the superior temporal sulcus of the monkey. Brain Res 342:91–102.

Beach FA (1940): Effects of cortical lesions upon the copulatory behavior of male rats. J Comp Psychol 29:193–239.

Ben-Ari Y (1981): "The Amygdaloid Complex." Amsterdam: Elsevier.

Brothers LA (1990): The social brain: A project for integrating primate behavior and neurophysiology in a new domain. Concepts Neurosci 1:27–51.

Brothers LA, Ring BD, Kling AS (1990): Response of temporal lobe neurons to social stimuli in *Macaca arctoides*. Soc Neurosci Abstr 00:000–000.

Bunnell BN, Sodetz FJ, Shalloway DI (1970): Amygdaloid lesions and social behavior in the golden hamster. Physiol Behav 5:153–161.

Chateau D, Aron CL (1988): Heterotypic sexual behavior in male rats after lesions in different amygdaloid nuclei. Hormones Behav 22:379–388.

Chateau D, Aron CL (1989): Lordosis behavior in male rats after lesions in different regions of the corticomedial amygdaloid nucleus. Hormones Behav 23:448–455.

Damasio AR, Tranel D (1988): Domain-specific amnesia for social knowledge. Soc Neurosci Abstr 516:3.

Delgado JMR (1967): Social rank and radio stimulated aggressiveness in monkeys. J Nerv Ment Dis 144:383–390.

Desimone R, Albright TD, Gross CG, Bruce C (1984): Stimulus-selected properties of inferior temporal neurons in the macaque. J Neurosci 4:2051–2062.

Dicks D, Meyers RE, Kling A (1969): Uncus and amygdala lesions: Effects on social behavior in the free-ranging rhesus monkey. Science 165:69–71.

Downer CJL (1962): Interhemispheric integration in the visual system. In Mountcastle VB (ed): "Interhemispheric Relations and Cerebral Dominance." Baltimore: Johns Hopkins Press.

Eleftheriou BE, Zolovick AJ (1966): Effect of amygdaloid lesions on oestrous behavior in the deermouse. J Reprod Fert 11:451–453.

Eleftheriou BE (1972): "The Neurobiology of the Amygdala." New York, London: Plenum Press.

Eslinger PJ, Damasio AR (1985): Severe disturbance of higher cognition after bilateral frontal lobe ablation: Patient EVR. Neurology 35:1731–1741.

Fleming AS, Miceli M, Moretto D (1983): Lesions of the medial pre-optic area prevent the facilitation of maternal behavior produced by amygdala lesions. Physiol Behav 31:503–510.

Fonberg E (1968): The role of the amygdaloid nucleus in animal behavior. In Asratyou EA (ed): "Progress in Brain Research," Vol 22. Amsterdam: Elsevier, pp 273–281.

Fuller JL, Rosvold HE, Pribram KH (1957): The effect on affective and cognitive behavior in the dog of lesions of the pyriform-amygdala-hippocampal complex. J Comp Physiol Psychol 50:86–96.

Gloor P (1986): The role of the human limbic system in perception, memory, and affect: Lessons from temporal lobe epilepsy. In Doane BK, Livingston KE (eds): "The Limbic System: Functional Organization and Clinical Disorders." New York: Raven Press.

Hansen S, Ferreira A (1986): Effects of bicuciline infusions in the ventromedial hypothalamus and amygdaloid complex on food intake and affective behavior in mother rats. Behav Neurosci 100:410–415.

Harper RM, Frysinger RC, Trelease RB et al. (1984): State-dependent alteration of respiratory cycle timing by stimulation of the central nucleus of the amygdala. Brain Res 306:1–8.

Harris VS, Sachs BD (1975): Copulatory behavior in male rats following amygdaloid lesions. Brain Res 896:514–518.

Herzog AG, Van Hoesen GW (1976): Temporal neocortical afferent connections to the amygdala in the rhesus monkey. Brain Res 115:57–69.

Hilton SM, Zbrozyna AW (1963): Amygdaloid region for defence reactions and its efferent pathway to the brain stem. J Physiol 16:160–173.

Iwai E, Yukie M (1987): Amygdalofugal and amygdalopetal connections with modality specific visual cortical areas in macaques (*M. fuscata, M. mulatta, M. fascicularis*). J Comp Neurol 261:362–287.

Jonason KR, Enloe LJ (1971): Alterations in social behavior following septal and amygdaloid lesions in the rat. J Comp Physiol Psychol 75:286–301.

Jürgens U, Ploog D (1970): Cerebral representation of vocalization in the squirrel monkey. Exp Brain Res 10:532–554.

Jürgens U, von Cramon D (1982): On the role of the anterior cingulate cortex in phonation: A case report. Brain Lang 15:234–248.

Kaada BR (1951): Somato-motor, autonomic, and electrocorticographic responses to electrical stimulation of "rhinencephalic" and other structures in primates, cat, and dog. Acta Physiologica Scand (1):24.

Kaada B (1967): Brain mechanisms related to aggressive behavior. In Clemente CD, Lindsley DB (eds): "Aggression and Defense: Neural Mechanisms and Social Patterns." Los Angeles: University of California Press, pp 95–124.

Kapp BS, Gallagher M, Frysinger RC (1981): The amygdala, emotion, and cardiovascular conditioning. In Ben Ari Y (ed): "The Amygaloid Complex." Amsterdam: Elsevier/North Holland, pp 355–366.

Keating GE, Kormann, Horel A (1970): The behavioral effects of stimulating and ablating the reptilian amygdala. Physiol Behav 5:55–59.

Kemble E, Blanchard CE, Takushi R (1984): Taming in wild rats following medial amygdaloid lesions. Physiol Behav 32:231–234.

Kirn J, Floody OR (1985): Differential effects of lesions in three limbic areas on ultrasound production and lordosis by female hamsters. Behav Neurosci 99:1142–1152.

Kling A (1962): Amygdalectomy in the kitten. Science 137:429–430.

Kling A, Coustan D (1964): Electrical stimulation of the amygdala and hypothalamus in the kitten. Exp Neurol 10:81–89.

Kling A (1965): Behavioral and somatic development following lesions of the amygdala in the cat. J Psychiat Res 3:263–273.

Kling A, Green PC (1967): Effects of amygdalectomy in the maternally reared and maternally deprived neonatal and juvenile macaque. Nature 212:742.

Kling A (1968): Effects of amygdalectomy and testosterone on social behavior of male juvenile macaques. J Physiol Psychol 65:466.

Kling A, Dicks D, Gurowitz EM (1968): Amygdalectomy and social behavior in a caged group of vervets (*C. aethiops*). Proceedings 2nd International Congress of Primates, Vol 1. Atlanta, New York: Karger, Basel, pp 232–241.

Kling A, Lancaster J, Benitone J (1970): Amygdalectomy in the free-ranging vervet. J Psychiat Res 7:191–199.

Kling A, Cornell R (1971): Amygdalectomy and social behavior in the caged stump-tailed macaque (*M. speciosa*). Folia Primatol 14:91–103.

Kling A, Dunne K (1976): Social-environmental factors affecting behavior and plasma testosterone in normal and amygdala lesioned *M. speciosa*. Primates 17:23–42.

Kling A, Steklis HD (1976): A neural substrate for affiliative behavior in nonhuman primates. Brain Behav Evol 13:216–238.

Kling A, Steklis HD, Deutsch S (1979): Radiotelemetered activity from the amygdala during social interactions in the monkey. Exp Neurol 66:88–96.

Kling A (1981): Influence of temporal lobe lesions on radio-telemetered electrical activity of amygdala to social stimuli in monkey. In Ben-Ari Y (ed): "The Amygdaloid Complex." Amsterdam: Elsevier, pp 271–280.

Kling AS, Lloyd RL, Perryman KM (1987): Slow wave changes in amygdala to visual, auditory, and social stimuli following lesions of the inferior temporal cortex in squirrel monkey (*Saimiri sciureus*). Behav Neural Biol 47:54–72.

Klüver H, Bucy P (1939): Preliminary analysis of functions of the temporal lobes in monkeys. Arch Neurol Psychiat 42:979–1000.

Lehman MN, Winans SS (1980): Medial nucleus of the amygdala mediates chemosensory control of male hamster sexual behavior. Science 210:557–560.

Leonard CM, Rolls ET, Wilson FAW, Baylis GC (1985): Neurons in the amygdala of the monkey with responses selective for faces. Behav Brain Res 15:159–176.

Lloyd RL, Kling AS (1987): Amygdaloid electrical activity in response to conspecific calls in squirrel monkey (*S. sciureus*): Influence of environmental setting, cortical inputs and recording site. In Newman JO (ed): "Physiological Control of Mammalian Vocalization." New York: Plenum Press.

Masco DH, Carrer HF (1980): Sexual receptivity in female rats after lesion or stimulation in different amygdaloid nuclei. Physiol Behav 24:1073–1080.

Miczek KA, Brycznski T, Grossman SP (1974): Differential effects of lesions of the amygdala, periamygdaloid cortex and stria terminalis in aggressive behavior in rats. J Comp Physiol Psychol 87:760–771.

Miller R (1968): Effects of amygdalectomy on sexual behavior in juvenile female monkeys (*M. speciosa*). Master's thesis, Illinois Institute of Technology.

Perrett DI, Rolls ET, Caan W (1982): Visual neurons responsive to faces in the monkey temporal cortex. Exp Brain Res 47:329–342.

Plotnik R (1968): Changes in social behavior of squirrel monkeys after anterior temporal lobectomy. J Comp Physiol Psychiat 66:369–377.

Price JL (1973): An autoradiographic study of complementary laminar patterns of termination of afferent fibers to the olfactory cortex. J Comp Neurol 150:87–108.

Price JL, Russchen FT, Amaral DG (1987): The amygdaloid complex. In Bjorklund A, Hokfelt T, Swanson LW (eds): "Handbook of Chemical Neuroanatomy, Vol. 5, Integrated Systems, Part I." Amsterdam: Elsevier.

Robinson BW (1967): Vocalization evoked from forebrain in *Macaca mulatta*. Physiol Behav 2:345–354.

Robinson BW, Mishkin M (1968): Penile erection evoked from forebrain structures in *Macaca mulatta*. Arch Neurol 19:184–198.

Rolls ET (1981): Responses of amygdaloid neurons in the primate. In Ben-Ari Y (ed): "The Amygdaloid Complex." Amsterdam: Elsevier pp 383–393.

Rosvold HE, Mirsky AF, Pribram KH (1954): Influence of amygdalectomy on social behavior in monkeys. J Comp Physiol Psychol 47:173–178.

Sawa M, Delgado JMR (1963): Amygdala unitary activity in the unrestrained cat. Electroencephalogr Clin Neurophysiol 15:637–650.

Scalia F, Winans SS (1975): The differential projections of the olfactory bulb and accessory olfactory bulb in mammals. J Comp Neurol 161:31–55.

Schreiner L, Kling A (1953): Behavioral changes following rhinencephalic injury in cat. J Neurophysiol 16:643–659.

Schreiner L, Kling A (1956): Rhinencephalon and behavior. Am J Physiol 184:486–490.

Schwartz NB, Kling A (1964): The effect of amygdaloid lesions on feeding, grooming and reproduction in rats. Acta Neuroveget 26:12–34.

Shealy CN, Peele TL (1957): Studies of the amygdaloid nucleus of the cat. J Neurophysiol 20:125–135.

Steklis HD, Kling A (1985): Neurobiology of affiliative behavior in non-human primates. In Reite M, Field T (eds): "The Psychobiology of Attachment and Separation." New York: Academic Press, pp 93–129.

Stephan H, Frahm HD, Baron G (1984): Comparison of brain structure volume in insectivora and primates: III. Amygdaloid components. J Hirnforsch 28:571–584.

Takahashi LK, Gladstone CF (1988): Medial amygdaloid lesions and the regulation of sociosexual behavioral patterns across the estrous cycle in female golden hamsters. Behav Neurosci 102:268–275.

Tarr RS (1977): Role of the amygdala in the intraspecies aggressive behavior of the iguana lizard, *Sceloporus occidentalis*. Physiol Behav 18:1153–1158.

Thompson C, Schwartzbaum JS, Harlow HF (1969): Development of social fear after amygdalectomy in infant rhesus monkeys. Physiol Behav 4:249–254.

Tigges J, Walker LC, Tigges M (1983): Subcortical projections to the occipital and parietal lobes of the chimpanzee brain. J Comp Neurol 220:106–115.

Turner BH, Mishkin M, Knapp M (1980): Organization of the amygdalopetal modality-specific cortical association areas in the monkey. J Comp Neurol 191:515–543.

Ursin H (1965): The effect of amygdaloid lesions on flight and defense behavior in cats. Exp Neurol 11:61–79.

Ursin H, Kaada BR (1960): Functional localization within the amygdaloid complex in the cat. Electroencephalogr Clin Neurophysiol 12:1–20.

Ursin H (1972): Limbic control of emotional behavior. In Hitchcock E, Laitinen L, Vaernet K (eds): "Psychosurgery." Springfield: Charles C. Thomas.

Vochteloo JD, Koolhaas JM (1987): Medial amygdala lesions in male rats reduce aggressive behavior: Interference with experience. Physiol Behav 41:99–102.

Weiner H (1977): "Psychobiology and Human Disease." New York: Elsevier, pp 140–143.

Wood CD (1958): Behavioral changes following discrete lesions of temporal lobe structures. Neurology 8:215–220.

Yamane S, Kaji S, Kawano K (1988): What facial features activate face neurons in the inferotemporal cortex of the monkey? Exp Brain Res 73:209–214.

The Amygdala: Neurobiological Aspects of Emotion,
Memory, and Mental Dysfunction, pages 379–399
© 1992 Wiley-Liss, Inc.

14

Learning and Memory in Rats With an Emphasis on the Role of the Amygdala

RAYMOND P. KESNER
Department of Psychology, University of Utah, Salt Lake City, Utah

INTRODUCTION

The literature on the neurobiological basis of memory in rodents is voluminous. On the one hand there are a large number of theoretical approaches aimed at the understanding of the neurobiological basis of memory, and on the other hand there are many neural regions that have been implicated as critical substrates of memory. Therefore, in this chapter there is an emphasis on only one theoretical approach, namely the attribute model of memory, and only one neural region, namely the amygdala. Based on the idea that there might be multidimensional representations of memory rather than a single or dual representation and that specific localizable neural regions can mediate or code for these multidimensional representations, Kesner and DiMattia (1987) have proposed an attribute model of memory (see Fig. 1).

Based on earlier suggestions by Underwood (1969) and Spear (1976), the attribute model proposes that any specific memory is composed of a set of features or attributes that are specific and unique for each learning experience. In animal memory experiments, a set of at least five salient attributes characterizes the structural organization of memory. These are labeled space, sensory-perception, time, response, and affect. A spatial attribute within this framework involves the coding and storage of specific stimuli representing places or relationships between places, which are usually independent of the subject's own body schema. It is exemplified by the ability to encode and remember maps and to localize stimuli in external space.

A sensory-perceptual attribute involves the encoding and storage of a set of sensory stimuli that are organized in the form of cues as part of a specific experience. A temporal attribute involves the encoding and storage of specific stimuli or sets of spatially or temporally separated stimuli as part of an episode marking or tagging its occurrence in time, that is, separating one specific episode from

Address correspondence to: Raymond P. Kesner, Department of Psychology, University of Utah, Salt Lake City, UT 84112.

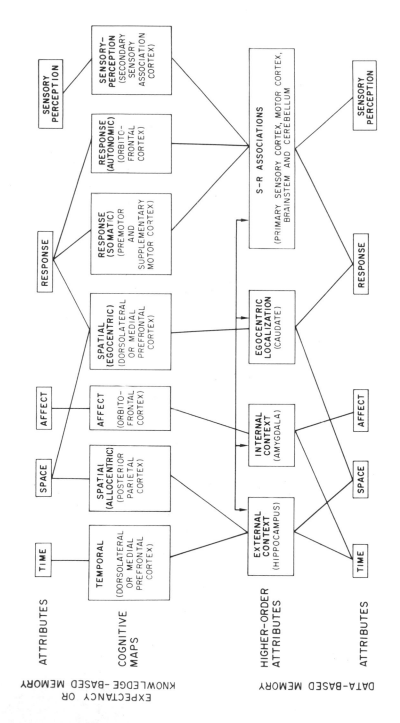

Fig. 1. Psychological and neural organization of data-based and expectancy or knowledge-based memory.

previous or succeeding episodes. A response attribute involves the encoding and storage of information based on feedback from responses that occur in specific situations as well as the selection of appropriate responses. An affect attribute involves the encoding and storage of reinforcement contingencies that result in positive or negative emotional experiences.

The organization of these attributes can take many forms utilizing both serial and parallel systems. Interactions between attributes can aid in identifying specific neural regions that might subserve a critical interaction. For example, the interaction between temporal and affect attributes can provide important information concerning the internal context (internal state of the organism), which is important in evaluating emotional experiences. It is assumed that the amygdala is critically involved in the coding of such affect-temporal attributes. Another important interaction involves the spatial and temporal attributes. In this case the interaction can provide for the external context of a situation, which is important in determining when and where critical events occurred. It is assumed that the hippocampal formation is critically involved in the coding of such spatial-temporal attributes.

In the attribute model it is not only assumed that specific memories are represented by a set of attributes, but they are also processed in data-based and expectancy or knowledge-based memory systems. The data-based memory system is biased toward the coding of incoming data concerning the present, with an emphasis on facts, data, and events that are usually personal and that occur within specific external and internal environmental contexts. In contemporary information-processing theory terms, the emphasis of the data-based memory system is on "bottom-up" processing. During initial learning there is a great emphasis on the data-based memory system, which will continue to be of importance even after initial learning in situations where trial unique or novel information needs to be remembered. It is assumed that the amygdala codes affect-temporal attributes only within the data-based memory system.

The expectancy or knowledge-based memory system is biased toward previously stored information and can be thought of as one's general knowledge of the world. It can operate in the abstract in the absence of critical incoming data. From an information-processing view, the emphasis of the expectancy or knowledge-based memory system is on "top-down" processing.

Memories within the expectancy or knowledge-based memory system are assumed to be organized as a set of cognitive maps and their interactions that are unique for each memory. The exact nature and organization of knowledge structures within each cognitive map need to be determined. The cognitive maps are labeled spatial (allocentric), spatial (egocentric), temporal, affect, response (somatic), response (autonomic), and sensory-perceptual, and are influenced by a set of attributes such as space, time, affect, response, and sensory-perception, as well as interactions between attributes such as space and response. Note that the same attributes are also associated with the data-based memory system. It is assumed that the neocortex mediates different sets of cognitive maps. Support for this assumption can be found in Kesner and DiMattia (1987).

The expectancy or knowledge-based memory system tends to be of greater importance after a task has been learned, given that the situation is invariant and familiar. In most situations, however, one would expect a contribution of both data-based and knowledge-based systems with varying proportion of involvement of one relative to the other.

Even though the attribute model is comprehensive and involves many neural regions, the emphasis here is placed on the amygdala. In addition, there is some discussion of specific neocortical regions and hippocampus. An attempt is made to illustrate with the use of a variety of behavioral paradigms the amygdala's assumed role in subserving memory functions within the attribute model of memory.

Within the attribute model, it is assumed that for the data-based memory system the amygdala subserves the interaction between affect and temporal attributes (internal context), but the amygdala does not play a role in coding somatic responses, spatial location, or sensory-perceptual attributes. The amygdala also does not play a role in representing knowledge-based memory for any of the proposed attributes.

A comprehensive review of the anatomy of the rat amygdala has been described (see Chapter 1, Amaral, this volume). Thus, it is not necessary to detail the connections to and from the amygdala. It is clear that there are a large number of neocortical, limbic, diencephalic, and brain stem interconnections with the amygdala. There are also many intrinsic connections among the subnuclei of the amygdala. Thus, the amygdala has the potential richness in anatomical organization and connections that is probably required for a critical role in mediating memory function.

WHAT INFORMATION IS CODED IN THE AMYGDALA

Does the amygdala code all attributes or a subset of critical attributes associated with memory? The attribute model assumes the amygdala codes primarily affect-temporal attribute information (internal context). Alternative views have been presented by LeDoux (1986), Aggleton and Mishkin (1986), and Murray (1990), who emphasize the importance of sensory-perceptual attributes in representing memory within the amygdala, and McGaugh (1989), who emphasizes the importance of peripheral feedback from the autonomic nervous system and hormones on the amygdala in modulating memory. I review herein some of the literature that pertains to the nature of information processing in the amygdala of the rat.

Affect Attribute

Before assessing whether the amygdala codes an affect attribute of memory, it is necessary to determine whether the amygdala is involved in the mediation of emotional experiences.

First, there are many reciprocal neuroanatomical connections between the amygdala (especially central nucleus), hypothalamus, and the autonomic nervous system (Kapp et al., 1984). Second, lesions of the amygdala in both animals and humans result in placidity, characterized by an almost complete lack of aggression, a markedly reduced emotional reaction to noxious stimuli, fearless exploration of novel and potentially dangerous stimuli, and a reduction in acquiring new learning based on fear (Goddard, 1964; Narabayashi, 1972; Kapp et al.,1984). Third, electrical stimulation of the amygdala in animals and humans can elicit a variety of emotional experiences (e.g., fear, rage, attack, flight, pleasure) with accompanying autonomic responses, including changes in heart rate, blood pressure, respiration, piloerection, and pupillary dilation (Mark and Ervin, 1970; Kaada, 1972). Fourth, rewarding self-stimulation can be obtained from the amygdala in both animals and humans (Wurtz and Olds, 1963; Heath, 1964). Fifth, unpleasurable emotional experiences in humans are often accompanied by changes in the amygdala EEG (Heath, 1964). Sixth, single cells within the amygdala of monkeys primarily respond to positive and negative stimuli and these responses can be altered depending on the significance and affective salience of the stimulus (Nishijo et al., 1988). Seventh, pre- or posttraining electrical stimulation, chemical stimulation, or lesions of the amygdala produce profound memory deficits in a variety of tasks in which reinforcement contingencies of sufficiently high magnitude are used. Some of the tasks include inhibitory (passive) and active avoidance, shock-motivated visual discrimination, taste aversion, fear-potentiated startle, and delayed matching-to-sample learning (McDonough and Kesner, 1971; Gold et al., 1975, 1976; Kesner et al., 1975; Todd and Kesner, 1978; Kesner and Andrus, 1982; Hitchcock and Davis, 1986).

On the basis of the above studies, which support a role for the amygdala in mediating emotional experiences, the attribute model proposes that the amygdala is critically involved in the encoding of emotional (positive and negative) attributes (internal context) of memory.

It should be noted that this idea is an extension of earlier theoretical notions that the amygdala is involved in the interpretation and integration of reinforcing stimuli (Weiskrantz, 1956), serves as a reinforcement register (Douglas and Pribram, 1966), or mediates stimulus-reinforcement associations (Jones and Mishkin, 1972). What triggers an affect attribute of memory? It appears to be activated by reinforcement, which, in turn, has sensory qualities and intrinsic incentive value, such as taste and nutrition in the case of food, and pain and fear in the case of footshock. However, the sensory qualities of the reinforcing stimulus such as taste, odor, visual appearance, or pain are not sufficient to trigger an affect attribute of memory; neither is the intrinsic incentive value of the reinforcement. It is assumed that there are two necessary conditions. First, reinforcement needs to be of sufficient intensity to elicit a strong emotional reaction as well as arousal and a variety of autonomic changes. Second, reinforcement needs to be attended to either because of the expectation of a subsequent memory test for the reinforcing stimuli or in anticipation of an important future event based on the presence of the reinforcing stimuli. The latter might involve an interaction with the coding of temporal attributes.

Once the internal context is represented in the amygdala, then an association can be made with external contextual stimuli and other attributes mediated by different neural regions.

One approach to test the proposed role of the amygdala is to vary the magnitude of reinforcement in situations involving either negative or positive reinforcement contingencies. As an example, Gold et al. (1975) showed that, in a passive avoidance learning situation, posttrial amygdala stimulation disrupts long-term retention when high footshock levels (2 mA, 2 sec) were used, but has no disruptive effect on long-term retention as compared with unoperated controls when low footshock levels (.5 mA, .5 sec) were used. [Electrical stimulation of the amygdala is thought to disturb its normal function (Kesner, 1982).]

In support of Gold et al.'s findings, other studies using high levels of footshock also have found a disruption of long-term retention following amygdala stimulation (McDonough and Kesner, 1971; Bresnahan and Routtenberg, 1972; Kesner and Conner, 1974; Baker et al., 1981); whereas in one study in which relatively weak footshock was used, amygdala stimulation failed to disrupt learning of conditioned emotional responses (Lidsky et al., 1970).

There are also data showing that amygdala-lesioned animals do not increase their running speed (frustration effect) following omission of a reward or otherwise alter their behavior as a function of increases or decreases in reward magnitude (Schwartzbaum, 1960; Kemble and Beckman, 1970; Henke, 1977).

A second approach is to test for a possible differential role of the amygdala in appetitive learning situations in which it is difficult to elicit a strong emotional arousal reaction compared to aversive learning situations in which it is easy to elicit strong emotional responses. Support for such a role was provided recently by Cahill and McGaugh (1990). They demonstrated that NMDA-induced amygdala lesions did not disrupt retention of place learning or odor conditioning when water consumption was used as an appetitive reinforcer or 0.2% quinine was used as a weak aversive stimulus. In contrast, retention was clearly disrupted in the same place learning and odor conditioning tasks when footshock was used as a strong aversive stimulus.

A third approach is to vary the expected value of reinforcement in anticipation of a specific magnitude of reward. Thus, Kesner and Andrus (1982) trained rats in a symbolic (one type of food) delayed spatial matching-to-sample task using an eight-arm radial maze. When the animals were provided with differential cues predicting a small or large reward, retention at a 23 hour delay was better for the large reward. It is assumed that a large reward results in greater affect. Electrical stimulation of the amygdala during 10 sec exposure to the appropriate food cue, which predicted a large reward, impaired performance. No disruptive effects were observed for the small reward. In this case amygdala stimulation appears to disrupt retention in the case where there is a magnitude of reinforcement effect; that is, fewer errors for the expectation of greater magnitude of reward. Thus, if it can be assumed that the expectation of a greater magnitude of reward results in stronger activation of positive affective attributes, then the above data provide support for amygdala involvement in the encoding of intense positive emotional attributes of specific events.

A slightly different variation of this approach was recently reported by Gallagher et al. (1990). In this experiment, rats with ibotenic acid lesions of the central amygdala were tested in an appetitive classical conditioning paradigm. The animals were presented with either an auditory or visual cue as conditioned stimulus (CS) prior to pairing with food reinforcement. Relative to controls, acquisition of a conditioned response in anticipation of food to the auditory cue (startle) or visual cue (rearing) was impaired, whereas acquisition of a conditioned response to the food reinforcement itself (standing motionless with head or nose in area of food delivery) was intact (see Chapter 10, Gallagher, this volume). In a different experiment Everitt et al. (1989) demonstrated that male rats with NMDA-induced basolateral lesions of the amygdala decreased responding maintained by a visual conditioned reinforcer when sexual reinforcement was presented under a second-order schedule. The lesions had no effect on sexual behavior elicited by the female rat. Thus, when rats needed to attend to specific stimuli in anticipation of reward, the amygdala appears to play a critical role.

A fourth approach is to facilitate attention to reinforcement information by training rats on a task in which successful performance requires memory for magnitude of reinforcement. To utilize this approach, Kesner et al. (1989) tested animals in a task in which memory for magnitude of reinforcement could be tested explicitly.

Rats received a single trial per day consisting of a study phase and a test phase. In the study phase, the animals received one or seven pieces (1/4 pieces of Froot Loop cereal) of food on different arms of the maze. After the study phase, the rats were delayed for either 10 seconds, 5 or 15 minutes. After the delay during the test phase the animals were allowed to choose between the two arms presented in the study phase. The correct response, leading to an additional Froot Loop reinforcement, was to select the arm in which the animal received the seven pieces of food. After training the rats received electrolytic lesions of the basolateral or central amygdala. After recovery from surgery, the animals were again tested for their ability to remember the correct arm at each delay. The results, shown in Figures 2 and 3, indicated that there were no deficits at any delay with basolateral amygdala lesions. In contrast, lesions of the central amygdala produced a marked deficit at the 5 and 15 minute delays, but no deficit at the 10 second delay.

In another study, Peinado-Manzano (1989) demonstrated that the lateral, but not central, amygdala lesions disrupted memory for a visual (dark-light) association with one or seven pieces of food (magnitude of reinforcement). In this case the association was between a visual cue and magnitude of reinforcement, whereas in the Kesner et al. (1989) study the association was between a spatial location and magnitude of reinforcement, which perhaps could account for differential involvement of lateral compared to central amygdala. Based on the assumption that memory for magnitude of reinforcement is a function of the activation of affective experiences, it can be concluded that perhaps the central or lateral, but not basolateral, amygdala is involved in the coding of positive affect information.

Thus, the amygdala appears to play a role in coding the affect attribute component of memory as triggered by attention to important reinforcement contingencies.

Temporal Attribute

The attribute model states that the amygdala is involved in the coding of the interaction between affect and temporal information, regardless of sensory

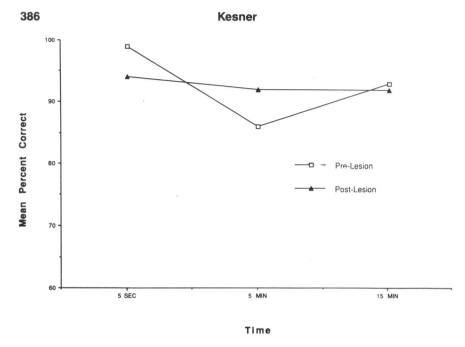

Fig. 2. Mean percent correct performance as a function of time (retention delay) before (prelesion) and after (postlesion) bilateral basolateral amygdala lesion.

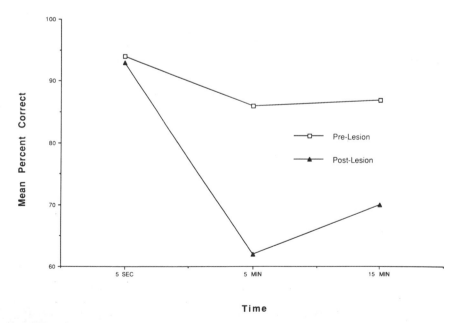

Fig. 3. Mean percent correct performance as a function of time (retention delay) before (prelesion) and after (postlesion) bilateral central amygdala lesions.

modality, within the data-based memory system. The amygdala is believed to code the time in which an affect-laden experience occurs relative to the occurrence of other affect-laden experiences. Thus, the attribute model suggests that the amygdala codes sequential processing of affect information. There is very little extant data aimed at addressing this specific question. Olton et al. (1987) demonstrated that large radiofrequency-induced amygdala lesions in rats did not alter the ability to remember duration of a previous stimulus nor did the rats have a problem remembering the onset of reinforcement. Thus, memory for duration does not appear to be mediated within the amygdala. There is some support, however, for memory for the sequential occurrence of events that involves order recognition memory for spatial locations targeted by specific food reinforcements. Details of the procedures used to assess order recognition memory can be found in Kesner et al. (1984). Briefly, for the order memory task, each animal was allowed on each trial (one per day) to visit all eight arms on an eight-arm radial maze in an order that was randomly selected for that trial. This constituted the study phase. Immediately after the animal had received reinforcement from the last of the eight arms, the test phase began. Only one test was given for each trial and consisted of opening two doors simultaneously. On a random basis either the first and second, fourth and fifth, or seventh and eighth doors that occurred in the sequence were selected for the test. The rule to be learned leading to an additional reinforcement was to choose the arm that occurred earlier in the sequence. After extensive training criterion performance (based on 24 trials with eight trials of each choice order) was achieved, animals received large electrolytic lesions of the amygdala or served as sham-operated controls. Following recovery from surgery the animals received an additional 24 tests with eight trials of each choice order. The results, shown in Figure 4, indicate that relative to controls, animals with amygdala lesions are markedly impaired for each choice order. Thus, the amygdala might indeed play a role in mediating sequential information. Clearly more research is needed to test further the role of the amygdala in mediating serial order information.

Spatial Attribute

The attribute model states that the amygdala is not involved in coding and processing of spatial information. Support for this idea comes from a variety of studies in which animals with large amygdala lesions were shown not to be impaired in the acquisition of a standard version of the Olton eight-arm maze (Becker et al., 1980), in the Morris water maze (Sutherland and McDonald, 1990), in the acquisition of a one-item delayed spatial nonmatching-to-sample task (Aggleton et al., 1989; Peinado and Manzano, 1990), and performance of a one-item delayed spatial matching-to-sample task (Kesner, unpublished observations).

In a more recent study (Kesner et al., 1990) rats were tested for recognition memory for a five-item list of spatial locations. Details of the procedures used to assess item recognition memory can be found in DiMattia and Kesner (1984). Briefly, for the item memory task, each animal was allowed to visit a sequence of five arms of an eight-arm radial maze on each trial (one per day), which was selected on a pseudorandom basis. This constituted the study phase. Immediately after the animal had received reinforcement from the last of the five arms, the test phase began. Only one test was given for each trial and consisted of

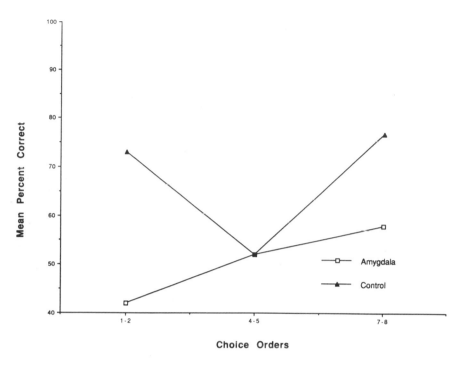

Fig. 4. Mean percent correct performance as a function of choice orders of spatial locations after amygdala or control lesions.

opening two doors simultaneously, with one door representing an arm previously visited for that trial and the other door representing a novel arm for that trial. The rule to be learned leading to an additional reinforcement was to choose the arm that had been previously visited during the study phase of the trial (win-stay). After reaching a high level of performance based on at least 40 trials with eight trials for each serial position, the animals received large electrolytic lesions of the amygdala or served as sham-operated controls. After recovery from surgery, the animals received 40 trials with eight trials for each serial position.

The results (Fig. 5) indicate that relative to controls, rats with amygdala lesions are not impaired in the spatial location memory task. Similar results were found in monkeys, in which amygdala lesions did not affect memory for spatial location information (Parkinson et al., 1988). Thus, in summary, the amygdala does not appear to code spatial information.

Sensory-Perceptual Attributes

Despite the need for sensory stimuli to contribute to the activation of an affect attribute of memory, the amygdala does not appear to code directly sensory-perceptual memory attributes triggered by the external environment.

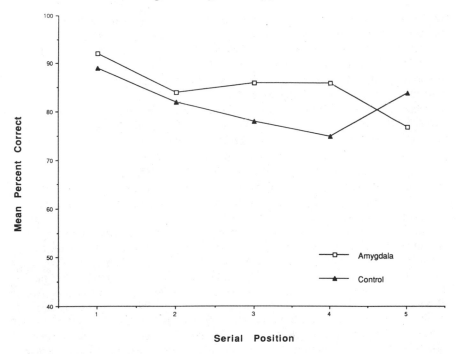

Fig. 5. Mean percent correct performance as a function of serial position of items (spatial locations) after amygdala or control lesions.

This is evident in the failure to disrupt (1) acquisition of an olfactory discrimination learning set in rats with radiofrequency-induced amygdala lesions (Eichenbaum et al., 1986), (2) performance of a delayed matching-to-sample task for visual and tactile cue information in rats with large radiofrequency-induced amygdala lesions (Raffaele and Olton, 1988), (3) acquisition of a delayed nonmatching-to-sample task for objects in rats with large ibotenic acid lesions of the amygdala (Aggleton et al., 1989), and (4) performance of a nonmatching-to-sample cross-modal (visual and olfactory cues) task in rats with large electrolytic lesions of the amygdala (Sutherland and McDonald, 1990). It should be noted that amygdalectomy in monkeys has been found to impair cross-modal associations (Murray, 1990). However, it is possible that the monkeys in that study sustained additional cortical damage which could have contributed to the observed impairment. Thus far, deficits have been found in rats in only one study (Peinado-Manzano, 1990). Peinado-Manzano reported that electrolytic lesions of the lateral amygdala disrupted the acquisition of a delayed nonmatching-to-sample task for visual or visual and tactile cues.

There are major differences between the Peinado-Manzano (1990) study and the other studies cited above in terms of the procedures employed. The major difference, however, might be that in the above studies most of the animals with amygdala lesions were the least likely to have damage to the lateral amygdala, whereas in the Peinado-Manzano study the damage was primarily seen only in the lateral amygdala. This observation would be consistent with LeDoux et al. (1990a), who showed evidence that the critical sensory input necessary for memory function of amygdala enters the amygdala primarily through the lateral amygdala nucleus. Since in the attribute model it is assumed that sensory-perceptual memory attributes are mediated via primary and secondary sensory areas of the neocortex, the failure to find a role for the amygdala in coding sensory-perceptual attributes is concordant with the model. However, it has been suggested that critical sensory information (visual, auditory, taste, and olfaction) for the evaluation and representation of affect can activate amygdala neurons directly (especially the lateral and central amygdala) via thalamic relay circuits and thereby bypass neocortical neural systems (LeDoux, 1986). Support for this idea comes from experiments that demonstrate that visual or auditory cue-mediated fear conditioning is not altered by visual or auditory cortex lesions, but rather by lateral or central amygdala lesions (LeDoux et al., 1990a,b). It appears that for certain types of tasks that do not involve high-order sensory analyses, the lateral amygdala can transfer sensory information to the other areas of the amygdala in order to represent an emotional or affective experience. Most likely, there are within the amygdala subcortically relayed sensory inputs that operate in parallel with neocortically relayed sensory-perceptual inputs to provide for possible associations of sensory-perceptual attributes with an evaluation of the emotional significance of information relayed via the internal state of the organism.

Even though the amygdala is not likely to represent most externally triggered sensory-perceptual information, it is likely to play a role in coding internally generated visceral sensory and hormonal information triggered by reinforcement (positive or negative) and arousal. This idea is consistent with Kapp et al.'s (1984) suggestion that the role of the amygdala in mediating arousal, affect, and learning is due to the responsiveness of the central amygdala to feedback from the autonomic nervous system. Evidence in support of the above suggestion comes from the observation that the vagus nerve (major component of the parasympathetic system) projects to the A2 norepinephrine containing neurons of the nucleus of the solitary tract (Loewy, 1990). In turn, the nucleus of the solitary tract projects directly to the central nucleus of the amygdala (Ricardo and Koh, 1978). Thus it should be the case that disruption of this pathway will result in decreased input into the amygdala with subsequent reduction in the elicitation of affect-laden experiences. In several studies, it was shown that severing of the subdiaphragmatic vagus disrupted in rats either the acquisition or retention of taste aversion learning, but did not alter retention of a conditioned emotional response (Coil et al., 1978; Kiefer et al., 1981). In another study in rats, stimulation of the vagus nerve concurrent with the presentation of a footshock disrupted a conditioned emotional response, suggesting that conditioned fear and arousal to the CS may have been reduced by the stimulation (Corwin and Slaughter, 1979).

Even though epinephrine is assumed not to cross the blood-brain barrier, posttrial injections of epinephrine can modulate retention within a variety of tasks. It is, therefore, assumed (McGaugh, 1989) that the effects of peripheral epinephrine are mediated via visceral afferents projecting to central nonadrenergic systems which, in turn, activate the amygdala. Support for this proposed feedback system comes from the findings that posttrial intracranial injections of β-adrenergic antagonists into the amygdala or cuts of the stria terminalis input pathway to the amygdala can block the effects of peripheral injection of epinephrine on retention. (For more detail, see Chapter 16, McGaugh, (this volume.) Thus, it appears that sensory-visceral feedback from the parasympathetic system to the amygdala might indeed play a role in the activation and subsequent memory representation of affect attributes. It is clear, however, that much more data are needed before one can be certain of the importance of sensory-visceral feedback in amygdala function.

Response Attribute

There are no published studies in rats in which the effect of amygdala lesions on memory for a specific somatic motor response has been investigated. The attribute model would not predict any deficits in somatic response memory following amygdala lesions. In order to test this prediction, rats were trained on a response memory task. In this task, there is a study and a test phase constituting a trial. In the study phase, a rat is placed at the end of a modified six-arm plus maze. The animal is given the opportunity to make a right or left turn, which is accomplished by opening the right or left door. After making the appropriate turning response, the animal is given food reinforcement in the arm. The rat is then removed from the maze, and within 10 seconds of 1 minute the test phase is begun. During the test phase, the rat is placed at the end of an arm opposite the arm that was selected in the study phase. In this case, both right and left doors are opened, and the rat is given the opportunity to choose between the right and left arms. A repeat of the turn made during the study phase results in reinforcement. Thus, if the animal makes a left turn during the study phase, it must also make a left turn during the test phase in order to receive reinforcement. The animals received six trials per day, five days per week. After reaching criterion of 75% or better performance on a set of 24 trials, the animals either received large electrolytic or ibotenic acid-induced lesions of the amygdala or sham control lesions. Following recovery from surgery, the animals were retested. The results indicate that there is no deficit following large amygdala or sham control lesions. It is of interest to note that animals with caudate lesions are impaired on this task. Thus, the amygdala does not appear to be involved in coding somatic motor response information.

Since the amygdala has reciprocal connections with a variety of brain stem areas, which in turn have reciprocal connections with the autonomic nervous system (Kapp et al., 1984; LeDoux, 1986; Loewy, 1990), the amygdala is likely to play a role in mediating visceral information to represent and influence the internal context. Even though one can often, albeit with difficulty, describe changes in the autonomic nervous system during an emotional or arousal experience, it is very difficult to assess the role of the amygdala in memory for specific autonomic responses, because one is often not consciously aware of any changes in the autonomic nervous system. Some indirect support for a role of the amygdala in responding to autonomic changes comes from a study with patient H.M., who had large bilateral removal of the temporal lobe including the amygdala. It was reported that H.M. is poor in monitoring appetite. He appears to have difficulty in detecting pain, hunger, or thirst (Hebben et al.,1985). Even though this implies that less information concerning the internal context might be available to this patient, its effects on memory for specific changes in the autonomic nervous system were not tested. More research will be needed to address the question of whether the amygdala is involved in memory for autonomic responses.

HOW INFORMATION IS CODED IN THE AMYGDALA

The attribute model suggests that the amygdala is directly involved in coding all new affect-temporal (internal context) information that is likely to be relevant in trial-unique situations, and could be of importance for all trials within a new learning task (data-based memory). In contrast, the amygdala is not involved in coding information based on expected nonvarying information in the form of maps, rules, strategies, and procedures (expectancy or knowledge-based memory). There is a variety of data that pertains directly to this question. Support for the idea comes from the observation that central amygdala lesions disrupt memory for magnitude of reinforcement in a task that emphasizes the importance of episodic, working or data-based memory (Kesner et al.,1989), but in a task that emphasizes the importance of knowledge-based or reference memory, large amygdala lesions do not impair preformance of a previously learned serial pattern based on differential magnitudes of reinforcement (Olton et al., 1984).

Since there is clearly more data input processing during the acquisition of new tasks (postlesion training) compared to retention of most previously acquired tasks (prelesion training), it is predicted that amygdala lesions would produce a greater deficit in the postlesion compared to the prelesion training condition. One example is provided by Peinado-Manzano (1988), who demonstrated that rats with lateral and central amygdala lesions were impaired in postlesion acquisition of a successive brightness discrimination, but were not impaired in the prelesion training condition. In another study, Thatcher and Kimble (1966) also reported normal performance of a previously learned avoidance response (prelesion training), but only when amygdala-lesioned rats were overtrained. When animals are undertrained, then amygdala lesions did produce retention (prelesion training) deficits (Thatcher and Kimble, 1966; Goldstein, 1974).

Additional support comes from studies demonstrating that retention of an inhibitory avoidance response is impaired by bilateral lesions of the amygdala shortly after training but not by lesions placed in the amygdala several days after training (Liang et al., 1982). Similarly, electrical stimulation, intracranial injection of protein inhibitors, as well as manipulation of the cholinergic, adrenergic, or opiate systems within the amygdala produce time-dependent retention deficits within a variety of learning situations (Gold et al., 1973, 1976; Berman et al., 1978; Todd and Kesner, 1978; Ellis and Kesner, 1983; McGaugh, 1989). These data suggest that the amygdala is involved in coding of new information, but is not the site of permanent representation of affect-laden information. If the amygdala is not the site of permanent long-term memory storage of affect attributes, then what other neural regions might subserve such a function? It has been proposed (Kesner and DiMattia, 1987) that the orbitofrontal cortex might represent such a neural region. There are reciprocal anatomical connections between the orbitofrontal cortex and amygdala (Aggleton et al.,1980; Porrino et al., 1981). Even though there is very little data on the role of the orbitofrontal cortex in rats, a case can be made for the above proposed role when one combines the rodent, monkey, and human data on orbitofrontal cortex function.

For example, humans with orbitofrontal cortex damage show a variety of personality changes characterized by facetiousness, euphoria, irritability, sudden depression, and impaired social judgment. Most patients so affected are unable to enjoy pleasurable experiences, especially when the rewards are social or intellectual. They seem to have a lack of appreciation of social rules, altered effect, and limited response to and experience of pain. In rats, orbitofrontal cortex lesions often cause changes in aggressive behavior (Kolb, 1974).

Orbitofrontal cortex-damaged animals have difficulty changing their behavior when the value of rewards is not consistent with expectations based on prior experiences. Thus, animals with orbitofrontal cortex lesions display prolonged extinction of a previously rewarded response (Butter, 1969; Butter et al., 1963), and they are impaired in visual discrimination and spatial tasks reversals (Butter, 1969; Iversen and Mishkin, 1970; Jones and Mishkin, 1972). Also, Thorpe et al. (1983) have found cells in orbitofrontal cortex that respond differentially to the expectation of a reward or a punishment.

Finally, in an unpublished study with rats, Kesner found that orbitofrontal cortex lesions disrupt performance on a five-item list in a spatial recognition memory task, when reward presented during the study phase consisted of only one piece of food. However, when four pieces of food were presented, the animals were no longer impaired, suggesting that the appreciation of reward is of critical importance to orbitofrontal cortex-lesioned animals. Thus, the data appear to support the idea that orbitofrontal cortex mediates affect information as it relates to social rules and the expectation of rewards and punishments.

Dissociations Between Orbitofrontal Cortex and Amygdala

The amygdala is assumed to code affect attributes of a memory based on episodic and varied incoming information and thus is an integral part of the data-based memory system. In contrast, the orbitofrontal cortex is assumed to code affect attributes of a memory based on information derived from an affect map in the form of reward strategies and rules. The model would predict deficits in subjects with orbitofrontal damage in situations where the expectations of reward or affect have been well established prior to injury. In this situation no deficits would be expected for amygdala-damaged subjects. There are two relevant studies that pertain to this prediction, even though neither study used rats as subjects. Brady et al. (1954) showed that after amygdala lesions, cats failed to acquire an active avoidance response, but showed no retention deficits when amygdala lesions were made after training. In contrast, cats with orbitofrontal cortex lesions made after training displayed a marked retention deficit. Jones and Mishkin (1972) found that both amygdala and orbitofrontal cortex-damaged monkeys had difficulty in learning object or place discrimination reversals. Based on an analysis of the early versus late trials of a reversal, they found that orbitofrontal cortex-damaged animals made most of their errors in the early stages of reversal training, while those with amygdala lesions made most of their errors in the later stages of reversal training. Based on these data, Jones and Mishkin (1972) suggest that orbitofrontal cortex-damaged animals cannot suppress prior expectations of reward, while amygdala-lesioned animals have a difficult time learning new stimulus-reward associations. Both sets of data support the idea of a dissociation of function between the amygdala and orbitofrontal cortex.

Dissociations Between the Hippocampus and Amygdala

Is the amygdala the only neural region that subserves information associated with the data-based memory system? The answer is clearly no, because the amygdala primarily mediates only affect and temporal attributes (internal context) of memory. There are likely to be other neural systems that mediate interactions between other attributes. For example, the attribute model proposes that the hippocampus codes new spatial-temporal (external context) information within the data-based working or episodic memory system. Data in support for an important role for the hippocampus in coding spatiotemporal attribute information have been presented elsewhere (Kesner, 1990). Thus, it is likely that each system (amygdala and hippocampus) contributes unique information to ensure that all aspects of a new experience are coded in the central nervous system in order to ensure optimal learning and memory of new tasks.

To what extent do the two neural regions (amygdala and hippocampus) interact with each other or operate independently of each other? Even though there are likely to be many functional interactions between the amygdala and the hippocampus, there is also some support for parallel and independent processing of attribute information. For example, lesions or electrical stimulation of the hippocampus impair performance on an eight-arm maze and impair memory for spatial locations, but have no effect on taste aversion learning or manifestation of the frustration effect as indicated by faster running following reward omission. In contrast, lesions or electrical stimulation of the amygdala impair taste aversion learning as well as manifestation of the frustration effect without altering eight-arm performance or efficiency of spatial location memory (Swanson and Isaacson, 1969; McGowan et al., 1972; Best and Orr, 1973; Plunkett et al., 1973; Nachman and Ashe, 1974; Kesner et al., 1975; Henke, 1977; Olton and Wolf, 1981; Olton, 1983; Murray, 1990).

Thus, there appears to be a double dissociation between the amygdala and hippocampus, implying that they can operate independent of each other.

Research with monkeys also revealed a double dissociation between the hippocampus and amygdala. The hippocampus appears to be involved in tasks that require memory for spatial locations of objects, whereas the amygdala appears to be involved in tasks that require memory for object-reward associations or object-object associations across modalities. Monkeys with lesions of the hippocampus, but not amygdala, have an impaired memory for object-place associations (Parkinson et al., 1988). In contrast, monkeys with lesions of the amygdala, but not hippocampus, have an impaired memory for object-reward associations (Spiegler and Mishkin, 1981) and cross-modal object-object associations (Murray and Mishkin, 1985; Murray, 1990). In conclusion, it appears that the hippocampus and amygdala can function independently as reflected by coding of different attribute components of memory.

SUMMARY

The amygdala in rats clearly plays a role in learning and memory. In order to organize the extant literature on the mnemonic functions of the amygdala, a role for the amygdala within an attribute model of memory was formulated. It is proposed that the amygdala encodes and processes affect and temporal (internal context) information within a data-based, working or episodic memory system. Furthermore, the critical conditions for the activation of an affect memory attribute within the amygdala is based on (1) presence of reinforcement of sufficient intensity to elicit a strong emotional reaction as well as arousal and a variety of autonomic changes and (2) attention to reinforcement either because of the expectation of a subsequent memory test for the reinforcement or in anticipation of an important future event based on the principle of reinforcement.

In addition, it is also suggested that (1) within the data-based memory system the amygdala does not encode spatial, somatic response, and sensory-perceptual attributes, but rather that other neural systems (e.g., hippocampus) encode some of these attributes and (2) within the knowledge-based memory system the amygdala does not encode or process affect information, but other neural systems (e.g., orbitofrontal cortex) might encode affect attributes.

ACKNOWLEDGMENTS

This work was supported by NSF award BNS 892-1532.

REFERENCES

Aggleton JP, Blindt HS, Rawlins JNP (1989): Effects of amygdaloid and amygdaloid-hippocampal lesions on object recognition and spatial working memory in rats. Behav Neurosci 103:962–974.

Aggleton JP, Burton MJ, Passingham RE (1980): Cortical and subcortical afferents to the amygdala of the rhesus monkey (*Macaca mulatta*). Brain Res 190:347–368.

Aggleton JP, Mishkin M (1986): The amygdala: Sensory gateway to the emotions. In Plutchik R, Kellerman H (eds): "Emotion Theory, Research, and Experience," Vol 3. New York: Academic Press, pp 281–299.

Baker LJ, Kesner RP, Michal RE (1981): Differential effects of a reminder cue on amnesia induced by stimulation of amygdala and hippocampus. J Comp Physiol Psychol 95:312–321.

Becker JT, Walker JA, Olton DS (1980): Neuroanatomical bases of spatial memory. Brain Res 200:307–320.

Berman RF, Kesner RP, Partlow LM (1978): Passive avoidance impairment in rats following cycloheximide injection into the amygdala. Brain Res 158:171–188.

Best PJ, Orr J (1973): Effect of hippocampal lesions on passive avoidance and taste aversion conditioning. Physiol Behav 10:193–196.

Brady JV, Schreiner L, Geller I, Kling A (1954): Subcortical mechanisms in emotional behavior: The effect of rhinencephalic injury upon the acquisition and retention of a conditioned avoidance response in cats. J Comp Physiol Psychol 47:179–186.

Bresnahan E, Routtenberg A (1972): Memory disruption by unilateral low level, subseizure stimulation of the medial amygdaloid nucleus. Physiol Behav 9:513–525.

Butter CM (1969): Perseveration in extinction and in discrimination reversal tasks following selective frontal ablations in *Macaca mulatta*. Physiol Behav 4:163–171.

Butter CM, Mishkin M, Rosvold HE (1963): Conditioning and extinction of a food-rewarded response after selective ablations of frontal cortex in rhesus monkeys. Exp Neurol 7:65–75.

Cahill L, McGaugh JL (1990): Amygdaloid complex lesions differentially affect retention of tasks using appetitive and aversive reinforcement. Behav Neurosci 104:532–543.

Coil JD, Rogers RC, Garcia J, Novin D (1978): Conditioned taste aversions: Vagal and circulatory mediation of the toxic US. Behav Biol 24:509–519.

Corwin JV, Slaughter JS (1979): Effects of vagal stimulation on the learning of specific and diffuse conditioned suppression. Behav Neur Biol 25:364–370.

DiMattia BV, Kesner RP (1984): Serial position curves in rats: Automatic versus effortful information processing. J Exp Psychol: Anim Behav Proc 10:557–563.

Douglas RJ, Pribram KH (1966): Learning and limbic lesions. Neuropsychology 4:197–220.

Eichenbaum H, Fagan A, Cohen N (1986): Normal olfactory discrimination learning set and facilitation of reversal learning after medial-temporal damage in rats: Implications for an account of preserved learning abilities in amnesia. J Neurol 6:1876–1884.

Ellis ME, Kesner RP (1983): The noradrenergic system of the amygdala and aversive information processing. Behav Neurosci 97:399–415.

Everitt BJ, Cador M, Robbins TW (1989): Interactions between the amygdala and ventral striatum in stimulus-reward associations: Studies using a second-order schedule of sexual reinforcement. Neuroscience 30:63–75.

Gallagher M, Graham PW, Holland PC (1990): The amygdala central nucleus and appetitive pavlovian conditioning: Lesions impair one class of conditioned behavior. J Neurosci 10:1906–1911.

Goddard GV (1964): Functions of the amygdala. Psychol Bull 62:89–109.

Gold PE, Hankins LL, Edwards R, Chester J, McGaugh JL (1975): Memory interference and facilitation with posttrial amygdala stimulation: Effect on memory varies with footshock level. Brain Res 86:509–513.

Gold PE, Macri J, McGaugh JL (1973): Retrograde amnesia produced by subseizure amygdala stimulation. Behav Biol 9:671–680.

Gold PE, Rose RP, Hankins LL, Spanis C (1976): Impaired retention of visual discriminated escape training produced by subseizure amygdala stimulation. Brain Res 118:73–85.

Goldstein ML (1974): The effect of amygdalectomy on long-term retention of an undertrained classically conditioned fear response. Bull Psychonom Soc 4:548–550.

Heath RG (1964): Pleasure response of human subjects to direct stimulation of the brain:

Physiological and psychodynamic considerations. In Heath RG (ed): "The Role of Pleasure in Behavior." New York: Harper, pp 219–243.

Hebben N, Corkin S, Eichenbaum H, Shedlack K (1985): Diminished ability to interpret and report internal states after bilateral medial temporal resection: Case H.M. Behav Neurosci 99:1031–1039.

Henke PG (1977): Dissociation of the frustration effect and the partial reinforcement extinction effect after limbic lesions in rats. J Comp Physiol Psychol 91:1032–1038.

Hitchcock J, Davis M (1986): Lesions of the amygdala, but not of the cerebellum or red nucleus, block conditioned fear as measured with the potentiated startle paradigm. Behav Neurosci 100:11–22.

Iversen SD, Mishkin M (1970): Perseverative interference in monkey following selective lesions of the inferior prefrontal convexity. Exp Brain Res 11:376–386.

Jones B, Mishkin M (1972): Limbic lesions and the problem of stimulus-reinforcement association. Exp Neurol 36:362–377.

Kaada BR (1972): Stimulation and regional ablation of the amygdaloid complex with reference to functional representation. In Eleftheriou BE (ed): "The Neurobiology of the Amygdala." New York: Plenum Press, pp 205–282.

Kapp BS, Pascoe JP, Bixler MA (1984): The amygdala: A neuroanatomical systems approach to its contribution to aversive conditioning. In Squire LR, Butters N (eds): "Neuropsychology of Memory." New York: Guilford, pp 473–488.

Kemble ED, Beckman GJ (1970): Runway performance of rats following amygdaloid lesions. Physiol Behav 5:45–47.

Kesner RP (1990): Learning and memory in rats with an emphasis on the role of the hippocampal formation. In Kesner RP, Olton DS (eds): "Neurobiology of Comparative Cognition." Hillsdale, NJ: Lawrence Erlbaum, pp 179–201.

Kesner RP (1982): Brain stimulation: Effects on memory. Behav Brain Biol 36:315–367.

Kesner RP, Andrus RG (1982): Amygdala stimulation disrupts the magnitude of reinforcement contribution to long-term memory. Physiol Psychol 10:55–59.

Kesner RP, Berman RF, Burton B, Hankins WG (1975): Effects of electrical stimulation of amygdala upon neophobia and taste aversion. Behav Biol 13:349–358.

Kesner RP, Conner HS (1974): Effects of electrical stimulation of limbic system and midbrain reticular formation upon short- and long-term memory. Physiol Behav 12:5–12.

Kesner RP, Crutcher KA, Omana H (1990): Memory deficits following nucleus basalis magnocellularis lesions may be mediated through limbic, but not neocortical, targets. Neuroscience 38:93–102.

Kesner RP, DiMattia BV (1987): Neurobiology of an attribute model of memory. In Epstein AN, Morrison A (eds): "Progress in Psychobiology and Physiological Psychology," Vol 12. New York: Academic Press, pp 207–277.

Kesner RP, Measom MO, Forsman SL, Holbrook TH (1984): Serial position curves in rats: Order memory for episodic spatial events. Anim Learn Behav 12:378–382.

Kesner RP, Walser RD, Winzenried G (1989): Central but not basolateral amygdala mediates memory for positive affective experiences. Behav Brain Res 33:189–195.

Kiefer SW, Rusiniak KW, Garcia J, Coil C (1981): Vagotomy facilitates extinction of conditioned taste aversions in rats. J Comp Physiol Psych 95:114–122.

Kolb B (1974): Social behavior of rats with chronic prefrontal lesions. Physiol Psychol 87:466–474.

LeDoux JE (1986): The neurobiology of emotion. In LeDoux JE, Hirst W (eds): "Mind and Brain Dialogues in Cognitive Neuroscience." New York: Cambridge University Press, pp 301–354.

LeDoux JE, Cicchetti P, Xagoraris A, Romanski LM (1990a): The lateral amygdaloid nucleus: Sensory interface of the amygdala in fear conditioning. J Neurosci 10:1062–1069.

LeDoux JE, Romanski L, Xagoraris A (1990b): Indelibility of subcortical emotional memories. J Cogn Neurosci 1:238–243.

Liang KC, McGaugh JL, Martinez JL, Jensen RA, Vasquez BJ, Messing RB (1982): Posttraining amygdaloid lesions impair retention of an inhibitory avoidance response. Behav Brain Res 4:237–249.

Lidsky TI, Levine MS, Kreinick CJ, Schwartzbaum JS (1970): Retrograde effects of amygdaloid stimulation on conditioned suppression (CER) in rats. J Comp Physiol Psychol 73:135–149.

Loewy AD (1990): Central autonomic pathways. In Loewy AD, Spyer KM (eds): "Central Regulation of Autonomic Functions." Oxford: Oxford University Press, pp 87–103.

Mark VH, Ervin FR (1970): "Violence and the Brain." New York: Harper.

McDonough JR, Kesner RP (1971): Amnesia produced by brief electrical stimulation of the amygdala or dorsal hippocampus in cats. J Comp Physiol Psychol 77:171–178.

McGaugh JL (1989): Involvement of hormonal and neuromodulatory systems in the regulation of memory storage. Ann Rev Neurosci 12:255–287.

McGowan BK, Hankins WG, Garcia J (1972): Limbic lesions and control of the internal and external environment. Behav Biol 7:841–852.

Murray EA (1990): Representational memory in nonhuman primates. In Kesner RP, Olton DS (eds): "Neurobiology of Comparative Cognition." Hillsdale, NJ: Lawrence Erlbaum, pp 127–151.

Murray EA, Mishkin M (1985): Amygdalectomy impairs crossmodal association in monkeys. Science 228:604–606.

Nachman M, Ashe JH (1974): Effects of basolateral amygdala lesions on neophobia, learned taste aversions, and sodium appetite in rats. J Comp Physiol Psychol 87:622–643.

Narabayashi M (1972): Sterotaxic amygdalectomy. In Eleftheriou BF (ed): "The Neurobiology of the Amygdala." New York: Plenum Press, pp 459–483.

Nishijo H, Ono T, Nishino H (1988): Single neuron responses in amygdala of alert monkey during complex sensory stimulation with affective significance. J Neurosci 8:3570–3583.

Olton DS (1983): Memory functions and the hippocampus. In Seifert W (ed): "Neurobiology of the Hippocampus." New York: Academic Press, pp 335–373.

Olton DS, Meck WH, Church RM (1987): Separation of hippocampal and amygdaloid involvement in temporal memory dysfunctions. Brain Res 404:180–188.

Olton DS, Shapiro ML, Hulse SH (1984): Working memory and serial patterns. In Roitblat HL, Bever TG, Terrace HS (eds): "Animal Cognition: Proceedings of the Harry Frank Guggenheim Conference, 1982." Hillsdale, NJ: Erlbaum, pp 171–182.

Olton DS, Wolf WA (1981): Hippocampal seizures produce retrograde amnesia without a temporal gradient when they reset working memory. Behav Biol 33:437–452.

Parkinson JK, Murray EA, Mishkin M (1988): A selective mnemonic role for the hippocampus in monkeys: Memory for the location of objects. J Neurosci 8:4159–4167.

Peinado-Manzano MA (1988): Effects of bilateral lesions of the central and lateral amygdala on free operant successive discrimination. Behav Brain Res 29:61–71.

Peinado-Manzano MA (1989): Intervention of the lateral and central amygdala on the association of visual stimuli with different magnitudes of reinforcement. Behav Brain Res 32:289–295.

Peinado-Manzano MA (1990): The role of the amygdala and the hippocampus in working memory for spatial and non-spatial information. Behav Brain Res 38:117–134.

Plunket RP, Faulds BD, Albino RC (1973): Place learning in hippocampectomized rats. Bull Psychonom Soc 2:79–80.

Porrino LJ, Crane AM, Goldman-Rakic PS (1981): Direct and indirect pathways from the amygdala to the frontal lobe in rhesus monkeys. J Comp Neurol 198:121–136.

Raffaele KC, Olton DS (1988): Hippocampal and amygdaloid involvement in working memory for nonspatial stimuli. Behav Neurosci 102:349–355.

Ricardo J, Koh ET (1978): Anatomical evidence of direct projections from the nucleus of the solitary tract to the hypothalamus, amygdala, and other forebrain structures in the rat. Brain Res 153:1–26.

Schwartzbaum JS (1960): Changes in reinforcing properties of stimuli following ablation of the amygdaloid complex in monkeys. J Comp Physiol Psychol 53:388–396.

Spear NF (1976): Retrieval of memories: A psychobiological approach. In Estes WK (ed): "Handbook of Learning and Cognitive Processes," Vol 4. Hillsdale, NJ: Lawrence Erlbaum.

Sutherland RJ, McDonald RJ (1990): Hippocampus, amygdala, and memory deficits in rats. Behav Brain Res 37:57–79.

Swanson AM, Isaacson RL (1969): Hippocampal lesions and the frustration effect in rats. J Comp Physiol Psychol 68:562–567.

Thatcher RW, Kimble DP (1966): Effect of amygdaloid lesions on retention of an avoidance response in overtrained and nonovertrained rats. Psychonom Sci 6:9–10.

Thorpe SJ, Rolls ET, Maddison S (1983): The orbitofrontal cortex: Neuronal activity in the behaving monkey. Exp Brain Res 49:93–115.

Todd JW, Kesner RP (1978): Effects of posttraining injection of cholinergic agonists and antagonists into the amygdala on retention of passive avoidance training in rats. J Comp Physiol Psychol 92:958–968.

Underwood BJ (1969): Attributes of memory. Psychol Rev 76:559–573.

Weiskrantz L (1956): Behavioral changes with ablation of the amygdaloid complex in monkeys. J Comp Physiol Psychol 49:381–391.

Wurtz RM, Olds J (1963): Amygdaloid stimulation and operant reinforcement in the rat. J Comp Physiol Psychol 56:941–949.

The Amygdala: Neurobiological Aspects of Emotion,
Memory, and Mental Dysfunction, pages 401–429
© 1992 Wiley-Liss, Inc.

15
Amygdala-Ventral Striatal Interactions and Reward-Related Processes

BARRY J. EVERITT AND TREVOR W. ROBBINS
Departments of Anatomy (B.J.E.) and Experimental Psychology (T.W.R.), University of Cambridge, UK

INTRODUCTION: THE LIMBIC SYSTEM AND EMOTIONAL BEHAVIOR

It is impossible to separate neuroanatomical from functional criteria in defining the limbic system. Structures such as the amygdala are referred to as "limbic" not only because their connections are intimately related to the original definition of a limbic circuit, but also because of their postulated role in the mediation of emotions. Such functional considerations place considerable weight on the analysis of what we mean by the term "emotion," a question, of course, that has been the subject of considerable philosophical debate and controversy in experimental psychology. One important debate concerns the specificity of the emotions and their differentiation (Buck, 1986; LeDoux, 1986a). Another useful distinction is between emotional experience and emotional behavior (LeDoux, 1986a,b; Rolls, 1990) which, in a sense, could be considered in terms of the distinction between perception and action, with emotional experience arising from the affective interpretation of sensory events (Schachter and Singer, 1962). However, it is emotional behavior that we wish to emphasize in this chapter, which is tantamount to considering the amygdala as the orchestrator of different types of response output. Commonly, emotional output has been understood in terms of integrated patterns of autonomic, endocrine, and unconditioned, reflexive behavior (Richardson, 1973; Swanson and Mogenson, 1981; Davis et al., 1987; Swanson, 1987). However, of course, much emotionally driven behavior is not reflexive, but voluntary, representing behavior instrumental in obtaining access to particular goals, such as a sexual partner or a safe place (Robbins et al., 1989; Everitt, 1990).

The importance of the goal in instrumental behavior is reflected in theories of instrumental performance which stress the role of learned associations

Address correspondence to: Dr. Barry Everitt, Department of Anatomy, University of Cambridge, Downing Street, Cambridge CB2 3DY, UK.

between environmental stimuli and goals, or actions and goals (Dickinson, 1980, 1989; Dickinson et al., 1983; Mackintosh, 1983; Dickinson and Dawson, 1989). To some extent, these theories, while accommodating the concept of an incentive stimulus that elicits approach (or avoidance), may supersede, or at any rate complement, the older behavioristic notion of the goal as a reinforcer that cements or consolidates connections made between stimulus and response.

There has been an entirely different tradition of research that has sought to identify the neural substrates of reinforcement or incentive [commonly called "reward" (cf. Wise, 1981, 1982, 1989a,b)] which has only marginally implicated the amygdala, or indeed, other limbic structures. This was originally inspired by the phenomenon of intracranial self-stimulation from medial forebrain sites (Milner, 1989; Shizgal, 1989). It has now focused on the likely role of dopamine-dependent processes of the ventral striatum (Koob and Goeders, 1989; Phillips et al., 1989) and has been extended by advances in understanding the neural and neurochemical mode of action of drugs of abuse such as the psychomotor stimulants and narcotic opiates (Phillips and Fibiger, 1987; Carr et al., 1989; Koob et al., 1989; Koob and Goeders, 1989; Robbins et al., 1989). There have also been suggestions that the ventral striatal system represents a final common element in all reward-related functions, including those of natural reinforcers such as food and sex (Blackburn et al., 1986; Phillips et al., 1989; Robbins et al., 1989; Everitt, 1990).

These advances to date have proceeded largely in parallel with the evolution of the concept that the amygdala is implicated in the processes by which environmental stimuli are invested with affective value (Weiskrantz, 1956; Jones and Mishkin, 1972; Richardson, 1973; Aggleton and Passingham, 1981, 1982; Kesner, 1981; Spiegler and Mishkin, 1981; Sarter and Markowitsch, 1985; Aggleton and Mishkin, 1986). It would seem that there are now grounds for integrating these different strands of research into a more general scheme of the neural basis of emotion. This integration at a functional level is especially warranted by the discovery of specific anatomical connections between the limbic system and the ventral striatum (see Groenewegen et al., 1991, and below).

Previously, the strong connections between the amygdala and the hypothalamus and autonomic brain stem have been emphasized in understanding its role in various aspects of emotional output (Swanson and Mogenson, 1981; Aggleton and Mishkin, 1986; Davis, 1986; Davis et al., 1987; Ray et al., 1987; LeDoux et al., 1988; Sananes and Campbell, 1989). An excellent example of this is the recent proposal that various aspects of anxiety, such as hyperventilation, cardiovascular change, freezing, and even facial expression, are mediated by specific projections from the central nucleus to the brain stem (LeDoux, 1986b; Davis et al., 1987). There are also data that strongly indicate that endocrine responses are similarly coordinated via this fractionation of outflow from the amygdala to the medial hypothalamus (Swanson and Mogenson, 1981; Beaulieu et al., 1986, 1987; Gray et al., 1989). Furthermore, *reflexive* responses, such as freezing, can interfere with instrumental behavior, as may occur via Pavlovian conditioning, for example, in the conditioned emotional response paradigm. However, it is difficult to imagine how the hypothalamic and brain stem connections of the amygdala alone can also account for voluntary aspects of behavior, such as of active avoidance.

LIMBIC-STRIATAL CONNECTIONS

During the past decade it has become apparent that limbic structures such as the subiculum, limbic frontal cortex, and, especially, basolateral parts of the amygdala richly project to the ventral striatum (Heimer and Wilson, 1975; DeFrance et al., 1980; Groenewegen et al., 1980, 1982; Nauta and Domesick, 1984; Russchen and Price, 1984; Haber et al., 1985; Alexander et al., 1986; Alheid and Heimer, 1988). Moreover, the termination of both amygdaloid and subicular neurons in the ventral striatum is closely related to the termination of the mesolimbic (A10) dopaminergic neurons (Kelley et al., 1982; Kelley and Domesick, 1982; Yim and Mogenson, 1982, 1983, 1989; Yang and Mogenson, 1984, 1985), which have long been studied in experiments on reward and incentive motivational processes (see above). Thus, the functions of limbic forebrain structures such as the amygdala have come to be viewed in a wider neuroanatomical context than was the case hitherto, with the hypothalamus and brain stem no longer being viewed as the sole route by which limbic processes come to determine emotional behavior.

Mogenson and his colleagues were the first to draw attention to the functional importance of such connections, which they termed a "limbic-motor interface" (Mogenson, 1984, 1987; Mogenson et al., 1984; Mogenson and Nielson, 1984). Thus, the ventral striatum was suggested to be a site at which affective processes occurring in the limbic forebrain may gain access to subcortical elements of the motor system and thereby affect action. The subsequent research of these workers has demonstrated that hippocampal and amygdaloid electrical stimulation affects the activity of ventral striatal neurons in a way that is also modulated by coincident manipulation of dopamine transmission there (Yim and Mogenson, 1982, 1983, 1989; Yang and Mogenson, 1984, 1985). Furthermore, locomotor responses induced by pharmacological stimulation of the amygdala or hippocampus, or by exposure to a novel environment, are also affected by manipulation of the ventral striatum or the targets of its outflow, namely the ventral pallidum or mesencephalic locomotor region (Mogenson, 1984, 1987; Mogenson and Nielson, 1984). Thus, a body of data exists that strongly indicates that simple locomotor responses generated by stimulation of forebrain limbic structures depend upon direct interactions between these structures and the ventral striatum. However, what is not clear from these important and elegant experiments is the nature of the processes occurring in the limbic structures and the circumstances under which this output system is recruited; in other words, the importance of this system for emotional response output remains to be established (Everitt et al., 1989a; Everitt, 1990).

To address this issue, the impact of experimental manipulations of the amygdala on aspects of emotional behavior other than those more readily ascribed to interactions of this structure with hypothalamic and brain stem autonomic targets must be considered. A considerable body of evidence, largely derived from experiments involving the destruction of the amygdala, indicates that it is fundamentally involved in aspects of reinforcement (Weiskrantz, 1956; Jones and Mishkin, 1972; Aggleton and Passingham, 1981; Kesner, 1981; Spiegler and Mishkin, 1981). For example, rats with bilateral electrolytic lesions of the amygdala do not respond appropriately to changes in the magnitude of reward (Kemble and Beckman, 1970; Henke et al., 1972; Henke and Maxwell, 1973; Kesner, 1981), while the control over behavior by secondary reinforcers is also impaired (Weiskrantz, 1956; Gaffan and Harrison, 1987; Gaffan et al., 1988, 1989; Aggleton et al., 1989; Cador et al., 1989; Everitt et al., 1989a; Everitt, 1990).

Weiskrantz (1956), in reviewing the body of data existing at the time, suggested that many of the behavioral changes following amygdala lesions may indicate an important and pervasive role in the association of environmental stimuli with a variety of biologically important aspects of events, thus mediating the impact of their reinforcing value. More specifically, a marked impairment in remembering stimulus-reward associations over short delays by monkeys with amgydala lesions, which was not due to difficulties in object recognition, has been demonstrated (Spiegler and Mishkin, 1981). Gaffan and Harrison (1987) have more recently demonstrated that bilateral amygdalectomy in monkeys profoundly disrupted the association of arbitrary stimuli (white noise) with the intrinsic, incentive value of a primary reward (in this case food), arguing that the amygdala is especially important in mediating the control over behavior by secondary (or conditioned) reinforcers (see Chapter 18, Gaffan, this volume).

In this chapter, we review our own recent experiments, which have investigated the importance of interactions between the amygdala and ventral striatum in the processes by which environmental stimuli gain affective value through their predictive association with primary goals and thereby come to control instrumental components of an integrated emotional response.

BEHAVIORAL PARADIGMS

The results of experiments using three different, but complementary, behavioral procedures for studying the neural mechanisms of reward-related processes are described (see Table I).

In the *acquisition of a new response procedure* (Taylor and Robbins, 1984, 1986; Cador et al., 1989; Robbins et al., 1989), thirsty rats are initially trained in an operant chamber to approach a dipper and drink in the presence of a discrete, visual conditioned stimulus (CS). Following this Pavlovian conditioning, the conditioned reinforcing properties of the CS are assessed by its ability to support the acquisition of a new response. Thus, in phase 2, water is no longer presented and two novel levers are introduced into the chamber. Responding on one of them, [the conditioned reinforcement (CR) lever] results in presentation of the light CS plus the noise made by the (empty) water dipper as it rises to the niche in the chamber where the subject previously drank water. Responses on the second lever [nonconditioned reinforcement (NCR) lever] have no programmed consequence and serve as a control for nonspecific changes in activation or motor activity. This is a stringent test of CR, since differential responding on the lever associated with the CR would not occur if the com-

TABLE I. Behavioral Procedures for Studying the
Neural Mechanisms of Reward-Related Processes.

Paradigm	Procedure
1. Acquisition of a new response with conditioned reinforcement	Phase 1: Pavlovian association of an arbitrary stimulus with primary reinforcement (e.g., water in thirsty rats). Phase 2: The conditioned reinforcing properties of the CS are assessed by its control over the acquisition of a new response in the absence of the primary reward.
2. Conditioned place preference	Phase 1: Repeated presentations of primary reinforcement (e.g., sucrose in hungry rats), or nothing, in one of two distinctive environments. Phase 2: The conditioned approach to the environment previously paired with reward is measured in a preference test in extinction.
3. Second-order schedule of reinforcement	Phase 1: Pavlovian association of an arbitrary stimulus with primary reinforcement (e.g., sexual interaction with an oestrous female). Phase 2: Acquisition of responding for the primary reinforcer presented under a second-order schedule: responding is maintained by the contingent presentation of the CS (which has gained conditioned reinforcing properties in Phase 1).

pound stimulus had not acquired motivational salience through prior association with primary reward.

The *conditioned place preference procedure* shows many similarities to the acquisition of a new response procedure, save that neither the stimulus nor the response is precisely specified (van der Kooy, 1985; White et al., 1985; Phillips and Fibiger, 1987). Thus, in the experiments to be described, hungry rats repeatedly have the opportunity to drink 10% sucrose in one discrete compartment of the apparatus that is made distinctive by the colour of its walls, the nature of the wood shavings on the floor, and its spatial location with reference to extra-apparatus cues. In an equivalent, equally distinctive second compartment the hungry rats do not experience an ingestive reward on days that alternate with exposure to the other side. In the test phase, animals are placed in a neutral start chamber and are allowed freely to choose either side of the compartment and spend their time there (see Everitt et al., 1991). Sucrose is no longer presented in this phase. Thus, the animals in displaying a preference for the side in which reinforcement previously had occurred demonstrate the control over approach behavior by the previously neutral cues which define the distinctive place. This procedure is frequently used to study the rewarding properties of a drug, since the test phase allows the measurement of responses to conditioned incentives in the absence of the drug, thereby eliminating its unconditioned effects which may nonspecifically interfere with the behavior being measured.

In the *second-order schedule of reinforcement* (Everitt et al., 1987; Everitt and Stacey, 1987; Everitt, 1990), naive male rats are initially allowed to interact sexually with an oestrous female in the presence of an arbitrary light in an operant chamber. In the second phase, the oestrous female is presented at the end of a (fixed interval 15 minutes) session, during which the light CS is presented contingent on a small fixed ratio (FR) of responses. We have established that the CS, which is formally equivalent to a CR, maintains responding during the fixed interval (FI), since its omission from the schedule is followed by a rapid collapse of responding for the primary reinforcer (Everitt et al., 1987). Indeed, it has proved impossible in many attempts to obtain a high level of instrumental responding by male rats directly for access to a receptive female, most probably because small "aliquots" of sexual reinforcement cannot be presented without profoundly disrupting the measurement of ongoing behavioral responses (see Everitt et al., 1987). For this reason, second-order schedules of reinforcement have been utilized with great success in studies of the reinforcing properties of drugs of abuse, such as psychomotor stimulants, which similarly disrupt ongoing instrumental behavior when administered during the test session (see Goldberg et al., 1976; Katz, 1979). A particular advantage of this procedure is that it allows the investigation of stimulus-reward associations in a more integrated and so less abstract behavioral context than does the acquisition of a new response procedure. Stable baselines of instrumental responding can be maintained over long periods, since neural and other manipulations are carried out after acquisition. Furthermore, the effects of each neural manipulation on conditioned behavior can be compared directly with those on unconditioned behavior within the same test session.

NEURAL MANIPULATIONS

The experiments reviewed here have been conducted in order to test the hypothesis that the amygdala—at least its basolateral parts*—and the ventral striatum (VS), including its dopaminergic innervation, form part of a neural system that is involved with aspects of emotional behavior. To do this, two types of neural manipulation have been used: first, coincident, bilateral manipulations of either structure; second, asymmetric (i.e., contralateral), unilateral lesions of each structure.

In the first case, we have in two experiments studied the effects of bilateral lesions of the basolateral amygdala (BLA) both alone and in combination with infusions directly into the ventral striatum of the dopamine-releasing drug,

---

*Throughout this chapter, the term "basolateral amygdala" (BLA) is used as a collective term for the lateral, basal magnocellular, basal parvocellular, and basal accessory nuclei (Price et al., 1987), since these structures are those generally damaged following excitotoxic lesions used in the experiments. We have not to date localized behavioral effects of BLA lesions to individual nuclei, although some authors have suggested this to be possible (e.g., Gallagher et al., 1990; Hiroi and White, 1991).

d-amphetamine, through chronically implanted cannulae. In this way, the impact of basolateral amygdala lesions, dopaminergic activation of the ventral striatum, and the way that the effects of the latter are modified by coincident basolateral amygdala lesions have been assessed within the same behavioral paradigm (Cador et al., 1989; Everitt et al., 1989a).

In the second case, we have in a further experiment compared the effects of bilateral lesions of either the ventral striatum or the basolateral amygdala within the same paradigm and then made a "disconnection" of these structures by making unilateral lesions of each structure, but on opposite sides of the brain. If the basolateral amygdala and ventral striatum are indeed functionally and serially interrelated, then the asymmetric lesions should have behavioral effects that resemble closely those followed by bilateral lesions of either structure alone (Everitt et al., 1991).

The cannulation procedures used to deliver d-amphetamine (and, indeed, other dopaminergic drugs) directly to the ventral striatum are straightforward and have been reported on in some detail elsewhere (Taylor and Robbins, 1984, 1986; Cador et al., 1989; Robbins et al., 1989). Briefly, bilateral guide cannulae are implanted chronically to lie just dorsal to the nucleus accumbens (NAS) region of the ventral striatum at about its midpoint anteroposteriorly. Infusion cannulae can then be inserted directly into the NAS itself and the drug infused in the freely moving animal. Observations begin within 5 minutes of the drug infusion.

Electrolytic, aspirative, or radiofrequency lesions of the amygdala have been widely used over many years in studies of its functions (Weiskrantz, 1956; Kemble and Beckman, 1970; Jones and Mishkin, 1972; Henke and Maxwell, 1973; Grossman et al., 1974; Kling and Stecklis, 1976; Dacey and Grossman, 1977; Aggleton and Passingham, 1981, 1982; Kemble et al., 1984; Davis, 1986; Simbayi et al.,1986; LeDoux et al., 1988, 1990; Hitchcock et al., 1989; Gaffan and Murray, 1990). These types of lesions not only destroy intrinsic amygdaloid neurons, but also axons passing through the structure, between the medial forebrain bundle/substantia innominata region and the temporal and insular cortex. In the studies reported here, we have adopted a different lesioning procedure involving the infusion of excitotoxic amino acids into the basolateral amygdala, which effectively destroys its intrinsic neurons, but generally spares those fibre bundles passing through it (Schwarcz et al., 1979; Köhler and Schwarcz, 1983; Dunn and Everitt, 1988). Our earlier work has indicated that such lesioning procedures are essential if valid conclusions are to be made concerning the localization to the amygdala of behavioral changes following its destruction (Dunn and Everitt, 1988).

This is perhaps best illustrated by reference to some of this earlier work. The impairment in conditioned taste aversion seen in many studies to follow amygdala lesions (Rolls and Rolls, 1973a; Nachman and Ashe, 1974; Aggleton et al., 1981; Simbayi et al., 1986; Dunn and Everitt, 1988) has long been presented as data in support of an important role of this structure in one aspect of emotional behavior: Namely, the modification of motivational responses to current goals in the context of past (in this case, aversive) experience (Rolls and Rolls, 1973a; Rolls, 1990). However, near-total destruction of the amygdala made by infusing N-methyl,D-aspartic acid (NMDA) had no effect on the acquisition of a conditioned taste aversion (Dunn and Everitt, 1988), a finding that has subsequently been confirmed (Cahill and McGaugh, 1990). We went on to show that the critical feature of electrolytic lesions that does disrupt conditioned taste aversion is the destruction of axons passing through the amygdala, to and/or from the insular, gustatory neocortex (Dunn and Everitt, 1988). This was confirmed by studying the retrograde transport of the fluorescent dye, True Blue, from the insular cortex to the hypothalamus and brain stem in rats with both types of lesions. Electrolytic basolateral amygdala lesions impaired both conditioned taste aversion and retrograde dye transport; NMDA-induced lesions had no effect on conditioned taste aversion and also did not affect the retrograde transport of the dye (Dunn and Everitt, 1988). Thus, the process by which associations between illness and tastes are made do not, as was earlier thought, depend on the basolateral amygdala. By contrast, step-down passive avoidance learning, which in the past has also been repeatedly shown to be affected by electrolytic basolateral amygdala lesions (Richardson, 1973; Grossman et al., 1974; Kesner, 1981; Sarter and Markowitsch, 1985), was also impaired by NMDA-induced lesions, suggesting that this type of fear-motivated learning is indeed dependent on the amygdala (Riolobos and Garcia, 1987).

Thus, to attribute functions to a structure on the basis of the consequences of its destruction requires, at the very least, that as optimal a lesioning procedure as possible be utilized. In the case of the basolateral amygdala, that procedure involves the use of excitotoxic amino acids. In the earlier experiments NMDA was employed. In later experiments, quinolinic acid was used since this resulted in more restricted and better controlled neuronal damage. However, it has rarely proved possible to restrict excitotoxic lesions to individual nuclei in the amygdaloid complex (but see Gallagher et al., 1990) and focal electrolytic lesions, viewed in parallel with axon-sparing lesions, may be used to good effect in localizing disrupted functions to discrete nuclei in some circumstances (see Hiroi and White, 1991).

Lesions of the ventral striatum, for similar reasons, have also been made by infusing an excitatory amino acid. In this case quisqualic acid, which is an agonist at the AMPA/Quisqualate (non-NMDA) receptor (Schoepp et al., 1990; Barnard and Henley, 1990; Watkins et al., 1990), has been used (Everitt et al., 1991). This excitotoxin destroys neurons intrinsic to the ventral striatum (including the NAS, ventromedial caudate-putamen, and, in some cases, the olfactory tubercle) while sparing adjacent fibres of passage, such as the anterior commissure.

Experiment 1: Acquisition of a New Response With Conditioned Reinforcement: Effects of Basolateral Amygdala Lesions and Ventral Striatal Infusions of d-Amphetamine

It is well known and of obvious adaptive value that arbitrary stimuli which predict reinforcement may, by conditioning, themselves eventually control behavior as conditioned reinforcers (Mackintosh, 1983; Dickinson, 1980). The data reviewed in this section indicate that this control may depend on associative mechanisms occurring within the basolateral amygdala that interact with the

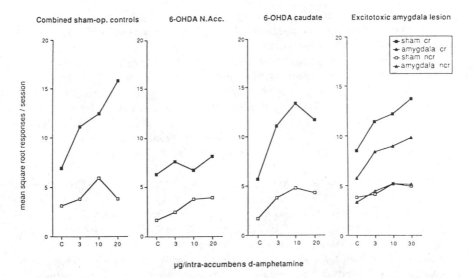

Combined sham-op. controls   6-OHDA N.Acc.   6-OHDA caudate   Excitotoxic amygdala lesion

μg/intra-accumbens d-amphetamine

Fig. 1. The effects of intra-accumbens d-amphetamine on responding with conditioned reinforcement in controls **(first panel)**, subjects with dopamine depletions from the ventral **(second panel)** or dorsal **(third panel)** striatum and subjects with excitotoxic lesions of the basolateral amygdala. The dose-dependent potentiation of responding selectively on the lever producing the conditioned reinforcer by intra-accumbens d-amphetamine can be seen in panel 1 (cr lever). This is completely prevented by 6-hydroxydopamine-induced dopamine depletion from the ventral, but not the dorsal, striatum (panels 2 and 3). Note that dopamine depletion does not affect selective responding on the lever producing the conditioned reinforcer under control (C) conditions (i.e., when vehicle alone is infused into the ventral striatum). By contrast, lesions of the basolateral amygdala reduce responding on the lever producing the conditioned reinforcer, but this occurs independently of the effect of intra-accumbens d-amphetamine, which continues to potentiate responding on the lever producing the conditioned reinforcer, but from a lower, lesion-induced baseline. There are no significant effects of any procedure on responding on the lever having no programmed consequence (control, or ncr lever). (N. Acc, nucleus accumbens). Data from Taylor and Robbins, 1984, 1986; Cador et al., 1989. The figure is reproduced from Robbins et al., 1989 with permission from Pergamon Press PLC.

ventral striatum in a way that is itself subject to modulation by dopaminergic transmission within the latter structure.

Using the acquisition of a new response procedure (Table I), it has long been apparent that psychomotor stimulant drugs, such as d-amphetamine and pipradrol, selectively increase responding with conditioned reinforcement (Robbins, 1976; Beninger et al., 1980). Subsequently, these potentiative effects were demonstrated to be dependent upon increased dopaminergic activity in the ventral striatum (Taylor and Robbins, 1984, 1986). Thus, intra-NAS infusions of d-amphetamine (Taylor and Robbins, 1984) (see Fig. 1), cocaine (Rosenzweig-Lipson et al., 1990), dopamine itself (Robbins et al., 1989; Cador et al., 1991), or directly acting D1 and D2 receptor agonists (Wolterink et al., 1989) all result in a significant, dose-dependent increase in responding on the lever providing CR, but have only minor and variable effects on the NCR lever. No such effects of d-amphetamine are seen after infusion into the dorsal striatum or thalamus, indicating a clear degree of neural site specificity (Taylor and Robbins, 1984). Behavioral specificity of the effects of these drugs is evidenced by the observation that they depend upon the predictive association of the CS with primary reinforcement (water in these experiments). Thus, random pairing of the unconditioned stimulus (US) (water) and CS resulted in no stimulation of responding on the CR lever following intra-NAS d-amphetamine (Taylor and Robbins, 1984; Robbins et al., 1989).

Depletion of dopamine from the ventral striatum by infusing the catecholaminergic neurotoxin 6-hydroxydopamine (6OHDA) completely prevented the dose-dependent potentiation of responding with CR that usually follows intra-NAS d-amphetamine (Taylor and Robbins, 1986) (see Fig. 1). By contrast, an equivalent degree of dopamine depletion from the dorsal striatum did not prevent the actions of d-amphetamine—except possibly at the highest doses used (Taylor and Robbins, 1986) (see Fig. 1). The reductions in ventral striatum noradrenaline content which result from 6OHDA infusions have been shown not to be an important variable in these results, since 6OHDA-induced dorsal noradrenergic bundle lesions, which noradrenergically denervate the ventral striatum by more than 95%, did not decrease the effects of intra-NAS d-amphetamine (Cador et al., 1991). Conversely, infusing noradrenaline itself into the NAS did not potentiate responding with CR (Cador et al., 1991) and this indicates that noradrenaline release following intra-NAS d-amphetamine is not important in the potentiation of responding with CR.

These data make it apparent that dopamine release or postsynaptic receptor activation in the ventral striatum mediate the control over behavior by conditioned reinforcers. However, until recently it has been unclear whether the conditioned influence on behavior also depends on the same neural substrate. Indeed, some evidence from the above studies indicated that it is not. Thus, although near-total depletion of dopamine from the ventral striatum abolished the *potentiative* effects of d-amphetamine on responding with CR, basal levels of responding, which were 5–10 times higher on the CR than on the NCR lever, in the control condition were completely unaffected (Fig. 1). This raised to us the possibility that information about conditioned reinforcers is not directly dependent upon activity of the ventral striatum and its dopaminergic innervation arising from the midbrain ventral tegmental area. We proposed that it might depend instead upon processes occurring in limbic structures—especially the basolateral amygdala, which had been proposed to be important in the formation of stimulus-reward associations (see above), as well as more specifically in conditioned reinforcement (Gaffan and Harrison, 1987) and which had also been demonstrated to project richly to the ventral striatum (Groenewegen et al., 1991) in a manner subject to modulation by dopaminergic transmission (Yim and Mogenson, 1982, 1989).

Therefore, we investigated the effects of bilateral, NMDA-induced lesions of the basolateral amygdala on the acquisition of a new response with conditioned reinforcement. The rats with lesions also were implanted with cannulae so that the effects of basolateral amygdala lesions on the potentiative actions of d-amphetamine on responding could also be studied.

The excitotoxic lesion of the basolateral amygdala resulted in a significant reduction in responding on the lever producing CR, but not on the NCR lever (Fig. 1). Thus the differential distribution in responding between CR and NCR levers that is usually seen was much reduced following basolateral amygdala lesions (Cador et al., 1989). However, intra-NAS infusions of d-amphetamine continued to dose-dependently potentiate responding in the animals with lesions, albeit from this lower baseline, such that levels of responding on the lever producing the conditioned reinforcer were only about half those seen following identical infusions in sham-lesioned subjects (Fig. 1) (Cador et al., 1989).

These data suggest, therefore, that the impact on behavior of conditioned reinforcers depends on two relatively independent processes: First, information from the amygdala concerning the conditioned association of the CS with reinforcement. This information determines the choice of lever under control conditions and, since it is preserved following dopaminergic denervation of the ventral striatum (Robbins et al., 1989), is relatively independent of dopaminergic transmission in this structure. Second, the effect of this latter dopaminergic input to the ventral striatum from the ventral tegmental area is apparently to amplify the basal differential responding on the two levers by selectively potentiating that occurring on the lever producing the conditioned reinforcer (Robbins et al., 1989).

The behavioral specificity of the effects of basolateral amygdala lesions is important to emphasize. First, although earlier studies using electrolytic lesions of the amygdala reported motivational deficits (Rolls and Rolls, 1973b; Box and Mogenson, 1975; Dacey and Grossman, 1977; Fitzgerald and Burton, 1981), these are not seen following the NMDA-induced lesions used here (Dunn and Everitt, 1988). Thus, in a 23 h deprivation test, for example, basolateral amygdala-lesioned and sham-operated rats drank similar volumes of water (Cador et al., 1989). Second, the basolateral amygdala lesion did not change locomotor activity under either basal conditions or in response to systemic d-amphetamine (Cador et al., 1989). Third, although impaired in the acquisition of a new response with conditioned reinforcement, basolateral amygdala-lesioned subjects were not impaired at all in the acquisition of an identical lever press response, under a variety of schedules, for the primary reinforcer, water (Cador et al., 1989). Finally, the basolateral amygdala lesions did not impair the discriminated approach to the water dipper that is signalled by the CS. The lesioned animals, then, appeared not to show any simple sensory impairment and were able to discriminate the CS effectively (Cador et al., 1989). It was only when serving as a conditioned reinforcer that the control over behavior by the CS was impaired (Robbins et al., 1989).

Taken together, the results of this experiment strongly indicated that the basolateral amygdala and ventral striatum interact under the conditions of this experimental paradigm to mediate the control over behavior by conditioned reinforcers; the basolateral amygdala appears to be important for the association between arbitrary stimuli and primary reinforcement and its subsequent influence over behavior is dependent upon interactions with the ventral striatum, where modulation by dopamine release can occur.

Experiment 2: Second-Order Schedule of (Sexual) Reinforcement: Effects of Basolateral Amygdala Lesions and Ventral Striatal Infusions of d-Amphetamine

The acquisition of a new response procedure, while providing a stringent test of conditioned reinforcement that, as we have shown, is of great utility in probing the neural mechanisms underlying stimulus-reward associations, is nevertheless a rather abstract one. Second-order schedules of reinforcement, on the other hand, allow the study of a more integrated pattern of behavior. Both instrumental measures, reflecting the control over behavior by conditioned reinforcers, and also unconditioned behavior that can be observed when the primary reinforcer is presented, can be quantified separately and in sequence.

Male rats can be trained to work for the presentation, under a second-order schedule, of a female in heat (Everitt et al., 1987). Acquisition of this response is relatively slow because test sessions can only be conducted twice weekly, but over a three month period (i.e., about 24 test sessions) rats achieve relatively stable and high rates of responding under a FR10 schedule for the contingent presentation of a CS (usually a light) that maintains behavior during an overall FI of 15 minutes. On completion of the first FR after the timing out of the FI, an oestrous female automatically enters the operant chamber and the male is allowed to interact sexually with her until the first intromission following ejaculation (Everitt et al., 1987).

Both instrumental and copulatory behavior are dependent upon testosterone, since castration significantly reduces the former and abolishes the latter; both are reinstated by systemic testosterone (Everitt and Stacey, 1987). It is important to note that the recovery of instrumental responding following testosterone treatment occurs before males have had the opportunity to interact sexually with females and thereby experience recovery of their copulatory ability. Testosterone, then, has an impact on sexual motivation that is not secondary to improvements in sexual performance (Everitt and Stacey, 1987; Everitt, 1990).

By contrast, bilateral lesions of the medial preoptic area—a structure of major importance in mediating the effects of testosterone on sexual behavior [see Everitt (1990) for discussion]—have no effect on instrumental responding under the second-order schedule, yet eliminate mounting, intromitting, and ejaculation (Everitt and Stacey, 1987). It seems, then, as if the rostral hypothalamus is important for the execution of copulatory responses, but not for the performance of appetitive behavior that is maintained and directed by environmental stimuli which have gained motivational salience through their predictive association with sexual interaction (Everitt, 1990). It seems reasonable to suggest, in the light of the results of Experiment 1, that the latter process might depend not on hypothalamic substrates but on the basolateral amygdala. Furthermore, it is well known that appetitive, but not performance, elements of sexual behavior in males are markedly affected by manipulations of dopamine in the ventral striatum (Everitt, 1990). Thus, using the second-order schedule, we have studied the effects of identical manipulations of the basolateral amygdala and ventral striatum to those used in Experiment 1 in order to gain further insight into interactions between these structures in the expression of emotional behavior.

Following acquisition, bilateral, NMDA-induced lesions of the basolateral amygdala resulted in a significant and permanent reduction in responding under a second-order schedule of presentation of an oestrous female. By contrast, when the female had entered the chamber, the sexual behavior of basolateral amygdala-lesioned males was no different from controls (Fig. 2; see Everitt et al., 1989a). Thus, the lesion disrupted appetitive sexual responses maintained by a visual conditioned reinforcer, but not the performance of copulatory responses elicited by the primary reinforcer, a female in heat. Infusion of d-amphetamine bilaterally into the ventral striatum of lesioned males increased instrumental behavior to levels similar to controls (Fig. 2), that is, this treatment tended to ameliorate the response deficit (Everitt et al., 1989a). Parameters of copulatory behavior were unaffected by this treatment, save that the latencies to mount and intromit were significantly reduced—but to an equal extent in basolateral amygdala-lesioned and control rats (Everitt et al., 1989a).

The effect of d-amphetamine to increase responding was critically dependent upon the presentation of the light CS. Thus, alteration of the schedule so that the light was no longer presented resulted in a marked reduction in responding in the control but not the basolateral amygdala-lesioned animals, such that the controls actually responded at a lower level than did lesioned subjects (Fig. 3). An explanation for this striking observation is that animals without the basolateral amygdala are less sensitive to alterations in stimuli associated with reward (Everitt et al., 1989a). The question then arises as to what maintained responding on the lower baseline following amygdala lesions. The answer is unclear at the moment, but it seems reasonable to suggest that the behavior of basolateral amygdala-lesioned subjects is subject to greater control by the primary reinforcer, i.e., the oestrous female, since she is visually, vocally, and olfactorily present in a Perspex trapdoor compartment in the roof of the chamber (Everitt et al., 1989a). Infusion of d-amphetamine into the ventral striatum under these conditions, when responding had decreased to low levels following removal of the CS, was without significant effect on responding in either control or lesioned rats (Fig. 3). Hence, the potentiation of responding when d-amphetamine is infused into the ventral striatum depends upon the conditioned reinforcement contingency (Everitt et al., 1989a).

Experiment 3: Conditioned Place Preference: Effects of Bilateral Basolateral Amygdala or Ventral Striatal Lesions, or Amygdala-Ventral Striatal Disconnection

The dopaminergic innervation of the ventral striatum has consistently been implicated as an important neural structure mediating conditioned place preference (Spyraki et al., 1982, 1983; Messier and White, 1984; van der Kooy, 1985;

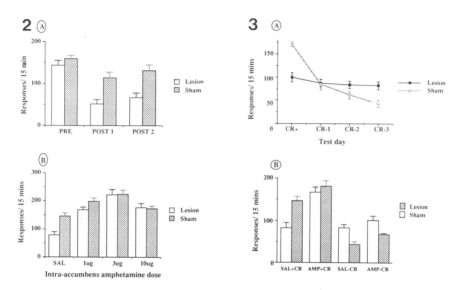

Fig. 2. A: The effects of lesions of the basolateral amygdala on responding by male rats for an oestrous female presented under a second-order schedule of reinforcement. Responding is significantly and permanently reduced by the lesions (data from two postoperative tests, one week apart, are shown here, POST 1 and POST 2; Pre, preoperative data; **B:** The effects of saline (SAL) or three doses of intra-accumbens d-amphetamine (1,3, and 10 μg in 1 μl) on responding by lesioned or sham-operated animals under the second-order schedule. It can be seen that d-amphetamine ameliorates the effects of the lesion on responding. (Data from Everitt et al., 1989a.)

Fig. 3. A: The effects of omitting the conditioned reinforcer (a light) on responding by amygdala-lesioned and sham-operated control male rats for an oestrous female presented under a second-order schedule. Note the marked decrease in responding in the controls such that they come to respond at a lower level than the lesioned subjects. CR +, responding with the conditioned reinforcer; CR-1, -2, -3, three consecutive days when the conditioned reinforcer was not presented during the test session (fixed interval 15 min); **B:** The effects of intra-accumbens d-amphetamine on responding under the second-order schedule with and without conditioned reinforcement. Note that the effect of d-amphetamine is greatly attenuated in the absence of the conditioned reinforcer. SAL + CR, AMP + CR, saline or d-amphetamine infusions, respectively, with the conditioned reinforcer being presented contingent upon completion of a fixed ratio of 10 responses, as usual; SAL-CR, AMP-CR, saline or d-amphetamine infusions, respectively, without the conditioned reinforcer being presented following each fixed ratio of responses. (Data from Everitt et al., 1989a.)

White and Carr, 1985; White et al., 1985; Phillips and Fibiger, 1987). Thus, not only do dopamine agonists, such as d-amphetamine, support the acquisition of a conditioned place preference when given systemically (Phillips and Fibiger, 1987), they fail to do so following 6OHDA-induced dopamine depletion from the ventral striatum (Phillips and Fibiger, 1987). Dopaminergic agonists also support the acquisition of a conditioned place preference when infused directly into the ventral striatum (Phillips and Fibiger, 1987). In addition, this substrate also seems to be important for the acquisition of a place preference conditioned by exposure to natural reinforcers such as sucrose, since dopamine depletion from the ventral striatum blocks the development of a conditioned place preference by repeated exposure to sucrose (White and Carr, 1985; White et al., 1985). However, on the basis of the data in Experiments 1 and 2 described above, it seemed reasonable to suggest that the basolateral amygdala might also be a critical structure in the formation of associations between stimuli characterizing a discrete place and the presentation of a primary reinforcer. Moreover, the relative simplicity of this behavioral procedure suggested it might be an ideal one to explore interactions between the basolateral amygdala and ventral striatum more directly.

In this experiment, a place preference was conditioned by allowing hungry animals to consume 10% sucrose in one distinctive half of a large, three-chambered apparatus. They never experienced an ingestive reward in the other large compartment. Following several pairs of conditioning days, animals received either (1), bilateral quinolinate-induced lesions of the basolateral amygdala, (2) bilateral, quisqualate-induced lesions of the ventral striatum, (3) bilateral, quisqualate-induced lesions of the ventromedial caudate-putamen, (4) bilateral, quisqualate-induced lesions of the dorsolateral caudate-putamen, and (5) contralateral lesions of the ventral striatum and basolateral amygdala—i.e., a basolateral amygdala-ventral striatum "disconnection." The effects of these neural manipulations on the expression of the sucrose conditioned place preference were studied (Everitt et al., 1991).

Significant preoperative place preferences were abolished in subjects receiving bilateral lesions of the basolateral amygdala (Fig. 4). A similar abolition of place preference followed bilateral lesions of the ventral striatum, both those involving the NAS (Fig. 4) and those involving the ventromedial caudate-putamen [data not shown, see Everitt et al. (1991)]. Unilateral basolateral amygdala or ventral striatum lesions, bilateral lesions of the dorsolateral caudate-putamen, and all sham operations had no effect on the previously established conditioned place preference. The asymmetric lesion procedure, which combined a unilateral lesion of the basolateral amygdala with a contralateral lesion of the ventral striatum, also significantly attenuated the conditioned place preference (Fig. 4), although the effect was somewhat less severe than that seen to follow bilateral lesions of either structure alone. The latter result strongly supports the view that the basolateral amygdala and ventral striatum interact serially in this behavioral context (Everitt et al., 1991).

The behavioral effects showed some specificity. Measures of the ingestion of sucrose following 23 h deprivation demonstrated that there was no deficit in

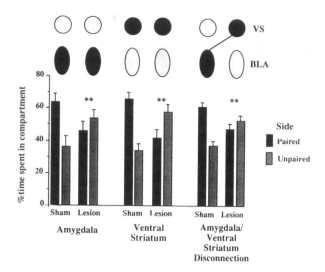

Fig. 4. The effects of bilateral, basolateral amygdala, or ventral striatal lesions, or asymmetric, unilateral lesions of each structure on a sucrose-conditioned place preference. Each lesion procedure abolishes the expression of the conditioned place preference. VS, ventral striatum; BLA, basolateral amygdala. The cartoon above each block of data indicates the lesion procedure used. In panel three, the nature of a "disconnection" resulting from asymmetric lesions of the basolateral amygdala and contralateral ventral striatum is shown. Paired, side of the apparatus paired with sucrose; Unpaired, side of the apparatus not paired with sucrose. (Data from Everitt et al., 1991.)

primary motivation following basolateral amygdala lesions and that this could not underlie the loss of the conditioned place preference (Everitt et al., 1991). Although there was a significant reduction in sucrose ingestion following ventral striatum lesions, this was minor and it is difficult to envisage it could underlie such a large impairment in conditioned place preference [in fact, sham-lesioned rats that were given a conditioned place preference test after free-feeding continued to show a place preference which was not significantly different from that observed when they were tested under mildly deprived conditions, suggesting that motivational factors do not greatly affect the expression of a conditioned place preference, at least under the testing conditions used here; see Everitt et al. (1991)]. No changes in sucrose ingestion followed other striatal or the asymmetric lesions.

In sham-operated controls, locomotor activity and rearing were differentially distributed between compartments during the preference test in that they reared more and were more active in the unpaired side when sucrose was no longer presented in the paired side; this presumably reflects an adaptive response to the nonpresentation of the sucrose in the test phase (Everitt et al., 1991). Rats with basolateral amygdala lesions showed no absolute change in activity and thus the impaired conditioned place preference could not be attributed to gross alterations in locomotor activity (Everitt et al., 1991). However, there were differences in the distribution of this activity between compartments in the apparatus. Thus, the basolateral amygdala-lesioned rats were less active in the unpaired side and also reared less in this environment than did controls (Everitt et al., 1991). Rats with lesions of the ventral striatum or ventromedial caudate-putamen similarly showed no gross change in levels of locomotor activity, but did show a quite different distribution of activity between sides in being significantly more active on the paired side during the extinction test, such that there was no difference between activity on paired and unpaired sides, as usually seen in controls (Everitt et al., 1991). Whereas basolateral amygdala-lesioned animals showed a simple loss of the differential distribution in activity between sides shown by controls, ventral striatum- and ventromedial caudate-putamen-lesioned animals showed an inappropriate increase in activity on the side where least activity was seen in controls. This may indicate an increase in activity independent of control by environmental contingencies (Everitt et al., 1991). No changes in activity were seen following lesions of the dorsolateral striatum or the asymmetric lesions. The latter observation is important since it suggests that the loss of conditioned place preference following asymmetric lesions reflects disruption of a discrete process subserved by interactions between amygdala and striatum, and that the hyperactivity seen following bilateral ventral striatal lesions may have been rather a nonspecific release phenomenon.

One possible explanation of the attenuation or abolition of place preference following the lesions is that it was consequent upon impaired discrimination by the animals of the sensory characteristics of the paired and unpaired compartments. The data on this point are not entirely straightforward, partly because measures of sensory discrimination or threshold usually depend upon reinforced discrimination which may be disrupted indirectly by the effects of amygdala lesions on stimulus-reward associations. However, the majority of the literature, as we have indicated in this chapter, is largely consistent with the latter interpretation (Weiskrantz, 1956; Jones and Mishkin, 1972; Spiegler and Mishkin, 1981; Sarter and Markowitsch, 1985; Gaffan and Harrison, 1987; Gaffan et al., 1988, 1989; see Everitt et al., 1991; Robbins et al., 1989 for discussion).

SYNTHESIS

The results of the three experiments described above provide converging evidence for a role of the basolateral amygdala in mediating conditioned (or secondary) reinforcement, in agreement with the conclusions of Gaffan and Harrison (1987). Thus, in Experiment 1 basolateral amygdala lesions attenuated responding with conditioned reinforcement, in the presence or absence of concomitant dopaminergic activation of the ventral striatum produced by intra-NAS amphetamine. In Experiment 2, the ability of a previously neutral stimulus paired with sexual reinforcement to maintain responding under a second-order schedule was similarly attenuated. Finally, in Experiment 3, the expression of a place preference conditioned to the presentation of food was abolished. It can be argued that the impact on behavior of the stimulus-reward association has been prevented by damage to this portion of the amygdala. However, there are inevitably issues raised by the comparison of these results obtained in rather different paradigms. For example, the reduction in responding for the conditioned reinforcer produced by basolateral amygdala lesions was incomplete in Experiment 1, whereas place preference conditioning was totally abolished. In the case of the second-order schedule, it is difficult to be precise about the exact degree of reduction obtained because of evidence that the rats with lesions responded at a higher level than sham-operated controls following repeated sessions in the absence of the conditioned reinforcer. This suggested that a degree of instrumental behavior was being maintained by the unconditioned reinforcer.

There are several obvious factors to bear in mind when attempting to reconcile these quantitative differences: First, the completeness of the basolateral amygdala lesion (however, this would not appear to be critical because lesions were of comparable magnitude in the three experiments described). Second, the precise nature of the behavioral paradigm employed; for example, the procedures could vary in their sensitivity in measuring the effects of conditioned reinforcement, and this can only be resolved by double dissociation studies. Third, each procedure used a different unconditioned reinforcer (respectively, water, sex, and sucrose). While the generally comparable results obtained are impressive in this light, it remains possible that some of the differences can be attributed to the nature of the primary reinforcer (see below for example). Fourth, although the effects of basolateral amygdala lesions were assessed at different stages of the procedure (in Experiment 1, after conditioning but prior to the acquisition of a new response, in Experiment 2, after conditioning and acquisition of the instrumental response, and in Experiment 3, after conditioning), subsequent unpublished data have indicated that the effects are similar in Experiment 1 if the surgery occurs prior to conditioning (Burns, Robbins and Everitt, to be published) and in Experiment 3, if it occurs prior to place preference conditioning (Everitt, unpublished observations; see also Hiroi and White, 1991). Finally, the processes governing the implementation of stimulus-reward associations are unlikely all to be vested within a single brain structure, and a degree of parallel distributed processing of stimuli with acquired affective significance would appear to be adaptive.

Comparisons of the present results with those from the published literature are made difficult by the paucity of relevant studies. The effects described by Gaffan and Harrison (1987) are clearly consistent and their maintenance of visual discrimination learning by secondary reinforcement is reminiscent of a second-order schedule. In the case of place preference conditioning, it has been reported that a place preference induced by systemic d-amphetamine, an effect known to depend on dopamine-dependent mechanisms of the ventral striatum (Phillips and Fibiger, 1987), is abolished by lesions of the basolateral amygdala (Hiroi and White, 1991). In the same study, there were no effects of lesions to the fimbria-fornix or ventral hippocampus and, moreover, specificity within the amygdala was suggested by the demonstration of no effects of central nucleus damage, and by localizing the deficit to the lateral amygdala (Hiroi and White, 1991).

There has been one study showing apparently discrepant results following large excitotoxic lesions of the amygdala on appetitive conditioning to an odor cue, assessed using a place preference (Cahill and McGaugh, 1990). While the reasons for this discrepancy are not immediately obvious, it is of considerable interest that the arbitrary olfactory stimulus (amyl nitrate) was in the same sensory modality as the reinforcer (sucrose). Given the suggestion that the amygdala is particularly implicated in cross-modal associations (Murray and Mishkin, 1985), it would be of considerable interest to manipulate this factor in further experiments with conditioned reinforcement. The companion experiment in the study by Cahill and McGaugh (1990) failed to show any effect of the amygdala lesion on the appetitive learning of a one-trial Y maze brightness discrimination for water. This is analogous to the lack of effect of basolateral amygdala lesions on discriminated approach in Experiment 1 reported above and does not rule out possible effects on conditioned reinforcement which were not tested.

What is not addressed by the present studies is the precise nature of the effect of the basolateral amygdala lesion; is it upon the associations between the erstwhile conditioned reinforcer and the unconditioned reinforcer that are compromised, or is it upon the association between the conditioned reinforcer and the instrumental response that the conditioned reinforcer comes to control? This question is difficult to answer because of course the easiest way of measuring the strength of conditioned reinforcement is to quantify its effect via an instrumental contingency. Even in the case of place preference conditioning, it is unclear to what extent the preference is maintained by voluntary instrumental responses to the food-paired side and to what degree the preference is determined by Pavlovian approach tendencies. These questions are also relevant to the functions of the ventral striatum and its interaction with the amygdala, but once again are yet to be addressed by experimentation.

It is likely that the detailed analysis of these and other simple behavioral paradigms will be required fully to elucidate the exact role of the amygdala in appetitive conditioning. For example, although we found the discriminated approach to a CS that signals the presentation of water is unaffected by the basolateral amygdala lesion, our recent evidence has shown small but significant effects on such responding conditioned to sucrose presentation in hungry rats (Everitt et al., 1989b), which may parallel possible impairments in approach seen in the place preference procedure.

Recent results have also suggested some dissociations between the effects of amygdala lesions on different aspects of appetitive behavior, but with a focus on the central nucleus rather than the basolateral amygdala (Gallagher et al., 1990). Excitotoxic lesions of this structure impaired the Pavlovian conditioned orientational response that occurs to either visual or auditory CSs predictive of food delivery, without impairing the (presumed Pavlovian) approach response to the food cup (Gallagher et al., 1990). This effect may represent a behavioral manifestation of the various components of the orientation reflex, including for example changes in cardiac rate, that may occur in response to significant stimuli (LeDoux, 1986a,b; Davis et al., 1987).

SPECIFICITY OF AMYGDALA-VENTRAL STRIATAL INTERACTIONS

We have begun to define the effects of just one of the sources of limbic afferents to the ventral striatum, but it is reasonable to raise the issue of what might be unique about this form of functional interaction. The ventral striatum receives afferents from the entorhinal, cingulate, and prelimbic cortex, as well as from the subiculum of the hippocampal formation, and it seems likely that these inputs too provide quite specific forms of interaction with striatal outflow (Groenewegen et al., 1991). Given the less than complete effects of basolateral amygdala lesions on conditioned reinforcement in its interactions with the ventral striatum, it is possible that these additional structures also mediate some of the processing of these stimuli.

However, most of the preliminary indications are that structures such as the hippocampus have quite different forms of interaction with the ventral striatum. For example, lesions of the ventral striatum produce deficits in several behavioral tests that appear to be more dependent upon hippocampal rather than amygdaloid influences. These include the induction of schedule-induced polydipsia, a possible expression of activating effects of the unconditioned reinforcer (Annett and Robbins, 1987; Robbins and Koob, 1980; Mittleman et al., 1990), and the disruption of spatial learning in the water maze (Annett et al., 1989), a well-established effect of hippocampal damage (Morris et al., 1982). Lesions of the amygdala have been reported to be without effect on spatial learning (Sutherland and McDonald, 1990), and similarly excitotoxic lesions of the basolateral amygdala have been found not to impair schedule-induced polydipsia (Cador et al., unpublished findings). Hence, it appears that there may be doubly dissociable limbic-striatal functional interactions that correspond to the compartmentalisation of the ventral striatum.

The possibility of double dissociation has recently been shown in sharper relief by the experiments demonstrating that, whereas basolateral amygdala lesions similar to those described above produce deficits in CS-shock conditioning, they have no effect on aversive conditioning to contextual cues inherent in the conditioning situation (Selden et al., 1991). By contrast, excitotoxic lesions of the hippocampus produced the symmetrically opposite pattern of effects (Selden et al., 1991). These experiments raise several issues; first, concerning the nature of the stimulus-reinforcer associations that are impeded by lesions of the amygdala, and second, the role of the amygdala-ventral striatum system in aversive conditioning.

In the study by Selden et al. (1991), contextual conditioning was assessed using a place preference procedure. Whereas the lack of effect of amygdala lesions was clear, it is to be contrasted with the considerable disruption produced in appetitive place conditioning alluded to above. This apparent discrepancy might depend upon the nature of the reinforcer, but seems unlikely to depend on the greater emotional arousal inherent in the appetitive procedure (cf. Cahill and McGaugh, 1990). More particularly, it might arise from an important difference between the nature of conditioning in the place preference procedure and that in contextual learning. Thus, as noted above, it is difficult to be sure in place preference conditioning whether the Pavlovian conditioning is in fact spatial in nature, depending on associations formed between the topographical interrelationships of the environmental stimuli, or whether it is to unspecified, discrete cues, much as occurs in conventional conditioning to explicit CSs. The observation that amphetamine-induced place preference conditioning survives fimbria-fornix transection (Hiroi and White, 1991), a procedure which is known to disrupt spatial learning in other paradigms, supports this interpretation.

POSSIBLE ROLE OF THE AMYGDALA-VENTRAL STRIATAL SYSTEM IN AVERSIVE CONDITIONING

Although we have shown a role for the basolateral amygdala in the mediation of appetitive conditioned reinforcement, it may also be implicated in its aversive counterpart, as exemplified particularly by punished behavior or responding with negative reinforcement (e.g., shock postponement schedules). The majority of experiments on the role of the amygdala in fear conditioning, by contrast, have studied the Pavlovian conditioned emotional response of freezing in anticipation of an aversive conditioning stimulus (Davis, 1986, 1989; LeDoux, 1986b; Jellestad et al., 1986; Davis et al., 1987; LeDoux et al., 1988, 1990). Such Pavlovian contingencies often confound the measurement of punished instrumental behavior, so that a disinhibition of such responding can sometimes result indirectly from a blockade of freezing. Thus the disinhibitory effects of intra-amygdaloid application of benzodiazepine drugs on punished responding (Petersen and Scheel-Kruger, 1982; Scheel-Kruger and Petersen, 1982; Petersen et al., 1985; Shibata et al., 1982, 1986; Thomas et al., 1985; Kataoka et al., 1987; Vellucci et al., 1988) may depend on a disruption of freezing, rather than a specific increase in punished behavior.

There has been a considerable consensus that the amygdala plays an important role in fear conditioning based largely on the effects of lesions (LeDoux, 1986a,b; Davis et al., 1987). Previously, much of the emphasis has been on the central nucleus, but recent studies of the effects of ibotenic acid lesions have failed to show substantial effects on passive avoidance learning (Jellestad and Bakke, 1985; Jellestad and Cabrera, 1986; Jellestad et al., 1986; Riolobos and Garcia, 1987) and the effects on various components of the aversive conditioned response have been reinterpreted by some (e.g., Gallagher et al., 1990) to represent effects on conditioned orientational or attentional functions. However, it is clear that excitotoxic lesions of the basolateral amygdala do produce robust effects on the conditioned emotional response (Selden et al., 1991), punished running (Cahill and McGaugh, 1990), and passive avoidance (Dunn and Everitt, 1988), although not on conditioned taste aversion (Dunn and Everitt, 1988). Furthermore, CS-induced freezing and lick suppression (as well as some associated autonomic responses) can be blocked by electrolytic lesions of the lateral nucleus (LeDoux et al., 1990), a structure in which long-term potentiation has been demonstrated (Clugnet and LeDoux, 1990).

Thus, it does appear that the basolateral amygdala or, more specifically, the lateral nucleus of the amygdala, plays some role in the formation of aversive associations between the conditioned stimulus and reinforcer and this may be viewed, therefore, in the light of the effects of amygdala lesions on conditioned appetitive responding summarized herein. What is far less clear is the way in which this aversive information may be used. The central nucleus is a possible effector structure for the autonomic, endocrine, and even certain somatotopic, reflexive responses (freezing, startle). However, it is as yet unknown whether the ventral striatum acts as an output station for the mediation of voluntary or instrumental aversively controlled behavior, as has been suggested for such behavior controlled by positive reinforcers.

SUMMARY

In this chapter, we have described how research on the functions of the basolateral amygdala and the ventral striatum, including its dopaminergic innervation, have converged in the context of the neural basis of reward-related processes that are integral to the expression of emotional behavior. Evidence has been presented that these structures are part of a neural system that is importantly involved in the mediation of voluntary elements of an integrated emotional response. However, it is also apparent that there is still some way to go before the nature of the psychological processes associated with the amygdala and ventral striatum, as well as interactions between them, is fully understood in both negatively and positively motivated situations.

It has for some time been appreciated that the amygdaloid complex cannot be treated as a single structure, being composed as it is of individual nuclei having markedly different developmental origins, patterns of neurochemical organization, and connectivity (Price et al., 1987). It more recently has become clear that the ventral striatum similarly must not be viewed as a unitary structure. It is a neurochemically heterogeneous structure with inputs and outputs organized, as in the dorsal striatum, in a compartmental manner (Groenewegen et al., 1991). The possible segregation of input/output lines (for example, involving hippocampal, amygdaloid, prefrontal cortical, and thalamic loops) at both anatomical and functional levels is an important area of future research. Acknowledging this complexity and attempting to address it psychopharmacologically is likely to be of the greatest utility in further understanding the role of limbic-striatal interactions in emotional behavior.

ACKNOWLEDGMENTS

The work summarised here was supported by grants from the Medical Research Council. We thank Dr. Michael Baum for his constructive criticism of the manuscript.

REFERENCES

Aggleton JP, Blindt HS, Rawlins JNP (1989): Effects of amygdaloid and amygdaloid-hippocampal lesions on object recognition and spatial working memory in rats. Behav Neurosci 103(5):962–974.

Aggleton JP, Mishkin M (1986): The amygdala: Sensory gateway to the emotions. Emotion: Theory, Research and Experience 3:281–299.

Aggleton JP, Passingham RE (1981): Syndrome produced by lesions of the amygdala in monkeys (*Macaca mulatta*). Physiol Psychol 95:961–977.

Aggleton JP, Passingham RE (1982): An assessment of the reinforcing properties of foods after amygdaloid lesions in rhesus monkeys. J Comp Physiol Psychol 96:71–77.

Aggleton JP, Petrides M, Iversen SD (1981): Differential effects of amygdaloid lesions on conditioned taste aversion learning. Physiol Behav 27:973–978.

Alexander GE, DeLong MF, Strick PL (1986): Parallel organization of functionally segregated circuits linking basal ganglia and cortex. Am Rev Neurosci 9:357–381.

Alheid GF, Heimer L (1988): New perspectives in basal forebrain organization of special relevance for neuropsychiatric disorders: The striatopallidal, amygdaloid and corticopetal components of the substantia innominata. Neuroscience 27:1–39.

Annett LE, McGregor A, Robbins TW (1989): The effects of ibotenic acid lesions of the nucleus accumbens on spatial learning and extinction in the rat. Behav Brain Res 31:231–242.

Annett LE, Robbins TW (1987): Ibotenic acid lesions of the nucleus accumbens block the acquisition of adjunctive behavior. Proceedings of the EBBS, Marseilles, France (Abstr).

Barnard EA, Henley JM (1990): The non-NMDA receptors: Types, protein structure and molecular biology. Trends Pharmacol Sci 11:500–597.

Beaulieu S, Di Paolo T, Cote J, Barden N (1987): Participation of the central amygdaloid nucleus in the response of adrenocorticotropin secretion to immobilization stress: Opposing roles of the noradrenergic and dopaminergic innervation. Neuroendocrinology 45:37–46.

Beaulieu S, Di Paulo T, Barden N (1986): Control of ACTH secretion by the central nucleus of the amygdala: Implication of the serotoninergic system and its relevance to the glucocorticoid delayed negative feedback. Neuroendocrinology 44:247–254.

Beninger, RJ, Hanson DR, Phillips AG (1980): The effects of pipradrol on responding with conditioned reinforcement: A role for sensory pre-conditioning. Psychopharmacology 69:235–242.

Blackburn JR, Phillips AG, Jakubovic A, Fibiger HC (1986): Increased dopamine metabolism in the nucleus accumbens and striatum following consumption of a nutritive meal but not a palatable non-nutritive saccharine solution. Pharmacol Biochem Behav 25:1095–1100.

Box BM, Mogenson GJ (1975): Alterations in ingestive behavior after bilateral lesions of the amygdala in rats. Physiol Behav 15:679–688.

Buck R (1986): The psychology of emotion. In LeDoux JE, Hirst W (eds): "Mind and Brain: Dialogues in Cognitive Neuroscience." Cambridge: Cambridge University Press, pp 275–301.

Cador M, Robbins TW, Everitt BJ (1989): Involvement of the amygdala in stimulus-reward associations: Interaction with the ventral striatum. Neuroscience 30:77–86.

Cador M, Taylor JR, Robbins TW (1991): Potentiation of the effects of reward-related stimuli by dopaminergic-dependent mechanisms in the nucleus of accumbens. Psychopharmacology 104:377–385.

Cahill L, McGaugh JL (1990): Amygdaloid complex lesions differentially affect retention of tasks using appetitive and aversive reinforcement. Behav Neurosci 104:532–543.

Carr GD, Fibiger HC, Phillips AG (1989): Conditioned place preference as a measure of drug reward. In Liebman JM, Cooper SJ (eds): "Neuropharmacological Basis of Reward." Oxford: Oxford University Press, pp 264–319.

Clugnet MC, LeDoux JE (1990): Synaptic plasticity in fear conditioning circuits: Induction of LTP in the lateral nucleus of the amygdala by stimulation of the medial geniculate body. J Neurosci 10:2818–2824.

Dacey DM, Grossman SP (1977): Aphagia, adipsia and sensorimotor deficits produced by amygdala lesions: A function of extra-amygdaloid damage. Physiol Behav 19:389–395.

Davis M (1986): Pharmacological and anatomical analysis of fear conditioning using the fear-potentiated startle paradigm. Behav Neurosci 100:814–824.

Davis M (1989): Sensitization of the acoustic startle reflex by footshock. Behav Neurosci 103(3):495–503.

Davis M, Hitchcock JM, Rosen JB (1987): Anxiety and the amygdala: Pharmacological and anatomical analysis of the fear-potentiated startle paradigm. In Bower GH (ed): "The Psychology of Learning and Motivation: Advances in Research and Theory." New York: Academic Press, pp 263–305.

DeFrance J, Marchand J, Stanley J, Sikes R, Chronister R (1980): Convergence of excitatory amygdaloid and hippocampal inputs in the nucleus accumbens septi. Brain Res 185:183–186.

Dickinson A (1980): "Contemporary Animal Learning Theory," Cambridge: Cambridge University Press.

Dickinson A (1989): Intentionality in animal conditioning. In Weiskrantz L (ed): "Thought Without Language." Oxford: Oxford University Press, pp 305–332.

Dickinson A, Dawson GR (1989): Incentive learning and the motivational control of instrumental performance. Q J Exp Psychol 41B:99–112.

Dickinson A, Nicholas DJ, Adams CD (1983): The effect of the instrumental training contingency on susceptibility to reinforcer devaluation. Q J Exp Psychol 35B:35–51.

Dunn LT, Everitt BJ (1988): Double dissociations of the effects of amygdala and insular cortex lesions on conditioned taste aversion, passive avoidance and neophobia in the rat using the excitotoxin ibotenic acid. Behav Neurosci 102:3–23.

Everitt BJ (1990): Sexual motivation: A neural and behavioural analysis of the mechanisms underlying appetitive and copulatory responses of male rats. Neurosci Biobehav Rev 14:217–232.

Everitt BJ, Cador M, Robbins TW (1989a): Interactions between the amygdala and ventral striatum in stimulus-reward associations: Studies using a second-order schedule of sexual reinforcement. Neuroscience 30:63–75.

Everitt BJ, Fray P, Kostarczyk E, Taylor S, Stacey P (1987): Studies of instrumental behavior with sexual reinforcement in male rats (Rattus norvegicus): I. Control by brief visual stimuli paired with a receptive female. J Comp Psychol 101(4):395–406.

Everitt BJ, Morris KA, O'Brien A, Burns L, Robbins TW (1989b): The effects of basolateral amygdala and ventral striatal lesions on conditioned place preference in rats. Soc Neurosci 15:490.11 (Abstr).

Everitt BJ, Morris KA, O'Brien A, Robbins TW (1991): The basolateral amygdala-ventral striatal system and conditioned place preference: Further evidence of limbic-striatal interactions underlying reward-related processes. Neuroscience 42:1–18.

Everitt BJ, Stacey P (1987): Studies of instrumental behavior with sexual reinforcement in male rats (Rattus norvegicus): II. Effects of preoptic area lesions, castration, and testosterone. J Comp Psychol 101(4):407–419.

Fitzgerald RE, Burton MJ (1981): Effects of small bilateral amygdala lesions on ingestion in the rat. Physiol Behav 27:431–437.

Gaffan D, Harrison S (1987): Amygdalectomy and disconnection in visual learning for auditory secondary reinforcement by monkeys. J Neurosci 7(8):2285–2292.

Gaffan D, Murray EA (1990): Amygdalar interaction with the mediodorsal nucleus of the thalamus and the ventromedial prefrontal cortex in stimulus-reward associative learning in the monkey. J Neurosci 10:3479–3493.

Gaffan EA, Gaffan D, Harrison S (1988): Disconnection of the amygdala from visual association cortex impairs visual-reward association learning in monkeys. J Neurosci 8:3144–3150.

Gaffan EA, Gaffan D, Harrison S (1989): Visual-visual associative learning and reward-association learning in monkeys: The role of the amygdala. J Neurosci 9:558–564.

Gallagher M, Graham PW, Holland PC (1990): The amygdala central nucleus and appetitive Pavlovian conditioning: Lesions impair one class of conditioned behavior. J Neurosci 10:1906–1911.

Goldberg SR, Morse WH, Goldberg M (1976): Behavior maintained under a second-order schedule by intramsucular injection of morphine or cocaine in rhesus monkeys. J Pharmacol Exp Therapeu 199:278–286.

Gray TS, Carney ME, Magnuson DJ (1989): Direct projections from the central amygdaloid nucleus to the hypothalamic paraventricular nucleus: Possible role in stress-induced adrenocorticotropin release. Neuroendocrinology 50:433–446.

Groenewegen HJ, Becker NEHM, Lohman AHM (1980): Subcortical afferents of the nucleus accumbens septi in the cat, studied with retrograde axonal transport of horseradish peroxidase and bisbenzimid. Neuroscience 5:1903–1916.

Groenewegen HJ, Berendse HW, Meredith GE, Haber SN, Voorn P, Wolters JG, Lohman AHM (1991): Functional anatomy of the ventral, limbic system-innervated striatum. In Willner P, Scheel-Kruger J (eds): "The Mesolimbic Dopamine System: From Motivation to Action." Chichester: Wiley, pp 19–60.

Groenewegen HJ, Room P, Witter MP, Lohman AHM (1982): Cortical afferents of the nucleus accumbens in the cat, studied with anterograde and retrograde transport techniques. Neuroscience 7:977–995.

Grossman SP, Grossman L, Walsh L (1974): Functional organization of the rat amygdala with respect to avoidance behavior. J Comp Physiol Psychol 88:829–850.

Haber SN, Groenewegen HJ, Grove EA, Nauta WHJ (1985): Efferent connections of the ventral pallidum: Evidence of a dual striato-pallidofugal pathway. J Comp Neurol 235:322–325.

Heimer L, Wilson RD (1975): The subcortical projections of the allocortex: Similarities in the neural associations of the hippocampus, the pyriform cortex and the neocortex. In Santini M (ed): "Golgi Centennial Symposium." New York: Raven Press, pp 177–192.

Henke PG, Allen JD, Davison C (1972): Effects of lesions in the amygdala on behavioral contrast. Physiol Behav 8:173–176.

Henke PG, Maxwell D (1973): Lesions in the amygdala and the frustration effect. Physiol Behav 10:647–650.

Hiroi N, White NM (1991): The lateral nucleus of the amygdala mediates expression of the amphetamine conditioned place preference. Brain Res (In press).

Hitchcock JM, Sananes CB, Davis M (1989): Sensitization of the startle reflex by footshock: Blockade by lesions of the central nucleus of the amygdala or its efferent pathway to the brainstem. Behav Neurosci 103(3):509–518.

Jellestad FK, Bakke HK (1985): Passive avoidance after ibotenic acid and radiofrequency lesions in the rat amygdala. Physiol Behav 34:299–305.

Jellestad FK, Cabrera IC (1986): Exploration and avoidance learning after ibotenic acid and radio-frequency lesions in the rat amygdala. Behav Neural Biol 46:196–215.

Jellestad FK, Markowska A, Bakke HK, Walther B (1986): Behavioral effects after ibotenic acid, 6-OHDA and electrolytic lesions in the central amygdala nucleus of the rat. Physiol Behav 37:855–862.

Jones B, and Mishkin M (1972): Limbic lesions and the problem of stimulus-reinforcement associations. Exp Neurol 36:362–377.

Kataoka Y, Shibata K, Yamashita K, Ueki S (1987): Differential mechanisms involved in the anticonflict action of benzodiazepines injected into the central amygdala and mammillary body. Brain Res 416:243–247.

Katz J (1979): A comparison of responding maintained under second-order schedules of intramuscular cocaine injection or food presentation in squirrel monkeys. J Exp Analyt Behav 32:419–431.

Kelley AE, Domesick VB (1982): The distribution of the projection from the hippocampal formation to the nucleus accumbens in the rat: An anterograde-and retrograde-horseradish peroxidase study. Neuroscience 7:2321–2335.

Kelley AE, Domesick VB, Nauta WJH (1982): The amygdalostriatal projection in the rat—an anatomical study by anterograde and retrograde tracing methods. Neuroscience 7:615–630.

Kemble ED, Beckman GJ (1970): Runway performance of rats following amygdaloid lesions. Physiol Behav 4:45–47.

Kemble ED, Blanchard DC, Blanchard RJ, Takush R (1984): Taming in wild rats following medial amygdaloid lesions. Physiol Behav 32:131–134.

Kesner RP (1981): The role of the amygdala within an attribute analysis of memory. In Ben-Ari Y (ed): "The Amygdaloid Complex," INSERM Symposium, No. 20. Amsterdam: Elsevier, pp 331–342.

Kling A, Stecklis HD (1976): A neural substrate for affiliative behavior in non-human primates. Brain Behav Evol 13:216–238.

Köhler C, Schwarcz R (1983): Comparison of ibotenate and kainate neurotoxicity in rat brain: A histological study. Neuroscience 8:819–835.

Koob GF, Goeders NE (1989): Neuroanatomical substrates of drug self-administration. In Liebman JM, Cooper SJ (eds): "Neuropharmacological Basis of Reward." Oxford: Oxford University Press, pp 214–263.

Koob GF, Stinus L, LeMoal M, Bloom FE (1989): Opponent process theory of motivation: Neurobiological evidence from studies of opiate dependence. Neurosci Biobehav Rev 13:135–140.

LeDoux JE (1986a): The neurobiology of emotion. In LeDoux JE, Hirst W (eds): "Mind and Brain: Dialogues in Cognitive Neuroscience." Cambridge: Cambridge University Press, pp 301–354.

LeDoux JE (1986b): A neurobiological view of the psychology of emotion. In LeDoux JE, Hirst W (eds): "Mind and Brain: Dialogues in Cognitive Neuroscience." Cambridge: Cambridge University Press, pp 355–358.

LeDeoux JE, Cicchetti P, Xagoraris A, Romanski LM (1990): The lateral amygdaloid nucleus: Sensory interface of the amygdala in fear conditioning. J Neurosci 10:1062–1069.

LeDoux JE, Iwata J, Cicchetti P, Reid DJ (1988): Different projections of the central amygdaloid nucleus mediate autonomic and behavioral correlates of conditioned fear. J Neurosci 8(7):2517–2529.

Mackintosh NJ (1983): "Conditioning and Associative Learning." Oxford: Clarendon Press.

Messier C, White NM (1984): Contingent and non-contingent actions of sucrose and saccharin reinforcers: Effects on taste preference and memory. Physiol Behav 32:195–203.

Milner PM (1989): The discovery of self-stimulation and other stories. Neurosci Biobehav Rev 13:61–68.

Mittleman G, Whishaw IQ, Jones GH, Koch M, Robbins TW (1990): Cortical, hippocampal and striatal mediation of schedule-induced behaviors. Behav Neurosci 104:399–409.

Mogenson G, Jones DL, Yim CY (1984): From motivation to action: Functional interface between the limbic system and the motor system. Prog Neurobiol 14:69–97.

Mogenson G, Nielson M (1984): Pharmacological evidence to suggest that the nucleus accumbens and subpallidal region contribute to exploratory locomotion. Behav Neural Biol 43:52–60.

Mogenson GJ (1984): Limbic-motor integration—with emphasis on initiation of exploratory and goal-directed locomotion. In Bandler R (ed): "Modulation of Sensorimotor Activity During Alterations in Behavioral States." New York: Alan R. Liss, pp 121–137.

Mogenson GM (1987): Limbic-motor integration. In Epstein A, Morrison AR (eds): "Progress in Psychobiology and Physiological Psychology," Vol 12. New York: Academic Press, pp 117–170.

Morris RGM, Garrud P, Rawlins JNP, O'Keefe J (1982): Place navigation impaired in rats with hippocampal lesions. Nature 297:681–683.

Murray EA, Mishkin M (1985): Amygdalectomy impairs crossmodal association in monkeys. Science 228:604–606.

Nachman M, Ashe JH (1974): Effects of basolateral amygdala lesions on neophobia, learned taste aversions and sodium appetite in rats. J Comp Physiol Psychol 87:622–643.

Nauta WJH, Domesick VB (1984): Afferent and efferent relationships of the basal ganglia. CIBA Foundation Symposium 107:3–29.

Petersen EN, Braestrup C, Scheel-Kruger J (1985): Evidence that the anti-conflict effect of midazolam in amygdala is mediated by the specific benzodiazepine receptors. Neurosci Lett 53:285–288.

Petersen EN, Scheel-Kruger J (1982): The GABAergic anticonflict effects of intra-amygdaloid benzodiazepines demonstrated by a new waterlick conflict paradigm. In Spiegelstein MY, Levy A (eds): "Proceedings of the 27th OHOLO Conference: Behavioral Models and Analyses of Drug Action." Amsterdam: Elsevier.

Phillips AG, Blaha CD, Fibiger HC (1989): Neurochemical correlates of brain-stimulation reward measured by ex vivo and in vivo analyses. Neurosci Biobehav Rev 13:99–104.

Phillips AG, Fibiger HC (1987): Anatomical and neurochemical substrates of drug reward. In Bozarth MA (ed): "Methods of Assessing the Reinforcing Properties of Abused Drugs." New York: Springer Verlag, pp 275–290.

Price JL, Russchen FT, Amaral D (1987): The limbic region. II: The amygdaloid complex. In Björklund A, Hökfelt T, Swanson LW (eds): "Handbook of Chemical Neuroanatomy, Vol 5: Integrated Systems of the C.N.S., Part 1." Amsterdam: Elsevier, pp 279–388.

Ray A, Henke PG, Sullivan RM (1987): The central amygdala and immobilization stress-induced gastric pathology in rats: Neurotensin and dopamine. Brain Res 409:398–402.

Richardson JS (1973): The amygdala: Historical and functional analysis. Acta Neurobiol 33:623–648.

Riolobos AS, Garcia AIM (1987): Open field activity and passive avoidance responses in rats after lesions of the central amygdaloid nucleus by electrocoagulation or ibotenic acid. Physiol Behav 39:715–720.

Robbins TW (1976): Relationship between reward-enhancing and stereotypical effects of psychomotor stimulant drugs. Nature 264:57–59.

Robbins TW, Cador M, Taylor JR, Everitt BJ (1989): Limbic-striatal interactions in reward-related processes. Neurosci Biobehav Rev 13:155–162.

Robbins TW, Koob GF (1980): Selective disruption of displacement behaviour by lesions of the mesolimbic dopamine system. Nature 285:409–411.

Rolls ET (1990): A theory of emotion and its application to understanding the neural basis of emotion. Cogn Emotion 4:161–190.

Rolls ET, Rolls BJ (1973a): Altered food preferences after lesions in the basolateral region of the amygdala in the rat. J Comp Physiol Psychol 83:248–259.

Rolls ET, Rolls BJ (1973b): Effects of lesions in the basolateral amygdala on fluid intake in the rat. J Comp Physiol Psychol 83:240–247.

Rosenzweig-Lipson S, Chu B, Delfs J-M, Kelley AE (1990): Microinjection of cocaine, buproprion and pipradrol into the nucleus accumbens septi enhance locomotor activity and potentiate responding for a conditioned reinforcer. Soc Neurosci 16 (Part 1):310.7.

Russchen FT, Price JL (1984): Amygdalostriatal projections in the rat: Topographical organization and fiber morphology shown using the lectin PHA-L as an anterograde tracer. Neurosci Lett 47:15–22.

Sananes CB, Campbell BA (1989): Role of the central nucleus of the amygdala in olfactory heart rate conditioning. Behav Neurosci 103(3):519–525.

Sarter M, Markowitsch HJ (1985): Involvement of the amygdala in learning and memory: A critical review, with emphasis on anatomical relations. Behav Neurosci 99(2):342–380.

Schachter S, Singer J (1962): Cognitive, social and physiological determinants of emotional state. Psychol Rev 69:378–399.

Scheel-Kruger J, Petersen EN (1982): Anticonflict effect of the benzodiazepines mediated by a GABAergic mechanism in the amygdala. Eur J Pharmacol 82:115–116.

Schoepp D, Bockaert J, Sladeczek F (1990): Pharmacological and functional characteristics of metabotropic excitatory amino acid receptors. Trends Pharmacol Sci 11: 508–515.

Schwarcz R, Köhler C, Fuxe K, Hökfelt T, Goldstein M (1979): On the mechanism of selective neuronal degeneration in the rat brain: Studies with ibotenic acid. Adv Neurol 23:655–667.

Selden NRW, Everitt BJ, Jarrard LE, Robbins TW (1991): Complementary roles of the amygdala and hippocampus in aversive conditioning to explicit and contextual cues. Neuroscience 42:335–350.

Shibata K, Kataoka Y, Gomit Y, Ueki S (1982): Localization of the site of anti-conflict action of benzodiazepines in the amygdaloid nucleus of rats. Brain Res 234:442–446.

Shibata K, Kataoka Y, Yamashita K, Ueki S (1986): An important role of the central amygdaloid nucleus and mammillary body in the mediation of conflict behavior in rats. Brain Res 372:159–162.

Shizgal P (1989): Toward a cellular analysis of intracranial self-stimulation: Contributions of collision studies. Neurosci Biobehav Rev 13:81–90.

Simbayi LC, Boakes RA, Burton MJ (1986): Effects of basolateral amygdala lesions on taste aversions produced by lactose and lithium chloride in the rat. Behav Neurosci 100:455–465.

Spiegler BJ, Mishkin M (1981): Evidence for the sequential participation of inferior temporal cortex and amygdala in the acquisition of stimulus-reward associations. Behav Brain Res 3:303–317.

Spyraki C, Fibiger HC, Phillips AG (1982): Attenuation by haloperidol of place preference conditioned using food reinforcement. Psychopharmacology 77:379–382.

Spyraki C, Fibiger HC, Phillips AG (1983): Attenuation of heroin reward in rats by disruption of the mesolimbic dopamine system. Psychopharmacology 23:843–849.

Sutherland RJ, McDonald RJ (1990): Hippocampus, amygdala and memory deficits in rats. Behav Brain Res 37:57–79.

Swanson LW (1987): Integrated systems of the CNS, Part I: The hypothalamus. Handbook Chem Neuroanat 5:1.

Swanson LW, Mogenson GJ (1981): Neural mechanisms for the functional coupling of autonomic, endocrine and somatomotor responses in adaptive behavior. Brain Res Rev 3:1–34.

Taylor JR, Robbins TW (1984): Enhanced behavioural control by conditioned reinforcers following microinjections of d-amphetamine into the nucleus accumbens. Psychopharmacology 84:405–412.

Taylor JR, Robbins TW (1986): 6-hydroxydopamine lesions of the nucleus accumbens, but not of the caudate nucleus, attenuate enhanced responding with reward-related stimuli produced by intra-accumbens d-amphetamine. Psychopharmacology 90:390–397.

Thomas SR, Lewis ME, Iversen SD (1985): Correlation of [^{3}H] diazepam binding density with anxiolytic locus in the amygdaloid complex of the rat. Brain Res 342:85–90.

van der Kooy D (1985): Place conditioning: A simple and effective method for assessing the motivational properties of drugs. In Bozarth MA (ed): "Methods of Assessing the Reinforcing Properties of Abused Drugs." New York: Springer Verlag, pp 229–240.

Vellucci SV, Martin PJ, Everitt BJ (1988): The discriminative stimulus produced by pentylenetetrazol: Effects of systemic anxiolytics and anxiogenics, aggressive defeat and midazolam or muscimol into the amygdala. J Psychopharmacol 2:80–93.

Watkins JC, Krogsgaard-Larsen P, Honoré T (1990): Structure-activity relationships in the development of excitatory amino acid receptor agonists and competitive antagonists. Trends Pharmacol Sci 11:25–33.

Weiskrantz L (1956): Behavioral changes associated with ablation of the amygdaloid complex in monkeys. J Comp Physiol Psychol 49:381–391.

White NM, Carr GD (1985): The conditioned place preference is affected by two independent reinforcement processes. Pharmacol Biochem Behav 23:37–42.

White NM, Messier C, Carr GD (1985): Operationalizing and measuring the organizing influence of drugs on behaviour. In Bozarth MA (ed): "Methods of Assessing the Reinforcing Properties of Abused Drugs." New York: Springer Verlag, pp 591–618.

Wise RA (1981): Brain dopamine and reward. In Cooper SJ (ed): "Theory in Psychopharmacology." London: Academic Press, pp 102–122.

Wise RA (1982): Neuroleptics and operant behavior: The anhedonia hypothesis. Behav Brain Sci 5:39–87.

Wise RA (1989a): The brain and reward. In Liebman JM, Cooper SJ (eds): "Neuropharmacological Basis of Reward." Oxford: Oxford University Press, pp 377–424.

Wise RA (1989b): Opiate reward: Sites and substrates. Neurosci Biobehav Rev 13:129–134.

Wolterink GM, Cador M, Wolterink I, Robbins TW, Everitt BJ (1989): Involvement of D1 and D2 receptor mechanisms in the processing of reward-related stimuli in the ventral striatum. Soc Neurosci 15(2):490.15.

Yang CR, Mogenson GJ (1984): Electrophysiological responses of neurons in the nucleus accumbens to hippocampal stimulation and the attenuation of the excitatory responses by the mesolimbic dopaminergic system. Brain Res 324:69–84.

Yang CR, Mogenson GJ (1985): An electrophysiological study of neuronal projections from hippocampus to ventral pallidum and subpallidal areas by way of the nucleus accumbens. Neuroscience 15:1015–1025.

Yim CY, Mogenson GJ (1982): Response of nucleus accumbens to amygdala stimulation and its modification by dopamine. Brain Res 239:401–415.

Yim CY, Mogenson GJ (1983): Responses of ventral pallidal neurons to amygdala stimulation and its modification by dopamine projections to nucleus accumbens. J Neurophysiol 50:148–161.

Yim CY, Mogenson GJ (1989): Low doses of nucleus accumbens dopamine modulate amygdala suppression of spontaneous exploratory activity in rats. Brain Res 477:202–210.

The Amygdala: Neurobiological Aspects of Emotion,
Memory, and Mental Dysfunction, pages 431–451
© 1992 Wiley-Liss, Inc.

16
Involvement of the Amygdala in Neuromodulatory Influences on Memory Storage

JAMES L. MCGAUGH, INES B. INTROINI-COLLISON, LARRY CAHILL,
MUNSOO KIM, AND K.C. LIANG
*Center for the Neurobiology of Learning and Memory and Department of
Psychobiology, University of California, Irvine, California (J.L.M., I.B.I-C.,
L.C., M.K.); and Department of Psychology, National Taiwan University,
Taipei, Taiwan (K.C.L.)*

INTRODUCTION

There is a general consensus that the amygdala plays a role in the formation of long-term memory. More specifically, the accumulated evidence strongly suggests that the amygdala may have a special role in emotionally influenced memories. There are, however, alternative views concerning the nature of the involvement. The findings of a number of recent studies suggest that the amygdala may be a locus of neural changes underlying the memory of affective experiences (Hitchcock and Davis, 1987; Chapter 9, Davis, this volume; LeDoux et al., 1988; Chapter 12, LeDoux, this volume). Other evidence suggests that the amygdala may have a general role in enabling the association between stimuli and rewards or punishments (Weiskrantz, 1956; Jones and Mishkin, 1972; Spiegler and Mishkin, 1981). Another possibility is suggested by the findings summarized in this chapter: The amygdala may serve to modulate the storage of information at other brain sites. According to this latter view, physiological systems activated by affective stimulation influence memory storage, at least in part, through effects mediated by the amygdala. Viewed from this perspective, the amygdala may be part of a brain system that serves to ensure that memories of significant experiences are well retained (McGaugh, 1989a, 1990).

ROLE OF ENDOGENOUS SYSTEMS IN THE MODULATION OF MEMORY STORAGE

The central hypothesis guiding the research summarized in this chapter is that memory storage is regulated by neuromodulatory systems activated by experiences. There is extensive evidence supporting this view (Gold and McGaugh, 1975; McGaugh, 1989a). Furthermore, as is summarized below, the findings of experiments from our laboratory provide strong support for the view that neuromodulatory influences on memory storage are mediated, at least in part, through influences involving the amygdala.

The view that neuromodulatory systems play a role in regulating memory storage is based on extensive evidence indicating that the retention of recently acquired information is altered by drugs and electrical stimulation of the brain administered after training (McGaugh, 1966; McGaugh and Herz, 1972). Such findings suggest that posttraining treatments affect retention by modulating memory storage processes (McGaugh, 1973). Evidence indicating that retention can be enhanced by posttraining administration of drugs (McGaugh, 1973, 1989b) suggested the possibility that the memory storage process may be regulated by endogenous physiological systems activated by learning experiences (Gold and McGaugh, 1975). It is well known that training experiences activate many hormonal, transmitter, and neuromodulatory systems. Furthermore, there is considerable evidence indicating that the retention of information can be enhanced (as well as impaired) by posttraining administration of hormones and drugs affecting transmitter and neuromodulatory systems activated by training experiences (McGaugh, 1989a,b; McGaugh and Gold, 1989). Such evidence is consistent with the view that endogenous neuromodulatory systems play an important role in the regulation of memory storage (Gold and McGaugh, 1975).

Research in our laboratory has focused primarily on the involvement of adrenergic, opioid peptidergic, and GABAergic systems in memory storage. The studies of Gold and van Buskirk (1975) were the first to show that posttraining systemic injections of the adrenergic hormone epinephrine produce dose-dependent and time-dependent effects on retention: Retention is enhanced by low doses and impaired by high doses, and epinephrine is most effective in influencing retention if administered shortly after training. And, of particular importance for the more recent findings reviewed in this chapter, the studies of Gold and van Buskirk (1978a,b) also suggested that the memory-modulating effects of epinephrine involve the release of central norepinephrine (NE). Subsequent research findings discussed below have provided extensive evidence supporting that view. Furthermore, our findings indicate that opioid peptidergic as well as GABAergic influences on memory storage also appear to involve the release of central NE. And, more specifically, recent findings indicate that these effects as well as those of epinephrine involve noradrenergic influences within the amygdala.

It is, of course, important to note that hormones and central neuromodulatory systems may also influence memory through mechanisms other than those explored in our experiments. For example, the findings of Gold (1988) suggest that the influences of epinephrine on retention may be mediated, at least in part, by the release of glucose. Vasopressin may affect memory through peripheral influences on blood pressure as well as through direct influences on the brain (Burbach et al., 1983; de Wied, 1984, 1991; Koob et al., 1991).

The findings of experiments using a variety of training tasks, including inhibitory avoidance, active avoidance, discrimination learning, and appetitive learning, have provided extensive evidence indicating that low doses of epinephrine administered systemically after training enhance the subsequent retention

(Izquierdo and Dias, 1985; Sternberg et al., 1985; Introini-Collison and McGaugh, 1986; McGaugh, 1989a; McGaugh and Gold, 1989). It is also clear from recent findings that epinephrine effects on memory storage are initiated at peripheral adrenergic receptors. The finding indicating that memory modulating effects of epinephrine are blocked by the peripherally acting β-adrenergic antagonist sotalol is consistent with evidence indicating that epinephrine does not readily enter the brain (Weil-Malherbe et al., 1959). The adrenergic drug DPE (dipivalyl epinephrine), which is less polar than epinephrine and thus more readily enters the brain when administered peripherally, and the β-adrenergic agonist clen-buterol, which readily enters the brain, produce effects on memory like those seen with epinephrine (Introini-Collison and McGaugh, 1991; Introini-Collison and Baratti, unpublished findings). Sotalol does not block the memory-modulating effects of either DPE or clenbuterol. However, the memory-modulating effects of epinephrine, DPE, and clenbuterol are blocked by propranolol, a β-adrenergic antagonist that readily enters the brain (Introini-Collison and McGaugh, 1991). These findings, considered together with evidence indicating that α-antagonists do not block the memory-enhancing effects of either epinephrine or DPE (Introini-Collison and McGaugh, 1991; Introini-Collison and Baratti, unpublished findings), clearly suggest that the memory-modulating effects of epinephrine, DPE, and clenbuterol are mediated by activation of central NE receptors. Thus, epinephrine effects on memory appear to be due to activation of central noradrenergic systems, presumably by stimulating adrenergic receptors on visceral afferents. These recent findings are consistent with those of earlier studies indicating that, in rats and mice, retention can be enhanced by posttraining i.c.v. administration of NE (Haycock et al., 1977; Meligeni et al., 1978).

INVOLVEMENT OF THE AMYGDALA IN ADRENERGIC INFLUENCES ON MEMORY

There is extensive evidence suggesting that epinephrine influences on memory are mediated by influences involving the amygdala. The findings of experiments examining retrograde amnesia induced by posttraining electrical stimulation of the amygdala were the first to suggest this possibility. The amnestic effect typically produced by amygdala stimulation administered to rats after training in inhibitory avoidance and active avoidance tasks (McGaugh and Gold, 1976) was not obtained in adrenal demedullated rats (Bennett et al., 1985). Retrograde amnesia was produced, however, if epinephrine was administered (i.p.) after the training, immediately prior to the brain stimulation (Liang et al., 1985). Thus, influences induced by peripheral epinephrine appear to be essential for the memory-modulating effects of amygdala stimulation. These findings, considered together with the evidence, discussed below, indicating that epinephrine effects on memory are blocked by lesions of the stria terminalis (Liang and McGaugh, 1983a), strongly suggest that epinephrine influences on memory involve the amygdala.

Other findings from our laboratory indicate that epinephrine effects on memory involve activation of NE receptors within the amygdala. In rats trained on an inhibitory avoidance task, posttraining intra-amygdala injections of propanolol

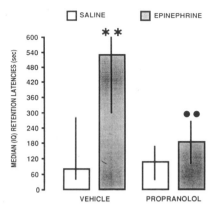

Fig. 1. Effects of posttraining intra-amygdala injections of propranolol (0.2 μg) on epinephrine-induced enhancement of retention of an inhibitory avoidance response. Epinephrine (0.1 mg/kg) was administered s.c. Retention was tested 24 h after training. **$P < 0.01$ as compared with the vehicle-injected control group. ●●$P < 0.001$ as compared with the epinephrine-injected control group. From Liang et al., 1986.

blocked the memory-enhancing effect of intraperitoneal injections of epinephrine administered immediately after the amygdala injections (see Fig. 1) (Liang et al., 1986). In addition, posttraining intra-amygdala injections of NE (see Fig. 7 below) or clenbuterol, administered alone, enhanced retention (Introini-Collison et al., in press a; Liang et al., 1986, 1990). Intra-amygdala injections of NE also attenuated the learning impairment produced by adrenal demedullation (Liang et al., 1986). These findings are consistent with those of Gallagher and her colleagues (Gallagher et al., 1981) indicating that rats' retention of an inhibitory avoidance response was impaired by posttraining intra-amygdala injections of the adrenergic receptor antagonist propranolol and that the memory-impairment was blocked by administration of NE together with propranolol (Gallagher et al., 1981).

INVOLVEMENT OF THE AMYGDALA IN THE
EFFECTS OF OPIATE ANTAGONISTS ON MEMORY

Experiments examining the effects of opioid peptide agonists and antagonists provide additional evidence suggesting that amygdala NE is involved in the modulatory influences of these treatments on memory. A large number of studies have reported that, in rats and mice, retention is enhanced by posttraining systemic (Izquierdo, 1979; Messing et al., 1979; Introini-Collison and McGaugh, 1987) as well as intra-amygdala (Gallagher and Kapp, 1978; Introini-Collison et al., 1989b) injections of opiate antagonists such as naloxone and naltrexone. In view of evidence indicating that opioid peptides inhibit the release of NE (Montel et al., 1974; Arbilla and Langer, 1978; Nakamura et al., 1982; Werling et al., 1987), such findings suggest that opiate antagonists affect memory by stimulating the release of NE. In support of this view, Izquierdo and Graudenz (1980) reported that propranolol blocks the memory-enhancing effects of naloxone. Naloxone-induced enhancement of memory is also blocked in animals treated with DSP4, an adrenergic neurotoxin (Introini-Collison and Baratti, 1986). The findings indicating that the memory-enhancing effects of systemically injected naloxone are not blocked by α-antagonists or by sotalol (Introini-Collison and Baratti, 1986) strongly suggest that the naloxone effects involve selective activation of central β-adrenergic receptors.

There is also extensive evidence indicating that naloxone effects on memory are due to influences on NE within the amygdala. In an extensive series of studies, Gallagher and her colleagues reported that, in rats given posttraining intra-amygdala injections, retention is enhanced by naloxone and impaired by opiate agonists (Gallagher, 1982, 1985; Gallagher and Kapp, 1978; Gallagher et al., 1981). Gallagher and her colleagues also found that neurotoxic-induced (6-OHDA) lesions of the dorsal noradrenergic pathway block the memory-enhancing effects of peripheral as well as intra-amygdala injections of naloxone (Gallagher et al., 1985; Fanelli et al., 1985). Our findings indicating that posttraining intra-amygdala injections of β-adrenergic antagonists block the memory-enhancing effects of systemic injections of naloxone provide additional evidence that naloxone effects on memory involve noradrenergic influences within the amygdala (McGaugh et al., 1988). In this experiment, rats were trained in an inhibitory avoidance task and β-antagonists (propranolol, atenolol, or zinterol) or a buffer solution were injected intra-amygdally via implanted cannulae immediately after training. Saline or naloxone was administered i.p. immediately after the amygdala injections. Figure 2 shows the retention performance one week after the training. As can be seen, intra-amygdala injections of the β-antagonists blocked the retention-enhancing effects of the systemically administered naloxone. The β-antagonists were effective only when administered to the amygdala: Injections into either the caudate-putamen or cortex dorsal to the amygdala did not block the memory-enhancing effects of naloxone. Furthermore, $α_1$-(prazosin) and $α_2$-(yohimbine) antagonists were also ineffective in blocking the effects of naloxone. Results highly similar to these were obtained in comparable experiments using a Y-maze position discrimination learning task (McGaugh et al., 1988).

These recent findings are consistent with the view that peripherally administered naloxone influences memory through effects involving NE within the amygdala. As was noted above, previous findings have indicated that retention is enhanced by posttraining intra-amygdala injections of naloxone (Gallagher et al., 1981). In recent experiments using both an inhibitory avoidance task and a Y-maze discrimination task, we found that the retention-enhancing effects of intra-amygdala injections of naloxone were blocked by propranolol injected concurrently with the naloxone (Introini-Collison et al., 1989b). Results obtained with the inhibitory avoidance task are shown in Figure 3A. As is shown in Figure 3B, naloxone did not affect retention when injected into the caudate nucleus or cortex dorsal to the amygdala. Thus, it is unlikely that the effects of intra-amygdala injections of naloxone were due to diffusion of the drug dorsally to other brain regions penetrated by the injection cannulae.

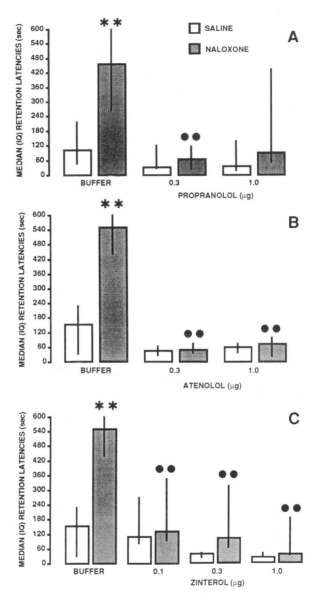

Fig. 2. Effects of posttraining intra-amygdala injections of β-adrenoceptor antagonists on naloxone-induced enhancement of retention of an inhibitory avoidance response. Naloxone (3.0 mg/kg) was administered i.p. Retention was tested one week after training. **$P < 0.01$ as compared with the buffer-injected control group. ●●$P < 0.01$ as compared with the naloxone-injected control group. From McGaugh et al., 1988.

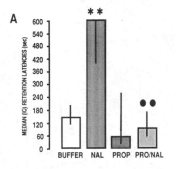 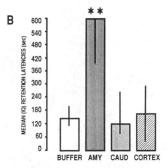

Fig. 3. (A) Effects of posttraining intra-amygdala injections of naloxone (0.1 µg) and propranolol (0.3 µg) on retention of an inhibitory avoidance response. Retention was tested one week after training. Propranolol blocked naloxone-induced enhancement of memory when the drugs were injected concurrently into the amygdala. **$P < 0.01$ as compared with the buffer group. ●●$P < 0.01$ as compared with the naloxone-injected group. **(B)** Enhancement of retention induced by posttraining injections of naloxone into the amygdala, but not in the caudate or cortex dorsal to the amygdala. **$P < 0.01$ as compared with the buffer controls as well as groups given naloxone injections into the caudate nucleus or cortex dorsal to the amygdala. From Introini-Collison et al., 1989b.

INVOLVEMENT OF THE AMYGDALA IN GABAergic INFLUENCES ON MEMORY STORAGE

Experiments examining the effects of adrenergic blockers have provided strong support for the view that epinephrine and naloxone effects on memory involve the activation of β-noradrenergic receptors within the amygdala. More generally, such findings suggest that the amygdala may be a site at which neuromodulatory systems interact in the regulation of memory storage. In support of this general hypothesis, other recent findings from our laboratory indicate that posttraining treatments affecting GABAergic systems also influence memory storage through effects involving the amygdaloid complex. Moreover, GABAergic effects on memory, like adrenergic and opiate effects, appear to involve NE receptors within the amygdala.

Findings of an early experiment (Breen and McGaugh, 1961) indicated that posttraining systemic administration of the GABAergic antagonist picrotoxin enhanced appetitively motivated maze learning in rats. Comparable effects have since been obtained in experiments using a wide variety of training tasks (Bovet et al., 1966; Brioni and McGaugh, 1988; McGaugh et al., 1990). Recent studies using aversively motivated training tasks have provided extensive evidence indicating that, in rats and mice, posttraining systemic administration of GABAergic antagonists, including picrotoxin and bicuculline, enhance retention and that GABAergic agonists (muscimol and baclofen) impair retention (Swartzwelder et al., 1987; Brioni and McGaugh, 1988; Castellano and McGaugh, 1989; Castellano et al., 1989a,b).

As the GABAergic agonists and antagonists used in these experiments readily pass the blood-brain barrier, it seems likely that they influence memory by

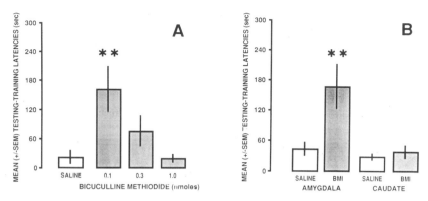

Fig. 4. Effects of posttraining injections of bicuculline methiodide (BMI) on retention of an inhibitory avoidance task. BMI facilitated retention of an inhibitory avoidance response when injected into the amygdala **(A,B)** but not when injected into the caudate (B) dorsal to the amygdala. Retention was tested 48 h after training. $^{**}P < 0.01$ as compared with the saline-injected control group. From Brioni et al., 1989.

acting on brain GABAergic systems. To examine this issue more explicitly, we examined the effect of bicuculline methiodide, a GABAergic antagonist that does not readily pass the blood-brain barrier. When injected i.p. immediately posttraining, bicuculline methiodide did not affect retention (Brioni and McGaugh, 1988). However, as is shown in Figure 4A, when injected intra-amygdally, bicuculline methiodide produced dose-dependent enhancement of retention of inhibitory avoidance. Injections administered to the caudate nucleus dorsal to the amygdala were ineffective (Fig. 4B). The findings of other experiments indicated that retention is impaired by intra-amygdala injections of the GABAergic agonists baclofen and muscimol (Brioni et al., 1989; Castellano et al., 1989b).

The findings of other recent experiments examining the effects of posttraining systemic injections on retention, in mice, of inhibitory avoidance training indicate that propranolol blocks the memory-enhancing effects of bicuculline and that muscimol does not block the memory-enhancing effects of clenbuterol (unpublished findings). Further, as is shown in Figure 5, propranolol also blocks the retention-enhancing effects of bicuculline when both drugs are injected into the amygdala after training.

INTERACTION OF NEUROMODULATORY INFLUENCES

The findings summarized above strongly suggest that GABAergic influences on memory, like those of adrenergic and opioid peptidergic systems, involve activation of NE receptors within the amygdala. Thus, these findings provide additional support for the general hypothesis that neuromodulatory influences on memory are integrated within the amygdala. Figure 6 summarizes the interactions of adrenergic, opioid peptidergic, and GABAergic influences on memory storage suggested by the evidence reviewed above. According to this general

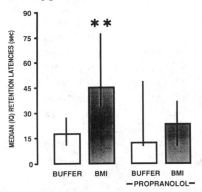

Fig. 5. Effects of posttraining intra-amygdala injections of bicuculline methiodide (BMI) (0.05 μg = 0.1 nmol) and propranolol (0.3 μg) on retention of an inhibitory avoidance response. Retention was tested 48 h after training. Propranolol blocked bicuculline-induced enhancement of memory when both drugs were administered concurrently. **$P < 0.01$ as compared with the buffer-injected control group. Unpublished data.

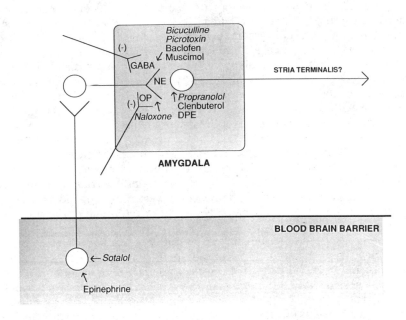

Fig. 6. Proposed interactions of hormones and neurotransmitter systems in regulating memory storage.

model, the memory-modulating effects of drugs affecting these systems are due to influences on the release of NE within the amygdala. As is indicated, the model assumes that epinephrine activates a central NE system projecting to the amygdala and that GABAergic and opioid peptidergic influences regulate the release of NE. Evidence indicating that retention is influenced by posttraining intra-amygdala injections of a dopamine antagonist suggest that dopamine influences on memory may also be mediated, at least in part, through influences involving the amygdala (Vu et al., 1989). However, other findings suggest that serotonergic influences on memory are not elicited in the amygdala. Although retention of inhibitory avoidance responses is enhanced by posttraining systemic injections of the serotonin uptake blocker fluoxetine (Flood and Cherkin, 1987; Introini-Collison et al., in press b), intra-amygdala injections are ineffective (Introini-Collison et al., in press b). It remains to be determined whether neuromodulatory influences on memory other than those examined to date are mediated by interactions involving the amygdala.

EFFECTS OF LESIONS AFFECTING AMYGDALA FUNCTIONING

If, as the findings discussed above clearly suggest, the influences of several neuromodulatory systems on memory are mediated by the amygdala, lesions of the amygdala should block such influences. There is extensive evidence supporting this implication. Several experiments have examined the effects of lesions of the stria terminalis, a major amygdala pathway. The findings indicating that stria terminalis lesions block the memory-impairing effects of electrical stimulation of the brain (Liang and McGaugh, 1983b) provided the first evidence suggesting an intact amygdala system is required for memory-modulating effects of treatments affecting amygdala functioning. The findings of that study also suggest that the memory-modulating effects of the amygdala stimulation result from influences in brain regions activated by the amygdala. Experiments examining neuromodulatory influences on memory have provided additional evidence consistent with this suggestion. Stria terminalis lesions block the memory-enhancing effects of systemically administered epinephrine and naloxone as well as the memory-impairing effects of posttraining β-endorphin (Liang and McGaugh, 1983a; McGaugh et al., 1986). Furthermore, stria terminalis lesions also block the memory-modulating effects of drugs affecting the cholinergic system (Introini-Collison et al., 1989a). These findings thus provide additional support for the general hypothesis that adrenergic, opioid peptidergic, and cholinergic systems influence memory storage through effects involving the amygdala.

However, as the stria terminalis carries both afferent and efferent fibres, it is not clear from the studies discussed above whether the effects of stria terminalis lesions are due to loss of amygdala afferents or to disruption of amygdala influences on other brain regions. The findings of a recent study examining the memory-modulating effects of posttraining intra-amygdala injections of NE in rats with lesions of either the stria terminalis or the ventral amygdalofugal pathway (VAF) provide some clarification of this issue (Liang et al.,1990). As is shown in Figure 7A, stria terminalis lesions blocked both the memory-enhancing effects of a low dose of NE as well as the memory-impairing effects of a high

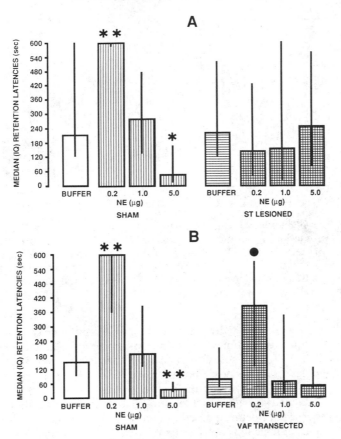

Fig. 7. Effects of stria terminalis (ST) lesions **(A)** and ventroamygdalofugal (VAF) pathway transections **(B)** on the effects of the intra-amygdala injections of norepinephrine (NE) on memory. ST lesions but not VAF transections blocked NE-induced enhancement and impairment of memory. Retention was tested 24 h after training. *$P < 0.05$ and **$P < 0.01$ as compared with the buffer-injected control group. ●$P < 0.05$ as compared with the buffer/VAF transected group. From Liang et al., 1990.

dose. However, as is shown in Figure 7B, VAF lesions did not block the memory-modulating effects of intra-amygdala NE.

These findings clearly suggest that the memory-modulating effects resulting from activation of the amgydala are due to outputs to other brain regions mediated by the stria terminalis. Other findings indicated that VAF lesions attenuated, but did not block, the memory-enhancing effects of systemically administered epinephrine (Liang et al., 1990). That is, in VAF-lesioned animals, a higher dose of epinephrine was required for enhancement of memory. These findings, considered together with evidence indicating that stria terminalis lesions block the memory-modulating effects of systemically administered epinephrine, sug-

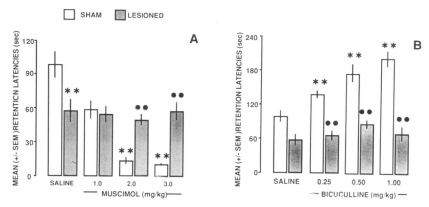

Fig. 8. Effects of muscimol (**A**) and bicuculline (**B**) on inhibitory avoidance retention in animals with lesions of the amygdala. Amygdala lesions blocked muscimol-induced impairment of memory as well as bicuculline-induced enhancement of memory. Retention was tested 24 h after training. $**P < 0.01$ as compared with the saline-injected control group. $\bullet\bullet P < 0.01$ as compared with the sham group receiving the same drug treatment. From Ammassari-Teule et al., in press.

gest that the VAF may partially mediate the central influences of peripheral epinephrine on amygdala functioning. In considering the implications of this evidence it is important to note that stria terminalis lesions selectively disrupt memory-modulating influences: These lesions alone do not markedly impair learning or retention. Thus, although the pathway is not critical for learning or memory, an intact stria terminalis does appear to be required for the regulation of memory storage by posttraining neuromodulatory systems.

Other recent findings indicate that neuromodulatory influences on memory are also blocked by lesions of the amygdala. NMDA-induced lesions of the amygdala block the enhancing effects of posttraining systemic injections of epinephrine on retention of an inhibitory avoidance response (Cahill, 1989). Further, in mice, electrolytic lesions of the amygdala block the memory-modulating effects of posttraining injections of GABAergic drugs (Ammassari-Teule et al., 1991). Figure 8 shows the effects of posttraining systemic injections of muscimol (Fig. 8A) and bicuculline (Fig. 8B) on retention in amygdala-lesioned mice. The lesions blocked the memory impairing effects of muscimol as well as the memory-enhancing effects of bicuculline. Interestingly, comparable effects were produced by lesions of the dorsal hippocampus. Lesions of the caudate nucleus, however, were ineffective. In this experiment as well as that of Cahill (1989) the amygdala lesions alone produced significant learning impairment. Thus the effects of amygdala lesions differ from those induced by stria terminalis lesions.

The evidence indicating that learning was impaired in amygdala-lesioned rats was, of course, not surprising, as there is extensive evidence indicating that amygdala lesions impair learning of aversively motivated tasks (e.g., Sarter and

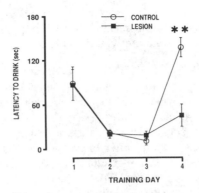

Fig. 9. Effect of NMDA-induced lesions of the amygdala on acquisition of one trial appetitive and aversive training. Amygdala lesions blocked acquisition of an aversively but not an appetitively motivated response. Mean (± SEM) latency to drink on each day. **$P <$ 0.01 as compared with day 4 amygdala-lesioned group. From Cahill and McGaugh, 1990.

Markowitsch, 1985; Hitchcock and Davis, 1987; LeDoux et al., 1988). More generally, the amygdala appears to be selectively engaged by training in tasks that elicit relatively intense affective responses (Kesner and DiMattia, 1987). A recent experiment comparing the effects of amygdala lesions on appetitive and aversive learning provides additional support for this conclusion (Cahill and McGaugh, 1990). Rats with NMDA-induced lesions of the amygdala were first trained to enter an alley in a Y-maze, where they received a water reward. Figure 9 shows that on the three days of training, the learning of the amygdala-lesioned rats, as indexed by latency to find and drink the water, was comparable to that of sham controls. Clearly, the amygdala lesions did not block the learning of an association between the water and the location of the water. On the third day, a footshock was delivered when the rats began drinking. As can be seen, the response latencies of both the sham and lesioned animals increased significantly on the fourth day, the day following the footshock. However, the amygdala-lesioned rats showed less effect of the punishment. That is, the lesion attenuated, but did not block, the effect of the footshock on subsequent response latencies. The findings of another experiment indicated that NMDA lesions also attenuated the learning of an association between an odor and footshock but did not prevent the learning of an association between an odor and a sucrose reward (Cahill and McGaugh, 1990).

Clearly, the findings of these experiments do not support the view that the amygdala is required for the formation of associations between stimuli and rewards associations. In both experiments the lesion selectively affected the aversively motivated learning. Furthermore, in both experiments the amygdala lesions attenuated but did not prevent the aversively motivated learning. Thus, the findings are consistent with the view that the engagement of the amygdala in learning depends upon the extent to which the training induces the activation of neuromodulatory systems (McGaugh, 1989a; Cahill and McGaugh, 1990).

Viewed in the context of the findings of studies discussed above, these results suggest that the lesions impaired learning by blocking the influences of endogenous neuromodulatory systems activated by the training.

EFFECTS OF NMDA ANTAGONISTS

Although our findings provide extensive evidence suggesting that the amygdala is involved in memory storage, they have as yet provided little evidence suggesting that the amygdala is a site of permanent changes underlying learning. Rather, the findings suggest that the amygdala is involved in regulating the storage of long-term memory in other brain regions. In other recent experiments addressing this issue we have examined the effects, on learning and retention, of intra-amygdala injections of NMDA antagonists.

There is substantial evidence suggesting that the mechanisms underlying long-term potentiation (LTP) may provide a basis for long-term memory (Teyler and DiScenna, 1984; Lynch et al., 1989). Recent findings indicating that LTP can be induced in the amygdala (Chapman et al., 1990; Clugnet and LeDoux, 1990) are consistent with the view that the amygdala may be a site of neural alterations mediating learning. Moreover, other recent findings (Miserendino et al., 1990) indicate that intra-amygdala injections of NMDA antagonists impair fear conditioning. As it is well established that the induction of LTP requires the activation of NMDA receptors (Collingridge et al., 1983), these recent findings suggest that the fear conditioning may be mediated by connections formed within the amygdala.

Recent experiments in our laboratory examined the effects of NMDA antagonists (d,1-AP5, d-AP5, CPP, and MK801) injected into the amygdala on the acquisition and retention of inhibitory avoidance (Kim, 1991). In these experiments rats were given intra-amygdala injections of NMDA antagonists prior to training on an inhibitory avoidance task. The animals were placed in the starting alley of a two-compartment straight alley and received footshocks each time they entered the other compartment. Training was continued until they remained in the starting compartment for 100 consecutive seconds. Each entry of the shock region was recorded as a training trial. A retention test trial was administered 48 hours later. Figure 10 shows the findings obtained in an experiment using d,1-AP5. As can be seen, the two lower doses of the drug did not affect the number of trials required for the original learning (Fig. 10A). However, the drug produced dose-dependent impairment of retention (Fig. 10B). Furthermore, significant retention impairment was produced by a dose (3 μg) that did not affect acquisition. In subsequent experiments the rats were given additional intra-amygdala injections of NMDA antagonists shortly prior to a second training session given two days after the original training. The effects of the second training session were assessed on a retention test two days later. The additional training improved retention performance of control animals as well as animals given the NMDA antagonists.

The findings of these experiments indicate that low doses of NMDA antagonists injected into the amygdala prior to training on a multitrial inhibitory avoidance task do not impair acquisition. Thus, acquisition of the inhibitory avoidance

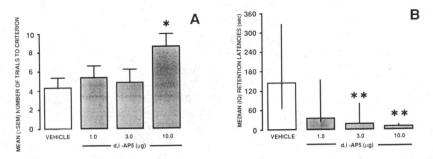

Fig. 10. Effect of pretraining intra-amygdala injections of d,1-AP5 on acquisition (**A**) and 48 h retention (**B**) of an inhibitory avoidance response. d,1-AP5 impaired retention at a dose (3.0 μg) that did not affect acquisition. (**A**) Mean (±SEM) number of trials to criterion. (**B**) Median (interquartile range) retention latency. Retention was tested 48 h after training. *$P < 0.05$ and **$P < 0.01$ as compared with the vehicle-injected group. Unpublished data.

response does not appear to involve NMDA-dependent mechanisms within the amygdala. Further, on the basis of the evidence indicating that NMDA antagonists impair but do not block the long-term retention of the training, it seems unlikely that NMDA-dependent changes within the amygdala provide the basis for long-term memory of the training in this task. The latter finding suggests the possibility that NMDA-dependent changes within the amygdala may provide a basis for the modulatory influences of the amygdala on long-term memory storage in other brain regions (Kim, 1991). These conclusions are consistent with the evidence discussed above (Cahill and McGaugh, 1990), indicating that lesions of the amygdala attenuate but do not block retention in this task.

CONCLUDING COMMENTS

The findings summarized in this chapter leave little doubt that long-term memory storage processes are subject to the modulating influences of hormonal and neurotransmitter systems. The findings also provide strong support for the hypothesis that several neuromodulatory systems influence memory storage through influences based on interactions affecting the release of NE within the amygdala. Although an intact amygdala appears to be required for the modulating influences, impairment of amygdala functioning induced by lesions of the stria terminalis or the amygdala, or by intra-amygdala injections of NMDA antagonists, does not block learning of the tasks used in these experiments. Thus, the findings are consistent with the view that the amygdala may be selectively involved in modulating memory storage in other brain regions. The evidence from our studies does not support the general view that the amygdala mediates the associations between stimuli and rewards: In our experiments amygdala lesions did not impair appetitively motivated learning, and attenuated but did not prevent aversively motivated learning. However, the evidence indicating that under other experimental conditions amygdala lesions can also impair appetitively motivated learning (Kesner and DiMattia, 1987; Chapter 10, Gallagher and Holland, this volume) clearly suggests that the amygdala is not exclusively involved in memory based on aversive experiences. Rather, findings from studies using a variety of training tasks suggests that the amygdala is engaged by stimulus conditions that evoke relatively intense affective responses (Kesner and DiMattia, 1987). The nature of the affect, whether positive or negative, does not appear to be critical. As we have emphasized, our evidence suggests that the role of the physiological systems activated by experiences is to regulate the storage of the experiences. And, in our view, the stored information does not necessarily consist of associations between the situation and the affect evoked. There is extensive evidence indicating that treatments affecting neuromodulatory systems affect learning (i.e., latent learning) that is not based on rewards and punishment (McGaugh, 1989b). However, it has not as yet been determined whether, as our hypothesis suggests, such effects are mediated by activation of the amygdala.

If it is the case, as our findings suggest, that the amygdala influences memory storage in other brain regions it should, in principle, be possible to determine the locus or loci of such modulating influences. Our findings suggest that brain areas activated by pathways in the stria terminalis should be of particular importance. We have not as yet examined that implication. We have, however, obtained evidence suggesting that the insular cortex may be a cortical site involved in the long-term storage underlying inhibitory avoidance as well as other types of learning (Bermudez-Rattoni and McGaugh, 1991). This evidence is of particular interest in view of the extensive evidence indicating that the amygdala and insular cortex are reciprocally interconnected (Otterson, 1982; Yamamoto et al.,1984). In recent experiments we found that reversible inactivation of the insular cortex by injections of tetrodotoxin impairs retention when administered either before or after training in inhibitory avoidance and spatial learning tasks (Bermudez-Rattoni et al., 1991). Comparable effects were not produced by tetrodotoxin administered to adjacent cortical areas. These findings indicate that the learning of these tasks involves time-dependent processes in the insular cortex and suggest the possibility that such processes may be modulated by activation of the amygdala. There are, of course, many other possible modulatory sites, as the amygdala projects to many brain regions. Further examination of the possible sites of modulatory influences should provide important clues to understanding how the amygdala is involved in ensuring that important events are well remembered.

ACKNOWLEDGMENTS

Supported by research grant MH12526 from NIMH and NIDA and ONR contract N000014-90-J-1626. We wish to acknowledge and thank Federico Bermudez-Rattoni, Jorge Brioni, Claudio Castellano, and Alan Nagahara for their contributions to the findings and interpretations summarized in this chapter and Nancy Collett for assistance in the preparation of the manuscript.

REFERENCES

Ammassari-Teule M, Pavone F, Castellano C, McGaugh JL (1991): Amygdala and dorsal hippocampus lesions block the effects of the GABAergic drugs on memory storage. Brain Res 551:104–109.

Arbilla S, Langer SZ (1978): Morphine and beta-endorphin inhibit release of noradrenaline from cerebral cortex but not of dopamine from rat striatum. Nature 271:559–561.

Bennett C, Liang KC, McGaugh JL (1985): Depletion of adrenal catecholamines alters the amnestic effect of amygdala stimulation. Behav Brain Res 15:83–91.

Bermudez-Rattoni F, Introini-Collison IB, McGaugh JL (1991): Reversible lesions of the insular cortex by tetrodotoxin produce retrograde and anterograde amnesia for inhibitory avoidance and spatial learning. Proc Nat Acad Sci 88:5379–5382.

Bermudez-Rattoni F, McGaugh JL (1991): Insular cortex and amygdala lesions differentially affect acquisition on inhibitory avoidance and conditioned taste aversion. Brain Res 549:165–170.

Bovet D, McGaugh JL, Oliverio A (1966): Effects of posttrial administration of drugs on avoidance learning of mice. Life Sci 5:1309–1315.

Breen RA, McGaugh JL (1961): Facilitation of maze learning with posttrial injections of picrotoxin. J Comp Physiol Psychol 54:498–501.

Brioni JD, McGaugh JL (1988): Posttraining administration of GABAergic antagonists enhance retention of aversively motivated tasks. Psychopharmacology 96:505–510.

Brioni JD, Nagahara AH, McGaugh JL (1989): Involvement of the amygdala GABAergic system in the modulation of memory storage. Brain Res 487:105–112.

Burbach JPH, Kovacs GL, de Wied D, van Nispen JW, Greven HM (1983): A major metabolite of arginine vasopressin in the brain is a highly potent neuropeptide. Science 221:1310–1312.

Cahill L, McGaugh JL (1990): Amygdaloid complex lesions differentially affect retention of tasks using appetitive and aversive reinforcement. Behav Neurosci 104:523–543.

Cahill LF (1989): The amygdala and emotional memory. Ph.D. dissertation, University of California, Irvine.

Castellano C, Brioni JD, Nagahara AH, McGaugh JL (1989a): Posttraining systemic and intra-amygdala administration of the gaba-b agonist baclofen impair retention. Behav Neur Biol 52:170–179.

Castellano C, Introini-Collison IB, Pavone F, McGaugh JL (1989b): Effects of naloxone and naltrexone on memory consolidation in CD1 mice: Involvement of GABAergic mechanisms. Pharmacol, Biochem Behav 32:563–567.

Castellano C, McGaugh JL (1989): Retention enhancement with posttraining picrotoxin: Lack of state dependency. Behav Neur Biol 51:165–170.

Chapman PF, Kairiss EW, Keenan CL, Brown TH (1990): Long-term synaptic potentiation in the amygdala. Synapse 6:271–278.

Clugnet MC, LeDoux JE (1990): Synaptic plasticity in fear conditioning circuits: Induction of LTP in the lateral nucleus of the amygdala by stimulation of the medial geniculate body. J Neurosci 10:2818–2824.

Collingridge GL, Kehl SJ, McLennan H (1983): Excitatory amino acids in synaptic transmission in the schaffer collateral-commisural pathway of the rat hippocampus. J Physiol 334:33–46.

de Wied D (1984): Neurohypophyseal hormone influences on learning and memory processes. In Lynch G, McGaugh JL, Weinberger NM (eds): "Neurobiology of Learning and Memory." New York: Academic Press, pp 289–312.

de Wied D (1991): The effects of neurohypophyseal hormones and related peptides on learning and memory processes. In Frederickson RCA, McGaugh JL, Felten DL (eds): "Peripheral Signaling of the Brain: Role in Neural-Immune Interactions, Learning and Memory." Toronto: Hogrefe & Huber, pp 335–350.

Fanelli RJ, Rosenberg RA, Gallagher M (1985): Role of noradrenergic functions in the opiate antagonist facilitation of spatial memory. Behav Neurosci 99(4): 751–755.

Flood JF, Cherkin A (1987): Fluoxetine enhances memory processing in mice. Psychopharmacology 93:36–43.

Gallagher M (1982): Naloxone enhancement of memory processes: Effects of other opiate antagonists. Behav Neur Biol 35:375.

Gallagher M (1985): Re-viewing modulation of learning and memory. In Weinberger NM, McGaugh JL, Lynch G (eds): "Memory Systems of the Brain: Animal and Human Cognitive Processes." New York: Guilford Press, pp 311–334.

Gallagher M, Kapp BS (1978): Manipulation of opiate activity in the amygdala alters memory processes. Life Sci 23:1973–1978.

Gallagher M, Kapp BS, Pascoe JP, Rapp PR (1981): A neuropharmacology of amygdaloid systems which contribute to learning and memory. In Ben-Ari Y (ed): "The Amygdaloid Complex." Amsterdam: Elsevier/North Holland, pp 343–354.

Gallagher M, Rapp PR, Fanelli RJ (1985): Opiate antagonist facilitation of time-dependent memory processes: Dependence upon intact norepinephrine function. Brain Res 347:284–290.

Gold PE (1988): Plasma glucose modulation of memory storage processes. In Woody CD, Alkon DL, McGaugh JL (eds): "Cellular Mechanisms of Conditioning and Behavioral Plasticity." New York: Plenum Press, pp 329–342.

Gold PE, McGaugh JL (1975): A single-trace, two process view of memory storage processes. In Deutsch D, Deutsch JA (eds): "Short-Term Memory." New York: Academic Press, pp 355–378.

Gold PE, van Buskirk R (1975): Facilitation of time-dependent memory processes with posttrial amygdala stimulation: Effect on memory varies with footshock level. Brain Res 86:509–513.

Gold PE, van Buskirk R (1978a): Posttraining brain norepinephrine concentrations: Correlation with retention performance of avoidance training with peripheral epinephrine modulation of memory processing. Behav Biol 23:509–520.

Gold PE, van Buskirk R (1978b): Effects of alpha and beta adrenergic receptor antagonists on post-trial epinephrine modulation of memory: Relationship to posttraining brain norepinephrine concentrations. Behav Biol 24:168–184.

Haycock JW, van Buskirk R, Ryan JR, McGaugh JL (1977): Enhancement of retention with centrally administered catecholamines. Exp Neurol 54:199–208.

Hitchcock JM, Davis M (1987): Fear-potentiated startle using an auditory conditioned stimulus: Effect of lesions of the amygdala. Physiol Behav 39:403–408.

Introini-Collison IB, Arai Y, McGaugh JL (1989a): Stria terminalis lesions attenuate the effects of posttraining oxotremorine and atropine on retention. Psychobiology 17: 397–401.

Introini-Collison IB, Nagahara AH, McGaugh JL (1989b): Memory-enhancement with intra-amygdala posttraining naloxone is blocked by concurrent administration of propranolol. Brain Res 476:94–101.

Introini-Collison IB, Baratti CM (1986): Opioid peptidergic systems modulate the activity of beta-adrenergic mechanisms during memory consolidation processes. Behav Neur Biol 46:227–241.

Introini-Collison IB, McGaugh JL (1986): Epinephrine modulates long-term retention of an aversively-motivated discrimination task. Behav Neur Biol 45:358–365.

Introini-Collison IB, McGaugh JL (1987): Naloxone and beta-endorphin alter the effects of posttraining epinephrine on retention of an inhibitory avoidance response. Psychopharmacology 92:229–235.

Introini-Collison IB, McGaugh JL (1991): Interaction of hormones and neurotransmitter systems in the modulation of memory storage. In Frederickson RCA, McGaugh JL, Felten DL (eds): "Peripheral Signaling of the Brain: Role in Neural-Immune Interactions, Learning and Memory." Toronto: Hogrefe & Huber, pp 275–302.

Introini-Collison IB, Miyazaki B, McGaugh JI: Involvement of the amygdala in the memory-enhancing effects of clenbuterol. Psychopharmacology (in press a).

Introini-Collison IB, To S, McGaugh JL: Fluoxetine effects on retention of inhibitory avoidance and water-maze spatial learning: enhancement by systemic but no intra-amygdala injections (in press b).

Izquierdo I (1979): Effect of naloxone and morphine on various forms of memory in the rat: Possible role of endogenous opiate mechanisms in memory consolidation. Psychopharmacology 66:199–203.

Izquierdo I, Dias RD (1985): Influence on memory of posttraining or pre-test injections of ACTH, vasopressin, epinephrine, or B-endorphin, and their interaction with naloxone. Psychoneuroendocrinology 10:165–172.

Izquierdo I, Graudenz M (1980): Memory facilitation by naloxone is due to release of dopaminergic and beta-adrenergic systems from tonic inhibition. Psychopharmacology 67:265–268.

Jones B, Mishkin M (1972): Limbic lesions and the problem of stimulus-reinforcement associations. Exp Neurol 36:362–377.

Kesner RP, DiMattia BV (1987): Neurobiology of an attribute model of memory. In Epstein AN, Morrison AR (eds): "Progress in Psychobiology and Physiological Psychology." New York: Academic Press, pp 207–277.

Kim M (1991): NMDA receptors in the amygdala in learning and memory. Doctoral dissertation, University of California, Irvine.

Koob GF, Lebrun C, Bluthe R-M, Dantzer R, Dorsa DM, Le Moal M (1991): Vasopressin and learning: Peripheral and central mechanisms. In Frederickson RCA, McGaugh JL, Felten DL (eds): "Peripheral Signaling of the Brain: Role in Neural-Immune Interactions, Learning and Memory." Toronto: Hogrefe & Huber, pp 351–363.

LeDoux JE, Iwata J, Cicchetti P, Reis DJ (1988): Different projections of the central amygdaloid nucleus mediate autonomic and behavioral correlates of conditioned fear. J Neurosci 8:2517–2529.

Liang KC, Bennett C, McGaugh JL (1985): Peripheral epinephrine modulates the effects of posttraining amygdala stimulation on memory. Behav Brain Res 15:93–100.

Liang KC, Juler R, McGaugh JL (1986): Modulating effects of posttraining epinephrine on memory: Involvement of the amygdala noradrenergic system. Brain Res 368:125–133.

Liang KC, McGaugh JL (1983a): Lesions of the stria terminalis attenuate the enhancing effect of posttraining epinephrine on retention of an inhibitory avoidance response. Behav Brain Res 9:49–58.

Liang KC, McGaugh JL (1983b): Lesions of the stria terminalis attenuate the amnestic effect of amygdaloid stimulation on avoidance responses. Brain Res 274:309–318.

Liang KC, McGaugh JL, Yao H-Y (1990): Involvement of amygdala pathways in the influence of posttraining amygdala norepinephrine and peripheral epinephrine on memory storage. Brain Res 508:225–233.

Lynch G, Granger R, Larson J, Baudry M (1989): Cortical encoding of memory: Hypotheses derived from analysis and simulation of physiological learning rules in anatomical structures. In Nadel L, Cooper LA, Culicover P, Harnish RM (eds): "Neural Connections, Mental Computations." Cambridge: MIT Press, pp 180–224.

McGaugh JL (1966): Time-dependent processes in memory storage. Science 153:1351–1358.

McGaugh JL (1973): Drug facilitation of learning and memory. Ann Rev Pharmacol 13:229–241.

McGaugh JL (1989a): Involvement of hormonal and neuromodulatory systems in the regulation of memory storage. Ann Rev Neurosci 12:255–287.

McGaugh JL (1989b): Dissociating learning and performance: Drug and hormone enhancement of memory storage. Brain Res Bull 23:339–345.

McGaugh JL (1990): Significance and remembrance: The role of neuromodulatory systems. Psychological Science 1:15–25.

McGaugh JL, Castellano C, Brioni JD (1990): Picrotoxin enhances latent extinction of conditioned fear. Behav Neurosci 104:262–265.

McGaugh JL, Gold PE (1976): Modulation of memory by electrical stimulation of the brain. In Rosenzweig MR, Bennett EL (eds): "Neural Mechanisms of Learning and Memory." Cambridge: MIT Press, pp 549–560.

McGaugh JL, Gold PE (1989): Hormonal modulation of memory. In Brush RB, Levine S (eds): "Psychoendocrinology." New York: Academic Press, pp 305–339.

McGaugh JL, Herz MJ (1972): "Memory Consolidation." San Francisco: Albion.

McGaugh JL, Introini-Collison JB, Juler RG, Izquierdo I (1986): Stria terminalis lesions attenuate the effects of posttraining naloxone and b-endorphin on retention. Behav Neurosci 100:839–844.

McGaugh JL, Introini-Collison IB, Nagahara AH (1988): Memory-enhancing effects of posttraining naloxone: Involvement of B-noradrenergic influences in the amygdaloid complex. Brain Res 446:37–49.

Meligeni JA, Ledergerber SA, McGaugh JL (1978): Norepinephrine attenuation of amnesia produced by diethyldithiocarbamate. Brain Res 149:155–164.

Messing RB, Jensen RA, Martinez Jr JL, Spiehler VR, Vasquez BJ, Soumireu-Mourat B, Liang KC, McGaugh JL (1979): Naloxone enhancement of memory. Behav Neur Biol 27:266–275.

Miserendino MJD, Sananes CB, Melia KR, Davis M (1990): Blocking of acquisition but not expression of conditioned fear-potentiated startle by NMDA antagonists in the amygdala. Nature 345:716–718.

Montel H, Starke K, Weber F (1974): Influence of morphine and naloxone on the release of noradrenaline from rat brain cortex slices. Arch Pharmacol 283:283–369.

Nakamura S, Tepper JM, Young SJ, Ling N, Groves PM (1982): Noradrenergic terminal excitability: Effects of opioids. Neurosci Lett 30:57–62.

Otterson OP (1982): Connections of the amygdala of the rat. IV. Corticoamygdaloid and intra-amygdala connections as studies with axonal transport of horseradish peroxidase. J Comp Neurol 205:30–48.

Sarter M, Markowitsch HJ (1985): Involvement of the amygdala in learning and memory: A critical review, with emphasis on anatomical relations. Behav Neurosci 99(2):342–380.

Spiegler BJ, Mishkin M (1981): Evidence for the sequential participation of inferior temporal cortex and amygdala in the acquisition of stimulus-reward associations. Behav Brain Res 3:303–317.

Sternberg DB, Isaacs K, Gold PE, McGaugh JL (1985): Epinephrine facilitation of appetitive learning: Attenuation with adrenergic receptor antagonists. Behav Neur Biol 44:447–453.

Swartzwelder HS, Tilson HA, McLamb RL, Wilson WA (1987): Baclofen disrupts passive avoidance retention in rats. Psychopharmacology 92:398–401.

Teyler TJ, DiScenna P (1984): Long-term potentiation as a candidate mnemonic device. Brain Res Rev 7:15–28.

Vu K, Introini-Collison IB, McGaugh JL (1989): Differential effects of pretraining and posttraining intra-amygdala administration of apomorphine on learning and memory. Soc Neurosci Abstr 15:467.

Weil-Malherbe H, Axelrod J, Tomchick R (1959): Blood-brain barrier for adrenaline. Science 129:1226–1228.

Weiskrantz L (1956): Behavioral changes associated with ablation of the amygdaloid complex in monkeys. J Comp Physiol Psychol 49:381–391.

Werling LL, Brown SR, Cox BM (1987): Opioid receptor regulation of the release of norepinephrine in brain. Neuropharmacology 26:987–996.

Yamamoto T, Azuma S, Kawamura Y (1984): Functional relations between the cortical gustatory area and the amygdala: Electrophysiological and behavioral studies in rats. Exp Brain Res 56:23–31.

The Amygdala: Neurobiological Aspects of Emotion,
Memory, and Mental Dysfunction, pages 453–470
© 1992 Wiley-Liss, Inc.

17

Medial Temporal Lobe Structures Contributing to Recognition Memory: The Amygdaloid Complex Versus the Rhinal Cortex

ELISABETH A. MURRAY

Laboratory of Neuropsychology, National Institute of Mental Health, Bethesda, Maryland

INTRODUCTION

Ablation studies examining the neural substrates of memory in nonhuman primates have repeatedly led to the suggestion that the amygdaloid complex, together with other medial temporal lobe structures such as the hippocampal formation* and the entorhinal cortex, is necessary for accurate recognition memory as measured by the delayed nonmatching-to-sample task (Mishkin, 1978; Murray and Mishkin, 1984; Saunders et al., 1984). Recently, however, the view that the amygdala contributes to recognition memory in monkeys has been challenged. Zola-Morgan and his colleagues (Zola-Morgan et al., 1989a,b) have proposed that damage to the cortical regions that surround the amygdala, rather than complete removal of the amygdala itself, is responsible for the exacerbation of the memory impairment that follows addition of aspiration lesions of the amygdala to hippocampectomy.

In the context of the more recent evidence that severe impairments in recognition memory in monkeys follow removal of cortical regions subjacent to the amygdaloid complex and hippocampal formation (Horel et al., 1987; Murray et al., 1989; Zola-Morgan et al., 1989b), the contributions of both the medial temporal lobe limbic structures to recognition memory need to be reevaluated. This chapter specifically addresses the topic of amygdala contributions to recognition memory but, because many of the arguments presented are relevant to both limbic structures, includes comments regarding hippocampal contribu-

Address correspondence to: Dr. Elisabeth A. Murray, Laboratory of Neuropsychology, National Institute of Mental Health, Building 9, Room 1N107, 9000 Rockville Pike, Bethesda, MD 20892.

*In this report the terms "hippocampal formation" and "hippocampus" are used interchangeably to refer to the dentate gyrus, hippocampus proper, and subicular complex.

tions as well. The first section provides a brief historical review of the events leading to the present controversy, and later sections explore the current evidence for and against the view that the amygdala participates in recognition memory. The aim of this chapter is both to clarify the issues and to promote discussion of experiments that may resolve the conflict.

EVIDENCE FOR AMYGDALA CONTRIBUTIONS TO RECOGNITION MEMORY: A REVIEW
Delayed Nonmatching-to-Sample

For the purposes of this discussion, recognition memory is defined as the ability to judge whether a given stimulus object or item has been experienced before. In the studies described below, monkeys were trained on visual delayed nonmatching-to-sample. In this task each trial is composed of two parts, a sample presentation and a choice test. First, a sample object, overlying the central well of a three-well test tray, is presented for familiarization and the monkey is allowed to displace the object to find a food reward hidden underneath. Following a 10 sec delay, the sample plus a novel object, both overlying the lateral wells of the test tray, are presented for choice; the monkey must learn to displace the novel (nonmatching) object in order to receive another food reward. This procedure is repeated with a new pair of objects for the next trial, and so on, until the 20 trials comprising a test session have been completed. When trained on this version of delayed nonmatching-to-sample with trial-unique objects at the rate of one session per day, five days per week, monkeys learn quite rapidly, in only 100–150 trials. When an animal has learned the task (i.e., mastered the nonmatching rule), its accurate performance at the time of the choice test presumably reflects proficiency in discriminating familiar from novel sensory events; at this time the monkey receives a selective surgical ablation, is allowed about two weeks for recovery, and then is retrained on the basic task with 10 sec delay. After the monkey has relearned, it is given a performance test that taxes memory in two ways. First, the monkey is required to remember each sample object for a longer period of time, an objective that is achieved by increasing the delay between the sample presentation and choice test from 10 sec to 30, 60, and finally, 120 sec, in blocks of 100 trials each. Second, the monkey is required to remember a list of 3, 5, or 10 objects, in blocks of 150 trials each. Because the precise training and testing methods for this task have remained stable for over a decade, most of the studies described below can be directly compared with one another.

Behavioral Findings

As discussed in the Introduction, numerous studies involving the ablation technique have led to the suggestion that the amygdala, together with other medial temporal lobe structures, contributes critically to recognition memory in monkeys (Mishkin, 1978; Zola-Morgan et al., 1982; Murray and Mishkin, 1984; Saunders et al., 1984). The studies were carried out with either rhesus or cynomolgus monkeys (*Macaca mulatta* and *M. fascicularis*, respectively), and in each of these studies, monkeys' visual memory for objects was inferred from their learning and performance scores on the delayed nonmatching-to-sample task described above.* In some of these studies, the behavioral effects of amygdala removal were directly compared with those following either hippocampal removal or combined amygdala and hippocampal removals. Removals of the amygdala alone were found to yield either slight (Mishkin, 1978) or moderate (Murray and Mishkin, 1984) impairment and, likewise, removals of the hippocampus were found to yield either slight (Mishkin, 1978) or no (Murray and Mishkin, 1984) impairment on the performance test. Combined ablations of the two medial temporal lobe limbic structures, however, yielded severe deficits in visual recognition memory (Mishkin, 1978; Murray and Mishkin, 1984). This effect appeared to be synergistic; the magnitude of the impairment following the combined lesion was much greater than that expected by simply summing the effects of the two lesions made separately. Monkeys with the combined removals of the amygdala and hippocampus performed accurately with the short (10 sec) delays between sample presentation and choice test, but their scores fell dramatically with the imposition of longer delays. Thus, the impairment could not be attributed to global changes in perception or to the inability of the operated animals to discriminate the objects. Instead, the impairment was specific to memory.

The studies described above suggested not only that the amygdala and hippocampus contributed critically to recognition memory in monkeys, but also that they contributed roughly equally. To investigate this further, Saunders et al. (1984) examined the behavioral effects of removal of three of the four medial temporal lobe limbic structures. One group of monkeys received bilateral amygdala removal plus unilateral hippocampectomy, and the other received bilateral hippocampal removal plus unilateral amygdalectomy. The scores of animals in these groups were compared to the scores of those in the earlier-prepared groups (Mishkin, 1978) that had received bilaterally symmetrical removals of either the amygdala or hippocampus, or of all four limbic structures. The two newly prepared groups, which did not differ significantly from each other at any stage, obtained performance test scores that fell about halfway between the scores of the groups with two structures removed and those with all four structures removed. So, this study, too, supported the idea that both the amygdala and hippocampus contributed critically to recognition memory in monkeys. In addition, the results suggested that there was a quantitative relationship between the magnitude of the recognition impairment and the amount of conjoint damage to the amygdala and hippocampus.

---

*The study by Murray and Mishkin (1984), like the other studies described in this chapter, used objects that were trial-unique within a test session. Unlike the other studies, however, this one used the same objects across days as well. Although this factor (total number of objects in stimulus set) did interact with lesion condition, the outcome does not alter any of the points presented in this chapter, and the study has therefore been included in the discussion. In addition, the study by Zola-Morgan et al. (1982) employed post- but not preoperative learning prior to the performance test.

Anatomical Considerations

Because the ablations in these studies were made by direct aspiration of tissue, some cortex ventromedially adjacent to the limbic structures was necessarily included in the lesions in order to gain access to the limbic structures. The intended lesions are shown schematically in Figure 1. With amygdala removals, approximately the anterior half of the entorhinal cortex was removed, as well as some piriform and periamygdaloid cortex. With hippocampal removals, approximately the posterior half of the entorhinal cortex was removed, as well as the cortex of the parahippocampal gyrus. As a result, only the combined amygdala and hippocampal removal included the entire entorhinal cortical area. Thus there was a logical possibility that damage to this periallocortical† tissue underlying the limbic structures might itself be responsible for the severe memory deficits that follow combined ablations of the amygdala and hippocampus.

To investigate this possibility directly, Murray and Mishkin (1986) carried out an experiment in which removal of this tissue was combined with either amygdalectomy or hippocampectomy. In this study, the periallocortical tissue included in the lesion comprised both the entorhinal cortex, which occupies the medial bank of the rhinal sulcus and extends medially onto the ventromedial surface of the temporal lobe, and the perirhinal cortex, which occupies the lateral bank of the rhinal sulcus and extends slightly lateral to the sulcus (Van Hoesen and Pandya, 1975; Amaral et al., 1987; Saunders and Rosene, 1988).‡ In the text that follows, the term "rhinal cortex" is used to refer collectively to the entorhinal and perirhinal cortical fields. In this experiment, as in the earlier ones, monkeys were trained on delayed nonmatching-to-sample with trial-unique objects. As illustrated in Figure 2, the animals with amygdala plus rhinal cortical ablations (A + Rh) were severely impaired on the performance test, whereas the monkeys with hippocampus plus rhinal cortical ablations (H + Rh) were not any more impaired than animals with hippocampal ablations (H) alone. Presumably, the rhinal cortical removal

---

†Stephan (1975) includes a variety of cytoarchitectonic fields under the rubric "periallocortex," not only the entorhinal cortex and perirhinal cortex, but also the retrosplenial cortex, the claustrum, a strip of cortex neighboring the corpus callosum including the subgenual cortex, and the pre- and parasubiculum. In the present report, I have adopted the term periallocortex because, of the terms available, it comes closest to encompassing all the structures that might serve as candidate neural structures involved in memory. Specifically, however, I mean to exclude from consideration the subicular complex, as it is an integral part of the hippocampal formation (see Amaral, 1987), but to include the other regions listed above, as well as the periamygdaloid cortex and piriform cortex, which are classified as paleocortex (Stephan, 1975).

‡Because the perirhinal cortex, like the entorhinal cortex, projects to the mediodorsal nucleus of the thalamus (Aggleton and Mishkin, 1984), the perirhinal cortex was included in the lesion to make the experiment a stronger test of the hypothesis that damage to this portion of the periallocortical region alone was responsible for the severe memory deficit.

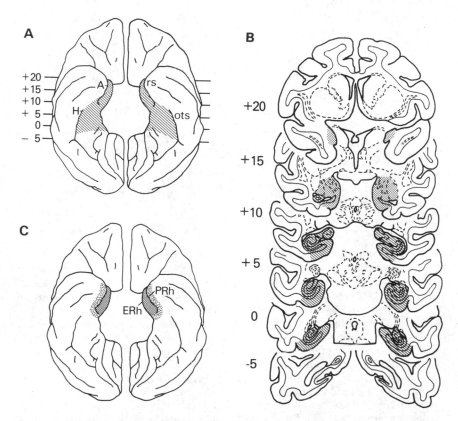

Fig. 1. A,B: Schematic diagram of the intended location and extent of amygdala lesions and hippocampal lesions shown on both the ventral view of the macaque brain **(A)** and coronal sections through the temporal lobe **(B)**. **C:** Ventral view of the brain showing locations of the entorhinal and perirhinal cortical fields. Compare and contrast A and C; note that the amygdala ablation includes roughly the anterior half of the entorhinal cortex, whereas the hippocampal ablation includes roughly the posterior half of the entorhinal cortex and the cortex of the parahippocampal gyrus as well. The piriform and periamygdaloid cortex are located on the rostral pole of the temporal lobe and are therefore not illustrated in this view. Abbreviations: A, amygdala removal; H, hippocampal removal; ERh, entorhinal cortex; PRh, perirhinal cortex; rs, rhinal sulcus; ots, occipitotemporal sulcus. Numerals indicate the distance in mm from the interaural plane (0).

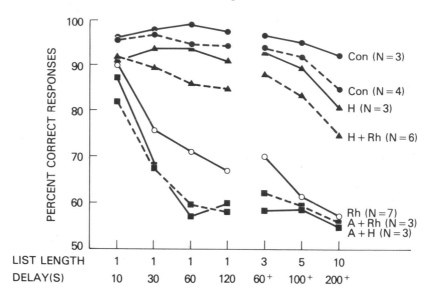

Fig. 2. Postoperative performance test scores on delayed nonmatching-to-sample. Curves on the left show the effects on recognition memory of increasingly longer delays between sample presentation and choice test. Curves on the right show the effects of increasingly longer lists of items to remember. Note that with list length testing, the delay between sample presentation and choice test for each item in the list necessarily increases. The number of items to be remembered, as well as the approximate delays for each of the items, is noted on the abscissa. Abbreviations: Con, unoperated controls; H, hippocampal ablation; H + Rh, hippocampus plus rhinal cortical ablation; Rh, rhinal cortical ablation; A + Rh, amygdala plus rhinal cortical ablation; A + H, combined amygdala plus hippocampal ablation. Dashed lines and solid lines indicate that groups were comprised of cynomolgus and rhesus monkeys, respectively. Data are from the work of Mishkin (1978), Murray and Mishkin (1986), and Murray et al. (1989). Note that the Rh removal employed in group "H + Rh" (Murray and Mishkin, 1986) is not as extensive as the Rh removal in group "Rh" (Murray et al., 1989) and group "A + Rh" (Murray and Mishkin, 1986). See Figure 3.

essentially deafferented the hippocampal formation from its sensory input; hence the behavioral effects of the amygdala plus rhinal lesion were similar to those of the combined amygdala plus hippocampal lesion. This result, too, clearly supported the idea that the amygdala, together with other medial temporal lobe structures, contributed critically to recognition memory. In addition, the lack of a severe impairment in the group with the hippocampus plus rhinal cortical ablation showed that removal of the rhinal cortex alone could not account for the profound deficits that followed combined amygdala and hippocampal removals.

RECENT EVIDENCE REGARDING CONTRIBUTIONS TO
RECOGNITION MEMORY FROM CORTICAL REGIONS IN THE
VENTROMEDIAL TEMPORAL LOBE

The periallocortical region removed by Murray and Mishkin (1986), as indicated previously, included both the entorhinal cortex and perirhinal cortex. The boundaries of the cortical portion of the lesions were based on the cytoarchitectonic analyses available at the time (Van Hoesen and Pandya, 1975); the rhinal cortical part of the lesions thus included the tissue lying along the banks of the rhinal sulcus from the base of the temporal pole, rostrally, to the end of the rhinal sulcus, caudally. Because the amygdala removal was made by a supraorbital approach to the temporal lobe, the amygdala plus rhinal cortical lesion included tissue on the rostral face of the temporal pole, along the line connecting the rhinal sulcus with the lateral fissure, whereas the hippocampus plus rhinal cortical lesion did not (see Fig. 3A,B).

Recently, Amaral and his colleagues have re-examined the connections and cytoarchitecture of the perirhinal cortex, and have suggested that the perirhinal cortex, in particular, extends much more rostrally than previously thought (Amaral et al., 1987; Insausti et al., 1987). If this is true, the amygdala plus rhinal cortical lesion of Murray and Mishkin (1986) included this rostralmost portion of perirhinal cortex (see Fig. 3D), but the hippocampus plus rhinal cortical lesion spared it. Further, this recently discovered difference in the extent of the perirhinal damage in the two experimental groups might account for some or all of the difference in the behavioral effects of the two ablations.

A natural consequence of this revised view of the full location and extent of the perirhinal cortex was the execution of a set of behavioral studies taking the redefinition into account. As illustrated in Figure 2, removals of the rhinal cortical region alone, this time including the tissue on the rostral face of the temporal pole (see Fig. 3C), have been found to result in severe impairments in recognition memory in monkeys (Murray et al., 1989). Further, Zola-Morgan and his colleagues (1989b) have found that ablations of the perirhinal cortex plus cortex of the parahippocampal gyrus also yields a severe deficit in recognition memory. Earlier, and consistent with the foregoing, Horel and his colleagues (1987) had found a severe impairment in delayed matching-to-sample following either ablations or reversible cooling lesions of the inferior temporal gyrus, which includes a large portion of the perirhinal cortex. These results collectively demonstrate that the periallocortical tissue in the ventromedial temporal lobe is contributing critically to recognition memory. Thus, damage to the rhinal cortical region clearly is sufficient to produce a severe impairment in recognition memory, and a corollary is that combined removal of the amygdala and hippocampus is *not* necessary to produce the impairment.

Despite the strong agreement across laboratories concerning the mnemonic contribution of this periallocortex, different views have emerged to explain the mechanisms underlying the impairment. Murray et al. (1989) removed both the perirhinal and entorhinal cortex, an ablation that substantially deafferents, i.e., disconnects from sensory inputs, not only the medial thalamic regions known

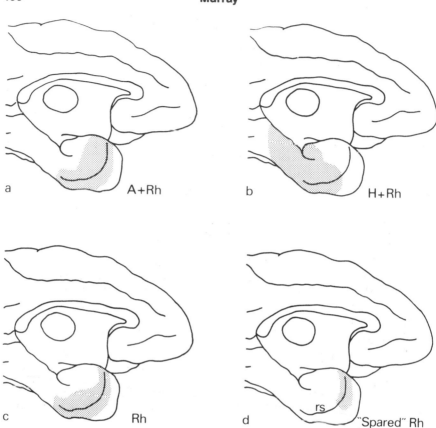

Fig. 3. Medial view of a macaque brain illustrating the intended location and extent of three different medial temporal lobe lesions (**a–c**). **a,b:** Stippled region shows the A + Rh and H + Rh ablations employed by Murray and Mishkin (1986). **c:** Stippled region shows the Rh ablation employed by Murray et al. (1989). **d:** Stippled region shows the extent of the rhinal cortical region spared in the H + Rh group prepared by Murray and Mishkin (1986). Compare and contrast b and c.

to be involved in recognition memory, but the amygdala and hippocampus as well; these investigators have suggested that such a disconnection of rhinal cortex from all three regions (i.e., amygdala, hippocampus, and medial diencephalon) may account for the behavioral effects of the rhinal cortical ablation. Interestingly, the amygdala is known to receive *direct* projections from many of the same modality-specific neocortical areas that project to the perirhinal cortex. Consequently, if the rhinal cortical lesions yield their behavioral effects in part by "deafferenting" the amygdala, one must posit that it is the sensory input reaching this structure indirectly via the perirhinal cortex that is necessary for recognition.

Zola-Morgan et al. (1989b) removed the perirhinal cortex and cortex on the parahippocampal gyrus in order to deafferent the entorhinal cortex, which serves as the main source of sensory inputs to the hippocampal formation. Because their lesions spared the rostral perirhinal cortex that projects heavily into the amygdala, these authors have argued that the behavioral effects of their lesions cannot be viewed as a deafferentation of the amygdala, but, instead, should be viewed as a deafferentation of the hippocampal formation that is exacerbated by the added perirhinal cortical removal. In any event, both the rhinal lesion alone and the perirhinal plus parahippocampal cortex lesion yield a behavioral effect that is much greater in magnitude than that which follows hippocampal removals by aspiration (i.e., which include parahippocampal cortex), so the idea that the hippocampal formation alone is critical for recognition memory can be rejected.

Finally, Horel et al. (1987) cooled or ablated the inferior temporal gyrus, which is comprised of a portion of visual area TE, laterally, and much of the perirhinal cortex, medially. He, too, has suggested that interaction of this cortex with other cortical and subcortical structures is critical for memory. Although it is hazardous to compare results across studies involving different test procedures, it is noteworthy that the animal in their study with the most severe recognition memory deficit had a bilaterally symmetrical lesion along the banks of the rhinal sulcus, one that appears to approximate the rhinal lesion of Murray et al. (1989) and Gaffan and Murray (in press). This finding is consistent with the idea that it is damage to the tissue lying on the medial part of the inferior temporal gyrus, i.e., perirhinal cortex, rather than the more laterally placed area TE on the gyrus that is primarily responsible for the recognition impairment in all three studies.

WHY WAS THE AMYGDALA THOUGHT TO BE IMPORTANT FOR RECOGNITION MEMORY?
Aspiration Lesions of the Amygdala

The foregoing analysis raises the question of how the amygdala came to be seen as contributing critically to recognition memory in the first place. The major reason of course is that the amygdaloid complex, of all the structures removed in the amygdala ablation by aspiration, possesses by far the largest volume, and so was quite naturally thought to be the structure responsible for the synergistic behavioral effect when its removal was combined with hippocampectomy. A corollary is that the small amount of piriform and entorhinal cortex that was included in the lesion was deemed unlikely to account for the behavioral effects. Further, the amygdaloid complex receives direct projections from the modality-specific neocortical processing areas and is the source of projections to other regions known to be important for memory, such as the medial portion of the mediodorsal nucleus and the orbital frontal cortex (Porrino et al., 1981; Aggleton and Mishkin, 1984; Amaral and Price, 1984), and this finding, too, is consistent with a role for the amygdala in sensory memory.

Nevertheless, it was still possible that the cortex underlying the medial temporal lobe limbic structures was instead responsible for the behavioral effects of the combined limbic lesions. As discussed previously, Murray and Mishkin (1986) directly examined this possibility and, because of the limited knowledge available at the time regarding the extent of the perirhinal cortex, came to the wrong conclusion concerning the contribution of the rhinal cortex to recognition memory. Their findings served to simultaneously strengthen the idea that the amygdala contributed critically to recognition memory, and to discredit the idea that the periallocortex in the ventromedial temporal lobe contributed critically to recognition memory.

The Question of Involvement of the Perirhinal Cortex

There is yet another factor complicating the interpretation of the effect of amygdala removals (by aspiration) on recognition memory in monkeys. Despite the fact that the perirhinal cortex (i.e., the cortical tissue occupying the lateral bank of the rhinal sulcus and the portion of the inferior temporal gyrus immediately adjacent to the sulcus) was not meant to be included in the combined amygdala and hippocampal lesions, some monkeys did sustain damage to this area. Indeed, Zola-Morgan et al. (1989b) have argued that this inadvertent damage to the perirhinal cortex is responsible for any behavioral effects on recognition of amygdala lesions. Their idea is based on the following: (1) Aspiration lesions of the amygdala result in direct damage to the perirhinal cortex in some animals; (2) selective radiofrequency lesions of the amygdala that spare the periallocortex, when combined with hippocampal removals, do not produce a more severe memory impairment than hippocampectomy alone; whereas (3) ablations of the perirhinal cortex combined with hippocampal removals *do* exacerbate the behavioral impairment.

Although some monkeys with amygdala removals made in conjunction with hippocampectomy do indeed sustain direct inadvertent damage to the perirhinal cortex, this direct damage is variable, and not always bilateral. Further, there are cases where negligible damage to the perirhinal cortex has occurred (Murray, unpublished observations), and yet the synergistic effects on memory are consistent and marked. Consequently, if loss of perirhinal function is to be held responsible for those effects, the dysfunction must arise in some other way. One possible explanation along these lines is suggested by anatomical studies of structures in the ventromedial temporal lobe. Aggleton and Mishkin (1984) described the rhinal efferents to the medial thalamus in monkeys as coursing adjacent to the amygdala to join the ventral amygdalofugal pathway near the dorsal amygdala, so one could posit that removal of the amygdala by aspiration damages this efferent fiber projection system of the rhinal cortex. Examination of the brain of a macaque monkey that received a large injection of tritiated amino acids into the perirhinal cortex reveals a sizable efferent fiber bundle hugging the lateral aspect of the amygdala (see Fig. 4). Although some of these fibers terminate in the amygdala itself, the majority of the projection fibers appear to terminate in the medial, magnocellular portion of the mediodorsal nucleus of the thalamus, orbital frontal cortex, anterior cingulate cortex, ventral striatum, and tail of the caudate nucleus plus ventral putamen, all structures that have been implicated in memory processes, and some of which are known to

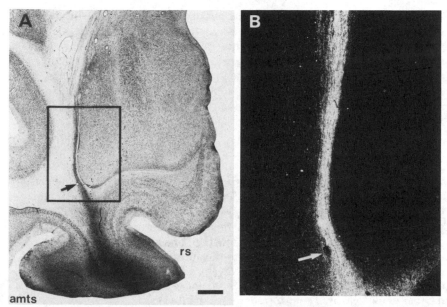

Fig. 4. A: Brightfield photomicrograph of a Nissl-stained coronal section showing the region of the ventromedial temporal lobe, including the amygdaloid complex, the entorhinal cortex, and the inferior temporal gyrus. Note injection site of tritiated amino acids (blackened area) centered in perirhinal cortex, lateral to the rhinal sulcus, and efferent fiber bundle traveling just lateral to the amygdaloid complex. Calibration bar = 1 mm. **B:** Higher-power darkfield photomicrograph of region indicated by rectangular outline in A showing the perirhinal efferent fibers hugging the lateral aspect of the amygdala. Arrows in A and B point to the same blood vessel. Abbreviations: rs, rhinal sulcus; amts, anterior middle temporal sulcus. (Anatomical material courtesy of Leslie G. Ungerleider.)

contribute specifically to recognition memory (Aggleton and Mishkin, 1983a,b; Zola-Morgan and Squire, 1985; Voytko, 1985; Bachevalier and Mishkin, 1986). Further, it seems likely that this bundle would indeed be damaged during aspiration lesions of the amygdala, and a review of published photomicrographs and reconstructions of amygdala lesions from a variety of studies bears this out (e.g., Fig. 2 in Spiegler and Mishkin, 1981; Figs. 4, 5 in Murray and Mishkin, 1984; Fig. 1 in Malamut et al., 1984; Fig. 1 in Overman et al., 1990; Fig. 2 in Gaffan and Murray, 1990). To date, there has been no direct examination of the possibility that perirhinal efferent fibers are transected in the process of amygdala removal, but presumably this question could be addressed directly through an analysis of the projection patterns of perirhinal/entorhinal cortex to some of the target structures (e.g., the medial portion of the mediodorsal nucleus of the thalamus) in animals with and without aspiration lesions of the amygdala.

Recently, removals of the perirhinal cortex alone have been found to yield substantial impairments in visual recognition memory in monkeys (Meunier et al., 1990). Monkeys with ablations of perirhinal cortex alone were found to attain a mean of 78% correct responses on the performance test (i.e., the three longer delays and the three list lengths), relative to the 67 and 97% correct attained by monkeys with rhinal ablations and unoperated controls, respectively. Consequently, if perirhinal efferent fibers are indeed consistently damaged during aspiration removals of the amygdala, and if these connections constitute part of a memory circuit (Mishkin, 1982; Bachevalier et al., 1985; Gaffan and Murray, 1990; see also Cirillo et al., 1989), then the amygdala contribution to recognition memory may well have been markedly overestimated.

Lesions of the White Matter Adjacent to the Amygdala

This section considers two experimental approaches that address, one directly and the other indirectly, the mnemonic function of fibers traveling immediately lateral to the amygdala. If aspiration lesions of the amygdala indeed damage the white matter at the lateral boundary of this structure, and if this fiber damage is responsible, at least in part, for the impairment in recognition memory that follows this kind of amygdalar lesion, then one would predict that damage to the white matter laterally adjacent to the amygdala would also yield impairments in recognition memory. The relevant studies examined the effects on recognition of transections meant to interrupt either: (1) the white matter of the temporal stem; or (2) the amygdalofugal pathways.

First, although temporal stem lesions placed immediately posterior to the amygdala, at the anteroposterior level of the hippocampus, fail to yield an impairment in recognition (Zola-Morgan et al., 1982), temporal stem lesions located at the level of the temporal pole and amygdala do yield the predicted impairment (Cirillo et al., 1989).* Because most of the rhinal cortex lies rostral to the hippocampus, the two structures overlapping for the rostral third of the hippocampus at most, these data are consistent with the idea that interruption of rhinal cortical efferent fibers, which would only be substantial following the more rostrally placed transection, is sufficient to disrupt recognition memory.

The second approach that will be considered is that of Bachevalier et al. (1985), who found that combined but not separate transections of the amygdalofugal pathways (AFP) and fornix in cynomolgus monkeys yielded an impairment in visual recognition memory. The AFP (both the ventral amygdalofugal pathway and the stria terminalis) were transected at the level of the dorsal amygdala, with the transection extending from the frontotemporal junction medial to the rhinal sulcus, medially, to the temporal horn of the lateral ventricle and

---

*Indeed, the present argument is consistent with the temporal stem hypothesis (Horel, 1978), which proposed that damage to fibers traveling in the white matter of the temporal stem was responsible for the impairments in learning and memory associated with medial temporal lobe damage or pathology in both humans and other animals. The present proposal differs from that of Horel's and his colleagues (Horel, 1978; Cirillo et al., 1989) in specifying that it is disruption of the projections of the periallocortical tissue lining the banks of the rhinal sulcus, and not of the neocortical tissue of the anterior inferior temporal cortex (Von Bonin and Bailey's area TE), that is critical in producing the amnesic syndrome.

the white matter of the temporal stem, laterally. Although the monkeys with the AFP transection did not perform at a level significantly different from that of the controls, there was some variability among the scores of the animals in the group. This suggested the possibility that the performance scores of the animals with the AFP lesions could be related to the amount of damage to the temporal stem white matter. A re-examination of the histology of the animals in this group shows that although the lowest-scoring animal in the group (AFP-3; τ = 83%) does appear to have the greatest amount of damage to the white matter lateral to the amygdala, the remaining two animals did not follow the trend. The monkey judged to have the least amount of white matter damage (AFP-1) scored a mean of 87% correct responses to the performance test, whereas the monkey with slightly more damage (AFP-2) scored 94%. Because AFP-1 also had the poorest preoperative learning score of the animals in this group, it is possible that this animal scored poorly relative to AFP-2 for reasons unrelated to the surgery. Consequently, the histology of the animals with AFP lesions, while not supporting the present hypothesis, are at least consistent with it.

EVIDENCE FOR AMYGDALOID CONTRIBUTIONS TO RECOGNITION MEMORY: A RECONSIDERATION

As indicated earlier, Zola-Morgan and his colleagues have suggested that amygdala does not contribute to recognition memory. Instead, they propose that damage to cortex adjacent to the amygdala, especially the perirhinal cortex, accounts for the increase in magnitude of the behavioral impairment when amygdala removals by aspiration are added to hippocampal removals (Zola-Morgan et al., 1989a,b). Their data are not entirely convincing because the amygdala ablations in their study (Zola-Morgan et al., 1989a) appear to be incomplete; the findings are provocative, however, and Zola-Morgan and his colleagues may nevertheless have settled upon the right answer.

On the other hand, there is some evidence that supports the idea of amygdaloid contributions to recognition memory, even in the context of the substantial rhinal cortical contribution; ablations of the amygdala plus rhinal cortex yield a more severe impairment in recognition than ablations of the rhinal cortex alone (see Fig. 2). Although the magnitude of the difference between the two impairments is relatively small, it is statistically significant. Whether one views the rhinal lesion as functionally disconnecting the amygdala from its sensory inputs or not, the difference in the impairments can be interpreted as evidence that the amygdala contributes to recognition memory. Presumably the small advantage of monkeys with rhinal ablations over those with amygdala plus rhinal ablations would reflect the slight contribution to recognition afforded by the direct neocortical projection system, perhaps acting in concert with other structures. We should keep in mind that the amygdala, like the rhinal cortex, projects directly to the medial portion of the mediodorsal nucleus of the thalamus (Porrino et al., 1981; Aggleton and Mishkin, 1984) and to the orbital frontal cortex as well (Porrino et al., 1981; Amaral and Price, 1984), and in this respect is just as likely to participate in memory processes as the rhinal cortex. There are at least three alternative explanations for the significantly different effects on recognition of the rhinal versus amygdala plus rhinal ablations, however, none of which necessitates an amygdalar contribution. First, our rhinal lesions might be somewhat incomplete. If so, fibers emanating from spared cells in the rhinal cortex might be damaged by the amygdala lesion, thus accounting for the difference. Second, other tissue that is included in the amygdala plus rhinal lesion but not the rhinal lesion (e.g., piriform cortex, periamygdaloid cortex) may account for the difference. And finally, emotional or attentional factors may account for the different behavioral outcomes of the two lesions.

At present, none of these three alternative possibilities can be definitively ruled out. We are in the process of evaluating our rhinal cortical lesions by reconstructing them onto flattened maps of the brain and are not, at present, in a position to determine whether they are complete. As far as I am aware, there are no data concerning the possible contributions of the piriform cortex to recognition memory in monkeys, although, like the rhinal cortex, this region has been reported to project to the medial thalamus (Gower, 1989), and might therefore be in a position to participate in memory processes (Mishkin, 1982; Bachevalier et al., 1985). Finally, although rhinal cortical lesions may produce some subtle changes in emotional behavior, only the amygdala removals by aspiration or by radiofrequency result in the marked emotional changes first described by Klüver and Bucy (Weiskrantz, 1956; Butter and Snyder, 1972: Aggleton and Passingham, 1981; Zola-Morgan et al., 1991; Bachevalier, Meunier, Murray, and Mishkin, unpublished observations). If the amygdaloid contribution to memory, over and above the rhinal contribution, is slight, then it becomes more plausible that any effects of amygdala removal on recognition scores can be accounted for by attentional or emotional changes of the operated animals (cf. Zola-Morgan et al., in press).

The marked impairments in recognition memory in monkeys that follow lesions restricted to the perirhinal cortex, together with the evidence that efferent fibers from this region are probably consistently damaged during aspiration lesions of the amygdala, suggest that inadvertent and indirect damage to the perirhinal cortex, in the form of interruption of its efferent fibers, may account to a large extent for the effects of amygdala lesions by aspiration. The rostral portion of the entorhinal cortex, a region which is always removed or damaged during aspiration lesions of the amygdala, also contributes to the impairment in recognition memory that follows amygdala lesions, though this region appears to make less of a contribution than the perirhinal cortex (Meunier et al., 1990). Given the power of the rhinal cortical lesions to account in this way for the effects of amygdala removals,* plus the direct evidence arguing against an amygdaloid contribution, it now seems reasonable to assign the periallocortex a sub-

---

*Additional support for the idea that rhinal cortical lesions can account for the effects of limbic lesions is found in a recent study by Gaffan and Murray, who showed that rhinal cortical lesions yield the same pattern of mnemonic deficits as combined amygdala and hippocampal lesions. Both ablations produce a severe impairment in recognition memory but spare the ability to learn new visual discriminations (Malamut et al., 1984; Gaffan and Murray, submitted).

stantial role in recognition memory and the amygdala a negligible one until such time as selective amygdala lesions are documented to significantly affect recognition. This documentation might take the form of repeating the Zola-Morgan et al. (1989a) study in which selective amygdala lesions were added to hippocampal removals, this time ensuring that the amygdala lesions are complete, or alternatively, could take the form of adding selective amygdala removals to rhinal cortical lesions. If the amygdala is contributing critically to recognition memory in the manner originally conceived, it should significantly exacerbate the effects on recognition memory of either hippocampal removals or rhinal cortical removals. Some caution is warranted in selecting a method to attack this problem. Perirhinal cortical (and perhaps entorhinal cortical or inferior temporal cortical) fibers may well pass directly through the dorsal amygdala (see Fig. 6 in Aggleton et al., 1986), so excitotoxic lesions may yield a different result from radiofrequency lesions. In addition, complete radiofrequency lesions of the amygdala, like complete aspiration lesions, may damage some of the immediately adjacent white matter, and this technique may therefore be contraindicated as the method of choice.

ADDITIONAL CONSIDERATIONS

Even if the amygdala does not contribute to recognition memory as originally conceived, this does not rule out the possibility that this structure makes *some* contribution to recognition memory. Nor does it rule out the possibility that the amygdala contributes to other kinds of memory, for example, to stimulus-reward associative memory (Spiegler and Mishkin, 1981; Gaffan and Harrison, 1987; Gaffan and Murray, 1990), cross-modal sensory-sensory associative memory (Murray and Mishkin, 1985), or to recency memory (Mishkin and Oubre, 1976; Murray and Mishkin, 1984). Because the studies listed above all involved aspiration lesions of the amygdala, however, the contribution of the amygdala versus surrounding cortex needs to be re-evaluated for these mnemonic processes as well.

Finally, although the present discussion has focused on an evaluation of amygdaloid contributions to recognition memory, arguments that parallel those employed here may apply to hippocampal contributions as well. For example, removal of the parahippocampal gyrus, which accompanies aspiration lesions of the hippocampus, may account for some of the impairment in recognition that follows the combined amygdala and hippocampal ablation. In the final analysis it could turn out that selective, combined ablations of the amygdala and hippocampus (i.e., ablations which leave the surrounding cortex intact) in monkeys actually have *no* measurable effect on recognition memory. Future studies will need to evaluate the contributions to memory of both these medial temporal lobe limbic structures as distinct from the underlying cortical regions.

SUMMARY

For the last decade, ablation experiments pointed toward an amygdaloid contribution to recognition memory in monkeys that, together with contributions from other structures, was critical. Recent evidence that the periallocortex in the ventromedial aspect of the temporal lobe contributes critically to recognition memory in monkeys, among other findings, has led a number of investigators to re-examine and reassess the amygdaloid contribution. Specifically, in one set of experiments carried out by Zola-Morgan and his colleagues (Zola-Morgan et al., 1989a,b) selective ablations of the amygdala failed to exacerbate the effects of hippocampal removal, whereas perirhinal cortical ablations did exacerbate the effect. Furthermore, other investigators have found that lesions restricted to the cortex in the ventromedial aspect of the temporal lobe near the rhinal sulcus severely disrupt recognition memory in monkeys (Horel et al., 1987; Murray et al., 1989; Meunier et al., 1990). Early estimates of the extent of the amygdaloid contribution to recognition memory, being based on aspiration lesions of this structure, were in all likelihood substantially inflated due to inadvertent damage to perirhinal cortical efferent fibers traveling just lateral to the amygdaloid complex, an idea consistent with the effects on recognition of lesions to the white matter placed lateral to the amygdala (Cirillo et al., 1989). Given the foregoing, plus the fact that there is little independent and direct evidence in support of a critical contribution to recognition memory by the amygdala, it now seems more plausible to explain the effects of amygdala removal by aspiration in terms of the concomitant rhinal cortical damage than to explain the effects of rhinal cortical damage as a disconnection or deafferentation of the amygdala. Although attention has focused on the role of the perirhinal cortex, and indirect damage to this structure may indeed account for much of what formerly has been ascribed to amygdala damage, it is now evident that the entorhinal cortex contributes to recognition memory (Meunier et al., 1990; Beason et al., 1990), and the piriform cortex and other periallocortical areas may contribute as well.

ACKNOWLEDGMENTS

I gratefully acknowledge the contributions of my colleagues: Jocelyne Bachevalier, Martine Meunier, Mortimer Mishkin, and David Gaffan. I also thank Mortimer Mishkin for his support in all phases of this work, and both Leslie Ungerleider and Mortimer Mishkin for their valuable comments on an earlier version of this manuscript. Leslie Ungerleider kindly provided the anatomical material shown in Figure 4.

REFERENCES

Aggleton JP, Desimone R, Mishkin M (1986): The origin, course, and termination of the hippocampothalamic projections in the macaque. J Comp Neurol 243:409–421.

Aggleton JP, Mishkin M (1983a): Visual recognition impairment following medial thalamic lesions in monkeys. Neuropsychologia 21:189–197.

Aggleton JP, Mishkin M (1983b): Memory impairment following restricted medial thalamic lesions in monkeys. Exp Brain Res 52:199–209.

Aggleton JP, Mishkin M (1984): Projections of the amygdala to the thalamus in the cynomolgus monkey. J Comp Neurol 222:56–68.

Aggleton JP, Passingham RE (1981): Syndrome produced by lesions of the amygdala in monkeys (Macaca mulatta). J Comp Physiol Psychol 95:961–977.

Amaral DG (1987): Memory: Anatomical organization of candidate brain regions. In Mountcastle VB, Plum F, Geiger SR (eds): "Handbook of Physiology, Section 1, The Nervous System," vol 5. Bethesda, MD: American Physiological Association, pp 211–294.

Amaral DG, Insausti R, Cowan WM (1987): The entorhinal cortex of the monkey: I. Cytoarchitectonic organization. J Comp Neurol 264:326–355.

Amaral DG, Price JL (1984): Amygdalo-cortical projections in the monkey (*Macaca fascicularis*). J Comp Neurol 230:465–496.

Bachevalier J, Mishkin M (1986): Visual recognition impairment follows ventromedial but not dorsolateral prefrontal lesions in monkeys. Behav Brain Res 20:249–261.

Bachevalier J, Parkinson JK, Mishkin M (1985): Visual recognition in monkeys: Effects of separate vs. combined transection of fornix and amygdalofugal pathways. Exp Brain Res 57:554–561.

Beason LL, Moss MB, Rosene DL (1990): Effects of entorhinal, parahippocampal, or basal forebrain lesions on recognition memory in the monkey. Soc Neurosci Abstr 16:617.

Butter CM, Snyder DR (1972): Alterations in aversive and aggressive behaviors following orbital frontal lesions in rhesus monkeys. Acta Neurobiol Exp 32:525–565.

Cirillo RA, Horel JA, George PJ (1989): Lesions of the anterior temporal stem and the performance of delayed match-to-sample and visual discriminations in monkeys. Behav Brain Res 34:55–69.

Gaffan D, Harrison S (1987): Amygdalectomy and disconnection in visual learning for auditory secondary reinforcement by monkeys. J Neurosci 7:2285–2292.

Gaffan D, Murray EA (1990): Amygdalar interaction with the mediodorsal nucleus of the thalamus and the ventromedial prefrontal cortex in stimulus-reward associative learning in the monkey. J Neurosci 10:3479–3493.

Gaffan D, Murray EA: Monkeys with rhinal cortex lesions succeed in object discrimination learning despite 24-hour intertrial intervals and fail at matching to sample despite double sample presentations. Behav Neurosci (in press).

Gower EC (1989): Efferent projections from limbic cortex of the temporal pole to the magnocellular medial dorsal nucleus in the rhesus monkey. J Comp Neurol 280:343–358.

Horel JA (1978): The neuroanatomy of amnesia: A critique of the hippocampal memory hypothesis. Brain 101:403–445.

Horel JA, Pytko-Joiner DE, Voytko ML, Salsbury K (1987): The performance of visual tasks while segments of the inferior temporal cortex are suppressed by cold. Behav Brain Res 23:29–42.

Insausti R, Amaral DG, Cowan WM (1987): The entorhinal cortex of the monkey: II. Cortical afferents. J Comp Neurol 264:356–395.

Malamut BL, Saunders RC, Mishkin M (1984): Monkeys with combined amygdalo-hippocampal lesions succeed in object discrimination learning despite 24-hour intertrial intervals. Behav Neurosci 98:759–769.

Meunier M, Murray EA, Bachevalier J, Mishkin M (1990): Effects of perirhinal cortical lesions on visual recognition memory in rhesus monkeys. Soc Neurosci Abstr 16:616.

Mishkin M (1978): Memory in monkeys severely impaired by combined but not by separate removal of amygdala and hippocampus. Nature 273:297–298.

Mishkin M (1982): A memory system in the monkey. Philos Trans R Soc Lond 298:85–95.

Mishkin M, Oubre JL (1976): Dissociation of deficits on visual memory tasks after inferior temporal and amygdala lesions in monkeys. Soc Neurosci Abstr 2:1127.

Murray EA, Bachevalier J, Mishkin M (1989): Effects of rhinal cortical lesions on visual recognition memory in rhesus monkeys. Soc Neurosci Abstr 15:342.

Murray EA, Mishkin M (1984): Severe tactual as well as visual memory deficits follow combined removal of the amygdala and hippocampus in monkeys. J Neurosci 4:2565–2580.

Murray EA, Mishkin M (1985): Amygdalectomy impairs crossmodal association in monkeys. Science 228:604–606.

Murray EA, Mishkin M (1986): Visual recognition in monkeys following rhinal cortical ablations combined with either amygdalectomy or hippocampectomy. J Neurosci 6:1991–2003.

Overman WH, Ormsby G, Mishkin M (1990): Picture recognition vs. picture discrimination learning in monkeys with medial temporal removals. Exp Brain Res 79:18–24.

Porrino LJ, Crane AM, Goldman-Rakic PS (1981): Direct and indirect pathways from the amygdala to the frontal lobe in rhesus monkey. J Comp Neurol 198:121–136.

Saunders RC, Murray EA, Mishkin M (1984): Further evidence that amygdala and hippocampus contribute equally to recognition memory. Neuropsychologia 6:785–796.

Saunders RC, Rosene DL (1988): A comparison of the efferents of the amygdala and the hippocampal formation in the rhesus monkey. I. Convergence in the entorhinal, prorhinal and perirhinal cortices. J Comp Neurol 271:153–184.

Spiegler BJ, Mishkin M (1981): Evidence for the sequential participation of inferior temporal cortex and amygdala in the acquisition of stimulus-reward associations. Behav Brain Res 3:303–317.

Stephan H (1975): Allocortex. In "Handbuch der mikroskopischen Anatomie des Menschen, Band 4, Nervensystem." Berlin: Springer-Verlag, pp 1–998.

Van Hoesen GW, Pandya DN (1975): Some connections of the entorhinal (area 28) and perirhinal (area 35) cortices of the rhesus monkey. I. Temporal lobe afferents. Brain Res 95:1–24.

Voytko ML (1985): Cooling orbital frontal cortex disrupts matching-to-sample and visual discrimination learning in monkeys. Physiol Psychol 13:219–229.

Weiskrantz L (1956): Behavioral changes associated with ablations of the amygdaloid complex in monkeys. J Comp Physiol Psychol 49:381–391.

Zola-Morgan S, Squire LR (1985): Amnesia in monkeys after lesions of the mediodorsal nucleus of the thalamus. Ann Neurol 17:558–564.

Zola-Morgan S, Squire LR, Amaral DG (1989a): Lesions of the amygdala that spare adjacent cortical regions do not impair memory or exacerbate the impairment following lesions of the hippocampal formation. J Neurosci 9:1922–1936.

Zola-Morgan S, Squire LR, Amaral DG, Suzuki WA (1989b): Lesions of perirhinal and parahippocampal cortex that spare the amygdala and hippocampal formation produce severe memory impairment. J Neurosci 9:4355–4370.

Zola-Morgan S, Squire LR, Mishkin M (1982): The neuroanatomy of amnesia: Amygdala-hippocampus versus temporal stem. Science 218:1337–1339.

Zola-Morgan S, Squire LR, Alvarez-Royo P, Clower RP (1991): Independence of memory functions and emotional behavior: Separate contributions of the hippocampal formation and the amygdala. Hippocampus 1:207–220.

The Amygdala: Neurobiological Aspects of Emotion,
Memory, and Mental Dysfunction, pages 471–483
© 1992 Wiley-Liss, Inc.

18
Amygdala and the Memory of Reward

DAVID GAFFAN
Department of Experimental Psychology, Oxford University, Oxford, UK

INTRODUCTION

It is well known that monkeys with bilateral amygdalectomy show reduced emotional responses to rewarding or aversive objects. For example, amygdalectomized monkeys show no alarm when the net with which animals are caught is put near to them. In the category of rewarding objects, food items provide a clear example. A normal monkey, even when satiated on diet chow, becomes quite excited when shown a highly desirable food item such as a banana, while the animal with bilateral amygdalectomy remains apparently indifferent.

In the light of these familiar observations it may seem obvious that the amygdala has an important role in reinforcement, that is, the process by which rewards and punishments affect what an animal learns to do. If an animal is indifferent to rewards and punishments, how can learning by reinforcement proceed normally? Indeed, in the first paper on the effects of selective amygdala lesions in monkeys, Weiskrantz (1956, p. 390) concluded that "the effect of amygdalectomy, it is suggested, is to make it difficult for reinforcing stimuli, whether positive or negative, to become established or to be recognized as such." This simple view is, we now know, not the whole story. There are many ways in which the amygdalectomized animal remains sensitive to rewards and punishments. If reinforcers were without effect then the animal would fail to learn any task motivated by reinforcement, but in fact, as we shall see, the animal learns many food-motivated tasks quite normally. It is therefore necessary to take a closer look at the various subprocesses that are involved in monkeys' memory for rewards and punishments. I argue that the primary function of the amygdala is not in emotion or in sensitivity to reinforcement in general, but instead in a specific associative function, namely the association of stimuli with reward value.

ASSOCIATING STIMULI WITH THE REWARD VALUE OF FOOD

Even in the case of familiar everyday items such as bananas, which reliably elicit emotional reactions from normal monkeys, it is important to remember that they do so as the result of a learning process. When first shown a palatable but unfamiliar food, a monkey displays little interest in it. It is only when the animal tastes it and associates its appearance with its taste that the sight of the food comes to evoke emotional reactions. Therefore, a deficiency of these emotional reactions, following amygdalectomy, may arise from a failure of associative memory.

Associative learning about a new food item, of as yet unknown palatability, is easy to measure by simple preference tests. Baylis and Gaffan (1991, in press) gave monkeys a series of binary choices between food items which, as captive animals, they had rarely or never tasted before: olive, lemon, apple, and beef. Normal animals rapidly established a stable order of preference among these items. Since the choice was a visually guided choice—two items were presented on each trial and the animal was allowed to pick up only one—the preference which develops reflects the acquisition of an association between an item's appearance and its palatability. Amygdalectomized monkeys performed quite differently at this task, showing only weak preferences. In this task therefore the amygdalectomized animals showed no evidence of associating the appearance of a food with its palatability. Thus, abnormal reactions to the sight of a familiar food on the part of amygdalectomized monkeys may, similarly, reflect a loss of the association between the item's appearance and its palatability.

This analysis can be extended to a wider range of learning tasks. The palatability of a food item determines how rewarding the food is to the animal, that is, the food's incentive value. Many experimental tasks require an animal to associate some arbitrary stimulus with the incentive value of a food reward. For example, an auditory secondary reinforcer in a food-motivated visual learning task is associated with the incentive value of the food reward. (The task works as follows: The monkey see two new stimuli and must learn which to choose. Choice of the correct stimulus produces clicks, but choice of the wrong stimulus produces white noise. Four correct choices in succession produce a food reward, but these stimuli are then discarded and the monkey must learn a new pair. Thus, within-problem learning is based on visual associations with the secondary reinforcer, clicks, not the primary reinforcer, food.) If clicks mean food and white noise means no food, is the learning of these meanings similar, in terms of amygdala function, to learning what the sight of a banana means? The experimental evidence shows that it is. Gaffan and Harrison (1987) found that bilateral amygdalectomy produced a severe impairment in the effectiveness of such auditory secondary reinforcers in visual learning.

Thus, there is ample positive evidence of impairment, following amygdalectomy, in associating stimuli with the reward value of food. However, animals do not cease to perform food-motivated tasks after amygdalectomy. Indeed, the motivating power of food rewards does not change, even when carefully measured by the "progressive-ratio" technique, which measures how much work an animal is willing to do for a variety of different food rewards (Aggleton and Passingham, 1982). Horel et al. (1975) and others have understandably found it paradoxical that amygdalectomized animals work normally for food rewards to which they appear to be emotionally indifferent. A brief consideration of strategies and memories in the normal monkey will make this fact seem less paradoxical.

STRATEGIES AND MEMORIES IN FOOD-MOTIVATED LEARNING

To understand the learning abilities of normal monkeys, it is necessary to distinguish between learning a strategy of how to get food, and remembering particular stimulus-food associations. The apparently simplest explanation of a monkey learning a series of straightforward visual discrimination problems for food reward is to say that the associations between discriminanda and food, which the animal demonstrably acquires in solving each problem, also directly produce the animal's choices in the task. However, this simple explanation is inadequate, because monkeys can easily learn to make choices guided by quite different memories, not the memory of food rewards, if the strategy of following some particular memory-dependent performance rule results in the animal getting food. The familiar tasks of delayed matching or nonmatching to sample illustrate this ability, since the animals learn in these tasks to use the memory of having seen an object before to guide food-motivated choices. These tasks show that monkeys can learn to use a memory other than the memory of food to guide food-motivated choices.

A more extreme example of the same kind of flexibility in the use of memories is offered by the task of "win-shift, lose-stay" (Gaffan, 1985). Here the monkey learns to choose whichever object had no food under it before, in preference to the object which did have food under it before. (The task works as follows: There are many stimulus objects, each presented twice. Half of the objects have food reward under them on their first presentation and not on their second, while the others have vice versa no food on their first presentation and food on their second. The monkey learns to choose, on the second presentation, whichever object he remembers as previously having had no food under it.) Unlike delayed matching or nonmatching, this task cannot be performed by staying with or shifting from the more familiar of two objects; instead, the task requires memory of the objects' association with food. The use to which these stimulus-reward associations are put, however, is opposite in this task to the use normally required in experimental tasks. This does not appear to pose any difficulty for the monkeys, who learn the task readily. Thus, we can conclude that the effect of stimulus-food associations upon the food-motivated choices of monkeys is not direct and unchangeable, but flexible; the use that the animal makes of these associations is determined by the strategy he learns for most effectively using memories in getting food.

Indeed, monkeys' use of stimulus-reward associations appears to be not just flexible, but completely flexible: They learn the principle of the win-shift, lose-stay task no slower than that of the more conventional "win-stay, lose-shift" task, where the correct choice is the object which evokes the memory of food; and performance as a function of memory load (the number of object-food associations to be retained, and the length of the retention interval) also shows no difference between the two tasks (Gaffan, 1985). In this respect monkeys differ from rats; rats learn the principle of win-shift lose-stay with difficulty, and their performance of it is much poorer than their performance of win-stay lose-shift (J.N.P. Rawlins, personal communication).

Clearly, this higher-order learning of a strategy for getting food is itself reinforced by food rewards. Therefore, we have to think of food rewards as having
two distinct and independent effects upon the learning systems of the normal
monkey. One is the formation of specific stimulus-reward associations; the other
is the development of a general strategy for getting food.

In this light, the effects of amygdalectomy on food-motivated tasks need not
seem paradoxical. We discussed above two examples of stimuli to which the
amygdalectomized monkey reacts abnormally: the sight of food, and a noise
which predicts the imminent delivery of food. To these can be added the case
of a visual stimulus which is associated with delivery of food reward; this is
discussed in the next section. All of these are discrete sensory events which
have a close spatial or temporal relationship to the consumption of a particular piece of food. The fact that the animals do not cease to perform food-motivated
tasks after amygdalectomy is by no means in conflict with these observations.
Rather, it shows that the amygdala is specifically important for associating discrete stimuli with food reinforcement, rather than generally important for all
effects of food reinforcement, including the learning of general rules or strategies for getting food. Following amygdalectomy, the animal retains the knowledge that eating is accomplished by putting things in the mouth, or that (in a
food-motivated experiment on visual learning) food is got by reaching out to
choose between visual stimuli. But the specific knowledge that a particularly
shaped and coloured food item has a particular value as food, or that a specific
noise or visual stimulus means that food delivery is imminent, is lost or impaired.

One question to ask about associative memory for rewards is, as we have
seen, the question of what the rewards are associated with: discrete stimuli or
general performance rules. An equally important question, however, is what elements of the food reward are remembered.

REMEMBERING THE ATTRIBUTES OF A REWARD EVENT

The operational distinction between primary and secondary reinforcers is
familiar. However, as discussed above, there are learned components in the
animal's response to a primary reinforcer, and the association between (for example) the sight of a banana and its reward value as food is similar to the association between an experimentally established secondary reinforcer and the reward
value of the food it predicts. Moreover, the whole event which is triggered by
the delivery of some particular primary or secondary reinforcer is clearly made
up of diverse components: sensory properties in various modalities, emotional
reactions on the part of the animal, physiological after-effects of consummatory behaviour, and so on. When the aim is to understand how monkeys remember rewards, rather than to describe how trainers use rewards, the distinction
between primary and secondary reinforcement is less relevant than the distinction among the diverse components or attributes of reward events.

In the case of delivering a food reward, there are three classes of component in this event as it affects the animal. First, there is the unlearned intrinsic
incentive value which the food has because of its taste, smell, and nutritive
content. Second, there are some sensory attributes of the delivery of food, such

as the food's visual appearance or the noise of a food dispenser, which have no intrinsic incentive value of their own. Third, in the case of a familiar reward event, there are the emotional responses which these sensory attributes evoke because of their association in memory with the reward's intrinsic incentive value. In the case of a banana, component 1 is represented by the banana in the mouth and stomach, component 2 by the yellow shape, and component 3 by the monkey's excitement at the sight of this yellow shape. A secondary reinforcer, for example, an auditory secondary reinforcer in a food-rewarded task, can be described in similar terms. In this case, component 1 is absent: This event has no intrinsic incentive value. Component 3, however, is present, since the noise (component 2) is associated with the intrinsic incentive value of the food reward it predicts, and it therefore elicits emotional responses. We have seen that the ineffectiveness, in any amygdalectomized monkey, of the sight of a banana or the noise of an auditory secondary reinforcer can be explained by the hypothesis that the fundamental deficit is in the associations between class 2 components and class 1 components—the associations which themselves in turn, in the normal animal, produce the class 3 components of a reward event.

This explanation of the deficit in visual learning for auditory secondary reinforcers relies, however, on the assumption that visual discrimination learning in this task reflects the acquisition of associations between visual discriminative stimuli and the emotional responses which the secondary reinforcer evokes. This assumption is now considered in more detail.

In visual learning for an auditory secondary reinforcer, the visual stimulus might in principle be associated either with the sensory properties of this reinforcer, or with the emotional reactions it evokes. However, it is very difficult for monkeys to associate visual stimuli with sounds, in the case when those sounds are emotionally similar to each other—that is, when different sounds are not differently associated with food reward (Gaffan and Harrison, 1991, in press). But when different sounds are given different associations with food reward, by playing the role of secondary reinforcer and secondary nonreinforcer, it is easy for the monkey to form associations between visual stimuli and these events (Gaffan and Harrison, 1987). Thus, an auditory secondary reinforcer's associability with visual stimuli arises from its own association with food reward; and if amygdalectomy destroys that association with food reward, the associability of the secondary reinforcer with visual stimuli will be reduced, as observed.

The case is quite different when the secondary reinforcer is itself visual. Associations between one visual stimulus and another, when the two stimuli are spatially and temporally close to each other, can be formed rapidly by monkeys, even when all the visual stimuli involved are emotionally similar to each other in the sense that they are all similarly predictive of food reward (Gaffan and Bolton, 1983). This difference between visual-visual and visual-auditory associative learning clearly implies that if a visual secondary reinforcer is presented close in space and time to the visual discriminative stimuli it is to be associated with, then learning can proceed either by visual-visual associations between the visual discriminanda and the sensory properties (class 2) of this reinforcer, or by visual-emotional associations between the visual discriminanda and the emotional responses evoked by the reinforcer. In this case, therefore, the amygdala is important for only one of two possible routes of associative learning. As expected, amygdalectomy had (Gaffan et al., 1989) only a slight effect on visual learning for a local visual secondary reinforcer, an effect significantly milder than its effect when the secondary reinforcer was auditory.

SIMPLE VISUAL DISCRIMINATION LEARNING

Many important early investigations of the effects of amygdalectomy were addressed to an apparently uncomplicated question: What is the role of the amygdala when simple two-choice visual discrimination learning is rewarded in the most straightforward fashion, with immediate delivery of food reward? These investigations produced inconsistent findings, with visual learning for food reward substantially impaired in some experiments (e.g., Schwartzbaum and Poulos, 1965; Barrett, 1969) but almost normal in others (e.g., Douglas et al., 1969; Horel et al., 1975). Clearly, the possibility needs to be considered that these different results arise from differences in the completeness of the amygdalectomy, but as Gaffan and Harrison (1987) conclude from a discussion of the early findings, this factor cannot be a complete explanation.

In view of the foregoing discussion of memory for the attributes of a reward event, it is easy to see that procedural variations in this apparently simple task could produce quite different associative structures in different experiments. Since food itself is a visual stimulus, visual-visual associations could easily be formed when the food is presented close to the discriminative stimuli. Many of the early experiments were conducted in an apparatus (the Wisconsin General Test Apparatus) where visual discriminative stimuli are placed directly over food rewards, which the animal reveals by displacing the object. It was in this apparatus that Gaffan and Bolton (1983) showed that monkeys could easily associate visual discriminanda with the purely visual properties of objects placed under them in the same way as food is. Thus, it is to be expected that in this apparatus, monkeys could remember that the positive object had something under it, and choose on that basis, rather than associating the positive object with the intrinsic incentive value of the food reward. This is the most probable explanation of the mild effects of amygdalectomy in at least some experiments on simple discrimination learning in this apparatus, therefore.

The more recent experiments which I have described above were conducted in a quite different apparatus. A touch-sensitive screen displayed visual stimuli, the animal chose between them by touching one, and food rewards were dispensed into a hopper which was some distance from the screen. In the experiment on visual secondary reinforcement, a correct choice was rewarded with the appearance of the visual secondary reinforcer adjacent to the chosen positive stimulis, while an incorrect choice immediately blanked the screen. But in other experiments we have ensured that there is no local visual feedback which could tell the animal whether a choice had been correct or incorrect; not only is there no explicit visual secondary reinforcer, but also the timing of the screen blanking is identical for correct and wrong choices. In these circumstances of no differential local visual feedback, visual-visual associative learning is not possible. Under these circumstances, visual learning for immediate food reward is severely impaired by bilateral amygdlectomy (Gaffan and Murray, 1990). Thus, results in this apparatus support the idea that after amygdalectomy, monkeys can associate visual stimuli only with the visual properties of a food object, not with its reward value.

The fact that amygdalectomy (even when combined with hippocampectomy) can be without effect upon simple two-choice visual discrimination learning in the Wisconsin General Test Apparatus has led Mishkin and colleagues to argue that this task depends on habit formation rather than stimulus-reward association (Mishkin and Petri, 1984). Habit formation, in this formulation, produces only the tendency to choose the correct object and is independent of the amygdala and hippocampus. There are several objections to this view, however. It is implausible to suggest that the monkey, displacing objects and finding food rewards underneath, does not form some sort of association between objects and food rewards. If it is suggested that, even so, correct choices rely on habit formation rather than on these stimulus-reward associations, then why does not habit formation equally produce correct responses independently of the amygdala in other similar two-choice discrimination learning tasks for immediate food reward, such as that studied by Gaffan and Murray? It seems preferable to allow that associations between the stimuli and the food reward are formed, and control the animals' choices, in all these tasks. The contrasting effects of amygdalectomy in different tasks can be understood, as I have indicated, as arising from the fact that the visual properties of the food reward are associated with the stimuli only when they are presented in close proximity to each other.

SUMMARY OF THE EFFECTS OF BILATERAL AMYGDALECTOMY ON FOOD REWARD

To summarize the argument so far, the effect of bilateral amygdalectomy on food-motivated learning in monkeys is to disrupt associations between discrete stimuli and the intrinsic incentive value of the food reward. These associations are important for maintaining the power of secondary reinforcers to elicit emotional reactions; for discrimination learning when the discriminative stimuli are associated directly with the reward value of a food reinforcement; and for making appropriate choices between food items. But food-motivated associative learning can proceed normally without the amygdala when visual discriminative stimuli are associated with a local visual feedback for the correct choice; this feedback can be an arbitrarily chosen visual secondary reinforcer, or can be the visual aspect of the food reward itself. Normal learning in these tasks shows not only that visual-visual associative learning can proceed normally without the amygdala, but also that the role of food reinforcement in shaping and maintaining the general rules for performing a food-motivated task (as opposed to specific associations with specific discrete stimuli) is independent of the amygdala.

ASYMMETRICAL ABLATIONS

The simple task I described at the end of the last section, visual discrimination learning for immediate food reward without any local visual feedback, relies both on the amygdala (Gaffan and Murray, 1990) and on the visual association cortex TE (Gaffan et al., 1986; E.A. Gaffan et al., 1986), since bilateral lesions in either of these structures produce a severe impairment in the task. In addition, it is known that within each hemisphere, TE projects heavily into the ipsilateral amygdala (Herzog and van Hoesen, 1976). Therefore, it is natural to suppose that in this task, the association of the visual stimuli with reward relies on the interaction of TE with the amygdala via this direct intrahemispheric projection. If so, then the task should be disrupted by crossed unilateral lesions, of the amygdala in one hemisphere and of TE in the other hemisphere; this procedure disconnects the normal direct interaction between these two structures by destroying the origin of the direct pathway in one hemisphere and its termination in the other hemisphere. E.A. Gaffan et al. (1988) showed that, as predicted by this account, crossed unilateral lesions of TE and the amygdala produced an impairment as severe as that which followed bilateral lesions of TE or of the amygdala in the same task.

Experiments with asymmetrical ablations, like that just described, are a powerful tool for anlaysis of the relationship between different brain structures in different tasks. In general (though with certain exceptions) unilateral ablations by themselves have little effect on memory in the monkey. In general also (though again with certain exceptions) the anatomical connections between different structures are largely or exclusively intrahemispheric. When these two conditions are met, asymmetrical ablations of structure X in one hemisphere and structure Y in the other hemisphere have the specific effect of disconnecting information flow between X and Y. This procedure need not produce the full effects, in all respects, of a bilateral symmetrical ablation in either X or Y; for example, unlike animals with bilateral amygdalectomy, animals with TE disconnected from amygdala show normal emotional reactions to tactile stimuli (they jump away when touched by the experimenter). But if the two structures participate in the particular task studied by passing information to each other, then in that specific task the effect of the disconnection will resemble the effect of either of the bilateral symmetrical ablations.

Still with the same task, Gaffan and Murray (1990) showed that again a severe impairment, as severe as that produced by bilateral amygdalectomy, followed bilateral lesions of either the dorsomedial nucleus of the thalamus or the ventromedial prefrontal cortex; and since, again, one of the main projections out from the amygdala is to the ipsilateral dorsomedial nucleus of the thalamus and from there on to the ipsilateral ventromedial prefrontal cortex, it is again natural to suppose [as have Aggleton and Mishkin (1983) and Bachevalier and Mishkin (1986)] that the function of all these structures in this task relies on these pathways of projection between them. In this case, however, the natural supposition is wrong. Gaffan and Murray (1990) found that crossed unilateral lesions of the amygdala in one hemisphere, and of either the dorsomedial thalamic nucleus or the ventromedial prefrontal cortex in the other, produced only a mild impairment, significantly milder than that which followed bilateral lesions of any of these structures.

In a further experiment, Gaffan and Murray (in preparation) showed that again only a mild impairment in this task was produced by crossed unilateral lesions of the amygdala and another of its main projection targets, the ventral striatum. However, they also found that a full impairment was produced by making crossed unilateral lesions of the amygdala in one hemisphere and of all three main projection targets of the amygdala in the other hemisphere: the dorsomedial thalamus and the ventromedial prefrontal cortex, and in addition the ventral striatum.

These experiments, taken together, clearly indicate that the route of information flow through the amygdala in this task, of visual learning for immediate food reward without local visual feedback, is from TE to the amygdala and then, by pathways which are in part independent of each other, to more than one outflow target of the amygdala. Furthermore, the role of these outflow targets in this task is not only to receive information from the amygdala, but also to participate in functions that are independent of the amygdala; this is the implication of the finding that bilateral lesions of the dorsomedial thalamus, for example, produce a more severe impairment than that which follows disconnection of the information flow from amygdala to that structure. The relationship between amydgala and dorsomedial thalamus, therefore, is not that of serial stages in an integrated memory circuit, as Bachevalier and Mishkin (1986) envisaged. Rather, the functions of these two structures are partly dependent on the information flow between them, but partly independent of each other.

Experiments with crossed unilateral lesions also have implications for understanding what kinds of associative learning rely on the amygdala. I have argued above that in visual learning for auditory secondary reinforcement, the amygdala maintains the association of the auditory secondary reinforcer with food reward. Gaffan and Harrison (1987) showed that, as expected from this account, crossed unilateral lesions of the auditory cortex in one hemisphere and of the amygdala in the other, disrupting direct interaction between these two structures, produced a severe impairment. Since visual stimuli, by contrast, are not associated with food reward in this task, the task should not require visual information to be passed to the amygdala. Gaffan and Harrison (1987) found that, in agreement with this analysis, crossed unilateral lesions of TE and the amygdala were without effect in visual learning for auditory secondary reinforcement. The contrast between this result and the severe impairment observed by E.A. Gaffan et al. (1988), with the same crossed unilateral lesions but in visual learning for immediate food reward with no local visual feedback, brings out very clearly the importance of the nature of the reward event in amygdalar function.

In visual learning for an auditory secondary reinforcer, I have argued that the visual stimuli are associated with the emotional reactions (either central or peripheral) which the auditory reinforcer elicits by virtue of its association with food delivery. One possible different account would suppose that the amygdala's interaction with the auditory cortex could enhance the reinforcer's auditory representation, in the auditory cortex, by an attentional mechanism. This enhanced representation could then be associated with the visual stimuli. The difficulty with this account, as noted above, is that when several different noises all predict food, it is difficult for the monkey to associate specific noises with specific visual stimuli (Gaffan and Harrison, 1991, in press). The interpretation I have favoured is strengthened by some further results of the experiments with crossed unilateral lesions. Gaffan and Harrison's (1987) animals with crossed unilateral lesions of the amygdala and of TE continued to learn visual discriminations for auditory secondary reinforcement quite normally, even when the corticocortical commissures connecting the two hemispheres were sectioned. Thus, the auditory cortex in the hemisphere with TE intact had no interaction with the amygdala, while the contralateral auditory cortex had no corticocortical interaction with TE. This finding rules out the idea that an auditory representation of the reinforcer, enhanced by interaction with the amygdala, could be associated with the visual stimuli analyzed by TE. Rather, it suggests that auditory information passed to the intact amygdala aroused widespread emotional reactions, which the visual stimuli analyzed in the hemisphere with TE intact were then associated with.

CROSS-MODAL LEARNING

Murray (1990) has put forward the view that the specific function of the amygdala is cross-modal learning. In many ways this idea makes the same predictions as the ideas I have put forward above. The reason is that the intrinsic incentive value of a food reward, its taste and smell and the physiological after-effects of eating it, is represented in gustatory, olfactory, and interoceptive modalities, while the discriminative stimuli I have used are visual and auditory. Associating these stimuli with the incentive value of food is therefore a cross-modal task. Visual-visual associative learning, on the other hand, which I have argued is responsible for much of the visual learning ability preserved intact after amygdalectomy, is of course within-modal, and thus would also be assumed intact according to the cross-modal hypothesis of amygdala function. However, there are several important differences between these two views. When a monkey associates a visual stimulus with the emotional reactions elicited by a secondary reinforcer, this is a cross-modal association; yet, as we have just seen, it can be learned normally even when the visual association cortex has no interaction with the amygdala. Furthermore, when the monkey learns a general performance rule in response to food reinforcement, cross-modal associations must be involved; yet, as we have seen, amygdalectomy does not prevent monkeys from learning and following general performance rules.

RHINAL CORTEX AND SHORT-TERM OBJECT MEMORY

The main positive evidence for the cross-modal hypothesis of amygdala function comes from an experiment by Murray and Mishkin (1985). They found that amygdalectomy produced a severe impairment in cross-modal (tactile to visual) delayed nonmatching. (In this task, an object is presented for the animal to feel but not see, and a few seconds later the animals must choose by vision a novel object in preference to the object he felt.) The impairment in within-modal tactile or visual delayed nonmatching was much milder.

However, the interpretation of this finding has been reopened by some recent experiments on the function of the cortex in the rhinal sulcus and medial to it. (The anatomy of the region is complex, but for present purposes this region can be briefly called rhinal cortex.) Rhinal cortex is adjacent to the amygdala, and a large part of it was intentionally removed in the amygdalectomized animals in Murray and Mishkin's (1985) experiment. In a subsequent experiment Murray et al. (1989) found that localized lesions in the rhinal cortex, sparing the amygdala, produced a very severe impairment in delayed nonmatching. Following up these findings, Gaffan and Murray (1992, in press) showed that rhinal cortex ablation produced a very severe impairment also in delayed matching, but was without effect upon a long-term memory visual discrimination task, where each object is seen only once each day. The tasks of delayed matching or nonmatching test a monkey's ability to remember objects over a few seconds or minutes. The contrasting results of rhinal cortex lesions in long-term and short-term tasks, and the severity of the impairments produced in the short-term memory tasks, strongly suggest that this cortex is specialized for short-term memory.

If so, then the possibility needs to be considered that Murray and Mishkin's (1985) results in the cross-modal delayed nonmatching task were the results of damage to the rhinal cortex or its inputs and outputs. Presumably, cross-modal short-term memory is a more difficult memory task than within-modal short-term memory, and thus puts a greater demand on the short-term memory mechanisms of the monkey brain.

In fact, recent work on rhinal cortex has called into question the interpretation of a whole series of experiments, which I have not reviewed here, on the effects of amygdalectomy with rhinal cortex damage in short-term one-trial memory tasks such as delayed matching and nonmatching or win-stay, lose-shift. The amygdalectomies in early experiments by Mishkin and colleagues on this type of task were intended also to remove the ventromedial cortex subjacent to the amygdala, which includes much of the rhinal cortex. This rhinal cortex damage was probably sufficient in itself to account for the effects seen in this type of task (see Mishkin, 1978; Spiegler and Mishkin, 1981; Zola-Morgan et al., 1989).

The amygdalectomies in my own experiments were not intended to include the rhinal cortex, and any unintentional damage to it was slight. However, it is in any case unlikely that rhinal cortex damage (intended or unintended) could explain the effects of amygdalectomy upon memory of reward that I have reviewed above. The animals with bilateral removal of the rhinal cortex, and with amygdala intact, show none of the emotional changes in everyday life which follow amygdalectomy. Furthermore, the effects of rhinal cortex lesions, as known so far, are selectively upon short-term memory, while the effects of amygdalectomy can be seen clearly with long-established memories such as the association between an auditory secondary reinforcer and its food reward. Finally, the important contrasts between tasks, which I have discussed above, are to do with the reward event in visual discrimination learning. In different experiments the timing of the presentation of visual stimuli, and thus the importance of any putative defects in short-term memory, are similar; but quite different effects of amygdala lesions are obtained, according to the nature of the reinforcer.

THE AMYGDALA IN CONTEXT

Historically, one view of associative memory is as a very general mechanism. This may be the best way to understand the associative mechanisms of the prefrontal cortex, but in the temporal lobe it appears to be more useful to think of associative memory as made up of a set of specialist mechanisms, each subserved by a specially designed anatomical system. One of the things that a monkey most needs to be able to learn, as rapidly as possible, is the kind of association I have argued the amygdala is specialized for, when a repeated stimulus reliably predicts an event that is of intrinsic value (positive or negative) to the animal. Some further important specialist memory mechanisms in the temporal lobe are the hippocampus, which is specialized for a certain kind of spatially organized memory (Gaffan and Harrison, 1989), and the cortex of the rhinal sulcus, which as we have seen appears to be specialized for short-term memory. More of these specialist mechanisms may remain to be discovered.

REFERENCES

Aggleton JP, Mishkin M (1983): Memory impairments following restricted medial thalamic lesions in monkeys. Exp Brain Res 52:199–209.

Aggleton JP, Passingham RE (1982): An assessment of the reinforcing properties of foods following amygdaloid lesions in rhesus monkeys. J Comp Physiol Psychol 96:71–77.

Bachevalier J, Mishkin M (1986): Visual recognition memory impairment follows ventromedial but not dorsolateral prefrontal lesions in monkeys. Behav Brain Res 20:249–261.

Barrett TW (1969): Studies of the function of the amygdaloid complex in *Macaca mulatta*. Neuropsychologia 7:1–12.

Baylis LL, Gaffan D (1991): Amygdalectomy and ventromedial prefrontal ablation produce similar deficits in food choice and in simple object discrimination learning for an unseen reward. Exp Brain Res (in press).

Douglas RJ, Barret TW, Pribram KH, Cerny MC (1969): Limbic lesions and error reduction. J Comp Physiol Psychol 68:437–441.

Gaffan D (1985): Hippocampus: Memory, habit and voluntary movement. In L Weiskrantz (ed): "Animal Intelligence." Oxford: Clarendon Press, pp 87–99.

Gaffan D, Bolton J (1983): Learning of object-object associations by monkeys. Q J Exp Psychol 35B:149–155.

Gaffan D, Harrison S (1987): Amygdalectomy and disconnection in visual learning for auditory secondary reinforcement by monkeys. J Neurosci 7:2285–2292.

Gaffan D, Harrison S (1989): Place memory and scene memory: Effects of fornix transection in the monkey. Exp Brain Res 74:202–212.

Gaffan D, Harrison S (1991): Auditory-visual associations, hemispheric specialization and temporal-frontal interaction in the Rhesus monkey. Brain 114 (in press).

Gaffan D, Murray EA (1990): Amygdalar interaction with the mediodorsal nucleus of the thalamus and the ventromedial prefrontal cortex in stimulus-reward associative learning in the monkey. J Neurosci 10:3479–3493.

Gaffan D, Murray EA (1992): Monkeys *Macaca fascicularis* with rhinal cortex ablations succeed in object discrimination learning despite 24-hr internal intervals and fail at matching to sample despite double sample presentations. Behav Neurosci: 106 (in press).

Gaffan D, Harrison S, Gaffan EA (1986): Visual identification following inferotemporal ablation in the monkey. Q J Exp Psychol 38B:5–30.

Gaffan D, Gaffan EA, Harrison S (1989): Visual-visual associative learning and reward-association learning: The role of the amygdala. J Neurosci 9:558–564.

Gaffan EA, Harrison S, Gaffan D (1986): Single and concurrent discrimination learning by monkeys after lesions of inferotemporal cortex. Q J Exp Psychol 38B:31–51.

Gaffan EA, Gaffan D, Harrison S (1988): Disconnection of the amygdala from visual association cortex impairs visual reward-association learning in monkeys. J Neurosci 8:3144–3150.

Herzog AG, Van Hoesen GW (1976): Temporal neocortical afferent connections to the amygdala in the Rhesus monkey. Brain Res 16:281–284.

Horel JA, Keating EG, Misantone LJ (1975): Partial Klüver-Bucy syndrome produced by destroying temporal neocortex or amygdala. Brain Res 94:347–359.

Mishkin M (1978): Memory in monkeys severely impaired by combined but not by separate removal of amygdala and hippocampus. Nature 273:297–298.

Mishkin M, Petri HL (1984): Memories and habits: Some implications for the analysis of learning and retention. In Squire LR, Butters N (eds): "Neuropsychology of Memory," 1st ed, New York: Guilford Press, pp 287–296.

Murray EA (1990): Representational memory in nonhuman primates. In Kesner RP, Olton DS (eds): "Neurobiology of Comparative Cognition." Hillsdale, NJ: Erlbaum, pp 127–155.

Murray EA, Mishkin M (1985): Amygdalectomy impairs crossmodal association in monkeys. Science 228:604–606.

Murray EA, Bachevalier J, Mishkin M (1989): Effects of rhinal cortical lesions on visual recognition memory in Rhesus monkeys. Soc Neurosci Abstr 15:342.

Schwartzbaum JS, Poulos DA (1965): Discrimination behavior after amygdalectomy in monkeys: Learning set and discrimination reversals. J Comp Physiol Psychol 60:320–328.

Spiegler BJ, Mishkin M (1981): Evidence for the sequential participation of inferior temporal cortex and amygdala in the acquisition of stimulus-reward associations. Behav Brain Res 3:303–317.

Weiskrantz L (1956): Behavioral changes associated with ablation of the amygdaloid complex in monkeys. J Comp Physiol Psychol 49:381–391.

Zola-Morgan S, Squire LR, Amaral DG (1989): Lesions of the amygdala that spare adjacent cortical regions do not impair memory or exacerbate the impairment following lesions of the hippocampal formation. J Neurosci 9:1922–1936.

The Amygdala: Neurobiological Aspects of Emotion,
Memory, and Mental Dysfunction, pages 485–503
© 1992 Wiley-Liss, Inc.

19
The Functional Effects of Amygdala Lesions in Humans: A Comparison With Findings From Monkeys

JOHN P. AGGLETON

Department of Psychology, University of Durham, Durham, England

INTRODUCTION

Experimental studies into the effects of amygdala damage have told us much about its likely functions. But while a considerable amount is now known about amygdala function in animals, comparatively little is known about the human amygdala. One reason for this discrepancy is the lack of a disease that affects just the amygdala. Although the amygdala may be involved in diseases such as herpes encephalitis and some dementias (see Chapter 23, Mann, this volume), and it may be damaged by ischemia, epilepsy, or tumors, these disorders do not produce circumscribed lesions. A possible exception may be Urbach-Wiethe disease, as there is recent evidence from imaging techniques that this illness may very occasionally result in selective amygdala damage (Tranel and Hyman, 1990).

Further information concerning selective amygdala damage in humans does, however, come from neurosurgical procedures directed at the structure. A number of patients have received either unilateral or bilateral amygdala lesions in an attempt to control epilepsy. In addition, the amygdala became a target for psychosurgical operations, most often in an attempt to modify aggressive or hyperactive behavior. Using information drawn primarily from surgeries directed at the amygdala, this chapter reviews the functional effects of selective amygdala damage in humans and, wherever possible, compares these findings with those from studies of monkeys.

It should be emphasized that in many clinical cases the surgery was added to an already abnormal brain. As a consequence some of the changes seen after surgery may differ from those observed when normal tissue is destroyed. This is most likely to be the case for epileptic patients or for those with a known neuropathology prior to surgery (e.g., encephalitis). Unfortunately these patients are not always identifiable. This is partly because many reports group together patients with different etiologies and partly because data from imaging techniques such as computerized tomography (CT) or magnetic resonance imaging

(MRI) have not been available or have not been published. The situation is further complicated by the fact that some patients may have an unsuspected or unproven neuropathology at the time of surgery. While this possibility has proved contentious for individual patients (Mark and Ervin, 1970; Valenstein, 1973), it is clear that in an unknown proportion of cases the amygdala surgery will have been added to an already abnormal brain.

A related problem is posed by the type of person undergoing neurosurgery or psychosurgery. A significant number of patients had very low IQs, while others were psychotic with severe behavioral disorders. In addition, some surgeons have performed relatively large numbers of operations on young children (Balasubramaniam and Ramamurthi, 1970; Narabayashi, 1977). As a consequence there are inevitable limitations on postoperative assessment. Nevertheless, this should leave a number of cases for whom useful psychometric data is available. Unfortunately there is a distressing lack of objective data for the large majority of patients who have undergone selective amygdala lesions. This shortcoming was highlighted in a review of the postoperative evaluation of psychosurgery (Valenstein, 1980, p. 146), where it was noted that of 34 articles on amygdala psychosurgery, 58.8% failed to specify any objective tests and only about 10% contained objective data on either personality, psychiatric symptoms, abstract thinking, or learning and memory. Furthermore, comparison data on unoperated subjects is almost never provided, often making it difficult to exclude other influences on postoperative behavior. Given the extra attention that is likely to be given to surgical cases, this may be an important omission.

SUBJECTS AND SURGERY

In the early 1950s, a number of surgeons attempted to relieve schizophrenia by removing the entire amygdala bilaterally (Freeman and Williams, 1952; Scoville et al., 1953; Sawa et al., 1954). For some surgeries ("uncotomy" or "uncectomy") an anteromedial approach was used and the amygdala and the adjacent prepiriform and periamygdaloid cortices were removed by aspiration (Scoville et al., 1953; Scoville and Milner, 1957). In other cases the middle temporal convolution was cut prior to aspiration of the amygdala (Freeman and Williams, 1952; Sawa et al., 1954). These amygdala surgeries were sometimes combined with other surgeries, such as a frontal lobotomy, orbital undercutting, or removal of the hippocampus. Among this last group is the series of patients described by Scoville and Milner (1957) that included the well-known amnesic H.M. Unlike the rest of the patients in that series, all of whom were psychotic, H.M. received bilateral resection of the medial temporal lobes in an attempt to cure epilepsy. His surgery involved the amygdala as well as much of the hippocampus, prepiriform gyrus, uncus, and parahippocampal gyrus (Scoville and Milner, 1957; Corkin, 1984). The frequent failure of these amygdala surgeries to relieve schizophrenia and the arrival of other forms of treatment led to the early demise of this form of psychosurgery, although surgeries have continued to be directed at parts of the medial temporal lobes for the treatment of intractable epilepsy.

The introduction of stereotaxic surgery led to a resurgence of interest in the amygdala as a target for psychosurgery. The first reports from Japan (Narabayashi et al., 1963) were followed by other descriptions of stereotaxic amygdala surgery in the United States (Heimburger et al., 1966), India (Balasubramaniam and Ramamurthi, 1970), and various European countries (Kim, 1971; Mempel, 1971; Hitchcock and Cairns, 1973). In this second wave of psychosurgery the patients came from a number of different categories, although the large majority could be described as either assaultative, aggressive, or hyperactive. In a smaller proportion of cases, amygdala surgery was used as a last resort in cases of self-mutilation, depression, suicidal tendencies, psychosis, and intractable pain. At the same time some patients received stereotaxic amygdala lesions in an attempt to control epilepsy. The distinction between the epileptic and nonepileptic cases often became blurred, however, as both epilepsy and behavioral problems could occur in the same person and it is unclear whether some operations were primarily to relieve epilepsy or to relieve the behavioral problems (Valenstein, 1973).

The procedures used in these stereotaxic surgeries show a surprising degree of variation. Some surgeons reached the amygdala via a transtemporal approach (Mark et al., 1972), while others used a dorsal approach (Narabayashi et al., 1963; Hitchcock and Cairns, 1973). The methods used to destroy amygdala tissue included radiofrequency, cryothermy, the injection of substances such as oil, wax, kaolin, or alcohol, and mechanical destruction with a loop (Heimburger et al., 1966; Jelasic, 1966; Narabayashi, 1972; Balasubramaniam and Kanaka, 1975; Siegfried and Reichenbach, 1976). While some of these operations, especially those for the treatment of epilepsy, involved only unilateral lesions, a large number involved either one- or two-stage bilateral lesions. In some cases the amygdala surgery was preceded or followed by other psychosurgical procedures.

The stated intention of many of these stereotaxic surgeries has been to destroy only part of the amygdala ("amygdalotomy" or "amygdaloidotomy"). In those cases with epilepsy, the choice of target region within the amygdala may be based on electrophysiological evidence. In those cases with behavioral or psychotic disorders, the choice of target region within the structure depended largely on the individual surgeon (Table I). Preferred target zones within the amygdala have included the basal and lateral nuclei (Narabayashi et al., 1963; Kim, 1971; Roeder et al., 1971; Ramanchandran et al., 1974), the anteromedial amygdala (Small et al., 1977), the medial amygdala (Hitchcock et al., 1973; Kim and Umbach, 1973), the corticomedial group of nuclei (Narabayashi and Shima, 1973), and the closely related fundus of the stria terminalis (Burzaco, 1973).

Just as the intended locations of these lesions have varied, so have their intended total size (Table I). When it has been specified, the intended lesion size has ranged from between one-third and one-half of the structure (Narabayashi et al., 1963), to three-quarters (Ramamurthi, 1988), to almost the entire structure (Lee et al., 1988b). It must be stressed, however, that there does not appear to be a single psychosurgical case in which the location or extent of the lesion has been confirmed after death. This being so, it is worth noting that Heimburger (1975) found evidence that the temporal landmarks used to locate the amygdala probably show the greatest variation in those very patients for which they are used. Furthermore, the actual extent of an amygdala lesion may

TABLE I. Summary of Amygdala Surgeries

Reference	Total No. of Cases	Aetiology/ No. of Cases	Surgery/Comments
Andersen, 1978	15	Epil	U, intended size 8 × 8 × 10 mm
Andy et al., 1975	2	Epil	1U, 1B
Balasubramaniam & Kanaka, 1975	235	81 Behav/Epil 80 Behav/Enceph 12 Schiz 62 Behav	28U, 207B, Primarily for treatment of behavioral disorders—aggression, rage, self-mutiliation
Chitonondh, 1966	7	Epil	6U, 1B, target medial amygdala
Freeman & Williams, 1952	5	Schiz	B, aspiration lesion, target all of amygdala
Heimburger et al., 1978	58	12 Behav 14 Epil 32 Behav/Epil	35U, 23B, target anteromedial amygdala
Hitchcock & Cairns, 1973	18	2 Behav 16 Behav/Epil	2U, 16B, target medial amygdala
Hood et al., 1983	71	18 Behavior 53 Behav/Epil	4U, 67B
Jacobson, 1986	1	Behav	B, following bilateral subcaudate tractotomy
Kiloh et al., 1974	18	13 Behav 5 Behav/Epil	3U, 15B, 8 mm diameter lesion
Kim, 1971	7	Behav/Epil	U, basal + lateral amygdala and ipsilateral fornix
Kim & Umbach, 1973	63	Behav/Epil	U & B, target medial amygdala
Lee et al., 1988a	1	Behav/Enceph	B, 15 × 15 mm, near complete
Luczywek & Mempel, 1976	46	Epil	3U, 36B, target dorsal + medial amygdala, + 7B with rostral hippocampus damage
Mark et al., 1972	10	Behav/Epil	3U, 7B, target medial amygdala
Mempel, 1971	16	3 Behav 13 Behav/Epil	8U, 8B
Mempel, 1972	30	Behav/Epil	30B target medial and dorsal amygdala, 5 additional unilateral temporal damage
Nadvornik et al., 1973	11	Behav	4U, 7B, all mentally subnormal plus aggression
Narabayashi et al., 1963	60	14 Behav 46 Behav/Epil	39U, 21B, 8–10 mm diameter lesion, target basal and lateral amygdala
Narabayashi & Shima, 1973	47	Behav/Epil	20U, 27B, target central and medial amygdala

TABLE I. Summary of Amygdala Surgeries *(continued)*

Reference	Total No. of Cases	Aetiology/ No. of Cases	Surgery/Comments
Ramamurthi, 1988	481	Behavior Behav/Epil	B, some followed by hypothalamic surgeries; lesion 600–900 mm^3
Sawa et al., 1954	11	5 Schiz 5 Epil 1 Hyperactive	B, aspiration lesion via middle temp. gyrus; aim to remove nearly all of amygdala
Scoville et al., 1953	5	Schiz	B, aspiration uncotomy, remove nearly all of amygdala
Siegfried & Ben-Shmuel, 1973	8	3 Behav 5 Schiz	B, intend to destroy ⅔ of amygdala
Vaernet, 1972	45	Epil	37U, 8B, 8 × 10 mm lesion
Vaernet & Madsen, 1970	12	Behav/Schiz	B, 10 × 10 mm diam. lesion; 2 previous cingulectomy; 5 previous frontal lobotomy

Abbreviations: B, bilateral surgery; Behav, surgery for behavioral disorders, e.g., aggression; Behav/Epil, surgery for behavioral disorder in patients with epilepsy; Enceph, postencephalitic; Epil, surgery for epilepsy; Schiz, schizophrenic; U, unilateral surgery. Unless otherwise stated all surgeries by stereotaxy with intention to destroy some but not all of the amygdala.

not resemble the intended size, as was found in a group of epileptics who received a temporal lobectomy after receiving a stereotaxic lesion of the amygdala (Adams and Rutkin, 1969).

The surgical procedures used for humans can be contrasted with those used in experiments on monkeys. In the large majority of these experiments the intention has been to remove or destroy all of the structure, i.e., perform an "amygdalectomy." For nearly all such amygdalectomies an anteromedial temporal approach has been used and the tissue removed by aspiration. These surgeries almost invariably result in some additional damage to parts of the prepiriform, perirhinal, prorhinal, and entorhinal cortices and as a consequence they most closely resemble the "uncotomy" (Scoville and Milner, 1957). In contrast, stereotaxic methods have been used in only a handful of experimental studies on monkeys (Turner, 1954; Butter and Snyder, 1972; Aggleton and Passingham, 1981; Zola-Morgan et al., 1989) and even fewer studies have set out to produce selective, subtotal "amygdalotomies" (Turner, 1954; Aggleton and Passingham, 1981).

SENSORY FUNCTION

There is no evidence that amygdala damage directly affects visual, auditory, or somatosensory systems. While much of this evidence appears to be informal, the lack of any visual impairment is borne out by the detailed studies on case H.M. (Corkin, 1984). Further evidence comes from the studies on a post-encephalitic patient who received very extensive bilateral amygdala lesions in an attempt to control rage attacks (Lee et al., 1988a) and those on a woman with Urbach-Wiethe disease (Tranel and Hyman, 1990). Likewise, with one exception (Andy et al., 1975), there are no reports that amygdala damage directly affects taste. Overall, this apparent lack of change in visual, gustatory, and somatosensory sensitivity is consistent with studies of amygdalectomized monkeys (Schwartzbaum, 1965; Ursin et al., 1969; Aggleton and Passingham, 1982).

The amygdala is regarded as part of the rhinencephalon as it receives direct inputs from the olfactory bulb (Turner et al., 1978). Indeed, the responsiveness of amygdala units to odors has been used to guide stereotaxic surgery in humans (Narabayashi et al., 1963; Andy and Jurko, 1975). Furthermore, there is evidence that the amygdala can activate olfactory auras and that this is independent of hippocampal activity (Andy et al., 1975). In spite of these findings it is generally reported that neither uncotomy (Scoville et al., 1953) nor amygdalotomy (Chitonondh, 1966; Narabayashi, 1977) disrupts the sense of smell, although testing details have not been provided. Exceptions to this generalisation are a patient (I.S.) who became anosmic following a bilateral uncotomy (Scoville and Milner, 1957) and a woman in whom an extensive bilateral amygdalotomy, which involved the entorhinal cortex in one hemisphere, led to an impairment in odor identification, although detection of odors was largely unchanged (Andy et al., 1975). In the first of these two cases it is most likely that the olfactory tracts were directly damaged, especially as other patients in the same series received more radical surgeries but did not become anosmic (Scoville and Milner, 1957). In the second case there was some recovery of olfaction and two years after surgery the patient regarded her ability to smell as having returned to normal, although formal tests still revealed an odor identification deficit (Andy et al., 1975). This deficit may be similar to that observed in H.M., who can detect weak odors and appreciate odor intensity but is severely impaired in odor discrimination, matching, and identification tasks (Eichenbaum et al., 1983). Given the lack of other patients with olfactory deficits, it is possible that in this second case it was the combination of damage to the amygdala and the entorhinal cortex that was important (Andy et al., 1975). While it has been shown that amygdalectomy does not produce anosmia in monkeys (Schuckman et al., 1969) there are no available data concerning odor detection thresholds or identification.

Interest has recently been focused on the amygdala and the ability to link together sensory information from different modalities about the same object (cross-modal associations). This follows from the discovery that amygdalectomy produces a very severe tactile-to-visual cross-modal recognition impairment in monkeys (Murray and Mishkin, 1985), while performance on intramodal recognition tasks (tactile-to-tactile and visual-to-visual) is good. This apparently critical role in cross-modal associations is consistent with the anatomical connections of the amygdala and it may help explain some of the features of the Klüver-Bucy syndrome that are seen after amygdalectomy (Murray and Mishkin, 1985). It will, however, be necessary to demonstrate whether damage to adjacent cortical regions is involved in this deficit (see Chapter 17, Murray, this volume).

In a recent attempt to test whether the human amygdala has a similar function, Lee et al. (1988b) examined the ability of a man who had received near-total amygdala lesions, confirmed by MRI, to perform both intramodal and cross-modal recognition tasks. The subject, however, showed no change in postoperative performance levels. A similar lack of deficit was found in a second patient who also received extensive bilateral amygdala lesions (Lee, personal communication). These findings have been taken to indicate that the critical locus for cross-modal associations may be the perirhinal and entorhinal cortices and not the amygdala (Lee et al., 1988b). A different possibility is that the subjects had given verbal labels to the paperboard nonsense shapes used in the study and that this strategy had aided performance. In an attempt to minimise verbal labelling by using the "Arc-Circle Test" (Nebes, 1971) evidence was found that postencephalitic subjects may be impaired on cross-modal but not intramodal matching (Shaw et al., 1990). Unfortunately it could not be confirmed whether these subjects had suffered bilateral amygdala damage. It therefore remains to be determined whether bilateral amygdalectomy can disrupt cross-modal associations in humans when verbal cues are excluded.

MOTIVATION

Occasional increases in food intake have been reported following amygdala lesions (Sawa et al., 1954; Kim, 1971; Mark et al., 1972; Burzaco, 1973; Kim and Umbach, 1973; Narabayashi, 1977). These changes are typically transient and last from a few weeks up to a few months (Mark et al., 1972; Burzaco, 1973). More consistent changes in food intake were reported by Narabayashi (1977), who noted that about one-third of 78 cases receiving either bilateral or unilateral amygdalotomy showed transient increases in appetite lasting a few weeks. In contrast, Kim and Umbach (1973) reported a general increase in appetite and weight following surgeries aimed at the medial amygdala.

Similar inconsistent changes have been reported in amygdalectomized monkeys. While many experimenters have failed to find any evidence of persistent alterations in food intake in monkeys (Anand et al., 1958), there are some reports of hyperphagia in adult monkeys (Schwartzbaum, 1961; Kling and Cornell, 1971; Kling and Dunne, 1976). Long-term studies on the effects of neonatal amygdala lesions have, however, found normal growth curves (Kling and Green, 1967; Thompson et al., 1969).

Temporary increases in sexual drive have also been reported in patients after amygdala surgery (Scoville et al., 1953; Kim, 1971; Kim and Umbach, 1973; Ramanchandran et al., 1974; Heimburger et al., 1978; Lee, personal communication). But with the exception of the patients reported by Kim (1971), in whom a unilateral fornicotomy was added to a bilateral amygdalotomy, such patients make up a very small minority of the total cases.

While sexual activity has been observed to increase after amygdalectomy in monkeys, this appears to depend critically on the type and extent of the environment. In small group-cages hypersexuality may be quite prevalent (Kling, 1968; Kling and Dunne, 1976), but it is not seen in more naturalistic settings (Kling, 1972; Kling and Dunne, 1976). This finding might help explain the rarity of such changes in humans.

EMOTION

The most dramatic consequence of amygdalectomy in monkeys is a loss of emotional responsiveness. This hypoemotionality, which is combined with a willingness to approach and examine previously frightening stimuli, may diminish with time (Walker et al., 1953; Weiskrantz, 1956) but it does not completely disappear. In spite of the hypoemotionality these animals are still able to make affective responses, but the threshold for such responses appears to be considerably higher (see Chapter 13, Kling, this volume). Amygdala lesions also result in a permanent disruption of normal social behavior (Kling, this volume). In considering the effects of human amygdala damage, attention will be given, where possible, to the size and location of the lesions, as there is evidence from monkeys that these factors help determine the extent of any emotional changes (Kaada, 1972; Aggleton and Passingham, 1981). Lastly, it must be remembered that in none of these clinical reports has adequate control data been provided, so there is the possibility that some of the postoperative changes are not a direct consequence of amygdala damage.

In the first series of stereotaxic amygdalotomies to be reported, Narabayashi et al. (1963) described 60 aggressive or hyperactive patients who received relatively small unilateral or bilateral stereotaxic lesions involving approximately one-third of the amygdala. It was reported that 51 (85%) of the patients showed a marked reduction in emotional excitability and a "normalization" of social behavior (Narabayashi et al., 1963). It was stressed that while many of the patients became calmer and more cooperative, they did not become emotionless or apathetic (Narabayashi et al., 1963) and that even patients with bilateral lesions could become angry or excited when appropriate (Narabayashi, 1977). In a review of 47 surgeries it was concluded that in order to achieve a calming effect it was probably best to place the lesion slightly to the medial side of the midline, i.e., involving the lateral part of the corticomedial nuclei (Narabayashi and Shima, 1973).

The effects of small medial amygdala lesions were also described by Hitchcock and Cairns (1973). These surgeries, which were either unilateral or bilateral, were carried out in a group of 15 epileptic subjects who showed abnormal aggressive behavior. Formal assessment schemes revealed evidence of clear decreases in destructive aand antisocial behavior in about half of the cases. More detailed examination of five cases indicated that the surgeries produced very few changes on the 16 Personality Factor Questionnaire (Cattell et al., 1970) and that high levels of hostility still persisted (Hitchcock et al., 1973).

More extensive lesions, probably damaging at least two-thirds of the structure bilaterally, were used by surgeons in Madras (Balasubramaniam and Ramamurthi, 1970; Ramamurthi, 1988). It may be indicative that the term "sedative surgery" has been used to describe these operations (Balasubramaniam and Kanaka, 1975). In a brief review of 320 cases it was reported that about one-third of the patients became very much more docile and given to only occasional outbursts (Balasubramaniam and Kanaka, 1975). In a more extensive review of 481 patients from the same surgical group (Ramamurthi, 1988) it was stated that approximately 70% of the patients showed a reduction in either restlessness or destructiveness, and that one-half of these remained calm and quiet even in the face of provocation. Similar changes in emotion were noted in a group of 12 aggressive psychotics who received bilateral amygdala lesions involving approximately three-quarters of the structure (Vaernet and Madsen, 1970). Likewise, in a report on 45 epileptic patients with either unilateal or bilatereal lesions, it was observed that decreases in emotional tension were constant and that postoperatively the patients became emotionally more indifferent and had a neutral mood (Vaernet, 1972). A number of other reports also emphasize how amygdalotomy can reduce levels of rage and aggression (Kim, 1971; Mempel, 1971; Mark et al., 1972; Kiloh et al., 1974; Lee et al., 1988b), although these effects may be inconsistent (Kiloh et al., 1974; Nadvornik et al., 1973; Siegfried and Ben-Shmuel, 1973).

Descriptions of amygdalotomy frequently imply that the lesions primarily affect aggression. In contrast, there is no evidence that either total or subtotal amygdala lesions in monkeys can bring about a selective decrease in aggression (Aggleton and Passingham, 1981). It must, however, be remembered that clinical reports inevitably focus on the behavioral disorder being treated, which very often involves aggression. Furthermore, some reports have relied on crude, subjective rating scales which provide little insight into the actual postoperative status of individual patients (Valenstein, 1973). In spite of these constraints it would appear that small amygdala lesions do not produce a global hypoemotionality (Narabayashi et al., 1963; Narabayashi, 1972) and may have a more selective effect. On the other hand, the use of words such as calm, placid, indifferent, or sedated to describe patients who have received more extensive lesions (Balasubramaniam and Ramamurthi, 1970; Vaernet and Madsen, 1970; Ramamurthi, 1988) strongly suggests that these amygdala lesions affect a wider range of emotions.

Attempts to remove the entire amygdala were largely confined to the surgeries performed on psychotic patients in the 1950s. While a flattening or change of affect was reported for some cases (Scoville et al., 1953; Williams, 1953; Sawa et al., 1954) it is also clear that for many patients the preoperative abnormalities in emotional and psychotic behavior persisted after the surgery (Freeman and Williams, 1952; Scoville et al., 1953; Sawa et al., 1954; Scoville and Milner, 1957). As a consequence it is very difficult to assess the effects of these surgeries on emotion. For this reason the changes in affect observed in patient H.M. are of interest even though his surgery extended caudally far beyond the amygdala (Scoville and Milner, 1957). It has been observed that one of H.M.'s most striking postoperative characteristics is that he rarely complains about anything, even if he is unwell (Corkin, 1984). He appears to be content and placid nearly all of the time. On rare occasions when stressed he can become angry but this dissipates quickly and he remains even-tempered with a preserved sense of humor (Corkin, 1984).

There are surprisingly few descriptions of how the emotional changes that may follow amygdala damage feel for the subject. One exception is the case of a woman who received a subcaudate tractomy, with little apparent effect, followed by a two-stage bilateral amygdalotomy for the treatment of chronic self-mutilation (Jacobson, 1986). The estimated size of the lesions was not given. One consequence of the surgery was a blunting of emotions that included a marked placidity and an absence of anger that extended across all social situations. The patient, who was described as having a dissociated affect, complained that her affects could "not be pigeon-holed into any familiar category" since the operation (Jacobson, 1986). Emotions as a consequence felt different and unfamiliar but not dull, although externally she appeared more placid.

It would appear therefore that amygdala lesions frequently result in some loss or change of affect and that these changes often extend beyond aggression. In addition, the extent or likelihood of any emotional change appears to depend on the size, and, possibly, the location of the lesion. The fact that these changes in affect are seen after both stereotaxic or aspiration lesions indicates that they are not dependent on the involvement of other medial temporal structures such as the perirhinal and entorhinal cortices. This is also the case for old world monkeys (Aggleton and Passingham, 1981; Zola-Morgan et al., 1989). Furthermore, these emotional changes are not simply a consequence of a reduction in epilepsy (Narabayashi et al., 1963; Ramanchandran et al., 1974). For example, despite claiming that 85% of a group of 54 amygdalotomized patients showed a marked emotional improvement, less than 50% showed any improvement in their abnormal EEGs (Narabayashi et al., 1963). This does not of course mean that an alteration in seizure rate might not contribute to any postoperative change in affect. Finally, while follow-up studies indicate that changes in emotion may be long-lasting, they will attenuate or disappear in some cases (Narabayashi and Uno, 1966; Kiloh et al., 1974) and that this may happen most frequently after unilateral lesions (Mempel, 1971; Mark et al., 1972).

In an attempt to see if these changes in emotionality extend to autonomic correlates, a study was made of a man who had received extensive bilateral amygdala lesions for the treatment of rage attacks following encephalitis (Lee et al., 1988a). The surgery, which produced a marked decline in aggression, also resulted in decreases in skin conductance, hand temperature, and frontal electromyography consistent with a fall in sympathetic arousal (Lee et al., 1988a). These changes bear obvious similarities with the depression in electrodermal responses and the lack of heart and respiratory rate components of the orienting response that follow amygdalectomy in monkeys (Bagshaw et al., 1965; Bagshaw and Benzies, 1968). In contrast, normal skin conductance responses have been found following bilateral amygdala damage as a consequence of either Urbach-Wiethe disease (Tranel and Hyman, 1990) or encephalitis (Tranel and Damasio, 1989). While the source of this discrepancy is unclear, it is only in the report by Lee et al. (1988a) that direct comparisons can be made before and after amygdala damage.

While the consequences of amygdala damage on emotional behavior in humans and monkeys bear many similarities, there are some possible differences. There is no evidence that unilateal amygdalectomy has an overt effect on behavior in monkeys (Downer, 1961). In contrast, there are reports that unilateral lesions can have a pronounced effect in humans, even in nonepileptic cases (Narabayashi et al., 1963). One possible explanation of this difference is that damage to a particular hemisphere is associated with changes in emotion. In order to examine this possibility the findings from two series of patients (Narabayashi et al., 1963; Narabayashi and Shima, 1973) have been combined. Using the authors' clinical rating scheme it was found that 77% (27 from 35) patients receiving a left amygdalotomy showed postoperative changes in emotional behavior rated as either A or B (A = greatly improved, B = moderately improved), as compared with 78% (18 from 23) receiving a right amygdalotomy. Clearly there were no hemispheric differences between the effects of these surgeries. As the very large majority of these patients displayed abnormal EEGs prior to surgery, a second comparison just considered those patients for whom the surgery had no effect upon epilepsy or EEG. The proportion of such patients rated as either A or B following left amygdalotomy was 77% (17 from 22) compared with 43% (3 from 7) who received a right amygdalotomy. In spite of the smaller numbers in this second comparison it would appear that again damage to either amygdala can produce a fall in emotion.

Other possible differences concern the severity of the effects seen after amygdala damage in humans and monkeys. Thus, in spite of observations that there is some return to more normal emotional behavior with time in monkeys (Walker et al., 1953; Weiskrantz, 1956) and that the effects may be less extreme in juvenile animals (Kling, 1972), it does appear that the consequences of bilateral amygdalectomy in humans are not as devastating as they are in many monkey species. A part of the explanation lies in the fact that when subtotal, stereotaxic lesions ("amygdalotomies") are made in monkeys, very minor changes in affect are observed and the full hypoemotionality is only seen when there is extensive bilateral damage (Aggleton and Passingham, 1981). Nevertheless, this still leaves a possible discrepancy between the almost total loss of emotions observed after amygdalectomy in monkeys and the changes observed in humans after extensive bilateral lesions. For example, although H.M. shows a clear attenuation of affect, he is not emotionless.

One explanation may be that in humans it is necessary to combine amygdala damage with temporal cortical damage to produce a severe loss of affect. Support for this proposal comes from the finding that those surgical cases with dramatic, global losses of emotion have often received large bilateral, temporal removals extending beyond the amygdala (Obrador, 1947; Green et al., 1951; Pool, 1954; Terzian and Ore, 1955). Furthermore, the "Klüver-Bucy" symptoms such as orality, dietary changes, and hypermetamorphosis that are seen following amygdalectomy in monkeys are normally only seen in people when there is both cortical and subcortical temporal lobe damage (Terzian and Ore, 1955; Gascon and Gilles, 1973; Marlowe et al., 1975; Lilly et al., 1983). While these components of the Klüver-Bucy syndrome are occasionally reported after amygdala lesions, such cases make up a very small minority, the only exception being a series of patients who received aspiration removals of the amygdala and subsequently displayed abnormal oral symptoms (Sawa et al., 1954). As the surgical approach was through the temporal gyrus (Sawa et al., 1954) it is possible that cortical damage contributed to these effects.

In summary, there appear to be many similarities between the emotional effects of amygdala lesions in humans and monkeys, and these similarities far outweigh the differences. It does, however, also appear that amygdala damage in humans rarely produces the extreme loss of emotional reactivity seen in monkeys and that in order to observe a similar hypoemotional state in humans it may be necessary to suffer additional temporal cortical damage.

COGNITIVE ABILITIES

It must be remembered that as a large proportion of patients who have received amygdala surgery also suffered from epilepsy, a successful surgery may improve cognitive performance as a consequence of alleviating the epilepsy (Andersen, 1978; Luczywek and Mempel, 1980). In this way any direct effects of amygdala damage may be obscured.

Intelligence and Language

There is consistent agreement that amygdala damage does not affect overall measures of intelligence. This conclusion is based on informal statements (Balasubramaniam and Ramamurthi, 1970; Vaernet, 1972; Hitchcock and Cairns, 1973; Kiloh et al., 1974; Ramanchandran et al., 1974; Narabayashi, 1977; Luczywek and Mempel, 1980; Ramamurthi, 1988) and, more importantly, on comparisons between pre- and postoperative psychometric assessments (Heimburger and Whitlock, 1965; Small et al., 1977; Andersen, 1978; Jacobson, 1986). While many of the above cases received only partial amygdala lesions, the finding that bilateral removal of the amygdala in case H.M. did not affect his IQ scores (Corkin, 1984) helps confirm the view that amygdalectomy need not disrupt overall levels of intelligence.

Similarly, there is little evidence that even extensive bilateral lesions of the amygdala can produce obvious language difficulties. While studies on subjects with unilateral damage have suggested that damage to the left, but not the right, amygdala may impair word fluency and the Vocabulary subtest of the WAIS (Andersen, 1978), other studies of cases with bilateral damage have failed to find any deficit in speech and linguistic function (Jacobson, 1986; Tranel and Hyman, 1990).

Learning and Memory

Although it is reported that a small proportion of patients receiving amygdala surgeries display transient memory losses (Kim, 1971; Hitchcock et al., 1973; Small et al., 1977; Heimburger et al., 1978), it is also typically stated that amygdala lesions do not produce permanent disturbances of memory (Balasubramaniam and Ramamurthi, 1970; Narabayashi, 1972, 1977; Vaernet, 1972; Small et al., 1977; Luczywek and Mempel, 1980). Unfortunately it is also often the case that these reports are not accompanied by test data.

In one of the few studies looking specifically at the effects of amygdala lesions on memory, Andersen (1978) compared the pre- and postoperative performance of 15 epileptic patients who had received unilateral lesions involving approximately half of the amygdala. Testing took place on average 12 months after the surgery. She found that the surgeries had not altered forward or backward digit span nor had they impaired the learning and retention of word pairs, short stories, or the reproduction of a complex design (Andersen, 1978). Indeed, there was evidence that the subjects with right amygdala lesions showed a significant improvement in story recall. The only evidence of a significant postoperative impairment was in the right amygdalotomy subjects, who performed poorly on the immediate recognition of a series of pictures. A recognition test carried out on the same material an hour later indicated that the amygdala lesions had not, however, also increased the subsequent rate of forgetting of the material (Andersen, 1978). Comparisons with a large, normal sample indicated that the amygdalotomized patients performed relatively worse on the visual-spatial than on the verbal tests of memory (Andersen, 1978).

Studies on cases with bilateral amygdala damage indicate that there are no obvious changes in digit span (Jacobson, 1986; Lee et al., 1988b, 1991), digit supraspan learning (Tranel and Hyman, 1990; Lee et al., 1991), paired associate learning (Jurko and Andy, 1977; Jacobson, 1986), memory for prose passages (Jacobson, 1986), the learning of verbal material (Luczywek and Mempel, 1980), the recognition of printed words (Jacobson, 1986; Tranel and Hyman, 1990), and the learning and retention of the Rey Auditory-Verbal Learning Test (Tranel and Hyman, 1990). Similarly in tests using more nonverbal material subjects with bilateral amygdala damage have performed within preoperative or normal limits on the Benton Visual Retention Test (Jacobson, 1986), the Graham Kendall Memory for Designs Test (Hitchcock et al., 1973), on the learning of a complex set of geometric figures in a fixed sequence (Lee et al., 1991), and on motor learning (Tranel and Hyman, 1990). Furthermore, a patient who had received a bilateral uncotomy obtained the high overall score of 125 on the Wechsler Memory Scale (Scoville and Milner, 1957) and so had presumably performed normally on a range of memory tasks.

In contrast, Tranel and Hyman (1990) reported that a woman with bilateral amygdala damage as a result of Urbach-Wiethe disease was impaired on the Bead Memory subtest of the Stanford-Binet Scales (a test of immediate nonverbal memory), the Benton Visual Retention Test (a test of immediate visual memory), and on the recall of the Rey-Osterrieth Complex Figure. These deficits, which contrasted with her normal performance on tests of verbal material, were taken as evidence of an impairment in nonverbal, visuospatial memory. Some support for this notion comes from evidence of a retention deficit for geometric patterns in a woman with a bilateral amygdalotomy (Jacobson, 1986) and from the findings of Andersen (1978) on subjects with unilateral amygdalotomies.

It can be seen, therefore, that while even large, bilateral amygdala lesions fail to affect the learning or retention of verbal material, there is the possibility that amygdala damage may produce a subtle impairment in visuospatial memory (Tranel and Hyman, 1990). Additional support for this possibility comes from those studies that have used the Warrington Recognition Test on patients with bilateral amygdala damage. While performance on the word recognition test consistently remains unaffected, performance on the face recognition test is either defective (Jacobson, 1986; Lee et al., 1991; Broks, personal communication) or considerably poorer than that for words (Tranel and Hyman, 1990). In addition, there is the rather tantalising comment from Hitchcock and Cairns (1973) that some of their amygdalotomized cases showed a subtle deficit in face recognition.

A particular study was made of the face recognition deficit in a patient who, after bilateral amygdalotomy following an earlier subcaudate tractotomy, developed persistent difficulties in recognizing faces but not objects (Jacobson, 1986). This patient showed borderline deficits in the perceptual matching of faces and clear deficits in the recall of previously unfamiliar faces and in the recognition of familiar faces from after the operations (Jacobson, 1986). The patient was, however, able to recognize family members and distinguish different facial expres-- sions. This evidence for the involvement of the amygdala in some aspect of facial recognition is consistent with the discovery of units in the monkey amygdala that appear to respond selectively to faces (Rolls, 1984; see Chapter 5, Rolls, this volume). Whether this deficit is restricted to faces or whether it reflects a more general problem with visuospatial information remains, at present, an unanswered question.

The effects of amygdala damage on memory have aroused considerable interest, as it is well known that bilateral damage to the medial temporal lobes can produce a permanent, anterograde amnesia. While it is accepted that damage to the hippocampal formation is necessary for this amnesia, there is controversy over whether amygdala damage contributes to the severity of the memory loss. Experimental support for this view comes from the finding that while hippocampectomy or amygdalectomy may have relatively mild effects on a range of recognition memory tasks in monkeys, combined removal of these two structures has a much more disruptive effect (Mishkin, 1982; but see Chapter 17, Murray, this volume). As we have seen, there is a limited amount of evidence that amygdala damage in humans can produce mild deficits on some tests of visuospatial memory, deficits not dissimilar to those found in amygdalectomized monkeys (Mishkin, 1982; Tranel and Hyman, 1990). In addition, there are a number of clinical cases with combined amygdaloid and hippocampal damage that do display a very dense, anterograde amnesia (Aggleton, 1991). It has, however, been argued that the additive effect of amygdala damage upon hippocampal damage in monkeys is due to entorhinal and perirhinal involvement and is not a consequence of the amygdala damage itself (Zola-Morgan et al., 1989; see Chapter 17, Murray, this volume). It therefore remains possible that rhinal damage may have contributed to some of the clinical findings.

Lastly, it should be noted that tasks which tax the ability to form a rapid association between an arbitrary stimulus and a reward can be severely disrupted after amygdalectomy in monkeys (Aggleton and Mishkin, 1986; see Chapter 18, Gaffan, this volume). It is therefore surprising that there have been no attempts to examine this ability in patients with selective amygdala damage. One starting point might be to examine the ability to remember whether a particular face had been shown with a happy or sad expression, having first ensured that this was not confounded by a face recognition deficit.

Other Cognitive Functions

Two tests designed to look at attention were given both pre- and postoperatively to patients with unilateral amygdala lesions (Andersen, 1978). No systematic changes were seen in the number subtraction task but there was evidence of a significant decline in performance on a task in which the subjects had to draw a repeated pattern (Andersen, 1978). In this second task the subjects received no visual feedback and so they had to continuously monitor their progress. In contrast, a study on hyperactive children indicated that amygdala damage could increase attention span, as measured by time spent with toys, and decrease hyperactivity (Narabayashi, 1972).

Lastly, deficits in "executive control" were reported in a patient with bilateral amygdala damage as a consequence of Urbach-Wiethe disease (Tranel and Hyman, 1990). These deficits were observed in tests of category formation, cognitive flexibility, and abstract reasoning. It is not, however, known whether these findings are peculiar to this disease, and hence this subject, or whether they apply more generally to the effects of bilateral amygdala damage.

OVERVIEW

In spite of the shortage of systematic data and the limitations imposed by the nature of many of the subjects, it is evident that there are many important similarities between the effects of amygdala damage in man and other primates. It can be seen that amygdala damage does not directly affect sensory systems, with the possible exception of olfaction, nor does it typically affect motivational systems. While a small number of subjects do show changes in eating habits or sexual behavior, such cases make up a small minority and it is unclear what the special features are in these cases. There is also general agreement that damage to the amygdala does not affect IQ.

There is, however, preliminary evidence that while amygdala damage does not disrupt verbal memory, it may impair some aspects of visuospatial memory. Furthermore, these impairments may mirror some of the mild deficits found in amygdalectomized monkeys. But in the light of the present controversy over the contribution of damage to the entorhinal and perirhinal cortices to "amygdaloid" effects in monkeys (Chapter 17, Murray, this volume), this issue remains unresolved both in humans and nonhuman primates.

There is, however, much more agreement that damage to the amygdala is responsible for changes in emotion. As is the case in monkeys, it is not that humans with amygdala damage are unable to make appropriate responses, it is that the threshold for such responses is altered. While there is reason to believe that there are differences in the extent of the emotional changes that follow amygdala damage in man and other primates, there are no grounds to suggest that these effects are qualitatively different. It would appear, therefore, that detailed studies of the monkey amygdala will continue to help us determine how the functions of the human amygdala are realised.

REFERENCES

Aggleton JP (1991): Anatomy of memory. In Peterson RC, Yanagihara T (eds): "Memory Disorders. Research and Clinical Practice." New York: Marcel Dekker.

Aggleton JP, Mishkin M (1986): The amygdala: Sensory gateway to the emotions. In Plutchik R, Kellerman H (eds): "Biological Foundations of Emotion." New York: Academic Press, pp 281–300.

Aggleton JP, Passingham RE (1981): Syndrome produced by lesions of the amygdala in monkeys (*Macaca mulatta*). J Comp Physiol Psychol 95:961–977.

Aggleton JP, Passingham RE (1982): An assessment of the reinforcing properties of foods after amygdaloid lesions in rhesus monkeys. J Comp Physiol Psychol 96:71–77.

Adams JE, Rutkin BB (1969): Treatment of temporal-lobe epilepsy by stereotactic surgery. Confin Neurol 31:80–85.

Anand BK, Dua S, Chhina GS (1958): Higher nervous control over food intake. Ind J Med Res 46:277–287.

Andersen R (1978): Cognitive changes after amygdalotomy. Neuropsychologia 16:439–451.

Andy OJ, Jurko M (1975): The human amygdala: Excitability state and aggression. In Sweet WH, Obrador S, Martin-Rodriguez JG (eds): "Neurosurgical Treatment in Psychiatry, Pain, and Epilepsy." Baltimore: University Park Press, pp 417–427.

Andy OJ, Jurko MF, Hughes JR (1975): The amygdala in relation to olfaction. Confin Neurol 37:215–222.

Balasubramaniam V, Kanaka TS (1975): Amygdalotomy and hypothalamotomy—a comparative study. Confin Neuron 37:195–201.

Balasubramaniam V, Ramamurthi B (1970): Stereotaxic amygdalotomy in behavioral disorders. Confin Neurol 32:367–373.

Bagshaw MH, Benzies S (1968): Multiple measures of the orienting reaction and their dissociation after amygdalectomy in monkeys. Exp Neurol 20:175–187.

Bagshaw MH, Kimble DP, Pribram KH (1965): The GSR of monkeys during orienting and habituation and after ablation of the amygdala, hippocampus and inferotemporal cortex. Neuropsychologia 3:111–119.

Butter CM, Snyder DR (1972): Alterations in aversive and aggressive behaviors following orbital frontal lesions in rhesus monkeys. Acta Neurobiol 32:525–565.

Burzaco JA (1973): Fundus striae terminalis, an optional target in sedative stereotaxic surgery. In Latinen LV, Livingston KE (eds): "Surgical Approaches in Psychiatry." Baltimore: University Park Press, pp 135–137.

Cattell RB, Eber HW, Taksuoka M (1970): "Handbook for the Sixteen Personality Questionnaire." Champaign, IL: Institute for Personality and Ability Testing.

Chitonondh H (1966): Stereotaxic amygdalotomy in the treatment of olfactory seizures and psychiatric disorders with olfactory hallucinations. Confin Neurol 27:181–196.

Corkin S (1984): Lasting consequences of bilateral medial temporal lobectomy: Clinical course and experimental findings in H.M. Sem Neurol 4:249–259.

Downer JLdeC (1961): Changes in visual gnostic functions and emotional behavior following unilateral temporal pole damage in the split brain monkey. Nature 191:50–51.

Eichenbaum H, Morton TH, Potter H, Corkin S (1983): Selective olfactory deficits in case H.M. Brain 106:459–472.

Freeman W, Williams TM (1952): Human sonar: The amygdaloid nucleus in relation to auditory hallucinations. J Nerv Ment Dis 116:456–462.

Gascon GG, Gilles F (1973): Limbic dementia. J Neurol Neurosurg Psychiat 36:421–430.

Green JR, Duisberg REH, McGrath WB (1951): Focal epilepsy of the psychomotor type. J Neurosurg 8:157–172.

Heimburger RF (1975): Stereotaxic coordinates for amygdalotomy. Confin Neurol 37: 202–206.

Heimburger RF, Small IF, Small JG, Milstein V, Moore D (1978): Stereotaxic amygdalotomy for convulsive and behavioral disorders. Appl Neurophys 41:43–51.

Heimburger RF, Whitlock CC (1965): Steroid changes following stereotaxic destruction of the amygdaloid nucleus in the human. Excerpta Medica Int Cong 110:767–768.

Heimburger RF, Whitlock CC, Kalsbeck JE (1966): Stereotaxic amygdalectomy for epilepsy with aggressive behavior. J Am Med Soc 198:741–745.

Hitchcock ER, Ashcroft GW, Cairns VM, Murray LG (1973): Observations on the development of an assessment scheme for amygdalotomy. In Laitinen LV, Livingston KE (eds): "Surgical Approaches in Psychiatry." Baltimore: University Park Press, pp 142–155.

Hitchcock ER, Cairns V (1973): Amygdalotomy. Postgrad Med J 49:894–904.

Hood TW, Siegfried J, Wiesel HG (1983): The role of stereotactic amygdalotomy in the treatment of temporal lobe epilepsy associated with behavioral disorders. Appl Neurophysiol 46:19–25.

Jacobson R (1986): Disorders of facial recognition, social behaviour and affect after combined bilateral amygdalotomy and subcaudate tractotomy—a clinical and experimental study. Psych Med 16:439–450.

Jelasic F (1966): Relation of the lateral part of the amygdala to pain. Confin Neurol 27:53–55.

Jurko MF, Andy OJ (1977): Verbal learning dysfunction with combined centre medial and amygdala lesions. J Neurol Neurosurg Psychiat 40:695–698.

Kaada BR (1972): Stimulation and regional ablation of the amygdaloid complex with reference to functional representations. In Eleftheriou BE (ed): "The Neurobiology of the Amygdala." New York: Plenum Press, pp 205–281.

Kiloh LG, Gye RS, Rushworth RG, Bell DS, White RT (1974): Stereotactic amygdaloidotomy for aggressive behavior. J Neurol Neurosurg Psychiat 37:437–444.

Kim YK (1971): Effects of basolateral amygdalotomy. In Umbach W (ed): "Special Topics in Stereotaxis." Stuttgart: Hippokrates Verlag, pp 69–81.

Kim YK, Umbach W (1973): Combined stereotactic lesions for treatment of behaviour disorders and severe pain. In Laitinen LV, Livingston KE (eds): "Surgical Approaches in Psychiatry." Baltimore: University Park Press, pp 182–188.

Kling A (1968): Effects of amygdalectomy and testosterone on sexual behavior of male juvenile macaques. J Comp Physiol Psychol 65:466–471.

Kling A (1972): Effects of amygdalectomy on social—affective behavior in nonhuman primates. In Eleftheriou BE (ed): "The Neurobiology of the Amygdala." New York: Plenum Press, pp 511–536.

Kling A, Cornell R (1971): Amygdalectomy and social behavior in the caged stump-tailed macaque (*Macaca speciosa*). Folia Primat 14:190–208.

Kling A, Dunne K (1976): Social-environmental factors affecting behavior and plasma testosterone in normal and amygdala lesioned *Macaca speciosa*. Primates 17:23–42.

Kling A, Green PC (1967): Effects of neonatal amygdalectomy in the maternally reared and maternally deprived macaque. Nature 213:742–743.

Lee GP, Arena JG, Meador KJ, Smith JR, Loring DW, Flanigin HF (1988a): Changes in autonomic responsiveness following bilateral amygdalotomy in man. Neuropsychiat Neuropsych Behav Neurol 1:119–129.

Lee GP, Meador KJ, Smith JR, Loring DW, Flanigin HF (1988b): Preserved crossmodal association following bilateral amygdalotomy in man. Int J Neurosci 40:47–55.

Lee GP, Loring DW, Meador KJ, Smith JR, Flanigin HF (1991): Mnemonic effects of bilateral amygdalar lesions in man. J Clin Exp Neuropsych 13:21.

Lilly R, Cummings JL, Benson F, Frankel M (1983): The human Klüver-Bucy syndrome. Neurology 33:1141–1145.

Luczywek E, Mempel E (1976): Stereotactic amygdalotomy in the light of neuropsychological investigations. Acta Neurochir (Suppl) 23:221–223.

Luczywek E, Mempel E (1980): Memory and learning in epileptic patients treated by amygdalotomy and anterior hippocampotomy. Acta Neurochir (Suppl) 30:169–175.

Mark VH, Ervin FR (1970): "Violence and the Brain." New York: Harper & Row.

Mark VH, Sweet WH, Ervin FR (1972): The effects of amygdalotomy on violent behavior in patients with temporal lobe epilepsy. In Hitchcock E, Laitinen L, Vaernet K (eds): "Psychosurgery." Springfield, IL: Charles C. Thomas, pp 139–155.

Marlowe WB, Mancall EL, Thomas JJ (1975): Complete Klüver-Bucy syndrome in man. Cortex 11:53–59.

Mempel E (1971): The effect of partial amygdalectomy on emotional disturbances and epileptic seizures. Polish Med J 10:969–974.

Mempel E (1972): The influence of partial amygdalectomy on emotional disturbances and epileptic fits in humans. In Fusek I, Kunc Z (eds): "Present Limits in Psychosurgery." Prague: Avicenum, pp 497–500.

Mishkin M (1982): A memory system in the monkey. Phil Trans R Soc (Lond) B298:85–95.

Murray EA, Mishkin M (1985): Amygdalectomy impairs crossmodal association in monkeys. Science 228:604–606.

Nadvornik P, Pogady J, Sramka M (1973): The results of stereotactic treatment of aggressive syndrome. In Laitinen LV, Livingston KE (eds): "Surgical Approaches in Psychiatry." Baltimore: University Park Press, pp 125–128.

Narabayashi H (1972): Stereotaxic amygdalotomy. In Eleftheriou BE (ed): "The Neurobiology of the Amygdala." New York: Plenum Press, pp 459–483.

Narabayashi H (1977): Stereotaxic amygdalectomy for epileptic hyperactivity—long range results in children. In Blaw ME, Rapin I, Kinsbourne M (eds): "Topics in Child Neurology." New York: Spectrum Publications, pp 319–331.

Narabayashi H, Nagao T, Saito Y, Yoshida M, Naghata M (1963): Stereotaxic amygdalotomy for behavioral disorders. Arch Neurol 9:1–16.

Narabayashi H, Shima F (1973): Which is the bettter amygdala target, the medial or lateral nucleus for behavioral problems and paroxysms in epileptics. In Laitinen LV, Livingston KE (eds): "Surgical Approaches in Psychiatry." Baltimore: University Park Press, pp 129–134.

Narabayashi H, Uno M (1966): Long range results of stereotaxic amygdalotomy for behavior disorders. Confin Neurol 27:168–171.

Nebes RD (1971): Handedness and the perception of the part-whole relationship. Cortex 7:350–356.

Obrador S (1947): Temporal lobotomy. J Neuropath Exp Neurol 6:185–193.

Pool JL (1954): The visceral brain of man. J Neurosurg 11:45–63.

Ramamurthi B (1988): Stercotactic operation in behaviour disorders. Amygdalotomy and hypothalamotomy. Acta Neurochir (Suppl) 44:152–157.

Ramanchandran V, Balasubramaniam V, Kanaka TS (1974): Follow up of patients treated with stereotaxic amygdalotomy. Ind J Psychiat 6:299–306.

Roeder F, Muller D, Orthner H (1971): Stereotaxic treatment of psychosis and neuroses. In Umbach W (ed): "Special Topics in Stereotaxis." Stuttgart: Hippokrates Verlag, pp 82–105.

Rolls ET (1984): Neurons in the cortex of the temporal lobe and in the amygdala of the monkey with responses selective for faces. Hum Neurobiol 3:209–222.

Sawa M, Ueki Y, Arita M, Harada T (1954): Preliminary report on the amygdaloidectomy on the psychotic patients, with interpretation of oral-emotional manifestation in schizophrenics. Folia Psychiat Neurol Jap 7:309–329.

Schuckman H, Kling A, Orbach J (1969): Olfactory discrimination in monkeys with lesions in the amygdala. J Comp Physiol Psychol 67:212–215.

Schwartzbaum JS (1961): Some characteristics of amygdaloid hyperphagia in monkeys. Am J Psychol 74:252–259.

Schwartzbaum JS (1965): Discrimination behavior after amygdalectomy in monkeys: Visual and somesthetic learning and perceptual capacity. J Comp Physiol Psychol 60:314–319.

Scoville WB, Dunsmore RH, Liberson WT, Henry CE, Pepe E (1953): Observations on medial temporal lobotomy and uncotomy in the treatment of psychotic states. Assoc Res Nerv Ment Dis 31:347–369.

Scoville WB, Milner B (1957): Loss of recent memory after bilateral hippocampal lesions. J Neurol Neurosurg Psychiat 20:11–21.

Shaw C, Kentridge RW, Aggleton JP (1990): Cross-modal matching by amnesic subjects. Neuropsychologia 28:665–671.

Siegfried J, Ben-Shmuel A (1973): Long term assessment of stereotactic amygdalotomy for aggressive behavior. In Laitinen LV, Livingston KE (eds): "Surgical Approaches in Psychiatry." Baltimore: University Park Press, pp 138–141.

Siegfried J, Reichenbach W (1976): Personal experiences in the stereotaxic surgery of psychiatric patients. In Umbach W (ed): "Special Topics in Stereotaxis." Stuttgart: Hippokrates-Verlag, pp 106–111.

Small IF, Heimburger RF, Small JG, Milstein V, Moore DF (1977): Follow up of stereotaxic amygdalotomy for seizure and behavior disorders. Biol Psychiat 12:401–411.

Terzian H, Ore GD (1955): Syndrome of Klüver and Bucy reproduced in man by bilateral removal of temporal lobes. Neurology 5:373–380.

Thompson CI, Schwartzbaum JS, Harlow HF (1969): Development of social fear after amygdalectomy in infant rhesus monkeys. Physiol Behav 4:249–254.

Tranel D, Damasio H (1989): Intact electrodermal skin conductance responses after bilateral amygdala damage. Neuropsychologia 27:381–390.

Tranel D, Hyman BT (1990): Neuropsychological correlates of bilateral amygdala damage. Arch Neurol 47:349–355.

Turner BH, Gupta KC, Mishkin M (1978): The locus and cytoarchitecture of the projection areas of the olfactory bulb in *Macaca mulatta*. J Comp Neurol 177:381–396.

Turner EA (1954): Cerebral control of respiration. Brain 77:448–486.

Ursin H, Rosvold HE, Vest B (1969): Food preference in brain lesioned monkeys. Physiol Behav 4:609–612.

Vaernet K (1972): Stereotaxic amygdalotomy in temporal lobe epilepsy. Confin Neurol 34:176–180.

Vaernet K, Madsen A (1970): Stereotaxic amygdalotomy and basofrontal tractotomy in psychotics with aggressive behavior. J Neurol Neurosurg Psychiat 33:858–863.

Valenstein ES (1973): "Brain Control." New York: John Wiley.

Valenstein ES (1980): Review of the literature on postoperative evaluation. In Valenstein ES (ed): "The Psychosurgery Debate." San Francisco: W.H. Freeman, pp 141–163.

Walker AE, Thomson AF, McQueen JD (1953): Behavior and the temporal rhinencephalon in the monkey. Johns Hopkins Hosp Bull 93:65–93.

Weiskrantz L (1956): Behavioral changes associated with ablations of the amygdaloid complex in monkeys. J Comp Physiol Psychol 49:381–391.

Williams JM (1953): The amygdaloid nucleus. Confin Neurol 13:202–221.

Zola-Morgan S, Squire LR, Amaral DG (1989): Lesions of the amygdala that spare adjacent cortical regions do not impair memory or exacerbate the impairment following lesions of the hippocampal formation. J Neurosci 9:1922–1936.

The Amygdala: Neurobiological Aspects of Emotion,
Memory, and Mental Dysfunction, pages 505–538
© 1992 Wiley-Liss, Inc.

20
Role of the Amygdala in Temporal Lobe Epilepsy

P. GLOOR
*Montreal Neurological Institute and Department of Neurology and
Neurosurgery, McGill University, Montreal, Quebec, Canada*

INTRODUCTION

Among epileptic seizure disorders, those of temporal lobe origin are the most common (Penfield, 1954; Gastaut et al., 1975; Engel, 1989). It has been known for a long time that the mesial structures of the temporal lobe which include the amygdala and the hippocampus play an important role in the pathogenesis of these seizures (Earle et al., 1953; Penfield, 1954; Penfield and Jasper, 1954; Cavanagh and Meyer, 1956; Gastaut et al., 1958; Falconer et al., 1964; Bancaud et al., 1956; Margerison and Corsellis, 1966; Wieser, 1983; Engel, 1989). This chapter reviews the role played by the amygdala in the pathogenesis and the symptomatology of temporal lobe epilepsy.

The specific involvement of the amygdala in seizures of temporal lobe origin was put into the limelight for the first time in 1954 by Feindel and Penfield's observations that sitmulation in the amygdaloid region in awake, locally anesthetized epileptic patients undergoing surgery for relief of their seizures could reproduce features of epileptic automatism. Subsequent experience suggests, however, that the amygdala is only one among several temporal lobe structures that are involved in temporal lobe automatism (Bancaud et al., 1966; Wieser, 1983).

Neurosurgeons who carry out temporal lobectomies for the relief of temporal lobe seizures often find the amygdala to be small, shriveled, and of increased consistency. It thus appears to be part of a common area of induration of brain tissue found during such procedures. This sclerotic lesion frequently includes, besides the amygdala, the hippocampus, the parahippocampal gyrus, the temporal pole, and the anterior portion of the first temporal convolution (Earle et al., 1953; Penfield, 1954; Penfield and Jasper, 1954). These findings are still only insufficiently clarified in precise neuropathological terms, particularly as far as the amygdala is concerned.

Studies on temporal lobe epilepsy have provided evidence that the amygdala is involved in many of the common symptoms and signs that occur in the course of temporal lobe seizures. This evidence rests on observations made during the EEG recording of seizures with stereotaxically implanted intracerebral electrodes, and on the reproduction of signs and symptoms of temporal lobe seizures through localized stimulation of the amygdala during stereotaxic explorations of the brain or acutely during temporal lobe surgery (Feindel and Penfield, 1954; Bancaud et al., 1966; Weingarten et al., 1976; Halgren et al., 1978; Gloor et al., 1982; Wieser, 1983). The observations made during these procedures support the notion that the amygdala is a key player in temporal lobe seizures. When carefully analysed, observations of this kind can also throw light on the normal functions of the temporal lobe, particularly those of the amygdala.

The involvement of the amygdala in temporal lobe epilepsy is therefore reviewed in this chapter from two vantage points: (1) that of amygdala pathology, both structural and functional, as a pathogenetic factor in temporal lobe epilepsy, and (2) that of the contribution of the amygdala to the symptomatology of temporal lobe seizures and to normal brain function.

AMYGDALA PATHOLOGY IN TEMPORAL LOBE EPILEPSY

Ever since neuropathologists have studied pathological changes encountered in patients suffering from epilepsy, particularly temporal lobe epilepsy, the amygdala has been treated like the proverbial poor cousin in relation to the hippocampus. This neglect derives from the fact that the hippocampus, in view of the striking orderly geometric organization of its structure and connections, is a much more tempting and rewarding target for anyone wishing to make precise observations relating pathological changes to well-defined morphological features. By contrast, the anatomical organization of the amygdala appears to be less orderly and less intelligible and thus remains to a large extent terra incognita. This relative neglect, from which the study of the neuropathology of the amygdala in temporal lobe epilepsy has suffered, has become accentuated in recent years because the increasing number of temporal lobectomies performed for the treatment of complex partial seizures has yielded a rich harvest of hippocampi resected more or less en bloc, while for technical reasons comparable samples of amygdala have not become available because it cannot safely be removed en bloc. Even when reasonably sized chunks of amygdaloid tissue are given to the neuropathologist to examine, it is often difficult to identify specific subnuclei in such specimens and to get a proper fix on the orientation of the sections. Also, much less precise anatomical background information is available on the amygdala than on the hippocampus, in the light of which questions could be addressed that are now commonly being asked about hippocampal pathology in temporal lobe epilepsy. Questions such as those for instance regarding the relationship of the cytoarchitectonic profile of neuronal vulnerability to that of the density of NMDA receptors and of the distribution of calcium-binding proteins, the vulnerability of some peptide-containing neurons, and the sprouting of new collateral pathways in response to seizure activity. In the hippocampus these questions have now been addressed successfully and with great precision in experimental as well as in human material (for reviews see Ben-Ari and Represa, 1990; Gloor, in press). It has been shown that in the hippocampus of temporal lobe epileptics, the distribution of the lesions exhibits an orderly pattern which reflects the underlying chemoarchitectonic organization of this structure, an example and vindication of the often forgotten pathoclisis concept enunciated early in this century by the Vogts (Vogt, 1925; Vogt and Vogt, 1937). This success story, however, has its risks. It has already led to the premature assumption that hippocampal sclerosis is the most important pathogenetic factor in temporal lobe epilepsy (Babb and Brown, 1987), an assumption that ignores some important issues. The first is that the classical topographical profile of the lesions in hippocampal sclerosis is most likely a consequence of prolonged seizures or status epilepticus, particularly when occurring in early childhood, and can therefore be regarded as a lesion induced by seizures rather than as a causative agent of an enduring seizure problem. Admittedly, this damage in its turn may contribute to epileptogenicity (for review, see Gloor, in press). Furthermore, the classical distribution of lesions in the hippocampus in mesial temporal sclerosis is a nonspecific feature. It can result from anoxia, ischemia, and hypoglycemia, and even other pathological conditions, all of which are not known to be common causes of temporal epilepsy (Spielmeyer, 1925; Vogt and Vogt, 1937), except perhaps when these factors act in early childhood (see Gloor, in press). Finally, other changes such as the sprouting of collateral pathways and changes in opiate peptides are known consequences of seizures (for review see Ben-Ari and Represa, 1990; Gloor, in press) and whether they could in turn be pathogenetic in epilepsy is still an open question.

The study of the functional pathology of temporal lobe epilepsy as analyzed in recordings through stereotaxically implanted electrodes has also put the emphasis on the hippocampus. Such recordings taken from the mesial temporal region, however, have a built-in bias in favor of the hippocampus, especially when taken with closely spaced electrode pairs that are not part of a long bipolar chain reaching beyond the confines of the mesial structures. Because the hippocampus is an eminently laminated cortical structure, it creates powerful open electrical fields that can be detected by volume conduction at some distance. The amygdala is not organized like cortex and its neurons, even though some are pyramidal-like, are not arranged in "polarized" layers as are those of the hippocampus or other forms of cortex. Electrical fields created by discharging amygdala neurons are therefore most likely closed or at least partially closed, with negligible volume conduction outside the structure itself. Unless recordings are taken with a referential technique, or with a bipolar technique in which only one of the electrodes of a pair is in the amygdala, such electrical fields may be missed for biophysical reasons (Gloor, 1987). This may lead one to overestimate seizure onsets in the hippocampus as opposed to those in the amygdala. Several studies have in fact suggested that focal onsets of seizure discharges are more common in the hippocampus than in the amygdala (Engel and Cahan, 1986; Quesney, 1986; So et al., 1989). However, the most common pattern of seizure onset is regional, involving both the hippocampus and amygdala simultaneously (Quesney, 1986; So et al., 1989).

We must therefore recognize that several factors may cause the importance of the amygdala as a crucial structure in the pathogenetic mechanisms of temporal lobe seizures to be underestimated. There are some indicators that could

be used to support the argument that the amygdala may perhaps be more important than the hippocampus in the pathogenesis of temporal lobe seizures. One of
these indicators is the observation that of all brain sites, the amygdala kindles
(see Chapter 21, Cain, this volume) much faster than any of the others, certainly
significantly faster than the hippocampus (Racine et al., 1986). The second indicator is the observation by Feindel and Rasmussen (1990) and Rasmussen and
Feindel (1990) that the incidence of a favorable clinical outcome of temporal
lobectomy in their hands was as high in patients in whom the amygdala had been
removed and the hippocampus spared (mostly out of concern for potentially
adverse effect on memory) than in patients in whom the uncal portion and
about half of the body of the hippocampus had been removed together with the
amygdala. Thus, in many patients, removal of the hippocampus seemed to add
little benefit to the removal of the mesial structures of the temporal lobe. The
extent of amygdala removal in the Feindel and Rasmussen (1990) series was
deliberately as radical as possible. These observations suggest that in many
patients the amygdala may play a more important role in the pathogenesis of
temporal lobe seizures than the hippocampus. With the new MRI techniques it
should now be possible to compare the surgical outcomes in a group of patients
in which amygdala removals were as complete as possible with those in another
where a significant amount of amygdala tissue has been spared. The region most
commonly spared is the dorsomedial portion of the amygdala, where no obvious
plane of cleavage exists to separate it from adjacent tissue.

Having stated the case that one should be open-minded about the possibility that amygdaloid pathology, both structural and functional, could be as important in the causation of temporal lobe seizure as the hippocampus, let us see
how much is actually known concerning this pathology. Several authors have
described cell loss, gliosis, and other changes (Sano and Malamud, 1953;
Cavanagh and Meyer, 1956; Falconer et al., 1964; Margerison and Corsellis, 1966;
Ounsted et al., 1966; Bruton, 1988). However, no specific patterns suggestive of
an amygdaloid pathoclisis in epilepsy, as is the case for the hippocampus, has so
far emerged. As mentioned before, this is most likely due to the difficulties
encountered in the amygdala to perform the precise neuropathological studies
that would be required for such an analysis. However, it is quite evident from
the neuropathological studies that have been done that, in the majority of specimens in which hippocampal sclerosis was present and the amygdala was available for histological study, significant pathology was also present in the amygdala.
Of the cases showing the characteristic hippocampal sclerosis, 50 to 76%, depending on the series studied, showed neuronal loss in the amygdala. Additional
cases showed amygdaloid gliosis without any obvious cell loss. Neuronal loss
was, however, somewhat less common in the amygdala than in the hippocampus. In Cavanagh and Meyer's (1956) series, amygdala cell loss was usually focal
and involved "the basal group." It should also be added that mesial temporal
sclerosis, the most common pathological substrate of temporal lobe epilepsy,
most often is not confined to the hippocampus and amygdala, but also involves
the parahippocampal gyrus and even temporal isocortex. Cavanagh and Meyer
(1956), furthermore, found that in patients with surgically treated temporal lobe
epilepsy caused by tumors, vascular, and other circumscribed lesions, amygda-

loid pathology was more severe and more common than hippocampal pathology. In these cases amygdala lesions were always present when amygdala tissue was available for analysis, while the incidence of hippocampal pathology was only slightly more than 50%. When temporal lobe epilepsy is caused by alien tissue lesions, such as hamartomas, these lesions are most often localized in the amygdala rather than elsewhere in the temporal lobe and sometimes the hippocampus shows no lesion in these cases (Falconer et al., 1964; Bruton, 1988).

A review of these neuropathological studies demonstrates that many questions regarding the relationship between structural pathology and functional pathological changes revealed by the occurrence of epileptiform discharge in these structures remain unclarified. Both hippocampal and amygdaloid pathology undoubtedly play an important pathogenetic role in temporal lobe epilepsy, but how structural pathology leads to epileptogenic hyperexcitability remains unclear. A comparison of the distribution of structural pathology with that of epileptogenic electrophysiological dysfunction characterizing seizure onset supports the notion that regional pathology, both structural and functional, involving the mesial temporal structures is the outstanding feature of temporal lobe epilepsy. This pathology involves the amygdala, the hippocampus, and the parahippocampal gyrus, but it is presently impossible to identify within this region one structure that more than any other plays a crucial role in causing seizures. Structural reorganization, anatomical and functional plasticity of the type revealed in recent studies on the hippocampus, probably involves more than this structure and may implicate other components of the mesial temporal lobe as well, among them the amygdala. This may lead to a destabilization of the region's electrophysiological homeostasis, thus rendering it susceptible to seizures.

Metabolic pathologies of the amygdala revealed by positron-emission tomography have only been studied incompletely. In deoxyglucose studies the amygdala appears to be part of the region of hypometabolism so frequently encountered in patients with temporal lobe epilepsy, but there seems to be nothing distinctive about the amygdala in this regard (Engel et al., 1982; Henry et al., 1990).

SYMPTOMATOLOGY OF TEMPORAL LOBE SEIZURES ATTRIBUTABLE TO AMYGDALA INVOLVEMENT: ANATOMICAL AND FUNCTIONAL CORRELATIONS
Anatomical and Physiological Background

The stage for understanding the role of the amygdala in the symptomatology of temporal lobe seizures may be set by considering its anatomical relations to other brain structures. The amygdala is situated at a crossroad of important streams of information flow, to and from the cerebral cortex on one hand, and to and from subcortical structures, particularly those involved in the control of autonomic and endocrine functions. (For a recent review of amygdaloid connections, see DeOlmos, 1990; Chapter 1, Amaral et al., this volume.) In primates, the amygdala receives massive inputs from temporal, frontal, insular, and cingulate association cortex (Whitlock and Nauta, 1956; Pandya et al., 1973; Herzog and van Hoesen, 1976; Aggleton et al., 1980; Mufson et al., 1981; van Hoesen, 1981; Iwai and Yukie, 1987; Turner, 1981; Turner et al., 1988) and returns even more widespread projections to these cortical areas, including even the peristriate and primary visual cortex (Nauta, 1961; Mufson et al., 1981; Tigges et al., 1982, 1983; Amaral and Price, 1984; Amaral, 1986; Iwai and Yukie, 1987). The amygdala is likewise reciprocally interconnected with the hippocampus, partly through the intermediary of the entorhinal cortex (Aggleton, 1986; Amaral, 1986; Insausti et al., 1987; Saunders and Rosene, 1988; Saunders et al., 1988). In nonprimate mammals there is profuse input from the olfactory and accessory olfactory system which extends to deep amygdaloid nuclei (Scalia and Winans, 1975; Ottersen, 1982; Russchen, 1982) that is very much reduced in primates (Turner et al., 1978; van Hoesen, 1981).

In addition, there are unidirectional descending connections of the amygdala to the mediodorsal nucleus of the thalamus, which establish an alternative, indirect route of projection to frontal cortex (Nauta, 1961; Porrino et al., 1981; Aggleton and Mishkin, 1984; Russchen et al., 1987). The cortical projections of the primate amygdala, particularly those to association cortex, are much more extensive than those in nonprimate mammals (Price, 1981). The bidirectional connectivity of the amygdala to association cortex and hippocampus opens up interesting possibilities of interaction which are important for higher cognitive processes, of which fragments are often evoked in the course of temporal lobe seizures, as discussed later.

The subcortical connections of the amygdala are also to a large extent bidirectional. It receives afferents from the hypothalamus and lower brain stem nuclei concerned with viscerosensory and gustatory functions (Aggleton et al., 1980; Mehler, 1980; Norita and Kawamura, 1980; Amaral and Veazey, 1982; Veazey et al., 1982; Kapp et al., 1989) and from the auditory system (LeDoux et al., 1985, 1990a,b). Efferent amygdala projections to subcortical structures are directed toward the mediodorsal thalamic nucleus (see above), the preoptic area, and the hypothalamus (Gloor, 1955; Nauta, 1961; Dreifuss et al., 1968; DeOlmos, 1972; Krettek and Price, 1978; Price and Amaral, 1981; De Vito, 1982; DeOlmos et al., 1985; Price, 1986), particularly the region of the ventromedial nucleus of the hypothalamus (Gloor, 1955; Dreifuss et al., 1968; Price, 1986), to the nucleus accumbens of the ventral striatum (Kelley et al., 1982; Russchen and Price, 1984; Russchen et al., 1985b; Aggleton et al., 1987), the magnocellular basal forebrain nuclei (Russchen et al., 1985b; Aggleton et al., 1987), and to the lower brain stem, particularly the vagal complex and neurons controlling masticatory movements (Gloor, 1955; Krettek and Price, 1978; Price and Amaral, 1981; Hopkins et al., 1981; Takeuchi et al., 1988a,b). The pattern of connections of the human amygdala appears to be similar to that seen in other primates (Klingler and Gloor, 1960).

There finally remains the question of whether the amygdala has access to the motor system. There are no direct projections to the motor cortex and any behavioral response initiated by amygdala activity that needs to be played out through the motor cortex has to gain access to this part of the motor system indirectly, most likely through the intermediary of several links in the frontal cortex (for references, see above). Another route to the motor system is provided by connections to the striatal grey matter of the nucleus accumbens in the ventral striatum (for references, see above). An interesting connection to a specialized portion of the motor system is that to the masticatory centers in the brain stem (Takeuchi et al., 1988a,b), which may be involved in the masticatory movements so frequently seen in the automatism of temporal lobe seizures.

Physiological and behavioral studies in animals indicate that the amygdala is involved in a variety of behavioral mechanisms such as avoidance, sexual behavior, feeding, and social behavior. Many of the autonomic and neuroendocrine responses mediated by the amygdala must be regarded as integral components of these elaborate behaviors (for reviews and references see Gloor, 1960, 1972, 1975b; Goddard, 1964; the volumes edited by Eleftheriou, 1972, and Ben-Ari, 1981; Spyer, 1989; and chapters in the present volume). In spite of its influence on autonomic and endocrine mechanisms, the amygdala should not be regarded as a structure concerned with the basic homeostatic regulation of autonomic and neuroendocrine controls, functions which are integrated in the hypothalamus and lower brain stem. Nevertheless, the amygdala through its connections to the hypothalamus and lower brain stem can play on this autonomic-neuroendocrine keyboard in response to inputs, which in nonprimates are predominantly olfactory and accessory olfactory (vomeronasal) (for references, see above) and in primates increasingly depend upon information channeled into the amygdala from a vast expanse of association cortex (for references, see above).

Contribution of the Amygdala to the Symptomatology of Temporal Lobe Seizures: General Principles

Before discussing in detail what contribution the amygdala makes to the symptomatology of temporal lobe seizures, one point must be emphasized: None of the symptoms and signs that characterize these seizures can be exclusively attributed to the involvement of the amygdala, or, for that matter, to any other constituent of the mesial temporal region or even the temporal isocortex (Gloor et al., 1982; Wieser, 1983; Spiers et al., 1985). It may be argued that this is so because seizure discharge rapidly spreads within the temporal lobe, the symptomatology of the seizure thus reflecting this rapid spread to diverse structures which subserve different functions (Bancaud, 1987). Although this explanation is undoubtedly valid, particularly for the noninitial manifestations of the seizure discharge, it nevertheless appears incomplete, for it cannot be reconciled with some of the data obtained by localized electrical stimulation of various temporal lobe structures. Thus, even when such localized stimulations fail to induce a spreading seizure discharge, as evidenced by the lack of an afterdischarge or by the evocation of one that remains confined to the stimulated structure, none of the responses evoked by such stimulations, which are identical with phenomena that occur in the course of seizures, exhibit an exclusive and consistent localization to a particular structure of the temporal lobe, even though they may be elicited preferentially from one structure, most commonly the amygdala (Bancaud et al., 1966; Gloor et al., 1981; 1982; study in preparation). Tentatively, this puzzling fact may be explained by the hypothesis that each of these responses reflects the seizure- or stimulation-induced activation of a specific widely distributed neuronal matrix and its connections, which includes limbic and isocortical components of the temporal lobe and possibly even some extratemporal structures (Gloor, in press, a). This hypothesis is discussed in more detail later in this chapter when the mechanism underlying the anatomical representation of experiential phenomena is considered.

Autonomic (Including Respiratory) and Viscerosensory Phenomena of Temporal Lobe Seizures

Viscerosensory or autonomic, including respiratory, mechanisms are often activated by temporal lobe seizure discharge (Penfield and Jasper, 1954; Feindel, 1974; Daly, 1975; Wieser, 1983; Spiers et al., 1985; Bancaud, 1987). Among the viscerosensory phenomena, the most common is a rising epigastric or chest sensation; others are nausea, palpitation, a feeling of warmth or cold, or even shivering. Some of these effects have been reproduced by amygdaloid stimulation in awake patients during stereotaxic exploration or neurosurgical procedures. None of them are, however, exclusively reproduced by amygdaloid stimulation, although the amygdala seems to be the most common site from which they are evoked (Penfield and Jasper, 1954; Jasper and Rasmussen, 1958; Bancaud et al., 1966; Halgren et al., 1978; Wieser, 1983; study in preparation).

Autonomic and respiratory changes that may occur in temporal lobe seizures are mydriasis, flushing or pallor (usually of the face), lacrimation, an increase in heart rate (that may be associated with the subjective feeling of palpitation), changes in the depth and frequency of respiration including temporary apnea, salivation, belching, borborygmi, passing of flatus, horripilation with goosepimples, sweating, urge to void or involuntary micturition, rarely defecation or diarrhea, and in some women vulvovaginal secretions, but only when associated with erotic psychosexual experiences (Penfield and Jasper, 1954; Daly, 1958a, 1975; van Buren, 1958; van Buren and Ajmone Marsan, 1960; Bancaud et al., 1970; Wieser, 1983; Rémillard et al., 1983; Spiers et al., 1985; Bancaud, 1987). A number of these autonomic and respiratory effects have been reproduced in humans by stimulation of the amygdala or adjacent areas (Kaada, 1951; Kaada and Jasper, 1952; Chapman et al., 1954; van Buren, 1958; Chapman, 1960; Bancaud et al., 1966; Wieser, 1983; study in preparation). These phenomena do not occur in all patients in whom the amygdala discharges during a seizure, nor are they elicited with all stimulations applied to that structure. Some of these viscerosensory and autonomic responses occur in isolation in the course of a temporal lobe seizure, while others are part of a more complex response, commonly within an appropriate behavioral, usually affective, context (Daly, 1958a). For instance, mydriasis, epigastric discomfort, palpitation, and pallor may occur together with a feeling of fear or the evocation of a fearful memory, or vulvovaginal secretion may occur in the context of ictal libidinous feelings. In one study, approximately 50% of the patients reporting fear also experienced a visceral sensation referred to the abdomen or chest (Gloor et al., 1982).

Experiential Phenomena and Related Behavioral Phenomena in Temporal Lobe Seizures

In some (but not the majority of) patients suffering from temporal lobe epilepsy, seizures are ushered in by a hallucinatory or illusionary experience occurring out of any appropriate context and having subjective qualities similar to those experienced in everyday life. This "experiential" quality is often very vivid. First studied by Hughlings Jackson in the last century (Jackson, 1879 [1958b], 1888; Jackson and Beavor, 1889; Jackson and Stewart, 1899), such experiential phenomena have attracted the attention of a number of investigators in the present century (Penfield and Jasper, 1954; Penfield, 1955a,b; Mullan and Penfield, 1959; Penfield and Perot, 1963; Daly, 1975; Weingarten et al., 1976; Wieser, 1979, 1983; Gloor et al., 1982; Gloor, 1986b, 1990, 1991; Bancaud, 1987). These experiences are embedded in the patient's feeling of personal identity in contrast to elementary sensory hallucinations elicited by discharge or electrical stimulation in primary sensory areas, as for instance paresthesiae or phosphenes, which strike him as alien. Experiential phenomena as seizure manifestations are virtually confined to temporal lobe epilepsy. They can be affective, perceptual, or mnemonic, or a combination of two or of all three of these. When occurring in such a combination the similarity with a real-life experience is particularly striking. They nevertheless differ from it by their fragmentary character and their lack of forward motion in time (Gloor et al., 1982; Gloor, 1990). The patient never mistakes them for being real. Subdividing experiential phenomena into affective, mnemonic, and perceptual phenomena is somewhat artificial, yet didactically useful. They are thus discussed here under these separate headings.

Affective Changes

The most common affect produced by temporal lobe epileptic discharge is fear (Macrae, 1954; Penfield and Jasper, 1954; Williams, 1956; Daley, 1958a, 1975; Gibbs, 1956; Mullan and Penfield, 1959; Weil, 1959; Gloor and Feindel, 1963; Gloor, 1972, 1990, 1991; Feindel, 1974; Gloor et al., 1982; Strauss et al., 1982; Wieser, 1983; Spiers et al., 1985; Taylor and Lochery, 1987). It arises "out of the blue." Ictal fear may range from mild anxiety to intense terror. It is frequently, but not invariably, associated with a rising epigastric sensation, palpitation, mydriasis, and pallor and may be associated with a fearful hallucination, a frightful memory flashback, or both. Fear can be reproduced in many patients by stimulation of the amygdala or its immediate vicinity (Penfield and Jasper, 1954; Jasper and Rasmussen, 1958; Mullan and Penfield, 1959; Bancaud et al., 1966; Gloor, 1972; Halgren et al., 1978; Gloor et al., 1981, 1982, study in preparation). Hippocampal or isocortical stimulation reproduces fear less often. Sometimes fear occurs only once seizure discharge arising elsewhere spreads to involve the amygdala (Gloor, 1972). The activation of a mechanism of fear in temporal lobe epilepsy is probably much more common than the incidence of subjective reports of this emotion indicates. This is suggested by the observation that some patients who do not report fear show at the beginning of an attack a facial expression or a change in voice suggestive of fear, or they may utter a cry equally suggestive of fear, or they may run away or behave in a defensive or fearful manner (Strauss et al., 1983; Spiers et al., 1985; study in preparation; unpublished personal observations). The lack of a subjective report of fear may in some instances at least result from anterograde amnesia occurring early in the seizure which prevents the subsequent recall of the emotion. Such changes in facial expression or vocalization suggesting fear are sometimes elicited by amygdaloid stimulation (Bancaud et al., 1966, study in preparation).

Animal experiments have shown that stimulation of the amygdala may elicit defensive or fearful behavior (Gastaut, 1952; MacLean and Delgado, 1953; Kaada et al., 1954; DeMolina and Hunsperger, 1959; Hilton and Zbrozyna, 1963; Kaada, 1972; Zbrozyna, 1972). The central nucleus of the amygdala has recently become the focus of interest in studies of fear-conditioning, suggesting that this structure in the rat at least is essential for such conditioning and for some of the autonomic effects of fear-induced stress such as stress ulcers of the gastric mucosa (Henke, 1980, Chapter 11, this volume; Kapp et al., 1981; Iwata et al., 1986; Hitchcock et al., 1989; Spyer, 1989). In order to induce a conditioned fear response the central nucleus seems to depend upon impulses relayed from the lateral amygdaloid nucleus, the latter acting as a "sensory interface" (LeDoux et al., 1990a,b). Although these recent studies in rats have provided solid neurophysiological, behavioral, and anatomical support for an important role of the central amygdala nucleus in mediating fear, other studies in a different species, the cat, have indicated that a defensive response of the kind that occurs under natural conditions when the animal faces a threat is mediated by the basal nucleus, particularly its magnocellular division (Hilton and Zbrozyna, 1963; Zbrozyna, 1972; Bonvallet and Gary Bobo, 1973). Assessment of the role of the central nucleus of the amygdala in mediating fear is further complicated by the fact that this nucleus has also been reported to be involved in rewarding experiences (Wurtz and Olds, 1963; Kesner et al., 1989; Gallagher et al., 1990). The problem of the anatomical organization of amygdaloid neurons mediating fearful behavior and its concomitants is thus still incompletely understood. To reconcile these differences, the suggestion has been made that the central nucleus is involved in the conditioned attention to meaningful events regardless of the rewarding or aversive nature of the unconditioned stimulus (Gallagher et al., 1990).

Fear is a negative, nonrewarding emotion and one may wonder whether temporal lobe seizure discharge or amygdala stimulation can elicit other kinds of negative emotions. This is indeed the case and patients at the beginning of seizures have reported such emotions as anger, disgust, guilt, depression, sadness, or loneliness (Penfield and Jasper, 1954; Weil, 1955, 1959; Williams, 1956; Daly, 1958a, 1975; Mullan and Penfield, 1959; Gloor and Feindel, 1963; Wieser, 1979; Gloor et al., 1982; Spiers et al., 1985; Gloor, 1991). Sometime the elicitation of such negative emotional states is suggested by an appropriate change in facial expression (Strauss et al., 1983) or voice, or by the utterance of expletives even though the patient may not report such an emotion, possibly because of ictal amnesia. Subjective and objective responses of this kind have sometimes been produced by amygdaloid stimulation (Gloor et al., 1981, 1982; Wieser, 1983; study in preparation), but again, not only stimulation of the amygdala can elicit these responses, as they have at times also been evoked from other parts of the temporoinsular region (Mullan and Penfield, 1959). Negative emotional states other than fear are, however, rarely elicited by temporal lobe seizures or amygdala or other temporal lobe stimulation. This is also true for anger and even moreso for directed aggressive behavior. An angry mood and its expression by appropriate vocalization or cursing is sometimes, but only rarely, elicited under such circumstances (Saint-Hilaire et al., 1980; study in preparation; unpublished personal observations). There is no convincing report in the literature suggesting that temporal lobe seizure discharge ever induced a well-directed and coordinated aggressive act against another human being, with the possible exception of one case reported by Saint-Hilaire et al. (1980). In this case the patient in the course of a temporal lobe seizure lashed out at the psychologist who was testing her. The other reported examples of ictal "aggression" and "violence" consist of an aimless running around, with kicking and destruction of objects (Ashford et al., 1980; Treiman and Delgado-Escueta, 1981). A similar episode of senseless "aggression" was elicited by Mark et al. (1972) with electrical stimulation of the amygdala in an epileptic patient having a history of violent, potentially homicidal, but unmotivated attacks which, however, to judge from the information reported, seemed to represent interictal episodes rather than true seizures. Nevertheless, the violent episode elicited by amygdaloid stimulation in this case was associated with stimulation-induced seizure discharge. This observation, however, appears to be unique. Nevertheless, the belief is common that temporal lobe epileptics are aggressive. It seems to be based on a misinterpretation of the reactive defensive behavior that patients may exhibit, rarely during the ictal and quite commonly during the postictal confusional state when well-meaning people interfere with the patient's freedom of action (Gloor, 1975a, 1991; Treiman, 1986).

Positive emotions are only rarely elicited by temporal lobe seizure discharge. They may consist of a feeling of happiness or exhilaration, mirth with laughter, or of erotic excitement (Williams, 1956; Daly, 1958a, 1975; Van Reeth, 1959; Gloor and Feindel, 1963; Bancaud et al., 1970; Stoffels et al., 1980; Rémillard et al., 1983; Spiers et al., 1985; Gloor, 1991). For reasons that are not readily apparent, true psychosexual responses, i.e., experiences with an appropriate libidinous content, have only been reported to occur in women (Remillard et al., 1983), with the possible exception of a single case in a male (Jacome et al., 1980).

As with the negative affective states, positive ones may sometimes be inferred from the patient's behavior even though he may at the end of the attack not recall having had any such experience. Such inferences may be drawn from the observation that the patient smiles, laughs, or hums a tune with a smiling facial expression or chuckles mirthfully in the course of a seizure (Gloor, 1986a; Strauss et al., 1983; study in preparation; personal unpublished observations). Animal experiments support the notion that the amygdala is involved in mechanisms of reward (Olds, 1956; Wurtz and Olds, 1963; Spiegler and Mishkin, 1981; Cador et al., 1989; Everitt et al., 1989; Kesner et al., 1989; Gallagher et al., 1990).

The special case of sexual emotions is interesting, because it suggests that the representation of psychosexual mechanisms in the human brain may be sexually dimorphic, at least in the temporal lobe, the important structure most likely being the amygdala (Rémillard et al., 1983). Indeed, with one possible exception (Jacome et al., 1980), there are no cases in the literature in which positive sexual emotions have been observed to occur in men during seizures. Sexual sensations and even autonomic changes such as erections have been observed in males during seizures (Stoffels et al., 1980), but they are devoid of libidinous psychosexual feelings. Such manifestations most likely are unrelated to amygdaloid discharge since they can occur with discharges involving the paracentral lobule and the "perisylvian" region (Stoffels et al., 1980). Manipulation of sexual organs reportedly occurs in frontal lobe automatism (Spencer et al., 1983; Williamson et al., 1985). In my opinion it does not qualify as genuine sexual behavior, since it is very similar to other forms of self-manipulation in epileptic automatism such as rubbing of the nose, hands, etc., and indeed has been reported to occur in automatisms of nonfrontal origin (Stoffels et al., 1980). By contrast, sexual auras in women are frankly libidinous. They are often associated with appropriate autonomic changes such as viscerosensory erotic sensations in the genital region, vulvovaginal secretions, and sometimes orgasms. In one of our patients, amygdala stimulation elicited libidinous sensations in the vulva and thighs which were associated with a memory flashback to the instance of her first sexual intercourse, which she had had at age sixteen (Gloor, 1986b, 1991).

Thirst or at least the urge to drink, not necessarily associated with a subjective feeling of thirst, is another phenomenon that might be called affective and sometimes occurs in the course of temporal lobe seizures (Bancaud et al., 1966; Gloor, 1975a; Rémillard et al., 1981; Cascino and Sutula, 1989). It has been elicited by amygdaloid stimulation (Bancaud et al., 1966). A feeling of hunger or eating is rarely elicited by temporal lobe seizure discharge. Only Gastaut (1955) reports its occasional occurrence under such circumstances.

Sometimes, even though the patient does not report an affective experience, his mood may change in response to a temporal lobe seizure or electrical stimulation in the amygdala. Such a mood change can be instantaneous in response to amygdaloid stimulation and can persist for quite some time (Stevens et al., 1969; personal unpublished observations).

Perceptual Phenomena

Various kinds of perceptual phenomena can occur in temporal lobe seizures. They may involve all sense modalities but to different degrees and not always in the form of true experiential phenomena, the latter being virtually confined to the visual and auditory modalities (Penfield and Jasper, 1954; Penfield, 1955a,b; Penfield and Perot, 1963; Gloor, 1972, 1986b, 1991, in press, a; Daly, 1975; Halgren et al., 1978; Gloor et al., 1982; Spiers et al., 1985; Bancaud, 1987; Taylor and Lochery, 1987). The amygdala is probably not involved in all of them, perhaps only in those having true experiential subjective qualities. Elementary auditory and visual hallucinations do not involve the amygdala and indicate discharge in the primary auditory and visual cortices. Somatosensory hallucinations occurring in temporal lobe seizures are usually of the elementary nonexperiential type. They differ, however, from those elicited from the postcentral gyrus by being poorly localized, often involving widespread, even bilateral, regions of the body. Vague cephalic sensations also commonly occur (Penfield and Jasper, 1954; Jasper and Rasmussen, 1958; Fcindel, 1974; Wieser, 1983). The anatomical substrate of these ill-defined somatosensory phenomena is unclear, but they are sometimes elicited by amygdaloid and other temporal lobe stimulations (Jasper and Rasmussen, 1958; study in preparation). Somatosensory hallucinations with an experiential quality are virtually never reported by patients (Penfield and Jasper, 1954; Daly, 1975; Gloor, 1986b). I am aware of only two instances that might qualify as an experiential somatosensory hallucination in response to amygdaloid stimulation. The first is a feeling which a patient likened to that of falling into water, upon which he later elaborated by saying it felt like something was covering his eyes and face (Gloor et al., 1982, 1990). The second is the erotic sensation in the vulvovaginal and thigh region which accompanied the re-experience of her first sexual intercourse reproduced by amygdala stimulation in the patient mentioned above and may be regarded as another example of a somatosensory experiential response.

Olfactory and gustatory hallucinations usually are not clearly experiential, inasmuch as the nature and quality of the smell or taste often remains ill-defined and is not clearly linked to common everyday experiences or memories. There are, however, occasional exceptions to this (Daly, 1958b). Olfactory and gustatory hallucinations are usually described as aversive and much more rarely as pleasant. Olfactory hallucinations are relatively uncommon manifestations of temporal lobe seizures (Penfield and Jasper, 1954; Feindel, 1974; Daly, 1958b, 1975; Spiers et al., 1985; Taylor and Lochery, 1987). Bancaud (1987) is of the opinion that olfactory hallucinations in seizures are not of temporal lobe origin, but are caused by discharge of the posterior orbital frontal cortex. Olfactory sensations are, however, sometimes elicited by amygdaloid stimulation (Penfield and Jasper, 1954; Jasper and Rasmussen, 1958; Gloor et al., 1982). Gustatory hallucinations are reported to occur in temporal lobe epilepsy (Daly, 1958b; Spiers et al., 1985; Hausser-Hauw and Bancaud, 1987). They are occasionally reproduced by amygdaloid stimulation (Hausser-Hauw and Bancaud, 1987). It has been argued that the amygdala and other temporal lobe structures are not primarily involved in the elicitation of these phenomena, but rather the centroparietal operculum and the adjacent insula (Penfield and Jasper, 1954; Jasper and Rasmussen, 1958; Hausser-Hauw and Bancaud, 1987).

Visual and auditory perceptual phenomena are undoubtedly those most commonly elicited by temporal lobe seizure discharge. Two perceptual phenomena must be distinguished: visual and auditory illusions on the one hand and visual and auditory hallucinations on the other (Penfield and Jasper, 1954; Penfield, 1955a,b; Mullan and Penfield, 1958; Penfield and Perot, 1963; Feindel, 1974; Daly, 1975; Gloor, 1972, 1990, 1991; Wieser, 1979, 1983; Gloor et al., 1982; Spiers et al., 1985; Bancaud, 1987; Taylor and Lochery, 1987). Illusions are distortions or alterations in the quality of actual percepts, while hallucinations are de novo

creations of perceptions within the brain without there being any correspond
ing set of external stimuli. Auditory illusions are changes in loudness of perceived sounds, as if for instance a sound source were moving closer or farther
away, or there may be the illusion of sound quality changing. In the visual modality there may be a distortion of shapes, of objects looming larger or becoming
smaller, as if moving further away from the patient, the perceived hue of colors
may change, or stereoscopic vision may become altered by becoming more vivid.
Recordings of seizures through stereotaxically implanted electrodes and stimulation studies suggest that most of these changes are attributable to discharge
in auditory and visual association cortex (Penfield and Jasper, 1954; Mullan
and Penfield, 1958; Wieser, 1983; Bancaud, 1987), but occasionally they can be
reproduced by amygdaloid stimulation (Gloor et al., 1982). These illusions frequently have experiential qualities.

Experiential quality is a consistent feature of complex visual, auditory, or
combined visual-auditory hallucinations. They may be experienced as seeing a
face, a person, a scene, or as hearing a voice or a piece of music being played
(Penfield and Jasper, 1954; Penfield, 1955a,b; Penfield and Perot, 1963; Gloor,
1972, 1990, 1991; Feindel, 1974; Daly, 1975; Weingarten et al., 1976; Halgren
et al., 1978; Wieser, 1979, 1983; Gloor et al., 1982; Spiers et al., 1985; Bancaud,
1987; Taylor and Lochery, 1987). Since commonly the content of these hallucinations is associated with a personal memory (Penfield, 1952, 1955a,b; Penfield
and Jasper, 1954; Penfield and Perot, 1963; Gloor, 1972, 1990, 1991; Bancaud,
1970), it behooves one to examine whether these hallucinatory phenomena are
truly perceptual or merely represent vivid memories. In cases of a strong association with a remembered past event or situation, true perceptual features may
be missing or at least be fuzzy. In other instances, a true perceptual content
seems to be present, but even under these circumstances it may be imprecise
(Gloor et al., 1982; Gloor, 1990, 1991). The vividness of the subjective experience that strikes the patient and contrasts with its perceptual imprecision is
thus not caused by clarity of perceptual detail, but by the feeling of experiencing a true lifelike situation or a true memory flashback which may be more
vivid than a commonplace reminiscence or voluntary recall. This subjective
vividness is caused by a feeling of "being there," as one of our patients put it,
rather than to perceptual or cognitive semantic detail, and thus appears to be
primarily affective in nature. In auditory hallucinations of hearing a voice, the
voice is commonly familiar and can sometimes be identified, but the patient is
virtually never able to report any semantic content. The anatomical substrates
of these phenomena and their evocation by electrical stimulation are discussed
below in conjunction with those of all experiential phenomena.

Memory Phenomena

Two kinds of mnemonic phenomena can be activated by temporal lobe seizure discharge or stimulation (Gloor et al., 1981, 1982; Gloor, 1991): (1) reactivation of a past memory, a memory flashback, or (2) a "feeling of reminiscence"
as Hughlings Jackson (1888) called it, a phenomenon more commonly known
as the "*déjà vu*" illusion.

Reactivation of a memory of the past is at times unmistakably autobiographical in the most restricted sense, or it may not strictly be so, but still personal, as for instance when the patient realizes that a voice he hears is that of a family member or a place he sees is one well known to him, for instance his home or place of work (Penfield and Jasper, 1954; Penfield, 1952, 1955a,b; Penfield and Perot, 1963; Halgren et al., 1978; Wieser, 1979, 1983; Gloor et al., 1982; Spiers et al., 1985; Gloor, 1990, 1991).

The feeling of reminiscence, the illusion of familiarity or "*déjà vu*" illusion elicited by temporal lobe discharge or electrical stimulation has no mnemonic content attached to it (Penfield and Jasper, 1954; Mullan and Penfield, 1958; Daly, 1975; Wieser, 1983; Gloor et al., 1982; Spiers et al., 1985; Gloor, 1990, 1991). The patient projects the feeling of reminiscence onto the surrounding he finds himself in at the time, even if that surrounding is totally novel and unknown to him; hence, the incongruous and illusionary nature of the feeling. The feeling of reminiscence or familiarity can be regarded as a quasi-affective component of the memory recall process. As the "*déjà vu*" phenomenon, it is an illusion of memory; under normal circumstances this feeling is part and parcel of the experience of recall which then of course also includes semantic content.

The Role of the Amygdala in Affective, Perceptual, and Memory Processes as Suggested by the Experiential Phenomena of Temporal Lobe Seizures

The anatomical substrates of these experiential phenomena are of interest because among all temporal lobe structures, the amygdala is the one from which they can most easily be elicited by electrical stimulation, even without inducing an afterdischarge, as is shown in Tables I–III (Gloor et al., 1981; 1982). This was a highly unexpected finding, particularly with regard to the evocation of complex visual and auditory hallucinations and of memory flashbacks, which Penfield had been able to elicit from stimulations applied to temporal isocortex (Penfield, 1952, 1955a,b; Mullan and Penfield, 1958; Penfield and Perot, 1963). The map of Penfield and Perot's (1963) stimulation responses shows that the points in the temporal isocortex from which auditory experiential phenomena could be elicited occupied the first temporal convolution, with only a few found immediately below the superior temporal sulcus. Visual experiential phenomena were elicited from more widespread areas of temporal isocortex, including temporo-occipital transitional cortex and some points in the first temporal convolution and supratemporal plane. This relative segregation of areas yielding auditory from visual responses agrees reasonably well with the known compartmentalization of temporal lobe isocortex into auditory and visual association areas that have emerged from experimental studies in nonhuman primates. Such studies have shown that the auditory association cortex occupies the first temporal convolution (Dewson et al., 1970; Cowey and Dewson, 1972; Neff et al., 1975; Pandya and Yeterian, 1985; Colombo et al., 1990), while visual association cortex is located in the more ventral parts of the temporal isocortex (Mishkin, 1966, 1972; Desimone and Gross, 1979; Gross et al., 1981; Ungerleider and Mishkin,

**TABLE I. Emotions Elicited by Electrical Stimulation
(Fear 42, Anger 1, Emotional distress 2)***

Stimulated Structure	No AD or AD Confined to Stimulated Structure	Afterdischarge (AD)		
		Limbic Spread Only	Limbic + Isocortical Spread	Isocortical Spread Only
Amygdala	17	3	3	—
Hippocampus	9	5	1	—
Parahippocampal gyrus	1	1	3	—
Isocortex	2[a]	—	—	—

[a]Probably limbic responses: stimulation was deep, applied near limbic structures from which identical, but stronger emotional response (fear) was evoked on stimulation.
*Tables I to III are reprinted with minor changes from Gloor et al., 1981, by permission of Elsevier Science Publishers.

**TABLE II. Perceptual Hallucinations and Illusions Elicited by
Electrical Stimulation (Visual 23, Auditory 3, Olfactory 2)**

Stimulated Structure	No AD or AD Confined to Stimulated Structure	Afterdischarge (AD)		
		Limbic Spread Only	Limbic + Isocortical Spread	Isocortical Spread Only
Amygdala	14	2	4	—
Hippocampus	1	—	4	—
Parahippocampal gyrus	—	—	3	—
Isocortex	—	—	—	—

**TABLE III. Mnemonic Responses Elicited by Electrical Stimulation
(*Déjà vu* 18, Memory recall 16)**

Stimulated Structure	No AD or AD Confined to Stimulated Structure	Afterdischarge (AD)		
		Limbic Spread Only	Limbic + Isocortical Spread	Isocortical Spread Only
Amygdala	14	—	6	—
Hippocampus	2	—	11	—
Parahippocampal gyrus	—	—	—	—
Isocortex	1[a]	—	—	—

[a]Deep temporal stimulation near limbic structures.

1982; Mishkin et al., 1983; Pandya and Yeterian, 1985). There is thus no doubt that the responses elicited from temporal isocortex as reported by Penfield and Perot (1963) do indeed tell us something that is valid about the anatomical organization of the cortical structures involved in higher auditory and visual functions in humans. This, however, only deepens the mystery of why in subsequent studies when the temporal lobe was more thoroughly explored in its deep-lying components, the limbic structures, the amygdala in particular, turned out to be the structures from which experiential phenomena of any type could most often be elicited (Gloor et al., 1981, 1982; study in preparation) (Tables I, II, and III). That affective responses would show a preferential localization to the amygdala was not unexpected (Gloor, 1972), but to find perceptual and mnemonic responses equally strongly represented there was highly unexpected, but proved to be a robust phenomenon. It is also of some interest that the hippocampus yielded fewer experiential responses than the amygdala and did not appear to be preferentially involved in the evocation of mnemonic responses. An explanation for these findings at the present can only be hypothetical and a specific hypothesis is stated below (Gloor, 1990).

Before presenting this hypothesis one must, however, first deal with the difficulty that arises from the observation that as crude an event as a naturally occurring epileptic discharge or an artificial electrical brain stimulation is capable of eliciting highly organized experiences having a subjective quality akin to those occurring in real life. It is commonly assumed that epileptic discharge can only elicit simple and unstructured positive phenomena, such as the contraction of some muscle groups in response to motor cortex stimulation, or crude sensory phenomena like paresthesiae, phosphenes, or unstructured noise in response to stimulation of the primary somatosensory, visual, and auditory cortices. Stimulation applied to areas of cortex subserving more complex functions often seems to interfere with the normal utilization of these areas, the best-known example being stimulation of speech cortex which never elicits speech, but paralyzes the patient's ability to speak (Penfield and Roberts, 1959). Some have therefore argued that the elicitation of experiential phenomena by temporal lobe seizure discharge or stimulation must also result from interference with a highly elaborate function and that experiential responses thus must represent some sort of release phenomenon (Ferguson et al., 1969; Halgren et al., 1978). This is an unconvincing explanation for two reasons: (1) If experiential phenomena resulted from seizure- or stimulation-induced paralysis of temporal lobe function, one would also encounter them in the postictal phase, where they are however absent, with the occasional exception of the lingering on of stimulation- or seizure-induced mood changes. Experiential phenomena occur at the beginning of temporal lobe seizures when seizure discharge is presumably still limited both in its anatomical extent and intensity. (2) It would be highly unusual that ictal paralysis of structures such as the temporal isocortex, the hippocampus, and the amygdala, which are known to be involved in visual and auditory perception and recall as well as in the affective responses to such stimuli, should activate the very processes known to be dependent upon the functional integrity of these structures.

We are thus forced to accept the notion that these phenomena are indeed positive, but then how are we to explain the fact that epileptic discharge in or stimulation of different structures such as the amygdala or temporal isocortex can elicit them? By drawing upon some modern concepts of telencephalic organization and of cognitive science, a hypothetical explanation of these puzzling facts can be envisaged. It has become increasingly evident that the primate brain is organized in the form of parallel-distributed networks (Goldman-Rakic, 1987, 1988a,b) with widely dispersed components of these networks cooperating in elaborating complex functions. Furthermore, theoretical concepts of parallel models of associative memory (Anderson and Hinton, 1981; Kohonen et al., 1981) and of parallel-distributed processing (Rumelhart and McClelland, 1986) have suggested ways in which cortical networks could elaborate higher cognitive functions. A hypothesis based on these concepts that could account for the observed experiential phenomena has been proposed (Gloor, 1990). We must first bear in mind that temporal lobe association cortex as well as some other cortical association areas in the frontal and parietal lobes are interconnected reciprocally with each other and with the amygdala and hippocampus, as has been summarized above. While the afferent inputs to the amygdala and to the hippocampus have been well known for some time, much less attention has been paid to the still-accumulating evidence that there are widespread return connections from the amygdala and the hippocampal system (in the latter case mostly through the entorhinal cortex and subicular complex) to widespread areas of association cortex and even, in the case of the amygdala, to the visual cortex (Nauta, 1961; Rosene and van Hoesen, 1977; Tigges et al., 1982, 1983; van Hoesen, 1982; Amaral and Price, 1984; Amaral, 1986, 1987; Insausti et al., 1987; Iwai and Yukie, 1987).

If we assume that the various components of this widespread system function as a content-addressable memory operating according to the principles of parallel-distributed processing, then we can envisage that a given experience is represented within the system by a specific distributed matrix of neurons linked together through synapses that have been strengthened by plastic changes according to a Hebbian rule. Each such matrix consists of widely distributed neurons, but is unique for a given experience, with individual neurons participating in many but not all matrices. It is important to realize that an experience is not represented by any one single neuron within the matrix, that none of its neurons responds exclusively to only one given experiential feature, and that each neuron participates in many but not in all matrices that embody various experiences. The strength of connections between neurons which is modifiable through repeated usage and reflects synaptic plasticity allows specific patterns representing specific experiences to be created. Thus, it is the unique pattern woven within a distributed neuronal network that represents an experience, not the excitation of specific neurons. If such a network operates according to the rules of parallel-distributed processing, two predictions can be made. First, the entire matrix once created can be reproduced by activating only a segment of it, and second, the matrix will resist serious degradation if parts of it become destroyed or inactive, or if noise enters into it (Rumelhart and

McClelland, 1986). There are of course limits to this resistance to degradation, but it seems that much of the matrix can be destroyed or overwhelmed by noise before the message embedded in it becomes unintelligible. The tolerance to noise is the most interesting aspect with regard to the interpretation of experiential phenomena in temporal lobe epilepsy. If we make the assumption that incipient epileptic discharge, for instance in the amygdala, but also possibly in the isocortex, can recreate a neuronal matrix that corresponds to an actual experience, then the mounting noise introduced by increasing epileptic discharge may initially induce a degree of degradation that can be tolerated without loss of intelligibility, although the information content may be coarsened. This may explain why experiential phenomena are commonly fragmentary, perceptual detail may be fuzzy, and recall partial. It may also explain the short-lived character of these phenomena which occur only during the aura of a seizure, for further degradation by the mounting noise of epileptic discharge will ultimately render the neurons embedded in the matrix incapable of representing anything. We then enter the paralytic phase of a temporal lobe seizure when temporal lobe function is severely disrupted, a phase that is clinically characterized by confusion, automatism, and anterograde amnesia, as is discussed below when considering automatism.

Let us now envisage what the specific contribution of the amygdala in this context may be. In the course of building up a matrix through experience in the course of everyday living, amygdaloid neurons receive inputs from the main sensory association areas involved in perception. Association of such inputs with actual aversive or rewarding stimuli will cause an affective dimension to be attached to the perceptual experience represented in the matrix. Such affective significance will also be attached if what is perceived occurs in the context of a previously learned psychoaffective constellation related to affiliative behavior (for instance, kinship ties), or other forms of social behaviors, familiar surroundings, or earlier aversive experiences. The involvement of the amygdala in such sociobiologically important functions is well documented (Kling, 1972) and has become a focus of interest in modern socioneurological thought (Brothers, 1990). When the amygdala is activated under such circumstances, three streams of amygdaloid output will be set into motion, one directed to the hypothalamus and brain stem, priming the autonomic and endocrine system to respond appropriately to the incoming perceptual message, particularly if its affective associations are strong. A second stream is directed to the hippocampus and serves to reinforce consolidation of perceptual information which has also entered the hippocampal system at the same time that it accessed the amygdala. Finally, a third stream projects back to the population of association cortex neurons that have initiated the message directed to the amygdala and hippocampus in the first place and probably also to some association areas beyond the confines of the originally involved population. This return amygdala message probably coincides with the arrival there of a return hippocampal message and the two can be expected to induce some plastic changes at that level, thus creating a pattern of strengthened synaptic connections among specific sets of cortical neurons. These sets are part of the emerging distributed neuronal matrix representing the experience as a whole, with other neurons that are part of the matrix being located in the amygdala and in the hippocampal system. Recall of the experience with concomitant reproduction of the matrix can occur in different ways. The impingement of a perceptual experience similar to a previous one can through the activation of at least part of the isocortical population involved in the original experience recreate the entire matrix that corresponds to it and call forth the memory of the original event and an appropriate affective response through the activation of amygdaloid neurons. Interplay between the amygdala and hippocampus can further reinforce its consolidation in memory. Impingement of some stimuli not necessarily identical with the original experience but sharing some similarity with it even at a relatively noncognitive (for instance, on an affective) level, may through the amygdala light up the original matrix and thus lead to full or partial recall of the original perceptual message associated with the appropriate affect. In this case the first step may be an initially rather nonspecific signal of familiarity which could be a purely amygdaloid response that under most normal circumstances would elicit full recall, including cognitive content, by reactivating the whole matrix. However, sometimes this widespread reactivation may not occur and the result then is the experience of a feeling of reminiscence, the "*déjà vu*" illusion without cognitive content.

Assuming that this model is valid, it is obvious that incipient epileptic discharge in the amygdala, but also in other parts of the system, or localized electrical stimulation could lead to the lighting up of a specific matrix which may have been reinforced by the frequent recurrence of identical seizure discharge in the past. The experiential aura would be the subjectively experienced correlate of the activation of the matrix. This would explain why experiential phenomena can be elicited from both limbic and isocortical areas.

These considerations suggest that one of the functions of the amygdala may be to provide an affective recognition signal that may initiate what one may call affective recall as opposed to, for instance, voluntary or semantic recall. Such a mechanism may be involved in some forms of "spontaneous" recall that may occur when one encounters a situation with specific affective connotations.

Role of the Amygdala in Epileptic Automatism

One of the first functional correlates of amygdaloid activity reported in humans was that stimulation of the amygdaloid area in awake epileptic patients undergoing surgery for temporal lobe epilepsy could reproduce the essential features of epileptic automatism (Feindel and Penfield, 1954). The concept of automatism introduced by Hughlings Jackson (1875) [1958a] is however imprecise, for under this heading are grouped a variety of functional disturbances which may not always occur together (Feindel and Penfield, 1954; Penfield and Jasper, 1954; Ajmone Marsan and Ralston, 1957; Bancaud et al., 1966; Feindel, 1974; Daly, 1975; Wieser, 1983; Bancaud, 1987; Gloor, 1991). The term owes its origin and popularity in the medical literature to the fact that the patient may appear to carry out relatively complex forms of motor behavior without obvious reference to the prevailing circumstances, without responding to verbal stimuli, and subsequently is amnestic for the entire episode. The underlying assumption therefore is that during the period of automatism, consciousness has been suspended and the patient acts like an automaton, an assumption that is sometimes patently incorrect (Gloor, 1986a). Even when defined in this broad way, states often classed as automatism may not satisfy all the criteria listed above. Thus the most common form of automatism, often called "oro-alimentary automatism" by the French authors (Bancaud, 1987), consists of mouth and throat movements in the form of rhythmic chewing, swallowing, or lip-smacking (what Hughlings Jackson called "tasting movements"; Jackson and Coleman, 1898). The patient is usually unresponsive during such an episode and subsequently amnestic for it (Magnus et al., 1952). The motor behavior is simple, stereotyped, and confined to movement patterns related to eating. Slightly more complex behavioral patterns, but still relatively simple, are those of self-inspection and self-manipulation by the patient. He again appears impervious to external stimuli or commands and is amnestic for the episode, while he may be plucking on his clothes, pulling on his bedsheets, or rubbing his nose or some other part of the body. There is a wide spectrum of motor behavior during the state of automatism which can range from the just-described simple motor patterns, to much more elaborate forms, like undressing, going to the bathroom to void, manipulating either properly or improperly objects within the patient's reach, or carrying out very complex behaviors, indeed sometimes within appropriate contexts. A justifiably famous example of this is Hughlings Jackson's patient Dr. Z, who examined a patient while having a temporal lobe seizure, wrote a note "pneumonia of left base," had no recollection of having done so and upon later verifying the diagnosis which he had made "unconsciously," found it to be correct (Jackson, 1888). This type of seizure should probably not be called automatism but an amnestic seizure, since Dr. Z was obviously not confused when examining his patient, but merely amnestic for having done so. It is thus apparent that it is hard to give a satisfactory unitary interpretation of what constitutes automatism.

We may, however, start with the proposition that it largely corresponds, in contrast to the experiential phenomena of epileptic seizures, to a state of ictal interference with temporal lobe function. In the case of amnestic seizures as in Hughlings Jackson's patient Dr. Z, the interference seems to be predominantly one with hippocampal function. The state of automatism thus would reflect paralysis of function of the temporal lobe and perhaps of additional cortical and subcortical areas to which seizure discharge has spread (Magnus et al., 1952). This is in line with the observation that ictal automatism is indistinguishable from postictal automatism except when a concomitant EEG recording allows one to determine at what point the seizure discharge has stopped (Magnus et al., 1952; Feindel and Penfield, 1954; Daly, 1975; Gloor, 1991). The postictal state is one of profound depression of neuronal function as evidenced from the slow-wave activity which dominates the EEG at that time. Since ictal automatism is essentially identical to postictal automatism, where neuronal function is severely depressed, it must be the consequence of a profound interference with temporal lobe function and perhaps with that of some related areas as well. Furthermore, electrical stimulation of the amygdala or other temporal lobe structures never produces automatism without inducing a seizure or a spreading afterdischarge (Magnus et al., 1952; Bancaud et al., 1966; study in preparation). During ictal automatism, seizure discharge is intense and widespread within the temporal lobe and often also invades adjacent structures. It undoubtedly also disrupts the function of subcortical structures. Moreover, in most cases such a spread of discharge is bilateral (Jasper, 1964; Bancaud et al., 1966; Gloor et al., 1980; Munari et al., 1980; Wieser, 1983). It is thus not surprising that states qualifying as automatism can be induced by both amygdala and hippocampal stimulation (Bancaud et al., 1966) or by seizures arising elsewhere in the brain or even by the generalized discharges of absence attacks (Feindel and Penfield, 1954; Penfield and Jasper, 1954; Magnus et al., 1952; Williamson et al., 1985; Gloor, 1991).

The symptomatology which characterizes automatism is one that one would expect to result from ictal paralysis of temporal lobe structures and of other areas of association cortex. There is anterograde amnesia, undoubtedly reflecting ictal interference with the function of the hippocampal system; there is a lack of the patient's ability to respond adequately to stimuli presented in his environment. This most likely indicates that there is interference with the clarity of perception, although not all perception is lost. The patient usually does avoid obstacles, he is certainly able to see objects, grasp them, and even manipulate them normally, but his overall behavior is highly inappropriate. He does not respond normally to social signals emanating from his environment and may therefore not interact in any socially insightful or appropriate way with persons around him and may in addition engage in socially unacceptable behavior like undressing in a public place. This probably indicates a combination of deficits that are partially perceptual, not at an elementary level, but rather on the level of relating environmental signals to the fund of personal memories and acquired social attitudes that guide our behavior in everyday living. This probably indicates a lack of proper interplay of temporal and frontal association cortex with the hippocampal system and the amygdala. Finally, there is no evidence that in this state the patient responds normally to affective signals from his environment, and his own affective behavior is highly deficient or dominated by a fearful or more rarely a mirthful attitude which may extend into the postictal phase and bears no relationship to the circumstances in which he finds himself. This may at first glance appear to partially contradict the assertion made earlier that experiential phenomena are only seen at the beginning of a seizure. However, seizure- or stimulation-induced mood changes, as is the case in everyday life, once engendered, especially when intense, have a long-lasting reverberation, probably because the stimulation of hypothalamic and brain stem structures which integrate basic motivational mechanisms may set into motion biochemical or neuroendocrine responses that may last for a long time (Stevens et al., 1969).

There remains one difficult problem in explaining the symptoms of temporal lobe automatism. These are the rhythmic masticatory and associated oropharyngeal movements of lip-smacking and swallowing which are so common in temporal lobe automatism. Could these represent positive effects resulting from amygdaloid discharge? One may be inclined to believe this in view of the recent anatomical evidence that the amygdala projects to a neuronal pool in the lower brain stem known to be involved in the integration of the masticatory motor program (Nakamura and Kubo, 1978; Takeuchi et al., 1988a,b). It is, however, not known whether the neurons that project to these brain stem areas involved in mastication exert an excitatory or an inhibitory effect. Stimulation of the amygdala or adjacent structures does not produce rhythmic masticatory movements unless a seizure or an afterdischarge is produced (Magnus et al., 1952; Bancaud et al., 1966; study in preparation). They are not present at the very beginning of a seizure and often continue into the postictal period. This suggests that these movements may represent the consequence of some seizure-induced release from an inhibitory control normally exerted by the amygdala upon neurons in the brain stem that control motor programs involved in chewing and swallowing. However, until the physiological significance of the descending amygdala connections to brain stem masticatory neurons are clarified, the question must remain open whether this motor component of automatism represents a positive or negative phenomenon of temporal lobe seizures.

SUMMARY

Two aspects of the involvement and role of the amygdala in human temporal lobe epilepsy are reviewed: (1) The role structural pathological processes involving the amygdala play in the pathogenesis of human temporal lobe epilepsy, and (2) the role of the amygdala in the clinical symptomatology of temporal lobe seizures. Consideration of the latter may afford some insight into the organization of affective, perceptual, and mnemonic functions in the human brain.

Pathological changes in the amygdala in the form of partial neuronal loss and gliosis are common in mesial temporal sclerosis, which is the most common pathological substrate of temporal lobe epilepsy. The main lesion in mesial temporal sclerosis is usually assumed to be that affecting the hippocampus. However, in contrast to what is known about the fine details of hippocampal pathology in this condition, no comparable data exist with regard to amygdaloid pathology. In particular, the question of lesion-induced plastic changes of the type known to occur in the hippocampus of epileptic patients has not been addressed in the amygdala. In patients suffering from temporal lobe epilepsy caused by lesions other than mesial temporal sclerosis, the amygdala is more commonly affected than the hippocampus. It is therefore concluded that the common view according to which hippocampal pathology is the crucial element in the pathogenesis of temporal lobe epilepsy is not fully supported by the presently available evidence. It is suggested that amygdaloid pathology may be as important in this respect as that of the hippocampus and deserves more intensive study.

The careful study of the electrophysiological features of recorded temporal lobe seizures and that of the responses evoked by the electrical stimulation of various temporal lobe structures suggests that the amygdala is in some way involved in almost all the classical manifestations that characterize those seizures, whether they are viscerosensory, autonomic, affective, perceptual, or mnemonic. This is, however, not only true for the amygdala but applies also to the other structures of the temporal lobe, such as the hippocampus, parahippocampal gyrus, and temporal isocortex. This at-first-glance disconcerting situation reflects the intimate and reciprocal anatomical interconnectivity of these various components of the temporal lobe. It does not mean that each portion is functionally equipotent, but it indicates that to function in a normal physiological context (but also in the elaboration of the complex experiential phenomena that occur in some temporal lobe seizures), the various structures of the temporal lobe must interact in an intricate and reciprocal way. A hypothesis developed more fully elsewhere (Gloor, 1990) is proposed to account for these phenomena. The amygdaloid contribution in the elaboration of these complex phenomena is probably particularly concerned with affective mechanisms and their autonomic repercussions as well as in some mechanisms of memory recall.

Epileptic automatism, which once had been attributed specifically to the activation of the amygdala, has turned out to have a less specific anatomical correlate. Automatism reflects a seizure-induced functional paralysis of the temporal lobe in both limbic and isocortical components, an interference which probably extends to extratemporal structures. Only one manifestation of temporal lobe automatism, rhythmic mastication, may have a more specific relationship to the amygdala. It may reflect the firing of amygdala neurons projecting to lower brain stem nerve cells known to be involved in the control of mastication. However, this effect is also probably a negative one, reflecting epileptic interference with these connections, although a positive effect consisting of active driving of masticatory neurons by amygdala discharge cannot be entirely ruled out.

REFERENCES

Aggleton JP (1986): A description of the amygdalo-hippocampal interconnections in the macaque monkey. Exp Brain Res 64:515–526.

Aggleton JP, Burton MJ, Passingham RE (1980): Cortical and subcortical afferents to the amygdala of the rhesus monkey (*Macaca mulatta*). Brain Res 190:347–368.

Aggleton JP, Friedmann DP, Mishkin M (1987): A comparison between the connections of the amygdala and hippocampus with the basal forebrain in the macaque. Exp Brain Res 67:556–568.

Aggleton JP, Mishkin M (1984): Projections from the amygdala to the thalamus in cyonomolgus monkey. J Comp Neurol 222:56–68.

Ajmone Marsan C, Ralston B (1957): "The Epileptic Seizure: Its Functional Morphology and Diagnostic Significance." Springfield, IL: Charles C. Thomas.

Amaral DG (1986): Amydalohippocampal and amygdalocortical projections in the primate brain. In Schwarcz R, Ben-Ari Y (eds): "Excitatory Amino Acids and Epilepsy." New York: Plenum Press, pp 3–18.

Amaral DG (1987): Memory: Anatomical organization of candidate brain regions. In Plum F, Mountcastle V (eds): "Higher Functions of the Brain. Handbook of Physiology, Part I." Washington, DC: Am Physiol Soc, pp 211–294.

Amaral DG, Price JL (1984): Amygdalo-cortical projections in the monkey (*Macaca fascicularis*). J Comp Neurol 230:465–496.

Amaral DG, Veazey RB, Cowan WM (1982): Some observations on hypothalamo-amygdaloid connections in the monkey. Brain Res 252:13–27.

Anderson JA, Hinton JE (1981): Models of information processing in the brain. In Hinton JE, Anderson JA (eds): "Parallel Models of Associative Memory." Hillsdale, NJ: Lawrence Erlbaum, pp 9–48.

Ashford JW, Schultz SC, Walsh GO (1980): Violent automatism in a partial complex seizure. Arch Neurol 37:120–122.

Babb TL, Brown WJ (1987): Pathological findings in epilepsy. In Engel J Jr (ed): "Surgical Treatment of the Epilepsies." New York: Raven Press, pp 511–540.

Bancaud J (1987): Sémiologie clinique des crises épileptiques d'origine temporale. Rev Neurol 143:392–400.

Bancaud J, Favel P, Bonis A, Bordas-Ferrer M, Miravet J, Talairach J (1970): Manifestations sexuelles paroxystiques et épilepsie temporale: Étude clinique, EEG et SEEG d'une épilepsie d'origine tumorale. Rev Neurol 123:217–230.

Bancaud J, Talairach J, Bonis A, Schaub C, Szikla G, Morel P, Bordas-Ferrer M (1965): "La stéréo-électroencéphalographie dans l'épilepsie. Informations apportées par l'investigation fonctionelle stéréotaxique." Paris, Masson et Cie.

Bancaud J, Talairach J, Morel P, Bresson M (1966): La corne d'Ammon et le noyeau amygdalien: Effets cliniques et électriques de leur stimulation chez l'homme. Rev Neurol (Paris) 115:329–352.

Ben-Ari Y (ed) (1981): "The Amygdaloid Complex." Amsterdam, New York: Elsevier/North Holland Biomedical Press.

Ben-Ari Y, Represa A (1990): Brief seizure episodes induce long-term potentiation and mossy fibre sprouting in the hippocampus. Trends Neurosci 8:312–318.

Bonvallet M, Gary Bobo E (1973): La réaction de défense amygdalienne. Données historiques, histologiques et neurophysiologiques. Arch Ital Biol 111:642–656.

Brothers L (1990): The social brain: A project for integrating primate behavior and neurophysiology in a new domain. Concepts Neurosci 1:27–51.

Bruton CJ (1988): "The Neuropathology of Temporal Lobe Epilepsy." New York: Oxford University Press, 158 pp.

Cador M, Robbins TW, Everitt BJ (1989): Involvement of the amygdala in stimulus-reward associations: Interaction with the ventral striatum. Neuroscience 30:77–86.

Cascino GD, Sutula TP (1989): Thirst and compulsive water drinking in medial basal limbic epilepsy: An electroclinical and neuropathological correlation. J Neurol Neurosurg Psychiat 52:680–681.

Cavanagh JB, Meyer A (1956): Aetiological aspects of Ammon's horn sclerosis associated with temporal lobe epilepsy. Br Med J 2:1403–1407.

Chapman WP (1960): Depth electrode studies in patients with temporal lobe epilepsy. In: Ramey ER, O'Doherty DS (eds): "Electrical Studies of the Unanesthetized Brain." New York: Paul B Hoeber, 334–350.

Chapman WP, Schroeder HR, Geyer G, Brazier MAB, Fager C, Poppen JL, Solomon HC, Yakovlev PI (1954): Physiological evidence concerning importance of amygdaloid nuclear region in the integration of circulatory function and emotion in man. Science 120:949–950.

Colombo M, D'Amato MR, Rodman HR, Gross CG (1990): Auditory association cortex lesions impair auditory short-term memory in monkeys. Science 247:336–338.

Cowey A, Dewson JH (1972): Effects of unilateral ablation of superior temporal cortex on auditory sequence discrimination in *Macaca mulatta*. Neuropsychologia 10:279–289.

Daly D (1958a): Ictal affect. Am J Psychiat 115:97–108.

Daly D (1958b): Uncinate fits. Neurology 8:250–260.

Daly DD (1975): Ictal clinical manifestations. In Penrey JK, Daly DD (eds): "Complex Partial Seizures and Their Treatment." Adv Neurol 11:57–83.

DeMolina FA, Hunsperger RW (1959): Central representation of affective reactions in forebrain and brainstem: Electrical stimulation of amygdala, stria terminalis, and adjacent structures. J Physiol (London) 145:251–265.

DeOlmos JS (1972): The amygdaloid projection field in the rat as studied with the cupric-silver method. In Eleftheriou BE (ed): "The Neurobiology of the Amygdala." New York: Plenum Press, pp 145–204.

DeOlmos JS (1990): Amygdala. In Paxinos G (ed): "The Human Nervous System." San Diego, New York, London: Academic Press, pp 583–710.

DeOlmos JS, Alheid GF, Beltramino CA (1985): Amygdala. In Paxinos G (ed): "The Rat Nervous System," Vol 1. New York: Academic Press, pp 223–334.

Desimone R, Gross CG (1979): Visual areas in the temporal cortex of the macaque. Brain Res 178:363–380.

De Vito JL (1982): Afferent projections to the hypothalamic area controlling emotional responses. Brain Res 252:213–226.

Dewson JH, Cowey A, Weiskrantz L (1970): Disruptions of auditory sequence discrimination by unilateral and bilateral cortical ablations of superior temporal gyrus in monkey. Exp Neurol 28:529–548.

Dreifuss JJ, Murphy JT, Gloor P (1968): Contrasting effects of two identified amygdaloid efferent pathways on single hypothalamic neurons. J Neurophysiol 31:237–248.

Earle KM, Baldwin M, Penfield W (1953): Incisural sclerosis and temporal lobe seizures produced by hippocampal herniation at birth. Arch Neurol Psychiat 69:27–42.

Eleftheriou BE (ed) (1972): "The Neurobiology of the Amygdala." New York: Plenum Press.

Engel J (1989): "Seizures and Epilepsy." Philadelphia: FA Davis, 536 pp.

Engel J, Brown WJ, Kuhl DE, Phelps ME, Mazziotta JC, Crandall PH (1982): Pathological findings underlying focal temporal lobe hypometabolism in partial epilepsy. Ann Neurol 12:518–528.

Engel J Jr, Cahan L (1986): Potential relevance of kindling to human partial epilepsy. In Wada JA (ed): "Kindling 3." New York: Raven Press, pp 37–54.

Everitt BJ, Cador M, Robbins TW (1989): Interactions between the amygdala and ventral striatum in stimulus-reward associations: Studies using a second-order schedule of sexual reinforcement. Neuroscience 30:63–75.

Falconer MA, Serafetinides EA, Corsellis JAN (1964): Etiology and pathogenesis of temporal lobe epilepsy. Arch Neurol 10:233–248.

Feindel W (1974): Temporal lobe seizures. In Vinken PJ, Bruyn GW, Magnus O, de Haas L (eds): "Clinical Neurology," Vol 15. Amsterdam, New York: North Holland/Elsevier, pp 87–106.

Feindel W, Penfield W (1954): Localization of discharge in temporal lobe automatism. AMA Arch Neurol Psychiat 72:605–630.

Feindel W, Rasmussen T (1990): Temporal lobectomy with amygdalectomy and minimal hippocampal resection: Review of 100 cases. Can J Neurol Sci (Suppl) (In press).

Ferguson SM, Rayport M, Gardener E, Kass W, Weiner H, Reiser MF (1969): Similarities in mental content of psychiatric states, spontaneous seizures, dreams and responses to electrical brain stimulation in patients with temporal lobe epilepsy. Psychosom Med 31:479–498.

Gallagher M, Graham PW, Holland PC (1990): The amygdala central nucleus and appetitive pavlovian conditioning: Lesions impair one class of conditioned behavior. J Neurosci 10:1906–1911.

Gastaut H (1952): Corrélations entre le système nerveux végétatif et le système de la vie de relation dans le rhinencéphale. J Physiol (Paris) 44:431–470.

Gastaut H (1955): Les troubles du comportement alimentaire chez les épileptiques psychomoteurs. Rev Neurol 92:55–62.

Gastaut H, Gastaut JL, Gonçalves e Silva GE, Fernandez Sanchez GR (1975): Relative frequency of different types of epilepsy: A study employing the classification of the International League Against Epilepsy. Epilepsia 16:457–461.

Gaustaut H, Vigouroux M, Fischer-Williams M (1958): Partial epilepsies with localized expression (still called "Jacksonian") and those with diffuse expression (still called "psychomotor"). In Baldwin M, Bailey P (eds): "Temporal Lobe Epilepsy." Springfield, Ill: Charles C Thomas Publishers, pp. 13–22.

Gibbs FA (1956): Abnormal electrical activity in the temporal region and its relationship to abnormalities of behavior. Res Pub Assoc Res New Ment Dis 36:278–292.

Gloor P (1955): Electrophysiological studies on the connections of the amygdaloid nucleus in the cat. Part I: The neuronal organization of the amygdaloid projection system. Electroenceph Clin Neurophysiol 7:223–242.

Gloor P (1960): Amygdala. In Field J, Magoun HW, Hall VE (eds): "Handbook of Physiology. Section 1: Neurophysiology. Vol II." Washington DC: American Psychological Society, pp 1395–1420.

Gloor P (1972): Temporal lobe epilepsy: Its possible contribution to the understanding of the functional significance of the amygdala and of its interaction with neocortical-temporal mechanisms. In Eleftheriou BE (ed): "The Neurobiology of the Amygdala." New York: Plenum Press, pp 423–457.

Gloor P (1975a): Electrophysiological studies of the amygdala (stimulations and recording), their possible contribution to the understanding of neural mechanisms of aggression. In Fields WS, Sweet WH (eds): "Neural Bases of Violence and Aggression." St. Louis: Waner H. Green, pp 5–40.

Gloor P (1975b): Physiology of the limbic system. In Penry JK, Daly DD (eds): "Complex Partial Seizures and Their Treatment." Adv Neurol 11:27–55.

Gloor P (1986a): Consciousness as a neurological concept in epileptology: A critical review. Epilepsia 27(Suppl 2):S14–S26.

Gloor P (1986b): The role of the human limbic system in perception, memory, and affect: Lessons from temporal lobe epilepsy. In Doane BK, Livingston KE (eds): "The Limbic System: Functional Organization and Clinical Disorders." New York: Raven Press, pp 159–169.

Gloor P (1987): Volume conductor principles: Their application to the surface and depth electroencephalogram. In Wieser HG, Elger CE (eds): "Presurgical Evaluation of Epileptics." Berlin, Heidelberg: Springer-Verlag, 59–68.

Gloor P (1990): Experiential phenomena of temporal lobe epilepsy: Facts and hypotheses. Brain 113:1673–1674.

Gloor P (1991): Neurobiological substrates of ictal behavioral changes. In Smith D, Treiman D, Trimble M (eds): Adv Neurol 55:1–34.

Gloor P: Mesial temporal sclerosis: Historical background and an overview from a modern perspective. In Lüders H (ed): "Surgery of Epilepsy." New York: Raven Press (in press).

Gloor P, Feindel W (1963): Affective behaviour and temporal lobe. In Monnier M (ed): "Physiologie und Pathophysiologie des Vegetativen Nervensystems." Stuttgart 2: Hippokrates Verlag, pp 685–716.

Gloor P, Olivier A, Ives J (1980): Loss of consciousness in temporal lobe seizures: Observations obtained with stereotaxic depth electrode recordings and stimulations. In Canger R, Angeleri F, Penry JK (eds): "Advances in Epileptology: XIth Epilepsy International Symposium." New York: Raven Press, pp 349–353.

Gloor P, Olivier A, Quesney LF (1981): The role of the amygdala in the expression of psychic phenomena in temporal lobe seizures. In Ben-Ari Y (ed): "The Amygdaloid Complex." INSERM Symposium No. 20. Amsterdam, New York, Oxford: Elsevier/North Holland Biomedical Press, pp 489–498.

Gloor P, Olivier A, Quesney LF, Andermann F, Horowitz S (1982): The role of the limbic system in experiential phenomena of temporal lobe epilepsy. Ann Neurol 12:129–143.

Goddard GV (1964): Functions of the amygdala. Psychol Bull 62:89–109.

Goldman-Rakic PS (1987): Circuitry of primate prefrontal cortex and regulation of behavior by representational knowledge. In Plum F, Mountcastle V (eds): "Higher Cortical Functions. Handbook of Physiology." Washington, DC: Am Physiol Soc 5:373–417.

Goldman-Rakic PS (1988a): Changing concepts of cortical connectivity: Parallel distributed networks. In Rakic P, Singer W (eds): "Neurobiology of Neocortex." Dahlem Workshop on Neurology of Neocortex, 1987. Berlin, Life Sciences Rep #42, New York: Wiley, pp 177–202.

Goldman-Rakic PS (1988b): Topography of cognition: Parallel distributed networks in primate association cortex. Ann Rev Neurosci 11:137–156.

Gross CG, Bruce CJ, Desimone R, Fleming J, Gattas R (1981): Cortical visual areas of the temporal lobe: Three areas in the macaque. In Woolsey CN (ed): "Cortical Sensory Organization. Vol. 2. Multiple Visual Areas." Clifton, NJ: Humana Press, pp 187–216.

Halgren E, Walter RD, Cherlow DG, Crandall PH (1978): Mental phenomena evoked by electrical stimulation of the human hippocampal formation and amygdala. Brain 101:83–117.

Hausser-Hauw C, Bancaud J (1987): Gustatory hallucinations in epileptic seizures. Brain 110:339–359.

Henke PG (1980): The centromedial amygdala and gastric pathology. Physiol Behav 25:107–112.

Henry TR, Mazziotta JC, Engel J, Christenson PT, Zhang JX, Phelps ME, Kuhl DE (1990): Quantifying interictal metabolic activity in human temporal lobe epilepsy. J Cerebral Blood Flow Metab 10:748–757.

Herzog AW, van Hoesen GW (1976): Temporal neocortical afferent connections to the amygdala in the rhesus monkey. Brain Res 115:57–396.

Hilton SM, Zbrozyna AW (1963): Amygdaloid region for defense reactions and its afferent pathways to the brainstem. J Physiol (Lond) 165:160–173.

Hitchcock JM, Sananes CB, Davis M (1989): Sensitization of the startle reflex by footshock: Blockade by lesions of the central nucleus of the amygdala on its efferent pathway to the brainstem. Behav Neurosci 103:509–518.

Hopkins DA, McLean JH, Takeuchi Y (1981): Amygdalotegmental projections: Light and electron microscopic studies utilizing anterograde degeneration and the anterograde and retrograde transport of horseradish peroxidase (HRP). In Ben-Ari Y (ed): "The Amygdaloid Complex." Amsterdam, New York: Elsevier/North-Holland Biomedical Press, pp 133–147.

Insausti R, Amaral DG, Cowan WM (1987): The entorhinal cortex of the monkey. II. Cortical afferents. J Comp Neurol 264:356–395.

Iwai E, Yukie M (1987): Amygdalofugal and amygdalopetal connections with modality-specific visual cortical areas in macaques (Macaca fuscata, M. mulatta, and M. fascicularis). J Comp Neurol 261:362–387.

Iwata J, LeDoux JE, Meeley MP, Arneric S, Reis DJ (1986): Intrinsic neurons in the amygdaloid field projected to by the medial geniculate body mediate emotional responses conditioned to acoustic stimuli. Brain Res 383:195–214.

Jackson JH (1958a): On temporary mental disorders after epileptic paroxysms. West Riding Lunatic Asylum Medical Reports 1875; 5:105–129. Reprinted in Taylor J (ed): "Selected

Writings of John Hughlings Jackson, Vol. 1: On Epilepsy and Epileptiform Convulsions." New York: Basic Books, pp 119–134.

Jackson JH (1958b): Lectures on the diagnosis of epilepsy. Lecture III, Medical Times and Gazette *1879*; 1:141–143. Reprinted in "Selected Writings of John Hughlings Jackson, Vol. 1: On Epilepsy and Epileptiform Convulsions." New York: Basic Books, pp 295–307.

Jackson JH (1888): On a particular variety of epilepsy ("intellectual aura"), one case with symptoms of organic brain disease. Brain 11:179–207.

Jackson JH, Beevor CE (1889): Case of tumour of the right temporo-sphenoidal lobe, bearing on the localization of the sense of smell and on the interpretation of a particular variety of epilepsy. Brain 12:346–357.

Jackson JH, Coleman WS (1898): Case of epilepsy with tasting movements and "dreamy state"—very small patch of softening in the left uncinate gyrus. Brain 21:580–590.

Jackson JH, Stewart JP (1899): Epileptic attacks with a warning of a crude sensation of smell and with the intellectual aura (dreamy state) in a patient who had symptoms pointing to gross organic disease of the right temporo-sphenoidal lobe. Brain 22:534–549.

Jacome DE, McLain LW, Fitzgerald R (1980): Postural reflex gelastic seizures. Arch Neurol 37:249–251.

Jasper H (1964): Some physiological mechanisms involved in epileptic automatisms. Epilepsia 5:1–26.

Jasper HH, Rasmussen T (1958): Studies of clinical and electrical responses to deep temporal stimulation in man with some consideration of functional anatomy. Res Publ Assoc Res New Ment Dis 36:316–334.

Kaada BR (1951): Somato-motor, autonomic and electrocorticographic responses to electrical stimulation of "rhinencephalic" and other structures in primates, cat and dog. Acta Physiol Scand 24(Suppl 83), 285 pp.

Kaada BR (1972): Stimulation and regional ablation of the amygdaloid complex with reference to functional representations. In Eleftheriou BE (ed): "The Neurobiology of the Amygdala." New York: Plenum Press, pp 205–261.

Kaada BR, Andersen P, Jansen J (1954): Stimulation of the amygdaloid nuclear complex in unanesthetized cats. Neurology 4:48–64.

Kaada BR, Jasper H (1952): Respiratory responses to stimulation of temporal pole, insular and hippocampal and limbic gyri in man. Arch Neurol Psychiat 68:609–619.

Kapp BS, Gallagher M, Frysinger RC, Applegate CD (1981): The amygdala, emotion and cardiovascular conditioning. In Ben-Ari Y (ed): "The Amygdaloid Complex." Amsterdam, New York: Elsevier/North Holland Biomedical Press, pp 355–366.

Kapp BS, Markgraf CG, Schwaber JS, Bilyk-Spafford T (1989): The organization of dorsal medullary projections to the central amygdaloid nucleus and parabrachial nuclei in the rabbit. Neuroscience 30:717–732.

Kelley AE, Domesick VB, Nauta WJH (1982): The amygdalostriatal projection in the rat. An anatomical study by anterograde and retrograde tracing methods. Neuroscience 7:615–630.

Kesner RP, Walser RD, Winzenried G (1989): Central but not basolateral amygdala mediates memory for positive affective experiences. Behav Brain Res 33:189–195.

Kling A (1972): Effects of amygdalectomy on social-affective behavior in nonhuman primates. In Eleftheriou BE (ed): "The Neurobiology of the Amygdala." New York, London: Plenum Press, 511–536.

Klingler J, Gloor P (1960): The connections of the amygdala and of the anterior temporal cortex in the human brain. J Comp Neurol 115:333–369.

Kohonen T, Oja E, Lehtiö P (1981): Storage and processing of information in distributed associative memory systems. In Hinton JE, Anderson JA (eds): "Parallel Models of Associative Memory." Hillsdale, NJ: Lawrence Erlbaum, pp 105–143.

Krettek JE, Price JL (1978): Amygdaloid projections to subcortical structures within the basal forebrain and brainstem in the rat and cat. J Comp Neurol 178:225–254.

LeDoux JE, Cicchetti P, Xagoraris A, Romanski LM (1990a): The lateral amygdaloid nucleus: Sensory interface of the amygdala in fear conditioning. J Neurosci 10:1062–1069.

LeDoux JE, Farb C, Ruggiero DA (1990b): Topographic organization of neurons in the acoustic thalamus that project to the amygdala. J Neurosci 10:1043–1054.

LeDoux JE, Ruggiero DA, Reis DJ (1985): Projections to the subcortical forebrain from anatomically defined regions of the medial geniculate body of the rat. J Comp Neurol 242:182–213.

MacLean PD, Delgado JMR (1953): Electrical and chemical stimulation of fronto-temporal portion of the limbic system in waking animal. Electroenceph Clin Neurophysiol 5:91–100.

Macrae D (1954): Isolated fear; a temporal lobe aura. Neurology 4:497–505.

Magnus O, Penfield W, Jasper H (1952): Mastication and consciousness in epileptic seizures. Acta Psychiat Neurol Scand 27:91–115.

Margerison JH, Corsellis JAN (1966): Epilepsy and the temporal lobes: A clinical, electroencephalographic and neuropathological study of the brain in epilepsy, with particular reference to the temporal lobes. Brain 89:499–530.

Mark VH, Ervin FR, Sweet WH (1972): Deep temporal lobe stimulation in man. In Eleftheriou BE (ed): "The Neurobiology of the Amygdala." New York: Plenum Press, pp 485–507.

Mehler WR (1980): Subcortical afferent connections of the amygdala in the monkey. J Comp Neurol 190:733–762.

Mishkin M (1966): Visual mechanisms beyond the striate cortex. In Russel R (ed): "Frontiers in Physiological Psychology." New York: Academic Press, pp 93–119.

Mishkin M (1972): Cortical visual areas and their interactions. In Karczmar AG, Eccles JC (eds): "Symposium on the Brain and Human Behavior." New York, Heidelberg, Berlin: Springer Verlag, pp 187–208.

Mishkin M, Ungerleider LG, Macko KA (1983): Object vision and spatial vision; two cortical pathways. Trends Neurosci 6:414–417.

Mufson EG, Mesulam MM, Pandya DN (1981): Insular interconnections with the amygdala in the rhesus monkey. Neuroscience 6:1231–1248.

Mullan S, Penfield W (1959): Illusions of comparative interpretation and emotion. Arch Neurol Psychiat 81:269–284.

Munari C, Bancaud J, Bonis A, Stoffels C, Szikla G, Talairach J (1980): Impairment of consciousness in temporal lobe seizures: A stereoelectroencephalographic study. In Canger R, Angeleri F, Penry JK (eds): "Advances in Epileptology." The XI Epilepsy International Symposium. New York: Raven Press, pp 111–114.

Nakamura Y, Kubo Y (1978): Masticatory rhythm in intracellular potential of trigeminal motoneurons induced by stimulation of orbital cortex and amygdala in cats. Brain Res 148:504–509.

Nauta WJH (1961): Fiber degeneration following lesions of the amygdaloid complex in the monkey. J Anat (Lond) 95:515–531.

Neff WD, Diamond IT, Casseday JH (1975): Behavioral studies of auditory discrimination: Central nervous system. In Keidel WD, Neff WD (eds): "Handbook of Sensory Physiology. Auditory System. Vol 5." New York: Springer Verlag, pp 307–400.

Norita M, Kawamura K (1980): Subcortical afferents to the monkey amygdala: An HRP study. Brain Res 190:225–230.

Olds J (1956): A preliminary mapping of electrical reinforcing effects in the rat brain. J Comp Physiol Psychol 49:281–285.

Ottersen OP (1982): Connections of the amygdala of the rat. IV Corticoamygdaloid and intraamygdaloid connections as studied with axonal transport of horseradish peroxidase. J Comp Neurol 205:30–48.

Ounsted C, Lindsay J, Norman R (1966): "Biological Factors in Temporal Lobe Epilepsy. Clinics in Developmental Medicine No. 27." London: The Spastics Society Medical Education and Information Unit in association with William Heinemann Medical Books Ltd.

Pandya DN, van Hoesen GW, Domesick VB (1973): A cingulo-amygdaloid projection in the rhesus monkey. Brain Res 61:369–373.

Pandya DN, Yeterian EH (1985): Architecture and connections of cortical association areas. In Peters A, Jones EG (eds): "Cerebral Cortex, Vol 4, Association and Auditory Cortices." New York, London: Plenum Press.

Penfield W (1952): Memory mechanisms. Arch Neurol Psychiat 167:178–191.

Penfield W (1954): Temporal lobe epilepsy. Br J Surg 41:1–7.

Penfield W (1955a): The permanent record of the stream of consciousness. Proc 14th International Congress of Psychology, Montreal. Acta Psychol 11:47–69.

Penfield W (1955b): The twenty-ninth Maudsley Lecture: The role of the temporal cortex in certain psychical phenomena. J Ment Sci 101:451–465.

Penfield W, Jasper H (1954): "Epilepsy and the Functional Anatomy of the Human Brain." Boston: Little, Brown.

Penfield W, Perot P (1963): The brain's record of auditory and visual experience—A final summary and discussion. Brain 86:595–696.

Penfield W, Roberts L (1959): "Speech and Brain Mechanisms." Princeton, NJ: Princeton University Press, 186 pp.

Porrino LJ, Crane AM, Goldman-Rakic PS (1981): Direct and indirect pathways from the amygdala to the frontal lobe in the rhesus monkeys. J Comp Neurol 198:121–136.

Price JL (1981): The efferent projections of the amygdaloid complex in the rat, cat and monkey. In Ben Ari Y (ed): "The Amygdaloid Complex." Amsterdam: Elsevier/North Holland Biomedical Press, pp 121–132.

Price JL, Amaral DG (1981): An autoradiographic study of the projections of the central nucleus of the monkey amygdala. J Neurosci 1:1242–1259.

Quesney LF (1986): Clinical and EEG features of complex partial seizures of temporal lobe origin. Epilepsia 27(Suppl 2):S27–S45.

Racine RJ, Burnham WM, Gilbert M, Kairiss EW (1986): Kindling mechanisms. I. Electrophysiological studies. In Wada JA (ed): "Kindling 3." New York: Raven Press, pp 263–282.

Rasmussen T, Feindel W (1990): Temporal lobectomy: Review of 100 cases with hippocampectomy. Can J Neurol Sci (Suppl) (in press).

Rémillard GM, Andermann F, Gloor P, Olivier A, Martin JB (1981): Water drinking as ictal behavior in complex partial seizures. Neurology 31:117–124.

Rémillard GM, Andermann F, Testa GF, Gloor P, Aubé M, Martin J, Feindel W, Guberman A, Simpson C (1983): Sexual manifestations predominate in women with temporal lobe epilepsy: A finding suggesting sexual dimorphism in the human brain. Neurology 33:323–330.

Rosene DI, van Hoesen GW (1977): Hippocampal efferents reach widespread areas of cerebral cortex and amygdala in the rhesus monkey. Science 198:315–317.

Rumelhart DE, McClelland JL, and the PDP Research Group (1986): "Parallel Distributed Processing. Explanations in the Microstructure of Cognition. Vols 1, 2." Cambridge, MA: MIT Press.

Russchen FT (1982): Amygdalopetal projections in the cat. I. Cortical afferent connections. A study with retrograde and anterograde tracing techniques. J Comp Neurol 206:159–179.

Russchen FT, Amaral DG, Price JL (1987): The afferent input to the magnocellular division of the mediodorsal nucleus of the thalamus in the monkey, *Macaca fascicularis*. J Comp Neurol 256:175–210.

Russchen FT, Amaral DG, Price JL (1985a): The afferent connections of the substantia innominata in the monkey, *Macaca fascicularis*. J Comp Neurol 242:1–27.

Russchen FT, Amaral DG, Price JL (1985b): The amygdalostriatal projections in the monkey. An anterograde tracing study. Brain Res 329:241–257.

Russchen FT, Price JL (1984): Amygdalostriatal projections in the rat. Topographical organization and fiber morphology shown using the lectic PHA-L as an anterograde tracer. Neurosci Lett 47:15–22.

Saint-Hilaire JM, Gilbert M, Bouvier G, Barbeau A (1980): Epilepsy and aggression: Two cases with depth electrode studies. In Robb P (ed): "Epilepsy Updated: Causes and Treatment." Miami: Symposia Specialists, pp 145–176.

Sano K, Malamud N (1953): Clinical significance of sclerosis of the cornu ammonis. Arch Neurol Psychiat 70:40–53.

Saunders RC, Rosene DL (1988): A comparison of the efferents of the amygdala and the hippocampal formation in the rhesus monkey: I. Convergence in the entorhinal, prorhinal and perirhinal cortices. J Comp Neurol 271:153–184.

Saunders RC, Rosene DL, van Hoesen GW (1988): A comparison of the efferents of the amygdala and the hippocampal formation in the rhesus monkey: II. Reciprocal and non-reciprocal connections. J Comp Neurol 271:185–207.

Scalia F, Winans SS (1975): The differential projections of the olfactory bulb and accessory olfactory bulb in mammals. J Comp Neurol 161:31–56.

So N, Gloor P, Quesney F, Jones-Gotman M, Olivier A, Andermann F (1989): Depth electrode investigations in patients with bitemporal epileptiform abnormalities. Ann Neurol 25:423–431.

Spencer SS, Spencer DD, Williamson PD, Mattson R (1983): Sexual automatisms in complex partial seizures. Neurology 33:527–533.

Spiegler BF, Mishkin M (1981): Evidence for the sequential participation of inferior temporal cortex and amygdala in the acquisition of stimulus reward associations. Behav Brain Res 3:303–317.

Spielmeyer W (1925): Zur Pathogenese örtlich elektiver Gehirnveränderungen. Z Neurol Psychiatr 99:756–776.

Spiers PA, Schomer DL, Blume HW, Mesulam M-M (1985): Temporo-limbic epilepsy and behavior. In Mesulam M-M (ed): "Principles of Behavioral Neurology." Philadelphia: FA Davis, pp 289–326.

Spyer KM (1989): Neural mechanisms involved in cardiovascular control during affective behaviour. Trends Neurosci 12:506–513.

Stevens JR, Mark VH, Erwin F, Pacheco P, Suematsu K (1969): Deep temporal stimulation in man. Long latency long lasting psychological changes. Arch Neurol 21:157–169.

Stoffels C, Munari C, Bonis A, Bancaud J, Talairach J (1980): Manifestations génitales et "sexuelles" lors des crises épileptiques partielles chez l'homme. Rev EEG Neurophysiol (Paris) 10:386–392.

Strauss E, Risser A, Jones MW (1982): Fear responses in patients with epilepsy. Arch Neurol 39:626–630.

Strauss E, Wada J, Kosaka B (1983): Spontaneous facial expressions occurring at onset of focal seizure activity. Arch Neurol 40:545–547.

Takeuchi Y, Satoda T, Matsushima R, Uemura-Sumi M (1988a): Amygdaloid pathway to the trigeminal motor nucleus via the pontine reticular formation in the rat. Brain Res Bull 21:829–833.

Takeuchi Y, Satoda T, Matsushima R (1988b): Amygdaloid projections to commissural interneurons for masticatory motoneurons. Brain Res 21:123–127.

Taylor DC, Lochery M (1987): Temporal lobe epilepsy: Origin and significance of simple and complex auras. J Neurol Neurosurg Psychiat 50:673–681.

Tigges J, Tigges M, Cross MA, McBride RL, Letbetter WD, Anschel S (1982): Subcortical structures projecting to visual cortical areas in squirrel monkey. J Comp Neurol 209:29–40.

Tigges J, Walker LC, Tigges M (1983): Subcortical projections to the occipital and parietal lobes of the chimpanzee brain. J Comp Neurol 220:106–115.

Treiman DM (1986): Epilepsy and violence: Medical and legal issues. Epilepsia 27:S77–S104.

Treiman DH, Delgado-Escueta AV (1981): Aggression during fear and flight in complex partial seizures: A CCTV-EEG analysis. Epilepsia 22:246.

Turner BH (1981): The cortical sequence and terminal distribution of sensory related afferents to the amygdaloid complex of the rat and monkey. In Ben-Ari Y (ed): "The Amygdaloid Complex." Amsterdam, New York: Elsevier/North Holland Biomedical Press, pp 51–62.

Turner BH, Gupta KC, Mishkin M (1978): The locus and cytoarchitecture of the projection areas of the olfactory bulb in *Macaca mulatta.* J Comp Neurol 177:381–396.

Turner BH, Mishkin M, Knapp M (1988): Organization of the amygdalopetal projections from modality-specific cortical association areas in the monkey. J Comp Neurol 191:515–543.

Ungerleider LG, Mishkin M (1982): Two cortical visual systems. In Ingle DJ, Goodale MA, Mansfield RJW (eds): "Analysis of Visual Behavior." Cambridge, MA: MIT Press, pp 549–586.

van Buren JM (1958): Some autonomic concomitants of ictal automatism: A study of temporal lobe attacks. Brain 81:505–528.

van Buren JM, Ajmone Marsan C (1960): A correlation of autonomic and EEG components in temporal lobe epilepsy. Arch Neurol 3:683–703.

van Hoesen GW (1981): The differential distribution, diversity and sprouting of cortical projections to the amygdala in the rhesus monkey. In Ben-Ari Y (ed): "The Amygdaloid Complex." Amsterdam, New York: Elsevier/North Holland, pp 77–90.

van Hoesen GW (1982): The parahippocampal gyrus. New observations regarding its cortical connections in the monkey. Trends Neurosci 5:345–350.

van Reeth PC (1959): Un cas d'epilepsie temporale autoprovoquée et le problème de l'autostimulation cérébrale hédonique. Acta Neurol 59:490–495.

Veazey RB, Amaral DG, Cowan WM (1982): The morphology and connections of the posterior hypothalamus in the cynomolgus monkey (*Macaca fascicularis*). II. Efferent connections. J Comp Neurol 207:135–156.

Vogt O (1925): Der Begriff der Pathoklise. J Psychol Neurol (Leipzig) 31:245–255.

Vogt C, Vogt O (1937): Sitz und Wesen der Krankheiten im Lichte der topistischen Hirnforschung und des Variierens der Tiere. I. Teil: Befunde der topistischen Hirnforschung als Beitrag zur Lehre vom Krankheitssitz. J Psychol Neurol (Leipzig) 47:241–457.

Weil A (1955): Depressive reactions associated with temporal lobe-uncinate seizures. J New Ment Dis 113:149–157.

Weil AA (1959): Ictal emotions occurring in temporal lobe dysfunction. Arch Neurol 1:149–157.

Weingarten SM, Cherlow DG, Halgren E (1976): The relationship of hallucinations to the depth structures of the temporal lobe. In Sweet WH, Obrador S, Martin-Rodriguez JG (eds): "Neurosurgical Treatment in Psychiatry." Baltimore: University Park Press, pp 553–568.

Whitlock DG, Nauta WJH (1956): Subcortical projections from temporal neocortex in *Macaca mulatta.* J Comp Neurol 106:183–212.

Wieser HG (1979): "Psychische Anfälle" und deren stereo-electroenzephalographisches Korrelat. Z EEG-EMG 10:197–206.

Wieser HG (1983): "Electroclinical Features of Psychomotor Seizure. A Stereoelectroencephalographic Study of Ictal Symptoms and Chronotopographical Seizure Patterns Including Clinical Effects of Intracerebral Stimulation." London: Butterworths.

Williams D (1956): The structure of emotions reflected in epileptic experiences. Brain 79:29–67.

Williamson PD, Spencer DD, Spencer SS, Novelly RA, Mattson RH (1985): Complex partial seizures of frontal lobe origin. Ann Neurol 18:497–504.

Wurtz RH, Olds J (1963): Amygdaloid stimulation and operant reinforcement in the rat. J Comp Physiol Psychol 56:941–949.

Zbrozyna AW (1972): The organization of the defense reaction elicited from amygdala and its connections. In Eleftheriou BE (ed): "Neurobiology of the Amygdala." New York: Plenum Press, pp 597–606.

The Amygdala: Neurobiological Aspects of Emotion,
Memory, and Mental Dysfunction, pages 539–560
© 1992 Wiley-Liss, Inc.

21
Kindling and the Amygdala

DONALD P. CAIN

Department of Psychology, University of Western Ontario, London, Ontario, Canada

INTRODUCTION

Kindling is an experimental model of epilepsy that results from the repeated application of electrical stimulation or pharmacological agents to brain tissue. The development of seizures in response to these treatments had been observed by many researchers during work on brain self-stimulation and other topics, but it was usually regarded as a curiosity or an annoyance. It was Graham Goddard (1964, 1969) who observed kindled seizures during studies on the effect on learning of electrical and pharmacological stimulation of the amygdala, and first realized the importance of the phenomenon as an epilepsy model and possibly also as a general model of plasticity in the brain.

The research that led to the discovery of kindling, and the first efforts to systematically study kindling itself, concentrated on the amygdala (Goddard, 1967; Goddard et al., 1969), which remains the most frequently studied structure in kindling to this day. I review here the basic phenomena and mechanisms of amygdala kindling and the role of the amygdala/pyriform region in kindling of the forebrain in the mammal. Comprehensive general reviews of kindling have been published (Racine, 1978; Wada, 1978; Goddard, 1983; McNamara, 1986; Corcoran, 1988).

METHODS FOR KINDLING

Goddard's original work defined the standard methods for the kindling of seizures, the most common of which is the application of a brief (1 or 2 sec) train of electrical pulses at 60 Hz once daily through a chronically implanted thin wire electrode. Less common but no less effective is the repeated application of small amounts of pharmacological agents (e.g., carbachol, pentylenetetrazol, opioid peptides) once every 24 or 48 h. The route of administration can be peripheral if the agent readily passes into the brain, or central if it does not.

Address correspondence to: Dr. Donald P. Cain, Department of Psychology, University of Western Ontario, London, Ontario N6A 5C2, Canada.

The prime feature of kindling is that an unvarying stimulus that initially does not provoke a behavioral convulsion comes to have that ability if it is repeated sufficiently. This was the criterion for kindling in Goddard's initial work because he did not routinely record electrographic activity during the procedure. However, early work by Racine (1972a,b) showed that when the EEG was monitored in the stimulated structure, epileptiform afterdischarge (AD) invariably accompanied the kindling procedure. Further, Racine (1972b) showed that the occurrence of AD was essential for kindling, and that stimulation that never evoked AD was completely ineffective no matter how many times it was applied. Today, the recording of AD in the stimulated structure is routine, and the usual kindling rate measure is the number of ADs required for the development of a generalized convulsion.

BASIC PHENOMENA OF AMYGDALA KINDLING

Kindling involves at least two plastic phenomena that occur progressively over trials in the kindling process. The first is the reduction in the threshold current required to evoke AD (ADT). This is a local phenomenon that occurs whether AD is evoked or not. Thus, stimulation that is above or below the initial ADT will gradually lower the ADT on subsequent sessions, but it will not lower the ADT in other, nonstimulated structures (Racine, 1972a). In the rat amygdala the initial ADT is typically in the range of 40–100 uA depending on the details of the experimental arrangements (type and duration of stimulation, electrode design, etc.), and is among the lowest in the brain. The amygdala undergoes a significantly greater ADT reduction after repeated electrical stimulation than the hippocampus (Racine, 1972a). Interestingly, sub-ADT stimulation appears to reduce the amygdala ADT more than supra-ADT stimulation (Racine, 1972a; Pinel et al., 1976). However, there is no relation between initial ADT or ADT reduction and the rate of kindling (Racine, 1972a). The ADT-reduction effect has received relatively little attention and little is known about its mechanism. Consequently, it is not discussed further.

The second phenomenon is the progressive growth and propagation of AD throughout much of the brain, culminating in behavioral convulsions, and it is this that is typically referred to by the term "kindling." Racine (1972a,b) pioneered the routine recording of AD and documented the changes that take place during the kindling process: increases in AD amplitude, frequency, complexity, duration, and propagation. In the rat amygdala the initial AD is typically 6 sec long, is confined to the stimulated amygdala, and causes little behavioral change apart from arrest of movement. The 12th AD is typically about 60 sec long and propagates widely, and also is accompanied by a sequence of convulsive behaviors involving automatisms of the facial musculature, headnodding, clonic movements of the forelimbs, rearing on the hindlimbs, and loss of postural control: a generalized stage 5 convulsion. During the intervening sessions the animal will have shown progressive recruitment of these behaviors in the order given, and these successive stages in convulsion expression have been labeled stages 1–5 by Racine (1972b). Although the behaviors displayed by larger mammals during amygdala kindling are somewhat more elaborate than those of the rat, they are similar in their basic elements, and they contrast sharply with seizures kindled from anterior neocortex (Burnham, 1978).

Although the behavioral endpoint in amygdala kindling in the rat is typically Racine's stage 5, Pinel and Rovner (1978a) have documented the emergence of stages 6–8 with running fits and tonic convulsions if the stimulations are repeated sufficiently.

Kindling appears to involve permanent changes in the brain's response to the stimulation. Early work showed that amygdala kindling persisted with relatively little loss after intervals of 3–12 months (Goddard et al., 1969; Wada et al., 1974; Wada and Osawa, 1976). More recent work has shown near-complete retention of amygdala kindling for periods as long as 868 days in primates (Wada, 1980), which is the longest period tested. In all reported cases of partial fallback from the maximal kindled response, significantly fewer additional stimulations were required for rekindling than for initial kindling. We have recently examined the permanence of partial amygdala kindling in the rat and found that partial kindling to stage 1 or stage 3 shows the same degree of permanence as full kindling to stage 5 (Dennison et al., 1989, 1990). Collectively, these results show that kindling persists for periods that are long in relation to the life span of the species being studied, and that kindling is substantially more long lasting than long-term potentiation (LTP), another prominent model of neural plasticity (Racine et al., 1983).

In contrast to the local nature of ADT reduction, kindling exhibits "transfer" to other sites in the kindled brain (Goddard et al., 1969; Racine, 1972b; Cain, 1986). That is, the kindling of one site will usually facilitate the subsequent kindling of another site in the same brain. This indicates that kindling involves transsynaptic changes at some distance from the initially stimulated site.

Two major forms of spontaneous epileptic event occur following amygdala kindling: interictal discharges (IIDs) and spontaneous seizures. Interestingly, in rats the amygdala-pyriform region appears to generate the bulk of IIDs even when the animals are kindled from other sites (Kairiss et al., 1984; Racine et al., 1988a). Spontaneous seizures have been observed in all mammalian species kindled in the amygdala in which an effort has been made to monitor adequately (Wada et al., 1974; Pinel et al., 1975a; Wada and Osawa, 1976; Pinel and Rovner, 1978a,b; Wauqier et al., 1979; Corcoran et al., 1984), although additional stimulation beyond the development of stage 5 appears to be necessary for spontaneous seizures in the rat (Pinel et al., 1975a). In kindled photosensitive baboons, spontaneous seizures are primary generalized, although there is no relation between the degree of photosensitivity, the rate of initial kindling, and the occurrence of spontaneous seizures (Wada and Osawa, 1976; Corcoran et al., 1984). More generally, there seems to be no clear relation between the rate of initial amygdala kindling and the propensity for spontaneous seizures across species. Thus, cats and photosensitive baboons kindle more slowly than rats, but show spontaneous seizures more readily than do rats.

ADVANTAGES OF AMYGDALA KINDLING

Amygdala kindling is an extremely robust phenomenon that occurs reliably in almost every individual animal that is properly prepared and stimulated, including preweanling rats (Gilbert and Cain, 1982; Moshe et al., 1986). Seizure development progresses gradually and predictably and is essentially under the control of the experimenter. Although much of the mammalian brain supports kindling, kindling in the amygdala and closely related sites (see below) appears to be more rapid and reliable than kindling in other forebrain sites such as anterior neocortex, hippocampus, and dentate gyrus (Racine et al., 1977; Burnham, 1978; Seidel and Corcoran, 1986; Grace et al., 1990). This reliability and the ease with which measures of seizure development can be taken has made it attractive as a model for the study of the epileptogenic or antiepileptic effects of substances (e.g., Babington and Wedeking, 1973; Schwark et al., 1985; Cain et al., 1989a) as well as for the study of basic epileptic mechanisms. An in vivo preparation for an electrophysiological form of kindling in the brain slice has been developed for study of the microphysiological events in kindling, but to date this has been applied only to the hippocampus (Stasheff et al., 1985). The application of this approach to the amygdala-pyriform area would complement the large body of work that has been done on this region in the intact animal.

SPECIES DIFFERENCES

Amygdala kindling has been studied in a variety of mammalian species and strains (see Table I). There is considerable variability across species and across

TABLE I. Amygdala Kindling in Various Mammalian Species

Species	Strain	Mean ADs to Generalized Convulsion	Reference
Mouse	DBA/2	2.2	Leech and McIntyre, 1976
	C3H/He	13.5	Leech and McIntyre, 1976
	Swiss-Webster	8.4	Cain et al., 1980
Gerbil	Seizure-sensitive	4.8	Cain and Corcoran, 1980
	Seizure-resistant	9.8	Cain and Corcoran, 1980
Rat	Long-Evans/RVH hooded	11.3	Racine et al., 1972b
	Sprague-Dawley	7.0	Racine et al., 1973
	Wistar	17.9	Racine et al., 1973
	Tryon maze bright	15.9	Zaide, 1974
	Tryon maze dull	9.8	Zaide, 1974
	Kindling-prone	11.0	Steingart, 1983
	Kindling-resistant	42.1	Steingart, 1983
Rabbit	Unknown	13.4	Tanaka, 1972
Cat	Unknown	25.5	Wada and Sato, 1974
Dog	Beagle	7 (median)	Wauquier et al., 1979
Rhesus monkey		400 +	Wada et al., 1978
Baboon			
Papio papio		72.2	Wada and Osawa, 1976
P. cynocephalus		71.3	Corcoran et al., 1984
P. hamadrayas		125 +	Wada and Naquet, 1986

strains within some species. Amygdala kindling rates differ by more than two orders of magnitude across all mammalian species studied, and by as much as half an order of magnitude across some strains within a species. However, the rate of kindling within strains is reasonably consistent. In the hooded rat, for example, it is rare for amygdala kindling to require fewer than 8 or more than 16 ADs (excluding sites in the cortical nucleus; see below). Evidence from our own experience with amygdala kindling in the rat also indicates that the rate is stable across time. In a retrospective study involving seven control groups studied during a period of six years, the mean rate of kindling for the groups fell within the range of 10.8–12.7 ADs (Cain et al., 1989b). This stability contrasts with the apparent inconsistency across time of kindling in rat striate neocortex (Racine, 1975; Cain, 1982).

Although suggestions have been made about an inverse relation between body size or phylogenetic scale position and kindling rate, the data in Table I suggest that only the crudest relation exists, if one exists at all. Leaving aside the problems of ordering these groups in terms of phylogenesis, there are major discontinuities, with dogs kindling appreciably faster than the smaller rodents, felines, and lagomorphs, and with baboons, which most observers regard as more intelligent than rhesus monkeys, kindling faster than the monkeys. Photosensitive baboons kindle both more rapidly and to a more advanced degree (symmetrical primary generalized convulsion, Wada and Osawa, 1976; Corcoran et al., 1984) than do nonphotosensitive baboons and rhesus monkeys (asymmetrical secondary generalized convulsion, Wada et al., 1978; Wada and Naquet, 1986). These facts, and other evidence indicating that kindling can interact with endogenous seizure states (see Table I), suggest that genetically determined predispositions to seizures can be major factors in amygdala kindling.

Although many researchers have speculated on the possibility of kindling in humans, there are no unequivocal data available to resolve the question, and there are no data on kindling in apes. However, in the few observations made on humans receiving chronic electrical stimulation of the amygdala and nearby structures, the observations are strongly suggestive of an increased epileptic or emotional response to an unvarying stimulus (Heath et al., 1955; Sramka et al., 1977; Monroe, 1982). Further, the fact that Jacksonian and posttraumatic epilepsy in humans often exhibit progressively more severe clinical manifestations over time, and that prophylactic antiepileptic drug treatment can significantly reduce the long-term incidence of posttraumatic epilepsy (Jackson, 1931; Wada, 1977; Servit and Musil, 1981), is consistent with the possibility of kindling in the human (Engel and Cahan, 1986). We are probably justified in expecting that the human brain can be kindled and that genetically determined predispositions to seizures would probably affect the kindling of the human brain, as they do in animals.

REGIONAL NEUROANATOMY OF KINDLING IN THE AMYGDALA

In their initial mapping study, Goddard et al. (1969) found that all amygdala nuclei were equally responsive to the stimulation. However, this study used number of electrical stimulations rather than number of ADs as the measure of rate of kindling, which might have allowed the authors to miss subtle differences in the true kindling rate of different regions of the amygdala.

Two studies have addressed this question using number of ADs as the dependent measure. Le Gal La Salle (1981) reported that the medial nucleus required significantly more ADs to kindle (18.0) than either the central nucleus (10.3) or the lateral nucleus (13.0) in the Wistar rat. We have noticed that among normal hooded rats showing particularly slow rates of amygdala kindling, most seem to have electrode placements in the cortical nucleus. In a study comparing kindling rate in this nucleus with that of the basal nucleus we found that the cortical nucleus required significantly more ADs (21.7) than the basal nucleus (12.7) to kindle (Gilbert et al., 1984). Based on this finding, it is now routine in our laboratory to exclude rats with electrode placements in the cortical nucleus from amygdala-kindled groups. Although Le Gal La Salle's finding of a significantly slower kindling rate in the medial nucleus has not been confirmed in other laboratories, it might be appropriate to consider excluding rats with such placements in the interest of reduced variability and more homogeneous amygdala groups with which to test experimental effects.

In a retrospective study on possible hemispheric differences in ADT and rate of amygdala kindling, no hemispheric differences were found (Cain et al., 1989b).

In the interpretation of their original mapping study, Goddard et al. (1969) concluded that within the olfactory-limbic region, structures seem to kindle at rates that vary directly with the degree of interconnection with the amygdala. Subsequent work has shown that structures that have large and direct connections with the amygdala kindle very rapidly, often at rates that are faster than that of the amygdala itself. Among these are the following, all of which have been reported to kindle at rates of 7.0–9.5 ADs: fibers of the bed nucleus of the stria terminalis, olfactory bulb, pyriform cortex, and deep prepyriform cortex (Racine, 1975; Cain, 1977; Le Gal La Salle, 1979; Cain et al., 1988a; Racine et al., 1988a).

There seems to be little question that the amygdala-pyriform cortex area is the most sensitive for kindling within the limbic region of the rat brain, but the precise delineation of an area that is crucial for limbic kindling, if there is one, has not yet been achieved. Much of the evidence points to the pyriform cortex as such an area. As was discussed above, the pyriform cortex is an extremely active site for the generation of IIDs, one of the hallmarks of potential and actual epileptogenicity. Work by Racine and colleagues has clearly identified this area as the prime generator of IIDs during the early stages of kindling in the rat, even when the kindling site is elsewhere (Kairiss et al., 1984; Racine et al., 1988a). However, it appears that, across rats, there is no specific generating site within the pyriform cortex for the generation of IIDs. Racine et al. (1988a) conclude: "Within the pyriform cortex, all sites seem capable of serving as a primary generator, although, in any given animal, this function tends to be restricted to specific zones."

Additional evidence for the great seizure sensitivity of the pyriform cortex comes from a variety of approaches. Status epilepticus develops readily when various limbic sites are stimulated for long periods, and a syndrome of severe damage usually develops. The damage predominantly involves the lateral amygdala and pyriform cortex, even when the stimulating electrodes are elsewhere (McIntyre et al., 1982; Milgram et al., 1985; Cain, 1987), which presumably reflects the high level of neural activation of those areas during the status. Metabolic mapping of the pathways activated during amygdala kindling by 2-deoxyglucose or iodoantipyrine autoradiography has shown that the pyriform cortex, as well as some other limbic areas, are preferentially active during the early stages of kindling, and that the pyriform cortex almost always shows more metabolic activity than the stimulated amygdala itself (Engel et al., 1978; Ackermann et al., 1986). Finally, McIntyre and Wong (1985, 1986) have shown in the amygdala-pyriform slice preparation that amygdala stimulation evokes much stronger burst activity in the pyriform cortex of slices taken from rats kindled in the amygdala than from slices taken from nonkindled control rats. Collectively these results suggest that pyriform cortex neurons might be more prone to bursting (and perhaps contribute more to the early stages of kindling) than amygdala neurons in rats, but there appears to have been no direct electrophysiological test of this idea.

Against this picture of the extreme epileptogenicity of pyriform cortex and amygdala neurons are the results of lesion work, which temper the view that either the pyriform cortex or amygdala are crucial for limbic kindling. Early lesion work by Racine (1972b) had shown that the originally kindled amygdala was not necessary for rapid transfer kindling of the contralateral amygdala, and that both lesioned and intact rats exhibited comparable transfer to the contralateral amygdala. This demonstrated that the transfer effect does not depend on activation of the originally kindled site during transfer kindling, and that, in a previously kindled animal, a single intact amygdala is sufficient for full expression of transfer kindling. More recently, Racine's group has approached the question of the importance of the amygdala-pyriform cortex area for limbic kindling more directly (Racine et al., 1988b). They found that large bilateral lesions of the pyriform lobe that included removal of most of the amygdala and pyriform cortex had a small but statistically significant retarding effect on the rate of septal kindling. However, all rats displayed apparently normal generalized convulsions, and otherwise differed from unlesioned controls only in having a shorter mean final AD duration. Other lesion studies have yielded similar results. We showed that amygdala lesions retard but do not block olfactory bulb kindling (Cain, 1977), and Le Gal La Salle (1979) obtained the same result for bed nucleus of the stria terminalis kindling. In another study Le Gal La Salle and Feldblum (1983) found that amygdala lesions do not affect dorsal hippocampus kindling, but the lesions were smaller than those made in some of the other studies discussed here and did not include all of the amygdala. It is possible that larger lesions that include damage to the pyriform cortex might retard hippocampal kindling. In any case, it is clear that although lesions of the amygdala-pyriform cortex area can retard limbic kindling, they do not block it or even markedly affect the expression of the kindled convulsions. Collectively, the data suggest that the amygdala-pyriform cortex area participates in and contributes to most if not all instances of limbic kindling, but that it is not essential for such kindling.

Racine et al. (1988b) attempted to determine the relative importance of the outflow from the stimulated amygdala for kindling by making knife cuts anterior, posterior, and medial to the amygdala. The medial cuts, which interrupted the ventral amygdalofugal pathway, had no effect on amygdala kindling. The posterior cuts, which interrupted fibers to the entorhinal cortex and the hippocampus, facilitated amygdala kindling. The only cuts that retarded amygdala kindling were the anterior cuts, which interrupted anterior-going fibers connecting with pyriform cortex and medial structures, again pointing to a contribution by the pyriform cortex to amygdala kindling.

A specific site in the deep prepyriform cortex anterior to the amygdala has been claimed by Piredda and Gale (1985) to be a crucial site for limbic epileptogenesis. Direct unilateral injection of picomole amounts of bicuculline (a GABA antagonist), kainic acid (an excitatory amino acid agonist), or carbachol (a cholinomimetic) into this site were reported to evoke first-trial bilateral clonic convulsions. Injection of a GABA antagonist into the same site was reported to prevent seizures induced by peripheral administration of a convulsant (Piredda and Gale, 1986). These reports generated great interest among researchers concerned with amygdala kindling, some of whom tested the claim by electrically kindling the site (which Piredda and Gale had not attempted), injecting drugs, and making lesions. Collectively these data indicate that, although the deep prepyriform cortex kindles readily, it does not kindle more rapidly than the other amygdala and pyriform sites tested, and that lesions of the site or injections of GABA agonists or N-methyl-D-aspartic acid antagonists into it do not affect amygdala kindling (Morimoto et al., 1986; Zhao and Moshe, 1987; Cain et al., 1988a). It appears that much of the pyriform lobe is strongly seizure-prone, but to date no site has been identified that is crucial for limbic seizures.

A final point relates to the role of the hippocampus in limbic kindling. In humans the hippocampus is identified as the site of an epileptic focus much more often than is the amygdala (Engel and Cahan, 1986). The animal kindling data present a different picture. In rats and cats, the hippocampus is one of the slowest kindling structures in the whole brain (Madryga et al., 1975; Sato, 1975; Racine et al., 1977; Le Gal La Salle and Feldblum, 1983; Lerner-Natoli et al., 1984), and lesions of the hippocampus typically do not affect kindling in other limbic sites (Sutula et al., 1986; Racine et al., 1988b). In cases in which hippocampal damage was reported to disrupt the kindling or the expression of previously kindled amygdala seizures, it was ventral hippocampal damage that had this effect (Dashieff and McNamara, 1982; Yoshida, 1984), and the ventral hippocampus has been found to be considerably more seizure-prone than the dorsal hippocampus (Racine et al., 1977, 1988a; Gilbert et al., 1985; see also Racine et al., 1988b for comment). In the only study in which primate hippocampus was kindled, the forebrain commissures had been transected prior to kindling, but still there was evidence of very slow kindling (Wada and Mizoguchi, 1984).

In summary, of the subhuman data on the regional susceptibility of the amygdala and other limbic sites to kindling, we can probably do no better than to quote the conclusions of Racine et al. (1988a) in their work on the generation of IIDs in limbic tissue: "We propose the following order of sensitivity to the development of chronic epileptogenesis: pyriform cortex, amygdala, entorhinal cortex, and ventral hippocampus" (p. 262).

AMYGDALA KINDLING AS A MODEL OF EPILEPSY

Early efforts to assess the validity of amygdala kindling as a model of epilepsy dealt with possible artifacts that could be responsible for the seizures. Given the tendency of the amygdala and some surrounding structures to exhibit epileptiform activity in response to damage, this was an important issue. The general conclusion has been that artifacts or damage resulting from kindling techniques are not the cause of kindling. Many control studies have shown that time-dependent damage effects, metallic ions, high current levels, massed stimulation, and other possible damage-related factors do not in themselves kindle seizures or accelerate normal kindling (Goddard et al., 1969; Racine, 1972b, 1978). Rather, the necessary and sufficient condition for kindling is the occurrence of AD. Further, transfer of kindling to sites far distant from the stimulated primary kindling site readily occurs (Cain, 1986), which indicates that kindling effects can occur based on the functioning of undamaged synaptic contacts. Pharmacological agents and other treatments can very effectively kindle seizures in the absence of electrodes and tissue damage, and the kindling then readily transfers to subsequent electrical kindling of the amygdala (Mason and Cooper, 1972; Cain, 1986). Finally, data reviewed above indicate that amygdala kindling can interact with natural seizure states. These observations suggest that amygdala kindling is not simply an artifact of the treatments used to induce it.

If amygdala kindling models epilepsy, what form of epilepsy is amygdala kindling a model of, and is kindling also a model of other forms of brain plasticity? Many researchers agree that amygdala kindling effectively models partial complex seizures ("temporal lobe" epilepsy). The evidence for this judgment comes mainly from the phenomena of amygdala kindling itself and the profile of antiepileptic agents that affect kindled seizures (Wada and Osawa, 1976; Albright and Burnham, 1980; Engel and Cahan, 1986; Loscher et al., 1986; McNamara, 1986). Amygdala kindling appears to be a valuable epilepsy model since partial complex epilepsy is the single most frequent type of human epilepsy and is the most resistant to drug treatment.

Whether kindling models other forms of brain plasticity is less easy to answer. Early speculation suggested that kindling might model normal learning processes (Goddard et al., 1969; Goddard and Douglas, 1976), but this approach is discussed rarely now, perhaps because of the emphasis that has been placed on kindling as an epilepsy model and the availability of LTP as a model of learning.

CLINICAL IMPLICATIONS OF KINDLING

The idea that amygdala kindling models partial complex epilepsy and is permanent has a variety of implications for our view of treatments involving repeated electrical or pharmacological stimulation of the brain. First is the obvious fact that electrical or pharmacological stimulation that evokes AD is not innocuous, and if repeated sufficiently will eventually kindle seizures. This can occur even if the stimulation is initially below the threshold for evoking AD, since the AD threshold can be reduced permanently by subthreshold stimulation (Racine, 1972a; Pinel et al., 1976). As was discussed above, the amygdala is one of the most kindling-prone regions in the brain, and even as few as four amygdala ADs have a lasting facilitatory effect on subsequent full kindling in the rat (Dennison et al., 1989, 1990). In principle, even a single brief AD should have a similar lasting effect, although this is somewhat difficult to demonstrate experimentally, and to my knowledge it has not yet been attempted. However, we have shown that a single pentylenetetrazol or hyperthermic convulsion in infant rats can significantly facilitate amygdala kindling in adulthood (Gilbert and Cain, 1985), which indicates that single seizure episodes can have a lasting effect on later susceptibility to seizures. Others have obtained similar results in rats that were slightly older (Moshe and Albala, 1982; Holmes and Weber, 1983).

As long ago as 1971, Goddard sounded a warning about the possible clinical consequences of repeated electrical stimulation of the human brain. Since that time additional research, some of which has been reviewed above, has reinforced the view that electrical or pharmacological stimulation of brain can lead to an enduring epileptogenicity. Further, the increased epileptogenic response is not necessarily limited to the original brain site or the original kindling treatment. Transfer of kindling frequently occurs between different sites and between different kindling or seizure-promoting treatments in the same brain. This means that a brain that has received focal or nonfocal (i.e., electroconvulsive therapy) electrical stimulation, or is treated in any way that results in seizures, might well be rendered permanently more responsive to a large variety of other seizure-inducing treatments. Transfer of kindling might manifest itself clinically as an increased susceptibility to seizures upon withdrawal from alcohol or barbiturate drug intoxication in a person who had previously experienced a series of electroconvulsive therapy treatments. Just such a result has been reported in rats: Repeated electroconvulsive shock can result in a kindling effect, which then renders the rats significantly more susceptible to seizures upon withdrawal from alcohol exposure (Pinel, 1980). Transfer has also been demonstrated between full electrical kindling of the amygdala, or even repeated subthreshold (for AD) electrical stimulation of the amygdala, and alcohol withdrawal (Pinel et al., 1975b), and between many other combinations of seizure-inducing treatments (Cain, 1985, 1986). Transfer of kindling is also a potential concern in the development of sensory substitution prostheses that operate by direct electrical stimulation of brain tissue (Cain, 1979).

Kindling has implications for basic research as well. The fact that AD thresholds can be as low as 40 uA in the rat amygdala suggests that in studies in which electrical stimulation is applied to the amygdala, AD easily could be evoked. Therefore it is advisable to record the electrographic response to the stimulation to determine whether this has occurred. The occurrence of AD in the stimulated site might lead to some degree of propagation to nearby sites, and if the measures taken in the study depend on neural activation it is possible that the propagated AD might affect the measures in ways that are different from the effect of stimulation that is subthreshold for AD. If the purpose of an experiment is to localize an effect of electrical stimulation, it is important to avoid evoking AD. Although 60 Hz pulses are most often used for evoking AD in kindling, pulses delivered to the amygdala at frequencies as low as 0.75 Hz can very effectively evoke AD and kindle seizures (Cain and Corcoran, 1981), indicating that a very wide range of stimulus frequencies can kindle seizures. As is discussed in the next section, electrical stimulation alone, as well as partial kindling, can affect nonconvulsive behaviors, and this should also be taken into account in studies involving electrical stimulation of the amygdala. As was pointed out above, partial kindling has been shown to last at least 12 weeks, and probably can last much longer. The occurrence of even a few ADs can have lasting effects on nonconvulsive behaviors well after the last AD. This topic is discussed in the next section.

KINDLING AND NONCONVULSIVE BEHAVIORS

It is clear that amygdala kindling can lead to changes in a variety of nonconvulsive behaviors between seizures, including behaviors related to learning and memory (Belluzzi and Grossman, 1969; McIntyre and Reichert, 1971; McIntyre and Molino, 1972; Boast and McIntyre, 1977; McIntyre, 1979; Lopes da Silva et al., 1986; Stone and Gold, 1988), sleep (Smith and Miskiman, 1975; Shouse and Sterman, 1981, 1983; Shouse, 1986; Stone and Gold, 1988), spontaneous motor behavior (Ossenkopp and Sanberg, 1979; Post et al., 1981; Ehlers and Koob, 1985), and predation and defensiveness in cats (Adamec, 1976; Adamec and Stark-Adamec, 1986). It is worth emphasizing that Adamec's work showed that partial kindling was effective in leading to behavior change in cats, and that full kindling to a generalized convulsion was not necessary. Recall also that partial kindling is as permanent as full kindling (Dennison et al., 1989, 1990), suggesting that the behavioral changes that result from partial kindling are probably permanent. However, amygdala or septum kindling does not lead to changes in predation, intraspecific aggression, or passive avoidance performance in the hooded rat (McIntyre, 1978; Bawden and Racine, 1979), although it increases predation (muricide) in the Wistar rat (McIntyre, 1978), suggesting that important species and strain differences probably exist. Kindling rate has also been reported to vary in relation to age and maze performance (Toledo-Morrell et al., 1984). Some of these results have been interpreted in terms of functional lesion effects (Boast and McIntyre, 1977) or changes in the manner in which circuits conduct neural activity between seizures (Adamec, 1976; Adamec and Stark-Adamec, 1983a,b, 1986). It is well known that kindling can produce striking changes in the transmission of single electrical test pulses applied well after the last seizure (Racine et al., 1972, 1975), a phenomenon known as kindling-induced potentiation (KIP). Thus, kindling can have lasting effects on the way the kindled circuits transmit nonepileptiform activity, and perhaps in this way affect the behaviors described above.

There is a large literature on the relation between epilepsy and behavior disorders such as dyscontrol, schizophrenia, and depression in the human (Monroe, 1970, 1982; Girgis and Kiloh, 1980). Some of the data suggest an inverse relation between the occurrence of seizures and psychosis (Flor-Henry, 1969), and an association between the presence of seizure states and depression (Post, 1983). Researchers aware of the gradual and progressive nature of kindling epileptogenesis have speculated whether a kindlinglike effect in the human brain could underlie the "ripening" of human epileptic states and the brain changes that might lead to eventual expression of interictal behavior disorders (Post and Kopanda, 1976; Monroe, 1982; Adamec and Stark-Adamec, 1983b; Post, 1983).

As was pointed out above, Adamec demonstrated changes in predation and defensiveness in cats as a result of partial kindling of amygdala or hippocampus, which were interpreted as changes in emotional bias or personality (Adamec, 1976; Adamec and Stark-Adamec, 1983a,b, 1986). The changes were always toward reduced predation and increased defensiveness and withdrawal, which appear to be the opposite of the increased aggressiveness of the dyscontrol patient. On the other hand, Pinel et al. (1977) reported increased resistance to capture and increased reactivity to a pencil tap on the base of the tail after amygdala and hippocampus kindling in hooded rats, but not after caudate kindling, a result which they interpreted as increased aggressiveness. McIntyre (1978) reported increased predation after amygdala kindling in Wistar rats. However, in our experience of kindling mice, rats, gerbils, and baboons, we have not noticed increased aggressiveness, and most kindling researchers do not report noticing increased aggressiveness or difficulty in handling the animals they kindle. In fact, a tendency toward increased docility, perhaps caused by the repeated handling necessary for the kindling procedure itself, seems to be the usual result. The changes seen by Pinel et al. might have resulted from the fact that their rats received as many as 150 high-intensity stimulations given up to three times per day. This regimen would have strongly overkindled the subjects and possibly led to changes not associated with normal kindling to stage 5. Overall, there seems to be little evidence for normal amygdala kindling resulting in an animal model of the aggressive dyscontrol syndrome seen in some epileptic human patients.

In an examination of the possible relation between epilepsy and psychosis, Sato (1983) found that amygdala kindling in the cat resulted in a significant and lasting (10-day) hypersensitivity to the behavioral and autonomic effects of methamphetamine. Amygdala kindling resulted in increases in stereotyped behavior as well as piloerection and other autonomic behaviors. Post et al. (1981) also reported an increase in the reactivity to apomorphine in rats kindled in the amygdala. These findings suggest that amygdala kindling can result in a lasting hypersensitivity to dopamine, which has been strongly linked to schizophrenic psychosis in humans (Wong et al., 1986), and which also results from chronic administration of methamphetamine in animal models of paranoid psychosis (Sato, 1979). Sato and Okamoto (1981) have also reported that amygdala kindling is retarded by chronic pretreatment with cocaine or methamphetamine and is facilitated by haloperidol or pimozide in cats, which is consistent with an inhibitory role for dopamine in kindling. However, as Corcoran (1981) has argued, dopamine does not appear to play a role in amygdala kindling in the rat, and in any case one would expect a *subsensitivity* of dopamine receptors to develop after chronic administration of dopamine agonists. Sato (1983) has argued that these differences might result from species differences. However, since Post et al. (1981) also reported an increase in reactivity to a dopamine agonist in the rat, the response of the rat and cat appear to be similar in this respect. The answer could be that the behavioral increase in response to dopamine after amygdala kindling is not due to changes in dopamine levels or receptor properties, but rather to KIP in dopamine circuitry. The cause of KIP is unknown, but conceivably it could be nonsynaptic in its mechanism (Racine and Zaide, 1978). If KIP is responsible for the increased response to dopamine agonists, it is of little consequence whether synaptic dopaminergic mechanisms play a major role in the establishment of kindling. The approach pioneered by Sato could provide an explanation for interictal changes in dopamine-mediated behaviors, and it deserves to be examined further, perhaps in primates kindled in the amygdala.

As a final comment on efforts to draw parallels between complex human behavior disorders resulting from epileptic states and animal models of those disorders, we would be well advised to proceed with caution. There are many possible mechanisms for behavior change after seizures, including increased efficacy of neural circuits (KIP), potentiation of inhibitory neurotransmission (Tuff et al., 1983), postictal depression, and continuing epileptic activity (epilepsy partialis continua), among others. Established epilepsy in the human appears to be associated with considerable neuronal loss in many cases, a result which has not been reported in normal amygdala kindling. Further, although the events of amygdala and other forms of limbic kindling are strikingly consistent and predictable from one experimental subject to another within subhuman species and strains, the same cannot be said for human epileptic states. In the human the spread of seizure activity from the active focus, the brain structures ultimately affected by the propagated activity, and the ultimate manifestations the seizure state might take are typically variable and unpredictable (Goddard, 1980; Engel and Cahan, 1986). This suggests that it will continue to be difficult to study the neural basis of the relation between epilepsy in the human and the behavior disorders discussed here, and that it likely will be difficult to link firmly amygdala kindling in subhuman species and the behavioral outcome of human epilepsy.

MECHANISMS OF AMYGDALA KINDLING

A complete review of the mechanisms of amygdala kindling is beyond the scope of this review. Much work has been done on the neuroanatomical, pharmacological, electrophysiological, and other mechanisms involved in amygdala kindling, and only a summary of some of these findings can be given here. Relevant reviews are cited where appropriate.

Morphological Changes

One of the earliest attempts to study possible anatomical changes in kindling was that of Goddard and Douglas (1976), who examined the kindled amygdala in rats using electron microscopy. They found that some axon terminals appeared to be larger in kindled than in control rats, but were not able to conclude that the difference was due to kindling rather than other uncontrolled factors. Examination of kindled neocortical tissue similarly failed to reveal consistent changes in presynaptic terminals (Racine et al., 1976; Racine and Zaide, 1978; Racine, personal communication). This lack of consistent morphological change after kindling is in striking contrast to the relatively robust changes reported after LTP, a nonepileptiform model of plasticity that uses weaker and briefer forms of electrical stimulation (c.g., Chang and Greenough, 1984). However, as kindling and LTP appear to depend on different mechanisms (see below), this is perhaps less surprising than it first appears. More recent work has demonstrated increases in presynaptic terminals and the size of postsynaptic densities associated with perforated synapses after perforant path kindling (Geinisman et al., 1988; Sutula et al., 1988), but this has not yet been examined in the amygdala.

Pharmacological Mechanisms

As might be expected, neurotransmitters that have an excitatory action in limbic tissue contribute to amygdala kindling. Direct injection of agonists of muscarinic cholinergic and excitatory amino acid receptors into the amygdala can kindle seizures, and antagonists of these receptors can retard electrical kindling of the amygdala. Much of this evidence has been reviewed (Corcoran, 1988; Cain, 1989b). The uniform conclusion has been that although excitatory neurotransmitters contribute to amygdala kindling, no single transmitter is crucial for kindling. Rather, their separate contributions seem to summate (Cain et al., 1987, 1988b).

Although opioid peptides have been known for some time to produce epileptiform EEG activity, it is only recently that appropriate work has been done to demonstrate that they are capable of true kindling. Many sites in the posterior portion of the amygdala can be kindled by repeated injection of mu, delta, or epsilon receptor agonists, but sites in the anterior portion of the amygdala are largely unresponsive (Cain and Corcoran, 1985; Cain et al., 1990b). However, the fact that broad antagonism of opiate receptors by naloxone does not retard electrical kindling of the amygdala indicates that opiate neurotransmission is not necessary for normal kindling (see Corcoran, 1988, and Cain, 1989b, for reviews).

Again, as might be expected, neurotransmitters that have an inhibitory action retard amygdala kindling. One of the first and most consistent findings in the pharmacology of kindling was that norepinephrine strongly retards amygdala kindling (Corcoran, 1981, 1988; McIntyre, 1981). GABA also retards amygdala kindling, as is shown by the fact that agents such as picrotoxin that block the chloride ionophore readily kindle seizures when administered systemically or directly into the amygdala, presumably by removing the check on neural firing that GABA normally maintains (Cain, 1987). Further, GABA-complex antagonists generally facilitate, and GABA-complex agonists generally retard electrical kindling of the amygdala (see Burnham, 1989 for review). The question whether a loss of GABA-mediated inhibition actually underlies kindling has been more difficult to assess. Early evidence based on receptor binding studies was mixed. However, more recent work using different techniques that measure "synaptic" GABA function show persistent decrements in GABA function after amygdala kindling (Burnham, 1989). However, amygdala kindling also *increases* GABA-mediated inhibition in certain structures (Tuff et al., 1983), suggesting that the involvement of GABA in kindling is complex.

Biochemical Mechanisms

Early attempts to study possible biochemical mechanisms of kindling that might involve the synthesis of new neuronal constituents made use of inhibitors of protein synthesis such as anisomycin and cycloheximide. The general conclusion has been that amygdala kindling is significantly slowed or largely prevented by these agents (Jonec and Wasterlain, 1979; Cain et al., 1980), suggesting that the ongoing synthesis of protein is necessary for normal kindling. Unfortunately, little more can be said about basic biochemical mechanisms in kindling. For example, attempts to identify neuronal phosphoproteins that are critical for kindling plasticity have yielded variable results (see Corcoran, 1988, for review). The more recent interest in immediate-early gene expression after seizures led to attempts to study possible genetic mechanisms of neuronal change that might translate genetic information in the nucleus of neurons into some permanent form of structural or functional change in neuronal physiology that might underlie kindling (Dragunow et al., 1989). Although early data suggested that induction of the immediate-early gene *c-fos* might be an important component of the kindling mechanism, recent work in our laboratory has indicated that induction of *c-fos* occurs in response to virtually all instances of neuronal activation in the amygdala, including conditions that do not result in the kindling of seizures (Teskey et al., 1990). Although this area appears to be promising in a search for mechanisms of neuronal growth and plasticity, it will require a great deal of further work to identify which genes are expressed and necessary for kindling plasticity. Critical in this attempt will be the need to identify enduring mechanisms of kindling itself, rather than mechanisms that might oppose the perturbing effects of seizures, or responses to the simple occurrence of the intense neural activity that constitutes the seizure.

Electrophysiological Mechanisms

One of the earliest findings about the enduring effects of kindling on brain function was the observation of an increase in the amplitude of potentials evoked in neuroanatomically related sites by single pulses applied to the kindled amygdala (Racine et al., 1972). Soon after this observation, Bliss and Lomo (1973) described a similar phenomenon, now called LTP. These reports were followed by the suggestion that an increase in excitatory synaptic transmission, reflected in potentiation phenomena such as these, might be the basic mechanism of kindling (Goddard and Douglas, 1976). Although this idea is parsimonious and appealing, it is almost certainly incorrect. Potentiation probably contributes to kindling under certain circumstances, but the many differences between the characteristics and mechanisms of kindling and LTP suggest that the two models have different underlying mechanisms (Cain et al., 1990a; see Racine et al., 1986, and Cain, 1989a, for reviews).

One obvious difference between kindling and LTP is that the former is an epileptiform model while the latter is not. Kindling requires that epileptiform AD be evoked, and it always results in epileptiform events, neither of which are true of LTP. Kindling results in the development of a tendency for neurons in the kindled circuits to fire in epileptiform bursts, even in the absence of normal synaptic inputs (Racine et al., 1986). It may be the development of the burst response, due to changes in intrinsic (nonsynaptic) neuronal properties, that holds the key to understanding the mechanisms of kindling epileptogenesis in a structure such as the amygdala, whose neurons have such a strong tendency to fire in epileptiform bursts in response to electrical or pharmacological stimulation. We have seen that, in the rat, neurons in the amygdala-pyriform area play a prominent role in the development of IIDs and the kindling of seizures. This prominence may reflect both the strong tendency of amygdala-pyriform neurons to develop the burst response, and a ready access of the epileptiform output to other pyriform lobe structures and to motor structures to drive convulsive behavior. This idea is more fully expressed in the comprehensive theory of kindling by Racine and Burnham (1984).

ACKNOWLEDGMENTS

This work was supported by a grant from the Natural Sciences and Engineering Research Council of Canada. I thank Michael Corcoran for helpful comments and suggestions.

REFERENCES

Ackermann RF, Chugani HT, Handforth A, Moshe S, Caldecott-Hazard S, Engel J (1986): Autoradiographic studies of cerebral blood flow in rat amygdala kindling. In Wada JA (ed): "Kindling 3." New York: Raven Press, pp 73–87.

Adamec R (1976): Behavioral and epileptic determinants of predatory attack in the cat. In Wada J (ed): "Kindling." New York: Raven Press, pp 135–153.

Adamec R, Stark-Adamec C (1983a): Partial kindling and emotional bias in the cat: Lasting aftereffects of partial kindling of the ventral hippocampus. Behav Neur Biol 38:205–222.

Adamec R, Stark-Adamec C (1983b): Limbic kindling and animal behavior—Implications for human psychopathology associated with complex partial seizures. Biol Psychiat 18:269–293.

Adamec R, Stark-Adamec C (1986): Partial kindling and behavioral change—Some rules governing behavioral outcome of repeated limbic seizures. In Wada J (ed): "Kindling 3." New York: Raven Press, pp 195–211.

Albright PS, Burnham WM (1980): Development of a new pharmacological seizure model: Effects of anticonvulsants on cortical- and amygdala-kindled seizures in the rat. Epilepsia 21:681–689.

Babington RG, Wedeking PW (1973): The pharmacology of seizures induced by sensitization with low intensity brain stimulation. Pharmacol Biochem Behav 1:461–467.

Bawden HN, Racine RJ (1979): Effects of bilateral kindling or bilateral subthreshold stimulation of the amygdala or septum on muricide, ranacide, intraspecific aggression and passive avoidance in the rat. Physiol Behav 22:115–123.

Belluzzi JD, Grossman SP (1969): Avoidance learning: Long-lasting deficits after temporal lobe seizures. Science 166:1435–1437.

Bliss TVP, Lomo T (1973): Long-lasting potentiation of synaptic transmission in the dentate area of the anesthetized rabbit following stimulation of the perforant path. J Physiol 232:331–356.

Boast C, McIntyre DC (1977): Bilateral kindled amygdala foci and inhibitory behavior in rats: A functional lesion effect. Physiol Behav 18:25–28.

Burnham WM (1978): Cortical and limbic kindling: Similarities and differences. In Livingston KE, Hornykiewicz O (eds): "Limbic Mechanisms: The Continuing Evolution of the Limbic System Concept." New York: Plenum Press, pp 507–519.

Burnham WM (1989): The GABA hypothesis in kindling: Recent assay studies. Neurosci Biobehav Rev 13:281–288.

Cain DP (1977): Seizure development following repeated electrical stimulation of central olfactory structures. Ann NY Acad Sci 290:200–216.

Cain DP (1979): Sensory kindling: Implications for development of sensory prostheses. Neurology 29:1595–1599.

Cain DP (1982): Kindling in sensory systems: Neocortex. Exp Neurol 76:276–283.

Cain DP (1985): Transfer of kindling: Clinical relevance and a hypothesis of its mechanism. Prog Neuro-Psychopharmacol & Biol Psychiat 9:467–472.

Cain DP (1986): The transfer phenomenon in kindling. In Wada JA (ed): "Kindling 3." New York: Raven Press, pp 231–245.

Cain DP (1987): Kindling by repeated intraperitoneal or intracerebral injection of picrotoxin transfers to electrical kindling. Exp Neurol 97:243–254.

Cain DP (1989a): Long-term potentiation and kindling: How similar are the mechanisms? Trends Neurosci 12:6–10.

Cain DP (1989b): Excitatory neurotransmitters in kindling: Excitatory amino acid, cholinergic, and opiate mechanisms. Neurosci Biobehav Rev 13:169–176.

Cain DP, Boon F, Hargreaves EL (1990a): Pharmacological dissociation between the mechanisms of kindling and long term potentiation by APV and urethane anesthesia. In Wada JA (ed): "Kindling 4." New York: Plenum Press, pp. 343–351.

Cain DP, Boon F, Bevan M (1989a): Failure of aspartame to affect seizure susceptibility in kindled rats. Neuropharmacology 28:433–435.

Cain DP, Boon F, Corcoran ME (1990b): Involvement of multiple opiate receptors in opioid kindling. Brain Res 517:236–244.

Cain DP, Corcoran ME (1980): Kindling in the seizure-prone and seizure-resistant Mongolian gerbil. Electroencephalogr Clin Neurophysiol 49:360–365.

Cain DP, Corcoran ME (1981): Kindling with low-frequency stimulation: Generality, transfer, and recruiting effects. Exp Neurol 73:219–232.

Cain DP, Corcoran ME (1985): Epileptiform effects of met-enkephalin, B-endorphin and morphine: Kindling of generalized seizures and potentiation of epileptiform effects by handling. Brain Res 338:327–336.

Cain DP, Corcoran ME, Desborough KA, McKitrick DJ (1988a): Kindling in the deep prepyriform cortex of the rat. Exp Neurol 100:203–209.

Cain DP, Corcoran ME, Staines WA (1980): Effects of protein synthesis inhibition on kindling in the mouse. Exp Neurol 68:409–419.

Cain DP, Desborough KA, McKitrick DJ (1988b): Retardation of amygdala kindling by antagonism of NMD-aspartate and muscarinic cholinergic receptors: Evidence for the summation of excitatory mechanisms in kindling. Exp Neurol 100:179–187.

Cain DP, Desborough KA, McKitrick DJ, Ossenkopp K-P (1989b): Absence of a hemispheric difference in seizure sensitivity in the rat brain. Physiol Behav 45:219–220.

Cain DP, McKitrick DJ, Desborough KA (1987): Effects of treatment with scopolamine and naloxone, singly and in combination, on amygdala kindling. Exp Neurol 96:97–103.

Chang FF, Greenough WT (1984): Transient and enduring morphological correlates of synaptic activity and efficacy change in the rat hippocampal slice. Brain Res 309:35–46.

Corcoran ME (1981): Catecholamines and kindling. In Wada JA (ed): "Kindling 2." New York: Raven Press, pp 87–101.

Corcoran ME (1988): Characteristics and mechanisms of kindling. In Kalivas P, Barnes C (eds): "Sensitization of the Nervous System." Caldwell, NJ: Telford Press, pp 81–116.

Corcoran ME, Cain DP, Wada JA (1984): Amygdaloid kindling in *Papio cynocephalus* and subsequent recurrent spontaneous seizures. Folia Psychiatr Neurol Jap 38:151–157.

Dashieff RM, McNamara JO (1982): Intradentate colchicine retards the development of amygdala kindling. Ann Neurol 11:347–352.

Dennison Z, Teskey GC, Cain DP (1989): Effect of a 12 week interval on permanence of 'partial' and 'full' kindling. Soc Neurosci Abstr 15:778.

Dennison Z, Tandan T, Teskey GC, Cain DP (1990): The effect of a 12-week interval on permanence of 'partial' (stage 1), 'full' (stage 5) and low frequency (3 Hz) kindling in the rat. Soc Neurosci Abstr 16:1266.

Dragunow M, Currie RW, Faull RLM, Robertson HA, Jansen K (1989): Immediate-early genes, kindling and long-term potentiation. Neurosci Biobehav Rev 13:301–313.

Ehlers CL, Koob GF (1985): Locomotor behavior following kindling in three different brain sites. Brain Res 326:71–79.

Engel J, Cahan L (1986): Potential relevance of kindling to human partial epilepsy. In Wada J (ed): "Kindling 3." New York: Raven Press, pp 37–51.

Engel J, Wolfson L, Brown L (1978): Anatomical correlates of electrical and behavioral events related to amygdaloid kindling. Ann Neurol 3:538–544.

Flor-Henry P (1969): Psychosis and temporal lobe epilepsy. A controlled investigation. Epilepsia 10:363–395.

Geinisman Y, Morrell F, deToledo-Morrell L (1988): Remodeling of synaptic architecture during hippocampal "kindling." Proc Natl Acad Sci 85:3260–3264.

Gilbert ME, Cain DP (1982): A developmental study of kindling in the rat. Dev Brain Res 2:321–328.

Gilbert ME, Cain DP (1985): A single neonatal pentylenetetrazol or hyperthermia convulsion increases kindling susceptibility in the adult rat. Dev Brain Res 22:169–180.

Gilbert ME, Gillis BJ, Cain DP (1984): Kindling in the cortical nucleus of the amygdala. Brain Res 295:360–363.

Gilbert ME, Racine RJ, Smith GK (1985): Epileptiform burst response in ventral vs. dorsal hippocampal sites. Brain Res 361:389–391.

Girgis M, Kiloh LG (eds) (1980): "Limbic Epilepsy and the Dyscontrol Syndrome." New York: Elsevier.

Goddard GV (1964): Amygdaloid stimulation and learning in the rat. J Comp Physiol Psychol 58:23–30.

Goddard GV (1967): Development of epileptic seizures through brain stimulation at low intensity. Nature 214:1020–1021.

Goddard GV (1969): Analysis of avoidance conditioning following cholinergic stimulation of amygdala in rats. J Comp Physiol Psychol 68 (monogr 2, part 2):1–18.

Goddard GV (1971): The kindling effect: A precautionary note on therapeutic applications of localized brain stimulation. In Reynolds DV, Sjoberg AD (eds): "Neuroelectric Research." Springfield: Thomas, pp 37–39.

Goddard GV (1980): The kindling model of limbic epilepsy. In Girgis M, Kiloh LG (eds): "Limbic Epilepsy and the Dyscontrol Syndrome." New York: Elsevier, pp 107–116.

Goddard GV (1983): The kindling model of epilepsy. Trends Neurosci 6:275–279.

Goddard GV, Douglas RM (1976): Does the engram of kindling model the engram of normal long term memory? In Wada J (ed): "Kindling." New York: Raven Press, pp 1–18.

Goddard GV, McIntyre D, Leech C (1969): A permanent change in brain function resulting from daily electrical stimulation. Exp Neurol 25:295–330.

Grace GM, Corcoran ME, Skelton RW (1990): Kindling with stimulation of the dentate gyrus: I. Characterization of electrographic and behavioral events. Brain Res 509:249–256.

Heath RG, Monroe RR, Mickle WA (1955): Stimulation of the amygdaloid nucleus in a schizophrenic patient. Am J Psychiat 111:862–863.

Holmes GL, Weber DA (1983): Increased susceptibility to pentylenetetrazol-induced seizures in adult rats following electrical kindling during brain development. Dev Brain Res 11:312–314.

Jackson JH (1931): A study of convulsions. In Taylor J (ed): "Selected Writings of John Hughlings Jackson," Vol 1. London: Hodder and Stoughton.

Jonec V, Wasterlain C (1979): Effect of inhibitors of protein synthesis on the development of kindled seizures in rats. Exp Neurol 66:524–532.

Kairiss E, Racine RJ, Smith G (1984): The development of the interictal spike during kindling in the rat. Brain Res 322:101–110.

Leech CK, McIntyre DC (1976): Kindling rates in inbred mice: An analog to learning? Behav Biol 16:439–452.

Le Gal La Salle G (1979): Kindling of motor seizures from the bed nucleus of the stria terminalis. Exp Neurol 66:309–318.

Le Gal La Salle G (1981): Amygdaloid kindling in the rat: Regional differences and general properties. In Wada J (ed): "Kindling 2." New York: Raven Press, pp 31–44.

Le Gal La Salle G, Feldblum S (1983): Role of the amygdala in development of hippocampal kindling in the rat. Exp Neurol 82:447–455.

Lerner-Natoli M, Rondouin G, Baldy-Moulinier M (1984): Hippocampal kindling in the rat: Intrastructural differences. J Neurosci Res 12:101–111.

Lopes da Silva FH, Gorter JA, Wadman WJ (1986): Kindling of the hippocampus induces spatial memory deficits in the rat. Neurosci Lett 63:115–120.

Loscher W, Jackel R, Czuczwar S (1986): Is amygdala kindling in rats a model for drug-resistant partial epilepsy? Exp Neurol 93:211–226.

Madryga FJ, Goddard GV, Rasmusson DD (1975): The kindling of motor seizures from hippocampal commissure in the rat. Physiol Psychol 3:369–373.

Mason CR, Cooper RM (1972): A permanent change in convulsive threshold in normal and brain-damaged rats with repeated small doses of pentylenetetrazol. Epilepsia 13:663–674.

McIntyre DC (1978): Amygdala kindling and muricide in rats. Physiol Behav 21:49–56.

McIntyre DC (1979): Effects of focal vs. generalized kindled convulsions from anterior neocortex or amygdala on CER acquisition in rats. Physiol Behav 23:855–859.

McIntyre DC (1981): Catecholamine involement in amygdala kindling of the rat. In Wada JA (ed): "Kindling 2." New York: Raven Press, pp 67–80.

McIntyre DC, Molino A (1972): Amygdala lesions and CER learning: Long term effect of kindling. Physiol Behav 8:1055–1058.

McIntyre DC, Nathanson D, Edson N (1982): A new model of partial status epilepticus based on kindling. Brain Res 250:53–63.

McIntyre DC, Reichert H (1971): State-dependent learning in rats induced by kindled convulsions. Physiol Behav 7:15–20.

McIntyre DC, Wong RKS (1985): Modification of local neuronal interactions by amygdala kindling examined in vitro. Exp Neurol 88:529–537.

McIntyre DC, Wong RKS (1986): Cellular and synaptic properties of amygdala-kindled pyriform cortex in vitro. J Neurophysiol 55:1295–1307.

McNamara JO (1986): Kindling model of epilepsy. Adv Neurol 44:303–318.

Milgram NW, Green I, Liberman M, Riexinger K, Petit TL (1985): Establishment of status epilepticus by limbic system stimulation in previously unstimulated rats. Exp Neurol 88:253–264.

Monroe RR (1970): "Episodic Behavioral Disorders." Cambridge: Harvard University Press.

Monroe RR (1982): Limbic ictus and atypical psychoses. J Nerv Ment Dis 170:711–716.

Morimoto K, Dragunow M, Goddard GV (1986): Deep prepyriform cortex kindling and its relation to amygdala kindling in the rat. Exp Neurol 94:637–648.

Moshe SL, Albala BJ (1982): Kindling in developing rats: Persistence of seizures into adulthood. Dev Brain Res 4:67–71.

Moshe SL, Ackermann RF, Albala BJ, Okada R (1986): The role of substantia nigra in seizures of developing animals. In Wada JA (ed): "Kindling 3." New York: Raven Press, pp 91–104.

Ossenkopp K-P, Sanberg PR (1979): Relationship of some open-field behaviors to amygdaloid kindled convulsions in Wistar rats. Physiol Behav 23:809–812.

Pinel JPJ (1980): Alcohol withdrawal seizures: Implications of kindling. Pharm Biochem Behav 13(Suppl 1):225–231.

Pinel JPJ, Mucha RF, Phillips AG (1975a): Spontaneous seizures generated in rats by kindling: A preliminary report. Physiol Psychol 3:127–129.

Pinel JPJ, Rovner LI (1978a): Experimental epileptogenesis: Kindling-induced epilepsy in rats. Exp Neurol 58:190–202.

Pinel JPJ, Rovner LI (1978b): Electrode placement and kindling-induced experimental epilepsy. Exp Neurol 58:335–346.

Pinel JPJ, Skelton R, Mucha RF (1976): Kindling-related changes in afterdischarge "thresholds." Epilepsia 17:197–205.

Pinel JPJ, Treit D, Rovner LI (1977): Temporal lobe aggression in rats. Science 197:1088–1089.

Pinel JPJ, Van Oot PH, Mucha RF (1975b): Intensification of the alcohol withdrawal syndrome by repeated brain stimulation. Nature 254:510–511.

Piredda S, Gale K (1985): A crucial epileptogenic site in the deep prepyriform cortex. Nature 317:623–625.

Piredda S, Gale K (1986): Anticonvulsant action of 2-amino-7-phosphonoheptanoic acid and muscimol in the deep prepyriform cortex. Eur J Pharmacol 120:115–118.

Post RM (1983): Behavioral effects of kindling. In Parsonage M (ed): "Advances in Epileptology: XIVth Epilepsy International Symposium." New York: Raven Press, pp 173–180.

Post RM, Kopanda RT (1976): Cocaine, kindling and psychosis. Am J Psychiat 133:627–634.

Post RM, Squillance KM, Pert A, Sass W (1981): The effect of amygdaloid kindling on spontaneous and cocaine-induced motor activity and lidocaine seizures. Psychopharmacology 72:189–196.

Racine RJ (1972a): Modification of seizure activity by electrical stimulation: I. Afterdischarge threshold. Electroencephalogr Clin Neurophysiol 32:269–279.

Racine RJ (1972b): Modification of seizure activity by electrical stimulation: II. Motor seizure. Electroencephalogr Clin Neurophysiol 32:281–294.

Racine RJ (1975): Modification of seizure activity by electrical stimulation: Cortical areas. Electroencephalogr Clin Neurophysiol 38:1–12.

Racine RJ (1978): Kindling: The first decade. Neurosurgery 3:234–252.

Racine RJ, Burnham WM (1984): The kindling model. In Schwartzkroin PA, Weal H (eds): "Electrophysiology of Epilepsy." New York: Academic Press, pp 153–171.

Racine RJ, Burnham WM, Gartner JG, Levitan D (1973): Rates of motor seizure development in rats subjected to electrical brain stimulation: Strain and inter-stimulation interval effects. Electroencephalogr Clin Neurophysiol 35:553–556.

Racine RJ, Burnham WM, Gilbert ME, Kairiss EW (1986): Kindling mechanisms: I. Electrophysiological studies. In Wada JA (ed): "Kindling 3." New York: Raven Press, pp 263–279.

Racine RJ, Gartner JG, Burnham WM (1972): Epileptiform activity and neural plasticity in limbic structures. Brain Res 47:262–268.

Racine RJ, Milgram N, Hafner S (1983): Long-term potentiation phenomena in the rat limbic forebrain. Brain Res 260:217–231.

Racine RJ, Mosher M, Kairiss EW (1988a): The role of the pyriform cortex in the generation of interictal spikes in the kindled preparation. Brain Res 454:251–263.

Racine RJ, Newberry F, Burnham WM (1975): Post-activation potentiation and the kindling phenomenon. Electroencephalogr Clin Neurophysiol 39:261–271.

Racine RJ, Paxinos G, Mosher JM, Kairiss EW (1988b): The effects of various lesions and knife-cuts on septal and amygdala kindling in the rat. Brain Res 454:264–274.

Racine RJ, Rose PA, Burnham WM (1977): Afterdischarge thresholds and kindling rates in dorsal and ventral hippocampus and dentate gyrus. Can J Neurol Sci 4:273–278.

Racine RJ, Tuff L, Zaide J (1976): Kindling, unit discharge patterns and neural plasticity. In Wada JA (ed): "Kindling." New York: Raven Press, pp 19–39.

Racine RJ, Zaide J (1978): A further investigation into the mechanisms underlying the kindling phenomenon. In Livingston KE, Hornykiewicz O (eds): "Limbic Mechanisms." New York: Plenum Press, pp 457–493.

Sato M (1975): Hippocampal seizure and secondary epileptogenesis in the "kindled" cart preparations. Folia Psychiat Neurol Jap 29:239–250.

Sato M (1979): An experimental study of onset and relapse mechanisms in the chronic methamphetamine psychosis. Psychiat Neurol Jap 81:21–32.

Sato M (1983): Long-lasting hypersensitivity to methamphetamine following amygdaloid kindling in cats: The relationship between limbic epilepsy and the psychotic state. Biol Psychiat 18:525–536.

Sato M, Okamoto M (1981): Dopamine kindling and electrical kindling. In Wada JA (ed): "Kindling 2." New York: Raven Press, pp 105–122.

Schwark WS, Haluska M, Blackshear P, Magana T (1985): Lifetime lead intoxication: Influence on the amygdaloid kindling model of epileptogenesis. Toxicology 36:49–60.

Seidel WT, Corcoran ME (1986): Relations between amygdaloid and anterior neocortical kindling. Brain Res 385:375–378.

Servit Z, Musil F (1981): Prophylactic treatment of posttraumatic epilepsy: Results of a long-term follow-up in Czechoslovakia. Epilepsia 22:315–320.

Shouse MN (1986): State disorders and state-dependent seizures in amygdala-kindled cats. Exp Neurol 92:601–608.

Shouse MN, Sterman MB (1981): Sleep and kindling: II. Effects of generalized seizure induction. Exp Neurol 71:563–580.

Shouse MN, Sterman MB (1983): "Kindling" a sleep disorder: Degree of sleep pathology predicts kindled seizure susceptibility in cats. Brain Res 271:196–200.

Smith CT, Miskiman DE (1975): Increases in paradoxical sleep as a result of amygdaloid kindling. Physiol Behav 15:17–19.

Sramka M, Sedlak P, Nadvornik P (1977): Observation of kindling phenomenon in treatment of pain by stimulation in thalamus. In Sweet WH, Obradoc S, Martin-Rodriguez JG (eds): "Neurosurgical Treatment in Psychiatry, Pain, and Epilepsy." Baltimore: University Park Press, pp 651–654.

Stasheff S, Bragdon A, Wilson W (1985): Induction of epileptiform activity in hippocampal slices by trains of electrical stimuli. Brain Res 344:296–302.

Steingart MO (1983): The selective breeding of seizure-prone vs. seizure-resistant rats based on amygdaloid kindling: Behavioral, electrophysiological and pharmacological measures. Unpublished Ph.D. thesis, McMaster University, Hamilton, Ontario, Canada.

Stone WS, Gold PE (1988): Amygdala kindling effects on sleep and memory in rats. Brain Res 449:135–140.

Sutula T, Harrison C, Steward O (1986): Chronic epileptogenesis induced by kindling of the entorhinal cortex: The role of the dentate gyrus. Brain Res 385:291–299.

Sutula T, Xiao-Xian H, Cavazos J, Scott G (1988): Synaptic reorganization in the hippocampus induced by abnormal functional activity. Science 239:1147–1150.

Tanaka A (1972): Progressive changes of behavioral and electroencephalographic responses to daily amygdaloid stimulations in rabbits. Fukuoka Acta Med 63:152–164.

Teskey GC, Atkinson B, Cain DP (1991): Expression of the proto-oncogene *c-fos* following electrical kindling in the rat. Behav Brain Res 11:1–10.

Toledo-Morrell L, Morrell F, Fleming S (1984): Age-dependent deficits in spatial memory are related to impaired hippocampal kindling. Behav Neurosci 98:902–97.

Tuff LP, Racine RJ, Adamec R (1983): The effects of kindling on GABA-mediated inhibition in the dentate gyrus of the rat. I. Paired-pulse depression. Brain Res 277:79–90.

Wada JA (1977): Pharmacological prophylaxis in the kindling model of epilepsy. Arch Neurol 34:389–395.

Wada JA (1978): Kindling as a model of epilepsy. In Cobb WA, Van Dujin H (eds): "Contemporary Clinical Neurophysiology." Amsterdam: Elsevier, pp 309–316.

Wada JA (1980): Amygdaloid and frontal cortical kindling in subhuman primates. In Girgis M, Kiloh L (eds): "Limbic Epilepsy and the Dyscontrol Syndrome." Amsterdam: Elsevier, pp 133–147.

Wada JA, Mizoguchi T (1984): Limbic kindling in the forebrain-bisected photosensitive baboon, *Papio papio.* Epilepsia 25:278–287.

Wada J, Mizoguchi T, Osawa T (1978): Secondarily generalized convulsive seizures induced by daily amygdaloid stimulation in rhesus monkeys. Neurology 28:1026–1036.

Wada JA, Naquet R (1986): Experimental model in a primate predisposed to epilepsy. In Schmidt D, Morselli PL (eds): "Intractable Epilepsy." New York: Raven Press, pp 39–59.

Wada J, Osawa T (1976): Spontaneous recurrent seizure state induced by daily electric amygdaloid stimulation in Senegalese baboons (*Papio papio*). Neurology 26:273–286.

Wada J, Sato M (1974): Generalized convulsive seizures induced by daily electrical stimulation of the amygdala in cats: Correlative electrographic and behavioral features. Neurology 24:656–574.

Wada JA, Sato M, Corcoran ME (1974): Persistent seizure susceptibility and recurrent spontaneous seizures in kindled cats. Epilepsia 15:465–478.

Wauquier A, Ashton D, Melis W (1979): Behavioral analysis of amygdaloid kindling in beagle dogs and the effects of clonazepam, phenobarbital, diphenylhydantoin, and flunarizine on seizure manifestation. Exp Neurol 64:579–586.

Wong DF et al. (1986): Positron emission tomography reveals elevated D2 dopamine receptors in drug-naive schizophrenics. Science 234:1558–1563.

Yoshida K (1984): Influences of bilateral hippocampal lesions upon kindled amygdaloid convulsive seizures in rats. Physiol Behav 32:123–126.

Zaide J (1974): Differences between Tryon bright and dull rats in seizure activity evoked by amygdala stimulation. Physiol Behav 12:527–534.

Zhao DY, Moshe SL (1987): Deep prepyriform cortex kindling and amygdala interactions. Epilepsy Res 1:94–101.

The Amygdala: Neurobiological Aspects of Emotion,
Memory, and Mental Dysfunction, pages 561–574
© 1992 Wiley-Liss, Inc.

22

The Amygdala and the Neurochemistry of Schizophrenia

GAVIN P. REYNOLDS

Department of Biomedical Science, University of Sheffield, Sheffield, UK

INTRODUCTION

Schizophrenia affects almost one person in 100 and yet very little is understood of its etiology. Genetic factors are probably important in approximately half of all cases, although various environmental influences (e.g., obstetric complications) have also been implicated. While many patients respond well to antipsychotic drug treatment, for perhaps one-third of cases the prognosis is of a lifetime of institutional care. The pattern of symptoms too can be variable, with "positive" symptoms (e.g., hallucinations, delusions, and thought disorder) predominating in some, while others have primarily the more "negative" symptoms that include withdrawal, loss of drive, and flattened affect (Crow, 1980). Patients with predominantly positive or negative symptoms have been labelled as type I or type II respectively (Crow, 1980). Lack of response to classical neuroleptic drug treatment is particularly apparent in the latter patient group, in whom there is generally more evidence of neuropathological abnormalities.

The identification of the various neuropathologies in the disease, some of which correlate with certain symptom profiles, along with the multiplicity of proposed causal effects and the variability in drug response, all suggest that schizophrenia may well be heterogeneous. This heterogeneity serves to confound research into the pathogenesis (or pathogeneses) of the disease. Nevertheless, a wide range of evidence is accumulating pointing to abnormalities in two particular regions of the brain. Imaging studies of blood flow and energy metabolism, along with neuropsychological and some limited neuropathological investigations, have indicated the frontal cortex as a site of dysfunction in schizophrenia. Other work, including a rapidly growing body of magnetic resonance imaging and postmortem morphological studies, suggests strongly the presence of structural deficits within the temporal lobe, particularly in the more medial regions of the left hemisphere. Whether the changes observed in these two parts of the brain are interrelated in any way, or whether (in the most extreme interpretation) they reflect different syndromes of the disease, is as yet unclear. Nevertheless, it is apparent that similar behavioral manifestations may well arise from pathological changes in different brain regions. Some of this evidence for structural abnormality, where it might throw light on the neurochemical pathology of schizophrenia, is reviewed below.

In this chapter, I hope to demonstrate that the amygdala may well be important in mediating (at least some of) the symptoms of schizophrenia. The neurochemical, pathological, and other evidence for this does not necessarily indicate that the amygdala is the only and primary site of dysfunction in the disease, but it may mediate the effects of pathology elsewhere, as well as provide a site of potential importance in antipsychotic drug treatment.

SCHIZOPHRENIA AND AMYGDALA FUNCTION

The amygdala is a component of the limbic brain, a system of interrelated structures that has been implicated in the pathophysiology of schizophrenia for many years (Stevens, 1973; Torrey and Peterson, 1974). The classic in-depth electrode studies of Heath (1954) demonstrated abnormal electrical activity from limbic brain structures (amygdala and hippocampus) of schizophrenic patients. The amygdala and several other limbic structures lie in the temporal lobe, and disorders of this part of the brain, notably temporal lobe epilepsy, are often associated with schizophreniform symptoms (Ounsted and Lindsay, 1981). In particular, temporal lobe epilepsy with a focus in the dominant hemisphere apparently predisposes to schizophrenia (Flor-Henry, 1969; Perez et al., 1985), an observation that has been the basis for the proposal that schizophrenia represents a dysfunction of the left temporal lobe. This proposal has been the subject of much investigation, especially using neuropsychological and electrophysiological techniques (Takahashi et al., 1987), although recently some supportive evidence has emerged from work with imaging techniques. In addition, there is evidence from neuropathology and neurochemistry of lateralised temporal lobe abnormalities in schizophrenia, which are also mentioned below.

With its multitude of interconnections with cortical regions, particularly those of the association cortex in the frontal and temporal lobes, the amygdala is thought to have a role in interrelating highly processed sensory input. Thus it is implicated in the selection of sensory information and in this respect it is notable that there has been much discussion as to how the attentional deficits found in schizophrenic patients might relate to a loss of this "filtering" of information (e.g., Hemsley, 1987). In addition, as Gloor (1986) states, the amygdala is involved in giving "an affective connotation to the perceptual information," presumably by relating and modulating this cortical input in concert with the transfer of information to and from subcortical structures such as the hypothalamus. In the dysfunctioning of such processes we have a mechanism for the blunted or inappropriate affect commonly seen in schizophrenia.

More than this has been gleaned from Gloor's work (Gloor, 1986) with amygdala stimulation in humans. Kling and Brothers (see Chapter 13, this volume) conclude that amygdala activity in the human is involved, at least in part, in the "neural representations of the dispositions and intentions of others." This is a succinct description of a process that is so clearly malfunctioning in the delusions of paranoid schizophrenia.

Thus there is much opportunity to postulate, on the basis of its functional neuroanatomy and involvement in complex behaviors, a role for the involvement of the amygdala in schizophrenia. Perusal of several other chapters in this volume will permit the reader to develop further hypotheses along these lines; however, such speculations are inevitably no more than circumstantial.

Do we have any direct evidence for abnormalities of the amygdala in schizophrenia? The recent developments in various imaging techniques and the application of quantitative morphometric and modern cytochemical methods to neuropathology has brought about great advances in the in vivo and postmortem study of the human brain. As yet, however, the amygdala has not attracted a large amount of attention; its size and position in the brain has made resolution a limiting factor in imaging studies and its anatomical complexity has probably inhibited neuropathological investigation. Nevertheless, there are some morphometric investigations describing changes in the amygdala and related regions of the brain in schizophrenia.

Consideration of the amygdala as a site of neuronal dysfunction in schizophrenia can be made in two ways. A structural abnormality within the region will inevitably be reflected by local changes in neuronal activity. However, neuropathological changes in other brain regions with projections to the amygdala may also induce effects on the activity of neurons in this region. That the amygdala innervates, and receives innervation from, a very wide range of other regions of the brain suggests that dysfunction in one of many parts of the brain could influence neuronal function in the amygdala. In this respect it is relevant to mention the emphasis that Poletti (1986) puts on the close interrelationship between the amygdala and the anterior hippocampus, describing one function of the amygdala as integrating and modulating the influence of the anterior hippocampus. Abnormalities of some of the structures which are closely related to the amygdala, particularly the hippocampus but also the frontal cortex, are certainly strongly implicated in schizophrenia. It is thus appropriate to consider the neurochemical and pathological changes in these regions too, since there are indications that these changes may influence amygdala function in the disease.

NEUROPATHOLOGICAL CONSIDERATIONS
The Medial Temporal Lobe

Of the recent advances in the neuropathology of schizophrenia, it is the study of the regions of the temporal lobe that has been most productive in identifying cellular and structural abnormalities of the brain. One key report is that of Crow et al. (1989), who showed, in a highly "purified" series of brains in which other pathologies were eliminated, an increase in volume of the temporal horn of the left lateral ventricle. Some magnetic resonance imaging studies provide in vivo support for these results (e.g., Bogerts et al., 1990) and, although they are not always confirmed in other neuropathological and imaging studies (e.g., Kelsoe et al., 1988), it would seem that there is strong evidence for a structural abnormality of the (left) temporal lobe in schizophrenia. There are certainly other reports in support of this interpretation.

In a study of a series of brains collected over 40 years ago from well-documented schizophrenic cases (the Vogt collection), it was found that the amygdala and hippocampus were substantially and significantly decreased in volume in comparison with a control series (Bogerts et al., 1985). It is notable that these studies were performed on single, primarily left, hemispheres. Further studies by this group indicated that the central and basolateral nuclei of the amygdala were the most affected parts of this structure (Falkai, unpublished).

Within the medial temporal lobe, the hippocampus and adjacent cortex have been better studied than the amygdala and yielded more evidence for a neuropathology in schizophrenia. A diminished volume of the hippocampus is mentioned above; neuronal counts have indicated that this may reflect a deficit of hippocampal neurons (Falkai and Bogerts, 1986; Jeste and Lohr, 1989). In addition, a disorientation of pyramidal neurons has also been reported (Kovelman and Scheibel, 1984), although the work of other groups (e.g., Christison et al., 1989) has demonstrated that both neuronal deficits and disorientation is not a consistent finding.

The adjacent entorhinal cortex also demonstrates pathological differences in schizophrenia. A unilateral (left hemisphere) thinning of the parahippocampal region has been found (Brown et al., 1986). The microscopic correlate of this observation might be found in the reports of neuronal deficits (Falkai et al., 1988) and a disorganisation of normal neuronal grouping in this area which has been interpreted as reflecting a developmental abnormality (Jakob and Beckmann, 1986).

The Frontal Cortex

Early imaging studies of the brain in schizophrenia have concentrated, partly for methodological reasons, on cortical structures. A repeated, although not invariable, observation is that cortical blood flow (Ingvar and Franzen, 1974), as well as more direct measures of energy metabolism (Weinberger and Berman, 1988), are relatively reduced in the frontal cortex. This "hypofrontality" has been found to correlate with various more negative symptoms of the disease (Ingvar, 1987).

There have been few morphometric studies of the cortex in schizophrenia, although one exception is the work of Benes et al. (1986), who reported that there were significant, and laminar-specific, neuronal deficits in the prefrontal cortex suggestive of losses in corticofugal pathways. No glial proliferation was observed, indicating that here too a developmental disturbance, and not an atrophic process, was responsible for the changes observed.

NEUROCHEMICAL STUDIES IN SCHIZOPHRENIA

Neurochemical studies using postmortem brain tissue are presently the major approach in understanding neurotransmitter involvement in the neuronal changes presumed to be present in, and associated with, schizophrenia (for recent reviews, see Owen and Crow, 1987; Reynolds, 1988, 1989). Various hypotheses of the disease have been followed up in this way, of which the "dopamine hypothesis" has attracted the most interest. This reflects the fact that pharmacological accentuation of dopamine neurotransmission by, for example, amphetamine administration can induce, or increase, schizophreniform symptoms and that the one action common to all major neuroleptic drugs is a blockade of dopaminergic neurotransmission. This latter observation points to the site of antipsychotic action but provides no direct evidence for an abnormal increase in the activity of dopaminergic neurons in schizophrenia.

More recently, an interest in amino acid neurotransmitter systems has yielded results, discussed below, that are beginning to provide neurochemical correlates of some of the abnormalities found in pathological studies. Nevertheless, a complete understanding of brain dysfunction in schizophrenia will require the integration of neurochemical and morphological findings with the pharmacological effects of antipsychotic drugs. This demonstrates the value of a continued consideration of dopamine systems in the disease.

AMYGDALA FUNCTION AND DOPAMINE

The amygdala receives a substantial dopaminergic innervation from several groups of brain stem neurons, notably (but not exclusively) the ventral tegmental area and the substantia nigra compacta (Takada, 1990). These innervations, which represent the major proportion of dopamine projections to the temporal lobe, are primarily to the central and lateral nuclei of the amygdala, where the dopamine concentrations are between 4 and 100 times greater than those in the other major nuclei (Kilts et al., 1988). These authors have also shown how the activity of dopamine neurons in these terminal regions of the rat brain is low, relative to striatal and cortical regions. This, however, may not be as true in the human brain since the ratios of the major metabolite of dopamine, homovanillic acid, to dopamine are substantially higher in the amygdala than those found in the caudate nucleus (Reynolds, 1987). On the basis of this and other biochemical and pharmacological evidence, Kilts et al. (1988) have shown that these neurons exhibit many differences from the dopaminergic innervation of other limbic structures (e.g., the nucleus accumbens).

Without an understanding of the intimate neuronal connections of the dopamine terminals in the amygdala, it is not possible to ascribe a role to these pathways in the control of dysfunctioning systems in schizophrenia. Nevertheless, it is conceivable that inhibitory dopaminergic neurons can modulate the various, and varied, complex inputs from the cortex. It is especially notable that substantial efferents to the highly dopaminergically innervated central nucleus of the amygdala derive from both of the areas particularly implicated in the neurochemical and structural pathology of schizophrenia: the hippocampus (Morrison and Poletti, 1980) and frontal cortex (e.g., Kapp et al., 1985).

Amygdala Dopamine and Laterality

Neuropathological and physiological evidence of the involvement of the temporal lobe in schizophrenia is increasingly implicating the left hemisphere. The human amygdala normally demonstrates a hemispheric asymmetry of volume

(Murphy et al., 1987) with the lateral nucleus (one of the two regions containing most dopamine) showing the strongest effect. Perhaps surprisingly, a functional laterality of the dopamine system of the rat amygdala has been reported (Bradbury et al., 1985). These authors observed that dopamine could induce a hyperactive response when delivered into the left amygdala of animals with a left-turning preference. This identified a subgroup of animals that may be equivalent to one of the two groups defined by Simon et al. (1988), who showed that amphetamine will induce increased activity in only a proportion of rats receiving a bilateral 6-hydroxydopamine lesion of amygdala dopamine neurons. This evidence for a laterality of dopamine function in the amygdala would be less interesting were it not for the indication that there is also a laterality of this system in schizophrenia, as described below.

AMYGDALA NEUROCHEMISTRY AND SCHIZOPHRENIA
Dopamine

In spite of the evidence implicating the medial temporal lobe and dopamine projection regions within the limbic system, past neurochemical studies have paid little attention to the amygdala as a potential pathophysiological site in schizophrenia. One major indication of a neurochemical abnormality in this region in schizophrenia was the finding of an increase in the concentration of dopamine in postmortem brain tissue from two series of patients (Reynolds, 1983). The increase was not reflected by changes in noradrenaline or markers for other mesolimbic neurons, nor was it observed in the caudate nucleus in the same cases. But, most importantly, it was found to be specific to the left hemisphere, not being found in the right amygdala. This asymmetric increase has been confirmed in further series of cases, in which a corresponding (albeit smaller) asymmetry of homovanillic acid was also found, with an increase in the left amygdala (Reynolds, 1987). A range of other neurochemical markers for monoamine neurons have also been investigated and show no changes or asymmetry in this region. While the finding appears to be relatively specific, the results could be due to an effect of neuroleptic treatment, although such a lateralisation of neurochemical response to drugs would still imply an interesting asymmetry of function in the amygdala. Nor is it clear whether an asymmetry of dopaminergic innervation or of neuronal activity might be responsible for the lateralised increase in amygdala dopamine. The latter interpretation could be a result of unilateral atrophy of another neuronal system which provides a controlling influence on amygdala dopaminergic terminals. There is evidence that such an effect might indeed occur and this is discussed below.

Neuropeptides

In two independent neurochemical studies, vasoactive intestinal polypeptide (VIP) was observed to be increased in the amygdala in schizophrenia (Roberts et al., 1983; Emson et al., cited by Bissette et al., 1986), the former group finding the effect in a type I subgroup of patients. An immunohistochemical study gave results consistent with these findings, observing a slight increase in the central nucleus of the amygdala in schizophrenic patients (Zech et al., 1986).

VIP coexists with acetylcholine in the neurons of this structure, and since an overall increase in amygdala choline acetyltransferase has not been observed (Reynolds, 1986), there may be a relative increase in the VIP synthesis and release in the amygdala. If this effect was not artifactual in being, for example, related to drug treatment, it could be secondary to pathological changes in other neuronal systems.

Some other neurochemical differences may well reflect deficits of specific neuronal populations, although here, as before, no account has been taken of possible hemispheric differences. Thus while cholecystokinin (CCK) is unchanged in several brain areas in acute psychotic patients (Kleinman et al., 1983), it has been found to be reduced in the amygdala from patients presenting with primarily negative symptoms (Roberts et al., 1983).

γ-Aminobutyric Acid

The close, and to some extent reciprocal, relationship between the γ-aminobutyric acid (GABA) and dopamine-containing neurons of the striatum and substantia nigra has led to the proposal that a reduction in the activity of the inhibitory neurotransmitter GABA may underlie an enhanced dopaminergic function in schizophrenia (Roberts, 1972). That such a relationship extends to the more relevant areas of the brain, the temporal lobe and limbic system, is not clear. Nevertheless there are indications of abnormalities in GABAergic systems in the amygdala and related structures.

The changes in CCK mentioned above provide some support. While CCK is found to coexist with dopamine in some mesolimbic neurons, by far the great majority of limbic and cortical CCK is present in GABAergic cells (Somogyi et al., 1984). Thus it is likely that the losses of CCK in the amygdala reflect deficits in a subgroup of GABA neurons. Measurement of the amino acid itself has been undertaken in a range of brain regions from chronic schizophrenics. GABA was found to be diminished only in the amygdala, as was tryptophan (Korpi et al., 1987). The fact that increased tryptophan concentrations in brain are an indicator of hypoxic terminal illness suggested to these authors that the changes in GABA too might be artifactual, although GABA concentrations are normally unrelated to agonal state. An earlier study also found a deficit of GABA in the amygdala of psychotic patients (Spokes et al., 1980), although not all investigations have been able to confirm this finding (Reynolds, 1987).

Since GABA concentrations in the brain rapidly increase postmortem by 100–200%, measurement of the amino acid is not always considered to be a particularly sensitive indicator of GABAergic neuronal integrity in human brain tissue. An alternative marker for GABAergic neurons is the GABA uptake site. Binding of radiolabelled nipecotic acid to brain tissue membranes gives a measure of these sites which presumably relates to the density of GABAergic terminals in brain (Czudek and Reynolds, 1990). The technique has recently been applied to amygdala tissue from schizophrenic patients; one report was of a significant 10–20% deficit below control values (Simpson et al., 1989). In another study, the use of an improved method gave consistent results demonstrating a 10–15% loss (albeit not reaching statistical significance) of these binding sites in the amygdala in schizophrenia (Reynolds et al., 1990). Most neurochemical studies of the amygdala have been unilateral; however, the last two reports above showed that the decreases were not particularly related to one hemisphere; a bilateral amygdala deficit was apparent.

It would appear that investigations of both neuropeptides and amino acids are consistent with a subtle deficit of (subtypes of) GABAergic neurons in the amygdala in at least some patients with schizophrenia.

Excitatory Amino Acids

Glutamate is the major excitatory neurotransmitter and is ubiquitously, if unequally, distributed throughout the central nervous system. Along with aspartate, the transmitter has effects on several subtypes of postsynaptic receptor and these receptors, along with presynaptic indicators of excitatory amino acid systems, have been studied in postmortem brain tissue in schizophrenia. As yet, no consistent changes in markers for glutamate synapses have been identified in the amygdala, although this is not true for other regions of the brain, and these are described below.

NEUROCHEMICAL CHANGES IN RELATED REGIONS
The Frontal Cortex

That dopamine turnover is increased in frontal (and other) cortical regions in schizophrenia is apparent from the increased concentrations of its major metabolite, homovanillic acid, in these regions in postmortem brain tissue. This is undoubtedly an effect of chronic neuroleptic medication (Bacopoulos et al., 1979); nevertheless it could conceivably result in changes in the activity of neuronal systems of the amygdala via an influence on the cortical output neurons innervating the structure.

There are also disease-related neurochemical pathologies of the frontal cortex, as indicated by the changes associated with glutamatergic synaptic transmission, although no chemical parallel of the pathological findings of Benes et al. (1986) has been identified. Two groups have reported increases in the kainate subtype of glutamate receptors, albeit in different cortical regions (Nishikawa et al., 1983; Deakin et al., 1989). One interpretation of increases in postsynaptic receptors is that they might be in response to presynaptic denervation; however, there is no evidence for glutamatergic deficits in this case since two presynaptic markers, glutamate concentrations (Reynolds, 1991) and ligand binding to glutamate uptake sites (Deakin et al., 1989), are both increased in orbital frontal cortex. If these findings are confirmed, they would be more consistent with a relative increase in the number of glutamatergic synapses in the frontal cortex in schizophrenia.

The Hippocampus

As has been mentioned above, it is the structures of the medial temporal lobe that have particularly been found to exhibit neuropathological abnormalities. These are apparent in the two adjacent structures of the hippocampus and parahippocampal gyrus, perhaps to a greater extent than the amygdala, although the complexity of the amygdala has made quantitative neuropathological investigations less straightforward than in the former laminar structures.

The morphological abnormalities found in the hippocampus in schizophrenia are found to have some neurochemical correlates. One is the observed decrease in binding to a kainate-sensitive subgroup of glutamate receptors in the left hippocampus (Kerwin et al., 1988), which could be interpreted in terms of a lateralised loss of neurons on which these receptors lie. Other evidence appears to indicate the identity of the affected neurons in terms of their neurotransmitter deficits. Both CCK and somatostatin are reportedly diminished in the hippocampus of patients presenting with negative symptoms (Roberts et al., 1983). Like CCK, somatostatin is found almost exclusively in GABAergic neurons in this area (Somogyi et al., 1984) and thus this result is indicative of a deficit in another subgroup of hippocampal GABA-containing cells.

Recently there has been more direct evidence in support of this conclusion. Two studies have identified a bilateral decrease in GABA uptake sites in the hippocampus in schizophrenic patients (Simpson et al., 1989; Reynolds et al., 1990), the latter report indicating an additional asymmetry with a greater deficit in the left hemisphere. This deficit in a marker for GABA neurons, with a more profound effect in the left hemisphere, is potentially related to the increased concentrations in dopamine in the amygdala. It was found that only in the left hemisphere of schizophrenic patients is there a correlation between amygdala dopamine concentrations and the numbers of hippocampal GABA uptake sites (Reynolds et al., 1990).

It is tempting to conclude that there might be a causal relationship in the correlation between hippocampal GABA uptake sites and amygdala dopamine in the left hemisphere. Such a relationship might imply that a neuronal deficit in the hippocampus could lead to an increase in dopamine in the amygdala, perhaps via a presynaptic effect on dopamine neuronal activity. Certainly there is a substantial innervation of the region of the amygdala containing the greatest amounts of dopamine, the central nucleus, by the anterior hippocampus (Morrison and Poletti, 1980). While this is excitatory and presumably not containing GABA, a deficit of local hippocampal GABAergic neurons could conceivably lead to a diminished inhibition of these output pathways. Such a relationship between hippocampal GABA and amygdala dopamine systems has yet to be tested in an animal model. However, some circumstantial evidence in support is found in studies of the influence of the GABA cotransmitter CCK on dopamine systems in the limbic brain. Suggestions have emerged that CCK and related peptides act via an inhibition of limbic dopaminergic activity, with behavioral effects following intracerebral injection in the rat that resemble those of the neuroleptic drugs (Van Ree et al., 1983). This implies that a loss of CCK-containing GABAergic neurons in schizophrenia could result in a disinhibition of limbic dopamine, an effect which in turn might be ameliorated by treatment with neuroleptic drugs.

AMYGDALA DOPAMINE SYSTEMS AND ANTIPSYCHOTIC EFFECTS

Although very speculative, this latter point is an important one. Any useful hypothesis for the cerebral abnormalities responsible for the symptoms of schizophrenia needs to be compatible with the antipsychotic effects of the neuroleptic drugs. Since these effects are most likely to be produced by antagonist action at dopamine receptors, the interaction between dopamine systems and any neuronal ronal deficits in the disease must be considered. Thus while the neuropathological evidence mainly implicates the medial temporal lobe, and perhaps the hippocampus and entorhinal cortex rather more than the amygdala, the fact that the amygdala contains by far the greatest dopaminergic innervation of the temporal lobe is a major factor in concentrating our attention on this structure. This argument applies more to the positive symptoms of the disease than to the more negative symptoms, which respond less well to classical dopamine D2 receptor antagonists.

It has been mentioned above how the dopamine neurons projecting to the amygdala appear to have properties differing substantially from other mesolimbic or mesostriatal neurons (Kilts et al., 1988). This includes the development of tolerance to the increase in dopamine turnover in response to chronic haloperidol administration. In the central and lateral nuclei of the amygdala this occurs to a greater extent than in striatal regions; in the frontal cortex the subsequent decrease in dopamine turnover is even less. A previous study (Matsumoto et al., 1983) showed the amygdala to demonstrate the greatest tolerance of all of 12 regions studied after 10 weeks haloperidol treatment. Although these authors suggested the lack of tolerance in the frontal cortex indicated that this region was important in the action of the neuroleptics, Kilts et al. (1988) propose the amygdala effect to be a critical mechanism in the antipsychotic action of these drugs, with the time course of the antipsychotic response (typically developing over several weeks) potentially correlating with this development of tolerance.

There has recently been a development in psychopharmacology that has permitted the pharmacological perspective of schizophrenia to develop beyond the simple dopaminergic hyperfunction model and to take a step toward compatibility with neuronal deficits in the disease. This is the observation that phencyclidine (PCP) can produce a syndrome in humans that resembles schizophrenia, exhibiting both the positive and the negative symptoms seen in the disease. Thus as a human model of schizophrenia, PCP is considered to induce a symptom profile closer to the disease than is the model provided by amphetamine-induced psychosis, in which the negative symptoms are not an important component.

PCP blocks the ion channel associated with the NMDA subtype of glutamate receptors as well as having effects on the little-understood sigma site. These actions are presumably responsible for the highly specific changes in dopaminergic activity that PCP is found to induce. After PCP administration, dopamine release is increased in the amygdala and cortical regions but not in the striatum (Rao et al., 1989). These effects presumably reflect differences between the systems regulating nigrostriatal and mesocortical/mesolimbic dopaminergic pathways. One explanation might be that glutamatergic systems have a modulatory effect (through NMDA receptors) on dopamine release in the amygdala and cortex, but no such influence in the striatum. If this were so, neuronal deficits might be expected to have similar effects. Thus losses of the equivalent glutamatergic neurons, or a deficit of the postsynaptic cells on which the receptor sites lie, could also induce PCP-like dopamine release in the amygdala and/or cortex and thereby produce, in humans, some of the symptoms of schizophrenia. As yet, a decrease in the numbers of PCP binding sites has not been identified in temporal lobe structures in schizophrenia, although these proposals would be compatible with the deficit of GABAergic interneurons indicated above.

CONCLUSION

We are still far from understanding the role of the amygdala in schizophrenia. Nevertheless there is substantial evidence in support of its (dys)function in at least some of the symptoms of the disease:

1. Neuropsychological investigations indicate its importance in the control of behaviors that are abnormal in schizophrenia;

2. It has a close anatomical and neuronal relationship with other structures (i.e., the frontal cortex and the other medial temporal lobe regions) implicated in these behaviors;

3. Chemical and morphological neuropathology of these structures, as well as (perhaps to a lesser extent) the amygdala itself, is apparent in brains of patients with schizophrenia;

4. Some evidence for a lateralisation of amygdala neurochemistry and its relationship to hippocampal neuropathology supports the suggestion of left temporal lobe dysfunction in the disease; and

5. The dopaminergic innervation of the amygdala provides a means of understanding the action of antipsychotic drugs in a disease with primarily temporal lobe pathology.

REFERENCES

Bacopoulos NG, Spokes EG, Bird ED, Roth RH (1979): Antipsychotic drug action in schizophrenic patients: Effects on cortical dopamine metabolism after long-term treatment. Science 205:1405–1407.

Benes FM, Davidson J, Bird ED (1986): Quantitative cytoarchitectural studies of the cerebral cortex in schizophrenics. Arch Gen Psychiat 44:1017–1021.

Bissette G, Nemeroff CB, Mackay AVP (1986): Peptides in schizophrenia. In Emson PC, Rossor M, Tohyama M (eds): "Progress in Brain Research," Vol 66. Amsterdam: Elsevier, pp 161–174.

Bogerts B, Meetz C, Schonfeldt-Bausch R (1985): Basal ganglia and limbic system pathology in schizophrenia: A morphometric study. Arch Gen Psychiat 42:784–791.

Bogerts B, Ashtari M, Degreef G et al. (1990): Reduced temporal limbic structure volumes on magnetic resonance images in first episode schizophrenia. Psychiat Res 35:1–13.

Bradbury AJ, Costall B, Domeney AM, Naylor RJ (1985): Laterality of dopamine function and neuroleptic action in the amygdala in the rat. Neuropharmacology 24: 1163–1170.

Brown R, Colter N, Corsellis JAN et al. (1986): Postmortem evidence of structural brain changes in schizophrenia. Arch Gen Psychiat 43:36–42.

Christison GW, Casanova MF, Weinberger DR, Rawlings R, Kleinman JE (1989): A quantitative investigation of hippocampal pyramidal cell size, shape and variability of orientation in schizophrenia. Arch Gen Psychiat 46:1027–1032.

Crow TJ (1980): Positive and negative symptoms and the role of dopamine. Br J Psychiat 137:383–386.

Crow TJ, Ball J, Bloom SR, Brown R, Bruton CJ, Colter N, Frith CD, Johnstone EC, Owens DGC, Roberts GW (1989): Schizophrenia as an anomaly of development of cerebral asymmetry. Arch Gen Psychiat 46:1145–1150.

Czudek C, Reynolds GP (1990): (^{3}H)-Nipecotic acid binding to GABA uptake sites in postmortem human brain. J Neurochem 55:165–168.

Deakin JFW, Slater P, Simpson MDC, Gilchrist AC, Skan WJ, Royston MC, Reynolds GP, Cross AJ (1989): Frontal cortical and left glutamatergic dysfunction of schizophrenia. J Neurochem 52:1781–1789.

Falkai P, Bogerts B (1986): Cell loss in the hippocampus of schizophrenics. Eur Arch Psychiat Neurol Sci 236:154–161.

Falkai P, Bogerts B, Rozemuk M (1988): Limbic pathology in schizophrenia: the entorhinal cortex—a morphometric study. Biol Psych 24:515–521.

Flor-Henry P (1969): Psychosis and temporal lobe epilepsy: A controlled investigation. Epilepsia 10:363–395.

Gloor P (1986): Role of the human limbic system in perception, memory and affect. In Doane BK, Livingston KE (eds): "The Limbic System." New York: Raven Press, pp 159–169.

Heath RG (1954): "Studies in Schizophrenia." Cambridge: Harvard University Press.

Hemsley DR (1987): An experimental psychological model for schizophrenia. In Häfner H, Gattaz WF, Janzarik W (eds): "Search for the Causes of Schizophrenia." Heidelberg: Springer, pp 179–188.

Ingvar, DH (1987): Evidence for frontal/prefrontal cortical dysfunction in chronic schizophrenia: The phenomenon of "hypofrontality" reconsidered. In Helmchen H, Henn FA (eds): "Biological Perspectives of Schizophrenia." Chichester: Wiley, pp 201–212.

Ingvar DH, Franzen G (1974): Abnormalities of cerebral blood flow distribution in patients with chronic schizophrenia. Acta Psychiat Scand 50:425–436.

Jakob H, Beckmann H (1986): Prenatal development disturbances in the limbic allocortex in schizophrenics. J Neural Trans 65:303–326.

Jeste DV, Lohr JB (1989): Hippocampal pathological findings in schizophrenia. Arch Gen Psychiat 46:1019–1024.

Kapp BS, Schwaber JS, Driscoll PA (1985): Frontal cortex projections to the amygdaloid central nucleus in the rabbit. Neuroscience 15:327–346.

Kelsoe JR, Cadet JL, Pickar D, Weinberger DR (1989): Quantitative neuroanatomy in schizophrenia. Arch Gen Psychiat 45:533–541.

Kerwin RW, Patel S, Meldrum BS, Czudek C, Reynolds GP (1988): Asymmetric loss of glutamate receptor subtype in left hippocampus in schizophrenia. Lancet 1:583–584.

Kilts CD, Anderson CM, Ely TD, Mailman RB (1988): The biochemistry and pharmacology of mesoamygdaloid dopamine neurons. Ann NY Acad Sci 537:173–187.

Korpi ER, Kleinman JE, Goodman SI, Wyatt RJ (1987): Neurotransmitter amino acids in post-mortem brains of chronic schizophrenic patients. Psychiat Res 22:291–301.

Kovelman JA, Scheibel AB (1984): A neurohistological correlate of schizophrenia. Biol Psychiat 19:1601–1621.

Kleinman JE, Iadarola M, Govoni S, Hong J, Gillin JC, Wyatt RJ (1983): Postmortem measurements of neuropeptides in human brain. Psychopharmacol Bull 19:375–377.

Matsumoto T, Uchimura H, Hirano M et al. (1983): Differential effects of acute and chronic administration of haloperidol on homovanillic acid levels in discrete dopaminergic areas of rat brain. Eur J Pharmacol 89:27–33.

Morrison F, Poletti CE (1980): Hippocampal influence on amygdala unit activity in awake squirrel monkeys. Brain Res 192:353–369.

Murphy GM, Inger P, Mark K, Lin J, Morrice W, Gee C, Gan S, Korp B (1987): Volumetric asymmetry in the human amygdaloid complex. J Hirnforsch 28:281–289.

Nishikawa T, Takashima M, Toru M (1983): Increased (^{3}H)kainic acid binding in the prefrontal cortex in schizophrenia. Neurosci Lett 40:245–250.

Ounsted C, Lindsay J (1981): In Reynolds EH, Trimble MR (eds): "Epilepsy and Psychiatry." Edinburgh: Churchill Livingstone.

Owen F, Crow TJ (1987): Neurotransmitters and psychosis. Br Med Bull 43:651–671.

Perez MM, Trimble MR, Murray NMF, Rieder R (1985): Epileptic psychosis: An evaluation of PSE profiles. Br J Psychiat 146:155–163.

Poletti CE (1986): Is the limbic system a limbic system. In Doane BK, Livingston KE (eds): "The Limbic System." New York: Raven Press, pp 79–94.

Rao TS, Kim HS, Lehmann J, Martin LL, Wood PL (1989): Differential effects of phencyclidine (PCP) and ketamine on mesocortical and mesostriatal dopamine release in vivo. Life Sci 45:1065–1072.

Reynolds GP (1983): Increased concentrations and lateral asymmetry of amygdala dopamine in schizophrenia. Nature 305:527–529.

Reynolds GP (1986): Amygdala dopamine asymmetry in schizophrenia: Neurochemical evidence for a left temporal lobe dysfunction. In Woodruff GN, Poat JAP, Roberts PJ (eds): "Dopaminergic Systems and Their Regulation." London: Macmillan, pp 285–291.

Reynolds GP (1987): Post-mortem neurochemical studies in schizophrenia. In Häfner H, Gattaz WF, Janzarik W (eds): "Search for the causes of schizophrenia." Heidelberg: Springer, pp 236–240.

Reynolds GP (1988): Post-mortem neurochemistry of schizophrenia. Psychol Med 18: 793–797.

Reynolds GP (1989): Beyond the dopamine hypothesis: The neurochemical pathology of schizophrenia. Br J Psychiat 155:305–316.

Reynolds GP, Czudek C, Andrews HA (1990): Deficit and hemispheric asymmetry of GABA uptake sites in the hippocampus in schizophrenia. Biol Psychiat 27:1038–1044.

Reynolds GP (1991): The neurochemical pathology of schizophrenia: Evidence for abnormalities in amino acid transmitter system. In Nakazawa T (ed): "The Biological Basis of Schizophrenic Disorders." Tokyo: Scientific Societies Press (in press).

Roberts E (1972): An hypothesis suggesting that there is a deficit in the GABA system in schizophrenia. Neurosci Res Prog Bull 10:468–481.

Roberts GW, Ferrier NI, Lee Y et al. (1983): Peptides, the limbic lobe and schizophrenia. Brain Res 288:199–211.

Simon H, Taghzouti K, Gozlan H et al. (1988): Lesion of dopaminergic terminals in the amygdala produces enhanced locomotor response to D-amphetamine and opposite changes in dopaminergic activity in prefrontal cortex and nucleus accumbens. Brain Res 447:335–340.

Simpson MDC, Slater P, Deakin JFW, Royston MC, Skan WJ (1989): Reduced GABA uptake sites in the temporal lobe in schizophrenia. Neurosci Lett 107:211–215.

Somogyi P, Hodgson AJ, Smith AD, Nunzi MG, Gorio A, Wu JY (1984): Different populations in the visual cortex and hippocampus of cat contain somatostatin or cholecystokinin-immunoreactive material. J Neurosci 4:2590–2603.

Spokes EGS, Garrett NJ, Rossor MN, Iversen LL (1980): Distribution of GABA in postmortem brain tissue from control, psychotic and Huntington's chorea subjects. J Neurol Sci 48:303–313.

Stevens JR (1973): An anatomy of schizophrenia? Arch Gen Psychiat 29:177–189.

Takada M (1990): The A11 catecholamine cell group: Another origin of the dopaminergic innervation of the amygdala. Neurosci Lett 118:132–135.

Takahashi R, Flor-Henry P, Gruzelier J, Niwa S-I (eds) (1987): "Cerebral Dynamics, Laterality and Psychopathology." Amsterdam: Elsevier.

Torrey EF, Peterson MR (1974): Schizophrenia and the limbic system. Lancet 2:942–946.

Van Ree JM, Gaffori O, De Wied D (1983): In rats the behaviour profile of CCK-8 related peptides resembles that of antipsychotic agents. Eur J Pharmacol 93:63–78. .

Weinberger DR, Berman KF (1988): Speculation on the meaning of cerebral metabolic hypofrontality in schizophrenia. Schiz Bull 14:157–168.

Zech M, Roberts GW, Bogets B, Crow TJ, Polak JM (1986): Neuropeptides in the amygdala of controls, schizophrenics and patients suffering from Huntington's chorea: An immunohistochemical study. Acta Neuropathol 71:259–266.

The Amygdala: Neurobiological Aspects of Emotion,
Memory, and Mental Dysfunction, pages 575–593
© 1992 Wiley-Liss, Inc.

23

The Neuropathology of the Amygdala in Ageing and in Dementia

D.M.A. MANN

*Division of Molecular Pathology, Department of Pathological Sciences,
University of Manchester, Manchester, UK*

INTRODUCTION

The amygdala, through its connections with the hippocampus, temporal association cortex, and basal forebrain (see Chapter 1, Amaral, this volume) occupies a strategic position in the circuitry of the limbic system. A collective degeneration of this part of the brain has long been recognized as fundamental to disorders such as Alzheimer's disease and Pick's disease. Although the nature of the structural and biochemical defects that characterize these conditions has (particularly in recent times) been intensely studied in neighboring temporal neocortical and hippocampal areas, the amygdala itself has received much less attention.

In this chapter I review the nature of the pathological changes that occur in the amygdala in ageing and in dementing disorders such as Alzheimer's disease and related conditions like Down's syndrome. I will also encompass less common conditions such as Pick's disease and other "frontal-lobe" type dementias. The mechanisms whereby the pathological changes underlying the disorders are brought about and progress are discussed, as are the contributions such changes might make to the causation of the complex clinical symptomatology that typifies these diseases.

THE AMYGDALA IN ALZHEIMER'S DISEASE

Early descriptions of the involvement of the amygdala in the pathology of Alzheimer's disease go back to 1928 (Grunthal, 1928) and 1938 (Brockhaus, 1938); this latter author noted that in an 82-year-old woman with Alzheimer's disease, neuronal loss, reactive astrocytosis, and senile plaques were widely present and showed preferential involvement of the cortical nuclei. Later, Hirano and Zimmerman (1962) and Jamada and Mehraein (1968) remarked upon the high

Address correspondence to: Dr. D.M.A. Mann, Department of Pathological Sciences, University of Manchester, Oxford Road, Manchester, M13 9PT, UK.

neurofibrillary tangle counts within this structure and both Corsellis (1970) and Hooper and Vogel (1976) stressed the severe degeneration that occurred in the cortical and medial nuclei, as opposed to the basal and lateral regions.

However, it has only been recently that the neuropathology (particularly) and neurochemistry of the amygdala in Alzheimer's disease have been systematically studied. Investigations have moved toward a quantitative base in order that the topographic pattern to the damage might be better understood. Given the heterogeneity of structure and connectivity of this complex region, such regional data can provide valuable clues toward unravelling the pathogenetic process and the manner of the progression of the disorder.

Gross Atrophy

A marked reduction in the size of the amygdala is usually conspicuous in most cases of Alzheimer's disease and this is especially so in those persons dying before the age of 75 years (Fig. 1); enlargement of the temporal horn of the lateral ventricle usually accompanies this atrophy. In quantitative studies (Table I) we have found, in formalin-fixed coronal slices of brain from 10 younger patients with Alzheimer's disease, that the cross-sectional area (when compared to age- and sex-matched controls) is reduced, on average, by 40% and by as much as 60% in some instances (Fig. 2). Brady and Mufson (1990), in a series of 12 patients aged 68–92 years, noted the average cross-sectional area of the amygdala to be 35% less than that of controls.

The atrophy is often apparently preferential for the medial and cortical nuclei, with relative preservation of the basal and lateral nuclei, such that on cross section the nucleus adopts a "spindle" shape (Fig. 1), rather than the customary roughly circular profile. The adjacent uncus (pyriform cortex) is also usually obviously atrophied (Fig. 1). In a study of four males, aged 70–78 years, with Alzheimer's disease, Herzog and Kemper (1980) noted an overall 26% decrease in *volume* of the amygdala; all regions showed a significant decline in volume, though greatest reductions were noted in the cortical and medial nuclei (38%). The relatively minor differences between our own estimates and those of Brady and Mufson (1990) and Herzog and Kemper (1980) may reflect sampling variations, sample size, or age differences within studied patients. In this latter context, gross atrophy of the amygdala is seen more often in younger (i.e., less than 75 years old) patients (Mann, unpublished observations), though within the limited quantitative data so far available, such an inverse relationship between age and degree of atrophy does not necessarily achieve statistical significance (Mann, unpublished data; Brady and Mufson, 1990).

These areal/volumetric changes are reflected by weight alterations; Najlerahim and Bowen (1988) reported the weight of the amygdala in six elderly (73–89 years) females with Alzheimer's disease to be reduced by 47% from a control value of 1.14 g to that of 0.60 g.

Nerve Cell Loss

Although in Alzheimer's disease a widespread loss of nerve cells, but particularly from cortical and medial nuclei, is often readily appreciated in either routine haematoxylin & eosin- or Nissl-stained sections (Mann et al., 1988a) or

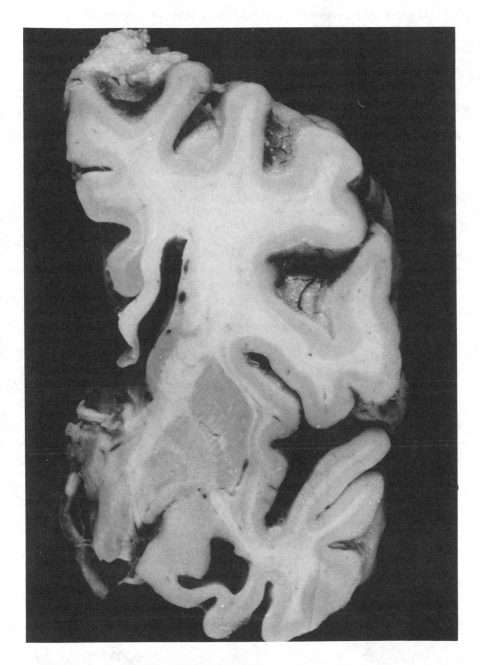

Fig. 1. Coronal section of cerebral hemisphere from a 65-year-old female with Alzheimer's disease. Note atrophy of the amygdala, especially within medial parts, and enlargement of the temporal horn of the lateral ventricle.

TABLE I. Atrophy of Amygdala in Dementing Disorders

Disorder	Case	Control	% Loss in Case
Alzheimer's disease (n = 10)	107.2 ± 29.5	173.6 ± 28.1	38.2
Pick's disease (n = 1)	56.3	186.0	69.7
Frontal lobe dementia (n = 7)	98.4 ± 38.5	174.2 ± 16.6	43.5
Frontal dementia with motor neuron disease (n = 5)	156.5 ± 21.8	188.0 ± 6.3	16.8
Huntington's chorea (n = 6)	119.6 ± 6.9	185.7 ± 30.5	35.6
Progressive supranuclear palsy (n = 2)	154.4 ± 9.3	180.0 ± 6.3	14.2

Mean (± SD) profile area of the amygdala in several dementing disorders, along with that from appropriate age-, and sex-matched control patients. Percentage reduction in profile area is given for each disorder. Number of patients is given in parentheses.

in acetylcholinesterase (AchE)-stained preparations (Rasool et al., 1986), only a single study (Herzog and Kemper, 1980) has attempted to quantify the extent of this nerve cell loss, either generally or on a regional basis. In this latter study these authors noticed a significant decrease in packing density of neurons in all subdivisions of the amygdala, though greatest reductions were found in cortical and medial nuclei (35–51%), whereas in lateral and basal nuclei the decreases ranged from 15–32%. When regional changes in volume were taken into account, these decreases in packing density translate into *absolute* reductions in neuron number of some 61–70% in cortical and medial nuclei respectively.

Losses of this magnitude at least match and probably exceed those reported for hippocampus (Ball, 1972; Mann et al., 1985), temporal cortex (Terry et al., 1981; Mountjoy et al., 1983; Mann et al., 1985), and nucleus basalis of Meynert (Mann et al., 1984), again emphasizing the serious involvement of the amygdala in the pathology of Alzheimer's disease.

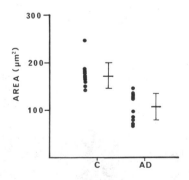

Fig. 2. Cross-sectional area of the amygdala in 10 patients with Alzheimer's disease (AD) and 10 age- and sex-matched non-demented controls (C). Mean (± SD) values are indicated for both patient groups.

Neurotransmitter Changes

In view of the extent of tissue atrophy and neuronal fallout, alterations in transmitter levels would be predictable. The amygdala receives a strong, cholinergic input from the nucleus basalis of Meynert (Carlsen et al., 1985), a noradrenergic input from the locus coeruleus (Farley and Hornykiewicz, 1977), a serotonin projection from the dorsal raphe (Wang and Aghajanian, 1977), and glutamatergic afferents from the neocortex. As such, the decreases in markers for acetylcholine (Davies, 1979; Rossor et al., 1982, 1984; Palmer et al., 1986) and 5-HT (Arai et al., 1984a; Cross et al., 1984) would be expected given the parallel degeneration of parent cell bodies located in the aforementioned cortical and subcortical areas and projecting to the amygdala (see Mann and Yates, 1986, for review). It is, however, of interest (see below) that in some patients with Alzheimer's disease, neocortical cholineacetyl transferase (ChAT) is little altered, yet within the amygdala of these same patients, ChAT is severely reduced (Rossor et al., 1981, 1984; Palmer et al., 1986) and AchE activity is grossly reduced only in cortical and medial areas (Rasool et al., 1986; Unger et al., 1988; Brashear et al., 1988).

Changes in amino-acid and peptide markers seem less clear. No significant alterations (or at least nonsignificant decreases) have been reported in whole nuclear preparations for somatostatin (Rossor et al., 1980; Arai et al., 1984b; Beal et al., 1986a), VIP (Arai et al., 1984b), CRF (Bissette et al., 1985), neurotensin, and TRH (Biggins et al., 1983). However, regional deficits of somatostatin within the basal nucleus (Candy et al., 1985) and of neuropeptide Y (NPY) within the central nucleus (Beal et al., 1986b) alone have been reported. Unger et al. (1988) noted many somatostatin and NPY immunoreactive neurons to be shrunken in Alzheimer's disease, though despite showing such apparently atrophic changes, a dense network of fibres not dissimilar from controls was maintained throughout all subregions and no obvious change in numerical density of neurons was observed. The lack of clear changes in many transmitter concentrations, however, may come about because of the effects of the severe atrophy and compacting down of surviving structures that often occurs (see above), which may mask an actual loss of *transmitter content* or fibre *length* and result in an apparently normal *concentration* or fibre *density*. Hence, nonsignificant alterations in concentration or density may actually reflect (given the extent of atrophy quoted earlier) a 40% or more decrease in content. Without compensation for atrophy it is still not clear in Alzheimer's disease what the true extent of transmitter losses from the amygdala might be, though given the degree of cell loss and tissue atrophy that is usually present, all are likely to be sizable.

Senile Plaques and Neurofibrillary Tangles

The presence of senile plaques (SP) and neurofibrillary tangles, in great numbers, within the amygdala in Alzheimer's disease has been commented upon on numerous occasions (Grunthal, 1928; Brockhaus, 1938; Jamada and Mehraein, 1968; Corsellis, 1970; Hooper and Vogel, 1976; Herzog and Kemper, 1980; Mann and Yates, 1981; Saper et al., 1985; Unger et al., 1988; Brady and Mufson, 1990); indeed it has been suggested (Jamada and Mehraein, 1968) that this is the region most damaged by such changes. However, in a quantitative study of senile plaque density within the amygdala, Brady and Mufson (1990) noted an overall plaque density (as detected by thioflavin S staining) of $7.1/mm^2$, compared with a value of $0.2/mm^2$ in controls. These values in terms of relative density, in fact, compare less favourably with the neocortex, where density values exceeding $20SP/mm^2$ often exist (Mann et al., 1985). However, because of the larger size of senile plaques in the amygdala (usually well in excess of 20 μm and often reaching 200 μm in diameter) compared to those in the neocortex (40–50 μm; Mann et al., 1988b), their appearance in the amygdala is obviously more striking and this assertion may indeed be borne out in terms of the proportion of surviving tissue they occupy.

Neurofibrillary tangles are numerous throughout most subdivisions of the amygdala; in some patients they may in fact be 10 times as numerous as senile plaques (Brady and Mufson, 1990). Counts of neurofibrillary tangles within the amygdala regularly exceed those in most cortical regions, except for hippocampus and pyriform cortex, with which they are on a par (Esiri et al., 1990).

Distribution of Senile Plaques and Neurofibrillary Tangles

The distribution of senile plaques within the subdivisions of the amygdala is clearly not uniform (Corsellis, 1970; Hooper and Vogel, 1976; Rasool et al., 1986; Mann et al., 1988a; Brashear et al., 1988; Unger et al., 1988; Brady and Mufson, 1990). Although it has been noted (Corsellis, 1970; Hooper and Vogel, 1976; Mann et al., 1988a) that cortical and medial parts are usually more heavily involved than basal and lateral regions, this distribution does not seem to follow a simple medial to lateral gradient.

For example, in thioflavin-stained sections, Brashear et al. (1988) noted a striking medial to lateral increase in senile plaques within subregions such as the basal nucleus and to a lesser extent in the accessory basal nucleus. The generalised high counts of senile plaques within medial structures such as the cortical nucleus and the cortical transitional area and pyriform cortex and the paucity of senile plaques in the white matter bordering the lateral edge of the amygdala gives the (spurious) impression of an overall and gradual medial to lateral increase. However, low numbers of senile plaques occur in the medial nucleus itself and numerous senile plaques occur in certain more lateral nuclei such as the central nucleus. A broadly similar distribution to this was also noted by Unger et al. (1988) and by Brady and Mufson (1990), again using thioflavin-stained sections, and by Rasool et al. (1986) using antipaired helical filament (PHF) immunostained sections.

A regional difference in senile plaque morphology is also noticeable. The so-called "classic" or "mature" type of senile plaque (Wisniewski and Terry, 1973) with abundant amyloid protein (Fig. 3a) associated with numerous degenerating neurites and reactive glia is most abundant in regions where senile plaques are most numerous (i.e., accessory basal, medial basal, and cortical nuclei) (Brashear et al., 1988; Brady and Mufson, 1990). "Primitive" senile plaques, without an amyloid core and with few degenerating neurites, are the predominant type among the fewer senile plaques located in more lateral regions (Brashear

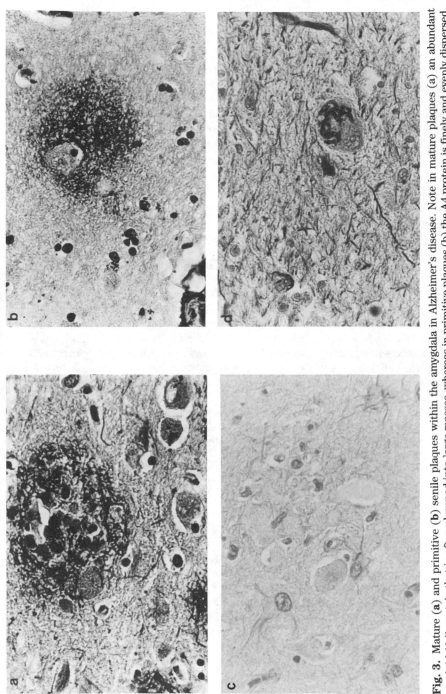

Fig. 3. Mature (**a**) and primitive (**b**) senile plaques within the amygdala in Alzheimer's disease. Note in mature plaques (**a**) an abundant amyloid (A4) protein that is often clumped into large masses, whereas in primitive plaques (**b**) the A4 protein is finely and evenly dispersed. An intense reactive astrocytosis (**c**) is associated with mature plaques. Globose neurofibrillary tangles are present in nerve cells of the amygdala (**d**). (a,b) Methenamine silver stain for amyloid (A4) protein; (c) phosphotungstic acid–haematoxylin for glial fibres; (d) Palmgren silver stain for neurofibrillary tangles. All figures, × 550 magnification.

et al., 1988; Brady and Mufson, 1990). Using antibody staining of the protein (anti-A4 immunostaining) that constitutes the senile plaque amyloid, Ogomori et al. (1989), like ourselves (Mann, unpublished data), noted numerous deposits of amyloid (A4) protein within the amygdala of all patients examined. In these deposits the A4 protein was usually diffusely distributed, often without a distinct core (Fig. 3b), though occasional cored deposits are present. The topographic distribution of these amyloid deposits (as opposed to thioflavin positive senile plaques) within the amygdala is not known, nor is it clear whether (as is the case in the cerebral cortex in Alzheimer's disease (see Ogomori et al., 1989) anti-A4 immunostaining reveals more sites of senile plaque formation than does thioflavin S, anti-PHF immunostaining, or silver (Palmgren, Bodian) methods. The question as to whether the distribution of such A4 protein deposits corresponds to that of senile plaques detected by these other techniques also remains unresolved.

Senile plaques within the amygdala, in contrast to those in the neocortex, are usually heavily invested with glial processes (Fig. 3c) and in some instances a dense feltwork of glial fibres exists particularly within cortical and medial nuclei.

Neurofibrillary tangles in the amygdala in silver stains appear as globular or fragmentary structures (Fig. 3d) and seem to have a similar immunoreactivity to their neocortical and hippocampal counterparts, being detectable using anti-PHF antisera (Rasool et al., 1986) or anti-tau antisera (Mann, unpublished observations). Like senile plaques, neurofibrillary tangles are not evenly distributed throughout all subdivisions of the amygdala; cortical, accessory basal, medial nuclei, and lateral nucleus seem preferentially involved (Rasool et al., 1986; Saper et al., 1985; Brady and Mufson, 1990). Tangle bearing neurons (i.e., intracellular tangles) seem to predominate within the cortical, medial accessory basal, and basal nuclei (Rasool et al., 1986; Brady and Mufson, 1990) whereas extracellular (ghost) tangles are most common in lateral and basal nuclei (Brady and Mufson, 1990).

The distributions of both senile plaques and neurofibrillary tangles do not seem to match those of any particular transmitter. For example, with acetylcholine, it has been demonstrated (Brashear et al., 1988; Brady and Mufson, 1990) that senile plaque and neurofibrillary tangle counts are highest in the normally AchE-poor regions of the amygdala (i.e., cortical and medial nuclei), whereas counts are low in the normally AchE-rich basal nucleus; only in cortical and medial regions is AchE activity obviously reduced. Although Unger et al. (1988) observed the presence of a few somatostatin and NPY immunoreactive fibres within senile plaque neurites, the *density* of immunostained fibres in senile plaque-rich areas (i.e., cortical and accessory basal nuclei) was similar to that in senile plaque-sparse (basal and lateral nuclei) regions.

Hence, it is unlikely that either senile plaque or neurofibrillary tangle formation is induced directly by abnormalities in either of these, or indeed any other, transmitter systems; neurons and their processes are probably destroyed unselectively within the progress of these lesions according to their pattern of connectivity (see below).

Other Changes

Granulovacuolar degeneration, a feature characteristic of hippocampal neurons, especially those of areas CA1 and subiculum (Tomlinson and Kitchener, 1972), is also common in cells of the amygdala (Hooper and Vogel, 1976), though the significance of this change remains unclear.

While anti-A4 immunostaining reveals in all patients with Alzheimer's disease numerous sites of amyloid (A4) protein deposition within the parenchyma of the amygdala, Ogomori et al. (1989) noted a vascular deposition of A4 protein to occur in only 5/14 (38%) patients.

Pathological Implications

Although the etiology of senile plaque and neurofibrillary tangle formation still remains enigmatic, it is widely believed that both of these destructive lesions evolve along a temporal sequence into the "end-stage" structures familiar at autopsy (or biopsy). The classical (mature) senile plaque develops from a more primitive form by the progressive deposition and fibrillary organization of the amyloid (A4) protein with an increasing degeneration of local nerve processes (neurites). It may eventually proceed into a compact or "burnt-out" form (Wisniewski and Terry, 1973) characterized by a core of amyloid with little or no neuritic change. Moreover, primitive senile plaques may be predated by a "pre-amyloid" form in which the "bare" amyloid (A4) protein is either nonaligned or only partially aligned into a fibrillar form and without a neuritic component being present. The continued accumulation of PHF within tangled neurons ultimately compromises their metabolism (Saper et al., 1985; Sumpter et al., 1986) with cell death and liberation of the residual indigestible tangle into the extracellular space as a ghost tangle ensuing.

Thus, the presence of classical mature senile plaques predominantly within cortical, accessory basal, and medial basal structures in Alzheimer's disease, while primitive senile plaques are mainly found in lateral and basolateral regions (Brashear et al., 1988; Brady and Mufson, 1990), implies that these former regions are damaged by senile plaque formation earlier in the course of the disease than are the latter. Indeed, the preponderance of extracellular neurofibrillary tangles within the lateral nuclei (which project medially to cortical and basal structures; Aggleton, 1985) with most intracellular neurofibrillary tangles being within cortical nuclei, would be consistent with this suggestion, if the proposal (Saper et al., 1985; Hardy et al., 1986; Pearson and Powell, 1987, 1989) is correct that neurofibrillary tangle formation is a secondary retrograde response to damage engendered at nerve terminals within the confines of the senile plaque.

It may be postulated therefore that in Alzheimer's disease, as far as the amygdala is concerned, the initial loci of damage occur within cortical, medial, accessory basal, and medial basal nuclei, with a later spreading to involve more laterally situated nuclei.

CHANGES IN DOWN'S SYNDROME

It is now well documented (see Mann, 1988, for review) that elderly persons with Down's syndrome (i.e., those over 50 years of age) almost invariably show within their brains the same neuropathological characteristics of Alzheimer's disease. Hence, a study of individuals with Down's syndrome dying before this age (in whom the full pathological picture of Alzheimer's disease predictably would have become manifest had they lived long enough) can help in understanding where the lesions of Alzheimer's disease commence, in what form they appear, and how they progress with time to culminate in that familiar form seen at autopsy in "end-stage" tissues.

We (Mann and Esiri, 1988, 1989; Mann et al., 1989) have noted that in such younger patients with Down's syndrome many classic mature senile plaques can be found in the amygdala (and particularly in cortical and medial nuclei) between the ages of 35 and 45 years. In such patients neocortical senile plaques are sparse and usually primitive and neurofibrillary tangles are rare, often being largely confined to the stellate cells of layer II of the entorhinal cortex. Deposits of amyloid (A4) protein without neuritic involvement are, however, widespread throughout the neocortex at these ages (Mann and Esiri, 1989; Mann et al., 1989; Ikeda et al., 1989; Giaccone et al., 1989; Rumble et al., 1989). Before 35 years of age, neuritic senile plaques are not seen, even in the amygdala, though again numerous amyloid deposits are present in the amygdala, hippocampus, and neocortex; neurofibrillary tangles are absent (Mann and Esiri, 1989; Mann et al., 1989; Rumble et al., 1989).

CHANGES IN NONDEMENTED ELDERLY PERSONS

It is well known that many elderly persons without clear evidence of dementia may show (relatively) few senile plaques and neurofibrillary tangles in their brains (Tomlinson et al., 1968; Dayan, 1970; Ulrich, 1985; Mann et al., 1987). In a study of 60 nondemented persons of all ages (Mann et al., 1987, 1988a, 1990) many amyloid (A4) protein deposits and mature senile plaques were detected in the amygdala of 15 patients aged between 39 and 84 years (12 of these were over 60 years of age). Again in many instances the cortical and medial nuclei were more severely affected and in these patients there was only minor involvement of the lateral nuclei. In the neocortex of these patients, senile plaques were usually sparse and contained few neurites, though amyloid (A4) protein deposits were more extensive; other patients were observed in whom an amyloid deposition alone was present only in the neocortex. A preferential involvement of the amygdala (and hippocampus) by typical senile plaques and neurofibrillary tangles was also noted by Ulrich (1985) in a series of 51 nondemented persons dying between the ages of 55 and 64 years.

However, the presence of (sometimes frequent) senile plaques and neurofibrillary tangles within the amygdala of many nondemented persons does not seem to be reflected by any major change in nerve cell density or amygdaloid volume. Herzog and Kemper (1980) noted only a 2% difference in the volume of the amygdala in four elderly males aged 67–76 years when compared with that in four males aged between 20–50 years; they also noted only slight (7–12%), though significant, decreases in cell packing density in medial, central, and cortical nuclei, with other regions being unaltered. Senile plaques and neurofibrillary tangles were stated to be only sparsely present.

CHANGES IN AGED AND NONHUMAN SPECIES

Struble et al. (1985) and Walker et al. (1990) have demonstrated that the brains of aged rhesus monkeys contain senile plaques (but not neurofibrillary tangles) and these are located preferentially within prefrontal and temporal lobes, with many being present within cortical and medial regions of the amygdala. Cork et al. (1988) noted neurofibrillary tangles to be present in the amygdala, hippocampus, and neocortex of aged brown bears, though no senile plaques were said to be present. Conversely, in an aged polar bear senile plaques were observed in the neocortex and hippocampus (whether senile plaques were also present or not in the amygdala is not stated) though no neurofibrillary tangles were detected. The neocortex of aged dogs often contains numerous deposits of A4 protein (Giaccone et al., 1990), though these authors did not comment on any involvement of the amygdala.

HYPOTHESIS

From observations on the topography and morphology of senile plaques and neurofibrillary tangles within the amygdala in Alzheimer's disease, it can be postulated that, for this particular region, lesions commence in cortical, medial, accessory basal, and medial basal nuclei, spreading later into other structures. This suggestion is supported by observations on younger persons with Down's syndrome (Mann and Esiri, 1988, 1989; Mann et al., 1989) and nondemented elderly persons (Mann et al., 1987, 1988a, 1990) who also show an early and preferential development of senile plaques (particularly) and neurofibrillary tangles within these same areas of amygdala. Even though, from observations based on these latter groups of individuals, it seems that deposition of amyloid (A4) protein commences widely and synchronously throughout the amygdala, hippocampus, and neocortex (Mann and Esiri, 1989; Mann et al., 1990), it is only in the amygdala that neuritic changes within senile plaques are initially located and these then "spread" to other brain regions. Because deposition of amyloid (A4) protein is an event that is widely seen in elderly persons with dementing disorders other than Alzheimer's disease (and Down's syndrome), such as Huntington's chorea, progressive supranuclear palsy, Parkinson's disease, frontal lobe dementia (Tan et al., 1988; Mastaglia et al., 1988; Mann and Jones, 1990), as well as in many aged nondemented persons, it becomes possible that amyloid deposition is a process that is more closely linked to ageing and genetics than to Alzheimer's disease per se (Mann, 1989). It is the neuritic degeneration that occurs in conjunction with amyloid deposition most commonly and most severely in Alzheimer's disease (and Down's syndrome) alone that characterizes the onset and progress of the "malignancy" of Alzheimer's disease and it is this that ultimately leads to neurodegeneration and clinical deterioration. In this latter context, the early and preferential involvement of the amygdala by neuritic changes (Mann and Esiri, 1988, 1989) assumes great importance since this implies that here the most destructive elements of the disease originate and subsequently disseminate.

ETIOLOGICAL CONSIDERATIONS

The etiological agent(s) responsible for the histopathological lesions of Alzheimer's disease are still not known, though from observations of the distribution of the degenerative changes (i.e., senile plaques and neurofibrillary tangles) throughout the brain, several authors (Pearson et al., 1985; Rogers and Morrison, 1985; Hardy et al., 1986; Pearson and Powell, 1987, 1989; Esiri et al., 1990) have argued that whatever the agent might be, the process of neurodegeneration is "spread" (possibly by retrograde transport) along connecting pathways, both within the cortex (by corticocortical connections) and to subcortical structures connected with the cortex (by subcorticocortical pathways). The distribution of the pathology in the cortex correlates well with the sequence of corticocortical connections passing out from the main sensory areas via the association areas in the parietotemporal and frontal lobes to the cingulate cortex and hippocampus (Pearson and Powell, 1989; Esiri et al., 1990). The areas at the end of this sequence (i.e., mesial temporal) are the most damaged and the sensory areas at the beginning (except olfactory; see below) the least, with intervening areas involved to intermediate degrees (Rogers and Morrison, 1985; Pearson et al., 1985; Pearson and Powell, 1989; Esiri et al., 1990).

In this context, the amygdala (and the parahippocampal gyrus) would occupy a pivotal role through their strong connections with the association cortex, hippocampus, and subcortical regions such as nucleus basalis and locus coeruleus. Indeed, the numbers of neurofibrillary tangles observed in patients with Alzheimer's disease in different neocortical areas closely parallels the density of connecting linkages between that area and the amygdala (Esiri et al., 1990). Hence, areas of brain that are heavily connected with both the amygdala and the parahippocampal gyrus would be more severely affected than those connecting with only one of these regions, these in turn being more affected than areas with no direct connections. Thus by this proposal, lesions would commence in cortical and medial nuclei of the amygdala, progress through basal and lateral nuclei and hippocampus, to involve eventually connecting association cortices and subcortical regions.

Several authors (Corsellis, 1970; Hooper and Vogel, 1976; Herzog and Kemper, 1980) have stressed that the sites of severe pathology within the amygdala (cortical and basal regions) appear ontogenetically earlier in formation of the amygdala than do the basal and lateral regions (Humphrey, 1972) and this might make them more susceptible to lesions (Corsellis, 1970). Rapoport (1990) pointed out that this part of the amygdala, along with certain connecting neocortical regions (association neocortex), the hippocampus, and subcortical areas such as nucleus basalis and septum, have all undergone "integrative phylogeny" during human (and higher primate) evolution (i.e., they have expanded synchronously and proportionately according to their increased functional capacity) and that this may have conferred a selective vulnerability to formation of Alzheimer-type lesions.

However, even if this is so, it does not explain why the amygdala (of all these regions) should apparently be the earliest to be involved. Neuroanatomy may again provide the clue. The cortical and medial regions of the amygdala are closely and reciprocally connected with the pyriform cortex and together these recieve fibres directly from the olfactory bulb. The pyriform cortex, like the amygdala but in contrast to other primary sensory regions, is *always* severely affected in Alzheimer's disease (Reyes et al., 1987; Mann et al., 1988a) and Down's syndrome (Mann et al., 1988a; Mann and Esiri, 1988, 1989) and is one of the most consistently damaged regions in nondemented elderly persons (Mann et al., 1987, 1988a). Hence, it is possible that the pathogenesis and progression of the lesions of Alzheimer's disease relate to the entry of a causative agent into the olfactory epithelium and its retrograde transfer along centrifugal fibres into the amygdala and pyriform cortex (Pearson et al., 1985; Pearson and Powell, 1987, 1989; Mann et al., 1988a; Esiri et al., 1990) with subsequent dissemination through associated brain structures, culminating in the distinctive distribution of lesions remarked upon earlier. This proposal does not, however, predict the nature of such an agent, though it is well recognized that neurotoxic substances such as aluminum or certain viruses (see Ferreya-Moyano and Barragan, 1989, for review) can indeed gain access to the brain by this route. Such facts might interplay with a phylogenetic/ontogenetic tendency toward degeneration to precipitate the cascade of pathological changes and clinical disordering that together we call Alzheimer's disease.

CHANGES IN OTHER DEMENTING DISORDERS

A consideration of Table I suggests that a degeneration of the amygdala may be a feature of dementing disorders, other than Alzheimer's disease (and Down's syndrome), such as Pick's disease and other "frontal lobe" dementias, Huntington's chorea, and perhaps also progressive supranuclear palsy (Steele-Richardson syndrome). In all these conditions there is a measurable overall atrophy of the amygdala that ranges from 14–70% of control values and presumably reflects the end-stages of a neurodegenerative process including this part of the brain. Although the histopathological features of these various disorders are, in general, well known as far as the cerebral cortex is concerned (see Tomlinson and Corsellis, 1984), there is sparse information relating specifically to the amygdala.

For example, although an involvement of the amygdala in Pick's disease has been briefly mentioned by several authors (Malamud and Waggoner, 1943; Neumann, 1949; Pilleri, 1966; Arima, 1989), only a single study has selected this region for special consideration (Cummings and Duchen, 1981). These latter authors, in a study of five patients with Pick's disease, noted that the amygdala was reduced in size in each instance (see also Table I) and that neuronal loss and atrophy and an intense gliosis affected all subdivisions equally; surviving neurons displayed an eccentrically placed nucleus and an abnormal accumulation of argyrophilic material (Pick bodies). As in Alzheimers disease, it is notable that in Pick's disease similar topographic brain regions are "selected" and again it has been suggested (Rapoport, 1990) that the integrative phylogenetic development of these related brain regions may confer pathological vulnerability. In patients with frontal lobe dementias (other than Pick's disease) (Neary et al., 1988, 1990) a variable atrophy of the amygdala is seen, sometimes profound, other times only mild. In those severely affected patients, the pathological changes mirror those of the cortex with a diffuse loss of neurons, a spongiform degeneration of the neuropil, and a mild astrogliosis being characteristic. In

Huntington's chorea and progressive supranuclear palsy, a mild to moderate atrophy of the amygdala is noted (Table I), though histopathologically no structural abnormality is seen; the atrophy here presumably reflects a loss of afferent projections from basal ganglia or other subcortical regions.

FUNCTIONAL CONSIDERATIONS

The precise role that amygdala lesions might play in the production and the progression of the syndrome of dementia has not yet been delineated. Experimentally, bilateral lesions affecting the temporal lobe, hippocampus, and amygdala (in particular) produce a behavioural pattern characterized by hyperorality, hypersexuality, emotional blunting, and defective visual recognition: Symptoms collectively known as Klüver-Bucy syndrome (see Cummings and Duchen, 1981). This type of behaviour seems typical of patients with Pick's disease (Cummings and Duchen, 1981) in whom amygdala pathology is prominent. However, it is also prominent among patients with "frontal lobe dementia" (Neary et al., 1988), especially when severe temporal lobe involvement is present. Such behaviour is not, however, characteristic of patients with Alzheimer's disease (though can occur irregularly and terminally in some patients; Sourander and Sjogren, 1970) despite the severe and universal pathological involvement of the amygdala in this disorder. The lack of such overt changes in Alzheimer's disease might be obscured or repressed by the many other intellectual and behaviour changes induced through the widespread neocortical, allocortical, and subcortical degeneration, though it is possible that the emotional lability common in Alzheimer's disease partially has its roots within amygdala damage.

Recent experimental work implies that the amygdala, through its close connections with the hippocampus, plays a role in memory processing and particularly that of recognition memory (see Brady and Mufson, 1990). Disconnection of these areas via neurofibrillary degeneration of neurons (in Alzheimer's disease) or through Pick-type lesions (in Pick's disease) may contribute to the totality of the memory deficit characteristic of Alzheimer's disease and the mnestic deterioration commonplace in Pick's disease. The observations of a permanent amnesic syndrome in patients following either resection of the medial parts of the temporal lobe (Scoville and Milner, 1957) or upon a selective degeneration of the hippocampus and amygdala (Duyckaerts et al., 1985) serve to emphasize this involvement.

ACKNOWLEDGMENT

The author wishes to ₊thank Mrs. B. Hunter for her careful preparation of this manuscript.

REFERENCES

Aggleton JP (1985): A description of intra-amygdaloid connections in old world monkeys. Exp Brain Res 57:390–399.

Arima K (1989): Involvement of subcortical nuclei and brain stem in Pick's disease: A topographical study of Pick bodies. Neuropathology 9:105–115.

Arai H, Kosaka K, Iizuka R (1984a): Changes of biogenic amines and their metabolites in post mortem brains from patients with Alzheimer-type dementia. J Neurochem 43:388–393.

Arai H, Moroji T, Kosaka K (1984b): Somatostatin and vasoactive intestinal polypeptide in post mortem brains from patients with Alzheimer type dementia. Neurosci Lett 52:73–78.

Ball MJ (1972): Neurofibrillary tangles and the pathogenesis of dementia: A quantitative study. Neuropathol Appl Neurobiol 2:395–410.

Beal MF, Mazurek MF, Svendsen CN, Bird ED, Martin JB (1986a): Widespread reduction of somatostatin-like immunoreactivity in the cerebral cortex in Alzheimer's disease. Ann Neurol 20:489–495.

Beal MF, Mazurek MF, Chatta GK, Svendsen CN, Bird ED, Martin JB (1986b): Neuropeptide Y immunoreactivity is reduced in cerebral cortex in Alzheimer's disease. Ann Neurol 20:282–288.

Biggins JA, Perry EK, McDermott JR, Smith AI, Perry RH, Edwardson JA (1983): Post mortem levels of thyrotropin-releasing hormone and neurotensin in the amygdala in Alzheimer's disease, schizophrenia and depression. J Neurol Sci 58:117–122.

Bissette G, Reynolds GP, Kilts CD, Widerlov E, Nemeroff CB (1985): Corticotropin-releasing factor-like immunoreactivity in senile dementia of the Alzheimer type. JAMA 254: 3067–3069.

Brady DR, Mufson EJ (1990): Amygdaloid pathology in Alzheimer's disease: Qualitative and quantitative analysis. Dementia 1:5–17.

Brashear HR, Godec MS, Carlsen J (1988): The distribution of neuritic plaques and acetylcholinesterase staining in the amygdala in Alzheimer's disease. Neurology 38: 1694–1699.

Brockhaus H (1938): Zur normalen und pathologischen Anatomie des Mandelkern-gebietes. J Psychol Neurol 49:1–136.

Candy JM, Gascoigne AD, Biggins JA, Smith AI, Perry RH, Perry EK, McDermott JR, Edwardson JA (1985): Somatostatin immunoreactivity in cortical and some subcortical regions in Alzheimer's disease. J Neurol Sci 71:315–323.

Carlsen J, Zaborsky L, Heimer L (1985): Cholinergic projections from the basal forebrain to the basolateral amygdaloid complex: A combined retrograde fluorescent and immunohistochemical study. J Comp Neurol 234:156–167.

Cork LC, Powers RE, Selkoe DJ, Davies P, Geyer JJ, Price DL (1988): Neurofibrillary tangles and senile plaques in aged bears. J Neuropathol Exp Neurol 47:629–641.

Corsellis JAN (1970): The limbic areas in Alzheimer's disease and in other conditions associated with dementia. In Wolstenholme GEW, O'Connor M (eds): "Alzheimer's Disease and Related Conditions." A Ciba Foundation Symposium. London: J & A Churchill, pp 37–50.

Cross AJ, Crow TJ, Ferrier IN, Johnson JA, Bloom SR, Corsellis JAN (1984): Serotonin receptor changes in dementia of the Alzheimer type. J Neurochem 43:1574–1581.

Cummings JL, Duchen LW (1981): Klüver-Bucy syndrome in Pick's disease: Clinical and pathological correlations. Neurology 31:1415–1422.

Davies P (1979): Neurotransmitter-related enzymes in senile dementia of the Alzheimer type. Brain Res 171:319–327.

Dayan AD (1970): Quantitative histological studies in the aged human brain. I. Senile plaques and neurofibrillary tangles in "normal" patients. Acta Neuropathol 16:85–94.

Duyckaerts C, Derouesne C, Signoret JL, Gray F, Escourolle R, Castaigne P (1985): Bilateral and limited amygdala hippocampal lesions causing a pure amnesic syndrome. Ann Neurol 18:314–319.

Esiri MM, Pearson RCA, Steele JE, Bowen DM, Powell TPS (1990): A quantitative study of the neurofibrillary tangles and the cholineacetyltransferase activity in the cerebral cortex and the amygdala in Alzheimer's disease. J Neurol Neurosurg Psychiat 53: 161–165.

Farley IJ, Hornykiewicz O (1977): Noradrenaline distribution in subcortical areas of the human brain. Brain Res 126:53–62.

Ferreya-Moyano H, Barragan E (1989): The olfactory system and Alzheimer's disease. Int J Neurosci 49:157–197.

Giaccone G, Tagliavini F, Linoli G, Bouras C, Frigello L, Frangione B, Bugiani O (1989): Down patients: Extracellular preamyloid deposits precede neuritic degeneration and senile plaques. Neurosci Lett 97:232–238.

Giaccone G, Verga L, Finazzi M, Pollo B, Tagliavini F, Frangione B, Bugiani O (1990): Cerebral preamyloid deposits and congophilic angiopathy in aged dogs. Neurosci Lett 114:178–183.

Grunthal E (1928): Zur hirnpathologischen Analyze der Alzheimerschen Krankheit. Psychiatr Neurol Wochenschr 36:401–407.

Hardy JA, Mann DMA, Wester P, Winblad B (1986): An integrative hypothesis concerning the pathogenesis and progression of Alzheimer's disease. Neurobiol Ageing 7:489–502.

Herzog AG, Kemper TL (1980): Amygdaloid changes in ageing and dementia. Arch Neurol 37:625–629.

Hirano A, Zimmerman HM (1962): Alzheimer's neurofibrillary changes: A topographic study. Arch Neurol 7:227–242.

Hooper MW, Vogel FS (1976): The limbic system in Alzheimer's disease. Am J Pathol 85:1–20.

Humphrey T (1972): The development of the human amygdaloid complex. In Eleftheriou BE (ed): "The Neurobiology of the Amygdala." New York: Plenum Press, pp 21–82.

Ikeda S-I, Yanagisawa N, Allsop D, Glenner GG (1989): Evidence of amyloid β protein immunoreactive early plaque lesions in Down's syndrome brains. Lab Invest 60:113–122.

Jamada M, Mehraein P (1968): Verteilungsmuster der seniles Veranderungen im Gehirn. Arch Psychiat Neurol 211:308–324.

Malamud N, Waggoner RW (1943): Genealogic and clinicopathologic study of Pick's disease. Arch Neurol Psychiat 50:288–303.

Mann DMA (1988): The pathological association between Down's syndrome and Alzheimer's disease. Mech Ageing Dev 43:99–136.

Mann DMA (1989): Cerebral amyloidosis, ageing and Alzheimer's disease: A contribution from studies in Down's syndrome. Neurobiol Ageing 10:397–399.

Mann DMA, Esiri MM (1988): The site of the earliest lesions of Alzheimer's disease. N Engl J Med 318:789–790.

Mann DMA, Esiri MM (1989): Regional acquisition of plaques and tangles in Down's syndrome patients under 50 years of age. J Neurol Sci 89:169–179.

Mann DMA, Jones D (1990): Amyloid (A4) protein deposition in the brains of persons with dementing disorders other than Alzheimer's disease and Down's syndrome. Neurosci Lett 109:68–75.

Mann DMA, Yates PO (1981): The relationship between formation of senile plaques and neurofibrillary tangles and changes in nerve cell metabolism in Alzheimer type dementia. Mech Ageing Dev 17:395–401.

Mann DMA, Yates PO (1986): Neurotransmitter deficits in Alzheimer's disease and in other dementing disorders. Hum Neurobiol 5:147–158.

Mann DMA, Tucker CM, Yates PO (1987): The topographic distribution of senile plaques and neurofibrillary tangles in the brains of non-demented persons of different ages. Neuropathol Appl Neurobiol 13:123–139.

Mann DMA, Tucker CM, Yates PO (1988a): Alzheimer's disease: An olfactory connection? Mech Ageing Dev 42:1–15.

Mann DMA, Yates PO, Marcyniuk B (1984): Alzheimer's presenile dementia, senile dementia of Alzheimer type and Down's syndrome in middle age form an age-related continuum of pathological changes. Neuropathol Appl Neurobiol 10:185–207.

Mann DMA, Yates PO, Marcyniuk B (1985): Some morphometric observations on the cerebral cortex and hippocampus in presenile Alzheimer's disease, senile dementia of Alzheimer type and Down's syndrome in middle age. J Neurol Sci 69:139–159.

Mann DMA, Marcyniuk B, Yates PO, Neary D, Snowden JS (1988b): The progression of the pathological changes of Alzheimer's disease in frontal and temporal neocortex examined both at biopsy and at autopsy. Neuropathol Appl Neurobiol 14:177–195.

Mann DMA, Brown AMT, Prinja D, Davies CA, Beyreuther K, Masters CL, Landon M (1989): An analysis of the morphology of senile plaques in Down's syndrome patients of different ages using immunocytochemical and lectin histochemical methods. Neuropathol Appl Neurobiol 15:317–329.

Mann DMA, Brown AMT, Prinja D, Jones D, Davies CA (1990): A morphological analysis of senile plaques in the brains of non-demented persons of different ages using silver, immunocytochemical and lectin histochemical staining techniques. Neuropathol Appl Neurobiol 16:17–25.

Mastaglia FL, Masters CL, Beyreuther K, Kakulas BA (1988): Deposition of amyloid (A4) protein in the cerebral cortex in Parkinson's disease. Alzheimer's Dis Assoc Disord 2:245.

Mountjoy CQ, Roth M, Evans JR, Evans HM (1983): Cortical neuronal count in normal elderly controls and demented patients. Neurobiol Ageing 4:1–11.

Najlerahim A, Bowen DM (1988): Regional weight loss of the cerebral cortex and some subcortical nuclei in senile dementia of the Alzheimer type. Acta Neuropathol 75:509–512.

Neary D, Snowden JS, Northen B, Goulding P (1988): Dementia of frontal lobe type. J Neurol Neurosurg Psychiat 51:353–361.

Neary D, Snowden JS, Mann DMA, Northen B, Goulding PJ, McDermott N (1990): Frontal lobe dementia and motor neurone disease. J Neurol Neurosurg Psychiat 53:23–32.

Neumann MA (1949): Pick's disease. J Neuropathol Exp Neurol 8:255–282.

Ogomori K, Kitamoto T, Tateishi J, Sato Y, Suetsugu M, Abe M (1989): β protein amyloid is widely distributed in the central nervous system of patients with Alzheimer's disease. Am J Pathol 134:243–251.

Palmer AM, Procter AW, Stratmann GC, Bowen DM (1986): Excitatory amino acid-releasing and cholinergic neurones in Alzheimer's disease. Neurosci Lett 66:199–204.

Pearson RCA, Powell TPS (1987): Anterograde VS retrograde degeneration of the nucleus basalis medialis in Alzheimer's disease. J Neural Transm (Suppl) 24:139–146.

Pearson RCA, Powell TPS (1989): The neuroanatomy of Alzheimer's disease. Rev Neurosci 2:101–122.

Pearson RCA, Esiri MM, Hiorns RW, Wilcock GK, Powell TPS (1985): Anatomical correlates of the distribution of the pathological changes in the neocortex in Alzheimer's disease. Proc Natl Acad Sci USA 82:4531–4534.

Pilleri G (1966): The Klüver-Bucy syndrome in man. Psychiat Neurol 152:65–103.

Rapoport SI (1990): Topography of Alzheimer's disease: Involvement of association neocortices and connected regions; pathological, metabolic and cognitive correlations; relation to evolution. In Rapoport SI, Petit H, Leys D, Christen Y (eds): "Imaging, Cerebral Topography and Alzheimer's Disease." Berlin: Springer-Verlag, pp 1–18.

Rasool CG, Svendsen CN, Selkoe DJ (1986): Neurofibrillary degeneration of the cholinergic and non-cholinergic neurones of the basal forebrain in Alzheimer's disease. Ann Neurol 20:482–488.

Reyes PF, Golden GT, Fagel PL, Fariello RG, Katz L, Garner E (1987): The prepiriform cortex in dementia of the Alzheimer type. Arch Neurol 44:644–645.

Rogers J, Morrison JH (1985): Quantitative morphology and regional laminar distributions of senile plaques in Alzheimer's disease. J Neurosci 5:2801–2808.

Rossor MN, Emson PC, Mountjoy CQ, Roth M, Iversen LL (1980): Reduced amounts of immunoreactive somatostatin in the temporal cortex in senile dementia of Alzheimer type. Neurosci Lett 20:373–377.

Rossor MN, Garrett NJ, Johnson AL, Mountjoy CQ, Roth M, Iversen LL (1982): A post mortem study of the cholinergic and GABA systems in senile dementia. Brain 105: 313–330.

Rossor MN, Iversen LL, Reynolds GP, Mountjoy CQ, Roth M (1984): Neurochemical characteristics of early and late onset types of Alzheimer's disease. Br Med J 288:961–964.

Rumble B, Retallack R, Hilbich C, Simms G, Multhaup G, Martins R, Hockey A, Montgomery P, Beyreuther K, Masters CL (1989): Amyloid (A4) protein and its precursor in Down's syndrome and Alzheimer's disease. N Engl J Med 320:1446–1452.

Saper CB, German DC, White CL (1985): Neuronal pathology in the nucleus basalis and associated cell groups in senile dementia of the Alzheimer type: Possible role in cell loss. Neurology 35:1089–1095.

Scoville WB, Milner B (1957): Loss of recent memory after bilateral hippocampal lesion. J Neurol Neurosurg Psychiat 20:11–21.

Sourander P, Sjogren H (1970): The concept of Alzheimer's disease and its clinical implication. In Wolstenholme GEW, O'Connor M (eds): "Alzheimer's Disease and Related Conditions." A Ciba Foundation Symposium. London: J & A Churchill, pp 11–36.

Struble RG, Price DL, Cork LC, Price DL (1985): Senile plaques in cortex of aged normal monkeys. Brain Res 361:267–275.

Sumpter PQ, Mann DMA, Davies CA, Yates PO, Snowden JS, Neary D (1986): An ultrastructural analysis of the effects of accumulation of neurofibrillary tangle in pyramidal cells of the cerebral cortex in Alzheimer's disease. Neuropathol Appl Neurobiol 12:305–319.

Tan N, Mastaglia FL, Masters CL, Beyreuther K, Kakulas BA (1988): Amyloid (A4) protein deposition in brain in progressive supranuclear palsy (PSP). Alzheimer's Dis Assoc Disord 2:264.

Terry RD, Peck A, Deteresa R, Schechter R, Horoupian DS (1981): Some morphometric aspects of the brain in senile dementia of the Alzheimer type. Ann Neurol 10:184–192.

Tomlinson BE, Corsellis JAN (1984): Ageing and the dementias. In Hume Adams J, Corsellis JAN, Duchen LW (eds): "Greenfields Neuropathology," 4th ed. London: Edward Arnold, pp 951–1025.

Tomlinson BE, Kitchener D (1972): Granulovacuolar degeneration of hippocampal pyramidal cells. J Pathol 106:165–185.

Tomlinson BE, Blessed G, Roth M (1968): Observations on the brains of non-demented old people. J Neurol Sci 7:331–356.

Ulrich J (1985): Alzheimer changes in non-demented patients younger than sixty-five: Possible early stages of Alzheimer's disease and senile dementia of Alzheimer type. Ann Neurol 17:273–277.

Unger JW, McNeill TH, Lapham LL, Hamill RW (1988): Neuropeptides and neuropathology in the amygdala in Alzheimer's disease: A relationship between somatostatin, neuropeptide Y and subregional distribution of neuritic plaques. Brain Res 452:293–302.

Walker LC, Masters CL, Beyreuther K, Price DL (1990): Amyloid in the brains of aged squirrel monkeys. Acta Neuropathol 80:381–387.

Wang RI, Aghajanian GK (1977): Inhibition of neurones in the amygdala by dorsal raphe stimulation: Mediation through a direct serotonin pathway. Brain Res 120:85–102.

Wisniewski HM, Terry RD (1973): Re-examination of the pathogenesis of the senile plaque. In Zimmerman HM (ed): "Progress in Neuropathology," Vol 2. New York: Grune & Stratton, pp 1–26.

Index

MARTINA COLE

THE FAITHLESS

headline

First published in Great Britain in 2011
by HEADLINE PUBLISHING GROUP

1

Cataloguing in Publication Data is available from the British Library

ISBN 978 0 7553 7553 0 (Hardback)
ISBN 978 0 7553 7554 7 (Trade paperback)

Typeset in Galliard by Avon DataSet Ltd,
Bidford-on-Avon, Warwickshire

Printed and bound in Great Britain by
Clays Ltd, St Ives plc

HEADLINE PUBLISHING GROUP
An Hachette UK Company
338 Euston Road
London NW1 3BH

www.headline.co.uk
www.hachette.co.uk

For my Freddie Fling Flang.

Love you, darling

Dolly R . . .

xx

Prologue

'Ain't It Grand To Be Bloomin' Well Dead'

Leslie Sarony
Song title

2009

'You are not going to make me listen to this shit, Gabriella. You are wrong, *very* wrong. Use your bloody head, girl! I loved that little boy with all my heart . . . and, as for your brother . . . I don't believe a word of it – they must have the wrong person.'

But Gabby could see the fear in her mother's eyes, and she knew that it was true. Every word of it.

'I met your old mate, Jeannie, today. That's how I know everything – she told me *all* about the house in Ilford.' She could see her mother's head working, trying to figure out exactly what she was saying, could almost hear her brain whirring as she tried to lie her way out of what they both knew was the truth.

'What the hell have you been taking this time, eh? What the fuck are you on, Gabriella, to make you come out with this shit?'

Gabby found she'd picked up a large bronze statue of a cat. As she held it in her scarred hands she felt the weight of it. Her mother kept talking. The world according to Cynthia Tailor who, along with God Himself, was almost omnipotent in the lives of her family, who ruled everyone around her with a rod of iron. She could see her mother's mouth moving constantly, but she couldn't hear what she was saying any more; all she was conscious of was a rushing noise in her ears. Then she struck her.

She lifted the bronze statue back over her head and hit her mother across the face with it, using all the force she could muster, and enjoying the feeling of total retaliation. She was

3

determined now, determined to shut her mother up once and for all.

Cynthia fell sideways on to the white leather sofa. The spray of blood that came from her mother's face was like a crimson mist. Gabby hit her again and again, each blow easing the knot inside her, each blow seeming to calm the erratic beating of her heart.

She looked down at the bloodied form and, for the first time in years, she felt almost at peace. Her mother's face was unrecognisable, a deep red gash that was pumping out blood at an alarming rate.

Gabby looked at the woman she had hated nearly all her life. Then she sat down on the ladder-backed chair her mother was convinced was an antique, put her face into her bloodied hands and cried.

Book One

Long is the way
And hard, that out of Hell leads up to light

Paradise Lost (1667)
John Milton, 1608–74

For the love of money is the root of all evil

1 Timothy 6:10

Chapter One

1984

'Come on, Jimmy, have another one. I'm celebrating.'

Jimmy Tailor grinned; he had an easy-going nature that some people took advantage of. He was a big man, big in all ways – over six feet and well built. Before his marriage he had been a body builder, and he still held traces of his former physique.

'Nah, better get home, Cynthia's waiting for me.'

It was Friday night and all his pals were going to have a few more pints before meeting their wives and girlfriends later on in a wine bar in the West End. He would have loved to have joined them, but he knew that Cynthia wouldn't come.

'Fucking hell, Jimmy, you're married, mate, not joined at the hip.'

This from his best friend Davey Brown. Davey thought Jimmy was a mug and that he should put his foot down with Cynthia, but Davey didn't understand her. No one did it seemed, except him. He smiled, but it was a tight smile. 'We're saving, what with little Gabriella and all.'

''Course, mate, you get yourself off.' Davey seemed immediately sorry for his jibe.

Jimmy left the pub a few minutes later, reluctant to go if he was honest, but even more reluctant to stay where he was. He walked along the road, feeling the cold hit him, making his face sting and, pulling up the collar of his overcoat, he made his way slowly home.

Chapter Two

Cynthia Tailor was pleased with herself. Her house looked lovely and festive – just how a home should look at Christmas time, from the scented pine tree, decorated in what she felt was a tasteful manner – no tinsel and no coloured lights – to the neatly wrapped presents underneath it. It couldn't be further away from the house she grew up in, with the dirt, the smell of frying bacon, and the garish, cheap hanging garlands. She shuddered inwardly as she thought of her mother's house. She had escaped from that life and there was no way she was ever going back.

Cynthia's sitting room was painted a pale cream, and the carpet was a thick Axminster. It had cost the national debt, but looked wonderful against the walls and the luxurious chocolate-brown velvet curtains at the windows. She knew her home was beautiful, and she never tired of cleaning it, or enhancing it. This was the first step on the ladder for them; they would go on from here, make their money on this place, and get bigger and better houses each time. She sighed with contentment at the thought.

James was a decent man, boring in some ways, but she knew that with his accountancy job in the city they would always be all right for money. And he was expecting some big news about a promotion any day now. Cynthia had come from a council estate in Hackney, and she had been determined from a young age that she wouldn't be staying there for longer than she had to. Now here she was, with a lovely semi in Ilford, and the chance to go onwards and upwards.

She walked out into her kitchen, and checked on the casserole she had bubbling on her new halogen hob. The kitchen was like something from a magazine, all white doors and stainless steel sinks. It was Hygena, and she knew it was far too good for the house, but she saw it as an investment. James had balked at the price but she had won him over. He always saw the sense of her arguments in the end; after all, she was the one stuck here all day, and she was entitled to have what she wanted around her – at least that was what she thought, anyway. And she had her ways to make sure he knew who was the boss under *this* roof.

She heard her daughter's cry and, sighing, she left the kitchen and made her way up the stairs.

Gabriella was a handful, and this was the only bugbear in her otherwise perfect life. She should be clean at night by now. The other kids at Gabriella's playschool were all clean, so why was her daughter so late?

She went into the child's room. It was decorated as a girl's bedroom *should* be decorated, with pale pink walls, and cream carpet. Cynthia loved this room. She had been brought up in a flat and had had to share her bedroom with her sister. It had been scruffy, cold and damp and she had hated every second she had spent in it.

The small night-light cast a rosy glow in the room. Kneeling down beside her daughter's cot, she looked at her child.

'What's wrong, Gabriella?'

The little blue eyes held a plea, and she knew immediately that her daughter had wet the bed again.

'Oh, Gabriella, why don't you call me, and I'll take you to the toilet.' She lifted her daughter out of the cot with a heavy sigh, and set about cleaning her up, without another word.

Gabriella allowed herself to be stripped, washed and re-dressed in a clean nightie without saying a word either. As young as she was, she could feel the tension filling the room. The unspoken disapproval and the knowledge she had done something wrong was enough to quieten her. She knew her mummy was cross, and she knew better than to aggravate her.

Ten minutes later, Gabriella was once more alone in her cot and, closing her eyes, she tried hard to get herself back to sleep.

Chapter Three

Jimmy came in as his wife was putting their daughter's pyjamas and bedding into the washing machine.

'Dinner smells good, Cyn.'

She didn't answer him. She could do that, just blank some-one, make them feel an outsider in their own home. It unnerved Jimmy. He was from a family who were boisterous, noisy, happy – not that Cynthia allowed him to see them any more. He wasn't used to long silences that had some kind of accusation in them, even though nothing was actually said. He wasn't sure how to deal with them. Turning abruptly, he went into the hallway and removed his coat. Careful to hang it up *properly* to make sure it didn't look untidy. Why this was a necessity when they were locked away in a cupboard under the stairs he wasn't sure. But Cynthia wanted everything perfect, so he did it anyway; it was easier in the long run.

As he went into the sitting room, he smiled at Cynthia's efforts. The room looked lovely, and he reminded himself how lucky he was to have a wife like her. She was not just pretty, she was like sex-on-legs. With her stunning blue eyes and thick sovereign-coloured hair, she turned heads everywhere she went. He knew that other men envied him his gorgeous wife. Every-where she went men looked at her, and she noticed them looking, he knew that. It pleased her, because it showed her that she was still attractive, even after having a child. It was important to Cynthia that she was wanted. Not that sex was her top

11

priority, unfortunately, but because she liked the power it gave her. She was a strange woman, cold – even towards their daughter. She only smiled when the child was doing what she wanted, acting as she felt a child should. Like him, poor Gabby had to behave just how Cynthia believed a daughter should, and not show her up. His wife had no room for reality, and that really worried him. Cynthia had two beliefs: that she was right, and that everyone else on the planet was wrong.

Now he had to give her some bad news and he wasn't looking forward to it. Not at all. No matter how he dressed it up, she frightened him; her colossal temper could erupt at any moment, and when it did she was like a madwoman. Most of the time she *acted* like a lady, he had to give her that. She was perfection personified – until you crossed her and told her something she didn't want to hear. Then she could swear like a docker and fight like the Irish. But then her family *was* Irish – not that she bragged about that.

He glanced at the TV set, but didn't put it on. Cynthia didn't think watching telly all the time was something *nice* people did. A good film or a documentary was fine, and *News At Ten* of course. But gameshows or comedy programmes were beneath her radar. She saw those as common, and common was what really sent her off her head.

It wasn't easy being married to her and, even though he told himself that he was lucky a girl like her chose him, it was getting harder and harder to keep up that pretence. They were over-stretched in every way – every half-penny was accounted for and, as much as he appreciated her housewifely acumen, he knew they were way over their heads in debt. Not that she wasn't good with money – she was – but, all the same, he felt they could have lived much better if she didn't feel this almighty urge to be something she wasn't. She had such exacting standards and, though he knew she wanted a better life for them all, he felt at times they'd be much better off if she spent the money in other ways, like on a night out or a day at the seaside, not just on *things* she felt were needed for the home. They had the best house in the street, but still that wasn't enough for her. She would never be content, he understood that now. The kitchen alone had cost a bloody fortune, and the carpets and curtains, all paid for on the weekly, were another drain on their resources.

Now she had the Christmas bug, had talked about having a goose and all other manner of expensive frippery. He knew she wanted the best for them, but it had to be stopped. She had to understand they couldn't go on like this.

Cynthia came into the room, slipping in quietly, as if she had materialised out of thin air. Her quietness had been what had attracted him; she had seemed so self-contained, yet so vulnerable. Not that he really believed *that* any more. It was getting harder and harder to convince himself that she was anything other than what she really was. A bully. His mother had warned him, but he had not been inclined to listen to her. Now he wished he had. But, as his old mum also said, hindsight was a wonderful thing.

Cynthia stood before him, her head slightly at an angle, and that tight little smile on her face. 'I'm dishing up.'

He sighed heavily, and barely nodded in reply.

'Are you all right?'

He sighed once more. 'Not really. Brewster got it.'

He saw her face freeze, and could see in her eyes, not pity for him – he could have coped with that – but disgust. Veiled disgust, but he saw it all the same. He knew what was going on inside her head. He tried to talk himself out of those kind of thoughts, but it was no good.

'And you just let him, I suppose.'

She was still standing there, only now her back was rigid, she was looking at him as if he had done it deliberately. He felt the air leave his body as if it had been punctured. He had been dreading this.

13

'I can't make my boss give me the position, Cynth. Be fair, love.'

She sighed heavily, her face set in a rigid mask of acceptance. ''Course not, I mean why would he give it to you, eh? Hardly setting the fucking place alight, are you? You know your trouble, don't you? You're weak. Weak as a bloody kitten.'

She left the room then, and her animosity went with her. The quiet was like a balm to his tortured spirit.

Willy Brewster was five years younger than him, and he was a dynamo. Jimmy liked him, you couldn't not. He was fun, clever and popular; he *did* set the place alight all right, with his energy and wit. Jimmy wasn't like that, and he didn't begrudge Willy for being something he wasn't.

He walked out to the kitchen, feeling better now he had actually said the words out loud. Had told her.

She was standing at the sink. Her shoulders were slumped and her hands were gripping the stainless-steel draining board so hard her knuckles were white. Her head was hanging, and he knew she was biting her lip. He could almost feel the hate coming off her in waves. Looking at her now, he felt a great sorrow for her, because he knew that there was a terrible kink in her nature. It was a mixture of loathing for her start in life, and a covetousness that made her envy everyone in her orbit. She would never be satisfied, because it wasn't in her nature. He hated that part of her, but he also pitied her for it. He understood that she had never known one happy day because she was always convinced that everyone else knew the secret of happiness, and it would always elude her. Yet if she could just once let herself be content with what she had, he knew she could find the thing she craved. If she could only understand that happiness had nothing to do with an expensive kitchen, and designer clothes, or being better off than the neighbours.

He placed his hand gently on her shoulder, willing her to turn to him, to just once let down her guard. He could feel the heat of her body through the thin material of her dress, and then when she turned towards him he felt his heart soar. He placed his arm around her slim waist, wanting to pull her towards him, comfort her, but she threw him off her with a strength that belied her slim frame.

'You fucking useless ponce.'

She was spitting out the words with fury, and the vitriol in them stunned him, as it always did when she exposed this side of herself. She never swore in front of the neighbours of course, she felt she was above that. But in private it was as if the swearing was a vent for her pent-up aggression. When she was angry with him or little Gabby her repertoire was never far away.

'You do realise what this means, don't you?'

She was looking into his eyes now, and he could see the first glimmer of fear amidst the anger and the disgust.

'Look, Cynthia, we won't starve.'

She pushed him away from her and, sighing, she shook her head sadly. 'No. No, you're right, we won't starve, but then again we won't be living the high life either, will we? It's make do and mend, it's thinking through every purchase. It's making ends fucking meet, and robbing Peter to pay fucking Paul. It's the life I grew up with, never being able to do anything . . . Never being able to just have what you want, when you want it. It's like admitting I've failed . . .' She turned from him, and her whole body seemed to have shrunk, as if the enormity of what she was saying had broken her somehow. 'It's being no one, no one and nothing for ever, that's what this all means to me.'

Jimmy looked at his wife, his heart in pieces. He couldn't understand why she was so upset. He looked out for her, he looked out for his family. 'You're wrong, Cynthia. We have a good life. The trouble with you is, it's never enough, is it? You always want more than you can have. You should never have married me; I can't give you what you want.' He had finally said it to her. Had finally said what was on his mind.

15

She laughed, a derisive little laugh. Then, facing him once more, she said quietly, 'Well, you got that much right anyway.'

For a split second she thought he was actually going to strike her and, in her heart, she knew no one would blame him if he did just that. Instead, though, he placed his hands by his sides, clenching his fists as if to stop himself.

'Maybe you're right, but do you know something, Cynthia? No one in the world could ever give you what you want, because it would never be enough. You want, want, want, and then when you get it you lose all interest in it, and you start wanting something else. Well, now you know the score, I'll have me dinner.'

He had never spoken to her like that, not once since she had set her cap at him, and she knew then and there that she would make sure he never spoke to her like it again. But she was trapped, trapped in this house, with his kid, and with his name. And, as if that wasn't bad enough, she had a terrible feeling she was pregnant again.

Chapter Four

'Oh, for fuck's sake, Cynthia! Cheer up, girl.'

Mary Callahan looked at the hard, set face in front of her and suppressed the urge to shake her daughter. Where she had got this one from she didn't know. Cynthia looked down her nose at everyone around her, had done since she could sit up on her own.

Gabby, bless her heart, was the antithesis of her mother. She looked like a little angel with her halo of blond hair and huge blue eyes. She was a gorgeous, loving little girl, but Mary knew that the poor child would not get that love returned from her own mother. Mary had accepted years ago that her daughter was capable of a lot of things, but love wasn't one of them. And as for that poor sap she had snared, and who she still had by the nuts . . . Mary wasn't an advocate of violence against women, but if ever a man should slap his old woman, poor Jimmy was that man. Cynthia rode him like a devil, and he let her, the poor bastard.

Mary glanced around her home; it was scruffy, granted, but it was clean enough. She was of the belief that a home was to be lived in, not just admired by fucking strangers. Unlike her daughter's gaff. She acted like fucking royalty was due round any minute. Cynthia's house was like the fucking library, you felt like you had to whisper, creep around it, as if noise of any kind was against the law.

She inwardly shook her head in sadness; her daughter would

17

never know a really happy day in her life, she wasn't built for joy. Still, that didn't mean little Gabriella shouldn't be happy. Not if Mary had any say in the matter, especially on Christmas Day. Turning to her granddaughter, she said cheerfully, 'Come on, Gabby, let's see what Santa left for you, shall we?'

The little girl ran to her nervously, worried as always that her mother would stop her in her tracks, give her a lecture about how little girls *should* behave.

Mary Callahan doted on her granddaughter. She was a little darling. Good as gold and pretty as a picture, with a lovely nature to boot. How her Cynthia had produced something so sweet she didn't know, but she had, and Mary prayed daily that her daughter didn't destroy this little girl's confidence with her constant criticisms.

Gabby sat in front of the plastic Christmas tree, her eyes glowing with happiness. She loved this house, from the garish tinsel everywhere, to the smell of cigarettes that permeated everything around her. She loved the whole 'Nana Mary experience'. And the constant noise – the TV was always on, as was the radio in the kitchen, and the record players upstairs. It was a jumble of sounds and smells. It was always full of people, there was always laughter, and any arguments were good-natured – unlike at home. She knew her mummy *liked* to leave her here sometimes and she knew, somewhere deep inside herself, that her mummy left her here for all the wrong reasons. But, for Gabriella Tailor, being here was enough.

Mary Callahan followed her daughter into the kitchen, wondering why she was even asking the question she knew her daughter would resent.

'Have you any idea how lucky you are, Cynthia? That man worships you, and he'd give you the earth on a plate if he could. Yet you still walk about with a face like a fucking wet weekend in Margate. What's your problem?'

Cynthia gritted her teeth in annoyance. 'Give it a rest, Mum, eh? You don't know the half of it.'

'Then tell me, child, maybe I can help?' It was a plea, and they both knew it.

Cynthia was tempted to turn to her mother and throw herself into her arms. She knew that, even after everything, she would be accepted, would be enveloped in her mother's love. But she couldn't do it. She could never admit to anyone, let alone this woman in front of her, that she had failed. Had made a grievous mistake. Had married a man who she had never loved, for a so-called decent life and who, nowadays, she had no respect for whatsoever, let alone any kind of warmth. He had let her down badly, and she was frightened of what the future held for them.

The worst of it all was she knew her mother would think that her feelings were not justified. She thought the sun shone out of James's arse. They all did. They thought *he* was a saint for putting up with *her*, and that rankled. They looked down on her for trying to get herself a better life, a decent life. James Tailor had promised her that, and he had reneged on his promise. At least that was how she saw it anyway. Instead she plastered a smile on her face. 'Nothing to tell, Mum, I'm just tired that's all.'

Mary Callahan grinned suddenly. 'You're pregnant again, aren't you?'

Cynthia closed her eyes slowly and nodded. 'Yeah, I think so. Just my fucking luck.'

Mary hugged her, even though the hug wasn't returned. 'That's what life is about, Cynthia! It's about having babies, and living your life as best you can. Millions of women do it every day.' She laughed then and said gently, 'And you, Cynth, have it easier than most, love.'

Cynthia shrugged nonchalantly. 'Well, that's as may be, but I want a bit more than this, Mum. I never signed on for cheap and cheerful, and I'm not settling for anything less.'

Her daughter's words wounded Mary, as she knew they were directed at her and the life she lived. The inference was that she had failed somehow, because the Callahans weren't rich or important enough for her elder child. Oh, she was itching to slap that beautiful face, but she wouldn't because she knew it would be pointless. She'd have a fleeting feeling of satisfaction, but it would also mean she wouldn't see her beloved grandchild until her daughter felt she needed to get away from the poor child once again. So Mary took a deep breath and said matter-of-factly, 'You got more than most women. Your trouble is you want the fucking earth on a plate. Well, as my mother used to say, you've made your bed, you better get used to lying in it.'

Looking around the kitchen as if it was the local dump, Cynthia replied, 'Well, you would know more about that than I would.'

Mary wanted to punch her daughter's lights out so badly she could almost taste it. Instead she said as coolly as she could, 'Do you know something, Cynth, one of these days you are going to push me too far, and when you do . . .' She was poking a finger into her daughter's face now, the anger rising inside her like a tide.

'Nana Mary, Granddad's here!'

Gabby, having run into the kitchen, was beside herself with excitement. After her nana Mary, her granddad Jack was the next best thing in her world.

Mary took a deep breath to calm her anger before she turned to Gabby, saying with forced joviality, 'Ah, sure, he'll be thrilled to see you, young lady!'

But Gabby could feel the tension in the small kitchen and, as always, it frightened her. She hated it when her mummy was like this, grim-faced and hard-mouthed. She wished her mummy would laugh more; she had a lovely laugh, like she had a lovely face.

20

'You better run, Mum, your better half just got home from the pub early. That must be a fucking first for you, eh?' Cynthia couldn't resist another jibe.

'Oh, you're a bitter pill, girl. At least your father *wants* to come home. More than you can say for poor Jimmy, I'm sure.' Mary knew it was a cheap shot but she couldn't help herself; sometimes Cynthia pushed you to the limit. Job himself would have struggled to be patient around her daughter.

Chapter Five

Jimmy Tailor liked all his in-laws. In fact, he was thrilled to be spending Christmas with them – anything was better than the silent dinner he would have had at home, with Cynthia sending him sneering, reproachful looks over the table. At least here he'd have a bit of fun and so would Gabby. Jimmy was especially fond of Celeste, his wife's younger sister. She was a really nice girl, not as beautiful as Cynthia, but still very attractive. She had a generous nature and kind heart too, and that made her a joy to be around.

'Hi, Jimmy, you look well.'

He grinned with pleasure. Celeste was always glad to see him. 'So do you, love. In fact, you look wonderful.'

She almost shone with pleasure at the compliment. Jimmy would never understand his wife's animosity towards her sister. It was beyond his comprehension. Jimmy didn't have a jealous bone in his body, so he never understood the naked envy in his wife's eyes when she looked at her little sister.

'Don't start her off, her head's big enough as it is.' He could hear the nastiness in his wife's voice.

Celeste smiled at her sister and said sweetly, 'You'd know all about that, Cynth. It's a wonder you can leave the fucking house!'

Everyone laughed. Cynthia watched them as they laughed at her expense. She hated that they were her family, hated that these people were her blood, hated that she needed them, that they were the only people who really knew her. It was the last place she wanted to be on Christmas Day but, then, she never missed an opportunity to lord it over them and look down her nose at them.

'Ha bloody ha ha. What are you so done up for?'

Celeste grinned once more, she was always so good-natured it made Cynthia want to hit her.

'Don't you mean for *who*? Didn't you tell her, Mum?'

Mary flapped her hand with feigned discretion. 'Why would I? It's your news to tell.'

'Come on then, Celeste, out with it.' Cynthia sounded bored now, as if anything to do with her sister was beneath her. Which, as far as Cynthia was concerned, pretty much summed up how she felt about Celeste and her excuse for a life.

'I'm seeing Jonny Parker, have been for a couple of months.'

Mary watched Cynthia as she digested this little bit of information, saw the shock as it occurred to her what that statement actually meant in real terms.

'He's too old for you.'

Celeste laughed, a happy, loud laugh, a natural laugh that made her look prettier than she actually was. She too had the arresting Callahan blue eyes and blond hair, although she didn't have the striking glamour of her sister. She might be a pale imitation in looks but Celeste's beauty came from within, from her nature. She had a wonderful lust for life, and she honestly believed that everyone was nice and kind, like her, and that if you treated people decently they would reciprocate.

'What you talking about, Cynthia? He's twenty-seven, and I'm nineteen. Eight years ain't much now, is it? It ain't like I'm thirteen and he's twenty-one. He's such a nice bloke, Cynth, treats me like a queen.'

Cynthia forced a smile on to her face; her sister couldn't know how this news was really affecting her. 'Well, you make sure he carries on treating you like that, OK?'

Celeste nodded happily, and Cynthia saw the genuine

pleasure on her face. She turned to her father. 'What do you think about it, Dad?'

Jack Callahan shrugged. He was already half cut, having been down the local pub for the best part of the day. He tried to focus on his elder daughter for a few seconds before saying amiably, 'What's to think? He's a nice enough fellow, and you can tell he thinks the world of her. Did you know he's bought the bookies on the high street? He's a dark horse, that one. He already owns a couple of pubs. This one here will be living the life of Riley if she plays her cards right!'

'Oh, Dad!'

Celeste was crimson with embarrassment at her father's words, and they all laughed at her discomfort at being the centre of attention, but knowing that she loved it really.

'Gabby can be your bridesmaid, she'd make a gorgeous little attendant!' Mary's voice was loud, and she watched her elder daughter carefully; if Celeste decided to settle down with Jonny Parker, and it looked more and more like that was going to be the case, Cynthia needed to accept it as soon as possible. Jonny and Cynthia had a history, not that Celeste knew that, but Mary knew that Cynthia had set her cap at him years ago. He had not been averse at first – no bloke was when she looked at them with her lovely face – but he had realised very quickly that Cynthia was seriously high maintenance and had dropped her so fast it had made her head spin. She was now hoping Cynthia would not feel the urge to enlighten her younger sister of that fact. Not that Celeste would be all that bothered, but Mary suspected from her reaction that Cynthia had never quite got over Jonny. And, as much as her elder daughter aggravated her, she still wouldn't like to see her hurt. But, more than that, she didn't want her younger child's happiness compromised because Cynthia was jealous. And jealous she might be, because Jonny Parker was going places, and that meant that Celeste would be going with him.

Mary Callahan looked at her granddaughter, the light of her life, and wondered, in the glow of her Christmas tree, what the future held for them all.

Knowing her elder child like she did, she knew that her younger daughter's life could be destroyed in an instant. But, if that ever happened, Mary would retaliate in a heartbeat because, if push came to shove, her younger child would win hands down. Cynthia had been given her chance with Jonny Parker many moons ago, and she had played it all wrong. Now he was fair game, and her Celeste was welcome to him. If Cynthia felt the need to challenge that, then Mary would be only too happy to put the fucker wise. Cynthia needed a wake-up call, and this might just be it.

Mary had two daughters, and she loved them both in her own way, but she wouldn't let one of them walk all over the other.

Chapter Six

'He's so handsome, Cynth!'

Mary wasn't surprised that her daughter didn't answer her, it was par for the course, but sometimes, like now, it grated. She looked down her bloody nose at them all, yet she still dumped the children on her parents on a regular basis. 'He's the image of Jimmy, but I can see you in him as well.'

Cynthia smiled but it wasn't a real smile. She was just going through the motions.

'We love having him over. Little Jimmy Junior!'

'He's James, Mum, he'll always be James.' Her daughter said it as if it was a matter of life and death. Which of course it was to her.

'Well, that's your call, love. He's your son after all.'

Cynthia nodded in agreement. 'Can you keep Gabriella for a few more days, just until I get into a routine?'

Mary nodded silently. She had been looking after Gabby for nearly six weeks now and, apart from Jimmy popping in most evenings to see his daughter, she might as well be an orphan, because Cynthia didn't bother with her at all.

James Junior was now a month old, and it looked like Cynthia was going to be the same with this child as she was with poor little Gabby. She fed him, changed him, and washed him, he was immaculately turned out, and well cared for in every way – outwardly that is – but she never picked him up unless she had to. Cynthia only did what she felt was expected of her. It was frightening to admit that his own mother, her daughter, had no real love for him. Because she knew that she didn't. She didn't truly care for either of her children. It was as if love was beyond her. Mary wished she knew how to stop it, how to make her daughter see the mistake she was making. Tell her how she saw through her – her life, her marriage and her sorry attempt at being a mother. She never comforted or played with her children, showed them any love or maternal instinct. Yes, she catered for their welfare, but she always kept her distance from them somehow. Cynthia always seemed to be on the periphery of their lives, never at the centre of it like she should have been.

Cynthia had always been a cold fish, she had never grasped the meaning of happiness. It seemed to have eluded her somehow, and Mary wondered at times if that was her fault. But she knew logically it wasn't anything she had done – in the beginning she had loved Cynthia as much as she had Celeste. She had loved both her girls with a deep and abiding passion from the minute she had given birth to them. But Cynthia had always had this wall around her, and nothing Mary had done had ever broken through it. So she had eventually accepted her daughter's personality, accepted that her Cynthia was not built for big displays of affection – in fact they troubled her, bothered her. Cynthia had always been a law unto herself, and it had been hard for Mary, a genuinely warm person, to be rebuffed by her own daughter from a young age. From then on, Cynthia had been a child who was difficult to love, really love. Mary had even disliked her sometimes, and now she wondered if that was why her daughter was such a hardcase. She'd tried to understand her daughter's personality but, if she was honest, it was beyond her. Cynthia had never been an easy child, and she was not an easy woman.

But now, her daughter's aloofness, and her complete indifference to her own children really worried her. She knew she couldn't do anything about it, because outwardly Cynthia was the perfect mother – who would believe her? But Mary worried that her grandchildren would suffer one day for their mother's lack of genuine affection.

Jimmy tried to make up for it, she knew, she saw that every day, and she wished she could tell him that she understood what he was going through. But voicing her worries would be tantamount to treason, would be criticising her own flesh and blood, and she just couldn't do that. It would be different if Jimmy came to her, and said it out loud. But she knew he would never do that. Cynthia had him well and truly under the thumb.

'Are you all right, Cynth? You look so down, love.'

Cynthia looked into her mother's eyes, the same deep blue eyes that her daughter had inherited, and she said in genuine bewilderment, ''Course I am! Why wouldn't I be?'

Mary smiled sadly. This was hard for her, really hard – she didn't know how she was supposed to deal with any of this.

Chapter Seven

Jimmy looked around the kitchen and made sure there wasn't a cup out of place. He wanted Cynthia to come home from her mother's to a spotless house and a nice meal. He had even cooked for them. He was looking forward to seeing her and his new son, of course. He just wished his daughter was coming home with them too.

Jimmy found he was shaking, and he *hated* that he was so nervous about something so normal. His wife had only been for a visit to her mother's – it wasn't as if that was something outrageous. But she was so difficult these days, even making a cup of tea was like a military operation around her. He loved his new son and he adored his daughter, but Cynthia made everything awkward, he felt unable to enjoy being with his own family. He hated that he was so weak, and he knew that *she* hated that he was so weak. But he didn't know how to fight her, he had never known how to fight for anything. That was the trouble.

He had always been the type of person who would do anything to keep the peace. That was all he had ever wanted, peace and quiet. How had it turned out so wrong? When did he realise that his life was a sham, and everyone had known long before he had that his wife was a nightmare?

As he heard the taxi pull up outside, he walked out into the hallway and said a silent prayer that his wife would be in a good mood for once. That she would walk into their house with a smile on her face, and tell him how much she had missed him.

But he didn't hold out much hope.

Chapter Eight

Jack Callahan was watching *Rainbow* with his granddaughter on his lap. He loved this little girl, and he was loathe to send her back home to her mother. He didn't think Cynthia was strange – he thought she was a complete fucking nut-job. And he was very vocal about his opinions, much to his wife's chagrin.

'Listen, Mary, the trouble with Cynthia is she's self-obsessed, always was, and always will be. There is nothing you can do about it, so let it go, will you?'

Mary didn't answer her husband; she knew from experience that he had said all he was going to say on the subject. Unlike her, he never made any allowances for his elder daughter, in fact, he was quite happy to denigrate her on an almost hourly basis. He had no time for Cynthia whatsoever and, as she had no time for him either, it was a very mutual arrangement. But it hurt Mary, because she loved her family, and she hated that her elder child had ruined everything with her toxic personality. She had left this poor child with them and, as much as she loved her, she knew that Cynthia should have wanted her own daughter at home with her, along with her new son. But Cynthia had never wanted Gabby, not really, and Mary knew she mustn't think about that too much. It just hurt her feelings, hurt her inside.

Thankfully she had her younger daughter to take her mind off it. Celeste had just got in from work, and she was beaming, as always, with happiness. Smiling widely in response, Mary

30

looked at her younger daughter and said with determination, 'You look happy!'

Celeste grinned back at her, and Mary decided that this child at least was going to be all right. Celeste was the antithesis of her older sister – she had no side to her, what you saw was what you got.

'I'm all right, Mum. I take it Cynthia hasn't taken poor Gabby home?'

Mary shook her head. 'I think she's still a bit tired after the birth of young Jimmy . . .'

Celeste frowned then, very theatrically, in a perfect imitation of her older sister, said 'Don't you mean *James*, Mum!'

They both laughed. Cynthia hated the child being called 'Jimmy'. She had given birth to a James, and James was his name, that was the end of it.

'Yeah, James! Like anyone will ever call him that.'

Celeste stopped laughing and said seriously, 'Cynthia will, Mum, you know what she's like.'

'That's true. Like anything else where the kids are concerned, we can only do what she wants.'

The laughter stopped completely then, even the pretence of it. They had often laughed about Cynthia and her ways, mocked her even – behind her back, of course – but suddenly it was as if they had decided to stop playing the game, as if they had all realised that, in reality, none of it was actually very funny. In order for Mary to see her grandchildren she had to go along with Cynthia's rules – they all did. She used the children like a weapon. And they let her, they *allowed* her to do it, because they knew that without them in the background the children would have nothing.

'Do you think she'll ever be all right, Mum? Because she seems to me as if she's getting unhappier by the day.'

Mary flapped her hand in annoyance. 'She'll never be happy, Celeste, it's not in her nature.'

'Well, that's as may be, Mum, but at least she has a husband, and a family who care about her.'

Mary smiled sadly. 'Well, for the time being anyway, eh, love?'

Jack Callahan, who had been listening to this exchange with half an ear, looked at his wife and daughter and shook his head in disbelief. Gesturing at Gabby, whose eyes were still glued to the TV, he said loudly, 'Look at this little one here, would you two rather she went home with that hard bitch?'

Celeste sighed heavily at her father's words. 'I think you should think a little about what you say in front of the child, Dad, you know.'

Jack Callahan laughed uproariously, amazed at his daughter's stupidity where her elder sister was concerned, and he said as much. 'Oh, fuck off, this little one here knows the score. For fuck's sake, she spends half her life here with us! As small as she is, she knows the score with that mad fucking whore.'

Mary Callahan shook her head in exasperation and, looking at her husband, she said seriously, 'Will you ever stop calling your daughter a *whore?*'

Jack Callahan took a deep breath and, after exhaling loudly, he said in a very quiet voice, 'And would you two ever fuck off? This child knows that she's safe here with me. Because her father, God forgive him, is as frightened of her mother as everyone else is. Well, *I* ain't, and I told him, poor fucker that he is, that if he was any kind of man he would batter her on a daily basis. Women like Cynthia need that. They are like poison, and you have to sort them out from the off. She looks down on us, and she looks down on *everyone* around her. If he had any fucking gumption he'd leave her, and do you know what? I'd be the first one to shake his hand if he did.'

Celeste looked at her mother and shrugged in resignation. Then Jack Callahan dropped his bombshell.

'And you, Celeste, had better watch your back because, mark

my words, she doesn't like what's going on between you and Jonny Parker. As long as she leaves this little one here with us, I'll swallow me knob, but I'm telling you now, I wouldn't trust her as far as I could kick her.'

Gabby looked up at her granddad and smiled happily. She knew that he would always stand up for her. As young as she was, she knew, deep inside, that her mummy didn't love her properly. She only felt truly loved and cared about when she was with her father, or her grandparents. Her daddy, she knew already, was too nervous of her mother to be trusted completely. Her granddad, though, would fight for her with everything he possessed. It was a good feeling, cuddled up with him, because she knew that he was the only person in her little world who wasn't scared of her mummy.

Chapter Nine

As Jimmy watched Cynthia kneel down at the altar, ready to receive Holy Communion, he wondered at how they had ended up like this. They were like strangers. She avoided him at every opportunity, slept in their spare room, and tried to convince him it was because it was easier to see to their son. She shrugged off any attempt he made to discuss their financial situation – which, thanks to her, was dire – and she continued to spend money at an alarming rate.

Looking at her like this, from a distance, he understood how he had fallen in love with her. She was still beautiful, her body was hardly changed by childbirth. If anything, she looked lovelier. She had filled out somehow, and her curves were all in the right places. But now he knew her properly, and that, in all honesty, meant he knew that inside she wasn't in any way beautiful. In fact, as far as her personality went, she was ugly. Ugly and hateful. Dissatisfied in every possible way with her life. And with him. She told him over and over again, how bored, disenchanted, and completely disillusioned she was with him and the life he had tried to give her. She made him feel as though everything he tried to do for her was pointless.

Now, as he watched her accept the communion host and look up at the cross of Christ, he wanted to slap her across the face. Of course he never would, he knew he wasn't capable of that kind of display of emotion, not outwardly anyway. He seethed inside though, and imagined slapping her across the face again and again. Oh, how he dreamt of that, how he dreamt of putting her firmly in her place. But he didn't know how to.

He waited for her to come back to the pew beside him and, kneeling down, he prayed to God to give him strength. The strength to fight against this wife of his, and the strength to fight for his children, because he knew that, if he wasn't careful, she would hurt them too, just as she had hurt him.

Chapter Ten

Jonny Parker looked at Celeste as she walked back to the table and sat down and wondered at how much his life had changed through meeting this girl. She was lovely, really lovely. It wasn't so much her looks – though she was certainly the prettiest in the pub tonight – but she was lovely *inside*. There wasn't a bad bone in her body. He loved that she saw the best in everyone, even that leech of a sister of hers. What a narrow escape he'd had there!

All those years ago he had been blinded by Cynthia's beauty, but then so had a lot of men. She had been cold-blooded though, so he'd had to get shot of her. In the end she went for a man she believed would give her the life she craved. Unfortunately, it seemed, she had made a serious fuck-up in that respect, and now she was tied to that poor bastard come hell or high water. But that wasn't his problem – he'd wiped her from his memory. His love for Celeste was completely different. Of all the women he had met, slept with, and gone through, she was the only one who had kept his attention, kept him interested, and kept him enthralled. He loved her with every fibre of his being. He just hated that he had been with her sister first, that Cynthia was a part of his life still, because she was there whether he liked it or not. And he didn't like it, not one bit.

He was making a name for himself, becoming a Face of sorts, making himself important to the right people. He could give Celeste a good life, a good home, and a good seeing-to as and when she needed it. He also knew that Celeste was the kind of girl who would appreciate that – and welcome it. She didn't have any hidden agenda, she just loved life itself. And he loved her for that.

His mother was a drama queen. He loved her of course, but he knew that he could never live with all that himself. Celeste was a real woman, as innocent and unassuming as she was. Jonny knew she would never understand how marvellous she really was. He also knew that Cynthia, her older sister, would never accept that he had chosen Celeste over her. But he had, and he would never regret that decision. Cynthia still bothered him though, if he was truthful. For some reason he knew that Cynthia would make them pay for their happiness. He didn't know how, or why, but he knew Cynthia would somehow extract her pound of flesh. It was in her nature. He had fallen for Cynthia, sexually and mentally, for a short while, but he never wanted Celeste to know that. Cynthia was poison, she was not someone anyone in their right mind would have kept in touch with. And she was dangerous, because she had no real care for anyone or anything, except herself. He had realised overnight how one person could change your life, not for the better, but for the worse. Because that was what people like Cynthia did, they tainted everyone around them, and they made sure that everything and everyone they touched would be as broken as they were.

Back then he would never have dreamt that he would one day meet her sister and fall so deeply in love with her. To be truthful, if he had known the connection that first night he met Celeste, he would have walked away. But it hadn't happened like that. He *had* met her, and he had fallen for her. And now he couldn't imagine being without her. If Cynthia caused any aggravation whatsoever, if she made his relationship with Celeste a problem in any way, he would happily wipe her off the face of the earth. Because, unlike Celeste, he knew the *real*

Cynthia, and he had no intentions of making any kind of excuses for her.

She had nearly got her claws into him once before, and he would never ever let her do that to him again.

Chapter Eleven

'Come on, Cynth, let's go out for a couple of hours? Your mum's happy to have the kids.'

Cynthia looked at her husband and stifled the urge to take him out once and for all. She pictured herself taking a knife from the wooden block she had paid so much for, and running him through with the boning knife. She knew she would never use the boning knife otherwise; after all, why would she ever feel the need to bone a piece of meat? That knife was obsolete, she would never use it, no more than she would use most of the other knives in the set. She had bought them because they were expensive, and would give her kudos should anyone visit her kitchen. But sometimes, like now, she felt that she could happily use a couple of the knives on her lawful husband.

She was getting more and more worried, because he had no idea about how much debt she was actually in. He didn't understand how hard it was for her when she wanted something new, because he couldn't earn enough money to keep them afloat. Oh, it was so unfair! Here she was laden down with two children, a house that had a kitchen worth more than their car, and a husband who was never going to go up in his world because he didn't have the fucking brains he was born with. She was now lumbered with a moron, who she had never really even liked, if she was totally honest, let alone loved, but who, until recently, she had believed would give her the life she craved. The life she had *deserved* because, after all, she was very beautiful and very shrewd, and she had made a point of looking out for a man she was certain would give her what she wanted – a life of luxury and ease.

Now, it seemed, she had sacrificed herself to a man who had no real ambition, and who was happy to stay at the bottom rung of the ladder of life. He actually thought that their son would make them happy – that having a second child made them some kind of family! And perhaps they would have been if he had reached his full potential. But he hadn't – James had lied to her, he had told her he would make something of himself, he had promised her he would give her the world. Instead, he had let her down spectacularly, while her little sister had snagged herself a fucking real grafter. A grafter *she* had actually been attracted to. How was it that fucking Celeste, that fucking stupid, sense-less, brain-dead idiot, was swanning around with Jonny Parker, like she was important or something. Celeste! Who was another fucking moron, who had the brains of a gnat. Who had no personality to speak of and no looks either really. Nothing to write home about anyway.

Cynthia looked in her bedroom mirror. She saw herself as a stranger would see her, looked at herself without any bias whatsoever, and she knew she still looked good. She had been lucky – most women after two children looked exactly like they had given birth to two children. She didn't; there wasn't a mark on her. That pleased her, because she knew that she would have to look around at some point for another husband.

Because there was no way she was going to stay in this marriage, no way she was going to waste herself on someone as pathetic as James.

Chapter Twelve

Celeste was happier than she had ever been, since Jonny had asked her to marry him. And it was obvious to anyone who knew her. She was genuinely thrilled at the direction her life had taken. As she looked at Jonny sitting at her mother's dining table, she felt the happiness well up inside her. Her love for him was so strong it was as if she could hold it in her hands.

She knew that Jimmy was thrilled for her; he was a really nice man, too good for her sister of course – not that she would ever say that out loud. But Cynthia somehow made you think awful things about her. It was as if she was only there to make you dislike her. She dumped her children here, at her parents' house, for weeks at a time. Not that she minded; in fact, like her mum and dad, Celeste actually felt happier when the kids were there, because Cynthia didn't seem to care about them really.

Now, though, as they all sat around the table for Sunday lunch, Celeste suddenly felt sorry for Cynthia, and that was a new experience for her. She had always felt she was beneath her elder sister somehow, because in many ways she was a hard act to follow. For a start Cynthia was movie-star beautiful, a head-turner, a real stunner. It had been difficult to grow up in her shadow, a watered-down version of Cynthia. People had often pointed out her sister's lovely face and perfect figure, and they had never realised how hard it had been for *her*, because no one ever talked about her in that way. It was as if, to them, she didn't exist. But, in fairness, she had understood why they had singled Cynthia out.

Things were very different now. With Jonny loving her like he did, and her life being so tremendous, Celeste felt for the first time ever that she could pity her sister. Because, no matter what, she knew that Cynthia wasn't happy at all, she was desperately *un*happy, and that saddened her. At the end of the day Cynthia was still her sister, she was still her flesh and blood. And she *did* want her to be happy. She wanted her sister to be as happy as she was, she wanted her sister – just once – to have a smile on her face that wasn't forced.

As Celeste looked at Jonny and saw his handsome face beaming at her, as she looked at little Gabby, all nervous twitches and tension, she wondered how anyone could give birth to a child, and not care for them in any way. It was clear to her suddenly that her sister didn't care about anyone, least of all her little daughter.

'What you thinking about, Celeste?' Cynthia's voice was low, but the question was serious. Everyone around the table went quiet, each interested in the answer.

Celeste shrugged nonchalantly, embarrassed as always to be the centre of attention. 'Nothing really, Cynth, nothing you'd be interested in anyway.'

Cynthia grinned then. 'Listen, Celeste, an original thought in your head would die of fucking loneliness.' She laughed at her own joke, a loud, harsh laugh.

Celeste couldn't help herself. She said loudly and honestly, 'If you're not careful, you're the one who'll die of loneliness, Cynth.'

Cynthia looked around the table, and she saw the shock on everyone's faces at her sister's words, a shock that was quickly followed by genuine laughter, and she knew then what they really thought about her.

'That told you, Cynth! The truth hurts, girl, don't it?'

Her father was looking at her with such loathing it made her realise just how disliked she actually was in her family. It was a real shock for her because she had been under the impression that she was better than them somehow, and she had believed that they had thought that too. She glanced at her husband, and saw the triumph in his eyes, even though he wasn't looking directly at her, and she knew then that, if she wasn't careful, she would be sidelined by this sister of hers.

She was the elder sister, *she* was the one who had dragged herself out of this dump, and *she* was the one who had bettered herself. And she would carry on bettering herself, because there was no way she would settle for anything less than the best.

Chapter Thirteen

'Oh, for crying out loud, James, are you stupid or what?'

Jimmy looked at his wife and wondered, not for the first time, how he had ended up tied to a woman who he had nothing at all in common with. In fact, he knew somewhere in his heart that she had nothing in common with anyone else in the world. She was a one-off, a complete enigma. No one liked her. Once that had saddened him, he had thought she was misunderstood and seen her as someone he could protect. Now, though, he knew that if anyone needed protecting it was him – him and his children. He had married a bully, an emotional bully, and he could no longer pretend otherwise. The last few months had shown him what his life was really like, and it wasn't pretty. He had finally admitted to himself that he *had* no real life, nothing even remotely resembling one. All he had was Cynthia and her wants and her moods. She had taken away everything from him: his dignity, his self-respect, his children.

He was also not blind to Cynthia's reaction to her sister's husband-to-be. Cynthia was almost ill with jealousy at Celeste's obvious happiness and, even though he hated his wife at times, hated her for her coldness and her complete disregard for everyone around her, there was still a part of him that longed for her to love him. Look at him in the way she looked at Jonny Parker. But he knew it would never happen.

They lived in this expensive mausoleum, and the saddest thing of all was that this house, which he had bought because she had loved it so much, was now her prison. They couldn't sell it, couldn't make their money back – she had spent so much on it that to try and sell it now would mean they would be thousands of pounds out of pocket. The expensive kitchen, which he had known at the time was too good for a semi-detached house in Ilford, had been paid for with what amounted to a second mortgage. When you added in to all that the carpets, curtains, the fitted wardrobes, the bathroom with its cast iron bath, and the new central-heating system, they were up to their eyebrows in hock.

'No, Cynthia, I ain't stupid. I *was* stupid, though, when I let you borrow money like it was going out of fashion. But I wanted *you* to be happy, and *you* were only happy when you were spending money. Well, we can't sell this drum and make a profit on it because the designer kitchen and bathroom that cost the national debt hasn't actually put a fucking bean on this place! It's still just a semi in Ilford, in Essex. *And* we still have to pay it all off. So, thanks to you, and your fucking wanting, we'll still be here when we're fucking seventy.'

Cynthia looked at her husband, and she felt the hatred rising up inside her. She looked at his weak features, his pale eyes, nondescript brown hair and his doughy body. She'd thought him handsome once. Now all she saw was that he was useless, useless and weak. She felt like her life was over. She had tied herself to a man who would never ever be even remotely important to her, or anyone else for that matter. She had two children, children who had half of this man inside them, children who, if she wasn't careful, would grow up to be as useless and nondescript as he was.

'We're insured, aren't we? I made sure of that much. Use your fucking loaf for once in your life!'

Jimmy looked at his wife and felt overwhelmed with despair. Life could not get much worse, surely? His children lived at his mother-in-law's and his home was a permanent battleground because his wife no longer hid her disdain for him. He was earning a good wage, but it still wasn't enough for what they owed. He had allowed her to do what she wanted, and he had stood back while she sunk them further and further into debt. He had not been man enough to put his foot down – in fact, he had not even thought about curbing her spending. But, now she knew he wasn't on the fast track, now she knew he wasn't going to become the boss of bosses, she treated him like dirt. Like he was nothing. And it hurt.

Chapter Fourteen

'Oh, Celeste, you'll look stunning in that, babe. I'm so proud of you.'

Jonny was thrilled at his fiancée's choice of dress for their engagement party. It wasn't cheap but, in fairness, it wasn't really expensive either. It was just like Celeste in many respects – quietly beautiful.

'Do you like it really, Jonny?'

He grinned happily at her and she caught her breath. He was so good-looking, with thick dark hair, and dark blue eyes, well built and always well dressed. Celeste wondered every day how she had been lucky enough to catch his eye.

Gabby grabbed her hand and she laughed delightedly. 'Don't worry, you. You'll be the chief bridesmaid.'

Jonny picked the little girl up, and threw her into the air. Gabby screamed with delight and, as he placed her back on to the ground, she said happily, 'Can I live with you two when you get married?'

Celeste looked into Jonny's eyes and she saw the sadness in her own mirrored there. She knelt down and hugged her little niece tightly. 'You can stay with us any time you want, right?'

Gabby nodded seriously, understanding that she wasn't being invited for any real length of time. But already in her short life she understood that people came and went. And often let you down. One thing she had learned was that everyone eventually let you down, *that* was real life, that was how it all worked. But it hurt her, because she would love nothing more than to become a part of her auntie's life. She would love to be a part of something that she felt would last for a long, long time.

She knew her daddy loved her, but he never came to get her any more from her nana's, and her mummy *never* came to see her, never gave her the time of day.

It was as if she had done something wrong and her mother was punishing her for it. But she hadn't done anything – she had tried her hardest to be a good girl. She tried everything in her power to make her mummy want her again, but nothing had worked in any way, shape or form. It was hard for her, because she didn't know what she was supposed to do. She didn't know *how* to make her mummy love her. She didn't know why she wasn't wanted by her mummy.

Her nana loved her, of that much she was sure. Because, no matter what happened to her, she always ended up back at her nana's, which was strange because, according to her mummy, her nana's house was a filthy shithole that she wouldn't let a dog live in. Gabby supposed that was why she couldn't have a puppy, though she would love one dearly. Her nana's house wasn't clean like her mummy's, but it felt better than her mummy's house because she didn't have to be on her best behaviour all the time. And the nicest thing of all was she never wet the bed at her nana's. Her granddad said that was because she could kip in peace without her mummy watching her every move. Her granddad also said that her mother was a stuck-up bitch, who needed a right-hander, and that her dad was a lovely bloke but he needed to toughen up and stop letting his old woman walk all over him like a second-hand carpet. He was funny, her granddad.

As she saw her auntie smiling and laughing, she felt warm inside. She loved her auntie Celeste, and she loved her uncle Jonny, and she wondered why her mummy didn't like them very much. She had the idea it was something to do with Uncle

Jonny. Her mummy always tried to get Uncle Jonny's attention, but she guessed that, like most people, he didn't want anything like that from her. She could understand it too – *she* didn't like being in her mother's eyeline either because all she did if you were was moan and complain.

Gabby pushed away the thoughts that troubled her and tried to bask in the sheer happiness of being with her auntie. So many of her thoughts worried her, and she didn't know how she was supposed to make them go away. As she forced a huge smile on her lovely face she suddenly felt the urge to cry, because times like this, the really good times, only made her more aware of the sadness inside her, the sadness that was always there.

'You all right, sweetheart?' Celeste knelt before her little niece and, seeing the tears in her eyes, she said brokenly, 'What are you crying about, you silly mare? You're with family, darling, family who love you.'

But Gabby couldn't tell her auntie that *that* was what was wrong with her. That was why she felt so sad. With this part of her family she felt loved and cared for, and she was always terrified that one day this would all stop.

Gabby realised then that she didn't want to go home ever again. She was far too happy here.

Chapter Fifteen

'You're not taking them, Cynth, and that's that.'

Cynthia looked at her father and sighed heavily. They all knew she had no intention of taking her children home with her. This was a game they played all too frequently; Cynthia faked a maternal interest and her parents pretended to talk her out of taking her children home with her. It was tedious, but they all saw it as a necessary evil. Cynthia could go back home content in the knowledge she had done her bit, and that her parents would be heartbroken if she removed the children from their care. It was a win-win situation as far as she was concerned.

Mary joined in the argument. 'I'm taking Gabby to the market with me tomorrow, and then we're going to get her fitted for her bridesmaid's dress. So it's not convenient really, unless you want to take her to that?'

Cynthia shook her head as if her mother had asked her to do something completely outrageous. 'No, thanks! Like I haven't got enough to do!'

This was another part of the pretence; that Cynthia had a busy life, that she was somehow too busy to do the usual things other women did like take her daughter for her fitting for her bridesmaid's dress. And yet this was the woman who wouldn't get a job if her life depended on it.

'They're all right here then, Mum, if you're sure.'

Mary Callahan barely kept the sarcasm from her voice as she replied casually, 'Oh, I'm sure, Cynth.'

Cynthia looked around the home she had grown up in, at the scuffed paintwork, and the old-fashioned wallpaper, and shuddered inwardly. How had these people spawned her? It was a question that had always baffled her, and always would. All her life she had wondered at how she had been brought up in this dump, and yet had somehow known the proper way to dress, eat and live. Her childhood had been all slapdash; it was beyond her how she had grown up so refined. She believed that somewhere, way back in the bloodline, there must have been someone just like her and, generations later, she had been the recipient of those good genes.

Cynthia looked at her daughter and saw her own beauty reflected in her face. She was a good-looking child, true, but she was too much like this lot. Happy with nothing, happy to eat crap and spend her life watching telly.

It even smelled, this house – all overflowing bins and dirty ashtrays, washing-up and bacon sandwiches, everything she had hated growing up here. It never changed – the smell of her father's work shirts and her mother's cheap perfume seemed to permeate the very walls. And then there was the gas fire that popped all night long, leaving its residue on the walls and the doors, the constant noise of a radio or the TV, no real conversation unless it was about someone they knew, never about what was going on in the world. It was like being caught up in a soap opera, except the people in the soaps had personalities – this lot had nothing of any interest going for them at all. Her mother was bad enough. She spent her whole life smoking her fags, drinking her tea and living for the next episode of *Coronation Street*. Her mother knew more about Emily Bishop than she did about her own family.

And now her sister was lording it up with a man who was a right Face, and a right earner. It was so unfair. If only she had used her loaf, waited a while, kept her options open. But, back then, she had been so *sure* about James. Now look where she was; stuck in a vicious circle of debt with two kids hanging round her neck. If James had kept his part of the bargain she would have had a nanny, or at least an au pair, to take the brunt of the work off her. She closed her eyes in frustration. She had to work out a way to get rid of the house and still come out quids in. Once she sorted *that*, they could get back on track. If she left it to James, they would still be in that dump of a street when they were drawing their pensions – if she could stand him for that long.

Now, here was Celeste, about to hitch up with a man who was obviously going places. It was like a kick in the teeth.

Her father lifted his leg and broke wind loudly, and she pursed her lips, knowing it was for her benefit. Her father enjoyed her discomfort at what she regarded as common behaviour. If she wasn't going to be so busy the next few days she would take Gabriella home with her just to teach him a lesson.

'Here, Cynth, do you want to stay for your tea? Jonny's coming round, and Jimmy Boy could come here as well. Be a nice family get-together.'

Her mother was smiling as she said it, and Cynthia realised that she genuinely meant it. Still, she was going to refuse because seeing Celeste and Jonny together made her feel even more depressed than usual.

'I would, Mum, but I've made arrangements . . .' Her voice tailed off and she forced a smile. 'Maybe another night, eh?'

Mary nodded, wondering why she had bothered asking Cynthia in the first place. Mary Callahan could see that this daughter of hers was eaten up with jealousy about Celeste and Jonny, and she also knew why, though she wouldn't bring it up in front of her husband. He'd love to go on about it, to use it as another stick to beat his daughter with. It was strange really because Cynthia had always been his favourite – until she was about thirteen. Then the fastidious ways that they had laughed at and her determination to act like the lady of the manor had ceased to amuse them. Jack had suddenly realised that his daughter was ashamed of him. Not only that, but she also despised him. Despised them all and wanted to be nothing like them. She had only stayed a Catholic because the nuns had beaten the religion into her, and it was the one thing she knew would cause a complete break from her parents. Jack Callahan was a lot of things, but he was a devout Catholic and there was no way he would countenance his daughter turning her back on her faith. And Cynthia, for all her airs and graces, was secretly frightened of having this front door closed on her once and for all. Mary could see that. And, deep down, she needed them more than they needed her.

Cynthia saw a momentary flicker of sadness on her mother's face, and stood up to put her coat on; she didn't want or need her pity. Just because she wouldn't settle for less than what she deserved didn't make her a bad person. In Cynthia's book it made her a winner, a fighter, a survivor. A council house and making do would never be her life, she was determined about that much anyway. She would sort out their financial problems, and put all this behind them.

When her mother left, Gabby sighed deeply. Her mother could even make the air seem heavier with her presence, but Gabby hadn't understood until then the force of certain people's personalities.

She was beginning to understand that only too well now.

Chapter Sixteen

Jimmy was tired and it showed. A lot of it was to do with being married to Cynthia; she had worn him down to nothing. It saddened him that none of his friends visited any more. Cynthia could cook a beautiful meal, pour them good wine, but her very nature stopped people from wanting to be in her company for any length of time. She only bothered with people she thought were class, with people she thought were a cut above. Unfortunately, those were the very people who saw through her like a pane of glass, much quicker than her own kind anyway. She was neither fish nor foul as his old grandmother used to say. She didn't really fit in anywhere.

Now, as he sat in the warmth of a pub in Dean Street, he wondered why he didn't come here more often. It was a great place, full of people, full of laughter. He was with Jonny Parker and his cronies and he was having a really fantastic time – he liked Jonny, and he liked Jonny's mates. He couldn't understand Cynthia's almost pathological hatred of him and all he stood for. Jimmy knew Jonny was a bit of a lad, but that was *his* business, certainly nothing for him to concern himself with. He swallowed another Scotch, and felt the warm glow as it hit his empty belly.

'How you doing, Jimmy Boy?'

Jonny was smiling at him, but Jimmy could feel his concern.

'I'm all right, Jonny, just thinking, mate. Drink can do that to a body.'

Jonny sat beside him and, leaning across the table, he grabbed his own drink and sipped it. Lighting a cigarette, he casually waved towards the bar for another round of drinks. They appeared only a few minutes later. Jimmy was very impressed; it was as if Jonny owned the place, and that's how it had been all night long.

'Here, Jonny,' said one of his mates, 'you heard about Black Micky?'

Jonny nodded and said nonchalantly, 'He knew the score. I warned him, but he wouldn't listen to me. He'll get an eighteen if he's lucky.'

The other men at the table all nodded sagely, the conversation had suddenly turned serious.

'His old woman's to blame,' someone else pitched in. 'Fucking want, want, want. She could spend money like a fucking Russian oligarch, or whatever they're called! That's what alerted the Old Bill – fucking BMWs outside the front door, the kids in private school, and him without a legal fucking earn to his name. Got to attract the wrong attention.'

Jonny nodded once more. 'I told him five years ago when he was first on a good earn – I was working for *him* then, I was only a kid meself – but I said to him, buy a few houses, rent them out, get a shop or a café, something to look like you're grafting. But you know him, thought he was sorted because he had a few Old Bill on his payroll. It was the serious crime squad who gave him the capture, not local fucking plod.'

Jimmy listened in amazement at the men's conversation.

'The SCS are all over the place lately. Someone, somewhere is earning a fucking wedge of some description from them, either getting a pass for their own dirty dealings, or picking up a serious rent. Either way, there's skulduggery afoot.'

Jonny laughed nastily then. 'Well, whoever it is, I wouldn't want to fucking be in their boots when it all comes floating to the top. And it will. You can't get away with that for any length of time. Someone will stumble eventually, that's the law of the streets.'

Trevor Carling, a small, dark-haired man, with eyes that were a deep violet-blue, leant forward and said conversationally, 'I hope I get first fucking refusal on the cunt. I'd keep him screaming for days – within the hour I'd have the ponce praying for a quick death.'

All the men laughed now, and Jonny grinned as he said, 'Fucking hell, Trevor, you'd glass your own granny if she owed you a fiver!'

Trevor laughed good-naturedly then, lightening the mood once more as he said, 'Nah, I love me granny and she's too intelligent to borrow money from me in the first place!'

Jimmy sat back in the chair, shocked at the conversation around him, and frightened now of the men who had welcomed him into their company and who he had liked and admired only a few minutes before.

Jonny saw the way Jimmy was reacting to their banter and he put an arm around his shoulders. Then, winking at the men around him, he said loudly, 'Enough! This is my soon-to-be brother-in-law, and he's straighter than a copper's parting.'

Trevor leant towards Jimmy and said with a chuckle, 'Oi, son, remember the old wartime slogan, careless talk costs lives!'

It was a serious warning, and Jimmy knew it.

'He won't say a word, he's sound is Jimmy.'

Jimmy saw that, with those few words from Jonny, he was accepted without a murmur. And he also thought he understood now why Cynthia had such a problem with her sister's intended. Jonny Parker was going places, and even Jimmy, who was as green as the proverbial grass where the criminal life was concerned, could see that much. It was also obvious that Celeste would be going with him, and that must be what was really causing Cynthia sleepless nights.

Jimmy knew then that Jonny Parker wouldn't be getting an

eighteen any time soon. He was too shrewd for that. Jimmy also knew that he liked him, even if those last few moments had surprised him. Still, whatever he might be, Jonny Parker was a nice bloke.

Chapter Seventeen

'You all right, Jimmy Boy?'

Jonny Parker was laughing as Jimmy emptied his stomach into the lay-by. He rubbed Jimmy's back and, when the retching eased off, he opened the boot of his Mercedes and got out a bottle of water.

'Here y'are, mate, get that down you, you'll feel better.'

Jimmy drank the cool water gratefully. 'I don't drink that much normally.'

Jonny laughed delightedly. 'I should fucking hope not and all, your liver must be praying for a transplant.'

Jimmy smiled and Jonny wondered at how this big man, who was a lump in many respects, had lumbered himself with someone like Cynthia. But he knew the answer to his own question; Cynthia was a looker, and she had that stuck-up way about her that attracted men. Jimmy had fallen for her, just as many a man before him had fallen for a prize bitch; it wasn't till they were safely married that they showed their true colours. Jonny should know – his own mother had been a ball-breaker, and his father, a Face in his own right, a hard man, had still never been hard enough to put her in her place. She had dripped her poison in his earhole all day, every day and, eventually, that kind of treatment could bring down even the toughest of men. This poor sap didn't stand a chance.

Jimmy sat on the kerb and took a few deep breaths; the world was finally coming back into focus, and he was grateful for that much at least. 'I really enjoyed tonight, Jonny, but I think the strippers had best be kept a secret if you know what I mean!'

'Well, I won't be broadcasting it to the nation, mate. Celeste is an easy-going girl, but she ain't that easy going!' Jonny lit a cigarette and pulled on it deeply before settling himself beside Jimmy on the dirty kerbside.

'She's a lovely girl, Celeste, you got a good one there, Jonny.'

'I know that, wouldn't be marrying her otherwise.'

Jimmy sighed heavily. 'She's kind is Celeste, very kind-hearted. My Gabriella loves her, which is just as well, because she spends more time with her than she does with her mother.'

Jonny could hear the bitterness in Jimmy's voice, and felt ashamed for the man's weakness. 'Well, Jimmy Boy, that's not really any of my business, is it?'

Jimmy shook his head; he appreciated Jonny's tact, but the drink had taken its toll and he wanted to talk to someone. *Needed* to talk to someone, say it all out loud, and he knew that Jonny would listen and not hold it against him.

'I know that, Jonny, but tonight I realised how much I've lost out on. You lot together, having a laugh, a few drinks. I miss that. Not that I ever did anything like tonight, but I used to meet the blokes after work in the West End, you know. Not any more, though, Cynthia has me on a bloody schedule. She knows my movements better than I do, plus I'm not running the firm, not even going upwards if truth be told. I haven't got what it takes for the office politics. I congratulate men younger than me when they get promoted over my head. My kids live at their grandparents' house. Not that *my* parents ever get a look in with the kids – they've never been allowed to see them. I just don't know how this all happened to me. I don't know how to make it all right.'

Jonny threw the cigarette into the road, and immediately lit another one. He was genuinely sorry for the man, even though he couldn't help feeling that the situation was all of his own making. Having been brought up by a woman who was like Cynthia, having seen the damage someone like her was capable of causing to the men who were unlucky enough to love them, he could understand the man's predicament. And he had been on the receiving end of Cynthia himself, when he had been enamoured with her and her lush body for a while. But, unlike James Tailor, he had seen her for what she was before it was too late. His father's example was always with him, and he knew that a big part of Celeste's attraction was that she was the complete opposite to Cynthia. He knew that with her he wouldn't have to fight for supremacy in the relationship; all he would have to do was love her and take care of her. That would be more than enough for her, and she would be loyal to him till her dying day.

'Look, Jimmy, I know the score, but you have to sort this out yourself. You have to put your foot down, let her know who's boss.'

Jimmy laughed then, and it was almost as if he really found the conversation hilarious. 'Easier said than done, Jonny! She has this knack of saying things in such a way you have to believe she's in the right. We are in so much debt, she spends money like it's going out of fashion and, when we discuss it, *I* end up feeling like *I'm* the one who's in the wrong. She convinces me that it's not *her* getting us into the debt in the first place that's the problem, but it's *my* inability to pay said debts which is.'

Jonny knew exactly where Jimmy was coming from; he could write the script. 'Well, Jimmy Boy, you either sort the debts out, though in my experience she'll just run up more, or you put the foot on her neck and rein her in once and for all.'

Jimmy didn't answer him.

Then Jonny said quietly, 'There is a third option, Jimmy.'

Jimmy looked up. 'What's that, Jonny?'

'You could do a bit of moonlighting. You're good with other people's money, and I could do with a creative accountant, if you get my drift?' As he said it, Jonny could have kicked himself. He blamed it on the whisky. Scotch always made him sentimental.

'Really, Jonny, could I make decent money from it? I mean real money?'

Jonny realised he had just answered this man's prayers. And ruined him into the bargain. 'If you can hide a good percentage of my earnings and still make it all look legit, you'd be an asset, mate. But before you go making any quick decisions, remember that you'll be breaking the law and if we ever get a capture you could go down for it. You'll be expected to keep your trap shut, and do your time without a whimper to anyone, especially not the Filth. I work for some very heavy people, so think long and hard about what you'll be getting involved in. Because if you step out of line, you'll be wiped off the face of the earth. Family or no family connections, you fuck up and I'll come after you meself.' Jonny hoped this advice, delivered with a threat and a promise of trouble to come, would be the decider for Jimmy Tailor, and make him see that this wasn't the life for someone like him.

Jimmy, though, saw this man as a saviour and saw the chance of a good earn doing what he was good at – working with money. Jimmy, in his desperation, believed that if he worked for Jonny Parker nothing bad could ever happen to him. After all, he would only be keeping the books, it wasn't as if he would be a real part of the business. He conveniently forgot about the conversations he had heard earlier in the evening, chose to forget that those were the very people whose money he would be responsible for. All he could see was a way out of the enormous debt they were in, and the look on Cynthia's face when she realised he had finally sorted it out.

'Thanks, Jonny. But I don't need to think about it. I'd be honoured to come and work for you. You won't regret it, I'll work my fingers to the bone . . . Twenty-four seven if needs be.'

Jonny held his hand up to stop the man's excited chatter. It occurred to him that Jimmy was not exactly *au fait* with what the job actually entailed, and he also knew that he would have to test the man's abilities before he gave him any kind of real money to work with. 'Hang on a minute, Jimmy Boy. You have to keep the day job, mate, that will be your blind for the future. Mr Respectable and all that. You'll do my number crunching in your spare time and keep it under your hat – don't even tell Cynthia until it's a done deal. I'll take you on trial for two months to see if you can do the job how I want it done, and to see if you can handle what the job entails. That way we can both decide if it's not what either of us want, OK?'

Jimmy nodded then as if he finally understood the situation, and Jonny Parker wondered how the fuck this idiot would cope with the stress that this new world he was becoming a part of would inevitably place on his rounded shoulders. But the damage was done now, and all Jonny could do was make sure he kept a beady eye on the situation.

As if he didn't have enough to fucking do.

Chapter Eighteen

1988

Cynthia was beside herself with annoyance, but she held her temper as she had learned to do over the last couple of years. Seeing Celeste with her detached house and her flash little sports car was bad enough, but that contented smile that was always on her moon face was the real bugbear.

Cynthia had finally got herself and her family out of the house in Ilford – and she had made sure they made their money back on that place. *Not* that she had ever told anyone the long and the short of *that* story – even that prat James was still none the wiser where that was concerned. He wasn't capable of understanding her logic. Also he was like all villains and, when all was said and done, he *was* now a villain, albeit a minor one. He believed you should never publicly break the law. It brought the Filth down on your head, and made them look at you a bit closer than you'd like. And, though they weren't exactly rolling in it, they were in a much better financial position than they had thought they would be – all thanks to her, of course. That prick would have sold at a loss, and they would never have got out of the debt. But, seeing how they were now getting an extra few quid courtesy of Celeste's husband, the high and mighty Jonny Parker, she had to watch herself these days and it was getting harder and harder to keep her opinions to herself.

Now, as they walked into the restaurant for another expensive party, to celebrate yet another feather in Jonny Parker's cap, Cynthia felt she could easily scream in utter frustration.

She caught a glimpse of herself in a mirror, confident she was easily the best-dressed and the best-looking woman in the place. That wasn't difficult – the competition wasn't exactly Crufts standard. She smiled at the simile. She could stop an articulated lorry in its tracks when she was wearing the right top and the right make-up. Yet she knew that to Jonny Parker she might just as well be invisible. He spoke to her, he was polite to her, but she knew that he didn't see her in any way that meant anything.

She, on the other hand, was always conscious of his presence; and he had just that – presence. It was no wonder he was doing so well in his chosen field – men as well as women were drawn to him. He was charismatic, dangerous and he knew the score better than the people around him. It was the one thing she could never get out of James, because no matter how much she kicked off, no matter how much she created, he would not, under any circumstances, tell her the extent of Jonny's businesses. In fact, he told her absolutely nothing. He was another one getting too big for his boots; since he had started working full time for Jonny he was getting far too clever for his own good.

Cynthia sat at the table beside her sister, aware that she looked much better than her, and the knowledge was like a balm. She saw a lot of the men giving her the once over on the quiet. She was wearing a plain black silk dress that had looked like a rag until she slipped it on, and then it hugged her ample curves in such a way it was almost obscene. But that was the whole point of it; she acted as if she had no idea of the way she looked, and she enjoyed the way the women reacted to her even more than the men. She knew they all envied her – two kids and she still looked better than any of them. She smiled tightly as her sister poured them both a glass of white wine.

'What do you think of Jonny's restaurant, Cynth? It's lovely, ain't it? Really upmarket.'

Cynthia nodded and forced herself to answer her sister. 'Beautiful, Celeste, really smart.'

Celeste knew that her sister was putting on an act, but she didn't mind; after all, this was preferable to her causing murders, and Cynthia was more than capable of doing just that. To Cynthia, a good fight was all in a day's work, and it was wearing at times. Celeste was a great believer in a quiet life. She could never understand her sister's need to make everything a drama. She had a mouth on her, and she knew how to say things so they were not just hurtful, but also seemed to hold a modicum of truth. That was how she justified what she said. She was a hard taskmaster – she could destroy a person's reputation with her insinuations.

She was vocal in her opinions on how kids should be brought up, and how women should act as mothers and wives, even though she never bothered with her own kids. She had an opinion on everything and everyone, yet she couldn't see herself clearly or how people perceived her. If Cynthia only knew how disliked she was by both women and men, she would be genuinely surprised – not that she had ever cared what women thought of her, Celeste knew. But she was aware that her sister assumed every man she encountered found her as fascinating as she herself did. She loved herself all right, and it was a shame that love didn't extend to the other people in her life. Maybe then she would be a happier person. Still, Celeste was shrewd enough to keep those thoughts to herself; she knew that everyone liked her because she didn't express the majority of the thoughts that came into her mind. She had learned very young that it brought you nothing but grief.

Cynthia, on the other hand, saw it as her God-given right to tell it like it is in a vicious and demeaning way. Cynthia didn't care if someone took it badly; she loved upsetting people, loved the negative vibe she created wherever she went. But it left a bad taste in everyone's mouth, and Cynthia was now basically *persona non grata* with just about everyone in her orbit.

'I wouldn't eat here if you weren't my sister, to be honest. It's a bit ostentatious for my liking.'

Celeste replied amiably, as always, 'Well, people seem to like it, Cynth, so I think we'll do all right.'

Celeste smiled as she spoke, and Cynthia felt the rage at her sister being the beneficiary of all this money and kudos. As the wife of a man of means she would always be afforded a great deal of respect, and it was that respect Cynthia wanted more than anything else. It was that respect that would have afforded her the life she felt she deserved, the life she should have demanded. But all she'd been given was boredom, a firm belief in the power of a good insurance policy and hope for an early death for the fucker she'd lumbered herself with. If it was left to her, James would have a massive heart attack and she could start all over again. Properly this time, and with the hindsight she wished she'd had at the outset.

'Well, Celeste, people always want what's new and different, although it soon wears thin. Still, in fairness, he's done a good job.'

The naked envy was evident and Celeste felt a deep sadness for this sister of hers who, if she would only relax and stop wanting the impossible, could enjoy her life like everyone else. Celeste smiled once more and suddenly hugged her sister to her. She said happily, 'Thanks, Cynth. If you like it then it must be good!'

Cynthia preened at the praise and, feeling magnanimous, said kindly, 'You're getting there, Celeste, so don't let it bother you too much.'

'I won't. Thanks for coming, mate, it means a lot.'

Cynthia was thrilled at how her sister saw her as the yardstick for her husband's new enterprises. It was another balm to her tortured soul. She felt she should be the one enjoying all this, not her younger sister. If only she had seen the truth of the situation years ago, she wouldn't have let him go, whatever the circumstances.

It never occurred to Cynthia that her sister was actually in the know where all that was concerned. Celeste was clever enough to keep that information close to her ample chest. Jonny had never said a word – he wouldn't, he was too nice a person – but she listened to gossip. It *had* bothered her that her sister had been there before her, but now she knew, deep inside, that Jonny loved her, *really* loved her, and she was woman enough to accept the truth of that. She only worried that her sister would find out that she actually knew the score, and thereby feel the humiliation of realising that Celeste knew and didn't care. With people like Cynthia you told them what they wanted to hear, because it was so much easier that way. If they ever saw themselves as everyone else did, it would be too much for them to take onboard. They lived in their own little worlds, it was what made them into the people they were.

Jonny Parker walked deliberately to the table that held his lovely Celeste, as always feeling the pull of her. She was worth fifty of any other woman in his world.

'You enjoying it, babe?'

'Oh, Jonny, it's wonderful.'

He looked into Cynthia's eyes as he said seriously, 'She chose all the décor, what a star, eh?' Tonight he wanted to get his first conversation with her out of the way, and he wanted it to be in front of his Celeste. He had nothing to hide and he wanted to make that plain.

Cynthia smirked as she answered him. 'That explains a lot, Jonny.'

The insult was clear and he knew it. More to the point Celeste knew it but, as ever, she chose to ignore the implication. Jonny loved her for her kindness and the fact that she only ever saw the good in everyone, including that ponce of a sister.

Cynthia looked at Jonny with her heavily made-up eyes; she could eat him as he was. Every time she saw him she could kick the fuck out of herself. What she could have had was evident in every move he made. She wanted him more than ever. If she had only known he would have achieve what he had, and in such a massive way, she would never have let him slip away from her. Unfortunately, she had believed he was no more than a fucking wanter, she had never believed he would be a getter. Just proved how wrong a girl could be. But Cynthia wasn't going to give up – she still believed she could change the future, and she wanted Jonny Parker back badly. She felt that if she fought hard enough she might just get him. After all, what was she up against? Her sister Celeste wasn't exactly a hard sell where she was concerned. She was a prat, and a prat of the first water.

Jonny watched the thoughts flicker over Cynthia's face and he could read her mind. He had no intentions of giving this vicious bitch what she wanted, what she expected. True he had felt something for her once, well, her body at least – that had been spectacular and what she had promised him and eventually delivered had been the best of the best. But it had not lasted. She had expected too much for far too little. She had been a great fuck, but even then that was only because he had been her first, and *that* had only happened because she had wanted what she *thought* he might have to offer. Cynthia was like a robot, she would fuck a table if it got her what she wanted. And, as luck would have it, he had realised that sooner rather than later, seen the seriousness of his dilemma. In fact, he now thanked fuck at every available opportunity for getting as far away from her as possible. That he had met and fallen in love with her younger sister he now saw as righteous retribution. It was as if Christ Himself was making amends.

'Come on, Celeste, let's go and meet our clientele.' This was said with enough arrogance for Cynthia to know that it was a barb aimed directly at her.

Cynthia watched as her sister walked away with the man of *her* dreams. If life was really fair it would have been her walking around like she was the dog's knob. Not her little sister. It was as if the world had gone mad, and somehow her little sister had been given the all clear, had been allowed to be somebody. Celeste, who was a no mark, a nothing, who was actually the recipient of her leftovers.

As they walked into the crowd, James came and sat beside her. He was full of it she could tell, loving the fact that they were a part of it all. Enjoying the whole experience. He made her sick. He was so grateful for nothing.

'What a great night, Cynth! And you know I'm a part owner now, don't you? If we play our cards right this could be the start of something big.'

He was made up, thrilled with the whole shebang, as her mother would say. But to her, he was no more than a pawn in what would eventually be her sister's pension. He had a minor stake in what would one day be a very lucrative business. After all, who stood to really gain from all these restaurants and pubs and nightclubs? Fucking Celeste, that's who. With *her* ninety-eight per cent share, as opposed to Cynthia's two per cent. Two per cent out of a hundred! And her husband thought that was something they should celebrate. While the rest would be Celeste's. Would be her sister's earn. Celeste, who couldn't fight her way out of a wet paper bag. Who was as much use as a fucking chocolate fireguard. Who, if the Filth came knocking, would not know how to answer their questions, wouldn't know how to protect her own. *She* would be the main earner. It was fucking outrageous, and here was *her* husband bragging because Jonny Parker had allowed him a tiny percentage. It was easier than giving him a proper wage! She knew that even if Mr fucking Know-It-All financial advisor didn't understand. It disgusted her that her husband, her James, could be pleased with *so little*. That he could allow Jonny Parker to insult him and still not see the reality of what was going on grieved her. He was obviously being offered a pittance – and she was convinced it was no more than that – and there was he, almost on his knees with gratitude and that, above all, was what really made her angry.

It should have been fifty-fifty at least. If her James had been given a stake he must have earned it, but Jonny Parker, being what he was, would never give anyone what they really deserved. It meant that her husband was being ripped off, another reason to make her feel hard done by. To make herself believe that they were being had over, were being taken for mugs. After all, her James was the person who kept these people *legitimate*. He was the money man, and knowing that made her feel much better about herself. It made her believe that all the hateful things she felt and she thought about had some kind of basis in fact.

As she looked around her, saw the people fawning over her sister and Jonny Parker, she was already wondering how she could bring them down and, more importantly, when.

She knew she could easily take them out without a second's thought if she opened her mouth to the right people, at the right time. She didn't know enough yet. But she would, eventually. She would bide her time and she would learn what she needed to know. And then bring them down she would, if it was the last thing she did in her life.

Chapter Nineteen

'Stop it, Cynth, we're earning a good wage. He gives us more than anyone else would.' Jimmy watched as his wife rolled her eyes dramatically and shook her head in abject disbelief.

'Huh, only you would say something that fucking stupid. *They* are the ones on a good earn, not us! They are making fucking mugs of us. You might be content with fuck-all, but I'm not.'

Jimmy looked at his wife and, for the first time in years, he knew he had to fight her, had to make her see sense. He knew that if he wasn't careful she would queer their pitch once and for all. This had been coming for a long time, and he knew he had to nip this latest tantrum in the bud. She was getting too outrageous even for him. If only she could understand their world like normal people, but he knew that was never going to be the case. So now he had to finally stop her in her tracks.

Jonny Parker had already said as much and, in fairness to him, he had a point. Cynthia was a liability, and he knew that better than anyone. She had a trap that was dangerous, she never knew when to *shut the fuck up*. He also knew that if he didn't sort her out then Jonny would have to make sure someone else did the dirty deed. They were all in it up to their necks, and he had no interest in being sidelined because his wife was a loose cannon.

'We are on a seriously good earn if only you would see that. We get a percentage of everything, Cynth. Where else would we get that, eh?'

Cynthia laughed derisively as if he was a complete fool, then shouted angrily, 'Oh, have a day off, James, will you, for fuck's sake! You're such a mug! We're not earning fuck-all in comparison to that lot, you're a fucking joke . . .'

'Don't, Cynth, not tonight, don't start now . . .'

Cynthia was shaking her head slowly and deliberately as if she was in the presence of the greatest moron since Benny off *Crossroads*. But Jimmy shook his own head then, and she suddenly realised that she was pushing him too far. Looking at him now, his face contorted with anger, his heavy body taut with rage, she saw that her constant criticism had finally hit home. He looked menacing and dangerous; after all, he had had a good teacher and she forgot at times how his life had changed. He was playing with the big boys now and picking up their bad habits. He was looking at her with distrust, with an anger she didn't know he possessed. He looked capable of anything, and she knew it was in her interests to leave it for a while. That she should temper her barbs, not make her anguish so plain.

After all these years she understood that she had finally pushed him too far. For the first time ever she actually felt afraid of the man she had married, felt the strength of him, saw the anger in his eyes. In fairness, she knew he was providing for them more than adequately, not that she would ever tell him that, of course. But that was not enough for her, would never be enough for her; she wanted what her sister had. The lion's share was all she would ever be content with, was all she would ever accept. Even she admitted to herself that at times her jealousy got out of hand, but she couldn't help the feeling that life was pissing on her from a great height. That seeing that mousy little sister of hers getting one over on her was all she could ever think about. She should have been the one to have achieved it; she had more brains and more savvy than Celeste would ever have. It was unfair, it was so unfair. Not that he would ever understand that, of course.

But as he looked at her now, disgust and dislike in his eyes, she knew they had somehow crossed a line. Never before had he fronted her up like this, it had always been the other way round. Something had given him some Dutch courage that he'd never previously had, and she had a suspicion what that something was.

'You, calling me stupid?' he said. 'You, who wouldn't know how to earn a crust if your life depended on it? *You*, who can't even bloody get yourself together long enough to take care of your own kids! *You* dare to question me, and what I do for this so-called family?'

She didn't answer him, didn't know how to.

'I fucking get up and go out twenty-four seven. And do you know what? *That's* why Jonny looks after us, you stupid mare. He offers me a taste, a bit of what he's doing and I am thrilled to take it. Because without him we'd be scratching a living, like we were before. So you had better wind your fucking neck in, shut your trap and be grateful for what you have got, instead of constantly harping on about what you think you *should* have. I've had it, Cynth. I've had you and your fucking wants till I'm dizzy.'

Cynthia looked at her husband in complete amazement; if someone had told her he would turn on her like this she would have laughed in their face. But she shouldn't have been so shocked; she had watched him getting too big for his boots, saw him blossoming as he became more and more successful in his chosen field. She had seen him become a man of renown almost, knew he was respected because he could hide a few quid from the tax man and the law. Now it seemed he thought he was better than her, the mother of his children. She also suspected that he had acquired a habit of sorts – a severe case of the sniffles. In fact he was often assaulted by a case of Colombian flu. She was pretty sure her goody-two-shoes husband was a bit of a cokehead.

Oh, how times changed.

'You can't talk to me like that! I won't swallow *you* of all people treating me like a fool.'

Jimmy laughed then and, pushing her backwards on to the sofa, he said seriously, '*Fuck you*, Cynth, do I look like I care what you think these days? I'm over you and your viciousness. You bring my kids back home or you can fuck off. I've had you up to my eyebrows. You're a vindictive cunt, and a bully. But I ain't swallowing no more, so you better sort yourself out.'

Jimmy couldn't believe what he had just said, let alone that it was to Cynthia! All the things he had dreamt of saying he had finally said. He knew it was because he had partaken of a few lines of cocaine. Lately he had found that he liked the way it made him feel. He didn't care what anyone thought of him after a few lines, and he felt invincible. He felt that he could do no wrong. He also knew that if Jonny Parker found out about it he would go ballistic. Jonny didn't like drugs, especially not in his personal circle of friends; he might sell them of course, and in large quantities, but that was just business as far as he was concerned. As long as Jonny didn't know about his newfound habit, Jimmy knew he was OK. He also knew that his wife, who he still loved after everything, was a woman who needed a serious slap. And, if she wasn't careful, the chances were she would get just that. He had had enough, in more ways than one.

Cynthia realised that it was not in her interest to pursue this conversation, and her instincts were telling her it was much better to retreat on this occasion. But she knew that if her husband had access to drugs – and he had to be on drugs otherwise he would never have dared to say the things he had – it was something she could use against him in the future. Oh, he was on the old Persian rugs all right. And he had been on them for a while. That had to be something to do with Jonny Parker and, as such, she knew that it could only be to her benefit in the long run. She would dig and dig until she found the truth, and then she would use the knowledge to her advantage. She had access to James's clothes and his wallet. Sometimes it was so easy, all you had to do was sit back and wait. Eventually it just came to you, without any real graft.

Her sister thought that her life was so fucking special, so fucking great. Well, Cynthia could end it with a phone call. One call and it would be over. That knowledge alone made her feel so good.

Chapter Twenty

'Well? What's happening then?'

Mary Callahan was annoyed. She hated this weekly argument – Cynthia acting like she had arranged to take the children out for the afternoon when everyone knew that was never going to happen. Cynthia never had the kids for more than a day, and even then it was as if she was doing them a favour in some way. She couldn't cope with both her children for more than a couple of hours anyway. She palmed them off on her parents with a relief that was almost tangible.

But today Cynthia seemed determined to cause some kind of aggravation, it seemed as if she had an agenda, and it was not the first time she had acted this way in the last few weeks. It bothered her mother. She knew this daughter of hers better than anyone else. In many ways she hated her daughter if truth be told. She knew that Cynthia was capable of great hate, and great treachery. She also knew that Cynthia was not averse to using her children to get what she wanted. She had been doing that since they had been born. But lately she wouldn't trust her daughter with anything – she knew that there was a hidden agenda, there was *always* some kind of hidden agenda with Cynthia. This time she knew exactly what that was.

'Look, Mum, if you don't want them, I'll take them back home with me . . .'

Mary was already holding her grandson in her arms, and her

granddaughter was clasping her around her legs. She knew she was never going to let them leave now.

'I never said that, Cynth, did I? But you seem like *you* don't want to leave them.'

Cynthia sighed heavily, rolling her large blue eyes, and Mary Callahan saw just how lovely her elder daughter really was. And it hurt her, knowing that this beautiful girl had no real care for anyone in the world, least of all her two children. And they needed her. James Junior had developed a bit of a temper lately. Every time Cynthia left the kids behind he threw a tantrum.

'Oh, Mum, I'm worried that's all, I know they are safe with *you*.'

Mary didn't react to her daughter's words, but she could hear the drama in them. Instead she said to her granddaughter, 'Come on, you, let's go and see Granddad.'

Cynthia looked at her mother and said seriously, 'Is that it, Mum? Are you not going to listen to what I've got to say?'

Mary looked into her daughter's eyes and said quietly, but seriously, and everything she really thought about her elder daughter was there for anyone to hear, 'No, Cynth, I'm not, and neither is your father or anyone else. The Old Bill has told Jonny about your little chat, and they have decided to overlook it. But I'm warning you now, girl, you've crossed the line. You want to be a grass you do it on your own because none of us are even remotely interested. In fact, if you were anyone else you'd be dead. So you listen carefully, and you listen good. You've gone too far this time. I wouldn't start celebrating just yet, if you get my drift.'

Cynthia walked from the house without another word. For the first time ever, she didn't know how to react. She knew she had been rumbled and she was frightened – she knew she had gone too far. Her hate had caused this situation. She had hoped Jonny and his cronies would all be taken away, so she never had to look at them again. She had tried to bring them all down, had tried to make them all see how vulnerable they really were. But instead she had found out how deeply entrenched they were with the police, and now she finally understood how dangerous a position she was in. She had wanted to take them out, her husband included – *especially* her husband if truth be told – but now she knew she had no chance of making that happen. They were involved in some deep shit, and she knew exactly how deep that shit was. So she'd told the Filth all she knew – for a price, of course. Instead *they* had served her up, the *Filth* had served her up like a fucking sacrifice. She would never get over the fact that the people who should have been hanging on her every word, who had been given the information they'd need to bring down some serious crooks, had turned it all around and had left her hanging in the wind, at the mercy of the very people she had tried to bring down.

She was now an acknowledged grass, a woman who would never be trusted again. Someone who would be a dead body if her sister had not been Jonny Parker's other half. She knew that she was tainted, knew that she would have to really prove herself at some point and, worst of all, she knew that she had brought this on herself. She was a jealous, vindictive bitch. She knew that better than anyone. But everyone around her knew that too. And that really irked her.

She felt sick with apprehension and she realised that feeling would never leave her.

Chapter Twenty-One

'You've asked for it, Cynth, all of it. You would have taken us all out – even me. Or should that be *especially* me?'

Jimmy Tailor had long ceased to be in awe of his lovely wife's tongue. Since she had brought the Filth breathing down all their necks, he had been decidedly rude where she was concerned, and with what he thought was good cause.

Cynthia put on her best, please-why-don't-you-believe-me voice as she said sadly, 'Look, James, I believed at the time I was doing it for the best. You were taking cocaine like it was going out of fashion! I was worried about you . . .' Cynthia was still trying to prove herself a year later, but she wasn't making any kind of inroad and they both knew it. 'I just want what's best for my family. I know you don't see it that way, none of you see it that way . . .'

'Oh, change the record, Cynth! Like you ever cared about me, or anyone come to that.'

Jimmy was fed up with her. He was already putting on his jacket, and she knew he would be out of the house having a good time while she sat here alone wishing she could be a part of it all once more. She was desperate to be a part of it, if she was really honest with herself. She needed some serious brownie points to get herself back in with the big boys.

'I was frightened for you, James, whatever you might think . . .'

Jimmy rolled his eyes in annoyance. 'You nearly fucked us all up. You know what you did and you also know if it wasn't for your sister you would be dead.'

Cynthia had tried to get the sympathy vote from her husband, but it wasn't working. In the last year she had been treated as a pariah – in fact she had hardly left the house. Watching her back had become part of her daily routine – even Celeste had given her the cold shoulder. The worst of it was she missed her sister. She actually physically missed her. Who'd have predicted that? When all was said and done, Celeste had always been there for her, and it had taken a year of being blacklisted to make Cynthia realise that.

In that year, her sister and her husband had become the local celebrities, always in the local papers, opening a new boxing gym, or attending a charity auction. They were like the poor man's Burton and Taylor. Cynthia understood that if she had not been so vindictive, she would still have been a part of that. Would still have had some kind of a real life. She missed the social aspect of it all, missed the nights out, the reflected glory of being Celeste's sister. If only she had understood then how lucky she had been.

To compound all that, James was doing really well. They were living better than ever before, and she knew that she was walking a thin line with him. She still didn't understand why he had never left her – even she wouldn't have blamed him if he had.

It never occurred to her that he might actually love her, care for her as the mother of his children and as his wife. All she saw was that James was loving his new role in the family set-up. He was the main breadwinner, but he was also finally the head of his own household, as hard as that was for her to admit. He came and went as he pleased now.

Cynthia couldn't kick up too much fuss – she needed him these days, far more than she had ever thought possible. In fact, it was outrageous just how much she now needed him. She had played a hand that she had believed was a winner only to find out it was the opposite. The Old Bill had listened to her and then served her up without a second's thought for her welfare. She should have guessed that Jonny would have them in his pocket; he was too shrewd not to.

If Cynthia had achieved her objective, her sister's husband would be banged up now for the duration, and she would have felt a distinct satisfaction about that. She would have watched them fall, and from a fucking great height at that. Instead, she had inadvertently sabotaged any kind of life that could have come her way. She had, in effect, chewed her own foot off, because she was paying a terrible price for her treachery.

Celeste, in fairness, *wanted* her to have nice things, *wanted* her sister to have money in her bin and Celeste, most of all, wanted her to be content. As if she could have ever accepted that, especially coming from her of all people! But now, though, Cynthia knew she had to make some kind of amends, she had to prove herself worthy in some way. And she would do just that. She had to put herself on the line, make sure she was seen as a person of worth – not to the Filth, but to her sister and her sister's husband.

It was all that was left to her.

Chapter Twenty-Two

'Have a guess who I just saw?'

Jack Callahan shook his head, uninterested in his wife's yammering.

'Shaw Taylor, that's who.'

Shaw Taylor was the star of a programme called *Police 5* from the early sixties, where he would ask the public nicely to grass up various members of their families or their communities. Shaw Taylor was also the nickname they'd given Cynthia since she had caused all the trouble a year before. If she knew she would be mortified.

'Was she on her way here?'

''Course not, she would have been here by now, stupid. She was going into the train station, so I assume she's going up west.'

Jack Callahan didn't answer; they all knew she didn't shop or go anywhere local any more. Her name was a byword for treachery and so it should be. Every time he thought of what she had done he felt a murderous rage that he had fathered her. If she wasn't so like his own mother in looks he might have accused his wife of all sorts after his daughter had grassed everyone within her orbit. That she was capable of something so fucking heinous, so disgusting . . . He shook his head once more in absolute disbelief.

'Poor old Celeste. She still feels guilty about it – after everything she still tries to make excuses for her sister.'

Jack Callahan didn't even bother to reply; Cynthia had been nothing but trouble since she could open that big painted trap of hers. He didn't want her anywhere near him now. As long as she left the kids here regular like, he couldn't give a toss whether he ever saw her again. Good job she didn't know what was going on now, or they'd all be up shit street. His son-in-law Jonny was coining it in, and sailing a bit too close to the edge, even by his standards. Truth be told, even Jack was getting a bit shirty at the lad's audacity. But Jonny seemed to know what he was doing. He had a knack for skulduggery, and he had the sense to temper it with legitimate enterprises, so he could at least explain where the houses and cars came from. But sneaking over to South London was a daring little escapade, and it could cause nothing but grief to everyone concerned. Not that anyone involved seemed to be bothered about that. It was as if the old standards had died, and anyone who still believed in them was classed as a dinosaur.

Well, maybe Jack *was* a dinosaur, but he felt that the old guard, with their boundaries and their guidelines, had it right. You can't go around taking other people's earns without a fight, no matter who you were. It was the principle of the thing. He had a bad feeling about these new premises. The men on the receiving end of Jonny's new enterprises would not take it lightly, he knew that much.

Jonny Parker was a clever boy, and Jack thought the world of him, but he believed he had crossed one too many lines with this latest rigmarole. Bloody drugs, they caused no end of trouble, whether it was for the dealer or the buyer. Look at Jimmy, he was snorting up that white powder like his life depended on it. Although living with that fucking daughter of his, he could feel sorry for him in many ways. But drugs were drugs, and Jack didn't like them, and he didn't like the mayhem they caused for all concerned. But he would keep his own counsel for now and see what occurred. The problem was, his

Celeste was in the firing line if it went tits up, and that was what was really worrying him.

In Jack's day, there was honour among thieves, as much as that sounded like a contradiction in terms. Not any more though – now it was every man for themselves. And Jonny Parker wanted it *all* for himself, every pavement, and every earn.

It was nothing more than a recipe for disaster.

Chapter Twenty-Three

Jonny Parker was not as worried as he probably should have been, and that fact pleased him no end. He was taking a big chance and he knew it; he was putting his life on the line. But if he didn't do this, he knew he would regret it one day. He had always gone with his instincts and they, so far, had never let him down. He could only hope that this was another one of his more lucrative ideas.

His instincts now were telling him the time was right. It worked on paper, admittedly, but paper never allowed for the reactions of the people involved. He was *always* wary of the reactions to his more outrageous business enterprises. But, where this one was concerned, he would do murder if necessary, because he was determined to see this one through to the very end.

He was a much harder fuck than people realised. But after this next coup – and it was a very audacious and dangerous scam – his real intentions and his real personality would be known to all and sundry. He had bided his time, and this was the moment he had been working towards. If he was honest, he was still a bit nervous about it but, as far as he was concerned, that nervousness was all to the good. It would ensure he didn't take anything for granted. Didn't let his guard down. It was when people became too sure of themselves that they tended to make mistakes, and he had no intention of fucking this one up.

'You all right, Jonny?'

Celeste looked worried, and he forced a smile of nonchalance on to his face.

'I'm fine, sweetheart, just thinking that's all.'

Celeste grinned then. 'You're always thinking! What's on your mind, mate?'

He cupped her face in his hand, amazed at the force of the love he felt for this woman. 'Nothing for you to worry about. Now are you sure you'll be all right tonight? I won't be out longer than necessary, I promise.'

'Stay as long as you want. I'm going round me mum's anyway – she's got the kids.'

Jonny grimaced and the look made her grin again.

'She's always got the fucking kids!'

Celeste was serious suddenly. 'Not any more. Be fair, Jonny, she doesn't have them half as much as she used to.'

It amazed him how this woman – because she was a woman when all was said and done, despite her childishness and her naivety – could still stick up for that sorry excuse of a sister. But, as his old mum always insisted, blood was thicker than water. Bollocks of course, but women seemed to think it was a valid excuse for their family's treachery and skulduggery. Personally, he thought her sister should be six feet underneath a golf course somewhere. But that was only his opinion and, where her piece of shit of a sister was concerned, his wife was not going to listen to any arguments he might put forward, no matter how valid they may be.

'I'll retreat on this occasion, darlin', because I don't want to row about it. She ain't worth rowing about, is she?'

Celeste shook her head, but he knew she was upset.

'So I'll see you later then, eh?' He kissed her and, as always, she responded to his embrace with all her being.

'I'll hold you to that!'

When the door shut behind him, Celeste sat down and lit a cigarette from her secret stash. Jonny hated her smoking, but she needed it to calm her nerves. She knew something big was going down tonight, and she feared in her heart that it was something that could go very, very wrong. She trusted Jonny, but she knew he was taking some big risks these days – at least as far as her dad was concerned he was, and her dad wasn't a spinner. If *he* was worried, there was something to worry about. Her dad might not be the sharpest knife in the drawer, but he heard anything that was worth anything, and her husband should listen to him now and again. In fact, he ought to understand that he *should* listen to the truth sometimes even if he wasn't in the mood for hearing it. She felt personally that it was always worth a quick listen to the local gossip. Nine times out of ten, they knew more than the Filth ever would and even more than the people involved in a scam. Gossip was a serious thing where they came from; it was the forerunner to a serious nicking. If it was known outside their workforce, it was dangerous to everyone involved. It meant that it wasn't as secret as they all assumed. In fact, it meant it was common knowledge, in the public domain, and that meant that someone in his personal circle had a big mouth and that big mouth could cause more fights than John Wayne. She couldn't talk to her husband about any of this because he saw local gossip as nothing more than fabrication, stupidity and idiocy. Those being his exact words.

Celeste loved her husband more than life itself, but she knew he wasn't exactly kosher. In truth, she knew a lot more than he gave her credit for. She also understood what he was capable of, and that frightened her. Not for herself – he would never hurt her, of that she was sure. But he was capable of murder, she had no doubt about that at all.

She smoked the cigarette with shaking hands. Tonight was going to be a long one.

Chapter Twenty-Four

Jonny Parker was excited, but the excitement was tinged with worry. He might be a Face to be reckoned with, but he knew he was dealing with people who would never give him a second chance if he didn't achieve his goal straight off. And the goal was to get what they had; he wanted every bit of it. He was legitimate enough to pass off his affluent lifestyle as above board. He also had a cache of fall guys who worked for him, unaware that if it went pear-shaped they would be the ones in the frame. That was the brainchild of his dear brother-in-law who, if it ever did go off, would be the first one nabbed by Lily Law. Jonny had enough safety features in place to keep himself out of stir. What he *didn't* have, at least not one hundred per cent, was the guarantee that he wouldn't be taken out before he achieved the more outrageous of his goals. But he was a planner and he was a plodder in many respects; he waited and he watched, and he thought through his business moves with precision. Still, you always had to allow for eventualities, such as the people you were dealing with being a bit fucked off that you were intending to wipe them out. That tended to give people the raging hump.

Jonny was respected for doing the majority of his dirty works himself; that was so people knew what they were dealing with. He never left a trail though, he was far too shrewd for that. But tonight was about some serious money, and meant having to cross some serious people. He was confident he could make the transition from supplier to managing director with no real trouble. If he took out the main men, he was laughing all the way to the bank.

It was the taking them out that was the tricky thing. Taking them out and making sure the people who worked for them understood the economics of the deal. After all, his education had taught him that as long as people earned, they would happily work for whoever provided that earn. They lived in a Thatcherite society; you give me a good wage, and I'll swallow my knob and work for you instead. It was the way things worked now. It wasn't the sixties any more, and the sooner people realised that, the better off they would all be. It was like living in a fucking bubble; the old values were all right in their day, but this was the eighties, and anyone with a sawn-off and a few quid could walk in anywhere and get a decent hearing. The days of gentlemen villains was long gone; they were banged up, and wouldn't see the light of day until the fucking Jews returned to Zion, that's how remote their release dates were. They had been put away for the duration, judges had taken it upon themselves to rid the country of some of its best earners. Legal earners at that; for all their skulduggery they had been proper earners as well – good, decent taxpayers. None of them had ever signed on the dole or asked for a fucking handout.

It was a new world, with a whole new set of rules and regulations; the old guard were gone and forgotten. This was really about the survival of the fittest, and Jonny Parker knew he was fitter than most. He was going to play them all at their own game, and they would understand that this was not a dress rehearsal, this was the real thing.

He had planned it down to the last detail, and all he had to do now was make sure it was executed with the minimum of fuss and the maximum of terror. Fear was the best way to ensure the complete devotion of everyone concerned. Fear had its own rewards – that cunt of a sister-in-law had learned that the hard way. Without realising it she had taught him a good lesson: it was the people nearest you who were the real danger. It was something he would never forget. The shock of her revelations to the Filth had made him take a step back and look at his workforce and their relatives very closely. In her own way, that two-faced ponce Cynthia had shown him the chinks in his armour. He had understood then just how easy it was for outsiders to know far too much about his businesses.

Not any more, though. It was now common knowledge that anyone who talked outside of their working circle would be treated with the response that such treachery deserved. Wives and girlfriends were now treated as scornfully as the Filth, were seen to be as dangerous as the law courts. They were not party to anything even remotely pertaining to the business of their husbands or partners. It was working out wonderfully. Jonny told his wife, the love of his life, fuck-all as well. She was a great girl but, like every woman, the less she knew the better.

Tonight he would be well and truly blooded; he was going to make his mark once and for all. He didn't want to do this because it would be bloody and callous and it would become legend. He *needed* to do it because once he had, no one would be in any doubt who was the main earner in the Smoke. Now it was time. Every businessman comes to a crossroads, where they decide what route they'll take – either the easy option (always the less lucrative), or the hard option, where they have to fight for what they really want. Well, he was going to fight, and fight with everything he had. He was going to make sure that no one, no one at all, would be left to queer his otherwise perfect pitch.

This was make or break time, and he was determined to break them, little by little, bit by bit.

Chapter Twenty-Five

Joseph Makabele was a large Rastafarian, who had not been near Jamaica even once in his long and eventful life. He was actually a Nigerian, who knew that his heritage would not help him in any way, shape or form. Not in the world of drug-dealing anyway. He knew the real Jamaicans were suspect about him, and that the white boys were even more so. Mainly because they had gone to school with the Jamaicans and the Tobagonians, and every other Caribbean boy in the neighbourhood; he had never gone to school with anyone who was worth anything. He looked the part and he talked the part, but he didn't have the creds.

Joseph knew that meant he would not get the loyalty he needed; people worked for him, but they didn't really trust him. He offered a good wage, but nothing more, because no one knew him years ago and, in London, unless you were able to hark back at least three generations, you were no one.

He understood that now, he also understood that if he didn't win tonight with Jonny Parker, local hero, and all round likeable cunt, he was finished. But he had allowed for something like this, and he was sure he had enough get-out clauses to last him at least one lifetime. Joseph was handsome, he was charismatic, and he could supply enough drugs to keep the whole of the South East high until the next millennium, and at half the usual going price. But he also knew that being the outsider would always be his weak spot.

People in the south of England had a blind spot, and that was for others of their ilk. If Joseph had been born and bred here, he knew he would be all right. But he wasn't, and he also knew that his pretending to be a Jamaican Rasta meant nothing to the people he had to deal with tonight. Jonny Parker was going to challenge him and that, in itself, was a serious challenge by anyone's standards.

Joseph had seen this coming for a long time, but he had hoped, like many before him, that a good earn and good fringe benefits would see him safe. He had played the Rasta man, but it was an act and, deep inside, he was aware that everyone who worked for him knew it.

He was frightened. Tonight was the real deal, and how he reacted to it all would affect the rest of his life. But he was ready for the fight. He had surrounded himself with the best of the best, paid them more than they were worth, and now he had to hope that that would be enough.

He shrugged. He was letting the demons get the better of him, as his old grandma used to say. He wondered wistfully if she was still alive. He had been brought over to England by his mother, who had swiftly abandoned him and, eventually, he had ended up a Barnardo's boy. Another reason he wasn't trusted; after all, if your own family didn't want you . . . Another East-End saying that he had to admit had the ring of truth to it.

He mentally shook himself. He had got this far, and he had the nous and the guts to get wherever he wanted to be. He had told himself that all his life, and it had worked up to now. He reassured himself that he had the right men beside him, and that they were paid enough to ensure their loyalty. That had to mean something. They knew as well as he did that Jonny Parker was not really meeting him to arrange a large shipment of drugs – he was meeting him to tell him that from now on his services would no longer be required. Well, Jonny Parker had a big shock coming to him, and in a way he was sorry about that, because he liked Jonny Parker, he was a nice bloke.

Joseph got into the back of his large black BMW. For protection he had a driver and two outriders, one of whom was his right-hand man, Linford Fargas, who had been his number two for over three years now and was the nearest he had to a real friend. The men were well versed in what they had to do this night, and were well armed.

'Shall I go straight to the depot?'

Joseph nodded almost imperceptibly. 'Is everything arranged?'

The driver nodded, even the back of his head had an arrogant look to it. Like him, the man was black, dreadlocked, and spoiling for a fight with the white boys. Joseph felt himself relax. He leant forward and pulled a large machete from under the driver's seat; it would take off a hand or a foot easily, the perfect weapon for incapacitating the enemy. It could also take a man's head off his shoulders if the blow was powerful enough. A machete was the weapon of choice for most of the Yardies except, in England, unlike Jamaica where it was classed as a work tool like a screwdriver or a pair of pliers, it was illegal to walk along the road with them.

'You nervous, Joseph?' asked Linford.

'Not at all. I feel good about it all. This was needed, even I saw that.'

Linford nodded sagely.

'Besides, I'm gonna take that fucker out.'

The driver then laughed heartily, saying loudly, 'A-fucking-men to that! You take the fucker out, boss.'

That caused them to start laughing, but they were all aware it was a nervous laughter. It occurred to Joseph that his men were even more nervous than he was, and he knew he had no choice but to show a true hand to them tonight. Then maybe, just maybe, it might go some way to making them see him as one of them after all. The thought pleased him, and he was glad now that this was happening; it might be just the thing he needed to ensure his place in this London black boy society. All of the men were well versed in the art of fighting, both with their fists and with weapons. And none of them were in the least frightened of guns – they'd been around them for the best part of their lives.

Joseph realised he had been worrying about nothing – in fact he could already taste his victory as he drove into his depot in Croydon. This was where he kept the majority of his arms, this was where he was safest, because only a few people knew he even owned it. That was another thing; he liked to keep his private dealings private, and that could only hold him in good stead at times like these. Only four people knew about this depot, and they were all in this car.

Linford jumped out and opened the gates, unlocking the huge padlock. Joseph looked around the yard and smiled grimly at its sameness. As they drove in, he saw Linford opening the door of the Portakabin that served as his offices. He had a good bottle of Irish whiskey in there, and he was going to pour himself a large glass before setting off for the festivities.

There was still two hours to the deadline, to the meeting with Jonny Parker that would determine the rest of his life. As he put his foot out of the car, it suddenly occurred to him that neither of his other men had moved, but it was only when he felt a boot shove him in the back and saw the dirt floor of the yard coming up to meet him that he realised something was amiss.

Then Jonny Parker was standing over him with a machete that made his own look like a penknife.

'Sorry, Joe, but you didn't honestly think I was going to negotiate, did you?'

The first blow took off the top of Joseph's head; the other blows were entirely unnecessary, but the brutality of the attack was what made the statement for Jonny Parker. When word got out about Joseph's demise, and get out it would, he would be seen in a new and entirely different light, and that is exactly what this whole exercise was about.

Linford Fargas watched the events with a nonchalant air; he prided himself on always backing the winning pony. Truth be told, poor old Joseph had never had a chance. He wasn't fish nor fowl. Now he was nothing.

Linford went inside the Portakabin and picked up his twenty grand – not bad for a night's work. If Joseph had used his considerable loaf and paid out over the odds for his loyalty, he might have been in with a chance tonight.

Now, though, Jonny Parker was king of the hill, and there would be no one capable of stopping him for a good few years. It would take that long for a new little crew to grow and develop, but he had a hunch that Jonny P, as he was now known, would still be a match for them. Jonny had what they called back in Jamaica the devil's want, and he wanted it all. Well, he was welcome to it, and the problems that came with it. Because this first hurdle might be over but he now had to deal with Kevin Bryant, never a man to cross lightly.

But time would tell; by tomorrow night one, or all of them, would be dead. That was Linford's opinion anyway.

Chapter Twenty-Six

Kevin Bryant heard the news of his business partner's untimely demise with his usual closed features. His expressionless face was his trademark in his world. He never looked angry, rarely looked pleased and had never in living memory laughed out loud at anything. Hence his nickname, Kevin 'No Face' Bryant. He liked the moniker, felt it put him above most of his contemporaries. His countenance, coupled with the fact he never spoke unless it was extremely necessary, only added to his criminal mystique.

His wife Sojin, a thirty-something living doll, told all and sundry that he was a different person at home with her and the kids, that he never stopped talking, but no one actually believed her, much to her chagrin. They thought Sojin was with him because of *who* he was; it never occurred to anyone that she might actually see a different side to him than everyone else. It grieved her that no one saw the ebullient, funny man she loved and adored, because adore him she did. From his size twelve feet, to his balding, endearingly ugly, head.

Kevin's second-in-command, a tall, frighteningly skinny man called Bertie Warner, was trying desperately to gauge his boss's reaction to the outrageous news that Joseph Makabele had been hacked to death by Jonny Parker and the Anthill Mob from Brixton.

'Do you hear me, Kev? They fucking nutted him, he was

chopped up like a fucking Friday night fish! Do you not have any interest in what the fuck I am telling you?'

Shrugging disinterestedly, Kevin said quietly, 'He's dead then?'

'Hello, earth to fucking Kevin! He is dead as a fucking dodo! For fuck's sake, *Monty Python*'s parrot has more life in it than him! He's a human fucking paper chase. Get onboard, for fuck's sake!'

Sometimes Kevin's attitude could be severely aggravating, and this was one of those times. Their main supplier was now scattered to all corners of the country, loaded into bin bags and dumped like a fucking treasure hunt for the Old Bill, and here was Kevin unconcerned and, to add insult to injury, not even remotely disgruntled about it.

'He had our protection, Kev, we fucking owe him, and everyone else who thinks we are watching their fucking backs.'

Bertie was realising how this would look to outsiders; everyone, including that cunt Jonny P, knew that Makabele worked ostensibly for them – it was his ticket to the big time. That meant they had to be *seen* to be doing something about it – otherwise they could kiss goodbye to their stranglehold on South London, that much was a fucking definite.

Kevin shrugged nonchalantly once more. 'And?'

It wasn't a question, it wasn't anything. It was annoying that's what it was. 'And! Fucking "and"? Is that all you've got to fucking say? We are fucking being mugged off like a pair of prize cunts, and all you can say is fucking *and*!'

But Kevin Bryant wasn't listening to his friend any more; he was already planning his next step, and he knew better than anyone that he had to box very clever. If Jonny P had made it this far then he was armed and extremely dangerous. Obviously he was being protected, and he would have made sure that this little exercise was going to work out in his favour. Anger was a fruitless exercise – not that Bertie would see it that way, of course. What was needed now was a long, hard, sensible *think*, and he wasn't going to be able to do that with Bertie wittering on like a fucking old fishwife.

'Bertie.'

'What!'

'Shut the fuck up.'

Bertie did as requested, but he was seething inside. If Jonny Parker was allowed a walk on this kind of calumny then the London they knew and loved would be his for the taking. This was a direct affront to them and everything they had achieved, and if Kevin didn't strike quickly it would be their turn for the machetes next. Fucking machetes! What was wrong with a common or garden sawn-off? Were these people fucking animals or what? Bertie shook his head in utter disbelief at the skulduggery of some people.

Unlike Bertie, Kevin Bryant knew exactly why the man had been taken out with machetes. This was a statement as well as a killing. It was telling him and everyone else that Jonny P had the black vote of confidence. That meant Brixton, Tulse Hill, Norwood, et al, were happy to be on his payroll. He was carving up the city and, in fairness to him, he was doing it very well. Credit where credit was due, he had worked a fucking blinder, and Kevin Bryant admired a shrewd business head. So few Faces possessed one; most were daydreamers who never saw the big picture, were shocked and outraged when they were taken out by a more superior intelligence. Anyone could get a decent earn – it was keeping the fucker that took the time and the trouble. A good earn was like an unfaithful wife; you loved them, you fucked them, but you kept watch on them twenty-four seven. Otherwise they fucked you over in more ways than one.

But Kevin Bryant wasn't finished yet; he still a few miles to go on his clock, and when he retaliated, he would retaliate big time. But it had to be perfect, it had to be well planned, it had to be executed with the minimum of fuss and the maximum of aggravation. He could put on a show as well as the next man, and he was determined to do just that.

Chapter Twenty-Seven

Jonny P was euphoric. He had taken out Joseph without any real resistance at all. But that was all well and good – now he had to either take out Bryant completely, or try to negotiate some friendly terms with him, whatever seemed the most viable option.

Personally, he felt it was best to take the man out. Kevin was a loose cannon. He was a hard fuck in his own way, and that was to be taken into consideration. No one *ever* knew what Kevin Bryant was thinking, so it was difficult to negotiate with him. No one played cards with him any more either, he had a legendary poker face. Years ago, Jonny had watched Kevin take a twenty-grand pot on a ten high. He had also been playing those cards with some very naughty boys, the very same bad boys they had both overtaken on their quest for the pavements of their youth.

It was important to run your own neighbourhood. It meant a loyalty that was almost guaranteed, providing, of course, you looked after your own, and they had both done just that. But, whereas Jonny was a likeable fellow, Kevin Bryant wasn't. Respected, yes, but liked? That was a different kettle of fish altogether. No one approached Kevin, he wasn't that kind of bloke, whereas Jonny was accosted wherever he went. He always made sure people had a few quid in their bins, and was known for paying for the endless rounds of drinks his hangers-on and supporters expected. He mediated between warring factions, and was known to give out rough justice to the less salubrious of his neighbours – burglars, nonces, liars and the like. He was a hard taskmaster with his workforce, but paid them well, and they understood he would not, under any circumstances, tolerate bullying, thieving off him or their own and, most importantly of all, he would not countenance slackness in either word or deed. He paid well, and expected the best they could offer him, and he saw to it that he got just that.

But this latest deal he was going after was as audacious as it was dangerous. It could either bring him untold riches, and untold power, or it could mean he was on his last few hours on God's good earth.

Jonny took a deep breath and exhaled slowly; he had read somewhere that it calmed the nerves and, despite appearances, he was actually as nervous as fuck. He looked up as his new best friend and confidant on this latest scam, Linford, walked into the small office quietly.

'Any news?'

'Not a fucking murmur anywhere on the pavements. News has got round, of course – you're the hero of the hour. No one liked Joseph anyway. But nothing yet from Kevin Bryant and nothing from his mouthpiece Bertie.'

So they were scheming, and that was to be expected. Jonny nodded and sipped at his whiskey. They had paid off the best part of Bryant's workforce, guaranteed them a bigger and better earn and, more to the point, they had put the fear of Christ up half of London with their antics this night. He had done all that could be done.

He could hear the riotous laughter coming from the pub he owned on the Mile End Road. He was surrounded by his best workmen and his most trusted friends. They were tooled up and ready for anything. All he could do now was wait, and he had a feeling on him that the wait was going to be a short one.

Kevin Bryant was a lot of things, but a mug wasn't one of them.

Chapter Twenty-Eight

Bertie was fast getting the raging hump.

Kevin was so laid back he might as well be in a fucking coma for all the good he was doing at this moment in time. Bertie's old woman had made more noise in the sack and that was saying something. His Deirdre was a lovely girl, an exemplary mother, and an all-round decent bird, but she wasn't exactly what you'd call a live-wire in the fuck department.

Bertie, on the other hand, was a doer by nature; if anyone fucked him over, he done them, simple as that. It was a credo he had lived by and which had kept him alive and kicking this long in a very dangerous game. All his instincts were telling him to go after Jonny P mob-handed, guns blazing, pickaxes swinging, and maybe even a few fucking machetes thrown into the mix just for the irony factor. And that was exactly what he was going to suggest to Kevin. He couldn't sit here like a fucking Victorian mistress any longer. It was, in effect, doing his head in.

Bertie liked Kevin; he probably knew him better than anyone else, and he respected him, and saw his good points as well as the bad. But this fucking silence was deafening; he could almost hear his own brain turning over, and at every little noise he expected to be overrun by a mob wielding giant machetes.

Kevin was watching Bertie placidly; he knew exactly what was going through his mind and, in a way, he could sympathise with him. Bertie didn't have the patience of a three year old, and when a bit of chastising needed doing he was the man to call on.

Unfortunately, he had the brains of a fucking gnat and, whereas Kevin had never been that loquacious, Bertie could talk for England. He never shut his fucking trap from the minute he got up till the moment he fell into a fitful sleep. Kevin would like to bet he was still talking even then.

'Get your coat.' As he spoke he stood up and his considerable bulk seemed to fill the small room to capacity.

Bertie smiled, this was more like it!

In the small outer office of his scrap-metal yard, Kevin opened the arms safe and, taking out a semi-automatic he had purchased from an old acquaintance, he proceeded to arm himself to the hilt.

'Shall I call the boys?' The excitement was already overflowing in Bertie's voice. He was thrilled at this turn of events; there was nothing he liked more than a good tear-up, a serious fucking straightener was always something to be enjoyed. Violence as far as he concerned solved *everything*, there was nothing like a good fucking tear-up to sort out the men from the wannabes.

Kevin shook his head. 'Not yet. Make a cup of tea.'

Chapter Twenty-Nine

Jonny was half-pissed and he was annoyed with himself because of it. But it had been a very strange night so far, and he knew that if his calculations were correct it could only get fucking worse. Much worse. He glanced at his watch – it was twenty past one and no news yet. But there was plenty of time; he would sit and he would wait. He could feel the sweat trickling down his back, and he wondered at how this night would eventually pan out.

Linford had poured himself a large brandy, and he downed it in one gulp. 'I needed that, bwoy,' he said reverting to his Jamaican patois.

Jonny grinned. 'You're about as Jamaican as I am fucking Irish.'

Linford laughed happily, he knew the truth of that statement. 'I left Jamaica as a baby. My mother came here looking for me father – she still hasn't found the bastard. But I grew up in a Jamaican household and, believe me, that's as good as being brought up in the home country. A bit like the Irish, eh?'

They laughed together, pleased that the change of topic meant that they were not waiting in silence any more.

'Very much like us actually. I feel more Irish than English at times. Catholic school will do that to you.'

Linford nodded sagely. 'That's the truth.' He took a ready-rolled joint from his jacket pocket and lit it ostentatiously, as only a true Rasta could. Toking on it a few times, he breathed the smoke in deeply before saying seriously, 'You know you've got to kill him, right?'

Jonny sighed deeply before he said sadly, 'Knew it from the off, mate.'

Linford grinned through the thick blue smoke. 'You know it makes sense. He can't be left standing, he's too proud a boy. Eventually he would have to come a-knocking.'

'Shame though, Linford. I always respected Kevin Bryant.'

Linford shrugged. 'Don't mean he ain't a bad motherfucker. Mark my words, you don't cancel him out this night, he'll just wait for his opportunity. Stands to reason. Now Bertie has to go either way – holds too many fucking grudges for his own good, that one.'

Jonny didn't answer; there was nothing more to say, the decision had been made.

Chapter Thirty

Celeste felt ill with worry, and couldn't settle at all. Why she had come to her sister's she didn't know – she just supposed that at certain times in your life, you needed your own. Even with family like hers. She couldn't go to her mum's what with her father muttering away about Jonny's front and her mother offering endless cups of tea. Instead, she had found herself on her sister's doorstep.

Her sister seemed both amazed and pleased to see her, that much was obvious, even at this late hour.

'Oh! Hello, sis.'

Cynthia had taken to calling her 'sis' and it sounded more false each time she heard it.

'All right, Cynth? I thought I'd pop in and give you a quick hello.'

Cynthia's eyes said 'not at this time of night you haven't', but she didn't question further. Instead she said brightly, 'Come through to the kitchen, I'll make a cuppa. Or I've a nice bottle of wine if you'd prefer that?'

Celeste followed her sister into the pristine kitchen and asked frankly, 'Got any vodka?'

Cynthia turned to face her sister and, smiling sadly, she said sympathetically, 'That bad?'

Celeste nodded.

Cynthia responded, 'That's why I'm still up and about too, James is on the missing list as well.' She poured them both large vodkas and, gulping deeply from hers, she grimaced in a comical manner before saying, 'I know you can't tell me what's going down, but I can guess from the fact you're here it's important. I know I done a wrong one, but it was only because I was frightened for James. He's a cokehead, you know that, don't you?'

Celeste didn't answer her, she didn't know what to say.

'He snorts it up like it's going out of fashion – out of his nut most of the time, he is. Now I know better than anyone that I'm not the greatest wife, or mother come to that, but I was jealous of you, and frightened for him. Does that make sense? I know now that what I did was wrong, was disgusting, and I'm paying the price for that. But you're still my little sister and I can see you're not right. You can confide in me if you like, or we can just sit here and talk about nothing. It's your call, Celeste. Either way, I'm here for you, OK?' It was said with honesty and humbleness.

Celeste knew that her sister really meant what she was saying. Her time in the wilderness had obviously hit her hard, but she knew what Jonny would say if he ever found out she'd told Cynthia *anything*. 'I can't talk about it, Cynth, I wish to fuck I could. But I just *can't*.'

Cynthia plastered a smile on her lovely face and said in a resigned manner, 'Fair enough. We'll talk about something else. Have you seen the dresses in that new shop in Ilford? I treated myself the other day.'

Smiling gently, Celeste listened as her sister prattled on, grateful for her company, and glad that they were back on some kind of even footing. But the worry was still there, and she wondered when this bloody night would ever end.

Chapter Thirty-One

Bertie was getting worried. He couldn't track down anyone of note on his payroll. He realised after the second phone call that they had been poached. All the minions were available, but the real deals, the hard men they relied on to administer their commands, were nowhere to be found. At first he had refused to believe it, hadn't wanted to doubt that he had their loyalty. Now, though, it was an absolute certainty and he felt the unfamiliar feeling of dread lying in his stomach like lead.

Kevin wasn't as surprised as Bertie; he knew that everyone had their price, and that no one was really a hundred per cent loyal – not in their game anyway. Everyone wanted to play for the winning side – that was human nature. But he was a bit fucked off that it had been done so easily and so sneakily. Neither he nor Bertie had even sniffed anything untoward going on, so that showed it was well planned and had been well executed. It also told him that they were on a losing streak. They had one chance to rectify this situation, and that was by taking out Jonny P once and for all. This was no longer just about revenge, it was about absolute survival, and that put a completely different complexion on things. This was now a fight to the death. And it was going to get dirty, very dirty indeed.

Kevin looked at Bertie Warner and he could see the fear and the disbelief in his eyes. Bertie had always believed that their blokes were sound, were unwavering in their loyalty.

'He's done us up like kippers, Bertie. We have to accept that.

But if I'm going down, then I'm taking something of Parker's with me.'

Bertie had never seen Kevin Bryant look so human in his life, and that worried him. For the first time in living memory he could see emotion on the big man's face. But it was his friend's words that really chilled him. He knew that Kevin, like himself, was not going out without a fight, and that was something he could understand.

'I'm right behind you.'

Chapter Thirty-Two

'Thanks for coming home with me, Cynth. I know it's silly but I get nervous here by meself.'

Cynthia didn't answer her sister. Instead she busied herself making a pot of tea. She wanted to be seen to be the administering angel when her brother-in-law arrived home. She wished she knew what was going on, but she knew better than to ask too much about it. If she played her cards right, she could at least start to get back into the family and their way of life.

That Celeste was this anxious told her that something big was going down. For the first time that night she wondered if her James was involved. She hoped so – whatever it was would be a big earn. All this worry wasn't for a lousy couple of quid, of that much she was sure. Her quick brain worked out that it had to be about taking something from someone – that was the only way a true Face could go forward in life. It was how you spread your workforce and made sure everyone was getting a nice earn.

Cynthia was a born criminal. She had the innate cunning needed for the job, and she also had the hard core inside her that was necessary when the time came to take out those who had outlived their usefulness. She didn't know that, but her instincts were nearly always spot on. Except when she was blinded by jealousy – then her instincts risked being overpowered by revenge. She had a taste for revenge, she had since a small child. In a man these would have been traits that could

110

have taken her to the top of her game; in a woman they were seen as a weakness. Men in her world believed that women were ruled by their hormones, and they could never respect a creature that had no real will of their own – it was as simple as that. Yet Cynthia knew she was ten times more intelligent than most of the men in her orbit, especially her ignoramus of a father, and that imbecile of a husband she had tied herself to.

As she looked round her sister's home, saw the luxury and the expense, she could once more kick herself metaphorically in the head. This could have been *hers*, this could have been *her* life. This *should* have been her life. Because, all that apart, Jonny Parker was the only man to ever ring her bells. When he had taken her she had finally felt whole, poor James couldn't compete with that. No man could compete with that. She had chosen respectability and where had that got her?

She had imagined herself presiding over dinner parties, where her James, not Jimmy, *James*, would bring his minions, and she would patronise them while stunning them with her food and her witty repartee. Instead she had chosen a man who couldn't decide whether to wear a tie without a fucking twelve-day postmortem on the subject.

She closed her eyes in anger and frustration. She hated her life so much, and the fact she had been the instigator of her own downfall was doubly frustrating.

Cynthia took the teapot to the table, and looked at her little sister. She was all eyes, all big blue eyes and anxiety. Even in her anger she felt a stirring of pity for her. 'He'll be OK, Celeste, stop worrying.'

'It's three in the morning and not even a phone call.'

Cynthia sat down and sighed heavily. 'James does this all the time. It's the nature of the game, nightclubs are called nightclubs because they are open at night!'

Celeste smiled then. But she was still guarded, not saying anything that might give the game away. But Cynthia acted as though she didn't care about any of that and was once more the solicitous sister.

'Shall I make you a bit of toast? You need to eat, love.'

Celeste shook her head. 'I couldn't, Cynth, thanks.'

'How about a biscuit? You always had a sweet tooth.'

Celeste stood up abruptly. 'Did you hear that?'

'What?' Her sister's panic was spreading to her now.

'That noise, there's someone outside.'

'You stay here, Celeste, and don't move.'

Cynthia walked silently from the big kitchen and checked all the downstairs rooms. As she looked out of the front-room window, she saw a large man walking towards the front door. Running back to the kitchen, she said to her sister in a whisper, 'Get down to the cellar. Don't argue, just go.'

'What's going on, Cynth?'

After dragging her sister none too gently, Cynthia pushed her into the back kitchen and, opening the cellar door, forced her inside. Following her, she bolted the door and groped around in the gloom till they reached the bottom of the steps, where they crouched as quietly as they could. It was almost pitch black, the only light coming from under the door above them.

'Is there a torch anywhere in here?' Celeste was clearly terrified now. Shaking her gently, Cynthia whispered, 'For fuck's sake, Celeste, is there a torch in here?'

Celeste walked unsteadily to a row of shelves and took down a small hand torch. Giving it to her sister, she waited like a young child to be told what to do next.

Turning on the torch, Cynthia looked around the unfamiliar space and, seeing a door that was obviously once the coal hole, she went towards it and made sure it was secure.

By now they could hear people walking around above them. It wasn't Jonny that was for sure – they could hear the doors being wrenched open upstairs, and they both realised that whoever it was wasn't visiting for any kind of social reason.

'What's going on, Cynth?'

Celeste's voice was rising and Cynthia went to her and said quietly but forcefully, 'Shut up, Celeste. Whoever it is mustn't know we are here, OK?' But even in the weak torch light Cynthia could see the hysteria rising in her sister's eyes and marvelled once more at how such a fucking coward could ever be enough for Jonny. She hugged her to her tightly saying in a soothing voice, 'Calm down, Celeste, we'll sort this out. Now, has Jonny any weapons hidden down here?'

Celeste was shaking so badly she could barely talk. 'I . . . I don't know . . . Probably . . .'

Cynthia looked around the large room and, spotting a large steel trunk, she went over to it. There was a large padlock protecting the contents. She sighed heavily. Looking round again, she grasped a large spanner from one of the shelves and attempted to break the chain with it. It was a fruitless exercise and the noise would alert them as to their whereabouts, but she tried anyway.

She could hear the men at the cellar door now, and she knew that the still-warm teapot would tell them that they might still be in the house somewhere. And now they knew where. She guessed they had come through the French doors in the lounge; they wouldn't risk the neighbours hearing them kicking in the front or back doors.

The cellar door was another thing altogether though. It was well inside the house, and they were now kicking at the lock with a ferocity that told her they would be through at any moment.

Celeste was crying openly – she wasn't even attempting to be quiet any more. Terror had taken her over and Cynthia knew that if they were to get out of this it would be down to her. Panic rising inside her, she gave the locked box one last wrench and, even though it didn't open, she saw that if she lifted the lid there was a four-inch gap – just wide enough to get her hand inside. She did that and, feeling around, she gripped the first thing that came to hand. A few seconds later she was holding a small calibre gun. Whether it was loaded she had no idea, but in her blind panic she pulled the safety back and then, leaving her sister crying in fear, she walked deliberately behind the stairway.

She was shaking herself now, she felt as if she was going to pass out. She took a few deep breaths and, when the cellar door finally crashed open, she waited for the visitors to come down the stairs.

The man was like the anti-Christ. His anger was so consuming he looked willing to rip them limb from limb with his bare hands.

Emerging from the stairway silently, Cynthia pointed the gun at the back of his huge head and fired.

He dropped to his knees, and she felt the bile rising inside her as she saw the gaping hole that was left after his skull and brains had been ripped open.

Twenty seconds later she heard a muttered 'Fucking hell', followed by the sound of the other man leaving the house as quickly as possible. She went over and looked down at the man's body. He wasn't quite dead yet and, kneeling down beside him, she removed the heavy shotgun from his reach. Then, pointing the gun once more at his head, she pulled the trigger again.

That was when Celeste started to scream.

Going to her sister, Cynthia slapped her as hard as she could across the face. Seeing that the girl was calmer, she walked her slowly up the stairs back into the kitchen. Then, the gun still in her hands, she closed the now-open front door before pouring both herself and her sister large brandies. She gulped hers and made sure her sister did the same. Next, she walked out into the hallway and, picking up the telephone, she rang around until she located James, only telling him that she was at Jonny's house and that Celeste needed her husband as soon as physically possible.

Then she sat at the kitchen table and waited, all the time talking calmly to her little sister and assuring her that everything was going to be all right. She wasn't sure she believed any of that herself, but she knew it was all she could do until the men arrived.

Chapter Thirty-Three

'I still can't believe it.' That much was evident in Jack Callahan's voice.

'Your daughter shot Kevin Bryant in self-defence, and she saved our Celly's life by all accounts.' Mary Callahan's voice choked up as she once more relived her daughter's close escape from death. There was no doubt in anyone's mind that Kevin had been going to take out Celeste to get back at Jonny P. A few of the more sceptical said he might have only used her as a hostage, but Mary strongly suspected his plan was always to wipe her baby out like a little boy would stamp on an ant. 'Well, you better believe it, she's the fucking hero of the hour by all accounts, and our Celly won't have a word said against her.'

Jack Callahan could hear the fear in his wife's voice and decided to keep his opinion to himself; she might be stunned by Cynthia's actions but he wasn't. She was like a bloke in a lot of respects, oh, not in her womanly body, but in her mind. There was something missing in his elder daughter, and he knew that, as hypocritical as it was, had she been a boy he would have been proud of her. Males could be like his Cynth and it would be seen as strength, in a woman it was seen as suspicious.

His daughter a murderer! Because that's what she was. She had waited behind the cellar steps and done Bryant from behind, using her sister as bait. That was the action of a man, that was a cold-blooded reaction. If she had had a lump of pipe instead she would have hammered his head in, he was sure. That his daughter had knelt down and finished the fucker off, was so distasteful to him he felt a moment's sickness in his belly. She was a fucking strange cove and no mistaking. 'How does Jonny feel about all this?' he asked curiously.

'Pretty much the same as everyone else.'

Mary was as amazed as her husband about the turn of events. In fairness, Cynthia had saved the day; if it wasn't for her the chances were Celeste would be dead now and the thought upset Mary so much she had to swallow down the urge to cry.

The mess had been cleaned up at the house by all accounts, but Celeste still refused to go back there. Well, she could understand that – what she couldn't understand was why Celeste was staying with Cynthia and not with her? They were like Siamese twins nowadays – where Cynthia went, Celly followed.

Jonny Parker was too wise to do anything about that just yet; he knew that Celeste needed time to get over what had happened to her. Plus, Mary guessed shrewdly, he would be grateful to have Celly off his hands while he cleaned up the mess he had caused by his greediness. For once Mary agreed with her husband. This was something that should have been avoided at all costs. It had left a bad taste in a lot of people's mouths.

Kevin Bryant might not have been liked, but he had been respected. It was only the fact that he had gone after a defenceless woman that had stopped the other crime bosses in London from retaliating on his behalf. She bet they were watching their backs now. They would need to and all; Jonny had half the Smoke at his disposal. Kevin Bryant was dead and his business partner Bertie Warner had disappeared completely. She suspected they were sharing the same grave somewhere and she hoped they would rot in hell for what they had tried to do to her poor daughter. Bastards, the pair of them. No one went after wives or kiddies – it was the unwritten law.

Chapter Thirty-Four

'No one has seen him, Jonny, it's like he dropped off the face of the earth.'

'What about his wife and kids?'

'House is empty, hardly even any clothes packed. I've got people keeping an eye out in Spain and Portugal but, in reality, he could be fucking anywhere.'

Detective Inspector Jones was as bent as a nine-bob note, and he knew that he was expected to give his main benefactor Jonny Parker something substantial for the money he was paid on a weekly basis, but there was nothing. It was the gospel truth – he had not been able to locate the man, or his family.

'Bertie would have a fallback plan, he probably had passports, et cetera waiting for just such an eventuality. All we can do is wait and see if anyone recognises him, or he commits a crime somewhere and we get wind of it. As I say, Jonny, he could be anywhere. South America, maybe? They would welcome the cunt with open arms – look at Biggsy.'

Jonny Parker knew the truth of this, but it wasn't enough for him. He wanted Bertie Warner's balls for this outrage and he wanted them now. If there was one thing he knew, it was not good practice to let Bertie have a swerve on this. It would make Jonny look weak and it also meant that someone was out there and they would have him and his family in their sights. It made him uneasy, even though he knew they were well protected. He had made the mistake of assuming his family was out of bounds, and he would never make that mistake again. Celeste was in bits, and why wouldn't she be? After what she had seen, he was surprised she wasn't in a nut-house.

But it was Cynthia who had amazed him the most. She had taken out Kevin Bryant and, from what he could gather, she had knelt down and finished the job. Either way, she had fucking scared Warner off – he must have thought they were waiting down there for him and wasn't prepared to take the chance of a bullet in his own bonce. None of it seemed to have affected Cynthia that much, she seemed a bit unnerved but that was about it. As he had looked at her comforting his wife, it had crossed his mind that she would have been a worthy mate for him, and he had hated himself for that thought even as he had acknowledged the truth of it. She was like a modern-day Boudicca, all hair and fiery sexuality. He was ashamed at how she had affected him, because he knew she was a two-faced, conniving whore, but somehow that just made her seem more intriguing.

Celeste was like a ghost of her former self; he had taken her to a doctor in Harley Street who was known to keep a closed shop, but all he had said was that she was suffering from shock. Well, Jonny could have fucking told the doctor that much, and *he* wouldn't have charged five grand. But the doctor had given her some happy pills and some sleeping tablets – both of which Jonny could have purchased in any pub in London for a millionth of the price – and sent them on their way. Still, Jonny felt better for having done *something* for her.

It was Cynthia who was on his mind, though – and the fact that she had taken Bryant out in such an audacious way. She had shown her mettle and, even though she had been an outcast over her last carry-on, she was now number one in everyone's books. She had more than redeemed herself; she had killed someone, and not just anyone either – she had killed the man who had been going after his wife, after Jonny P's wife, and that

119

counted for a lot in their world. She had been a ruthless and efficient killing machine and for some strange reason that turned him right on. He liked a bit of fire in a woman, and she had it in abundance. Cynthia was a stroppy mare, she was arrogant, and she was dangerous. All those things in a man would have been great, but in a female they were a worry. Females bled every month, they lived on their emotions, and they were as unreliable as a bent Filth, so what was the attraction suddenly?

He knew what it was all right, she was a goer in every way was Cynthia Tailor, and it was Cynthia Tailor he wanted under him. Not Cynthia Callahan. He wanted the woman she was now, not the girl he had bedded all those years ago. Her face that night it had happened had been a revelation to him; she was almost triumphant she had killed a man and she was determined not to let it affect her too much. He could see her forcing the terror out of her body, saw it being replaced by pride, and she had never looked lovelier to him than at that moment when she had conquered her fear. She had stared him in the eyes and it had been a challenge; she was daring him to turn away from her, and she knew, and he knew, he couldn't. She had protected his most treasured possession, his wife, and she had seen to it that the person who had been a threat to them was no more.

Even Linford had been impressed and, though the clean-up operation had been long and laborious, they knew it could have been much worse. It had been a long night, but it had been a lucrative one. More than that, it had been a night that had given him an itch, a terrible itch that he knew he could only assuage by bedding his wife's sister. Even though he knew it was a madness inside him, he couldn't deny the strength of it. Every time he thought of her kneeling down and putting one right in Bryant's ugly face he felt a tightening in his groin, and he knew that he would get no relief until he had her under him and crying out his name. It was madness but, like many a man before him, any caution was all but gone to the wind.

Jonny forced his mind back to the matter at hand and, looking straight at DI Jones, he said seriously, 'So I am paying you a serious fucking wedge to be told sweet fuck-all? Bertie Warner could be hiding under this table for all you know, is that it?'

Jones sighed heavily, he knew he was on borrowed time. 'That's about the strength of it, yeah. As I say, unless he shows up somewhere . . .' His voice trailed off, it sounded futile even to him.

'Get this fucking muppet out of here.'

Jones didn't need telling twice, he couldn't wait to get out the door.

Linford was laughing as the man left the room shamefaced. 'I hate bent Filth, worse than a fucking grass. They fuck up their own. Give me a straight copper and a fair nick every time.'

Jonny nodded his agreement, most of his associates felt the same.

'How's Celeste?' Linford asked.

Jonny shrugged. 'How'd you think? Scared, frightened, timid.' Even he could hear the irritation in his own voice, and Linford raised his eyebrows but didn't comment.

He knew Jonny blamed himself and a man would not forget that he, and he alone, was responsible for his wife's condition. He had left her hanging in the wind, and that was something no man could live with easily. Of course, luckily, Cynthia had come up trumps. Linford found what she had done admirable but distasteful, if he was honest. A woman who could do that and not even feel remorse was not a woman to him. Jimmy Tailor was welcome to the hard-faced bitch; he wouldn't want to lie beside her of a night – who knew what she was capable of if you fucked her off? No, thank you. He thought Jimmy should out her at the first available opportunity. After all, she wasn't a wife who inspired love and affection, and she had the mothering skills of a fucking demented hyena. At least hyenas looked after their young; by all accounts Cynthia dumped hers at her mother's for weeks at a time. Jimmy was a fucking cokehead, and that was because he had nothing to go home to. That pristine mausoleum was not a home, it was a show place. Linford had been there twice and each time he had felt as welcome as a sausage at a Bar Mitzvah. No, he didn't envy poor Jimmy Tailor in the least.

Linford liked his women clean and uncomplicated; he also liked them living at a separate address so they never got too big for their boots. Once they started cleaning his drum up after a night of revelry they were out the door and gone from his life. He had too many things to do, places to see, and strangers to bed for one woman to do anything for him. He looked after any kids of his that arrived, and he saw that they were looked after very well, but there was no way he was tying himself to one woman. That, as far as he could see, was a mug's game.

It was cut and dried to him; he saw, he conquered, and he came. Then he went home. Unlike Jonny, he liked to keep his life as uncomplicated as possible.

Chapter Thirty-Five

'Come on, Celeste, have a bit of lunch – you'll feel better for it.'

Celeste smiled gratefully, and dutifully ate her salad sandwich. She liked it at Cynthia's house; it was clean, and it was orderly, and best of all she couldn't smell the blood here. She couldn't get that smell out of her nostrils and she couldn't get the picture of Kevin Bryant out of her mind. The fact that her sister had killed him didn't bother her one bit; she knew Cynthia had done it to save her life, and that she could brutally kill a man wasn't something she thought about. Cynthia was her saviour and that was that.

Today, with her mum there too, and the kids squabbling on the kitchen floor, she felt the best she had felt since it had happened. Gabby got on to her lap and Celeste hugged the child to her tightly. She needed the warmth of these children to make her believe that life was normal once more, even though inside herself she knew it could never be normal again.

Jonny was looking for a new house for them because she refused to ever set foot in that other one again as long as she lived. She knew that Jonny was annoyed with her, not that he said anything of course, but she could feel his impatience with her. But she wasn't like him, she couldn't shrug this off as if it was an occupational hazard – it might be for him, but for her it was a nightmare he had brought on her and she didn't know if she could ever forgive him. She hoped so, because she loved him with all her being. But his actions had caused this

123

turmoil and upset, and she couldn't quite get over that yet.

Gabby seemed to sense her auntie's upset and she snuggled into her like she was trying to take it on herself. Celeste hugged her little body as if it was a life raft. James Junior watched them silently, and Celeste felt the tears prick once more, at the innocence of these children. The same innocence she had once possessed, and now it was gone from her. She had seen death in its rawest form, and it had blighted her life.

Crying silently, she didn't see the look that was exchanged between her mother and sister. She didn't understand that they thought it was time she let it go and sorted herself out. Celeste had never been strong like them, and that was why she couldn't forget the sight of Kevin Bryant with half his head gone, the blood seeping out of his body and making a heart shape on the concrete floor. For the thousandth time, she wondered what his wife and children were going through, and how they would ever come to terms with his disappearance. Four little children and a wife. Everyone said Kevin Bryant's wife was a nice girl. Why was it always the nice girls who had their hearts broken?

Gabby was trying to wipe her auntie's eyes, as she felt herself being lifted off her lap. It was obvious her nana was going to take them back to her house, but Gabby wanted to stay here. So did James Junior, who was beginning to kick up his usual fuss. For once though her mum was being nice to him and wasn't shouting at him. In fact, her mum was being nice to everyone and they were calling Cynthia a 'Brahma', and she knew that the way they said it meant it was something good. But Gabby allowed her nana to put her coat on, and take her and her sobbing brother back to her house. After all, she was a kid and she had to do what she was told.

Whether she wanted to or not.

Chapter Thirty-Six

'Come on, Celeste, you have to at least look at the new house.' Jonny's voice was gentle but there was a steely undertone that wasn't lost on anyone in the room. He had stopped the cajoling weeks ago, and he was getting more and more aggravated by the day. But Celeste, as weak as she was in many ways, was adamant about this one thing. She would not leave her sister's house for anything. She had not stepped across the door since she had entered it that night, the night Bryant had been taken out.

Jimmy Tailor was heart-sorry for his sister-in-law, but he knew it would be futile to interfere. Also, in a selfish way, he wanted her gone from his home. It had been nearly three months now, and he wanted his wife back, though he never thought he would ever be saying that.

'You go, Cynthia,' said Celeste. 'You go and then come back and tell me about it.'

Cynthia looked at her husband and shrugged. 'It doesn't matter what I think, love, it's what you think that matters.'

'No, you go, Cynth. I'll wait here with the kids, and Jimmy, Jimmy will stay here with me, won't you?' She didn't want to be alone.

Cynthia walked out into her hallway and Jonny followed her. 'If I go with you, we can come back and tell her how lovely it is, and then I can get her to come with me tomorrow, I'm sure of it.'

Jonny looked into her eyes and knew, as she did, that if they went to the house together they wouldn't be doing much looking at it, not at first anyway. He felt the excitement in his groin and wondered at how such a change could come over a man.

'If you think so.' His voice was noncommittal; no one listening to them would ever guess at the turmoil inside him.

Cynthia was elated, she knew he was prepared for what was going to happen. 'I'll go and freshen up, get my coat.'

He nodded, not trusting himself to speak.

Thirty minutes later they were naked, they were sweating and they were both aware that no one else would ever fulfil the strange need that they both shared.

'Tell me, tell me what it was like to kill him, Cynth.'

As she bit into his shoulders and spewed her filth into his ears, Jonny Parker felt, for the first time in years, that he was well and truly, *finally* home. That he was betraying his wife, the so-called love of his life, didn't bother him one iota. Every time he looked at Cynthia's full breasts and long legs, he saw her kneeling down beside Kevin Bryant and taking him out once and for all. There was no woman on this earth who could compete with that, and they both knew it. They were a match made in hell, and the knowledge only made them desire each other more.

Chapter Thirty-Seven

'It's lovely, Celeste, I bet you're glad you came home, aren't you?' There was genuine warmth in Cynthia's voice and it wasn't lost on anyone in the room. Even Jack Callahan was beginning to warm to this strange daughter of his. Jonny and Celeste's house was like a mansion and, where normally that would eat at Cynthia like a cancer, she seemed to be genuinely pleased at her sister's good fortune.

''Course I am, Cynth.' It was forced and everyone ignored that fact.

Cynthia was like a different person, everyone remarked on it. She was almost playful with the kids, and she was always in a good mood, even Jimmy didn't get the tail end of her tongue as often as he had before. She seemed happier than anyone had ever seen her, and it made their lives so much easier. She still left the kids with her mother for weeks on end, but these days she was happy to have them around during the daytime. She had started taking a Cordon Bleu cookery course, and Jimmy was eating better than ever. She never questioned his late hours any more. She saw him off to work with a cheery wave and a big smile. It was as if she was born again, and this time God had given her a heart. Celeste loved her with a passion and Cynthia seemed to reciprocate those feelings.

But Cynthia lived for the stolen time with Jonny Parker.

That her killing Bryant had appealed to him so strongly was a real eye-opener. If she had known that, she would have gone on a fucking killing spree a long time ago! Kevin Bryant's death didn't bother her, it wasn't an issue where Cynthia Tailor was concerned. It had got her the one thing she wanted more than anything in her life, Jonny, so she saw it as a good thing – nothing to lose sleep over. She enjoyed telling Jonny all about it; it turned her on as much as it did him. She relived it over and over again, and she didn't feel the least bit sorry about it.

She had never questioned that she was capable of great violence. Inside she had always known it; from a child she had been consumed by violent rages. When she was really angry she knew she was capable of almost anything, she knew she could easily stab someone if they thwarted her. She saw it as part of her strength and now she saw it as part of her allure. She looked like butter wouldn't melt when, in reality, she was capable of carrying out serious harm.

That Jonny Parker loved that about her was the bonus, of course. She had always known they were meant to be together, she had made a big mistake once by letting him get away and she wouldn't be making that mistake again.

The strangest thing of all was she realised she loved Celeste – really loved her. Now she wasn't a rival any more, Cynthia could find it in her heart to pity her. With her big house and her endless supply of dosh, *she* now had the one thing Celeste really wanted. She had Jonny Parker, and she was not going to let him go.

She would kill him first.

Chapter Thirty-Eight

Gabby watched in amazement as her mother laughed and joked with them all. She was like a new person, and it was wonderful.

Gabby had at last stopped wetting the bed, and stayed Sundays and Mondays at her mum and dad's house. It was wonderful. They ate a lovely meal together then watched the telly. Sometimes her mum still got impatient with them, though never too much, even when James Junior was really naughty. She loved her school, and she was making friends and, all in all, life was good. Now she had Christmas to look forward to as well. Everyone was going to come to their house! Her grandad said it was unheard of, though somehow Gabby knew she mustn't say that to anyone or it would cause trouble. There was a big tree up, and the mantelpiece was decorated with a huge piece of pretend holly. Her nana said it looked like a Victorian Christmas card, and her mother had liked that so it must have been a compliment. Never had Gabby looked forward to something in her life as much as she looked forward to this coming Christmas Day. The turkey was massive, the veg was all prepared, and her nana was going to bring the Christmas pudding. She had actually helped her mum ice the Christmas cake, and she and James Junior had been allowed to make a chocolate log. It was magical.

As Gabby lay there wondering at how lucky she was, her mother came into her bedroom and sat down on the side of her bed. This was something else she was beginning to like – her mother had started chatting to her like a real person, like the mummies in the books at school. She didn't just tell her off all the time.

'You comfortable, love?'

'Yes, thank you.' She still knew enough to watch her Ps and Qs.

'Looking forward to Christmas, I bet?'

She nodded, her face shining with happiness.

'Well, remember that Santa only comes to good boys and girls.'

'I will, Mummy, and I've been good. Sister Angela said I had been impressive, that was the word.'

Cynthia laughed then, a real laugh. 'I remember her – tall, ugly old cow.'

Gabby grinned at this blasphemy. 'She said I looked just like you at the same age.' She had also said that her mother was a heart-scald if ever there was one, and that she had been nothing but trouble from the day she walked into the Sacred Heart School. But Gabby wisely kept that bit of the conversation to herself.

Cynthia looked down on her lovely daughter – she really was lovely, she was beautiful. 'You're a good kid, Gabs.'

This was another new thing, the shortening of her name to "Gabs", this from her mother who always insisted everyone got their full title.

Gabby felt the tears sting her eyes then, it was not often her mother was this kind to her. 'I try, Mummy.'

Cynthia smiled. 'I know you do, mate. I know you do.' She kissed her daughter's brow then and, making sure the bed was tidy, she left the room, whispering, 'Good night,' softly before shutting the door behind her.

When Cynthia went into her front room, she sat down and sipped at her wine. They would both be off to sleep soon, she had made sure of that – she had crushed half a sleeping tablet into their hot milks. James was off out, overseeing the books in a club in Romford, and she had a small lamb casserole in the oven simmering away ready for when Jonny got here. She felt the pull of him already, hence the drugged children; nothing or no one would interfere with her time with him.

It was strange the way it had panned out. She felt a sorrow for Celeste that was so deep, and so sad it was almost tangible. She knew that Jonny could never leave her sister, and she was content with that for the moment. All she wanted was him, inside her, in her bed where she gave her husband a mercy fuck often enough to allay his suspicions. All she wanted was what she had. And that was tonight, because there was no way they would be able to get together over Christmas.

She had put on her new underwear, she had made her face up so it looked more exquisite than ever, and she had put on her old clothes, because there was nothing that turned him on more than ripping them off her as he walked through the door. She felt the thrill of him inside her once more and, settling herself in the comfortable armchair, she awaited his arrival.

Life didn't get much better than this; a drink, a sit and the anticipation of a good fuck into the bargain. This was what she lived for, what kept her going. This was the stuff that dreams were made of.

Chapter Thirty-Nine

Jonny Parker was on his way to Cynthia's with a bottle of Dom Pérignon, and a diamond pendant that she would dismiss as a knock-off from the market like she had everything else he had bought her. He felt the tug of her as he drove sedately through the London traffic.

He liked to savour the journey to her house – always *her* house, never Jimmy's. He liked the knowledge that she would be waiting for him, would fuck him like an animal, and then feed him a wonderful supper and talk as if they were no more than good friends. She knew what a man wanted, a real man, and he felt sorry for Jimmy Tailor, who would never be enough for the woman who was his wife.

Jonny was the king of the world; he had outed Bryant, he was now the main man in the Smoke, and all that was left for him to do was find that cunt Bertie Warner. And find him he would, if it was the last thing he did in this life. He would find him, and he would crush him like a fucking beetle under his shoe. He owed Celeste that much, if nothing else. He had put her in danger and, if it hadn't been for Cynthia, she would be dead. Then he would never have found out what really made him tick.

No woman had affected him like Celeste – she was pure and clean and good. But, thanks to Cynthia, he saw that she was not enough for him. Without *her* he would never have understood that he had a real lust for blood, and that blood lust would take him places he had never dreamt possible, both mentally and sexually.

London was his, and he was going to own it all. The man who could take it off him hadn't been born yet. He had a slice of everything – from blags to betting shops to nightclubs, market stalls, shops, even the bingo halls, the list was endless. He had finally made it, was finally the top banana, and now came the hardest part of all.

Staying there.

Book Two

The half is greater than the whole

Hesiod, ca. 700 BC

Chapter Forty

1994

Cynthia was tired after her long day's work but happy; these days she was working for Jonny along with her husband and she loved it. They were getting a serious earn now, and if her husband wondered at the change in their status he was either too shrewd or too stupid to say so. She had a feeling it was the latter, but she never asked him, she didn't really want to know the answer. Jonny had gone from strength to strength in the last few years and was now the undisputed and, more importantly, the unchallenged king of London town. He was the main man, and he was loving it. That Cynthia was the main woman thrilled her even as it worried her. It was a miracle they had not been found out and that made her think people knew but weren't talking about it. Jonny Parker wouldn't look kindly on any gossiping, and she was not about to let her life be ruined over it either.

She was known as a killer in their circle, and she felt the respect from the men, and the fear from their women. The story had been repeated and built up over the years until it was nothing like the real events. The younger ones even thought it had been planned. It amused her how stories really did get stretched in the telling, and how a story, true or otherwise, could impact on a person's life. Everyone was wary of her these days and that helped her in her new-found career.

All except Celeste, of course. Celeste was still treating her like she was the second coming or something and, though she was sorry for her little sister, she didn't feel in any way guilty. She now believed that what had happened was inevitable, believed that she and Jonny Parker were meant to be. Like all great loves, theirs had not been an easy road.

She tolerated poor James, and she knew that he was grateful to her for her affection, scant though it was. His attempt at being the head of the household was long over; now he deferred to her as he always used to, only these days she didn't provoke him as she once had. In fact, she believed he was happy in his own way. Jonny saw to it that they were well looked after, and well compensated, and who would have thought she had a knack for the betting shops? She ran them all with military precision, and the percentage she took was no small amount.

All in all life was great – except for one thing. As good as she looked, time was beginning to take its toll on her. Lately she had noticed that Jonny, while still as ardent as ever when they were together, wasn't as eager to meet up as he used to be. Whereas once it had been every day, sometimes twice a day, often a quick coupling in the back of a car because they only had an hour, now he seemed as if he was stepping back from her somehow, and that was not something she was prepared to accept. That he had a lot more on his mind she understood and accepted, but what she wouldn't accept was another woman in his life – other than Celeste, of course. Celeste was no threat, but the advent of the lap-dancing clubs had made Cynthia aware that, unlike the nightclubs where young girls were in abundance but ultimately looking for a man on a permanent basis, the lap dancers were all out for what they could get. Their brazenness alone was something that would appeal to her Jonny. *She* should know, she was brazen enough herself, and that was what he wanted from her. She knew that this was a jealousy brought on by insecurity; she was still a good-looking woman, but she was just that – a woman, and these were girls. Very *young* girls at that.

Jonny had embraced the lap-dancing clubs and made them the jewel in his rather large crown. He also spent a lot of his free time in them, though he said it was work and she had to believe that, didn't she? But, as good as life was, she felt that he was somehow slipping away from her, and that was something she could never countenance.

No one, not her kids, her family, nobody on this earth meant as much to her as Jonny Parker, and she would see him dead before she saw him with someone else. That wasn't even a threat, that was a promise. Without him she would wither away and die. He was like a drug to her and, though she knew it was unhealthy, that their attraction was wrong in so many ways, she embraced it because she could not live without it.

Chapter Forty-One

Jonny Parker had changed over the last few years, and he was as aware of it as the people who worked for him. He would not be gainsaid and he would not listen to advice from anyone; he was unable to take any kind of criticism and he severely punished those who he felt were being disrespectful. It was said by a few that he was getting far too big for his boots – but not within his earshot naturally. Nevertheless, there were the beginnings of dissent, and it was something he should have been aware of, and should have done something about.

The old affable Jonny P, always ready to buy a round of drinks, always the first with a good joke, and always the first to arrange a big party, was long gone. He was a serious, rather dour man now, who occasionally reverted to his old ways while in his cups. He had still never touched a drug – alcohol being his only real vice – and he took his job and its responsibilities very seriously indeed. As his father-in-law always said, getting to the top was the easy part, it was staying there that took the real hard graft.

The truth of the statement was not lost on Jonny now as he sat working. He had fought to get the top prize and it was getting harder and harder to hang on to it. London in the nineties was run by him and a few other Faces – they had minor roles, of course. But it was being swamped by Eastern Europeans, Russians, and the like. They were like no other adversary seen on these turfs before; they had unlimited money and they were

140

ruthless, and that meant *he* had to become more ruthless. That was the law of their game, but it was a hard graft all the same.

The girls in many of his clubs were Eastern European. The men he dealt with had a constant supply, and the girls were brought over, relieved of their passports, and then told they had to work off their debts. Jonny also had fingers in more than a few pies concerning some Eastern-European brothels. These were constant money-spinners and, though he had found the whole thing distasteful at first, he knew if he didn't become a part of it some other enterprising fucker soon would. That would mean a serious rival for him and he could not allow that.

All the same he didn't like the business – but then he didn't bet and he still had plenty of betting shops. Betting was a fucking mug's game as far as he was concerned; only fools and bigger fools thought they could really beat the odds. If they had a win, it was rarely enough to cover the years of spending in his shops that preceded it. Still, each to their own and if the Good Lord had not invented lust, greed and all the other vices, he would not have been able to live the life of a biblical king. And live like a king he did, though he was clever enough not to live *too* ostentatiously. He did though have property all over the world, and that was thanks to his Eastern-European connections. They were masters at the long game and he was learning shitloads of stuff from them.

Jonny bought properties for cash, and laundered the money by remortgaging them, not just in England but all over the world; it was like a licence to print legal dosh. He was also amazed at the amount of money to be made in whoring, because it was the whoring that had been the most lucrative of all his new ventures. The only real drawback was that he had no real control over the money and, if caught, the sentences were heavy. That was because the girls were there against their will and that often led to charges of white slavery – even though many of the girls were West African – and kidnapping. It was costing a fortune to grease the right palms but, thanks to his connections, they were pretty safe. At least as safe as those kind of deals can be. It was taking its toll though, and he knew that the happiness he should have been feeling from all he had achieved was not there.

The reason for this was his Celeste. Yes, she was better than she had been, but she was still scared of her own shadow. In fact, the only time she was remotely happy was when they were out in Spain. She loved their house in Majorca and she seemed to relax there. It was up in the mountains, and the greenery and the dramatic views seemed to calm her soul. Personally, he liked it for the first week and then felt he was going stir-crazy, but he knew she needed the time there.

They had not yet had children, though Celeste had suffered miscarriages, and they both said there was plenty of time, but he guessed that deep down she was frightened of it all. He wanted children, but he was in no hurry. And perhaps that was just as well because he couldn't see how Celeste would cope with a baby. He loved her with all his heart, and he still cared for her, but now she was more like a sister. Although, in all honesty, that could be the result of the guilt he felt for what he was doing with her sister . . .

Now *there* was a woman, though she was getting harder and harder to keep in line. She was like a man in many respects; she thought like one, she worked like one, and she could fight like one when the fancy took her. The only downfall was her mouth. Cynthia never knew when to let something alone, and she would push an issue to the hilt. Lately, that had begun to irritate him; he had enough going on without having a five-point crisis every time he saw her. He understood her loathing of the lap-dancing clubs – most women disliked them. And yet the brothels didn't bother her one iota. She was a strange, contradictory creature. He cared for her deeply, but she was hard work; 'high maintenance' was the expression men used about women like her these days, and it described her totally.

All the same, when he was with her, deep inside her, was the only time he really felt content, the only time he felt fulfilled. He didn't analyse these thoughts, he just knew them to be true. What it was about her he could never put his finger on. All he knew was she drew him to her like a moth to a flame. And he hated that it was being spoilt by her constant wanting for more and more of his time.

He shrugged the thoughts away and concentrated on what he was doing. He glanced at his watch and realised he was already late for a meeting. Where did the time go, and why was he still working fifteen hours a day? But he knew why; he didn't trust anyone around him to do the job properly. He was wary of delegating too much of the big stuff; once you took your finger off the pulse you lost the beat of the world you were in, and that was a dangerous situation to be in. You only had to look at the likes of Kevin Bryant to see the truth of that statement.

Chapter Forty-Two

Gabby hated her life. She hated school and she hated the nuns there. She was thirteen, and her whole existence was a big drag, at least it was this week anyway.

But there was one high spot, and his name was Vincent O'Casey. He was seventeen and he was gorgeous. She had met him at Chrisp Street Market last Saturday and she was seeing him again tomorrow. She couldn't wait.

Like all her friends, Gabby's Saturdays were for doing the markets – the Roman Road, East Ham, Chrisp Street, Romford of course and, occasionally, Soho Market – not that they bought there, but it was wonderful to look at all the strange things. Sundays were for 'the Lane', as Petticoat Lane Market was called. Romford was Gabby's favourite though; she loved that it was far away from her mother, because her mother was a giant pain in the arse.

She frowned as she thought this, and she wondered at how on earth she had been lumbered with such a woman. These days, she went home for whole weekends, when she would prefer to be there only on Sundays and Mondays as it used to be. But her mother wasn't stupid. She wanted her there because she wanted to make sure she didn't go '*out* out', as she called it. That meant with boys, although it was never actually stipulated. It was fine for her to go with her friends to the markets – it was what her mother had done, after all – but when the evening drew in she had to be indoors like an errant school kid.

Well, she would be fourteen soon – she wasn't a baby any more. With her already ripened body she knew she could pass for eighteen with the right clothes and make-up. Christ Almighty, she could get in to see any film she wanted, and that was no mean feat. Some of her friends still looked younger than they were, but she was like her mother – all tits and legs, as her grandfather was forever saying. Gabby knew that she was pretty, knew that boys looked at her. Men did as well, though they made her uncomfortable. But they looked all the same – even some of her friends' dads, and that was absolutely gross.

Her dad was great but, as always, he had to do what her mother wanted, so Gabby got no support from him. She felt sorry for him, because he seemed so sad a lot of the time, and yet her parents lived in a lovely house and, to an outsider, it would seem they had a nice life. But Gabby knew instinctively that her mother didn't love her dad, not like he loved her, and that was why he was so sad inside. It was in his eyes, and it was tragic to see. Sometimes she looked at him and felt the urge to cry, he looked so forlorn, so lonely. But how could he be lonely when he had her and James Junior?

Her dad knew that they preferred it at their nana's house – at least there they could be themselves. He knew that their mother was sometimes inordinately hard on them both, and he tried in his own way to make up for that. He ruined them, according to her mother, gave in too quickly, but she saw her father was sensible enough to appreciate that if you let a child be free, they would come back to you of their own accord. All her mother's draconian measures seemed to do was make her want to break away, get away, as far away from the source of her unhappiness as possible.

But now she had Vincent to think about, and he was absolutely gorgeous, from his dark hair, his blue eyes, and his muscular physique, to his great big feet. She felt her pulse race as she thought of his body and wondered why she felt suddenly so shy and awkward. She knew she wanted to kiss him, but she would not let her mind imagine any more than that. She did think about him all the time though, alone in her bed at night, and the feelings she had then were exciting and frightening. She knew her mother would have a heart attack if she knew about them! Her biggest problem at the moment was how she could swerve her mother so she could meet him one night. Like her mother, she was very resourceful and very determined. And, like her mother, she would not, under any circumstances, be thwarted.

Unlike her mother, Gabby had a truly kind heart, and an even kinder nature. She was happy in her own way, and enjoying the act of defiance that meant her meeting up with her heart-throb Vincent O'Casey behind her mother's back. She couldn't wait.

Chapter Forty-Three

'The sap's rising in her, she's just growing up. She wants to be with her friends and not have us standing over her the whole time.'

'She's only thirteen, Dad.'

Celeste sounded upset and Jack Callahan retreated on this occasion. Celeste agreed with everything her sister said, and if Cynthia said that her daughter was not to move across the doorstep then that was that.

Personally, he felt sorry for the child. She was liked a caged lion, and eventually caged animals turned on the person who caged them in the first place. He could see the dislike and the irritation in his granddaughter's eyes for her mother, and he felt deeply sorry for her. Plus, she was a nice kid and a trustworthy kid at that, which was more than could be said about her mother at the same age.

Cynthia had been round the turf more times than a National winner by the time she was fifteen, although he wasn't supposed to know about that, of course. That was the problem with daughters, they got into trouble; boys were just the cause of their downfalls. Even in these so-called enlightened times, a girl in trouble was still looked down on where they lived, the doings of a load of braless fucking lesbians and their shouting about equality didn't cut much ice in the East End of London. Fucking feminism! A load of old cobblers as far as he was concerned. All it meant was that girls were getting like men, and what good would that do in the long run? Bullshit baffles brains all right, but where his granddaughter was concerned he hated to see her locked up like some kind of prisoner. Jack hated Cynthia at times, really loathed her. She was a piece of work. He knew about her and Jonny, but what could he do? If it ever came out it would be like one of those IRA bombs exploding in the heart of his family. And Jonny was *not* a son-in-law he could give a tug to, pull to one side and put the hard word on. Jonny was the local fucking Face – and how Jack would like to shove his fist into Jonny's face at times. He knew Jonny loved Celeste, loved her deeply, but he also knew that his Cynthia was in his blood. A woman could take a man like that and get under his skin. Jack had seen it before; when it hit a man he was helpless to fight it. Some women had the power to make a man go against all he believed in, go against his basic instincts, walk away from his family, his job, his life. And the worst thing of all was that these women were never worth it. Hindsight was a wonderful thing, as Jonny would one day find out. For now, as long as Celeste didn't get hurt, Jack had to go along with it.

He wondered how much his old woman knew. Mary was a shrewd old bird, and she could also keep her own counsel; she wouldn't air something so potentially dangerous unless she had to. She *had* to know but, like him, her first thoughts were for Celeste and her fragile state of mind.

All that mess years ago had left its mark on them, and the seed of hatred that he had always felt for his elder daughter had grown into something much deeper. He hated feeling useless, hated that he was in no position to do anything for his family. Jonny paid for all their lives now, he had them in the palm of his large and treacherous hands and, at bottom, that was what really bothered Jack. He was helpless to do anything and, for a man like Jack Callahan, that was a terrible position to be in. But one day Jonny would get his comeuppance, of that much he was sure.

Chapter Forty-Four

Mary Callahan was watching her grandson James Junior as he gazed at the television. She liked to think she had a special bond with him, but she worried that he wasn't *right* somehow. He could barely count to fifty, and he struggled to read the comics he bought by the dozen. He seemed to be away with the fairies half the time, and spent hours staring at the TV screen. Lately she had begun to wonder if he actually took in what he was watching. All he seemed interested in at the moment was getting a kitten. They couldn't have one here – she was too old for all that palaver – and there was no way Cynthia would have one in that surgically clean house of hers. But it was all James Junior went on about. His schoolwork was clearly suffering, though she had a feeling he just couldn't do it and that it was too advanced for him. He needed a private tutor or something.

Mary had broached the subject with Cynthia who had shrugged and said he was 'as thick as shit' and 'he'll snap out of it.' At nearly nine, James Junior was larger than other lads his age, but he hardly spoke a word unless spoken to first. Unless he *really* wanted something – then he would pester and annoy everyone till he got what he wanted. Look at all that about the kitten. James had flown into such a rage when he was told he couldn't have one. They had been amazed at the intensity of it. And the language! Kicking and spitting out filth the like of which she'd never heard before. Jack had eventually given him a good clump, and that seemed to have sorted him out. But again, the ferocity of his anger was all wrong, too deep and too hateful for a child of his age.

He seemed to have no friends either and she believed it was because he didn't seem to want any. That, to her mind, was unnatural in a child, and she knew that someone should address these problems but she didn't know who that should be. It wasn't as noticeable to everyone else, they just thought he was quiet. But Mary felt instinctively that there was something radically wrong with the boy, and that frightened her. If only she could talk to Cynthia, voice her concerns about his school-work, his indifference to other people. A kitten might be just what he needed, a little friend of sorts, something to love.

The doorbell rang, and she got up to answer it, leaving the young lad with her husband.

Roy Brown, their neighbour for over twenty-five years, was standing there with his little grandson Tyrone and, in his arms, he was holding a dead kitten and a Tesco carrier bag, blood everywhere.

Her evident surprise turned to shock when Roy Brown, his huge face twisted in disgust, said angrily, 'Get young James out here. Look what he did to the kitten. He cut the little fucker's throat.' He was roaring in his anger, and this brought Jack out into the hallway.

'What the fuck's all the shouting about?' He was looking at Roy Brown and the crying Tyrone in utter amazement.

'Your grandson, that fucking weirdo James, has cut my Tyrone's kitten's throat. Cut the little cat's throat, the wicked little bugger.'

Jack Callahan was looking at his old friend as if he had just grown another head in front of his eyes. 'What the hell are you on about, man?'

Little Tyrone Brown was only five years old but, with the acumen of men ten times his age, said tearfully, 'He did, he did, I saw him, he made me watch . . .'

Jack was staring from one person to another in utter disbelief. 'That's bollocks! Our James loves cats. For fuck's sake, he's been driving us mad about getting one for weeks.'

Roy interrupted him then saying, 'That's why he did this.' He thrust the dead body of the kitten towards Jack who instinctively stepped backwards. '*He* couldn't have one, so he didn't want my Tyrone to have one either, the murdering little fucker.'

Jack was shaking his head; he refused to believe his grandson was capable of such an act. He was stunned into absolute silence.

Roy handed him the carrier bag saying, 'Open that, go on, see whose knife it was that cut the animal's throat.'

Jack opened the carrier bag and peered inside. There, bloodstained and covered with the cat's tabby hair, was their bread knife. He knew it was theirs because it had a white bone handle – it had been Mary's mother's and she treasured it. Sometimes, as she cut up a loaf, she would remark at how long the knife had been in use and how it must never go into the dishwasher, but be cleaned lovingly by hand.

Now it had been used to kill this poor child's little pet and, staring into the blood-stained carrier bag, Jack Callahan felt the rage boiling up inside him. The wicked, feral little bastard. That he was capable of something so heinous, so barbaric was unthinkable. Yet the knife was there, and the only person who could have taken it out of this house was James.

Young Tyrone was looking at him with the sad, soulful eyes of an honest boy, and Jack knew he was telling the truth. Where was the culprit though? He must have heard all this commotion. Jack called his name out loudly and, when the boy didn't appear, he went into the front room. Lifting him bodily from where he was crouched on the sofa, he physically dragged him into the hallway.

'Did you do this? *Did you?*'

James was terrified and, for a few seconds, even Roy Brown

was almost sorry for the boy. Jack Callahan's temper was legendary in their street – he didn't go often but when he blew, he really lost it.

Snatching the dead kitten from Roy, Jack pushed the corpse into his grandson's face, smearing him with blood and hair, all the time shouting, 'You did this, didn't you? You vicious little fucker . . .'

Pulling away roughly, James screamed, 'It's not fair! *I* wanted a kitten, that should have been *my* kitten! Not his bastard kitten . . . But no, I couldn't have him, could I? Not me, I never get fucking anything off you bastards . . .'

The blow, when it landed, knocked James across the hallway and into the small table where they kept the phone. The table collapsed, and the phone was sent sprawling along with the boy, who was now attempting to cover his head, protect his skull from the rain of punches that was being administered by his granddad.

Eventually, Roy Brown stepped in and pulled Jack off, shocked at the severity of the beating. He could see that if it went on for much longer Jack would surely kill the child. The hallway was spattered with blood. Roy looked at Mary Callahan and, seeing the utter horror on her face, he wondered if he could have perhaps handled the whole situation better somehow.

Young Tyrone Brown was watching in morbid fascination, knowing this was wrong even though to him it felt right. His little cat Bullet had had its throat cut by James and he felt he should pay for that. Being too little and too young to fight James, he had gone to his granddad because he knew he was big enough to do what he couldn't. He had loved his little cat, and he didn't want to see it die like that. He started crying then, a high-pitched keening that seemed to jerk Mary Callahan to life.

'Come here, child, come to me.'

But Tyrone had had enough, and he left the hallway sobbing, his granddad following him in a bewildered state, shocked at the day's events, and wondering if he had any hard stuff in the house.

Picking up the dead cat, Jack Callahan threw it at his now inert grandchild and said scathingly, 'Clear this lot away. You'll bury that little lad's cat for him, and you'll do it properly and with an apology, you rotten little fucker. The shame you've brought on this house today, you murdering little bastard. You're your mother's son all right.'

It wasn't until much later when he went over the events again in his mind that it occurred to him that his wife had not once leapt to her grandson's defence. That alone spoke volumes.

Chapter Forty-Five

'It was a fucking cat, Jonny. Anyone would think he'd murdered Mother Teresa the way they're carrying on.'

Jonny had heard the story – it was all people were talking about. The school had got wind of it and had said that James Junior should see a psychiatrist. The general consensus was that the school was right; cutting a kitten's throat wasn't exactly a boyish prank for all Cynthia tried to make it out like that. It also seemed that her boy James was getting a name for himself as a weirdo, for want of a better word. The school had been concerned about him for a good while, and he knew that was what was really getting up Cynthia's nose. She didn't have any real interest in the children unless they were reflecting well on her – then she was proud, or at least acted proud. She played the part of an exemplary mother and housewife, but it was all a façade. Now this latest incident had brought out the mother lioness in her, and she was determined to make sure it was seen as a youthful indiscretion and no more. But even hardened criminals were shocked at the child's antics. Cutting that poor kitten's throat because he couldn't have one of his own was seen as something sinister, not quite acceptable. Not for a nine year old anyway.

'Still, Cynth, it's a bit OTT don't you think? Cutting its throat with a bread knife? Not exactly tit for tat, is it?'

Cynthia could feel the anger burning away inside her and she

154

held it in check. 'I should have let him have the cat, I didn't realise how much it meant to him.'

Jonny knew she was genuinely bewildered and believed that the reaction to James Junior's antics was overboard. 'Well, if you want my opinion, he needs a shrink now, before it's too late.'

Cynthia laughed then. A harsh, derisory laugh. 'Oh . . . hark at Doctor fucking Spock! What you know about kids I could write in block capitals on the back of a postage stamp. He's nine, fucking nine and, like any nine year old, he overreacted . . .'

Jonny was laughing now, really laughing. 'Overreacted? For fuck's sake, Cynth, can you hear yourself? Use your loaf and let this die down. Get him help – that's what normal people do for their kids.'

Cynthia knew that Jonny was trying to help not just her but James Junior too. But she couldn't accept what he was saying; she felt strongly that the general consensus was way off base. He was a kid, and kids did stupid things. Somewhere deep inside her she knew she should be worried; it wasn't because she believed it, but her common sense told her that when the opinion of the majority was against you, the chances were you were wrong. But he was a child, and children were cruel – how many times had she heard that expression? What was annoying her more than anything was that this man, who she actually loved in her own strange way, was also ridiculing her and calling into question her mothering skills. She knew she would never win any awards, but she prided herself on having the cleanest, best turned-out children anywhere.

She would not be criticised by *anyone* about *anything* – especially not where her kids were concerned. But what really rankled was Jonny talking about psychiatrists for her son, when his wife, her sister, was madder than a box of frogs. Not that she would ever point that out to him of course; she knew he blamed himself, and so he fucking should.

Celeste wandered around that big house like the Orphan of the Storm. She could barely leave the house these days, not that anyone pointed that out, of course, but there was a word for it – agoraphobia. Still, in all honesty, it made their lives easier and that suited her down to the ground. The only time Celeste left the house under her own steam was to go to Majorca and their house there, but even that was getting harder to achieve. He should leave her out there, let her enjoy the weather and the different surroundings.

Cynthia knew that she had to save this situation from getting out of hand, so she hid her true feelings and forced a smile on to her lovely face. 'Well, not a lot I can do. You'll be pleased to hear he's going to see a shrink on Tuesday, the school's insisting on it.'

Jonny felt the relief as a physical thing. Cynthia had to understand that *her* problems were not *his* problems, even though at times like this he felt he had to try and talk some sense into her. It wasn't easy reasoning with Cynthia. She had a knack of sounding right all the time – he assumed that was because she believed with all her heart that she *was* right all the time.

'Well then, darling, how about a drink?'

Cynthia smiled her assent, but the magic had gone out of the night and they both knew it. James Junior's so-called escapade was having far-reaching repercussions, and both suspected that the shrink would not be the end of it.

Chapter Forty-Six

Celeste was worried, but then that was nothing new. She was permanently worried these days. Since the night of Kevin Bryant's death she had never been the same. Every time she closed her eyes she saw his face, every time she opened her eyes she saw his face. And it was a horrible face, twisted up in anger and agony. Over the years he had grown in size, until now, all these years later, he was like some kind of giant in her mind.

She crept around her house, her lovely big house that should have made her happy, half-expecting his ghost to be behind her, expecting at any moment a tap on her shoulder and his decaying, rotten hand to touch her.

She poured herself another glass of vodka and downed it in one gulp. Alcohol was the only thing that stopped her from hearing the whispers and the noises that she was convinced came from the grave, the grave of Kevin Bryant. A constant whispering sound, it was reminiscent of when she had been a kid on a school trip to St Paul's Cathedral, and they had dutifully listened to the teacher in the Whispering Gallery, hearing the words travel around the structure, and all pretending to marvel at such a device in such an old building. She had not liked it in there with dead people everywhere you walked. So what if they were poets? They were still fucking dead and she was sure they would have much rather been buried in peace – somewhere a crowd of bored school kids wouldn't be taking the piss out of their names, and sniggering about their lives.

She closed her eyes against the negative thoughts. She had read somewhere that you had to force negative thoughts from your mind and think positive. But think positive about what? What did you think about when there was nothing positive in your life? When your whole world was built on quicksand and could be snatched from you in a millisecond?

Her husband loved her, that was a positive she supposed, but he could be shot dead, stabbed, maimed or disappear at any given moment. She knew better than anyone that that was the kind of world they lived in. So it was hard to think positive about that. She had a nice home and a caring family, but then so did a lot of people, so that wasn't really that big a positive when you analysed it properly. That was more of a human right, surely?

Celeste sighed heavily and looked at herself in her bedroom mirror. It was a large, very expensive mirror from France, and it made you look slimmer. But she knew it was just a trick of the glass so that, too, was built on a lie. Her whole life was built on lies and deceit, and she was powerless to do anything about it. She studied herself for a few moments. It was rare she ever looked at herself; she loathed what she was, what she had become. Outwardly she still looked OK. If she was on a bus – not that she ever got buses these days – she knew she would fit in with people's general opinion of someone normal. They couldn't see the blackness inside her, the rottenness that was at her core, and that bothered her. Really bothered her. It proved to her that you could never really trust anyone, because you couldn't see inside of them. You couldn't really ever know what was in their minds or, more importantly, their hearts.

Like James Junior killing that poor kitten. He looked like an angel that child, but he was filthy, putrid just like the rest of them. She was relieved now about her miscarriages, that she didn't have any children. How would you ever know what they were really like? Imagine having a baby which grew up to be a monster, a killer? By then you already loved it, had made plans for it, and then it turned around and kicked you and all your hard work right in the teeth.

Oh no, that wasn't for her – that was for the likes of Cynthia. She had the strength to deal with things. Cynthia was the only person Celeste trusted. Cynthia would always look out for her, would always save her from danger. She was like a modern day Penthesilea, an Amazonian woman who could fight like a man, and think like a man. She could always depend on her, she knew that much. Like she would sort out little James, and steer him towards the right path.

Celeste was surprised to find herself in the kitchen, and wondered vaguely how she had got there. She opened the huge fridge and took out a chunk of cheese. She bit into it and savoured the strong cheddar taste, the saltiness on her tongue. Then, replacing it, she went to the countertop and poured herself another vodka. It occurred to her that she had not left the house for over a week, but she shrugged off the thought. Inside the house was bad enough, but it was nothing compared to the dangers on the streets.

She settled herself at the kitchen table and began to peruse the papers they had delivered every day. She looked for stories of death, pain, serial killers and genocide. These stories made her feel safe, made her feel that her take on the world was the true one. Even Spain, her beloved adopted country, wasn't immune. It was filling up with gangsters and murderers, including Majorca where she had believed life was simpler and therefore better. The papers were full of it nowadays, all kinds of death and destruction, the whole world over.

Those facts, those stories she read, assured her that her thoughts were not wrong, that her life as it was could not be any other way. It was comforting to know that the world outside was just as she believed. That was the only positive thought she possessed, and she hung on to it like a dog with a bone.

Chapter Forty-Seven

Jimmy Tailor was understandably upset at his son's behaviour and, what was worse, he didn't know how to address it. He could see that the hiding had meant nothing to the boy. To compound these feelings of worthlessness, he was aware of the look of contempt for his family in the boy's eyes too. It was a strange thing, but he really disliked his son now. Knowing he was capable of something so shocking and so heinous, and was not the least bit concerned about his actions, had shown Jimmy the true state of the boy's mind. He knew that in his hands he was now holding a potential threat to society.

That Jimmy could have fathered a child so devoid of love, so devoid of care bothered him. In his heart of hearts he feared that while the boy may resemble him physically, the personality of his mother had come to the fore. The fact that Cynthia didn't think that the event was in any way catastrophic, really brought home to Jimmy just what he had tied himself to. Like Cynthia, James Junior looked as if butter wouldn't melt, whereas inside him was a seething cauldron of hate and viciousness. The school had regaled him with his son's other sins which had all come out after the affair with the cat had become public knowledge; from bullying to stealing, it seemed his James was capable of anything. No wonder he didn't have any real friends.

As he sat in the psychiatrist's waiting room, Jimmy looked at his son properly. He was reading a comic – always a comic never a book – and he looked unfussed about his surroundings and the reason why he was even here.

Most people here at the clinic looked like throwbacks from the sixties, all long hair and abundant moustaches. The rest were the opposite, well-tailored clothes and iron-grey hair, their countenances unreadable and their eyes cold and appraising. Not the most auspicious beginnings for the saving of this son of his.

A young girl sat opposite them. She looked to be about fourteen, with dyed hair and make-up. She smiled at him as he caught her eye and said, as if in answer to a question, 'I'm old enough to come on me own. Anyway, me mum's never up in time.' She shrugged as if this was a normal, everyday conversation.

Jimmy looked at her, wondering how the hell he had ended up in a place like this. He had been brought up in a nice home by nice people, and he had been happy in his job – the job which had displeased Cynthia because it had not provided enough for her and what she wanted from life. When she had chosen him – and he made no bones about it, *she* had set her cap at *him* and she had got him – he had envisaged a lovely life like his own parents had, a nice, secure kind of life. Holidays every year, and a couple of nice, normal kids.

Instead, he had become a criminal. He had been sucked into a world he would never understand although, in fairness, he sometimes quite liked. It was glamorous at times and it was lucrative. Once Cynthia had realised he would never run the company he worked for the rot had set in, and she was not a woman to compromise from what she wanted.

He wiped a hand over his face. He needed a line but he guessed this was not the place to have one. He knew he had a problem with the coke but it made him feel invincible, made him believe that he was living a good life. At least these days he got acceptance, if not respect, from his wife. She didn't go on at

161

him like she used to and, now she had her own 'career' as she referred to it, they were financially better off than they could have ever hoped to be. In a way he wished she had never been invited back into the fold; after her attempts to bring the family down, his life had been much easier. She had needed him then, she had needed what he could offer her.

Now she was like a phoenix risen from the ashes; she had all but become the main person in the businesses. He knew that Jonny liked her and her acumen. He said she was perfect for their world – she looked like an angel and thought like the devil, a simile that had made Jimmy shudder inwardly. It summed his wife up perfectly, and it also summed up his son.

When they were finally taken into the office and introduced to Dr Wendell, Jimmy started to relax. She looked like someone's nan, not at all as intimidating as he had expected.

After a few preliminary questions she looked into young James's face and said seriously, 'Why did you cut the kitten's throat, James?'

To which he answered truthfully, 'I don't fucking know, do I? That's why I was sent here.'

It was obvious to everyone in the room that the boy thought there was a moron among them and it certainly wasn't him.

Chapter Forty-Eight

Gabby was watching Vincent from inside the Golden Egg Cafe as he walked in to meet her. He looked very handsome and a little bit vulnerable. It was their third date and, thanks to her brother, she was now well and truly dispatched back to her nana and granddad's house – her mum didn't seem to want anything to do with either of them now. Though she hated what little James had done, she couldn't help but take advantage of the situation it had left them in.

Gabby liked Vincent even more when he wasn't trying to impress her, when he wasn't trying to act older than he was and more knowing. Inside, she knew he was as bewildered as she was about the feelings they had for each other. She had never felt like this before in her life. Never had she felt a pull from the gut like she did when she saw him walking towards her. It was almost primitive, and she instinctively knew that this was real love, not kids playing about at grown-up feelings and emotions. As young as they were, they were both completely sure that they were destined to be together. It wasn't something they had ever really discussed – it just was.

Vincent was dressed well – he always dressed like a man. At weekends he was suited and booted; like all his contemporaries he knew the value of a decent bit of clobber. She tried to dress for him now with longer skirts, tailored jackets, decent high heels. One good thing about it all was her mother had stopped frowning at her these days, believing it was *her* good taste that

163

had made her daughter opt for more conservative clothing. Good job she didn't know it was because she wanted to look older, more sophisticated, more adult and that meant not looking like Madonna or Cyndi Lauper. It meant looking like a grown woman should look. Clean, fresh and well appointed. She had read that in a magazine and it had become her mantra.

As Vincent O'Casey spotted Gabby sitting in the Golden Egg waiting for him, his heart soared with love and, he admitted, a great deal of lust. But this was Jonny P's niece and he was ever aware of that. This was also the daughter of Cynthia Tailor, a legend in her own lunchtime, and he was acutely aware of that too.

That aside, he loved this girl with all his being. At seventeen, and Gabby not yet fourteen, he knew he was playing with fire. But she was like a woman, a woman beyond her years, for all her schoolgirl chatter and smoking. She knew instinctively what he needed and she provided it for him. He knew that was rare in a couple and that what they had was special.

Vincent understood the loneliness Gabby felt inside, knew that her mother was the bane of her life, and everyone else's for that matter – his included. Because if Cynthia Tailor ever found out about him he knew he would be warned off, and not in a polite way either. He would get the kicking of a lifetime, which was why they were meeting so out of the way of their usual haunts. It was also why he was cultivating the friendship of certain young men who could give him an in to the kind of life he wanted to be a part of. If he could get some respect – and not just as a little local hard nut, but as an earner – Vincent knew it would sweeten the pot where her family was concerned. He had plans and he had dreams, and he was determined to see that they were fulfilled at some point in his life. Because this girl was going to be the mother of his children and that, he knew, was a fact.

As he walked over to the table, he saw the love shining out

of her eyes and, like many a man before him, he believed that would be enough for them. He was still too young to know that determination was only the half of it. It was the hard graft that was the really difficult part. Life was like that, he would find out much too late. It let you think you had the upper hand when all along it knew you were heading for disaster.

For the moment, anything seemed possible. They were happy just to be together, and that was more than enough for them.

Chapter Forty-Nine

Jonny Parker had spent a not entirely disagreeable afternoon with Cynthia, and was now on his way to visit one of his clubs. It was a very worthwhile enterprise which housed sixty different lap dancers over a two-week period. The girls were young, ultra fit and up for literally anything. Just the kind of girls needed for the West End of London. Even better, they were all well within the legal age, and had a vested interest in staying at that particular club. Jonny paid them *very* well, and they were in a position to meet men of all classes and colours who had one thing in common – serious amounts of dosh. Wonga was the girls' god, and they got it by the thankful. The men were vetted and they were, for one reason or another, interested in privacy more than the girls themselves.

A private club was a boon in many respects, because it afforded a level of safety that many of the men concerned needed in their daily lives – their work lives – and particularly in their night lives. Jonny had them all – from top businessmen to politicians and Old Bill to serious Faces, and he made sure any sojourn at the club was as secret as it was enjoyable. There was a lot of money in keeping people clean; he had tapped into a market that was not just lucrative money-wise but also gave him contacts who owed him.

This club was the first of many, and he was in negotiations to do the same thing in Liverpool, Manchester and Glasgow. The girls earned too much to open their traps, and they were also aware that one wrong word and they would never work anywhere again. This wasn't just a threat that they would be black-balled as such, but that their lives would be tragically cut short. No kiss-and-tell from *his* lap dancers. If they did, it would be the last thing they ever said and they were well aware of that.

Tonight hc had a meeting with a local up-and-coming Face by the name of Derek Greene. Derek was also known as 'Derek the Red' because he had no trouble spilling blood. He was thirty-one years old, built like the proverbial brick shithouse and had been educated at a private school thanks to his father, a notorious bank robber who thought his son should grow up in the straight world. Derek Senior was now doing a twenty-five, and his son, then seventeen, had been left penniless and with no real qualifications except his extreme strength, his short temper and the nous that living around a villain had ingrained into him. He had risen in the ranks and become a man to be reckoned with.

Now he wanted a meet, and Jonny was very interested in what he had to say. The boy had a good rep, and he liked him. Always open for a bit of naughty, he was happy enough as he walked into the dim foyer of the Madison Avenue Private Members Club. It was a great space and it looked fantastic – understated and with an abundance of glass and chrome. No one looking inside would believe what its respectable façade hid. It could be the offices of a banking corporation, but once through the heavy wooden doors it was the epitome of sexual gratification. All reds, purples and creams, the girls' outfits, albeit very small, were colour-coordinated to match the surroundings that were reminiscent of a brothel the Pre-Raphaelites would have frequented. It was upmarket trash, and it was making Jonny untold money.

It was quiet now, though. Early evening just had the serious drinkers in, the ones who needed the Dutch courage to actually approach the girls, and a few of the local Faces ready to have a meet in more luxurious surroundings than their local boozers, where everything they said was overheard and repeated. The club was for people who had an agenda, and that agenda was wholly their own.

Jonny spied young Derek sitting alone and smiled to himself; the boy was learning the art of confidence. Never discuss business in front of anyone who might have an interest in it, either for themselves or other people. It was a good rule to live by and he liked that the younger man had appreciated his need for privacy in all in his dealings.

He motioned for a bottle of Scotch and two glasses and, when the drinks were poured and the ice was clinking amiably, they began their meeting.

'So, young Derek, what can I do you for?'

Derek smiled, his huge face handsome in a dangerous kind of way. Jonny knew certain women would be attracted to it because looking at Derek you could tell this was a man capable of great cruelty and there were women who admired that.

'Nice set up, Mr Parker, really fucking impressive.'

It was said with genuine approval and Jonny felt himself relax. He liked this kid, though, in reality, he wasn't a kid, he was a large and very dangerous man. 'Glad you approve, Derek. And how goes your businesses? I hear tell you're knocking over more banks than the Luftwaffe.'

Derek grinned. 'Not too bad a business as it goes, Mr Parker. With my old man it stands to reason I would know the general economics of such an industry.'

They both laughed at his choice of words.

'True. I hear your little ones are well too.'

Derek almost blushed then; it was true what Jonny had heard – this was a family man beyond excellence. He had a lovely wife and three little ones, all daughters, who he doted on with a passion. The youngest had been born brain-damaged and it was rumoured that he had moved heaven and earth and serious amounts of poke to make sure she got the best treatment on offer. This was not seen as a weakness by the men in their world, but as a strength. You looked after your own before and above anyone else. It was another reason that Jonny felt he could work with the lad. He was decent and kind when appropriate, and a ruthless fucker when required. A lethal but necessary combination in a business partner.

Jonny hoped that the lad had a good proposition for him, one that would make it worth his while to take an interest in this fellow, because he would rather have him where he could keep an eye on him. There wasn't that much difference in their ages but, whereas Jonny had his creds, this boy was still paving the way for his own. If it was a bollocks proposition he would make a point of giving him a bit of collar – nothing too important but enough to give him a good earn. That way he could keep him close.

'So, back to where we began, what can I do for you?'

Derek smiled and it changed his whole face, he looked almost affable. 'It's holiday villas. Spain, Portugal, Florida. All above board and legal, and none of it really exists, at least it only does on paper. You need do fuck-all except advance me a few quid, and there is minimal risk as the businesses are owned off-shore by private investors. I have the people to sell, I have the wherewithal to get the relevant paperwork to make us kosher. I also know that, when we have enough poke, we shut down and start up again somewhere else. The Spanish are good like that; you can rip off anyone, as long as you have the relevant paperwork. I have the land, I own the fucking land and, one day, I will build on it, but no villas or apartment blocks naturally. It would take the average Joe twenty years of his life to follow the paper trails and, when they find the end of that particular rainbow, we will all be long gone.' He sat back in his seat and sipped delicately at his Scotch and water.

'Can I see an outline?'

'I had it biked to your offices this morning. I have also taken the liberty of enclosing a share scheme showing you exactly how much your investment will bring you on return, depending on your initial outlay, of course. You have my word that I am in this in a serious capacity and just want us all to earn a good crust, and walk away with the minimum of fuss.'

Jonny Parker liked this kid more and more. He had some initiative and didn't sit there with his plans in his hands explaining it all in an hour. He had biked the details over and now Jonny could peruse them at his leisure. He had made a good judgement call on this Derek Greene, and he was pleased.

'Fair enough, Derek, I'll look them over and I'll speak to you soon. Now, how's your old man?'

Derek shrugged. 'Truth is, Mr Parker, fifteen years behind the door takes its toll on a man but, all in all, he's doing OK. He's happy enough with his lot, swallowed his knob, can't do anything else, can he? We all visit. Me mum's waited, bless her heart. She spent the best years of her life travelling all over the fucking country. But she's a good old bird, and she deserves to see him home at some point. Brief reckons another two, three years, he'll be back in the bosom of his family.'

'Fucking harsh the sentences handed down. Fucking rapist would have been out now.'

'At least then he would have had a unit where he could wander about and watch telly in his cell. Fucking nonces and their VPUs. Vulnerable Prisoners Units – have you ever heard the fucking like? 'Course they're vulnerable, who wouldn't want to kick their fucking heads in?'

They both nodded, pondering the futility of a legal system that protected the scum of society, and locked away men like Derek's father for the duration. It was a fucking melon scratcher all right.

Chapter Fifty

'Go away, you weirdo.'

Cynthia Tailor rolled her eyes at the ceiling as she bellowed, 'Stop calling your brother a weirdo!'

Gabby grinned. 'But he is, Mum. Even his shrink thinks so.'

Cynthia wanted to laugh then; Gabriella was funny when she wanted to be.

James Junior looked around the table at his family silently. He was a large lad, and he had the look of his father's family. Staring at his sister, he smiled sneakily. 'How's Vincent O'Casey, Gabby?'

Cynthia looked at her son in shock, and he laughed at her as he said, 'Didn't you know, Mum? It's the romance of the century by all accounts.'

Cynthia looked at this son of hers that she was finding it increasingly difficult to like and said coldly, 'Not Bridie O'Casey's Vincent?'

Gabby thought she was going to faint with fright at her mother's words, and her eyes pleaded with her brother to not do this.

He grinned nastily as he said loudly, 'The very same.'

Gabby was out of her chair in a second, screaming at her brother, 'You cat-killing ponce! You rotten little bugger!'

Cynthia looked at her two children and wondered which one to slap first. Her instincts won and she knocked her son off his chair with a sideswipe. 'Get out of my sight, you.' Then, when

171

he had scrambled up off the floor and fled the scene of his crime, she turned to her daughter and said quietly, 'Is this true?'

Gabby knew it was pointless denying it, and so she nodded her head slowly.

When her mother's hand shot out and grabbed her hair she stifled a scream, knowing it was best to take whatever she dished out as quietly as possible. Begging annoyed her, as did screaming in agony, trying to escape, and attempting to talk your way out of things. Once her mother had you by the hair, you were all but finished.

'How long? How long have you been going behind my back?' This was her mother all over, not 'how long have you been seeing him' but 'how long have you been going behind my back'.

'A while, nearly a year . . .' Gabby had to be honest now she'd been caught; it was the only way out for her. If she lied now she was as good as dead. Her mother was not a woman to buy lies of any description. Once sussed out, all that you had left to redeem yourself in any way was the truth.

Cynthia screwed up her face in complete and utter amazement. A year! This had been going on for a *year*, and no one had guessed? No one had told her more like. The bastards. An O'Casey – a family so low down on the social stratum they might as well be fucking cavemen. Bridie O'Casey was a lazy, feckless trollop who couldn't even keep her kids clean, let alone her home. And the father! Paddy O'Casey, the local drunkard. It was beyond her comprehension.

'All I've done for you kids, and this is how you repay me? Your brother up there on the road to becoming a fucking serial killer and you well on your way to whoring! Well, lady, this stops here. You're coming home for good. No wonder you're always round your nana's! I bet she's encouraging him, fucking vicious old bag that she is . . .'

She punched her daughter in the mouth, sending her reeling

across the room. Gabby landed on the floor by the dining-room door, and it was as if Cynthia was seeing her properly for the first time in years. The long, shapely legs, the high breasts, the tiny waist. This was a woman in the making and, if her boyfriend had seen his way fit to helping her along the road, she would kill the fucker with her bare hands.

Terrified, Gabby pulled herself up off the floor. She knew from experience that this was now about damage limitation. Taking a deep breath she said in her most humble voice, 'I'm sorry, Mum, I should have told you, but I knew how you would react . . .'

Cynthia was shaking her head at the two-faced skulduggery of this daughter of hers. 'A fucking O'Casey? Is that your fucking limit? Barbie's Ken has got more brains than him! The whole family is a bit touched. And you are going out with him! You shouldn't be out with *any* boys, you're too young.'

The slap was resounding, and Gabby felt the fury coming out of her mother's pores. She also felt her own anger mounting; she would not give him up no matter what her mother said.

'Who's next, Benny fucking Hill? You stupid little mare, you better not have been doing something you shouldn't! If he's mounted you I'll cut his fucking throat.'

Even Cynthia in her rage could see the absolute shock on her daughter's face at the suggestion and thanked the powers-that-be that at least the girl hadn't gone that far. But she could also see that her daughter had no intention of giving this idiot up, and that was what was really upsetting her. She would make sure this family of hers would not go to the bad, and would not show her up.

Such was the thinking of Cynthia Tailor.

Chapter Fifty-One

Mary and Jack Callahan listened to their granddaughter, Mary with a sympathy that belied the fact she agreed, in part, with Cynthia's take on this state of affairs. Gabby was well and truly older than her years in looks, but not in any emotional capacity. She was all legs and make-up at the moment, and that was to be expected at her age. What the girl couldn't see was that a few choice words on Vincent's part, and her life as she knew it could be over and she'd be left holding a baby. Mary had never thought she would agree with that mad bitch of a daughter of hers, but on this she was right behind her. The boy was too old and too knowing by half. He was also too good-looking for his own good.

It would do Gabby good to go home for a while. In all honesty, since the episode with the kitten, Mary didn't want the lad here either. He was a strange boy, with his vicious trouble-making and she pondered long and hard at how he had become so callous without her or anyone noticing. She supposed that was the way of the world these days. TV was to blame in her opinion. It made children adults before they were ready – even the soap operas were full of sex and violence, and the kids watched them as avidly as she did herself. Though, at least she was scandalised by what she saw. Mary closed her eyes; she felt very tired suddenly and her granddaughter's voice was going through her head like a ninety-pound hammer.

'Well, you should have thought of all this, Gabby, when you were sneaking around meeting that lad.'

'But it's so unfair, Nana, my mum is the . . .'

'Don't say it, Gabby, she's still your mother.'

'I hate her, I hate her guts.'

Jack heard his granddaughter ranting and raving about her mother, his daughter, and he felt a terrible urge to join in with her. But he didn't. How they had come to this state of affairs he didn't know, all he knew was it was Cynthia's fault. Everything she touched she destroyed. Her own children included.

Chapter Fifty-Two

Derek Greene was a happy man. He had had the go ahead from Jonny P, and he knew his future was secure. He also knew that, if he played his cards right, his father's future would be secure too. He loved a bit of skulduggery, thrived on it in fact. 'Walk Like An Egyptian' by The Bangles came on Melody FM and he turned it up; he liked the beat of the record.

In the back of his car he had a small armoury, and he was delivering it to a friend in need. He was, therefore, driving within the speed limit, with his seatbelt on, and his face a mask of pure innocence. It annoyed him when people got a tug for a stupid traffic violation while endeavouring to carry out their illegal business. It was a pointless nicking and it led to far too much trouble. While he was pursuing his nefarious businesses, he acted, drove and lived by the letter of the law. Why attract unwanted attention to yourself?

Pulling up at the scrapyard in Bow, he got out of the car and stretched for a few seconds. The Bangles had been replaced by David Bowie singing 'Ashes To Ashes' and he hummed along for a few seconds before walking nonchalantly to the Portakabins that served as offices.

He liked the yard. It was a place he had played in as a kid, and it was owned by his dad's old mate Phillip Gardener, a prince among men. He had come to Derek's rescue after his father's untimely nicking, having heard about their financial position, and he had stepped in to help them out. Derek had a feeling

Phillip would have liked to help his mother out in a more personal fashion and she had knocked him back. He didn't blame the man for trying, and he respected his mother for her refusal; she was a decent old bird when all was said and done. His father had better remember that when he finally got out. Derek remembered his father had liked a bit of extra-marital interest, and that would *not* be tolerated this time round – his mother should be treated better than that. He would see she got the respect she deserved.

Phillip was a nice geezer, all bonhomie and kind nature most of the time, but he could also kick the shit out of men three times his size and he wasn't small by any standards. What Phillip had was a refusal to admit defeat, and young Derek understood that because he had a similar trait running through his veins. No matter how many times he was knocked down, he would get up again, making the opponent wonder just how long the fight would have to go on, and worrying how long they could keep up with the nutter in front of them.

Phillip watched Derek walking towards the offices and put the kettle on, he knew the lad liked a cup of tea. He drank gallons of the stuff day and night. He heard him come into the Portakabin and called out a greeting from the little cubby hole where drinks were made and hands were washed. Unhygienic, but unfortunately needs must and all that. Phillip was quite a fastidious man in his own way.

Phillip was a fixer. He fixed things for people and he had a knack of knowing how a fix should be executed. It was a very lucrative living for him and, when anyone was in a position they were not sure of, they came to him for advice – for a price of course. He was like the grave – he never discussed his own business so it was only right he never discussed anyone else's. He knew where the bodies were buried, and that meant literally as well as theoretically, so he was left alone, but was very well respected. No kids or wife had come his way – he had a large house that was looked after by his large, ugly, kind and very capable cousin, Marge. He quite liked his solitary existence, loving Belinda Greene from a distance and treating her son as his own.

The lad was a good study, and he learned quickly. He would make a good fixer himself one day, but first he had to learn the economics of this kind of work. One wrong word and the world he had so carefully constructed could tumble down on him in an instant.

Now they had a bit of work and they needed to make sure it was planned out and executed properly. Derek knew a small part of what was being undertaken, but that was all; even in his honoured position he would not get the full facts until it was deemed necessary. Phillip brought out the two teas and, as was his wont, he poured a small amount of brandy into his own mug.

Derek was sitting on the leather banquette, patiently as always, his face a study of earnest concentration. Oh, Phillip liked this kid. He was a pleasure to teach and a fine example of how a young man could be trained if under the right guidance.

'Did he swallow it?'

Derek smiled, a wide, amiable smile. 'Hook, line and fucking sinker.'

'He's a slippery cunt Jonny P, and he can smile while he cuts your nuts off, so don't let your guard down even once, you hear me?'

Derek nodded, exasperated at how careful Phillip could be at times, even as he understood why the man was chary. Jonny P was a force in his own right, but not for much longer.

'Let him stew a while, and get him onside, then we'll arrange the final meeting.'

Derek nodded his assent. 'My thoughts entirely, Phillip. Then we can meet our mutual friend and get the deal done sooner rather than later.'

'It's going to cause chaos, you know that, don't you?'

Derek nodded.

'You can walk away any time you like, son. This is a dangerous operation, and you have a young family.'

'I know, mate, but I'm in over me head now, and I feel confident we can pull it off.'

Phillip smiled, one of his rare, real smiles. 'Good lad. I knew you wouldn't let me down.'

Chapter Fifty-Three

'Well, maybe if you took more notice of him he might not be such a fucking strange one, James. If you didn't snort up that shit like there's no tomorrow . . .'

Jimmy Tailor looked at his wife and wondered as he often did what she would do if he slapped her across her lovely mouth. He never would, but it didn't stop him dreaming about it. 'Shut up, Cynth, for once in your fucking life, just shut up.'

It was evident that she was momentarily shocked at his words, but she recovered her composure in about three seconds. Her shouting could be heard all over the house and, in her bedroom, Gabby put her hands over her ears. She was sick of it, and she was sick of being held prisoner like she had done something wrong. She could hear James Junior next door, kicking the wall as loudly as possible, and wondered at how she wasn't as mental as him.

She turned her CD player up to drown out the noise of her family's madness. She lay on her bed and thought about Vincent, which was all she did these days – even her schoolwork was suffering. But he was like a obsession, growing more powerful by the day. She wondered if he would be at the school gates tomorrow? She hadn't seen him today and it had worried her. Maybe he was fed up with the situation. Who could blame him? It was all *her* fault. She couldn't bring herself to use the word mother, or mum. She was just *her* now, and Gabby hated her.

Downstairs, the shouting was reaching its crescendo.

'You! You're not a fucking man, James Tailor, you're a fucking *boy*, an innocent, a laughing stock as well!' Cynthia was in full screaming mode now, her life as she knew it was in tatters, and this idiot she had tied herself to was as much use as a handbrake on a canoe.

'He's fucking going, Cynthia. If it will help him he has to go, can't you see that?'

Cynthia was swallowing down the urge to smash this man over the head with the nearest chair. He was quite happy for their son, their child, to go into a psychiatric assessment centre, a place where he would be labelled a nut-bag, and he thought she would happily say it was OK. What fucking planet was he on? As always, her mind was not on the poor child, but on what his actions would look like to the outside world, what people would think of her.

'It's only for a few weeks, and then he'll be home, and he'll get the help he needs.'

'Over my dead body.'

'Well, from what the shrink said that's an option, Cynth. She said he's on his way to becoming a full-blown Looney Tunes. Or, in her words, he has no idea of the effect his actions have on the people around him. He is only interested in the world as it pertains to him and his wants. He cannot empathise with others, and has no understanding of the needs of others. Quote, unquote. Remind you of anyone, Cynth?'

'You ponce! Don't blame me for all this! This comes from your side, all fucking weird your family. Your mother's about as with-it as a three-legged camel.'

Jimmy sighed heavily. 'Can't you see that he has to go away, before he does anything terrible. It's for his own good as well as everyone else's. Anyway, we ain't got no say in it. If we refuse, the social workers will intervene and we'll have no control over his life at all.'

In her heart, Cynthia knew what her husband was saying was true, but it hurt her to admit that her child was 'not right', and she knew that people would blame *her*. They always blamed the mother in these cases. She felt the tears stinging her eyes and blinked them away rapidly. Why was this happening to her? What had she ever done to deserve this?

She needed to see Jonny and she needed to see him soon. He was another one – she could feel he was different, knew that all this with James Junior had pissed him off. She had gone on about it too much but, in all honesty, she couldn't see what they were up in arms about. He was ten years old, and they were labelling him already. He was highly strung that was all, and now tomorrow morning, they were supposed to take him to a child psychiatric unit in Kent and leave him there. Suddenly that didn't seem such a bad thing; with James Junior gone all she had left was Gabriella – that had to make life easier surely? He was a handful was young James and, as his father said, he would be in the best place.

She smiled grudgingly suddenly. 'If you're sure, James.'

Jimmy sighed with relief. She had finally seen sense and now the boy could get the help he so desperately needed.

He poured them both a stiff drink and, as she took hers from her husband, Cynthia was pondering how she could get rid of her daughter as well. She could do with a break; after all, she was the first to admit, she wasn't really the maternal type, and now she had her job. She would board her daughter in a good, strict school, where they would watch the little mare like a hawk. That would put a stop to her gallop, and give her the time she needed to pursue her other interests. James Junior killing that cat was like a gift from the gods really, it had turned out to have unexpected benefits. She felt a rush of excitement at having her life to herself once more, and it was very hard not to stop a wide grin from splitting her seriously concerned face.

Jimmy guessed what was really going through her mind; he

knew her better than anyone. But he didn't say a word, all he could do was make sure his son got the best treatment available and hope against hope that it worked. Being brought up by Cynthia Tailor had to have some kind of repercussions, and he had a feeling this was just the start of them for both his children. He didn't worry as much about Gabby though. She had a thick skin where her mother was concerned, and he was glad about that. She was going to need that thick skin for a while yet; she was growing up and turning into a beautiful girl and it wasn't something his wife was going to accept graciously. That Cynthia was jealous of the girl was evident – not that she would ever admit it – but Gabby was really going to be a beauty, and that was something Cynthia was going to find difficult to tolerate. It was her way or no way – how many times had he heard her say that to the kids over the years?

Well, this was the upshot of her mothering and, while he hoped that it taught her a lesson, he doubted very much that it would. Cynthia didn't care about anyone or anything enough to change her ways, and that thought, along with his kids' problems, depressed Jimmy further still. He knew he should leave, take his daughter now and go, but where? Cynthia would let them go, of that he had no doubt, but he knew that with his lifestyle and his little habit, he wasn't going to be much use to his kids. It was a cop out, but he didn't want the responsibility of those two by himself. Like his wife, he was too caught up in the world he lived in to make those kind of changes. It was a vicious circle, and every one of them was caught up in it. The kids more than any of them, because they lived at the whim of their parents, and he knew he and Cynthia were not parents anyone would choose to be lumbered with.

Still, he consoled himself with the fact he had fought her to get James Junior the help he so desperately needed, so at least he had done that much. A voice in his head was telling him it was too little, too late. But he ignored that, and left the house quick smart. Cynthia could do the boy's packing – she was better at things like that than he was.

An hour later he was coked out of his nut, and working on long columns of figures. Only numbers made any sense to him these days, and he lost himself in them like a drowning man grabbing on to a lifeboat.

Chapter Fifty-Four

Vincent O'Casey was waiting for Gabby outside the school gates the next morning and, seeing him, her heart rose in her chest.

'How's everything?' He genuinely cared, and that meant so much to her.

'I'm on me own today because me mum has to take me brother to some kind of kids' looney bin in Kent. I'll skip school, shall I? We can go somewhere and be together.'

Vincent knew he should refuse, but he missed her. Never had he felt like this about a girl before. Gabby was under his skin and, with the certainty of young love, he knew she always would be. She came from a dangerous family, and he was nervous about that, but it was her, Gabby, who filled his days and his nights. If he was honest, she was like a virus infecting every part of him, and he knew that she felt the same about him.

'I've got a motor round the corner, borrowed it off me mate Petey. He's working for your uncle Jonny actually, and he might get me onboard. I'm thinking of going into the banking business.'

Gabby smiled with pride. Once settled in the rather knackered Ford Capri Ghia, Gabby lit a cigarette and said earnestly, 'What bank will you work for? Barclays?'

Vincent grinned then and said mischievously, 'Sometimes, depends what bank we'll be robbing, don't it!'

Gabby laughed, but she felt the first fingers of fear inside her belly. She forced it away; he was older than her, and he knew what he was about. It was too late for her now, he was in her blood, and nothing he did would make her feel anything other than love for him.

'What, with guns?'

He nodded as he pulled out into the traffic. ''Course. Bit pointless trying to rob a bank with a fucking lolly stick!'

'But what if you get caught?'

'I won't get caught, it's a doddle really. Now, let's drop that, shall we? Where do you want to go? Victoria Park? How about Barking Park? We can go on the boats.'

She grinned shyly. 'How about Southend? I love Southend.'

'Southend it is.'

As they picked up the A13, she was quiet for a few moments. 'I know this ain't been easy, Vince, but my mum's a tough one you know.'

Vincent laughed then. 'Fucking understatement of the year that! She's harder than most blokes. I mean, you have to admire her, don't you? She saved her sister from certain death, girl, and, from what I heard, she took out Kevin Bryant quick as anything.'

Gabby didn't answer; she had heard the stories, and they all differed in some way. She was astute enough to know that the whole truth had been scrubbed out a long time ago. She also knew her mother was capable of anything. And not in a good way. It occurred to her that maybe Vincent was with her for her family connections. She could see that her family could be a big draw to a certain kind of people. The thought saddened her, and she wondered if this man, this young boy who she loved so much, was seeing her as a way into the firm. She felt she had to say something.

'I wouldn't give stories too much credence, Vince. Me mum's got a hard side, and she don't like you. So any thoughts you've got about getting an in with her and me uncle Jonny through me won't happen. She thinks you're leading me astray.'

Vincent was serious now. 'Listen, Gabby, I've got in with a

nice little firm, and they ain't nowhere in your uncle's league, or your mother's come to that. But I can tell you this, I know I won't be welcomed with open arms by your mum and dad. I'll sit it out until you're old enough to make your own mind up, and we can tip them bollocks, OK?'

At his words, Gabby felt the sun come out for her once more. He wanted her for *herself*, she was sure of that. She laughed gently and turned up the radio; Simply Red were singing 'Remembering The First Time', and they both grinned.

'Our record, eh?'

She laughed with him, happy to be beside him, happy to forget that she was playing truant and happy to forget about her mother. Today was just for them, and they were going to enjoy it.

Chapter Fifty-Five

Jonny Parker was pleased with the villa scam. Everyone he had spoken to was of the same opinion – it was a good time for something like this. Package holidays were affordable for most people these days and Spain was booming. From Calpe to Marbella, Brits were flocking in their thousands, and they all wanted a little bit of Spain for themselves. 'The Dorm', as Benidorm was affectionately known, was kicking nine months of the year. It was cheap, and it was crowded, and that was exactly what the punters wanted.

So, as he drove to Cynthia's house, he was a happy man. It was as if he could do no wrong, and everything he touched turned into golden coins. In this case, of course, it was pesetas, but the principle was the same. He was glad they were meeting at her house; it wasn't far for him to go home from there, and he was knackered.

As he pulled up outside the door, he felt a small twinge of apprehension. Cynthia was getting more and more insistent about their 'relationship' as she called it, and he had a feeling she would soon be asking him to call time on his marriage, and that was never going to happen. But, ever the optimist, he hoped he was wrong; they still had great sex and that was basic-ally what their 'relationship' had always been about. Knowing what she was capable of still rocked his boat, and he knew that he was playing with a very dangerous adversary. That was part of the thrill. But he knew, when all was said and done, that as hard as she was, he was harder and, if necessary, he would show her that, and put the frighteners on her once and for all. He hoped it wouldn't come to that of course, but he had to watch his back.

As he walked through the door he had to smile. She had more front than Brighton, sitting on the kitchen table, legs splayed and a beatific smile on her face.

'I thought you'd never get here!'

'It's your birthday tomorrow – as if I would forget that.' He was undoing his trousers as he spoke and she laughed with him.

An hour earlier she had fed her husband and daughter at this very table, knowing that once they were out for the evening, she would be entertaining Jonny. James had taken Gabriella out late night shopping to get her birthday present – like she believed they were going to the pictures! – but it was sweet of James to still play the part of the caring husband. She knew that her daughter didn't want to go. Gabriella's idea of a birthday present for her mother would be a milkshake full to the brim with deadly nightshade if it had been left to her. After all, today she had found out about the boarding school; the look on her daughter's face! It was true a picture was worth a thousand words – Gabriella's face had been worth that and more.

But that was forgotten now her Jonny was inside her and, as always, for both of them, it was all they really needed. When they were together like this, it was as if the rest of the world had disappeared, and it was just them.

Unfortunately, Jimmy Tailor had only had to go as far as his mother-in-law's to collect his wife's very expensive Rolex watch. Jack had got it for him cheap and, having spotted Jonny's car outside, as he and Gabby walked back through the front door, he expected to see Jonny Parker in his front room sipping a drink. But, strangely, it was in darkness. Moving through to the kitchen, his daughter by his side, Jimmy instead walked into a scene he would never in a million years have envisaged.

189

Even in his own distress, he still knew he should remove his daughter from the kitchen and get her away from what was happening on his kitchen table. The table where an hour earlier they had all eaten together like a normal family, like a real family. As if that had any truth in it. But, instead, he grabbed his wife's hair and dragged her off the table, and on to the floor.

He could hear screaming, but was that Cynthia or was it Gabby?

It was all happening so fast.

Chapter Fifty-Six

'Calm down, child, and tell me what's happened. Is it James Junior? Has something happened to him?'

'It's me dad, he's attacked me mum . . . You've got to come, Granddad.' Gabby was imploring Jack with her eyes while her nana tried to get some sense out of her.

'Me mum was on the table with . . . Me dad's gone berserk.'

Suddenly her words hit home and her grandparents both groaned as if in pain.

'Jesus Christ, what was she thinking! In her own home, the fucking whore.' Jack Callahan was fuming. 'I knew this would happen one day! I knew it. I warned her about being so brazen, I only wish I'd talked to him too. But you know Jonny Parker, no talking to *him*, is there? Too high and mighty for the likes of us . . .'

'Will you shut up, Jack!' hissed Mary.

It was only then he remembered that Celeste was there too, and she was looking at them as if they had all miraculously appeared before her in a vision.

Gabby looked from one to the other, and realised just how far-reaching the repercussions of her mother's actions would be. She had stopped herself saying Jonny's name, because her aunt had enough on her plate as it was. This was the night Celeste came round here for her dinner, and what her nana referred to as a 'catch up'. Now it was out, and Gabby felt it was her fault, but she had not known where else to go.

191

Her father had been like a maniac and, when she had left, her uncle Jonny was beating down on her dad in order to get him away from her mum. It was like a nightmare, only she was wide awake and it was really happening, and her dad would never be the same again. She had seen and heard the hurt inside him. The strange thing was, he seemed more upset with her uncle Jonny. And her uncle Jonny she could tell was ashamed, ashamed and frightened. But then so he should be, he had done the dirty on them all. She hated him now just as much as she did her mother. They were both of a kind, both selfish, both believing that the world was only there for *them* and what *they* wanted.

Celeste was in her nana's arms now, and she followed her granddad out of the house, wondering what this night would bring them all, and aware that it wouldn't be anything good, that much was for sure. It never was with her mother. She was sending *her* away to school in the middle of nowhere so she couldn't be with Vincent, and all the time *she* was having an affair with her uncle Jonny!

Gabby still couldn't believe what she had seen, still couldn't get over her father's reaction. Her poor dad, her poor, poor dad. She was crying again, and she hoped that her mum was dead on the floor when they got back home. She wanted her dead so badly. If she died she couldn't hurt them any more.

Even James Junior might be in with a chance if *she* was gone, because her mother infected everyone and everything around her, and she destroyed anyone who stood in her way, just as she beat down anyone who disagreed with her.

Gabby hated her, even more than before if that was possible. Her mother had more or less called her a whore today, smugly telling her she was going away to school, where there would be no boys. Well, she herself would know what a whore was – no one could know better. In fact, she was worse than a whore, because she had done the dirty on her own sister, and that was something only the lowest of the low could be capable of.

Gabby hoped her dad killed her, she hoped he had killed them both. They deserved it, the pair of them.

Chapter Fifty-Seven

'Oh, shut up, Cynthia. Shut the fuck up!' Jack Callahan was disgusted with them, both Cynthia and Jonny, and it showed. He looked at his son-in-law and, sneering, he said, 'Where's Jimmy gone?'

Jonny had the grace to look shamefaced and that placated Jack a little bit. Even his son-in-law's fearsome reputation wasn't cutting any ice with him this night. He thought these two before him were lower than the lowest, they were carrion to him now. If he never saw either of them again it would be too soon.

'I don't know, Dad.'

'Don't you call me "Dad", you fucking slag! After this night is over I never want to see your face again. All this time you were fucking him did you think of your sister?' He looked pointedly at Jonny then. 'That's my daughter Celeste, your fucking wife, in case you forgot her name. Did either of you think about that poor girl, eh? Between you you've sent her off her chump, but then you sent your little James off his head and all, didn't you, Cynthia? Quite a track record you've got now. Well, you better find your husband. Who knows what he's capable of in his state of mind! He might be sitting with Lily Law bringing you down. Funny what a man's capable of when he's been fucked over by his mate and his wife.'

Jonny Parker was looking around him as if he was drunk; he felt as if he was in a stupor. 'Does Celeste . . .'

194

'Oh, she knows, Jonny. You'll have a job talking her round after this little debacle.'

Jonny Parker felt physically sick at what he had caused. Looking at Cynthia now, her eye black, dried blood on her face from her husband's fists and boots, the ferocity of the attack was what had shocked him more than anything. Jimmy was a big man, and he had shown that he wasn't as docile as his wife had believed. He had even given Jonny a few good thumps before he had left the house, his car roaring off like something from the Grand Prix.

But it was young Gabby who really made him see what damage they had caused. Her eyes were on him and, if hate had been a tangible thing, he would have been knocked to the floor by now. And Celeste! His Celeste! She knew!

'Celeste . . . Is she still at yours, Jack?'

'If you mean does she know *everything*, yes, she does. Now maybe she'll get away from you and start living her life. As for you, Cynthia, you keep away from her. She thought the world of you, always did.' He looked at his elder daughter then, before saying, 'I hope you never know another happy day, Cynth. I hope you stew in your own hate and your own greed. You wanted what she had. Couldn't stand it, could you, that she got him, and you got poor Jimmy. Well, you're welcome to each other now, because I'm finished with you, lady. Finished with the pair of you.' With that he walked out of the house.

Cynthia was quiet as she watched her father walk away from her. Then, turning to Jonny, she said defiantly, 'I'm glad it's come out, now we can be together . . .'

Jonny was looking at her in utter amazement now. 'What the fuck are you on about, you silly bitch? Glad it's come out! Are you off your fucking trolley? If you were the only woman left in the world, I wouldn't have you now. Can't you see what *we've* done? What *we've* caused? I love Celeste, I always will. I couldn't love you . . . No one could. Face it, Cynth, you're a lot of things, girl, but lovable ain't one of them.' He looked at the woman who had been like an itch to him for so long, and was pleased to see that it was one itch that had well and truly been scratched raw. 'I need to find Jimmy, and make sure he doesn't do what your father suggested. But first I need to see my wife, and try and repair some of the damage I've done to her.' He looked at Gabby. 'Look after your mum . . .'

Gabby laughed, and she looked years older than fourteen as she said, '*You* look after her. As far as I'm concerned me granddad has the right idea, she's dead to me and all.'

She left the house, and ran to catch up with her granddad who, putting his arm around her, said sadly, 'I shouldn't have left you there, Gabby; I'm not thinking right tonight.'

She slipped her hand into his, and together they walked back to her nana's in silence.

Chapter Fifty-Eight

'Did you know about all this, Mum?'

Mary Callahan looked at this lovely daughter of hers and decided that only the truth would suffice now. 'Everyone knew, I think. But how could we interfere, lovie? I kept hoping it would burn itself out . . .'

Celeste nodded; inside her brain somewhere she realised she had known too – not about Cynthia, but she had always known there was someone else. Jonny wasn't a man to go without anything he wanted, it was what had attracted her to him and, if it hadn't been for that night when Kevin Bryant had come gunning for her, she knew instinctively that none of this with Cynthia would ever have happened. That night had changed them all somehow, her more than any of them. For Cynthia it had been her re-entry into the world she loved, the world Celeste had only ever really tolerated. But she had loved her sister so much, had felt so grateful to her, and all the while she had been sleeping with her husband.

Celeste felt the bile rising up inside her, wondering how many times he had slipped into their bed and held her, when earlier he had been holding her sister. Touching Cynthia, tasting her. It was sickening. She was actually heaving now, and her mother led her into the toilet, and held her daughter's head as she brought up everything she had eaten and drunk over the last twenty-four hours.

Mary Callahan knew that if she had her elder daughter in

197

front of her now she would take her out without a moment's hesitation. Cynthia had always been trouble and she knew she had always been jealous of this sister of hers despite the fact that Celeste was a watered-down version of her in every respect. Where Cynthia was beautiful, Celeste was pretty; where Cynthia had the body of an Amazon, Celeste, bless her, was only half the woman her sister had ever been. Yet, where it really counted, Celeste was worth a hundred of Cynthia, a thousand of her, because Celeste was a good girl, a decent, kind girl.

She rued the day Jonny Parker had met both her daughters. He had brought them nothing but trouble and heartache.

Chapter Fifty-Nine

Left alone after Gabby had followed Jack, Jonny Parker looked at Cynthia and it was as if he was really seeing her for the first time ever. She looked awful, and he could see the lines around her eyes and mouth, see the bitterness and ugliness that was inside her. He shook his head and turned to go.

'You're not walking away from me, Jonny. No one walks away from me,' Cynthia spat. Even now, after all this, she still couldn't bow her head in shame and hold her hand up to what they had done.

'No one walks away from you! Who the fuck do you think you are?'

'I'm the woman who took out fucking Bryant, that's who I am, mate – and don't you ever forget it.'

Jonny grinned. 'Who the fuck cares, eh? Can't you just once in your miserable life admit to being in the wrong? I would give anything for this not to have happened. My Celeste is everything to me and between us we've destroyed her. Could you honestly see her dragged down even further?'

Cynthia nodded, and said with her usual arrogant honesty, 'Yeah, why not? Pity is no basis for a marriage. You need a woman who is as strong as you, you need a woman who knows the score . . .'

Jonny looked at her for long moments before saying, 'You're off your fucking head if you think I would ever contemplate throwing my hat in the ring for you. Celeste means the world to me, and I thought you were sensible enough to know that. I have fucked you for years, but that's it, Cynth. We *fucked*. If Celeste outs me, and I wouldn't blame her if she did, I still wouldn't want you and all you entail.'

That was when she attacked him, when he knew the sooner he got away from her, and sorted out his life, the better it would be for them all.

Her strength was no match for his and, violently shoving her away from him, he said, 'Now I'm going to my wife, and I hope to Christ she forgives me, Cynthia, because until now I never realised just how much I needed her, how much she meant to me.'

Cynthia heard the front door close behind him and then she finally cried. She knew that her Jonny, her Jonny Parker, was gone from her for good. Other than herself, he was the only person she had ever cared about in her whole life. Jonny Parker was her true mate, her perfect match, and she had believed, in her heart of hearts, that he felt the same as she did.

Looking around her at the ruin that had been her kitchen, she experienced for the first time ever a feeling of loss – deep, emotional loss – and she was surprised at how badly it was affecting her. She knew that her old life was over, that from now on she would be alone, and that frightened her. But she also understood that it was somehow her own doing.

All her life she had taken whatever she wanted, without a real thought for the consequences. Now, though, she knew that her mother's words were true. Everything in life had to be paid for, and mostly it was paid for with bitter tears. She had never believed that those words could ever be used in conjunction with her, but she saw now how true they were. And, for the first time ever, she cried those bitter tears.

Chapter Sixty

Jimmy was drunker than he had ever been before and, to make things worse, he realised he had run out of gear. He searched his car until he found half a gram under the driver's seat mat. He snorted it straight from the wrap, and felt the tingling in his nose which told him it was good stuff. He laughed pitifully to himself. Then he took another long pull on the bottle of vodka. It was nearly empty.

He staggered out of the car, and the smell of his vomit hit him; he remembered vaguely throwing up earlier. He realised now he had knelt in his own vomit and felt the urge to throw up once again.

He looked around him then, and saw the lights of London twinkling everywhere. He was at the top of a multi-storey car park, and he felt the breeze as it brushed gently against him. His gaze drifted to the night sky, and he saw the Plough. He remembered his dad teaching him about the stars on a camping trip to France. He smiled at the memory. He had been lucky in that anyway – he had had a good childhood, not like his poor kids, dragged up by that cunt he had married.

Why had he stayed? He knew why really. Somewhere deep down he had always loved her, had hoped that inside her there was a nice person trying to escape. The last few years had been bearable. She had seemed happier, but now he knew the reason for that; she was trumping dear old Jonny Parker. Mate, family friend, brother-in-law and two-faced piece of shit. On his table where they ate their dinner every night, for Christ's sakes.

He heaved again at the thought. How often had they fucked on that table? Her calmly feeding them, knowing what she had done. She was beyond being a whore even – at least they didn't pretend to be other than they were. What she had done was so outrageous it was unbelievable. And the worst of it was the fact he had never even suspected anything, so what did that make him? Did they laugh at him behind his back? Did they joke about what a fucking fool he was? He had trusted them – well, Jonny; he had trusted Jonny.

He could hear music floating on the wind, and he strained to hear the song, he knew the melody, and then it came to him. Eddy Grant singing 'Baby, Come Back'. The irony was not lost on him, and he grinned then. He hated her now, really hated her for what she had done to him. Done to them all. Poor Celeste – she was not good at the best of times. Now she would have to deal with all this. He wondered if Mary and Jack had known about it all along. In fact, did everyone know, except him? He felt the shame burning through him as he thought of the people he knew, all of them aware he was being cuckolded, and not by just anyone, but by the most dangerous man in London.

Jimmy looked over the edge of the concrete barrier. The ground was a long way away. It was funny really – all this time he had believed he was a man, if not of renown, at least to be respected. But it seemed he had been wrong about that, as he had been about so many things.

He was sitting on the barrier now and, sighing deeply, he dropped off the side. His last thought as he plummeted was whether or not his son was actually his child.

He hoped not.

Chapter Sixty-One

'You happy now, Mum? He's dead, me dad's dead.'

Gabby was in tears, weeping silently. She felt as if her heart had been ripped from her body, and the only thing inside her was this deep, dark sorrow. She had loved her dad. He had been good to her, and he had loved her, genuinely loved her. Now he was gone. He had killed himself because of her mother, her mother who had never cared for anyone or anybody in her whole life except herself.

'Get your stuff, Gabriella, you're coming home with me.'

Mary Callahan looked at her elder daughter and wondered for the thousandth time how she had ever bred this excuse for a woman.

'Get yourself away, Cynth, you're not welcome here any more.'

'I want my daughter, Mum.'

'Well, you can't have her. She doesn't want to go with you.'

Cynthia looked at the woman who had borne her, and who she had loved and hated throughout her life, and she said snidely, 'Well, we'll have to see about that, won't we?'

Shutting the door in her daughter's face, Mary said sadly, 'Yes, Cynthia, I suppose we will.'

She put her arm around her granddaughter then and, hugging her, she said kindly, 'Come on, lovie, I'll make us a hot chocolate.'

'I ain't got to go back there, Nana, have I?'

Mary sighed heavily, then said in all honesty, 'I hope not, Gabby. I hope not.'

Jack Callahan was sitting drinking his beer; the telly was off, and the room was quieter than Gabby had ever experienced before. It was as if the events of the last few days had wiped out every bit of their energy and their happiness. Her auntie Celeste was back at home with her husband; he had, as always, talked her round. Jonny was sorry, there was no doubt about that, but her dad was dead because of him, and that wasn't something that could be forgotten overnight. She would never forgive either of them. Her dad had been one of the few people who had ever really cared for her, and she wished now, more than anything, that she had told him just how much he had meant to her. Now her mother was determined to get her back home, and had not shown even the slightest remorse at her husband's suicide, or acknowledged that she was the cause of it. As always it was about her mother, not anyone else. Her granddad and nana had aged before her eyes, and even James Junior was out of the picture. It felt as if her family had been dismembered, and she didn't know how to cope with it all.

The only bright spot was Vincent; he had been fantastic. Her granddad said he could come to the house, and that was wonderful. Just being near him, and feeling his love for her, was enough to make her feel she might, just might, get through all this heartache one day.

Her mum was bad, toxic – she destroyed everything she touched, and she didn't care who she hurt in her quest to get what she wanted. Gabby knew that she had been trying to get her uncle Jonny to go and see her. Phoning the house at all hours, until he had changed the number. It had made her nana and granddad furious. Her granddad said that it was common knowledge now, that the neighbours were having a field day. He also said that, if Jonny Parker had any sense, he would shoot Cynthia Tailor down like a rabid dog, and do them all a favour.

She agreed with her granddad about that; she would gladly shoot her mother herself.

That Jonny was back in favour didn't surprise Gabby. She understood that her grandparents had turned their back on one daughter, but that they could never do it to the other one. Celeste needed her family, and they needed her. It galled her, though, that Jonny Parker had walked away more or less scot-free – that wasn't right. He was as much to blame for her dad's death as her mother was.

Her poor dad, that he would kill himself like that! She felt the tears once more. It seemed as though her whole life had suddenly been destroyed, and she didn't know how to make it better. She would never see her dad's face again, never hear his voice. While her mother, the main cause of it all, seemed no different than usual. She was acting like her life hadn't even really been affected. Even today, she didn't look remotely bothered that her husband was dead, that he had dropped six storeys and landed on a set of metal railings. She looked like she always looked – angry, dissatisfied and bitter. It was so unfair.

Chapter Sixty-Two

Derek Greene was chatting to Vincent O'Casey, and they were getting on very well indeed. That young Vincent was seeing the teenage daughter of Cynthia Tailor was common knowledge as was the fact that he wanted an in with Derek and his crew. The boy had potential, that much was evident. He could steal almost any car to order, and he had a natural knack with engines of any kind. He would make a good driver, and that was a very important part of the bank robber's plans.

A good driver knew the roads like the back of his hands – the side streets and short cuts – and would not get flustered under pressure. Three burly blokes with sawn-off shotguns and a pile of cash, high on adrenaline, were not liable to be too kind to someone who didn't know where he was going. So a good driver was considered an asset.

From what Derek had seen and heard about this kid, he seemed like just the kind of lad they were looking for. More to the point, he had first-hand knowledge of what was going down with Jonny Parker, and that alone gave him an in where Derek Greene was concerned.

Vincent O'Casey, for his part, was only too happy to tell Derek Greene anything he wanted to know. He was flattered by the man's interest, and pleased that he had finally found himself a proper in to the world he so admired, the world he was determined to make his own one day. Jonny Parker's indiscretion with his wife's sister was the main topic of conversation around the campfires. It seemed he was not as clever as he thought and people were picking up on his skulduggery.

As far as Vincent was concerned, seeing his Gabby so torn up inside was like a physical pain to him. He loved the girl and, as young as they were, he knew in his heart that they would be together for ever.

'I hear that Jonny Parker's old woman has had him back?'

Vincent nodded. 'Yeah, she ain't all the ticket though, by all accounts. But Cynthia Tailor's out of the loop for good now. Even her own kids don't want her.'

Derek nodded sagely. 'And who could blame them? Six fucking storeys! That was not a cry for help – he was determined to top himself.'

'My thoughts entirely, Derek. It's my Gabby I feel sorry for. She's lost her dad, her brother's away in a nut-house, and her mother is about as much use as a fucking pork chop in a mosque. Her life as she knew it is over, and now she's got to try and pick up the pieces. Did I tell you her mother is having her put into care? Won't even let her go to her nana's. She's arguing that Gabby's out of control and that her grandparents aren't strong enough to cope with her.'

After shaking his head at the shocking revelation, Derek said conversationally, 'Could you find out Jonny Parker's movements next Friday for me? I have to have a meeting with him, and I could do with a heads up. On the QT, like.'

Vincent O'Casey almost swelled up physically with pride as he answered, ''Course I can, my Gabby can find that out for me.'

Derek Greene grinned then. 'I was hoping you'd say that.'

Chapter Sixty-Three

Gabriella Tailor was heartbroken; they had finally buried her father, and it had been a distressing few hours. Seeing her mother, in full make-up, her head covered with a black lace mantilla and her body encased in a figure-hugging black silk sheath dress, Gabby had felt the urge to tear her apart. *She* had played the part of the grieving widow to perfection, and it was just that – a part she played. Her whole life was an act.

Now, back at her nana's, Gabby wondered at parents in general. Her father's family had not shown, but then they never really had much to do with them anyway, her mother had seen to that. Suicide was a strange thing; people seemed ashamed of it. Some would rather see their loved ones waste away with cancer, or get killed in a car. To Gabby, suicide meant her father finally bailing out on her, once and for all.

She had felt so lonely, so vulnerable in the crematorium, unused to the strange smells and subdued chatter. Quite a few people had turned out, but the majority of them were what her nana termed 'sightseers'. People who came to tragic events out of a morbid fascination with other people's troubles. But her heart had soared when Vincent had slipped into the back pew, and the wink he had given her had lifted her troubled spirits.

Her mother, though, had stood alone, and she had wept alone. A forlorn figure, who wasn't fooling anyone who really knew what she was like. Not one person had acknowledged her, and that must have shown her what people really thought of her. Still, knowing her mother, Gabby supposed she probably didn't give a shit. Why change the habits of a lifetime?

Now she had to face the truth of the situation, because a social worker, a Miss Bellamy, was telling her grandmother that her daughter, Mrs Tailor, had signed the papers to put her daughter into care. Her nana and granddad were arguing with her, but somehow she knew there was nothing they could do – not at the moment anyway. By the sounds of it, they had to go to court and get a judge to grant a temporary custody order, and *then* they might get their granddaughter back. It wasn't a surprise to any of them; it was as if her mother had decided that if *she* couldn't have her family then *no one* could have them.

Still dazed from the events of the last few weeks, Gabby didn't have the strength to argue that she didn't want to go. Instinctively, she knew that if she caused problems with Miss Bellamy now it would affect her in the future.

She seemed a nice woman – well, girl. She looked a cliché of a social worker, all flat sandals and fat ankles. Her thick dark hair looked like a furze bush, but she had kind brown eyes, and that gave Gabby hope.

'Do I have to go?'

Miss Bellamy looked at the pretty girl with the long blond hair and blue eyes and sighed inwardly. She had not liked the mother of this child, who had seemed overly adamant that the child should not be left with her grandparents. Most parents would prefer their children with family – it was rare that they opposed that – but Mrs Cynthia Tailor had been convinced she was in no fit state to care for the child herself. Since her husband's suicide she had been on medication and suffering from depression – understandable, of course. But she had also stipulated that *her* parents were not fit role models; as well as their advanced ages, they were also supposedly drinkers, smokers and gamblers, among other more sinister things, not said but hinted at.

So, as always, these cases had to be investigated and, in the interim, the child would be taken into the care of the local authority. Just going on this initial visit though, Miss Bellamy felt the girl would be all right here. The house was clean and well kept, the couple, though old and smokers, were agile enough, and there was genuine affection between them. There was also undisguised animosity against the child's mother, and that was coming from every one of them.

That there was a brother in a secure unit also had to be taken into the equation. The mother had washed her hands of him, saying he was far too disturbed for her to deal with under the present circumstances. James Junior had had a meltdown when told about his father's death and had attacked everyone around him. And the next day he had knifed an orderly. He would not be going anywhere for a good while.

Miss Bellamy shook her head at the state of some people's lives. There was money in this family, good looks and wonderful homes, yet she wouldn't leave her dog with any of them for the day, let alone allow them to procreate. But such was life; you needed a licence to own a dog or a TV, and you were fined if you didn't have one, whereas there wasn't anything to regulate who had a child. It was scandalous really, but there was nothing she could do about any of it. Except pick up the pieces when it went wrong.

'Who would you like to stay with, Gabriella?'

Gabby smiled then. 'I'd like to stay here. I've been here for the best part of my life – I only lived at home recently.'

Mary chimed in then as if on cue, 'My daughter was never what you would call the maternal type, if you know what I mean.'

'That's an understatement, girl. A rat could do a better job of rearing its young than her.' Jack's voice was low and hard.

'She killed my dad, you know that, don't you?' Gabby added. 'He caught her with her boyfriend, my auntie's husband, her own *sister*'s husband. I was there, and they were on the kitchen table . . .'

Miss Bellamy had heard the gossip; who hadn't? It had lit up the offices for days. It was the talk of East London, and the man Mrs Tailor had been caught with was a local villain, so that just added grist to the mill. Not that there were any laws against villains having families, in fact many of the so-called villains were good parents. It was a contradiction in terms really.

'Please let me stay here.'

It was a genuine plea and, smiling, Miss Bellamy said gently, 'I'll do all I can, but you need to go through the proper channels. Can you pack a few things, Gabriella? Then we'll be on our way.'

'But I ain't long cremated my dad, I won't know anyone . . . I'm frightened, I want to stay here with my nana and granddad . . .' Gabby could hear the panic entering her voice. She didn't want to leave here, this was her home, the only home she had ever really wanted to be in. It was so unfair – once more her mother was controlling them all, even when she wasn't around she could still call the shots. Gabby ran into her grandmother's arms and Mary held her, soothing her as if she was a small child, not a growing girl.

'It won't be for long, if we cause trouble now it will go against us. Look at poor Hannah from across the road, they took all hers away because she fought with them. You do as you're told, child, and we'll have you back home quick smart. I'll let Vince know where you are, child, so don't fret.'

That was what she wanted, needed to hear and, after a little cry and a few more hugs, Gabby did as she was bidden, but with a heavy heart.

Chapter Sixty-Four

'Listen, Celeste, it was madness – I was caught up in a madness. You know what Cynthia can be like.'

Celeste still hadn't spoken to Jonny, not a word since Jimmy's funeral. It was as if she had left her body behind and gone some place no one could reach her.

'Please talk to me, love.'

She stared at him, her eyes unblinking. It was a clear, honest gaze and it made him feel even more ashamed than he already did. Celeste could do that, she could make a person feel they were in the wrong with a look, a look that was more powerful than a politician's maiden speech. He knew it was because of her and the way she lived her life. Straight as a die was his Celeste. Decent, *honourable*. He had thought he was honourable too, once. Now, with the flak coming at him from all sides, he knew that word would never be used about him again, ever.

Jimmy's death had caused him a lot of problems. Men were wary of dealing with him now. A thief was acceptable, though not a gas-meter bandit or a robber of council houses or sheltered accommodation. But an honest to goodness blagger – a bank robber – was respected for the time and effort that went into such an enterprise. Liars were never welcome. Liars were dangerous people you avoided at all costs, because eventually their lies caught up with them, and everyone around them was tarred with the same brush. Even the Bible had a section about liars, as it did about adulterers.

Many people had guessed about Jonny and his sister-in-law – the delectable but definitely off-her-rocker Cynthia – and they had not voiced their opinions, not in public anyway. After all, it *was* Jonny P they were talking about.

But Jimmy topping himself had left a bad taste with all and sundry. Suicide was not something the criminal world embraced – unless it was a grass, of course. *They* were expected to do it; it was a much easier death than if they were found by the people they had grassed. But that was beside the point. Since Jimmy's death, people had began to question Jonny P's other activities, the general consensus being if you were capable of something *that* sleazy you were capable of anything. To add fuel to the fire, there were a few new kids on the block and they were not helping by questioning the integrity of Jonny Parker.

Jonny had made many enemies on his way up the criminal ladder, and it was these people who were only too glad to see him reap what he had sown. The wives whispered about a man who could treat his wife so, a man who could happily cuckold someone who worked for him. Jimmy was now remembered as a paragon. People said that it was no wonder he had been a drunk and a cokehead with a wife like Cynthia, and her up to all sorts with her sister's husband, the man who employed him and paid his wages. That her children were now in care was the most scandalising thing of all. The boy, it was rumoured, was not all the ticket; he had killed a neighbour's cat, cut its throat of all things! The girl was supposedly a nice little thing. Now that she was in a home, some of the women speculated that Cynthia hadn't liked the competition from her daughter. The girl was a beauty and that hard-faced bitch had unloaded her like she did everyone who got in her way, her husband included. Some even hinted that it was planned, that finding them like that on the kitchen table had been deliberate.

It didn't take long for Jonny Parker's carefully garnered reputation as a good guy to be forgotten. He was now definitely deemed to have become too big for his boots or, as some of the cruder men said, he thought his shit didn't stink, and that could only cause him problems in his various enterprises.

It had shocked him as well that many of the Eastern Europeans he worked with, especially the Russians, saw what he had done as something akin to genocide. They were actively cold-shouldering him, and that was a worry in itself.

Yes, he had had an affair. So what? It wasn't his finest hour, even he admitted that, but the backlash had been astronomical. Jimmy Tailor killing himself had really sealed his fate, and he felt the weight of his guilt pressing down on him more and more each day.

Now he had the added torture of seeing Celeste, who he loved, really cared about, become, through his machinations, a shadow of her former self.

He wondered at times how the fuck he had allowed this to happen. But he knew the answer as well as the next man. He had always taken what he wanted, that was the trouble, and where that had once been seen as a strength, now it was a weakness. All he could do now was try and live it down. It was harsh and it was not going to be easy, but that was what he had to do. He had to get up and go to work as usual, look his critics in the eye and earn back his reputation little by little.

Celeste was still staring at him as he said slowly, smiling crookedly, 'I'm sorry, love. I'm so very sorry.'

She put her hand out and laid it on top of his. 'I know.'

He lowered his head and fought back the urge to cry.

Chapter Sixty-Five

Derek Greene was happy, but then he was a man with a happy disposition. He had a lovely family, a nice life, and he had a shrewd head on his rather large shoulders. Today he was happier than ever. Today was the day he finally came into his own, and he couldn't wait for the fireworks to start. It had been a long haul, but he was content enough to wait a few more days to get his bonus. And what a bonus.

Jonny Parker was champing at the bit, and that was *exactly* where Derek wanted him. Considering the man's troubles, he was conducting his business with his usual acumen and Derek had to admire that, even if he did think Jonny needed a moral compass for his dinner now and again to remind him what was acceptable behaviour and what wasn't. But that was then and this was now.

'You look happy, Del Boy.'

He grinned at his wife. 'That's because I am, my princess.'

She looked at him shrewdly; they had been together since they were thirteen and she knew him better than he knew himself. 'What you up to?' She was suspicious now; her biggest fear was that he would do something silly and get a serious lump like his father.

'Just a bit of graft, nothing too serious but a good earner. Who are you then, the police?'

She grinned back. She loved her husband with all her being, and she knew, without a shadow of a doubt, that he loved her back. Three kids, numerous stretch marks, and a boob job later, she and Derek were still together. She knew she was lucky and she appreciated her luck. She would never take him for granted – that was how you lost your man. She still ran his bath for him, and massaged his shoulders, he was a king in his domain. That was how you kept your man in his home, and stopped him from being tempted to visit someone else's. Men were like kids – when they got bored they moved on to the next game. Well, that wasn't going to happen to her and Derek; she would see to that.

'You going to be late tonight?'

He shrugged. 'Depends, love, but if I'm gonna be later than usual I'll call, OK?'

She nodded. She knew he would call, and that was enough for her.

Chapter Sixty-Six

'Come on, Linford, you know it makes sense.'

Linford Fargas grinned, but it wasn't his usual friendly grin, and Jonny knew it would be a long while before they were once more back on their old footing. Linford had worked often with Jimmy; he had liked him and had been grieved at Jimmy's demise. To kill yourself was a terrible thing, and Linford had first-hand knowledge of that as his brother had hanged himself in Brixton while on remand. It was still a sore point with him, and he believed wholeheartedly that nothing could ever be so bad that you would take your own life. Life was something precious – your own life especially. You had one crack at it and you had a duty to yourself to make that life the best it could be. He resented Jonny's part in Jimmy's death, and that resentment lingered, unspoken, between them now.

All Jonny could do was make up for what he had done by carrying on and not rocking anyone's boats.

'It's a scam, ain't it?'

Jonny nodded. He felt Linford's anger bubbling away beneath the surface. 'Yes but we can rake it in with minimal outlay, and that can only be a good thing.'

Linford shrugged. 'Sounds good. The figures look good, Jimmy said—'

He stopped himself then, and Jonny said quietly, 'Yes, Jimmy said it was a good earner. We can mention his name, you know.'

Linford shrugged again. 'I liked him, he was a good man.

But, like all good people, he didn't understand how bad the world could be.' This was the closest Linford had ever come to insulting his boss and they both knew it.

Jonny was silent for a few moments before saying earnestly, 'Look, Linford, if I could turn the clock back, don't you think I would? I lie awake at night pondering how the fuck I let her get under my skin like that. Truth be told, I never even really *liked* her. I can't explain the hold she had over me, and I know that sounds weak, and it sounds like I'm blaming her, and I'm not. After she outed Bryant, she fascinated me; she's dangerous, seriously fucking dangerous. She looks like an angel, but she's base. She fucks like an animal – it's almost primal. And I liked that. I know it sounds terrible, but I really liked that about her. She's like one of those devil dogs – you know, those fighting dogs? They can turn on you at any moment, but you still want to own one. I knew no good could come of it, but it didn't stop me. All I can say now is that my attraction to her is well and truly buried. I can't even stand the sight of her. Did you know she had the fucking audacity to turn up for work as if nothing had happened?'

Linford nodded.

'I think that was it. Her turning up at the betting shop really made me realise what I was dealing with. I know her, I know how she thinks, she is capable of anything. Literally anything. I've paid her off, what else could I do? She had to be given something, but it galled me. In my heart, I'd like to see her scrabbling in the fucking dirt, but then I can't talk, because I'm as bad as her – worse really – because I actually do genuinely love my wife. Celeste's forgiven me – well, sort of – and now I have to prove to her that she hasn't backed a loser. And I will. If it's the last thing I do, I'll make her see that the only person I will ever want is her.'

Linford believed Jonny was speaking the truth and, in a strange way, he almost understood where he was coming from.

But Linford also knew that, for all Jonny's protestations, there had also been an element of 'I want her, so I'll have her' to it as well. He had taken her because he could, and he had not cared about the consequences until they had jumped up and bitten him on the arse. *Jonny* was responsible for all this mess, because it was believed in their world that men were stronger than women. That men should have the strength to turn away from temptation, whereas women were too weak to resist.

'Well, she turned out to be a very expensive pastime, Jonny. She cost Jimmy his life, and everyone else around you two has been infected with your games. You more than anyone, because this has cost you your good name. You're the butt of jokes and the cause of idle gossip. It will die down, but it will always be there, and you have to live with that knowledge. People love nothing more than to see the mighty fall, and you have fallen a fucking long way in people's estimation.'

Jonny sighed heavily. Linford was honest, he'd give him that. Whoever said the truth hurt was a clever fucker, but he would ride this storm as he had others. Look at Kevin Bryant – he had taken that on, and it had worked for him up until the end. He would get through this, he was determined.

'Well, now we've got that out of the way, shall we get back to work? I'm meeting with the villa geezers tonight. Are you coming or not?'

Linford nodded. 'I'll be there, don't worry.'

'Good. Now what's next on the agenda?' Jonny felt depressed, but he knew what he had to do was show his face and act as if everything was normal, then eventually, in the not too distant future, it would be. At least, that's what he hoped anyway, although the way things were going, he worried it might take longer than he had first believed.

Chapter Sixty-Seven

Vincent O'Casey was thrilled to be in on his first ever piece of real skulduggery. He just hoped it all went as planned. At eighteen, he was a good-looking lad, and he had a nice way about him – not pushy, but not passive either. Anyone looking at him would know he could take care of himself if the situation demanded it. He was very respectful, called people 'Mr' when appropriate, and he had a reputation for being good with cars, and reliable into the bargain.

Derek Greene had seen his potential and, for that reason alone, he would always have young Vincent's loyalty and appreciation.

Vincent liked Derek. He was a man who was going places, but he listened to Vincent, and advised him on the many pitfalls of the criminal lifestyle. Vincent O'Casey came from a family of no-hopers – his father and brothers were nothing more than ice-cream freezers. Local geezers, thieves, sold a bit of knock-off, played the hard men to the neighbours. Talked the talk, but would need a glass to hand in a real fight. They were the kind of people that Vincent was determined *not* to be – local bully boys who thought the world began and ended on their council estate. He wanted more than that. Vincent knew he had the nous, the inborn cunning, necessary to achieve in the world he wanted to be a part of. Now he had a champion of sorts in Derek Greene, and this was his one and only chance of breaking free of his background and environment. If this all went tits up he would be like his father and brothers – just another fucking mook from East London, a blockhead, and he was not going to let that happen without a fight.

Tonight he was washed, shaved and in his best clobber, ready for literally anything. As he drove into the scrapyard in Bow, he was whistling with suppressed excitement. He was driving an old but spotless 2.8 litre Ford Capri, which had been a nice silver colour, until he had stolen it three nights previously. Now it was dark blue, and the plates were not the originals. The plates were actually off a 4.2 litre Jag, but that was nothing to worry about.

He parked up as arranged by the side of the Portakabin and, shutting the engine off, he waited as he had been told to do. He didn't even light a cigarette, unsure whether it would attract attention.

There were already a couple of cars there, and the lights were on inside. He felt a rush of adrenaline as he realised he was finally a real part of this world, and the pride he felt inside him was overpowering. If only his family could see him! He was on the periphery, he knew, but this was just a start for him. Once he proved himself, he would be given bigger and better jobs, and with those jobs would come the wonga and the prestige. He would make sure the O'Casey name would become something to be reckoned with.

When his Gabby was old enough, he would marry her and give her the life that she deserved. He hoped she was all right in that care home. He still felt enraged at what her mother was capable of. Even his mum – and she wasn't up to much – looked like the mother of Our Lady by comparison. At least *his* mother was loyal to her family, would lie to the Old Bill for them, would even stand up in court and do so if need be. Not like that unnatural whore poor Gabby was lumbered with.

No, he would see to it that Gabby had a good, decent life, and he would make that his purpose. He wanted a nice little house, and a nice little family, in a nice neighbourhood, where the kids would go to a good school, and have a bit of a chance in life. He worried about Gabby and where she was. He knew about care homes, had seen the inside of a few himself over the years. But that had been his own fault not his mum's; he had been a bit of a tearaway as a youngster, and that had been the cause of him being put away. That wouldn't happen to *his* kids, not on your Nelly. He would be there for his little ones, not half-pissed all the time, or in the betting shop like his old man.

So intent was Vincent on his day-dreaming that he didn't notice that the Portakabin was gradually filling with people.

Chapter Sixty-Eight

Cynthia Tailor was home alone, but that didn't bother her – she liked being alone. She glanced around the room, and felt the anger burning once more. She would have to sell up; the house was mortgaged to the hilt, and the insurance wasn't going to pay out.

She couldn't believe that she was in this position, and she blamed her husband and Jonny Parker. Thinking of her sister in that enormous house, with Jonny dancing to her every whim, made her almost apoplectic with rage. Everyone was acting as if it was *her* fault – he had walked away from it without any real damage. It was so unfair. She had wanted him like she had wanted no one else in her life and she had him for a time as well. But he had been a flake, just like the rest. Now where was she? He had paid her off, but it was a pittance considering what she was used to. She would have to get rid of this place and start again. Even Cynthia knew she couldn't stay around here after what had happened. But then maybe getting a fresh start was what she needed. She could buy a nice flat somewhere while she was still young enough and still good-looking enough to attract attention from men.

As for that daughter of hers, *she* would need her one day and, when she did, Cynthia would take great pleasure in shutting the door in her face, just like it had been shut in hers. Her mother and father were dead to her – they had acted as though *she* was the main culprit. But then Jonny was still keeping them, so they *would* have to take his part in it all. Like Celeste, they would do whatever he told them to do. Well, he would rue the day he dumped her as well. Just who the hell did he think he was? She still loved him, though. He was the only man to ever make her feel alive, and she would miss that more than anything.

She could feel the tears coursing down her cheeks, and she brushed them away angrily. For the first time in her life she knew what it was to lose someone she cared about, and she didn't like the feeling one bit.

Cynthia glanced around the room, remembering when they first came here, seeing the kids when they were still small enough to do as they were told, before they turned into a pair of scheming bastards like their father.

James had killed himself to spite her, she was convinced of that. Deep down she thought he had done it to teach her a lesson. She grimaced through her tears. Well, he had wasted his time, because she felt no guilt where he was concerned. None whatsoever.

She wiped her eyes carefully, then she went up her beautiful staircase and ran herself a bath. She had never been one for regrets. Instead, she would do what she had always done – look after number one.

Smiling now, she sank into the scented water, and planned her next move. The past was the past – she had a future to look forward to, and that future was going to be as a young widow with no kids, no ties, no nothing.

Fuck Jonny Parker, and fuck her family. She could get along without any of them, and that was exactly what she intended to do.

Chapter Sixty-Nine

Jonny had always enjoyed the food at the Greek restaurant in Dagenham. He liked the owners and it served good food. He particularly loved the kleftiko. As he ate there with Linford Fargas before their meet about the villa scam, he pondered on how a life could change overnight, and not always for the good either.

'Do you reckon she'll go on the trot, Jonny?' Linford asked.

He shrugged. 'Who? Cynthia? Yeah, I do. She won't stick around where she ain't wanted. Anyway, if she doesn't, I'll give her a nudge in the right direction.'

Linford nodded. 'I'll nudge her if you like, with my boot in her arse!'

Jonny grinned. 'She did have a great arse, I'll give her that.'

Linford snorted, saying disdainfully, 'No arse is worth all that, mate, not even Madonna's.'

They were quiet again for a few moments before Linford said, 'When's the meet in Bow again?'

'For fuck's sake, Linford, how many times? Eleven thirty, at a scrapyard. We meet all the other investors then, and get the run down on how much is in place. I think there's a chance of shifting some more gear as well. That little Derek was asking me about puff and I told him we could accommodate anyone for any amount. He seemed interested. Nice young fella, he is – I like him. But then his old man was on the up – well liked, by all accounts. Should get a walk in the next few years.'

Linford grimaced. 'All that time behind the door. Fucking disgraceful really. I couldn't do it.'

''Course you could. It's just getting your head around it, that's all.'

Linford didn't answer, but he wondered how well Jonny Parker would do in the same position. The *threat* of a great big lump and actually having to *do* a great big lump were two completely different things altogether. Jonny would have an easy ride being who he was. But Linford wondered at how well he would take his liberty being curtailed. That was why his brother hanged himself, he was sure of it. He had been looking at a twenty at least, and funky Brixton wasn't exactly hotel standard. But Jonny Parker was like a lot of the men in the game; they were too far removed to ever get a big capture. Too many smaller fish to catch before them. In a way, Linford supposed, he was in a similar position.

'Derek's dad was a real hard case in his day, wasn't he?'

'So the stories go, real, serious hard man – took no prisoners.'

Linford remembered hearing a story about him, but he couldn't remember what it was. Shrugging, he said carefully, 'As long as you're sure about this scam, that's all. Derek is young, and he hasn't got any real reputation yet. From what I've heard, he was only a whipping boy for a long time.'

Jonny sighed. Linford could be an old woman at times. 'Look, I've done me homework, and he's a kosher kid, OK? He's had a few good earns and this is his big one. He's getting a good little rep and I want him where I can see him, and that means working for me.' Jonny was getting pissed off now and, seeing two young men at another table watching him, he snapped at them, 'Had your fucking look? Want a photograph do you?'

The young men looked away. They knew who he was, and that was what had aroused their interest. Jonny was a name to them, he was famous. They dreamt of being him one day. The difference was that, at their age, Jonny would have challenged anyone who had spoken to him like he just had, no matter who they were.

The owner of the restaurant came over then. 'Everything all right, gents?'

Jonny nodded. 'Yeah, sorry, mate, feeling a bit fragile today.'

The owner smiled coldly. 'Well, that's understandable, ain't it?'

Jonny's fist, when it hit him, was so unexpected he took the full force of it. Linford was out of his chair and holding his friend back in seconds. The other diners in the restaurant were watching in fascination and terror.

Jonny knew he had done a wrong one, but he was sick of the way people were judging him; they didn't know him, they didn't know the half of it. This little story would be all over Silvertown by the morning and he was glad. It was about time people remembered just who they were dealing with. He was sick to death of it and, right now, anyone was fair game. He had been too nice; he should have shown his strength from the off. He had tried to play Mr Nice Guy because he had been feeling guilty. Well, that was then and this was now, and he wasn't going to take it lying down any more.

Outside the restaurant, Jonny looked over the A13 towards the concrete jungle that was Ford Motor Works and, spitting on to the pavement, he said angrily, 'Fucking shithole this place, can't believe we even bother to come out this far.'

Linford opened the car doors and, once inside, said calmly, 'Like we've said before, things like what you've done leave a nasty taste, and thumping all and sundry ain't going to help matters, is it?'

Jonny laughed. It was his old laugh, loud and raucous. 'Fuck them, Linford my boy. Fuck them all. Now let's get to Bow and be done with this lot. I've had enough.'

'Whatever you say, boss.'

Linford started the car and they made their way to their meeting with Derek, neither of them saying a word, both lost in their own thoughts.

Chapter Seventy

Jack Callahan was laughing to himself as Mary watched him in amazement.

'Are you feeling the ticket, Jack? Laughing away there all on your Jack Jones.' She was pleased to see him happy if she was honest; it was a long time since there had been any merriment in this house.

Jack looked at his wife and said seriously, 'I have a lot to be cheerful about, my lovely, but I can't say too much just yet. Once it's over you'll know soon enough.'

Mary was nonplussed at his answer, but she kept her own counsel; there were some things you were better off not knowing, and this sounded like one of those things. Jack had not been right since he had seen young Vincent earlier in the day, and whatever they had been talking about had cheered him up no end.

She smiled to herself; young Vincent was a nice boy and now she was pleased he was seeing her granddaughter. She had revised her earlier opinion of him. She had met Jack when they were teenagers and they were still together, so she wasn't against young lovers like Cynthia was.

She pushed thoughts of Cynthia out of her mind; she was done with her and she didn't want her taking up any more of her time or her life. It was the shame that was the hardest to bear, although the fact that people knew she had outed her daughter permanently had helped them get over that. But it was the effect this had had on her grandchildren that really rankled. James Junior was still locked up in a secure unit. She didn't even know what that meant until Miss Bellamy had told her, and the shock had really knocked her for six. But it was the best place for him. He wasn't right that child; to do what he had done was not natural.

Still, at least Mary had heard from Gabby. She didn't sound thrilled at her new accommodation but she didn't sound too down about it. She was going to school at least, and she said it wasn't that bad. Well, it wouldn't be for very long. Miss Bellamy thought they had a good chance of getting custody of her, but it was down to the courts now. Mary sighed; she was too old for this drama.

It was Jack she really felt for though. He had taken it much worse than she had believed possible. He had liked Jimmy, despite his weaknesses. For all he came from a different background and environment, they had got on very well together. She suspected that Jack had felt sorry for the man, but then hadn't they all? They would have felt sorry for anyone who had taken on Cynthia knowing her as they did.

And then there was Celeste to worry about. Mary had hoped she would finally walk away from Jonny after the last little lot, but it wasn't to be. She thought Celeste should have seen him for what he really was, but the girl wasn't right and hadn't been right for many a long year.

As Mary walked into the kitchen, she felt an enormous pain. It hit her chest and travelled down her left arm. She was suddenly breathless and, as she leant out to grab hold of a chair for support, she collapsed on to the floor, knocking over the tea things on her way.

Jack rushed out to see what the commotion was and, seeing his wife's grey face and shallow breathing, he phoned immediately for an ambulance, all the time cursing his elder daughter, and blaming her for her mother's collapse. It was a wonder this hadn't happened before now; she'd had more than enough on her plate the last few years, and this was the upshot. If he lost his Mary, he would do for that whore of a daughter himself, and that was a promise.

Chapter Seventy-One

Linford pulled in to the scrapyard in Bow, and parked between a new Daimler Sovereign, and an old stacked-head Mercedes. The Portakabin was ablaze with lights and, for a few seconds, Linford felt apprehension envelop him. He didn't know what it was, but something about this whole set up stank.

He had tried to voice his opinion to Jonny but he wouldn't budge. He was gagging for this villa lark, and who could blame him? It was the maximum return for the minimum outlay. It was all about renting offices, and looking the part. Once people parted with their dosh that was that. Over, done with, gone.

But it was Derek Greene who bothered him, and he could not for the life of him work out why. Then, as they walked into the Portakabin, it became as clear as day what had been niggling at the back of his mind. Now it was too late to do anything about it.

Chapter Seventy-Two

As she sat with her father by her mother's hospital bed, Celeste breathed a sigh of relief. She was bad, but she would pull through. A heart attack the doctors said and, looking at her mother now, tubes everywhere and her face devoid of colour, Celeste wondered at how vulnerable she suddenly looked. Her mum had always been there for her. She had been a good mum, had loved her and cared for her, made her smile when she was down, gone without so her daughters could have things. Celeste felt the tears once more and choked them back. How had everything gone so wrong?

Her mum and dad blamed Cynthia but, although she was a part of it, in reality it was Jonny who had caused the trouble. As much as she had loved him – and she realised the significance of the past tense – she should have known that he was trouble. He was a violent criminal and she had swallowed that, believing love could conquer all. Well, it couldn't. He had taken her sister and he had destroyed many lives.

She had gone back to him out of fear, fear of being alone, of having to earn a living, of going back out into the world; the world frightened her, the world was dangerous. Well, so was being in your own home she had learnt. Her house scared her; it was too big, too empty, and she longed for the bedroom of her youth.

She would give anything to be able to go back and do it all again, but that was impossible. She knew that if she had not married Jonny Parker her mother wouldn't be lying in this bed, and her father wouldn't be sitting opposite her, terrified of losing the person he had loved his whole life. Poor Gabby wouldn't be in care, and young James wouldn't be in a lock-up unit for kids.

She had brought this down on their heads by bringing Jonny into their lives. Celeste wasn't sure she would ever be able to forgive herself, but one thing she did know was that she would not go back to that house. She would go home and look after her dad, and then her mum when she finally came back from hospital. Jonny thought that he had done everything for the best reasons, but she knew that he had done everything he had for no other reason than that he could. Seeing her mother like this brought home to her just how useless her life had been up until this moment. It was time to grow up and take responsibility for herself, and those around her who she cared about, starting now.

'Can I get you a cup of tea, Dad?'

Jack looked at his daughter as if he'd forgotten she was there, then he just shook his head sadly and went back to watching his wife.

Jack knew that without Mary he would have nothing; he remembered everything she had done for him over the years, and was ashamed that he had never even made her a cup of tea. She had slogged and grafted to keep them all clean, fed and watered. He wondered how many meals she had cooked every-one over the years, how many beds she had made, how many shirts she had ironed. It was true what they said – you didn't know what you had till it was gone. Never was a truer word spoken.

He glanced at his daughter and saw the fear in her eyes that he knew was mirrored in his own; like him, she had taken her mother's presence in her life for granted. They all had at one time or another, especially that Cynthia – Mary had brought her children up for her, been there for her in the good times and the bad. He knew how hard it had been for his Mary to turn her back on her elder child, and the result of their daughter's actions was this heart attack.

Well, things were going to change, he was going to see to that himself. He never wanted to live through anything like this ever again, because he knew that if she went he would not be far behind her. A world without his Mary in it would be no world at all.

Chapter Seventy-Three

Bertie Warner was smiling, but it did not make him look in any way amiable. Jonny Parker's shock was apparent, and that made Bertie a very happy man.

'Surprised to see me, are you, Jonny?'

Jonny looked around him and, seeing the serious looks on the men's faces, he felt truly afraid for the first time in years. Not that he would let this lot know that.

'Well, well, well, if it ain't Bertie Warner back from the dead.' He injected as much humour as he could into the words.

But it was Bertie who got the laugh when he said, 'No, not the dead, Jonny, me old son. Grenada.' He looked at Linford then as he said seriously, 'You'd like it there, son. A lot of fucking machetes, if you know what I mean.'

Jonny knew then he was on borrowed time and he said nonchalantly, 'So you had a swerve. That's all water under the bloody bridge now. What are you back for, fucking revenge?'

Bertie laughed now himself. 'Oh yes, revenge, and to take back what was mine. Well, mine and Kevin's anyway. He was my best mate, was Kevin. Me and him even did our National Service together, bet you didn't know that? Back in the fifties when we were only kids. That's where he got the nickname "No Face". Playing poker in the stockade. But he was a good mate, a loyal friend, which is why you never approached me to have him over, you knew I wouldn't swallow that. You knew I would

236

chop your arms off, and then put you in the boot of a scrapped car and crush you alive.'

Jonny laughed at Bertie but it was a thin laugh. 'You're joking! That kind of thing went out in the sixties with all the old Mustache Petes. You can't touch me without recriminations, you stupid old cunt.'

'Oooh, hark at her! I can do what the fuck I like, mate, and the sooner you get your fucking thick head around that the better.'

Jonny Parker had forgotten how ferocious Bertie Warner could be. Bertie was a known headcase; he also had a taste for torture, and that had always been his ace card. No one had ever wanted to cross him, because the consequences were dire. He had once burnt a man alive for cutting him up in his motor. Linford was worried, Jonny could tell, and it seemed that history was repeating itself. Young Derek wanted what *he* had, so he was teaming up with the man that he had originally taken it from. It was like a fucking nightmare, and Jonny knew the chances of him leaving this room alive were minimal at best. But he was not going out without a fight, that was for sure.

He glanced around him at the men in the room; all were heavies, ready for anything, especially young Derek Greene. How could he have been so dense? Linford had smelled a rat and he should have listened to his friend's instincts. But, in fairness, it had been an eventful few weeks, and he was not exactly at the top of his game because of that.

Bertie grinned, and he looked like a death's head. 'Come on then, Jonny, if you think you're hard enough.' He looked at the men around him and said almost gleefully, 'You can see his brain working, can't you? He's wondering which one of us to take out first. Then he's planning how to get out that door, and do a runner. Well, Jonny, me old son, that ain't going to happen. Sorry for the inconvenience and all that.' He walked behind the small wooden desk which was used by the secretary three days a week, and picked up a large machete. 'See this? See the irony of it, do you? Well, this is going to remove your arms, and then you are going into a motor, and you are going to be crushed. I've been planning this for fucking years, Jonny Boy, and, now the time has come, I feel quite excited about it.'

Derek Greene's eyes were glittering with the prospect of serious violence. Like Jonny before him, he believed they would take it all over and there would never be any pretenders to their thrones.

Jonny read what was going on in Derek's head and laughed. There would always be another young buck like Derek, waiting in the sidelines for what he saw as his golden opportunity. Just as Jonny was finding out. That, unfortunately, was the way of the world they had chosen, and it was a foolish man who didn't watch out for it, and expect it, even from his closest allies. And foolish he had been.

'Look, man, it was nothing personal . . .'

Bertie's voice cut him off. 'Nothing fucking personal? Is this cunt for real? You murdered my mate, well, not you as such. That little matter was done by a *female*, a woman who was protecting her sister, that I can swallow. She was doing what anyone would have done, and my Kevin, as much as I loved him, and love him I did, done a wrong 'un going to your house. I hold me hands up to that. I didn't like it, but I had no choice – he was determined. What I am so irritated about is that you challenged us like we were *nothing*. You treated us like we were amateurs. Well, I'm back, lads, and you two are over with. You're finished, you're fucking done!'

As Jonny looked at Bertie and saw the maniacal look in his eyes, he knew this was it. His life would end in a Portakabin in Bow. Not the most salubrious ending to a life, but an ending all the same.

'Shove it up your arse, you silly old cunt! Bring it on! I ain't going without a fucking tear up.'

'I was hoping you would say that!'

Bertie swung the machete, a machete which had been sharpened into a lethal blade. It landed on Jonny's shoulder and, as Bertie had promised, it took his arm off.

The blood was spraying everywhere, and Derek Greene felt the thrill that hunters feel when they finally take an animal down.

Linford watched in horror as his friend was butchered before his eyes. One thing in Jonny's favour though, was he never screamed once, and that was remarked upon by all the men in the room. Even as they carried him, still alive, to the waiting car that was to be his tomb. He was slung into the boot like rubbish, and he was still cursing them loudly as they put the crushing machine in motion.

Linford watched every second with mounting dread; he had known this was not a kosher operation, had felt it in his water. It had all seemed too glib, too structured to be real. He looked into the blood-spattered face of Bertie Warner and accepted the inevitable.

Bertie took Linford's head off his shoulders with one hefty slice of the machete. As it rolled across the dirty ground of the scrapyard and eventually stopped in a small hole, Bertie shouted gleefully, 'Look, guys, a fucking hole in one!'

They were all laughing now, stacked up on adrenaline and the knowledge that their main adversaries were out of the picture. All that was left now was for them to take what they felt was rightfully theirs.

Young Vincent had watched it from the sidelines, and he felt the nausea rising up inside him. Of all the things he had expected of the night, this was not one of them. He was party to murder now, and he knew then and there that this kind of skulduggery wasn't for him. He just wanted to be a blagger, a bank robber, nothing more and nothing less.

Linford's body, minus its head, was bundled into the boot of Vincent's car, and Derek Greene climbed in the passenger seat, saying happily, 'We're gonna dump this outside their main offices, then we lose the motor and get as far away from the scene as possible, OK?'

Vincent nodded.

'You are part of a new guard tonight, mate, in on the ground floor.'

And, as Vincent thanked Derek, he wondered at just what he had signed himself up for. This was far too much for him; all he had wanted was to drive a few getaway cars. Now he was a witness to the murders of two of the most dangerous men in London. Life could be such shit at times.

It was only later on, lying in his bed at his mum and dad's flat, that it occurred to him he had been used; he had told Derek Greene everything he had needed to know about Jonny Parker, but he didn't know the half of what Derek was planning. It wouldn't be the first time he was used, and it would not be the last, of that much he was sure. He was in over his head, and he knew that he could not walk away from any of it. This had been far too big a night for him to be able to pretend it had never happened. It would go down in East-End folklore and, in a way, he knew that he would enjoy people knowing he had been a part of it. Derek Greene had hand picked him for the job and that was a compliment, surely? If he used his loaf he could get a fucking decent earn, and be a part of a new regime.

He was aware he was trying to convince himself that everything would be all right. But another thing he had found out this night was that he had no stomach for murder and, no matter what the score, that had been murder at its worst; cold-blooded and messy. He was part of it now, and he knew he had to do what was expected of him. But he regretted getting involved in it all. Whatever Jonny Parker was or he wasn't, it didn't change the fact that Vincent had been a part of the crew who had outed his Gabby's uncle.

Chapter Seventy-Four

Celeste didn't report her husband missing for three days, but she knew, like everyone else, including the police, that he was dead. Linford's headless torso had been a message, and that message had been received and understood. She had thought the news would destroy her, but instead, for the first time in years, she felt free. The house and most of the other properties were in her name, as were a majority of the bank accounts, so she was a very wealthy woman. Jonny being gone didn't really affect her that much in the long run.

She also knew intuitively that her father had guessed what was going to happen; he had not seemed surprised by the turn of events. She wondered how Cynthia was feeling and if she mourned Jonny. Celeste hoped so, because *she* couldn't mourn him. She was glad he was gone, glad he was away from her, glad she was finally able to walk away from the life he had given them. Her mum was on the mend, and her life was once more her own.

She had loved Jonny Parker once with all her heart, but she had not loved what he had become. What he had tried to be. The violence he had embraced had finally turned back on him. What goes around comes around, how many times had she heard that expression? She knew his body would turn up one day and, until then, she would live her life as quietly and as decently as humanly possible with her mum and dad. She had

had enough of the so-called good life; it had never been much good to her.

From that day, Celeste Parker never left her mother's home, not even for a few hours.

Book Three

As is the mother, so is her daughter

Ezekiel 16:44

It is not what a lawyer tells me I may do; but what humanity, reason, and justice tell me I ought to do

Edmund Burke (1729–97)

Chapter Seventy-Five

1998

'What's the matter with you, child?' Mary was worried about her granddaughter, she was very quiet these days, as if the light had gone out of her, and had been ever since coming out of care.

'I'm all right, Nana, I just don't feel that great lately.'

'You're not sickening for anything, are you?'

Gabby laughed at that. It was Irish for 'Are you pregnant?'

'Don't worry, Nana, *that's* not what's wrong with me.'

She saw the palpable relief on her grandmother's face and sighed inwardly. She wished she *was* pregnant; it would be lovely to have a baby of her own. Something to love and care for. A little person who loved you back unconditionally. Gabby craved love like other people craved water or food. It was because of her upbringing – God knows, the new social worker had told her that enough times. She grimaced at the thought of Miss Byrne; though she liked the woman, she could be hard work.

But that wasn't what was bothering her. How could she tell her grandmother that after nearly three years her mother wanted contact again? Of all the things she had expected that had not been one of them. And Miss Byrne was all for it! She said it would give Gabby 'closure'. What a crock of shit! What it would give her was untold aggravation, which was all her mother had ever brought to anyone in her life.

245

Still, she couldn't deny her interest was piqued. She was curious to see how her mother had fared since she had disappeared, and she would love to ask her how she could have dumped her two kids so unceremoniously without a second's thought. Then why ask the road you know? She knew the answer to that question already. Cynthia had walked away because that is what she did; she made a mess and she ran from it as soon as it got out of hand. Her husband had killed himself and what had she done? Left her children to cope with the fall-out.

'Are you going to answer me, madam?'

Gabby was brought back to the present by her grandmother's harsh words.

'Am I talking to myself here or what?' Mary was clearly irritated.

'Sorry, Nana, I was miles away.'

Kissing her nana's cheek, Gabby left the room and went to her bedroom. She sat on her bed and looked around. It was pretty enough; she liked the pale pinks and greens in the curtains and bedspread, the cream walls left unadorned – not a pop star or film star to be seen. She'd made it almost clinical, and she knew that was the result of years of being in her mother's house where there was *never* any mess whatsoever. She could still hear her mother's voice: 'Do you know how much that wallpaper cost a roll? And you want to put fucking Sellotape on it!' She had heard it many times, and it had always made her angry inside. Other girls had posters, pictures of ponies, whatever on their walls, but not her.

She pushed the thoughts from her mind; she was only thinking about her mother because the social worker had told her she wanted to see her. That was it. It was a natural reaction but, still, it was stirring up unpleasant memories.

Gabby looked in the small dressing-table mirror at herself, wondering what her mother would think of her now. At sixteen she was a beauty, or so everyone kept telling her. She was also the living image of Cynthia. She stared into her deep-blue eyes, framed by dark lashes, and looked at her mouth, the wide-lipped mouth that was so fashionable at the moment. She was prettier than most girls, and that wasn't her being big-headed – it was a fact. Anyway, she knew that looks really meant nothing in the grand scheme of things – it was brains and contentment that mattered. And being loved.

She *was* loved, by her nana and granddad and by Vince, and even her auntie Celeste – though *she* was getting stranger by the day. She had never left this house since the day she had walked back into it after Jonny was killed. Agoraphobia, the doctors called it though Auntie Celeste said that was shite, she just didn't like going out and that was her human right. She had a point, albeit in a weird and wonderful way. All she did was eat and watch TV. She was rich as Croesus by all accounts, but even that didn't have any impact on her; she gave most of her money away to charity or anyone who came and told her a sob story.

Gabby knew it drove her granddad mad, but he was powerless to do anything about it. Celeste was as right as the mail; that was an undisputed fact, even the doctors had told them. She had 'retired' from the world, that was how her nana put it, adding that that didn't mean Celeste was a nut job. But could she eat! She was half the size of the house nowadays, all chins and chafed thighs, but she had a good heart, and her eyes were alive with love when she looked at her family. In fact, if Gabby was honest, she actually believed that her auntie was one of the happiest people she knew. Go figure that one, Oprah.

But it was still her mother who was occupying Gabby's thoughts now. She couldn't rid herself of the terrible urge to meet with her, just to see what she was like now. Maybe she *had* changed, maybe she *was* a different kind of person, and if Gabby didn't go to see her she would never know.

Gabby didn't actually believe that for a moment, but it was a nice fantasy. Other kids took parental love for granted; some mothers stood by their kids through everything – even a rapist or a murderer often had the support of their parents, though Gabby suspected that was because they didn't want to believe their child was capable of such heinous crimes. But neither she nor James Junior had ever had their mother's love, and that hurt. Look at what had happened with poor James. He had got even worse and had ended up being sectioned. Gabby wondered if *she* had been in touch with him as well.

She sighed heavily again, and lay back on her bed. This had stirred her up inside, and made her think of times gone by that she would rather not remember. She turned her head and looked at the photo of her and her father she kept on her night table. It had been taken the Christmas before he died and he had his arm around her and they were both laughing into the camera. It was a lovely photo and anyone looking at it would never guess at the real Christmas they had endured that year – had endured every year with her mother in control, telling them what Christmas *should* be like. Cynthia thought Christmas was about having all the trappings. With all the wisdom of her age, Gabby knew that was where her mother always went wrong. Christmas was about people, about family – not things, not well-dressed trees and expensive presents, and a roast turkey that could feed a family of fifteen and still have enough left over for sandwiches. It was about enjoying the day, enjoying your family. Her mother had never known what it was to enjoy being with her family, that had always been the trouble.

Now she wanted to see Gabby, and Gabby didn't know what to do about it.

She was meeting Vincent later, so she would ask his advice; he might not be the sharpest knife in the drawer but he had a good heart. And he loved her, and she loved him, and that was what really mattered.

Chapter Seventy-Six

Vincent was thrilled. He had a good little earner thanks to Derek Greene, and he had just been recruited as a driver on his first ever bank job. He was almost sick with excitement, though he had been sure not to let that show. He had driven Derek and a few of his cronies over the last few years and he had made a name for himself as a good little runner. He always canvassed where they were going beforehand, making sure he knew the route better than anyone who was born and bred there. They never got lost on their way there, or their way home, and he knew that was valued. Some of the meetings had been in very out-of-the-way locations, that being the nature of the job involved, and he had always done his homework. It had been much appreciated, and he had got himself quite the reputation.

Well, it was paying off now; he was going to do such a fuck-off job he would soon be in demand. That was his goal in life – to be the best driver in London. Good drivers had a very important place in the scheme of things, and they were paid handsomely for their abilities. Another year or two and he could marry his Gabby, and they could start the family they were both looking forward to. They talked about it all the time; how they would decorate their house, what names they would give their kids, what kind of schools they would attend. They were going to have children who would be somebody in the straight world, and they would both work their arses off to achieve that for them.

As he parked his BMW convertible in the scrapyard, the same scrapyard where he had witnessed the demise of Linford and Jonny P, Vincent shuddered. It didn't matter how many times he came here – and that was frequently since Derek now owned it – he still felt the chill of apprehension as he drove through the large wrought-iron gates. It amazed him that the machinery in here was worth millions – it looked like a load of old tat. But he supposed it cost a fair bit to buy a machine that could gobble up cars – and people – and turn a large vehicle into a small block of metal, two foot by two foot.

He walked into the Portakabin, a large smile on his handsome face.

'All right, Del Boy?'

Derek Greene smiled back widely. He'd always liked Vincent O'Casey, and it had been a pleasure watching the boy flourish under his watchful eye. He was trustworthy and loyal, all the assets needed for this kind of life. Not exactly a contender for *The Krypton Factor*, but a shrewdie just the same.

'Sit down, mate, the others will be here soon. They're a little firm out of Manchester, and I have talked you up, so don't let me down, OK?'

It was a friendly warning and Vincent swallowed down his nerves as he said nonchalantly, 'I'm easy, looking forward to it. It's been a long time coming.'

Derek grinned again. 'Easy, tiger! I had to make sure you were ready before I sent you out into the big bad world!' Then, in a kinder voice, he said seriously, 'Look, everyone gets nervous, it's what gives you the edge. The day you don't get nervous on a jump is the day it goes wrong. I read a book once about Laurence Olivier, a very talented actor, but he said that he threw up every time he went on stage. See what I'm saying? It's the nerves that give people the edge. You'll be all right, Vince, you'll do good.'

Vincent smiled with pleasure at the man's words.

'Now, did you find them a hotel where they can get tooled up?'

Vincent nodded. 'It's in Southend. Small place off the front, where a crowd of men from Manchester won't be too noticeable.'

Derek grinned his usual amiable grin, the one that hid the hard man inside him. 'Good lad. We can't have them noticed by Lily Law around this gaff, know what I mean? They want to get in and out in a few days. You know the route, and we'll talk them through it together, OK? But they are relying on you to get them away. Have you arranged the chop?'

Vincent nodded. He'd already put everything in place to exchange the main motor for a more sedate model that the police would not be looking for. It was an honest motor, a family saloon, but with a revved-up engine in case of emergencies, such as the police recognising them and giving chase. 'All sorted, and all in place.'

'Excellent. I think you're going to be a useful addition to this oufit, young Vincent.'

Vincent was beaming at the praise. 'Thanks for the chance, Derek, I appreciate it.'

As he spoke, Bertie Warner pulled up outside. Bertie had taken on the mantle of boss with ease, and he was now at the top of this very lucrative game. As he swaggered into the small Portakabin, he was all good-natured bonhomie.

'Afternoon, my old mockers! I heard a great joke today: Why do brides wear white? Because all fucking kitchen appliances are white!'

Vincent and Derek both laughed, as was expected.

'My mate Peter Bailey is a funny man, no doubt about it. Shame he didn't go on the stage really – he could give that Jimmy Jones a run for his money.'

The phone rang and Derek answered it; he listened for a few seconds then passed the phone to Vincent saying, 'Fucking hell, no wonder they need a good driver. They can't even find their way to the Bow Road!'

As Vincent directed the men to the Portakabin, he felt the rush of adrenaline. This was the life, this was the life he had always craved, and it was within his grasp at last. He felt like the luckiest man alive.

Chapter Seventy-Seven

Cynthia Callahan – she had dropped the name Tailor after she had left East London – looked around her flat and felt the rush of pride her home always gave her. She was living in a new development called Chafford Hundred, and she had a penthouse that looked over the Thames. She could see the boats plying their trades, and the shores of Kent. It was a lovely setting.

She had bought this place for yet another new start; as usual she had become involved with a man, who had eventually walked out on her. But not until she had bled him dry. She smiled to herself, the smile that made her look like an angel, but actually hid the fact she was a devil in disguise. Amoral as ever, she had understood the need to leave the South Downs, where she had been living previously, sooner rather than later. She had bought this place after reading the advertising blurb and was now awaiting the sale of her small house in Sussex.

Sussex had been good to her; she had quite liked it there – especially Brighton. Brighton had been the nearest thing to London, so she felt at home there. Now, out here in the Essex countryside, she was near enough to London to visit, but not close enough to be a part of it all. That suited her down to the ground. She had the best of both worlds really, and she did like her solitude.

She had already met a few of her neighbours. In the penthouse opposite her was a man called David. In his mid-fifties, he was getting over a bitter divorce – just the kind of man she liked.

Old enough to appreciate her, and young enough to think they had a future together. He had a few quid, drove a decent car, and his furniture was expensive and tasteful. He would be her new conquest, and she was looking forward to the chase.

She opened her bedroom closets and looked at the large array of clothes. She would play the part of a retired career woman for him and, when she finally had him within her grasp, she would start borrowing money from him – just until her money arrived from the Cayman Islands of course. That would be her story. By the time he realised it was all lies, it would be too late.

She laughed with delight. It was so easy to get these men to part with their cash, and they never pressed charges – they were too embarrassed. Lying came easy to her, and she had discovered she was exemplary at it. It was said people who lied needed good memories, which was true! She had a patter, and she never deviated from it. She would talk in telephone numbers, insist on paying her half of any bills or holidays, and she would casually mention all the different business deals she had on the go. It was so easy she could con them in her sleep. Eventually she would need a cash injection, and they would give it to her unquestioningly.

It was only when it started to dawn on them that she wasn't all she said she was that the rot set in, but by then she was already making plans for her flight. She'd be unavailable on all her phone numbers and gone from her home that they eventually found out had been rented and not owned by her. The truth was she *did* own it, but through a holding company and she rented it to herself. Oh, she was a clever little girlie. No paper trails, no actual criminal act, she just borrowed money. It happened all the time. The police had never once interviewed her, and so she had no qualms about continuing. It was lucrative, and it was easy – perfect in fact.

So why had she felt this sudden longing to see her daughter? She truly *wanted* to see her, see what she looked like, how she had turned out. Gabriella would be sixteen now, on the cusp of womanhood. Did she look like her or did she now resemble James? Cynthia had a feeling it would be her; she always had, even from a baby.

Cynthia had no interest in James Junior; he was already too far gone from her to be of any interest. But Gabriella had possessed the same spark that she herself did. What she was feeling was in no way maternal, it was simply curiosity.

She knew Gabriella was with her mother and father, and she shuddered at the thought of how she would be living. They lived like tinkers – all TV sets and boiled food. Cynthia had hated it as a child, aspired to a better way of life than the working men's clubs they frequented. She felt almost sick with shame about her upbringing.

Yet Celeste had loved all that, so had James when she had taken him to the club for the first time. He said it was a great place for meeting up with friends – like he had ever had any friends! To her it had always felt like slumming, but then she was above all that kind of shit. A good restaurant, decent wine and intelligent conversation were beyond these people's comprehension – they had thought she was a snob, and she knew she was. She was proud to be one. Who in their right mind would want to live like *them*? Hand to mouth, eating food that had more preservatives in it than Joan Collins? Their main topic of conversation was what was going on in *EastEnders*.

If she had one regret, it was leaving her daughter to live like that. But then what would she have done with her? She had her own life, and a good life it was. Nevertheless she was curious to see her again. It never occurred to her though that her daughter might not *want* to see her, that what she had done to her family might not be forgiven, let alone forgotten. As far as Cynthia was concerned, she had summoned her daughter to her side and what else could her daughter do, but answer that call? To Cynthia Callahan, that was simple logic.

Chapter Seventy-Eight

'You're joking, Celly?'

Celeste shook her head, and said seriously, 'No, I'm not, Mum. She's frightened to tell you and Dad, and who can blame her?'

Mary felt sick at what she had heard, and if Jack found out there would be murder done. That Cynthia thought she could waltz back into her daughter's life after all this time was outrageous. 'She's not thinking of going, is she?'

Celeste, one eye on the *Trisha* show and one eye on her mother, said honestly, 'I think she's just curious, Mum, you know. But I don't think she wants to go for any other reason than that.'

Mary nodded, but her heart was beating too fast for her own good. She sat on the sofa and bit her lips in consternation. Her first thought was that Cynthia might have changed, but she dismissed that idea as soon as it arrived. This was something far more sinister, she knew that in her waters. If Cynthia wanted to see that child there *had* to be an agenda. So, what could it be? And why hadn't Gabby discussed it with her?

'When did this happen, Celeste?'

Celeste shrugged her huge shoulders. 'A few days ago.'

That explained the child's demeanour recently anyway. 'What do you think, love?'

Celeste closed her eyes for a few seconds before saying, 'I think she should run as far away from her mother as possible and, before you ask, I told her that.'

Mary nodded in agreement.

'Cynthia is trouble; she's a liar, and she's dangerous. But, at the end of the day, she *is* Gabby's mother.'

'More's the fucking pity. Well, I'll have to wait and see if she asks me about it, won't I?'

But Celeste wasn't listening any more; the woman on *Trisha* was confronting her demons, which were drink and drugs, and Trisha as always was sympathetic but firm. Celeste liked Trisha, she had a nice way about her.

Mary watched the screen blankly, her mind in turmoil. Cynthia plus Gabby added up to a disaster, and she knew she had to make sure that any meeting between them was monitored. By herself if possible. None of this was good for her heart, she knew, but it was something that had to be addressed and at the earliest possible opportunity. Her daughter Cynthia was like Jaws – just when you thought it was safe to go back into the water . . . back she came, like the proverbial bad penny.

One thing was for sure though – Jack must never know about any of this. He would see his elder daughter dead before he let her back in this family again.

Chapter Seventy-Nine

Terry Marchant was a Mancunian with a loud laugh and an even larger thirst. Vincent liked him and, along with his two cronies Patrick Miles and Anthony Dawes, he was good company. They were blaggers extraordinaire, and they roamed the country robbing banks and building societies with gay abandon. They did the stealing, and then relied on a good wheelman to get them out of the way. Which is where Vincent came in; he got ten per cent of the load, and all he had to do was drive. It was a doddle.

Now, sitting in a pub on Southend Seafront drinking orange juice, Vincent was getting a real insight into the men he would be dealing with. Terry Marchant was a hardcase, that was obvious to anyone. He had the look, the build and the carriage of a man who it would be foolish to mess with. Vincent had learnt that over the years – you could tell from looking at certain people whether or not you could fuck with them. Terry Marchant was a definite no-no in that respect. But he was a lot of fun, and he had a great personality. His two colleagues were small-time, but nice blokes all the same. Vincent felt he would enjoy working with them.

Terry Marchant, for his part, was pleased to see that the lad was not drinking alcohol. Even though the blag wasn't for a few days, he appreciated that the kid wasn't stupid enough to get a tug for driving over the limit. It meant he was sensible, and unlikely to get himself on the police radar, so to speak. Derek had spoken highly of the boy, and that should have been enough for him, but Terry still preferred to look the drivers over and form his own opinion of them before he gave the nod. Buyer beware and all that. He was weighing out a nice wedge for Vincent, and their livelihoods depended on him doing a good job.

It was strange really; no one ever understood that robbing was the easy part – it was the disappearing act afterwards that was hard. Once people saw a sawn-off, they tended to do as they were told. The Old Bill, on the other hand, were not so amenable. They hated blaggers with a vengeance; there was nothing so annoying to a Filth than a bank being knocked over in their jurisdiction. Fucking muppets! What were banks for? Sitting there, full of wonga, and no real security. Done properly it was a piece of cake.

He and the boys had sussed out the lay of the land already. It was a good little set up and the bank would be full of dough as it had all the wages for the surrounding areas waiting to be picked up. It was on a quiet road too – just the kind of place he liked. They'd do a final check but he was sure they'd covered all the bases and they'd be in and out, quick as a flash.

Terry ordered more drinks and started to tell a story about an old mate from Warrington who had robbed a bank while drunk as a cunt. It was a funny story but it was also a bit of an allegory. It showed the stupidity of people while in the throes of alcohol, and how badly things could go against you if you weren't careful.

He noticed that young Vincent listened raptly, and he knew then that he had got his point across with the minimum of fuss. He didn't like aggro and he didn't like heroes. He liked people to do their jobs and forget about it. Seemed that this kid had all the attributes he needed.

So, finally, Terry Marchant relaxed and was able to enjoy the rest of his stay in Southend.

Chapter Eighty

'I told the social worker I didn't want to see her, Nana.'

Mary relaxed, breathing out a heartfelt sigh of relief. 'You did the right thing, child. She wouldn't have wanted to see you for any other reason than trouble. God forgive me for saying that about my own daughter, but it's the truth. Everything she touches she destroys, and we both know that, don't we?'

Gabby nodded. 'I'm sorry I never told you, Nana. I didn't want to upset you. But when I came in and saw your face I knew then Auntie Celly had to have said something.'

Mary smiled sadly. 'She did it for the best, lovie.'

Gabby nodded, but her eyes were filling with unshed tears. 'I know, Nana, but I wanted to see her a bit, just a little bit. She *is* my mum.'

Mary held her granddaughter close and comforted her as best she could, all the time cursing her elder daughter. Why couldn't she have just stayed away? Why did she want to upend this child's life on a whim? With Cynthia she had no doubt it *would* be a whim. No good could come of it.

Chapter Eighty-One

Vincent was waiting patiently outside the bank in Essex. It was twenty past ten in the morning, and Terry Marchant and his two accomplices had just walked into the bank, ski masks over their heads and sawn-offs in their sports bags.

Vincent watched through the window. The bank didn't get busy until lunchtime and so at nearly ten thirty it was more or less empty with just the three tellers inside and a couple of young mums paying their electric bills. He watched the pantomime unfold inside and, five minutes later, the men were on their way to the car and he was already getting ready to drive away. It had been so easy – too easy really. He was around the roundabout and on his way to Basildon before the first sirens were even heard in the distance.

At Basildon he turned off towards the train station, and the three men, now devoid of ski masks and without their distinctive red tracksuit tops – which were all the bystanders would remember – were relaxed and laughing. The adrenaline rush was over, and their job was done without so much as a hiccough. They chopped the cars with the minimum of fuss, leaving everything behind them except the money, and they were back in Southend within the hour.

Never had Vincent O'Casey had such a spectacular day. And never had he believed that a blag could be that fucking simple. They had netted just under a hundred grand, and he went home ten thousand pounds better off; it was like all his Christmases and birthdays had come at once. The best thing had been that he had loved it, loved every second of it. And tonight he was going to have the greatest night out of his life.

Chapter Eighty-Two

Gabby had never seen so much money before in her life, and her eyes widened in disbelief. Vincent loved seeing her reaction as he showed her his cut.

Gabby looked at him in amazement. 'Ten grand!'

He grinned. 'Yes, ten thousand pounds, and keep your voice down or we'll have your nana and granddad in on top of us in a minute.'

'They're out, you div – they've gone to bingo with Mrs Jacobs over the road. And Auntie Celly ain't gonna come in here, she's watching her soaps. A fucking bomb couldn't get her away from the telly when Grant Mitchell's on.'

Suddenly they were both quiet, realising what that meant. Then, grabbing her, Vincent started to kiss her, and it was unlike any kiss they had ever had before. Gabby was in her dressing gown and, as he slipped it off her shoulders, she knew that she wouldn't stop him, this time she would let him. When he lay her down on her little single bed, and she felt the money beneath her body, she knew that this was meant to be, that they were meant to be together.

Two big events in one day, and Vincent felt like he was the king of the world.

Chapter Eighty-Three

'I'm telling you, the kid's good, Del. He didn't even break a sweat, and I know more experienced men who still collapse under that kind of pressure.'

Derek Greene was pleased at Terry's praise of his protégé. He had a good nose for talent, and he prided himself on nurturing that talent and finding a role which suited the person best.

'No, Del, he's a good one. I was well impressed.'

'How was your hotel? All right?'

'Perfect – small, out of the way, and run by an old couple who couldn't describe their own arses without a picture of it in their hands. Nice grub and all. It was a good little overnighter.'

Derek was thrilled. Terry Marchant was a Face of Faces in Manchester, but he still liked to work. He was a natural-born blagger, it was in his blood. It wasn't as if he even needed the money – what Terry needed was the rush. Just like his own father, Terry Marchant liked the thought of getting one over on the banking system and the Old Bill.

'So you would use him again, then?'

'In a heartbeat. He's got a natural talent for it, and that's rare in this day and age. Too many young lads can't keep their fucking traps shut. Also, he's a nice kid, easygoing, never saw him drink once, only orange juice. That tells me he has a bit of savvy about him. I'll spread the word when I get back to Manchester, you'll get more calls for him.'

Derek nodded, pleased with the result. He had his cut nicely stashed in the safe at the scrapyard – that was what he called his petty cash. His beer and entertainment money. He had a feeling he would be getting quite a bit more of that kind of money from hiring out young Vincent in the near future. He only hoped the kid didn't go splashing out on motors and watches he should not have been able to afford, thereby bringing down on him the interest of Lily Law.

The Filth were always aware when a local boy had a new car, or too much money in their pockets; it was what alerted them to potential Faces. Derek's dad had drummed that into his head – always have a legitimate business on the go. A real business could explain away houses, cars and holidays. It also let you live a legal life with mortgages, loans, etc. But he had explained that to young Vincent, and he was a sensible kid; Derek was sure he would have taken it onboard. But he knew better than anyone how money in the hand could burn a hole as big as the Ritz in certain people's pockets, so all he could do now was wait and see. He wasn't too bothered about it. He had a feeling that Vincent O'Casey had an agenda of his own, and that agenda was about that bird of his. Pretty little thing she was as well. Nice face, shame about her mother! He smiled at his own wit. Well, only time would tell with Vincent, and Derek Greene had all the time in the world.

Chapter Eighty-Four

Cynthia watched her daughter leave the house and get into Vincent O'Casey's car which was parked outside her parents' home. She was in her own car, a small BMW convertible, but she was wearing a scarf and it was dark, so she wasn't worried about being noticed.

Vincent, however, had parked under a lamppost, so she had a good view of her daughter and her beau. She was surprised it was still Vincent O'Casey – surprised and annoyed. Didn't Gabriella have any idea at all? Had she learned nothing from her mother? But then, this was *her* mother's influence, she was sure. Get the first boy that gives you any attention and marry him before someone else does. Cynthia was actually gritting her teeth with annoyance and she made a conscious effort to relax herself.

It was odd, being back in the old neighbourhood; she hated it even more now than she had then. It was so scruffy and so depressing, no wonder the women who lived here looked defeated and so *old*. It was as if they had given up on themselves, which of course they had. Cynthia prided herself on her skin, on her trim figure and she dressed to impress – these women dressed to go up the shops!

But her Gabriella was a beauty, she would give her that. She was just like Cynthia at the same age – all tits, legs and slim waist, and she held herself and walked well. That was important to a woman, walking well. Her old nanny used to say 'Walk into

266

a room like you own it and the chances are one day you will.'
Pity Mary had never listened to her own mother – how different
things might have turned out. Imagine still living in the first
house the council gave you! That was her mum and dad all over;
no fucking ambition, no desire for something better. Just
grateful for being alive. How she would love to knock on that
door, and give them the fright of their lives. She knew it would
be her mother who put the kibosh on her daughter seeing her.
Her mother would not want to lose the girl now she had her.

In truth, Cynthia was amazed at how much the refusal had
hurt her. Why should she care about it so much? Her pride
had definitely been hurt. And that social worker had irritated
her with her fake sympathy and platitudes. Silly bitch – like she
gave a flying fuck what she thought.

Still, she had made the woman promise to keep her up-to-
date on her daughter's life, and she had agreed to that. Fucking
cheek! This was *her* child, *she* had given birth to her, not that
fucking old bitch of a mother of hers, or that dried-up stick of a
social worker. No, it had been her, Cynthia Tailor that was, who
had endured nine months of hell and eighteen long, hard hours
of labour. She bet her mother had had a field day, advising her
granddaughter to keep away from her own flesh and blood.

Well, fuck them. This was all she had really wanted – a quick
peek, just to see what the girl had turned out like. And wouldn't
you know, she was exactly as she had expected. A foolish girl
who had no desire to make anything of herself. She would live
the life of her nana, without anything of real value, and without
any idea of the world that was going on outside the confines of
this council estate.

Cynthia lit a cigarette and pulled on it deeply; she allowed
herself three a day, otherwise all the hours she spent in the
gym keeping in shape were pointless. She had a better body
now than before she had had her kids. But that was the beauty
of living alone, you could do those kind of things; go to the

gym, eat well, take yourself off to a health spa for long weekends. Children stopped that, like they stopped anything good in your life.

Gabriella and Vincent were kissing now, and Cynthia shook her head in consternation. What a fool she had bred, what a complete and utter fool! Gabriella would settle for a life of petty dramas and no money, a life of cleaning and cooking for a man who, once the initial sexual thrill eased off, would use her like an animal while in drink. It was so predictable really, and fucking irritating. She had brought this girl into the world, surely there had to be at least a little bit of her in the child? She reasoned her mum and dad would have made sure whatever spark the girl might have would be repressed. The last thing they would want was another child under their roof with a bit more liveliness than they could cope with, a girl with the chance to make something of her life, instead of emulating them, just existing.

Cynthia drove away quietly, not even glancing into the car where her daughter was telling her boyfriend that she thought she was pregnant and that her nana was going to kill her.

Chapter Eighty-Five

'Calm down, Gabby. It's a shock, but it ain't exactly unheard of in this day and age, is it?'

Gabby couldn't believe how well Vincent was taking the news. She had thought he would be furious with her. 'I'm only sixteen, Vince!'

He laughed. 'We'll get married, so stop worrying about it, OK? I'll tell your nana and granddad with you. They won't be too thrilled but they'll come round eventually. So please, stop worrying.'

Vincent made it sound so easy and, in a way, she supposed it was. She'd tell them and be damned. But she still felt that she had let them down somehow, had broken their trust. She had a bad feeling on her, although that could just be her hormones.

Vincent felt a rush of love for this girl of his. She was having his baby and she was frightened, but surely she knew that he would always look out for her, always take care of her? She meant everything to him, and she always would.

'Look, Gabby, once the balloon's been dropped, you can start planning the wedding, OK? Once your nana knows about that she'll see we're serious about each other.'

Gabby nodded, feeling slightly happier but still apprehensive. It was as if a weight was bearing down on her, almost as if her mother was nearby, watching and judging her. Yet she knew that was stupid – what would her mother be doing here? She hated it here, always had. But for a while there she had felt her presence nearby. It had reminded her of when she was a kid and she had wet her bed, and she knew her mother would be coming into her room. Her mum had a way of letting you know she was near; it was hard to explain but she had almost felt her mother's closeness. But that was gone now, and she shook herself back to reality.

Vincent was right – it had happened now, and they had to make the best of it. She wondered if it would be a girl or a boy? She didn't care, she just wanted something to love of her own.

'Come on, we'll go up and tell your auntie Celly. She'll be our buffer until your nana and granddad come round.'

'Do you think they will come round, Vince?'

He grinned. 'Take my word for it, once this baby arrives they'll be over the moon.'

She hoped he was right. She wanted this baby badly, and she *wanted* it to be wanted, not just by her, but by everyone. She knew what it was like to feel unloved, and she was determined no child of hers would feel like that, not ever. It was the worst feeling in the world.

Chapter Eighty-Six

Mary was disappointed, as was Jack, but they both knew there was nothing they could do about any of it. At least Vincent was standing by her, and that was something they supposed. But Gabby was so young, and they both knew how hard it was rearing a child, especially in this day and age. And that social worker, Miss Byrne, had not even looked shocked – it was as if she had been expecting it. In fairness to her, maybe she saw something they hadn't. She had more experience than they did with children of all kinds, at least that was Mary's reasoning.

At the moment, though, her main worry was Celeste. The weight was dropping off her, and that would have pleased Mary if she didn't look so unwell on it. What was strange was that the girl was eating as much as she ever did. She was like some kind of human waste disposal unit, her mouth constantly in motion. Crisps, chocolate, take-aways – she ate anything at any time. And, to crown it all, she would not even go to the hospital, assuring them she was fine. She certainly didn't look fine – she looked awful but, as the doctor said, there was little anyone could do.

Mary felt plagued with anxiety nowadays, and that was not good for her heart, not good for it at all. Still, she had her tablets, and she didn't overdo it if she could help it.

'That girl's not well, Mary, but she won't admit it.'

Mary just stopped herself from berating her husband for his uncanny ability to state the bleeding obvious. Instead she said gently, 'I know, Jack, but what can we do? Like Doctor Morgan says, if she doesn't want to see him there's nothing he can do about it, and neither can we.'

Jack nodded, and Mary saw that, like herself, he was getting old. They were only in their late sixties but they were both in poor health. It was their dirt over the years; smoking, drinking, but also the worry. Oh, they had had their fair share of worry all right. She wondered for the thousandth time if Celeste should be forced from the house; after all, the reason she wouldn't go to a hospital for tests was because she wouldn't leave the house. Even the thought of the outside world sent her into a panic. How had this happened to her family? It was a familiar refrain these days, and Mary lay all the blame with Jonny Parker and her elder daughter.

She remembered Celeste as a young girl. She had been full of life, a nice girl without big ambitions – not like her sister in that way. No, Celeste had been a decent kind of person – she still was. But she had never had the toughness needed to survive in a world peopled with the likes of Jonny Parker and Cynthia Tailor.

When she heard that Cynthia had gone back to her maiden name, Mary had wondered briefly if there was any way they could stop her from doing that. Callahan was a good, decent Irish name, and it was meant for better than the likes of Cynthia. At times she loathed her daughter so intensely she felt sure the girl must sense it, no matter how far away she was. She believed that hate could be felt, even if the person wasn't in the room with you. She hoped her daughter felt her contempt as if it was a living thing; that was what she prayed for.

Since she had tried to get back into Gabby's life, she had stirred them up in different ways. Gabby had wondered if her mother had changed and was now capable of loving her at least a little. Mary thought she had more chance of getting a wank off the Pope than *that* ever happening. Still, she knew the girl had wanted it badly – needed it, in fact. She wanted to feel that her mother loved her at least a little. Well, Cynthia wasn't capable of love. Even her relationship with Jonny Parker had not been about love – it had been about taking what her sister had, and believing she had got one over on her in the process. Now, with Cynthia back in the picture, Celeste had been reminded of everything she had tried so hard to forget.

Celeste was tied to this house, frightened of the world itself. And it was understandable; after all; it had never done her any favours, had it? Now she lived in these few rooms content, in her own way, with her TV programmes and her films about other people's lives. Even the house in Spain which she had loved so much was now sold. It seemed she would travel only once more in her life, and that would be out of this house in a coffin.

Her daughter's existence caused Mary no small amount of pain. Knowing her lovely vibrant daughter had been reduced to this wreck of a woman was hard to bear at times. But bore it she did. What else could a mother do? Oh, Cynthia had a lot of things to answer for.

Even that poor demented boy, James Junior, was still in care. Mary didn't want to see him though, as she had explained to the social workers. She had more than enough on her plate to last her a lifetime. Plus, she had been a bit frightened of James Junior since the kitten incident. Gabby had been kind and written letters to him with all the news, he was her brother after all, despite everything. He had never replied though. But she hadn't given up.

'Can I make you a cuppa, girl?'

She nodded at Jack and smiled faintly. 'That would be lovely.'

Since her heart attack he was like the tea boy, always offering to make her a cup, or get her a few biscuits. She knew it was love and guilt, both of which, unlike Cynthia, he seemed to have in abundance.

Chapter Eighty-Seven

Vincent had done two more jobs for Derek and he had another couple lined up. Piece of piss, as his father would say. And that was just it – it was so easy. He drove like other people ate or slept – it came naturally to him. From the moment he drove his first stolen car at thirteen it had been instinctive. Now his talent was making him a fortune, and he would need it as well, what with the baby coming and everything else. He was considering buying into a garage; it would be a legitimate business, and explain away any money he weighed out. He had listened earnestly to Derek and he knew that the man was giving him sound advice. He wanted to be kosher, at least outwardly anyway, and a garage would be ideal for him. He loved nothing more than tampering with cars so, all in all, it would be a win-win situation.

As he sat in the pub in Wapping waiting for Derek Greene to bring his new employers to meet him, he saw a girl watching him. Smiling at her, he realised she was familiar, only he wasn't sure where he knew her from. She wasn't local anyway. Pleased that such a nice-looking girl was eyeing him, he sipped at his orange juice, before turning his attention to the door.

The girl was already gone by the time he looked back, and he forgot about her immediately and got on with waiting. He was a patient lad in that respect, and in his job that was what you had to be – patient and calm. Luckily, he possessed both traits in spades.

It was ten minutes later when he saw Derek walk over that it came to him where he had seen the girl before. Getting up, he looked at Derek and said quietly, 'Fuck off *now*, Del Boy. I think I was just eyeballed by one of the staff of the bank we blagged in Essex. I'm sure I recognised her from our recce.'

Derek didn't need telling twice, and he left immediately. Phoning the other two people who should have been on the meet he told them it was off, grateful that Vincent had the nous not to drag everyone else into his business. He went back to the yard and telephoned Terry Marchant; he had to give him a heads-up, and assure him that young Vincent would not be swayed. He only hoped that what he was saying was the truth, and the lad didn't succumb to the police offering him a deal. He didn't think the boy was capable of that kind of treachery, but you never really knew anybody until the chips were down. Harder men than him had served up their mates at the thought of a big lump.

He was sorry for the kid really; he had a pregnant girlfriend and a promising career. It was the girlfriend that bothered him. Would Vincent keep it shut in the face of leaving her to fend for herself? They would soon know, of that much he was sure.

But it was a bastard of an inconvenience; Terry had a few good jobs lined up for him. On the bright side, maybe the girl didn't recognise him; after all, he was a nice enough looking lad to attract some female attention. But if she *had* seen him on his recce of the bank, and she remembered him, it was all over. And he had remembered her, so it was definitely related, as the Filth would say. One thing was for sure though. If Vincent fingered any of them, he was a dead man, and that was a promise.

Chapter Eighty-Eight

'What do you mean arrested?' Mary Callahan was looking at Vincent's father as if he was an attraction in a zoo.

'What I say, Mary. He's been nicked for bank robbery.'

'What! Vincent?'

Paddy O'Casey sighed in annoyance. 'Look, is Jack about?'

She opened the door wider and invited the man inside. What was she thinking keeping him on the step like that? It was the shock she supposed.

Jack Callahan was watching the news with his daughter. When he saw Paddy come into the room, he knew there and then that it was not good news. He stood up and shook the man's hand. 'What's up? Is it Vincent?'

Paddy nodded. 'He's been pinched, Jack, armed robbery.'

'When? He's been here every day . . .'

Paddy waved a hand in annoyance. 'It was ages ago. He was seen by one of the girls from the bank in a pub and the Filth have him on CCTV a few days before the robbery. Fucking eejit, he is. Anyway, he's bang to rights and, with a bit of luck, he might make bail. But the brief ain't too hopeful. The girl in the bank was not the only one to pick him out of a line up – the manager did too. He'll keep stumm about who was in it with him and, if he pleads guilty, he might get off with a ten stretch.'

'Jesus, Mary and fucking Joseph, this will destroy Gabby! She's banking on him being there when the child's born.'

Paddy O'Casey sighed once more. 'I know, but we can't

always have what we want in life. She might as well learn that lesson now – this is as good a time as any.'

Hearing the defeat in the man's voice, Mary Callahan felt an urge to slap him across the face. This was his son's life, and he was acting as if it was nothing more than an inconvenience. No wonder young Vincent spent so much time round here. Well, he wouldn't be coming back for a long time, and she had to tell her granddaughter that at some point this evening. She would be devastated, and rightly so. Why were they being plagued with this bad luck? It just seemed to be one thing after another. Now Gabby was pregnant and alone. What a state of affairs.

Chapter Eighty-Nine

'You've got to snap out of this, Gabby, it's not good for you or the baby.'

Gabby knew that her nana was right, but it was hard. She was eight months pregnant, and her baby's father was doing nine years in Parkhurst. He would be out in four with good behaviour. He had not grassed up or implicated anyone else and the men thought he was wonderful, a real mate, and a right diamond geezer. Well, Gabby didn't share that opinion. *She* thought he should have told the Filth everything he knew, and got himself out a lot sooner. She shook her head as if she was clearing it. She didn't really mean it; she knew he had to take the fall. Grasses were not welcome in their world. Grasses were not welcome anywhere.

On top of everything else, his dad and brothers had found his hidden stash of money and taken it for themselves, so she was also skint into the bargain. They had jumped on that money like a monkey on a banana tree, and that had hurt. They had basically taken the food out of her baby's mouth. The O'Caseys had had a new TV and a good few parties on what should have been *her* money. Vincent was furious. That money was for her and her baby. But there was nothing he could do about it. Not from where he was sitting.

'I just miss him, Nana.' Her voice was a plaintive cry now.

''Course you do, child, it wouldn't be natural if you didn't.'

Her nana's no-nonsense approach made her smile at times,

even though it could annoy her too. Mary Callahan's attitude was, it's happened, get over it. But then her nana had had a lot of experience where being let down was concerned, she supposed. It didn't stop Gabby from feeling lonely and abandoned once again though.

Her baby kicked and she smiled; at least her child was strong and healthy, that was something she supposed. She was determined to be the antithesis of her own mother; everything her mother had done for her and James Junior, she would do the opposite. She figured that at least that way, she would have to be doing *something* right. But having a baby was a scary thing. A little person was going to depend on her for everything, from being fed and changed, to being loved and wanted. Well, this child would have all of that and, even though its father wasn't around, it wasn't because he didn't want to be. It was legally impossible for him to be there, and she would explain it just like that when the time came. It was so much better than being told your father had been nicked.

She was due soon, and she knew it would not be pleasant. In all honesty, she was frightened of what it entailed. She wished she had a mum to turn to. Her nana was great, but she was so old and, in truth, Gabby didn't want to worry her more than she had to. Her nana and granddad seemed to have aged almost overnight, and she knew it was because of her auntie Celeste.

Celeste was a shadow of her former self, and the really worrying thing was she didn't eat a thing now, she just lay there, on her bed, watching her programmes. Her granddad called her the *Radio Times*, because she knew every TV schedule, even Sky's back to front, making them all wonder if she ever actually slept. She believed the BBC was quality programming, but she claimed to prefer the shows that didn't make her feel like they were being condescending to her. She loved American talk shows, especially *Oprah*, and believed Jerry Springer had a place in that society, albeit not at the top end. It was surreal talking to her, because unless she had watched it on a TV programme she wasn't sure it was really true. She talked about Dr Phil as if he had come to the house and diagnosed her himself. She was really big on self-diagnosis. According to an episode of *Oprah*, she was losing weight because her good angel was helping her. After all, angels were real, weren't they? Celeste bought it all, hook, line and fucking sinker. She claimed to understand forensic pathology as well as if she had studied it at university, and was sad that most murder cases she read about in the papers didn't have access to the same resources that they did on TV shows. And why not? she demanded. Where was Dr Sam Ryan when you needed her?

Did these programmers never allow for people like her aunt, who believed all that shit without question? Or did they depend on them? What came first; the TV or the viewer? Did the people really have a chance against those boffins at TV stations around the world? That, Gabby realised, remained to be seen.

Even her granddad Jack had to acknowledge that Celeste wasn't right these days, and seemed to be becoming more and more entrenched in her TV world by the minute. She talked about Trevor McDonald as if he was an old friend, and she argued that Michelle Collins was not a bad person, she was *just* Cindy Beale.

Now that she rarely got out of bed, the smell was not good. She was not even forty years old but she looked sixty at least.

As she went into her aunt's bedroom, Gabby wrinkled her nose at the odour; it was sweet, but overpoweringly so. Gabby knew it was the Parma Violets her aunt sucked all day long, but it still made her want to heave.

'Fancy a take-away, Auntie Cel? You name it, I'll eat it!' This was getting boring; she did the same thing every night now, and each time she got the same answer.

'Nothing for me, sweetie. How're you and junior doing?'

Gabby sat on the edge of her aunt's bed and she said sadly, 'We're doing fine. And you?'

Celeste looked into her niece's eyes and saw the beauty in her face; it was the same innocent beauty her mother had possessed, except with Cynthia, it had masked her true nature. 'I nearly had a baby once, but I lost it. I lost a few actually. I thought it was terrible at the time, but now, well, how lucky was I, eh? I never had to tell them the truth about their father, never had to lie to them either.' She coughed gently before saying earnestly, 'I'm dying, Gabs, I have cancer of the uterus. I told the doc not to tell your nana. You know how she flaps about everything. But I'm telling you in case I don't see this little one born. No, don't be sad, I *want* to go. What kind of life is this for anyone, eh? But I want you to know I will miss you, and I loved you like you were me own.'

Gabby looked down into her aunt's face which still held the vestiges of her former prettiness and, choking down a sob, she held her to her breast as if she was the mother and her aunt was the child.

'I'll miss you, Auntie Celeste.'

Celeste smiled through her tears. 'No, you won't. When I go it will be a relief for you all, but not as much as it will be for me. My life was a waste, don't let that be *your* life. Promise me, darling, you'll make your life mean something.'

'I'll try, Auntie, I'll try.'

But even as she said it her heart and her waters were breaking.

Chapter Ninety

Vincent O'Casey was tired out. He had been in the gym all morning and then cooked all afternoon. One good thing about Parkhurst – on the SSB unit at least you weren't on constant lock up. It was still hard though. Knowing that Gabby was due at any moment, he was like a cat on a hot tin roof. All the other lags were chafing him, but he took it in a good-natured way. The fact that he had not named names had gone a long way to making his stay in nick quite easy. It wasn't ideal, but it was bearable, and Derek Greene had made sure of that, as had Bertie Warner. The Manchester boys treated him like some kind of mascot, and he appreciated it – it showed him that what he was enduring was not for nothing. The hardest thing to bear was that his little baby would be born without him, and he knew his Gabby needed him. She had no one really, except her old grandparents and they were fucking ancient. Nice people, but not exactly in the first flush of youth.

It was pointless dwelling on it now. The first thing he had learned was that the outside world was something you had no control over, therefore you must not let it do your head in. He knew better now than to let his thoughts wander too far from the normal. But with his Gabby on the verge of giving birth to his first child, a child he would not see until visiting day, it was getting harder and harder to pretend it was happening to someone else.

He consoled himself with the thought that he had not

dropped anyone in it, that he could hold his head up. But it still didn't make up for being banged up in here while his girl was alone and pregnant on the outside.

As he was walking back to his cell, a screw called his name and number. He stood to attention as was required and the screw, one of the few who was a nice enough geezer, said to him happily, 'You got a daughter, lad – eight pounds nine ounces. Congratulations!'

'A girl? Oh my God, I got a fucking daughter!' Vincent was jumping up and down, his face a picture of happiness, his voice louder than it had ever been before.

The commotion had brought all the lags out of their cells, and Vincent felt his hand being shaken, and his shoulders being hugged, but it was like a dream to him. A little girl – he had a little girl. He hoped his Gabby had not had too bad a time of it. According to half the men in here, the first one was a piece of piss – except George Palmer whose wife had died in childbirth, but that was twenty-five years ago. Things were so much different these days.

The screws congratulated him, and one gave him a pack of cigars, while another gave him two bottles of decent Scotch. He knew this lot was really from Derek Greene but he was grateful nonetheless. When all was said and done, he would much rather have been beside Gabby and seen his little baby for himself. The men on the wing understood that, and they did their best to help him forget. He was grateful to them because he wasn't sure he could have coped with it alone.

Chapter Ninety-One

Celeste died just two hours after Gabby's baby was born. Little Cherie Celeste Mary Tailor entered the world screaming, and it was a sound that her mother cherished from the first moment. She was a big lusty child with thick blond hair and the Callahan blue eyes. She was adorable, and Gabby fell instantly in love with her, as did her great-nana and granddad.

Jack looked at the child as if he had never seen a baby before. He wondered if it was the fact she was a great-granddaughter and he never thought he would live that long, or if it was because the baby was exquisite. He decided it was most probably a mixture of the two.

It was a night of celebration, and a night of mourning. As his Mary had pointed out, God takes one and leaves another in its place. A load of old cobblers really, but he wanted to believe it this night. Wanted to believe that his poor Celeste might live again through this child. He sat there for a long moment, the child in his arms, the fourth living generation of Callahans, and he wondered what kind of life this child would have. He prayed it would be a good life, a really good life. His old mum had often said, 'Life at its longest is short, make the most of it while you still can.' How true that was. But with this baby's start in life, a very young mother and her father doing a big lump for armed robbery, he couldn't really see any good coming of it. He hoped against hope that he was wrong.

Chapter Ninety-Two

Cynthia looked down at the baby who was, to all intents and purposes, her grandchild. She had taken the call about the birth from a girl she had known at school, and with whom she had resumed a rather sketchy relationship. The girl was a drinker and she supplied a few quid in exchange for news about Cynthia's family. Now she was at the hospital, and looking at her daughter's little girl.

The baby was very pretty – a robust, yet delicate-featured little girl, with thick blond hair and what already promised to be strong blue eyes. Oh, she would have the Callahan eyes all right, not those insipid Tailor eyes that James Junior had inherited.

Looking through the glass of the baby unit, Cynthia Callahan felt, for the first time in her life, a stirring inside her. Try as she might to force it away, she knew she would never be able to deny it. This child affected her on a primal level. Even her own children had never made her feel this deep a connection.

The child was looking straight into her eyes as if it knew she was its grandmother. Never had she seen a child so beautiful, so utterly gorgeous. And she looked exactly like her! The child was Cynthia all over.

The strength of her emotions shocked her. It occurred to her now that this was the *next* generation. She had given birth to this child's mother and, if it wasn't for *her*, this child would never have even been here. That was a very powerful thought. It made her feel invincible, like Methuselah in the Bible, who had lived for nine hundred years – well, *he* hadn't but his offspring had. She finally understood family, and it had taken this baby to make her see what that really meant.

Her first attempt had been lousy – she had been too young and she had had her children with the wrong man – but now, with this little one, she felt she had a chance to redeem herself, make her life mean something. She could turn this child into a good person. If she was left with her mother she would end up like her mother. A teenage unmarried mum, a fucking waster, worth nothing – nothing of value anyway. Not as far as Cynthia was concerned.

The baby was like a magnet, and she felt a pull that she had never felt before in her life. She wanted this child. And she would move heaven and earth to get it.

Chapter Ninety-Three

'She was my sister, Mum. I have every right to be here.'

Mary looked into her daughter's face and wondered what was the real reason this girl of hers had turned up on her doorstep at Celeste's wake. She could hazard a guess, but she was sure she would be wrong. Cynthia had not even wanted her own children, so why would she want a grandchild? Mary had felt she had no choice but to let her into the house and then she had seen the naked hunger in Cynthia's eyes as she had looked at little Cherie in her bassinet.

When Cynthia marched into the sitting room and immediately bent over the cradle to pick the baby up somehow Mary knew that her daughter had seen the child before, and she had felt as if she was witnessing a crime. Never had Cynthia been that gentle with her own children.

'If you're feeling maternal why don't you go and visit your son? I'm sure *he* could do with a bit of motherly interest.'

Cynthia held the child to her as she said dreamily, 'Why don't you have a day off, Mum? I know I made mistakes, but this is my grandchild and, whether you like it or not, that is the truth of the matter. She reminds me of my Gabriella at the same age. She's such a lovely child.' Cynthia knew that Gabby could hear her from her bedroom and she continued in a hurt voice, 'I hope you don't alienate this child from Gabriella like you alienated her from me. I was already aware I had made a big mistake marrying James, but it was you my kids wanted, wasn't it, not me. You made sure of that.'

Mary was incensed. 'How dare you! I took your kids in when you got fed up with them. I loved them like my own.'

Cynthia knew that was the truth, but she ignored it and said in a placating manner, 'Please, Mum, it's Celeste's funeral. Have a bit of respect.'

Mary was so furious at the words of her daughter she was rendered speechless. How could she say that to her, after all she had done! Her daughter was a manipulator who used everyone around her. Well, she would not use *her* any more, those days were long gone.

'You are welcome only to pay your respects. After that you can piss off.'

'I must say, Mum, that is you all over.'

Cynthia hugged the child to her; from her first contact with it she knew that this was a child that was meant to be with her. She loved it. The child was perfect in every way, like her little Gabriella when she was born, except now Cynthia was older and wiser, and she finally understood what flesh and blood meant. What made women kill for their kids, and what life was all about. She had never realised until this moment. The moment she had held her grandchild in her arms.

Cynthia was looking at the child with such love that even Mary wondered if she had been wrong about her daughter. Could it be that she wanted a second chance at motherhood?

Watching Cynthia, Gabby was completely convinced that there was genuine love in her mother for this child of hers. It hurt, knowing that she hadn't felt that way about her or her brother, but she was glad she felt like that about little Cherie. The baby had so few people in her little life – her father was banged up, his family had no interest, and this was the day of her great-auntie's funeral. Her family was shrinking by the day.

So, as useless as her mother was, Gabby would welcome her

into her daughter's life and take whatever her mother had to offer, for as long as it lasted. Gabby was so desperately lonely, and she needed other people in her life. At this point, even her mother was preferable to no one. She knew her nana would think she was mad, but what could she do? This was Cherie's grandmother and she owed it to her to try and build a few bridges. As bad as her mother could be, she appeared to be enamoured of her grandchild. That was enough for Gabby, who, alone in the world with a new baby, was desperate to have a family again.

They had buried Celeste, and they felt her loss keenly, especially Mary who had always had a soft spot for her younger child. She had tried, in her own way, to make their lives easier. Now Mary had to watch her granddaughter forge some kind of relationship with her mother – the same woman who was responsible for the death of the daughter Mary had buried this day.

Chapter Ninety-Four

'It's not like that, Nana!'

Mary shrugged aggressively. 'How is it then, Gabby? Tell me and your granddad. We're interested. Only your mother was never what we would call a frequent presence in your life, so we're amazed at how often you seem to be seeing her.'

Gabby couldn't explain how hard it was to walk away from her mother these days. She believed she had genuinely changed, and she wanted to make amends. But her nana and granddad couldn't see that. She knew they had reason to feel like they did, but this was still her mother they were talking about, Cherie's nanny. In producing this child she felt, for the first time in her life, like she had done something good in her mother's eyes, and she was enjoying that feeling. It was almost as if Cynthia was loving *her* through her baby, and that felt good. All her life Gabby had felt there was something wrong with her; if her own mother couldn't love her, then who could?

'Oh, Nana, I know you think I'm wrong, but she *has* changed. She loves little Cherie like we do! Please, Nana, don't ruin this for me.'

Mary was shocked at those words. As if *she* would ever ruin anything for this girl, or the child she had produced. The only person who had ever ruined anything for her she was now welcoming back into her life with wide open arms. And no good could come of it, she would lay money on that.

She understood why Gabby was desperate to make some kind

of connection with her mother, even after everything had happened. When all was said and done she was her closest kin. Mary was being forced to sit back and wait and then eventually pick up the pieces, because unfortunately she knew, as sure as she knew her own name, that this reunion could only end in tears.

Chapter Ninety-Five

As Jack Callahan looked at his wife, he felt the power of her, as he always had. She was stronger than he would ever be and it had taken her heart attack to make him appreciate just what a good woman he had bagged all those years ago.

Now he could see she was hurting. She had buried a child – something no parent should ever do. It was the wrong order of things; a child should bury its parents, not vice versa. And it had upset her that Gabby was all over her mother like a cheap suit.

'It can't last, Mary. You know Cynthia like I do – she'll fuck it up and Gabby will see her for what she is.'

Mary shook her head sadly; if only that was the case. But she had seen Cynthia looking at her grandchild, and she recognised that look. She had felt it herself many years ago. Cynthia saw an opportunity to make up for her mistakes; all the wrongs she had committed counted for nothing now that child was there. She thought of that baby as a new page to be written on, a new canvas to paint in her own image. Cynthia would not let this baby go, not now. Not when she had an in on its life.

Mary had felt the same when Cynthia had produced Gabby and James Junior. It was like a second chance at motherhood. When you became a grandparent, it was like God handing you a child without the pain of bearing it. And you were given something that was even more precious than your own kids, because it was *your* kids who had produced it in the first place.

It hurt a great deal to see Gabby forgetting what her mother was capable of and welcoming her with open arms. But what could she do?

Cynthia was on full charm offensive, and that was not an easy thing to ignore. She was playing on the fact that Gabby needed her mother, but Mary knew that Cynthia would soon lose interest. She always did, leaving a trail of death and destruction wherever she went.

Life was hard for a lot of people, Mary knew, but it seemed at times her family had it much harder than most. Cynthia saw to that; she had always been responsible for their problems.

'She will eat her up and spit her out, Jack. Cynthia wants that child, but she doesn't want its mother.'

Jack nodded in agreement. ''Course she does. Think about it – she's kicking forty, she has nothing in her life – *never* had anything in her life if she's honest with herself. A baby will be something new to her; after all, it won't know her, will it? Not like everyone else does. A baby loves whoever feeds it.'

'That's what worries me, Jack. Not the baby so much, but our Gabby – she has always wanted her mother to love her, admire her, care for her.'

'That's human nature, Mary. But Gabby ain't a mug – she will see that this is all a fucking act, and she'll aim her out of it.'

'But I'm not so sure she will, Jack. She needs Vincent, needs him by her side. She's missing him, she's all hormones and wanting. She wants to be loved, and she wants to be loved by the people who matter. But I hope you are right, mate. I really hope you are right.'

Chapter Ninety-Six

'Look at her go! She is as clever as a bag of fucking monkeys.'

Gabby could hear the pride in her mother's voice and she swelled with pride herself. Seeing her mother with her little daughter made her wish that she had been like that with her once. Cynthia certainly seemed a happier person now though. In fact, Gabby had never seen her mother like this before. She was lighter in herself, almost like a normal person. She *almost* seemed to enjoy her daughter's company, and it was no secret she couldn't get enough of her granddaughter's. Gabby knew her nana didn't like it, but she couldn't help herself – the pull of her mother was too strong. She had dreamt of having this kind of relationship with her for years. Daydreamed that they went shopping together for clothes, had lunch together, had fun together. Now they were finally doing those things, and it was all because of Cherie.

Cherie was gorgeous. She had a wonderful smile as well and, now she was crawling, she was becoming a little person – a little person who looked at her grandmother with love and happiness.

'Come to me, my little angel.' Cynthia picked the child up and carefully laid her on the changing table. As she expertly changed her nappy, she crooned away in her own particular brand of baby talk, before saying to Gabby, 'Leave her here tonight and have a night off, love. Go and visit your mates, have a few hours to yourself – young mums need that.'

Gabby wasn't sure.

'Look, Gabs.'

Her mother had taken to calling her that again and she liked it, it made her feel she was finally a part of Cynthia's life.

'You can have a nice bath in peace, do your hair and, best of all, you can have a full night's sleep. This little one is teething, and I haven't got any plans tonight. You can pick her up tomorrow.'

It did sound tempting, she had to admit. Gabby looked around the spare room in her mother's penthouse, which was kitted out like a movie star's nursery, and she was awed by it. It was pale lemon and white, and it even had stencilling on the walls. It looked wonderful. A lot nicer than the bedroom the baby shared with her at her nana's. She knew that Cherie would be OK here, but she still wasn't sure about leaving her. Her nana would go mad if she left her overnight; she seemed to think Cynthia was up to no good. She wished they could see her and Cherie together – it was sweet to watch.

Cynthia was not going to take no for an answer. 'When was the last time you were a young girl, eh? When was the last time you got your gladrags on and had a night out with your mates? Had a few drinks, let your hair down? It's not good for you being stuck in with a baby all the time, even one as lovely as our Cherie. We'll be here waiting for you.' She smiled at the baby in her arms. 'Won't we, darling? We'll wait for mummy, won't we? How's that mate of yours, the one I always thought was a bad influence?'

'Christine Carter? Oh, she's still around, pops in to see me sometimes. Now *she* is always out somewhere!'

Cynthia laughed with her daughter. She knew exactly what Christine Carter got up to – she was a byword for whoring and drug-taking, by all accounts.

'You should ring her, go out with her. You're not a kid any more, are you? I bet she'll show you a good time!'

'I could I suppose, she does love a night out. But Vince . . .'

'*Vince* is in the nick, love, and I'm sure that if *he* had the chance of a night out he would take it without a second's thought for you or anyone. Blokes are like that, love. Anyway, you're not married to him and, while he's away, why should you be locked up too? He should have thought of that, love; if you want *my* opinion, I think you *deserve* a night out.'

Cherie gave one of her big gummy grins and the matter was sealed.

A little later on, Cynthia handed her daughter fifty pounds in cash. 'Have a good night, sweetheart, and don't worry about little Cherie – she'll be safe as houses.'

Gabby hugged her mother then, overwhelmed by her generosity and, when her mother hugged her back, she felt as if she had won the rollover on the lottery.

Chapter Ninety-Seven

'Where the hell have you been?'

Mary's voice was angrier than Gabby had ever heard it and, putting the pillow over her head, she groaned. 'Not now, Nana, I'm tired out.'

Mary opened the curtains and dragged the quilt and pillow from her granddaughter's bed. ''Course you're tired out – you've been out on the lash for two days. It's Sunday, love, and you are getting up and you are going to go to your mother's and you are going to get your baby. Remember your baby? *Cherie*, ten months old, little bundle of happiness?'

Mary saw the ravaged look on the girl's face and sighed heavily. The last few months she had started going clubbing – whatever the fuck that was – and Gabby had apparently taken to it like a duck to water. She was out more than she was in, and the upshot was that Cherie now spent more time with her grandmother than she did with her own mother.

That Cynthia was behind this newfound freedom, Mary had no doubt but, at the moment, Cynthia could do no wrong in Gabby's eyes. She was all 'me mum this', and 'me mum that'. Like Cynthia was suddenly the fucking oracle or something.

Mary was even more worried because she had found little pills in Gabby's bedroom drawer, and she guessed they were those things called Es they were always talking about on the news. They were dangerous – people had died taking them.

She looked at her granddaughter's emaciated body; she had

297

lost a lot of weight, and she often appeared spaced out, that was the only way she could describe the vacant look on the girl's face. That was Christine fucking Carter's fault; she was known on the estate for everything from drugs to thieving. Now Gabby thought that Christine Carter was the epitome of council house chic.

Gabby was already asleep again, and Mary sighed, knowing it was pointless trying to talk to her while she was like this. In a way she sympathised. Gabby was little more than a child herself and she was tied down with a baby, with the father locked up on the Isle of Wight. With her mother on the scene, she felt her baby was being well looked after – it was with its nanny after all who doted on the child – so Gabby could go out and have a good time. Mary wasn't so old she didn't understand human nature, and if it was once a week she would have encouraged it. But it was now nearly every night. It was as if once Gabby had tasted freedom, she was hooked and wanted more and more of it, but at the expense of her baby daughter. Cherie had not been to their house in ten days, and that bothered Mary. The social worker was not impressed either, and that did not bode well.

She walked slowly from the room and, making a cup of tea, she wondered at how this would all finally pan out.

She didn't have long to wait for the answer to her question.

Chapter Ninety-Eight

'My mum's too old to have the baby full time and so Cherie would be much better off here. I think Gabriella would prefer it too.'

Miss Byrne nodded in resignation; as nice as this woman seemed there was something off about her that she couldn't quite put her finger on.

'Are the police sure *she* was selling the drugs?'

'Quite sure. She sold them to an undercover policewoman,' Miss Byrne responded bluntly.

Cynthia rolled her eyes in annoyance. 'For God's sake, what was she thinking! She has a little baby to care for and she does something that stupid. I admit I had my suspicions – I mean, she's always out. I knew she was taking something, I just didn't know what.' She gave the baby a rusk then fastened her into her high chair. 'She's so young, too young really to have a baby. I would have suggested an abortion but my mother would have none of that, of course. And now this little darling is here we wouldn't be without her, but . . .' She left the sentence unfinished but Miss Byrne actually felt herself agreeing with the woman's opinion.

'So you are happy to keep the child until we deem Gabriella capable once more to take over as the primary carer?'

Cynthia wondered if the woman had swallowed a dictionary; she bet that kind of talk went down a bundle on the council estates. 'If you mean will I take on my granddaughter until my Gabriella is on her feet again, then yes.'

Miss Byrne agreed. 'Quite. Well, everything seems fine here and, I must say, the nursery is lovely. She really is a lucky little girl.'

Cynthia preened at the praise and, after she had shown Miss Byrne to the door, she picked up her granddaughter and said in an excited voice, 'It's just me and you, kid! Just me and you!'

Hugging the child to her, she made a mental note to give Christine Carter a few quid; after all, without her none of this would have been possible.

Chapter Ninety-Nine

'What possessed you, child?'

A couple of nights in the cells had certainly sobered Gabby up, no doubt about that. She looked terrified.

'Drug-dealing! That I should live to see the day!' Mary was heartbroken at the news, and it was this that made Gabby feel worse than ever.

'I wasn't, Nana – at least, that was the first time I've done it. Christine asked me to do it for her because she felt ill. I only did as I was asked, I know it was stupid . . .'

Mary shook her head in disbelief; how could this girl be so stupid? 'First time, or fiftieth time, it will make no difference to the courts. And you had drugs in your system – that's all come up on the blood tests. So you've lost your daughter. Guess who has her at this moment? Your mother, and I can tell you now you will have a hard time getting her back.'

Gabby groaned with shame and hurt. This was like a nightmare, a nightmare of her own making. Sitting in that stinking cell had made her think about her life, and she was not impressed with herself, so God knew what her mother must think of her. But then, her mother had encouraged her to go out and enjoy herself – she even gave her the money to go out and have a good time.

It was odd, but from that first night out clubbing, she had felt for the first time in years like a teenager. Surrounded by music and other young people, she had felt she belonged. This

301

was what she *should* be doing. If she had used her head she could have been doing it without the responsibility of a baby and, as much as she loved little Cherie, she missed her freedom. She had known she was safe with her mum who loved the child. It wasn't wrong to leave the baby with its grandmother, was it?

But she had to be honest with herself now. It wasn't leaving her there that was the problem, it was that she left her there so often. Pretending that it was just because she knew her mother loved it, she had allowed her to become Cherie's main carer. Cherie didn't even want to come to Gabby any more, she just wanted her nanny. And who could blame her? Oh, she had been such a fool! And now she had a conviction for drug-dealing hanging over her. She felt sick.

'Will I go to prison, Nana?'

Mary shook her head in despair. 'I don't know, Gabby, I honestly don't know.'

Chapter One Hundred

Vincent O'Casey read the letter with growing anger and resentment. That his Gabby had been so foolish was one thing, but to find out that his child was now in the sole custody of Cynthia Callahan was quite another. After what Gabby had told him about her upbringing, he was not at all happy that his child was now at that woman's mercy. Yet, according to this letter, her mother was now a changed character, and she was helping her daughter to get back on her feet.

Gabby, he kept reminding himself, was very young, and she had made a very stupid mistake. He could forgive her that – of course he could – but he could *not* forgive her abandoning their child like this. She was promising to come and see him in a few weeks. She had missed the last few visits, and her letters had been sparse as well. Now he fucking well knew why.

He had missed Gabby, but he had also missed the baby. He hadn't seen her many times but he loved that child. She was a pretty contented little thing, always smiling and beautifully turned out.

This was the worst bit about being in prison; the world outside carried on, and there was nothing you could do about that. When things went wrong, like this trouble with Gabby, he couldn't help because he was stuck in here. Being helpless to do anything for the people he loved was worse than anything else he could think of.

Chapter One Hundred and One

'Look, Cherie, look at the pictures with Mummy.'

But Cherie wanted to get off her mother's lap, and sit with her nanny. Cynthia was holding a drink of apple juice, which she knew was Cherie's favourite treat at the moment. She picked up the child and sat her on her knee smiling at her daughter's crestfallen countenance.

'Listen to me, Gabriella – kids are amoral. They go to whoever feeds them. It's nothing personal, darling.'

Gabby smiled but her heart wasn't in it.

'I'll have to get her ready soon, love. She goes to a playgroup a few hours a day now, three times a week. She's making friends, bless her heart. While she's there, I nip up the shops, or go to the gym. I love her, darling, but she's a handful.'

Gabby felt she was being dismissed; she knew her mother was telling her she had better go soon. She made her feel as if she was holding the pair of them up somehow, was in the way. In fact, she realised that her mother had not even offered her a cup of coffee. She had only been there twenty minutes, if that, and she was already being asked, albeit politely, to leave.

'I can wait at the playgroup with her . . .'

'I don't think that's a good idea, Gabs, and, to be honest, I think you unsettle her. She has got into a routine, and Miss Byrne thinks she needs more structure in her life. Plus, I've arranged for her to go to tea with one of the little girls there. Dear little thing too, though not a patch on our Cherie!'

Gabby tried another tack. 'But I'm taking her to visit Vincent tomorrow – he'll expect to see her.'

Cynthia grinned then, and it was the old Cynthia for a few moments. 'Well, not a lot he can do about that, girl, is there? He should have thought of that before he got himself banged up.'

'But he wants to see her.'

'Well, then, in that case, he'll know what it's like to want, won't he? I promised Miss Byrne that I would do whatever is right for this baby and, at the moment, I don't think you should be around her. Not until you've sorted yourself out. Drug addicts are—'

Gabby interjected, shocked at her mother's choice of words, 'Drug addict! I ain't a fucking drug addict . . .'

Cynthia shrugged. 'Drug *dealer* then. Let's not split hairs, love. I don't think it's fair on this child to drag her from pillar to post, OK? It's not about what you want or what I want for that matter, it's about what is best for this little child.'

Gabby couldn't argue with that, but it was all wrong somehow. She was Cherie's mother, and she loved her baby. She had made a silly mistake, but she was already paying the price for that. Gabby was confused; her mother was pushing her away again, and she had a sneaking suspicion that somehow she had played right into Cynthia's hands and lost Cherie. Now her baby had a new mummy, and that was Cynthia Callahan. Suddenly, with stunning clarity, Gabby could see that her nana had been right – Cynthia had only wanted the baby, and she had used Gabby to get what she wanted. She felt as if someone had slapped her in the face.

'I'll ring you, Gabs, and we'll make arrangements for you to come over next week, eh?'

Cynthia was standing with the child in her arms, and Gabby knew she had been outfoxed, outmanoeuvred, and was now surplus to requirements.

Chapter One Hundred and Two

'She can't take our child for good, Gabby. Use your loaf.'

Gabby was sitting opposite Vincent and her heart felt like lead in her chest. 'But I realise now me nana was right about her. All her interest in me was for one reason only – to get Cherie.'

Vincent wasn't in the mood for this today. He was feeling out of sorts anyway; he had a cold coming, and he was suffering from cabin fever. It came on most long-timers two or three times a year. Especially the younger ones. Being banged up was hard work, and you had to get your head around it.

He took a deep breath and counted to ten like the gym instructor had told him to when he felt the urge to lash out. After he had exhaled slowly he said, 'I can't do this today, Gabby, I really can't deal with you moaning. You had a capture, you fucked up. We've all done it. All you can do now is make sure you sort it out, and sort yourself out while you're at it. But I can't help you, and the more you tell me, the harder it is for me, because I can't walk out that door and come to your aid. And that is difficult for me to admit. You reckoned your mum had turned over a new leaf? Maybe she has. Maybe she has that child's best interests at heart. But Cherie's *our* daughter. So all I can say is get the court case over with, plead guilty and do a deal. Then work at getting Cherie back. Prove to your mum, the social workers, King Street Charlie if

306

necessary, that you are back on track, and it will turn out right in the end. OK?'

She nodded then, her lovely face white with apprehension.

'Now, how's your nana and granddad?'

Chapter One Hundred and Three

David Duggan was very impressed with his neighbour Cynthia Callahan, especially when she told him her daughter was a recovering addict, and she now had to bring up her little grand-daughter. From what she'd said, it seemed the daughter was like her father – weak willed and always looking for the easy option. Poor Cynthia told him she'd done everything she could, but the girl was a lost cause, and she could not allow that to happen to her granddaughter, which he thoroughly agreed with. The child was a delight too, and he felt they were becoming quite the little family unit.

He had taken to staying over a few nights a week; the sex was unbelievable, and the breakfasts the next morning with the little girl crowing and making them laugh had become the highlight of his existence. He didn't know what he would do without Cynthia now – she had become such a big part of his life. She was also a fabulous cook, and she had taken to letting herself into his flat and doing his washing and ironing for him.

That she used those opportunities to rifle through his desk, and get her hands on his bank books he had no idea. She always gave him back his keys, so he had no way of knowing she had already had a set made for herself.

David Duggan felt that he was a very lucky man to be given a second chance at happiness at this stage of his life. And he thanked God every day for bringing Cynthia Callahan into his comfortable, but rather dreary, life.

Chapter One Hundred and Four

Cynthia adored her granddaughter and the feeling was entirely mutual. As she walked her in the park, Cynthia planned the child's life; a good school, private of course, and nice friends. Once she had fleeced David she would move on, this time to a nice London suburb. A place where the child would be surrounded by the finer things in life.

Oh, it was as if she had been given a second chance at happiness, and she was grateful to the powers-that-be for giving it to her. The only problem was Gabriella; she would always have to put up with her having some kind of role in the child's life, but she would make sure that her input was minimal at best. It irritated her but there wasn't a lot she could do about it. Well, not for a while anyway.

The social services thought she was the dog's bollocks, and she had made sure of that by being the picture of kindness and generosity. They agreed that her daughter was still too immature to look after a child, and she pointed out how well Cherie had settled with her, which was not a lie either. Cherie was very happy, and why wouldn't she be? She was waited on hand and foot, clean and well fed. She had only the best clothes and shoes too; she was like a little doll, and Cynthia loved to dress her up.

The doorbell rang and she went to answer it; she hoped it wasn't David, expecting a cup of coffee and a quick feel – she really wasn't in the mood today. Opening the door, a smile plastered on her heavily made-up face, she was amazed to see her mother standing there.

'Hello, Cynth, aren't you going to invite me in? The social worker's just parking the car.'

Then, walking past her speechless daughter, Mary went into the large lounge and, kneeling down, she opened her arms to little Cherie and said happily, 'Hello, my little lovely, your great-nana's here to see you.'

Chapter One Hundred and Five

Miss Byrne had a feeling that something was not right between Cynthia Callahan and her mother, but she couldn't put her finger on exactly what that might be. They were polite enough to each other, but it was forced, as if they were both playing a part. Which, of course, they were.

Mary couldn't help but be impressed with Cynthia's home; although it was clean as clean could be, it still had the smell and feel of a real home. Cherie's toys were scattered all over the place, something that she had never seen in Cynthia's house when Gabby and James Junior were little. The poor things had been terrified of making a noise, let alone a mess.

Cherie looked well cared for and happy and that was what really hurt Mary Callahan. Why couldn't Cynthia have been that way with her own children? Watching how the girl put her arms up to her grandmother to be picked up, and seeing Cynthia, her daughter Cynthia, smiling at the child with genuine affection, even love, Mary knew then that Gabby was going to have a fight on her hands to get that baby back. Cynthia was besotted with the child, and she had never seen her besotted by anything or anyone before – except maybe Jonny Parker, and look at how that had turned out.

The social worker was watching the interplay with fascination; this was a mother and daughter who obviously had issues. At least contact had been established though. She felt she was reuniting this family, and was quite pleased with herself because of it. Suicide, she knew, could divide families, as had clearly been the case here, but with a little help and some counselling, who knew what might be achieved. When she said as much a few minutes later, she was amazed at the way the two women laughed as if they were never going to stop.

Chapter One Hundred and Six

'Jesus, Jack, she's living like a fucking queen! The place is beautiful, and I hate to say this, but little Cherie is thriving. That's the only way I can put it – positively thriving.'

Jack Callahan listened with growing dismay. It seemed that his Mary had been right all along and, as he looked at young Gabby, he raised his eyes as if to say, well, you were warned this would happen.

Gabby swallowed back the tears that were threatening to fall. 'Did she look all right then, me mum? Was she all right about you going round there?'

Mary laughed gently. 'She had no choice. I had the social worker with me, and you know your mother – she could get an Oscar for her acting. I hate to say I told you so, but I did, didn't I? She wanted that child and now she's got her, and there ain't a thing you can do about it.'

'But *I'm* her mum!'

It was the petulant cry of a child, which, in reality, was all Gabby was. For the first time Mary Callahan wondered if Cherie might be better off where she was, but she forced that thought out of her head. Cynthia wasn't a person you could trust in the long term, she never had been.

'Well, all we can do is go through the proper channels and hope in the meantime that your mother gets fed up playing happy families. But I wouldn't bank on the latter, Gabby. I can honestly say I've never seen her so happy. I never saw a woman so obsessed with a child in my life. She won't let go easily.'

Gabby felt the weight of her mother crushing down on her; she felt like she had as a small child, unable to fight back against the might that was her mum, against the self-righteousness that her mother cloaked every word in. She knew she had been a very stupid girl. Caught up in Christine Carter's lifestyle, she had been too busy enjoying herself and forgotten her responsibilities. She wouldn't lie to herself about that. Lonely without Vincent she had liked pretending to be a carefree young girl, clubbing, having a drink, a few laughs. She had also enjoyed taking the Es, and smoking a bit of dope with people her own age. She had even liked the attention she got from boys, although she had never succumbed to any of their advances – at least she had that going for her. She knew Vincent had heard rumours, and he was desperately disappointed in her, but she also knew he understood that she was young and she had been foolish and he had forgiven her.

Well, she had to get herself together – work towards getting Cherie back and creating some kind of life for them both. It wouldn't be easy, but she knew that if she tried, she could do it.

Jack Callahan hugged his granddaughter to him as if he knew exactly what she thinking, and she wondered for the thousandth time how she could have been taken in by her mother. Even knowing everything she did about her, all she was capable of, she had still trusted her. Well, she would never make that mistake again.

Chapter One Hundred and Seven

2003

Cherie looked at her mother and shook her head petulantly. 'I'm staying at Nanny's. We're going to a party tomorrow.'

Gabby, at twenty-one, was used to these kind of conversations with her little daughter; Cynthia always arranged lots of trips and parties when she was due to have her for the weekend. Gabby had learned a long time before to ignore the child's wide-eyed pleading. Once she was out of her mother's house, the girl was a different child.

'No, you're not. You're coming with Mummy.'

Cherie glowered at Gabby, saying loudly, 'But I hate it at your house, and Nana Mary smells bad.'

Gabby was itching to put her hand across her daughter's arse but she restrained herself with difficulty. Her mum would be straight on to the social workers, reporting child abuse, beatings and anything else she could think of.

Cynthia watched the exchange with a small satisfied smile on her lips. She had to give it to her daughter, Gabby was resolute. Well, she got that from her but, unlike her, she wouldn't be able to keep it up indefinitely.

'Nana Mary does not smell bad, and you know that.'

Cherie didn't answer, she was waiting to see what occurred between her mummy and her nanny first. She knew they didn't like one another. It worried her sometimes, but at other times it

315

worked in her favour; it meant they vied with each other to give her what she wanted.

Gabby changed the subject. 'Your daddy will be home in a few weeks.'

Cherie brightened up then. She loved her daddy, and she truly believed that he was training to be a fighter pilot. Like a lot of kids she had been told that story, it explained away the uniforms everywhere on the visits. Cherie opened her mouth but, after a dark look from her nanny, she shut it again.

'The three of us will be together all the time then, and you can stay at Nanny's at weekends, *sometimes*.'

Stick that one up your arse, Mother, and smoke it.

Gabby knew that Vince was determined to get them back on track, and he had been a diamond. He had given Derek Greene a tug, and money had miraculously appeared every week, as had a nice council flat and new furniture. She was now established as a blagger's wife, and she was treated as one by everybody. It was amazing what the friendship of Greene and Warner could do for a body, and she was grateful for their help. She knew it bothered her mother as well, and she knew *why* it bothered her so much. But, as Vince said, he had earned his keep, he'd kept his trap shut and taken the fall for everyone. They *owed* him.

He was a very different Vincent these days; he was a man now, a big, handsome man and, like her, he had grown up quickly. She knew her mother would get the shock of her life when he came home, and she couldn't wait. He would put her well and truly in her place, and she wanted to be there when he did it.

The social workers were still hanging round like a bad smell, and she had heard through the grapevine that her mother told them exaggerated stories about Gabby's wild ways, and how she was still worried that her daughter was too immature to take care of Cherie on a regular basis. But Gabby was biding her time – she knew that fighting this woman was pointless. She knew the social workers wondered where all her money *really* came from, but they could go and fuck themselves; she was cleaner than a whistle. All she claimed was her Family Allowance and the minimum of benefits – that was it. But the drug conviction which, thanks to a good brief, had got her probation and one hundred and twenty hours community service, was still being held over her head like the sword of Damocles.

It was amazing really – if her mother had just kept out of it, she would be happily ensconced with her daughter now, and it would all be in the past. But that hadn't been her mother's plan. Right from the start, she had been determined to get the child, and she would stoop as low as she needed to make sure that happened. She had not allowed for the fact that Gabby was as stubborn as she was, when necessary, and so they were still playing this game.

'Has he got his release date, then?'

Gabby smiled, and Cynthia saw what a very beautiful young woman she was. It pained her to see herself as she had been twenty years earlier. She envied this girl her youth, and they both knew it.

'Yep.'

Cynthia would not lower herself to ask when that was; she would find out soon enough. 'Bet you can't wait.'

'Nope, I can't. You wait till you see him, Mum, you'll get the surprise of your life.' It wasn't exactly a threat as such, but she knew her mother was worried at the implication. 'Now come on, Cherie – I've got the car outside and we are going to Mackie D's for our dinner!'

Cherie was thrilled; she loved a McDonald's. Her nanny said they were too fattening and full of crap, but she didn't care. She was happy now to put her coat on and go with her mother, especially when she promised, 'Then we are going to watch whatever you want on TV.'

As her granddaughter got herself ready, Cynthia fought back the urge to take her daughter by the hair and batter her to death.

'Say bye bye to Nanny, darling.'

Cherie kissed and hugged her nanny, but it was obvious she was impatient now to be on her way.

'Don't let her watch anything frightening, she's too small.'

Gabby sighed heavily; this was a constant refrain. You'd think she let the child watch horror films day and night. 'As if I would.'

Cynthia replied, all self-righteous in her anger, 'Well, if I find out she's been glued to those American detective shows there'll be murders.'

'Well, you'd know all about that, wouldn't you, Mum?'

Cynthia was fuming at the inference, and the fact that her daughter felt confident enough to say it spoke volumes. The news of Vincent's return had given her girl an edge, an edge Cynthia would take great pleasure in blunting. She still had a few tricks up her sleeve.

Gabby smiled. 'See you.'

Cynthia smiled back, adding nastily, 'You can guarantee it.'

Chapter One Hundred and Eight

'He's going to want a bit of work at some point.' Derek Greene was glad Vincent would soon be out.

Bertie Warner grinned. 'Well, of course he will, but not for a few months. He's got four years of shagging to catch up on first, as well as getting used to being on the out. We'll have a party for him; after all, the boy's been a fucking diamond. Bung him a few grand to tide him over and see what occurs – he might want to go straight.'

Derek laughed loudly at that one.

Bertie made a *moue* with his lips, then said in a serious manner, 'It has been known!'

'Not Vincent, it's in his blood. I've had great reports about him, done his time like a fucking man, and he's a big lad by all accounts. But then six hours a day in the gym will do that to a body. No, I think we should find him a good earner, get him back in the fold. He done a big favour for us and all concerned, and I respect him for that. Only eighteen and put on the island, and he made his mark there and all. Well liked, but didn't take any nonsense.'

Bertie agreed with his friend, and he said jovially, 'I bet that little bird of his is champing at the bit, eh? Four years with no nookie! Not heard a detrimental word about her either, have you?'

'Not for a long time. Had a bit of trouble when he first went away, selling Es of all things, and to an undercover Filth.

319

Something dodgy there – I could never put me finger on it, but it all smelt wrong, you know? That slag Christine Carter was behind it – she's a fucking skank, that bird.'

Bertie was quiet for a moment. 'Will young Vincent want to pay back any debts, do you think? You know, settle any scores?'

'Wouldn't blame him if he did. She nearly lost the kid over it.'

'Her mother's got the kid now, ain't she?'

'Most of the time, from what I can gather. Fucking Cynthia Callahan – Tailor, that was. Who would let that whore near an innocent child?'

Bertie shook his head at the stupidity of the social services; you read about those mad fuckers every day in the papers. They left kids with complete nut-bags who murdered them, starved them, or took them off nice people. No fucking sense in any of it. 'Well, if he wants to hammer the fuck out of Cynthia, I bagsy a ringside seat.'

Derek grinned at that. 'I'm with you there.'

'But, Del Boy, she was fuckable when she was young. Arse like two boiled eggs in a handkerchief, tits that pointed at the ceiling, and she had a walk which could reduce a grown man to his knees. Well, you would want her on *her* knees, if you get my drift.'

Derek was really laughing now. 'Young Gabby looks like her then, spitting image.'

Bertie grinned. 'Yeah, but she ain't got that air of danger that her mother always had. And she was one mad cunt – she shot my mate, and I could never get back at her, because she was only defending herself and her sister. It's a bastard, but it's the truth. If Parker had come after *my* old woman, I would have wanted Cynthia Tailor on her team, know what I mean? But he was a silly fucker was, Kevin. He wanted revenge, and revenge is something you do at your leisure – not in the heat of the moment.'

Derek nodded at the truth of the other man's words. 'Well, none of them have had any real luck, have they? Jimmy Tailor killed himself, we removed Parker from the equation, and the son's in some kind of home for the mentally incapable. Fucking great family to be marrying into, that lot! Makes the fucking Borgias look like the Mickey Mouse Club.'

Bertie laughed. 'Well, young Vincent will soon make up his mind about them all once he's out from behind the door.'

Derek agreed with his old friend and said seriously, 'Amen to that.'

Chapter One Hundred and Nine

Mary loved little Cherie, she was an endearing little thing, but she could see a lot of Cynthia in the child and she had to admit that bothered her. She had the same selfish streak and the same arrogance that had been Cynthia's trademark all her life. She had her great-grandfather twisted around her little finger, but Cherie, Mary knew, understood, even at four years old, that her great-nana Mary wasn't as enamoured of her as she should be. Consequently, the child was a bit offish towards her. She was a little manipulator, but then she would be; after all, she had a great teacher.

'You all right, Nana?'

Mary nodded. 'I'm fine, love, just tired that's all. Did Vincent phone today?'

Gabby nodded and grinned. 'This morning. I can't wait, Nana, I've missed him so much.'

'He's a lucky lad. He got a result when all was said and done. Only four years . . .' Jack's voice was full of pride and, hugging his granddaughter, he continued, 'I hear he is very well thought of. I went in the pub the other day and everyone, and I mean *everyone*, was buying me drinks, and asking about him. Saying what a diamond geezer he is. You done well there, Gabby – he's got a great future ahead of him, that boy.'

Gabby glowed at the praise and, smiling, she said happily, 'I know. Bertie Warner came round today and dropped off a few quid, as he put it, to get Vincent back on his feet. It was ten grand! They're having a party for him as well – Vince will love that.'

Mary sniffed disdainfully and said sarcastically, 'Ten grand, eh? What's that work out at? About two and a half grand a year? Vincent would have been better off getting a job as a postman – at least he would have been home every night.'

Gabby rolled her eyes in annoyance, 'All right, Nana, we get your drift, but what's done is done, and I just want to put it behind me. Once Vince comes home it will all be different.'

'Well, hopefully he'll sort your mother out.'

'I think we can guarantee that much, Granddad. He hates her.'

Jack Callahan laughed then. 'Like me then! The only way I'd talk to her now is if it was through Doris Stokes!'

Even Mary laughed at that, though the joke saddened her. Cynthia had caused too much trouble for them, and she was still pulling their strings after all this time.

Chapter One Hundred and Ten

James Tailor Junior looked around him with wary eyes, and wondered if the girl sitting in front of him on the bus was worth chatting up. She had nice hair, long and dark, seemingly her natural colour, but you could never tell, never be sure about anything.

As he stepped off the bus, he noticed the changes that had occurred in the area; if anything it looked even more run down than it had when he had come here as a child. Walking along the road, he saw that the traffic had increased twofold, and the shops were now all either take-aways or cheque-cashing facilities. He knew that when the pawn shops moved into an area, it meant the work was on the way out. It was common sense – rich people didn't need pawn shops. They suited him though; they would take a TV set without asking too many questions and, as for most junkies, those shops were a godsend.

He was smiling to himself now, and he wondered at what kind of reaction he would get at his nana's house. Not a fucking visit from them in years – a birthday card or Christmas card had been the sum total of their interest in him. Which, in fairness, was more than he could say about his mother. He had not heard a fucking peep out of her since he had been taken away. When they had said he could go home, she had said, 'No, thank you, he's not my responsibility any more.' What a fucking diabolical liberty! Who the fuck did she think she was? Well, he was going to go and see her as well, and when he did she would know about it.

The only one who had ever kept any real contact was his sister. Gabby had written to him at least three times a year, and he had appreciated that. In fact, sometimes he wished he had written back, but what could he tell her? That he was still on a lock down? Still in trouble? Still fighting everyone?

He had learned to play the game, though. Eventually it had occurred to him that he had to change to get out of that place and that is what he had done. He had acted the way they wanted him to act, and the psychiatrists had patted themselves on the back – look how well we've done with him, he can join the real world again, mix in society and blend in!

Fucking morons. He had gone from a group home to his own bedsit at sixteen. He was still classified as mentally ill, but not violent any more. It was in the bedsit he had first encountered heroin. He had not been able to believe it was illegal – it was the best thing he had ever experienced in his life! And he had been on more drugs than fucking Kurt Cobain! Anti-psychotics – you name them, he'd had them. He had spent most of his life higher than a jumbo jet. Now he knew what it was to be mellow, and he liked it. He still had violent fantasies, but the heroin helped to subdue them much better than those fucking pills they had shoved down his throat ever had.

So, finally, he was going to visit the family. He was going to see just how the land lay and, more important than anything else, where that skank of a mother of his lived.

As he walked towards his nana and granddad's house, he saw Roy Brown, and nearly said hello. The cat incident had long been buried away in his mind, but now he remembered it and was sure his nana would remember it too; it wasn't exactly something you forgot, he supposed.

It all came back to him – the look on his nana's face when she had seen her bread knife, the precious antique bread knife she thought was so fucking marvellous. The memory made him laugh; she had looked so funny with that surprised look on her face.

Then he remembered the hammering his granddad had given him and suddenly he wasn't smiling any more. He was scowling, brooding. He'd like to see the old bastard try that now; he'd wipe the floor with him, and laugh while he did it.

James took a few deep breaths; he had to calm himself down, he had to look like he was a nice lad now. It was like pretending to the shrinks and the social workers – as long as you told them what they wanted to hear, and acted like they wanted you to act, you were all right.

Life, he had sussed out, was nothing more than an elaborate game; you played the role required, and you watched and waited for your opportunity. It was simple really.

As he approached his nana's house he felt the first stirrings of excitement mixed with apprehension. But it had been ten years since he had seen any of them, and that, he surmised, was to be expected.

Chapter One Hundred and Eleven

'Come on, Mummy, I want to go to Mackie D's!'

Cherie was already bored with being at her great-nana Mary's. All her great-granddad wanted to do was watch the horse racing; she had picked out his winners for him and, as one had come in, she was now the queen of the horse world. At least that was what her great-grandad was calling her anyway. But it was stifling here, and she wanted to go out, go somewhere else. It smelt of cigarettes, chip fat and furniture polish, and she hated it. So did her nanny Cynthia; she had said the house was like a tomb, and then explained it was a place for dead people. Cherie didn't really understand that, but she imagined that the smell of her nana Mary's was that of a dead person's house and she didn't like the thought of that. Dead people were scary.

She liked it at her mummy's flat because it was bright and cheerful. But Nanny Cynthia said that her mummy wasn't a proper mummy, and the police wouldn't let her stay there all the time because her mummy sold drugs and her daddy was in prison. She didn't believe her daddy was in prison, and she tried to explain that he was training to be a fighter pilot and go to the war. But her nanny Cynthia said it was lies and she should remember that. It was confusing really; she had to remember so much and it was very hard to understand.

But one thing she did know for sure was that her nanny Cynthia loved her more than anyone else in the world. She knew that must be true, because her nanny Cynthia was the person she had to live with.

As they were leaving, the doorbell rang, and Gabby went to answer it. Cherie saw her mummy stumble backwards, and she was immediately alert to the fact something was happening. And she knew she had to tell her nanny Cynthia *anything* and *everything* that she heard or saw.

A large man was standing there, and Cherie looked at him with interest; he was smiling, but it looked wrong on his face. He had long, dark blond hair, and he was dressed like the boys who hung around on her nana Mary's estate. He had on a black Puffa jacket and baggy jeans, and on his feet were scuffed white Adidas trainers. Scruffy was what her nanny Cynthia would call him. He looked scary somehow, and the main thing she noticed about him was how bad his teeth looked.

She listened with rapt attention as the man said, 'Hello, Gabby, long time no see.'

Chapter One Hundred and Twelve

When Mary Callahan went to find out what was going on she thought she was going to pass out with the shock of seeing her grandson standing in her hallway. She knew she should tell him to go away but how could she do that to him? He must have been deemed all right, or they would not let him roam the streets surely?

'You look like you've seen a ghost, Nana.'

He was smiling at her and she saw that whatever else had changed about him, he still had those dead eyes. The smile looked genuine enough, but it didn't reach his eyes. They reminded her of a dead fish, no emotion there whatsoever. He was the image of his father, but bigger somehow, she felt the threat of him invade her and she moved back instinctively.

She noticed that Gabby had moved behind her with little Cherie in her arms.

It was Jack who took over. He walked into the hallway and looked the boy up and down before saying quietly, 'What do you want?'

James grinned. 'I don't want nothing, Granddad. I was in the area . . .'

'You ain't welcome here, son. I'm sorry, but it's best to tell you straight off.'

Mary and Gabby both breathed a sigh of relief. James was not a person to invite into your life. It was sad, it was tragic, but they knew what was best. James was on medication, but that didn't guarantee anything. His 'psychotic episodes' as they called them – even though it was apparently some time since his last one – were still not something anyone in their right mind would want to be on the receiving end of.

James wasn't surprised at his granddad's words, but he had to swallow down the urge to take the old fucker by the throat and teach him a lesson. Instead he shrugged nonchalantly. 'Just as I expected, but I thought I would say a quick hello.' He turned his gaze to his sister and, smiling at Cherie, he said, 'She's beautiful, Gabs. Looks just like Mother, but I won't hold that against her. I'm thinking of visiting her next, but no one will give me her address. Don't suppose you've got it, have you?'

At that Jack Callahan laughed. 'I'll write it down for you, son, I'm sure you two have a lot of catching up to do.'

Chapter One Hundred and Thirteen

Vincent lay in his cell and counted down the hours till he could walk out the doors of this dump and retake his place in society. It was a different lad who would be going home, and he knew that himself. He hoped that his Gabby was as excited as he was. Even though they had a child together, they had never actually spent the night in the same bed, let alone lived in the same house. It was going to take a bit of getting used to for them both.

He knew he had a lot of things to sort out. First and foremost, was that ponce Cynthia. His being banged up had been all the ammunition she needed to keep his daughter by her side. Well, she was going to get a fucking big shock once he was out from behind the door. Poor Gabby had been treated abominably, not just by that cunt, but by his own family. His dad and his brothers had skanked his dough and blown it, without even giving Gabby a few bob to tide her over. He had left her, a sixteen-year-old girl, to contend with it all and that had eaten at him like a cancer over the last four years.

He had done the right thing by keeping his mouth shut, but now he wanted compensation for that – and he intended to get it. It was true what they said in here – the last few weeks were the worst. At least when you didn't have a release date you didn't dwell on it too much. Once that date was set though, it was like time was crawling, every day was like a fucking month.

But *tempus fugit* and all that, it *would* eventually fly for him, and he would be on the out.

The next cunt he was going to collar would be his old man. He was going to cut him, mark him for fucking life. That drunken Irish ponce had not even given him time to get sentenced before he had taken his stash and blown it. He intended to make them understand from day one that he was *not* a man to be mugged off, and that anyone who crossed him would pay the consequences. And they would pay dearly.

He had four long fucking years to plan it, and lying in the dark making those plans had kept him sane in this shithole. He was desperate to get out and make his mark in the world. He was a grown man now and, like the Bible said, he had put away childish things. He was determined to get a garage, a legit business, and he was going to become the best driver the Smoke had ever seen.

Derek Greene had already had a message delivered about how he would help him get on his feet, and he would see that the man followed through on his promises. Not many young lads would have been as tight-lipped as he had, leaving their little girlfriend alone and pregnant and prey to the world.

It had been hard watching poor Gabby try and get it together. He had understood her going off the rails a bit – she was a young girl and young girls needed someone to keep them on track. All that was forgiven and forgotten now. Her nana and granddad had been fucking diamond, and he would reward them for their kindness and their loyalty to his little family.

But he was itching to get out and start paying back the debts he knew were his and his alone. When he had finished with the people he felt had mugged him over, his name would be a byword for fucking retribution. And he would guarantee that no one, not *one* fucking person would ever think they could have him over ever again.

Prison was a strange place – it either broke you or it made

you stronger. Well, he was stronger now both physically and mentally than he had ever been before in his life. He had read books until eventually he had understood them, he had trained daily to keep both his body and his mind from stagnating and he was ready for literally anything.

He thought of Gabby on her last visit; she was a fucking beautiful woman now, everything and more he would ever want. His feelings for her had never wavered. He would give her the earth on a plate, and he would enjoy giving it to her. Together they were capable of great things. Of that much at least he was sure.

Chapter One Hundred and Fourteen

'I think we should have warned her.'

Jack Callahan had no such qualms and he said as much to his wife. 'Fuck her! He's *her* son, she sent him on the turn, so let her, for once in her life, deal with her own mess.'

'Supposing he hurts her . . .'

Jack shrugged nonchalantly. 'Well, we can only hope, love. Now, make me a cup of tea, and stop worrying.'

Mary went to the kitchen and put the kettle on, but she was worried. There was no telling what James Junior was going to do and, whatever Cynthia might be, she herself would not want something like that on her conscience.

In her heart she had always known that James would one day turn up at their door. It was natural that he would eventually want to seek out his kin. She had just *hoped* that he wouldn't, if she was honest.

Many years ago someone had asked her if she thought tragedy stalked some people, and if that person asked her the same question now she would say yes. Tragedy and evil had plagued her family, and they were helpless in the face of it.

She made the tea and carried it through to her husband; he took the proffered mug and sipped on it without a care in the world. She admired him in many ways, nothing really fazed him. He saw everything in black and white, did her Jack. No grey spots for him.

Chapter One Hundred and Fifteen

Bertie Warner decided to have the party for young Vincent at his pub on the Bow Road. He had arranged all the food and drink himself and it promised to be a great night. He couldn't wait to bring that young lad back into the fold.

As he looked at young Gabriella, who had come over to discuss the music for the party, he saw what had attracted the boy to her. She was exquisite, and she had waited for him – that was always a good sign in a bird as far as he was concerned. She reminded him of his old woman, sensible and calm, which were good traits in a villain's wife. If the Filth kicked the door in at three in the morning with a search warrant in one hand and a sniffer dog in the other, it was always handy to have a wife who took it in her stride, and kept the kids away from it. Occupational hazards and all that – every job had them.

'You must be looking forward to seeing him back on the outside, love.'

Gabby nodded happily. 'It will be great! And I'd like to thank you, Mr Warner, for your help, it's really appreciated.'

He felt choked, and was surprised that he could still be touched like that after all these years. Most women in her position would be complaining they couldn't manage on what they were getting; after all, they owed the girl's old man a huge debt of gratitude. But this little lovely was actually grateful. Wonders would never cease.

'You're welcome, love. It doesn't even begin to cover it. You got a good one there in Vince.'

She beamed at the praise and said honestly, 'You don't need to tell me that, Mr Warner. I've always known my Vince was special. But I have missed him. I was only sixteen when he got banged up, we've never even spent the night together! And now he's finally coming home to live in our house! How mad is that?'

Bertie Warner felt the urge to actually break down and cry. This lovely little girl had shown him that no one was ever so hard they couldn't appreciate a real sob story when they heard one. She wasn't even after a bit of sympathy, she was just being honest.

'He's a lucky man to have you, darling – I wish you both a long life of happiness.' She was smiling with excitement and he thought again how lovely she was. He envied young Vincent coming home to her. 'You book a DJ or whatever it is you have these days, and just bill it to the pub, all right, love?'

She nodded; this was like a dream to her, one she had been having for four very long years. And it was finally coming true.

Chapter One Hundred and Sixteen

'Mum, listen to me. Vincent wants his daughter at home and, no matter what you tell the social workers, they are already putting in place a residential order for her to come back home full time. Now, if you push me on this, I will leave it to Vincent to sort you out.'

Cynthia knew that she was on the losing side. She had to take this well because if she kicked off now she would lose all contact with little Cherie and that must never happen. She just had to bide her time. This pair of fucking muppets would ruin it all by themselves and when that happened she would make sure she was there to pick up the pieces. So she plastered a fake smile on her face and said, 'I know, love, and I was going to say that now you are back together, you should be a proper family. The social worker has already explained that you are on track, and that they are confident that you will be able to cope with motherhood in an adult and confident way.'

She had mimicked Miss Byrne so well that even Gabby had to laugh at her.

'That is exactly what she said to me as well! In that exact voice!' She was so happy that Vincent was coming home she could even be nice to her mother.

'Look, Gabriella, it wasn't anything personal, you know, me having Cherie here. It was for your own good. You were sixteen and alone, and I know I wasn't the best mother in the world to you or your brother, but it was different with Cherie. I felt older

337

and wiser. I was ready for the responsibility of a child and, truth be told, was trying to make up to you for everything that had happened in the past. If I had left her with you, you would have fucked up big time. You were just too young, love.'

Gabby smiled at her mother even though she didn't believe a word the woman was saying. She was backing off gracefully, and that meant she was more dangerous than ever, because she would be scheming. Well, let her scheme. Vincent would be there this time to protect her.

'Thanks, Mum. By the way, have you seen anything of James?'

For a second, Cynthia was nonplussed. Then Gabby watched as it dawned on her who she was talking about.

'No. Why, have you?'

Gabby enjoyed her mother's discomfort and that saddened her, because this was, after all, her mother. 'Yeah, he turned up at Nana's last week. He was asking after you. I didn't know if he'd been in touch.'

Cynthia shook her head violently, and Gabby could see she was rattled, far more than she had expected her to be.

'How did he look?'

'Scruffy, still strange. I think he was on something to be honest. His teeth were rotten. I was shocked at the sight of him – he looked really manic, but Granddad aimed him straight out the door. I felt a bit sorry for him.'

Cynthia didn't answer her.

'I tell you something, Mum, I'm glad my Vincent will be home soon. I wouldn't want James hanging around. Though I always wrote to him, a few times a year, like. He never answered a letter, but I still felt he should have some kind of contact with us, you know?'

Cynthia's mind was working overtime; on a couple of occasions lately she had felt as if she was being watched. Especially late at night when she parked her car, and now it seemed she might have been right to feel that way. Her son was back out on the streets, someting she had not envisaged ever happening. After all, he was as mad as a fucking March hare. But so-called care in the community meant all sorts were let out these days. Cynthia, being Cynthia, did not see his condition as anything to do with her; as far as she was concerned, he was just born like it. And that, as she was wont to say, was that. But she knew that he had a particular dislike of her after his father's death. The doctors had warned her of that, and the feeling was mutual. She would keep her eyes open, and take the appropriate precautions. If he came on too strong she would report him without a moment's guilt. She had a baseball bat she kept for emergencies, and she would happily wrap it round his head if the need arose. She had known he was on the out, but it had not occurred to her he would want to see her or, more to the point, confront her. But at least she had a heads up now, thanks to this daughter of hers. The same daughter who was happily taking away from her the only person she had ever truly cared about.

She forced another smile on to her face. 'Well, he knows where I am, I suppose.'

'Oh yeah, he knows where you are all right, Granddad told him.' Gabby smiled at her mother, and the fear in her eyes was like a balm to her tortured soul. 'So, I will take the last bits of Cherie's stuff tomorrow, if that's OK?'

''Course it is. I hope you'll still let her stay here sometimes. I mean, once Vincent is home, he's going to want you to himself I should imagine.'

'Oh, he'll have me *and* his daughter. That's all he wants, Mum.'

'Of course.'

Gabby wondered why, after everything her mother had done to her over the years, she still felt bad when she scored a point over her. And no one was more shocked than her as she heard herself say, 'You're coming to his party, Mum, aren't you? It's going to be great.'

339

All the way home she could have kicked herself, because she knew that her mother, being her mother, would come to the party all right and it would be the fucking party's death knell. She sighed in frustration. It was always the same – her mother had a knack of making *her* feel in the wrong and, consequently, she felt she had to make it up to her. Well, Gabby decided, if she turned up, she would act like she didn't know anything about it. That was pretty much all she could do.

Then it occurred to her that her brother could turn up too, and suddenly the whole thing just seemed too complicated and troublesome. James was her brother and she loved him. At least she loved the boy he had once been. He had serious mental issues, and when he wasn't taking his drugs he was violent. No one could have that kind of person too close to them. The thought of him near little Cherie made her blood run cold. He was so unpredictable. When he had suffered his violent bouts, the doctors had said there had been no warning, he had just snapped. And he had been like a steam train; whatever the person who'd supposedly wronged him had done, real or imagined, had made him almost murderous with his unsuppressed rage.

So why had they let him out? It made no sense. Her granddad said it was the arrogance of doctors – they believed they could tame people like James when in fact nothing could tame him. A chemical cosh only worked while the person involved was taking those chemicals. What happened if they decided to stop? Apparently James enjoyed hurting people, he *liked* it. So how on earth was he supposed to fit into normal society with normal people? He didn't know how to act, or what was acceptable behaviour.

Vincent would go mad if he caused any trouble, and she had a feeling that her brother would have met his match in her Vincent. She had to stop these negative thoughts. She had her daughter back, and her Vincent was coming home too. She had to stop looking for problems where there weren't any. The trouble was, when your whole existence had been a struggle, you started to think that was all it would ever be.

Well, her life was picking up, and she was finally getting everything she had ever wanted from it. And that was a cause for celebration.

Chapter One Hundred and Seventeen

James Tailor had been watching his mother and, even though he hated her, she still fascinated him. She was still a good-looking woman, and she still had that walk she had always had, as if she was the only person in the world of any note. Which, in her eyes, was God's honest truth.

When he had been a little kid she had seemed almost omnipotent, but now, watching her, he realised she was nothing really, nothing to be scared of anyway. In fact, he thought she was quite sad these days. Ageing, which he knew would be killing her. Having seen how beautiful Gabby had become, he knew that would be like a knife in her ribs, and that pleased him. He hated her with a vengeance, even while he loved her.

He felt that disconnection with the world once more; it was the best feeling in the world to him. His trouble had always been that he cared *too* much. Things made him angry, really angry, and that anger all but consumed him. It was like a storm that raged in his blood, and the only way to settle it down was through a bout of violence.

But he knew his anger had been the cause of him being locked away, so he had to try and control it. The heroin helped him enormously, and he was glad he had found something to dampen down those angry feelings. It couldn't quieten the voices completely, but it did calm them sometimes. He had stopped taking his medication, as it had interfered with his enjoyment of the drugs he injected into his body.

Watching his mother had become his hobby. The psychiatrist said he needed something to concentrate his mind on, and he was concentrating on her all right. He was watching her every move, and he found it enjoyable. He liked that he was spying on her and she didn't know he was there.

His dad had killed himself over her, which was sad because she really wasn't worth it. She was the shit on his shoes; his father had been worth fifty of her. She certainly wasn't worth dying for, but then his dad had never really understood just what he had lumbered himself with. But James could have explained – he understood it all now.

The psychiatrist had once asked him to describe his feelings for his mother, and he had thought about the question for a while before answering honestly that she was 'toxic'. She was like Agent Orange – it sounded quite nice but was full of hidden dangers, and it destroyed everything it touched. Just like Cynthia Tailor. Just like *him*. That was the one thing he had inherited from her; the urge to destroy things, destroy people.

Now it looked as if she was after Gabby's little girl, and that was something he could not allow to happen. Gabby was the only person he even remotely cared about; unlike the rest of his so-called family, she had always kept in touch with him, dropping him a line to tell him about herself and her life. Telling him everything he needed to know.

Gabby was a nice person and, although he thought she was a mug, she was the only person to have ever given him a thought. That was the worst of it, knowing they didn't even think about him, none of them did. Especially not his mother. She had dumped him faster than a cow dumped its pile of shit. She had walked away from him without even a backward glance.

Well, she would pay for her negligence, and she would pay dearly, of that much he was determined.

Chapter One Hundred and Eighteen

Vincent was packed and ready to go. It was amazing that after four years everything he owned fitted neatly into two carrier bags. But he didn't care about possessions; all he cared about was that he was on the out at last. In a few moments he would be outside, in the fresh air, in the real world. He felt almost sick with anticipation. Though underneath all the excitement ran a rich vein of apprehension; it was hard walking out of such a controlled environment. For four years he had not been on a bus or walked down a street, he had not even turned off a light switch. But he brushed away his nerves, and forced himself to relax. Not long now, and soon this would be a distant memory.

His Gabby was waiting out there for him and, for the first time ever, they could be together as adults, and that was heady stuff. He wanted to touch her, *really* touch her, feel her next to him, smell her hair . . . He felt almost dizzy with the thought.

He had been given a right royal send off, and for a moment he had almost been sorry he was leaving, but that had not lasted long. A couple of screws had arranged for a few bottles of Scotch and a bottle of brandy to arrive on the wing, courtesy of Derek Greene, and he had enjoyed the drink, appreciating the way his friends in there had been so glad that one of them was going on the outside.

It had been a great night; all the lags in there had reminisced about times past, about what they saw in their futures. And he had enjoyed listening to them as the Scotch loosened their tongues, and stories long forgotten had been told, and the laughter had been loud and free. That was the best bit – hearing that laughter, so uncontrolled and so natural. It was only then that he had realised that he had forgotten what laughter sounded like.

Usually on the wing everything was subdued somehow and people were always on their guard. You had to be – it was the way of this kind of world. Men banged up together could get into fights literally over nothing at all, small offences were allowed to fester until they became huge insults, and only violent retribution could assuage the injured party's ego. Men became different when they were isolated from family and friends; their children were growing up without them, and it was hard at times to deal with those kind of emotions.

Occasionally a man would come on to the wing who was an enemy on the outside for whatever reason, but the rule of thumb was you patched up your differences in nick. It was you against the screws, and it worked most of the time. But there was always the man who could not forget past mistakes, and then the wing became a subtle battleground. Tempers flared, and no one was safe. The main thing was learning to look after yourself. You had to watch your back constantly, watch what you said, and exercise a little diplomacy. He had seen the big mouths arrive, all bravado, with stories of how hard they were, only to become gofers within a week.

Gofers were the mugs who ended up doing the shit work – cleaning people's cells, making the tea. It was 'Go for this', or 'Go for that'. Vincent had found himself a niche there; it was well known he had been captured and had kept very quiet – not landing anyone in it but doing the time for them all. That had earned him a great deal of respect, especially as he had been so young. He had worked up from there, proving himself in small ways, and gaining a reputation for being a hard little fucker as well as a good companion. It was not an easy life, and it was hard for them all, but he had managed to overcome it. He had kept his head down, served his time and, now he had repaid his so-called debt to society, he was finally going home.

As he stepped out of the prison, he felt a rush of panic because, right up until this second, he had believed that it would go wrong somehow, and he would be stuck in there for good. As he acclimatised himself to the natural light, he saw a large black Bentley and, standing by it waving at him, dressed in a short black dress, was his Gabby.

He ran to her and picked her up in his arms. Her body fit into his perfectly as if they had been made for each other and, kissing her deeply, he felt at last like he was out. He was really on the other side of the wall.

'Oh, Gabby, you fucking gorgeous girl, this is like a fucking dream!'

Gabby was nearly speechless with happiness. 'Come on, mate, get in! We're finally going home.'

Vincent could feel her tears mingle with his as he kissed her over and over, afraid to let her go in case it all was a dream.

In the car, she handed him a bottle of Champagne, and said shyly, 'You'd better open that, mate, it's from Bertie Warner. He's waiting for us – there's a big party, and it's all for you!' She was beside herself with excitement.

The driver, a large, usually dour man called Peter Bates, turned and shook his hand saying jovially, 'I am going to put the glass up. Nothing personal, but I think you two might like a bit of privacy.'

Two minutes later the glass divide was up, and the curtains were drawn. Looking at his Gabby, at how nervous she seemed, Vincent knew then that this would be the happiest day of his life. As he slipped her dress over her head, he felt how shy and timid she was, and he would always remember this moment. Because she was, without doubt, the love of his life, and he knew that she felt the same way about him. All his fears about them finally being together were gone. It felt as natural as walking or talking. He also knew that if anyone ever hurt her, he would kill them without hesitation. He had left behind a schoolgirl, and had come out to find a woman, his woman. His Gabriella.

Chapter one Hundred and Nineteen

'The motor's here, it's just driven into the car park.'

The pub was packed with people, and little Cherie was the queen of the night and loving every second of it. Her daddy was coming home at last, and she was thrilled at the prospect. It was like a dream to her; the noise, the people, the dancing! And it was all for her daddy.

Her great-nana Mary and her great-granddad Jack were sitting at a table proud as punch, and she picked up on the way people deferred to them. Nanny Cynthia though looked cross and she didn't know why. Her daddy's family was also there, and she sensed that they were *not* as welcome as everyone else. It was a wonderful night, and everyone was telling her how pretty she looked, and how lovely she was. It was a great feeling being so important, so special. Her daddy must be somebody to have all this done for him, and she was proud to be a part of it.

As Vincent walked into the pub with his arm around Gabby's shoulders, Cherie ran to him, and he picked her up and threw her into the air. She hugged him tightly, her slim little arms locked on to his neck, and he kissed her hair, savouring the clean smell of her, and the feel of her slight little body in his grasp. For the first time ever he felt that he had a family, a real family.

As he looked across the room he saw his father and brothers standing up toasting him, raising their glasses with everyone else and, passing his daughter to her mother, he walked straight over to the table that held his family.

'Welcome home, son.' Paddy O'Casey extended his hand to Vincent, but his brothers all hung back, shy now that he was finally home, and aware of how far he had come up in the world. They knew they had not been as good to his little girl as they should have been, and they were nervous.

Vincent sensed all this in a heartbeat and, ignoring his father's proffered hand, he grabbed the man by the scruff of his neck and, in front of everyone, physically dragged him across the small dance floor and out into the car park. There he proceeded to hammer his father with his fists until he was pulled off by Bertie Warner and Derek Greene.

Looking at his father lying in the dirt he said quietly, 'You robbed me, you treacherous old cunt. You took money that should have been for my Gabby and my baby. If I ever clap eyes on any of you I'll fucking kill you, you got that? And that goes for you lot as well,' he said to his brothers, who had followed him out to the car park.

The men nodded their heads, humiliated and ashamed.

Turning to Derek and Bertie, Vincent then said jovially, 'Come on, lads, we've got a party to go to!'

The two men followed him inside, acutely aware that a young boy might have been sent down, but a very dangerous man had returned in his place.

Chapter One Hundred and Twenty

'You must be mad, Gabby!' Cynthia was beside herself with anger and it showed. That her daughter could be pregnant again so quickly was a source of irritation to her.

'Thanks for the congratulations, Mum, really appreciate it.'

Cynthia stopped herself from retaliating, instead saying levelly, 'You're only young, why tie yourself down again?' But she didn't mean a word of it; her daughter's happiness was eating away at her, and the fact that Vincent was making a great name for himself was galling.

'My Vincent and me want another baby – he's missed so much of Cherie's life, and we want to be a family, a proper family.'

The inference was not lost on Cynthia and she seethed with indignation. Vincent, however, was not a man to fuck, as the Jamaicans would say. He had already put the hard word on her, told her that if she pushed her luck he would come after her without mercy. He had explained in a quiet and patient voice that if his Gabby did not get the respect due to her, he would hunt her down like a dog. Those had been his exact words, and it had been hard swallowing, but she knew she had to. If she wanted to see little Cherie she would really have to restrain herself, and she was willing to do that for the child. She adored that little girl, and she knew that Vincent saw this love as her only redeeming feature.

The social worker was well off the scene now that Vincent

had got his little garage, and was a productive member of society. She couldn't tattle in the social worker's ear any more about rumours and stories of her daughter's wild ways, and how worried she was about her granddaughter's moral welfare. Those days were long gone, and she knew it.

She forced herself to smile. If Gabby was pregnant she would need more help with Cherie, it stood to reason. This might actually work in her favour.

'I just don't want to see you losing your freedom, love, that's all. Old before your time.'

That made sense to Gabby, and she smiled faintly, her eyes softer now. 'It's what we both want, Mum. Vince is thrilled.'

Cynthia didn't answer; instead she put the kettle on. 'Well, why don't you leave Cherie with me, and have the weekend off to celebrate, eh?'

Gabby nodded. It was what she had hoped her mother would say, and she felt a hypocrite in many ways; after all, it wasn't that long ago that she didn't want the child anywhere near her mother. But that was before, when she didn't have Vince by her side, and was at this woman's mercy. Those days were long gone.

It would be nice to have a weekend alone with Vince. Cherie was a handful, constantly wanting her father's attention. But that was to be expected – he had not been in her life properly until now, and Cherie, the little madam, was making the most of him being there. For his part, Vince loved his pretty little daughter, and she knew he was happy at the prospect of another baby.

'Thanks, Mum. I'll pick her up on Sunday afternoon.' Gabby walked into her daughter's bedroom which her mother had decorated to perfection, and hugged the little girl to her. 'You be a good girl for your nanny, OK?'

Cherie nodded happily. She loved it here; she was the centre of attention from the minute she opened her eyes until she fell asleep. For a child like Cherie that was heady stuff, and Cynthia indulged her shamelessly.

'Go on, get yourself away. I'm sure that man of yours is champing at the bit to see you.'

'He is, he always is.'

Gabby left the flat and walked to her car. As she unlocked it, she saw her brother standing at the corner of her mother's road, and felt troubled. After all, her Cherie was in the flat with her, and she didn't want James going there and causing trouble in front of her.

She drove to the corner and, stopping beside her brother, she said, 'What you doing here, James?'

He smiled absently at his sister, then he said, 'I hear your Vincent is doing well for himself.'

She ignored him and said again, 'What are you doing here, James? You know Mum doesn't want to see you.'

He shrugged and she saw how emaciated he had become. Vincent had heard he was an addict and, seeing him now, she believed it. He looked thin, drawn, and very run down. The weather was just turning cold and all he had on was a thin jacket over an even thinner T-shirt.

She looked into his face and was heart-sorry for the way his life had turned out. If he had not been her brother she certainly wouldn't have approached him. If she was honest, she had avoided him like the plague since he had been back on the scene. She had seen him from a distance a few times, and she had driven past him without stopping to even say hello. He made her nervous; anyone looking into his eyes could see that he was not quite right. He could easily be mistaken for a rapist, or a serial killer from a film. He was dirty, unkempt, and basically just odd. The trouble with James was that he was literally capable of anything, and she had to make sure he wasn't going near her mother's house while her daughter was there.

'My baby's in that flat, my Cherie, and if Vince finds out you've been near there, or that you scared her . . .' She left the sentence unfinished and she saw her brother's eyes widen. 'You are taking your medication, aren't you, James?'

The question threw him, and she could see it had also annoyed him.

'Are you?' she repeated.

He shuffled his feet for a few seconds, unable to meet her eyes. 'What do you care?'

She sighed then, a sad, drawn-out sigh. 'You're still my brother, James . . .'

He didn't answer her so she tried again.

'Where are you living? Locally?'

He shrugged. 'Why the interest suddenly?'

Gabby could smell the foetid breath of the junkie and she felt her stomach heave.

'Because you are hanging round Mum's street, and you aren't exactly her biggest fan, are you?'

He looked awful, like he had been sleeping on the streets, and she wondered at how her father would feel seeing him like this. Seeing what had happened to them all, for that matter. She wondered if, had he known what their fates would be, he would have left them like he had, at the mercy of a woman who had no real care for anyone except herself, and now also little Cherie.

Neither Gabby or James had had the best start in life. They had been little children at the mercy of an adult who had no real care for anyone or anything but what she herself wanted. It was an abortion really, all of it.

'It's a free country, Gabby. I can go where I like, and I like to watch Mother. I can promise you this though; if I decide to have a word with her, I'll make sure she's alone, OK? I can't be fairer than that, can I?'

Gabby looked at this man who was still her brother despite the fact they felt like strangers and, shaking her head, she said sadly, 'Please tell me where you're living, James. I just want to help you if I can.'

He didn't answer her; instead, he gave her his usual enigmatic smile and walked away.

She sat in the car for a while wondering if she should warn her mother about him. But she guessed that she knew he was there already. She wasn't a fool – she would have noticed him surely? Yet, turning the car around, she went back to her mother's flat anyway. While her Cherie was there she wanted to feel the girl was safe, and she made up her mind to tell Vincent about her worries.

Chapter One Hundred
and Twenty-One

'I need a good earner, Bertie. I've got another baby on the way and, though the garage does OK, I need some real money to get a mortgage, et cetera.'

Bertie Warner grinned laconically; he had wondered how long it would be before Vincent wanted more. It was indisputable that he was on a fucking good earn, but he would still never feel he was getting enough money – that was just this boy's nature. He seemed to think the world owed him a living. True, he had done them all a big favour, but, by the same token, he had already been handsomely recompensed, and he had earned the respect of everyone into the bargain. It was too soon for Vincent to be out on the rob and Bertie said as much.

'Calm yourself down, lad. If you go out too soon you'll get another fucking capture. They will be keeping an eye on you for a good while yet. They will be aware of your known associates and they will even be monitoring your calls. Now, you remember what I told you about mobiles, don't you? Never, and I mean *never*, use your mobile for work – you always talk business from a fucking public phone or an untraceable pay as you go. The Filth are using scramblers and all sorts to listen in on conversations, so be aware.'

Vincent could barely keep the impatience out of his voice as he answered heavily, 'You have mentioned that before, Bertie.'

Bertie Warner, annoyed now, said sarcastically, 'I'm sure I have, clever bollocks, but just in case you are a bit dense I thought I would mention it again. Only you lot seem to think you are technological wizards because you can fucking dial a phone number. Well, *my* technological wizards, who are shrewder than you lot put together and then some, have warned me of the pitfalls of tapping. The signal is winging its way through the air, and can be intercepted at any time. Now, I may not be Alexander Graham fucking Bell, but I know enough to listen to the people who *do* know about these things. So if you ever ring me cold again like you did today, I will see to it that your fancy new mobile gets shoved so far up your jacksie you'll have to shove your hand down your throat to answer a call!'

He was bellowing now; he could be heard all over the scrapyard. And it took Vincent O'Casey all his considerable willpower not to knock the man on his arse. But he knew that for the mug's game it would be – Bertie would have him sliced and diced without a second's thought. Bertie was a lot of things, but even-tempered was not one of them. He could be moved to tears at the plight of a starving child in Africa one moment, only to become murderous if the noise of a child's actual crying interrupted him watching the news. He was a mass of contradictions, and it was best to let him get his anger out of his system.

'And for the fucking record, Mr Big fucking Earner, *you* work for *me*, and *I* say when, and if, you go back out on the street.'

Vincent licked his dry lips, and bit back the retort he was dying to make. Instead, he bowed his head, feeling like some kind of errant schoolboy.

Satisfied by the boy's outward deference, Bertie lowered his voice and said amiably, 'I done a lump and half, son, and I know how you're feeling, but believe me when I say you have to lie low for a while. I mean, be honest, do you want to get captured again? Because this time, mate, it will be a lot longer than four years behind the door. Next time round you become what the courts call a serial offender, and they'll throw away the fucking key, son. So, tighten your belt. You're on a fucking decent earn – many men work a month to earn the poke you get a week – and the garage will pay off. Take my advice and stop giving it the large – you've plenty of time for all that when you're properly established.'

Although Vincent knew he was getting sound advice, he still couldn't let his wants go. He liked the life of a criminal; he liked the kudos and, most of all, he liked the money. He was determined to get some serious poke if it was the last thing he ever did in this life.

When he left, Bertie Warner sighed in annoyance. He had seen them all come and go – real hitters who, if they had a bit of patience, could have gone right to the top of their game. Impatience, Bertie had learned, was the scourge of the villain; it was the downside of easy money. So many of these young lads blew their wages in a week and were soon looking for another earn; if they saved a bit for the rainy days they would be quids in. He watched them in the pubs and clubs – big diamond Rolexes and eighty-grand motors and they were still signing on, for fuck's sake! The naïvety of these young men was laughable. He blamed the education system – they taught them how to add up, but not how to invest their money and save the bastard, or at least some of it, anyway.

Bertie lived well, but not as well as he could, and that was because he knew the Old Bill loved nothing more than someone who lived it large with no real means of employment. A local Face driving a prestige car, with all the rent paid, while still on fucking Jobseeker's Allowance did tend to raise the red flag. But these young lads wouldn't listen, none of them.

Well, he had said his piece – it was up to Vincent O'Casey now. But he hoped the lad used his noodle. He really had a knack for the driving and, if he could just wait a while, he would be set like the proverbial jelly.

Bertie decided to have a talk with young Derek and see what he thought about the situation. If the boy got a tug, he didn't want it coming down on them. The trouble was, the mood Vincent was in, he was liable to go outside for his work if *they* didn't give it to him. Vincent was like all this generation, they wanted everything in five minutes, but they needed to learn that it took a long time and a lot of effort to bring off any decent job. Planning was the key, planning for every and any eventuality. That, unfortunately, was the bottom line. Haste meant mistakes, and a mistake on this lad's part could get him a big lump inside, and another kid meeting their father only once a month.

Chapter One Hundred and Twenty-Two

James was squatting in Hoxton with three others – two girls in their late teens, and a man in his forties called Dougie McManus. As he looked at the three of them sprawled out on the floor, he wondered at how he had got himself in this mess.

Dougie was a hustler, a panhandler, and not a very good one. With his long straggly hair and beard, he resembled Christ in a good light. But he also looked like a junkie, and people either threw a few pence at him or told him to fuck off. But he could score anything from anyone.

The girls were relatively new, and would not last more than a week at most. They were runaways, drifters, and Dougie was already freaking them out; they were not interested in his sexual advances, and were already sick of his high stories. James had noticed that all junkies talked about was the last high, or a spectacular high from the past. Dougie's tales always involved a stash he had bought once, or stolen from someone, or found the Holy Grail of skag, always the best high ever.

Normally, James just tuned him out, but now he was getting angry, because the money he had hidden in the squat had miraculously disappeared, and Dougie and the girls were stoned out of their tiny – emphasis on the tiny – minds. So, putting two and two together, he made the usual four.

He looked down on their sleeping forms and thought about

359

how he'd ended up in this place. He had left his bedsit because he had wanted to. He believed that the woman in the next house could read his mind through the walls and he could feel her interfering with his thoughts day and night. She was very old, and she had a foreign accent, but he knew that was all just an act. She was working for his mother and reporting back to her.

He had been very clever. He had got dressed one day, and walked out of his bedsit without anything, as if he was just going to the shops, and he had never gone back. That's when he had shaken off the authorities – they were all a part of the conspiracy anyway, giving him tablets to stop him knowing the truth. He was a lot of things but a moron wasn't one of them.

Ha! He had shown them all, and he would carry on showing them all. Now here he was in a den of thieves, living with *actual* thieves. What was it his father had always said? Never steal off your own – and yet that was exactly what this lot had done. As bad as they had tried to make him out, he had never stolen unless he was at rock bottom. He prided himself on that.

Now these pieces of scum had robbed him. He could smell the sourness of the girls' bodies and wrinkled his nose in distaste. One of the girls, Alicia, was quite nice. She was very posh and had gone to an expensive school, but her parents had washed their hands of her, and who could blame them? She was a thief, and thieves never prosper.

He sat down on the hearth of the old-fashioned fireplace; it was filthy, overflowing with cigarette butts, roaches, and the usual detritus of a junkie's lair. Needles, wraps, and sooty tinfoil burned and wrinkled, McDonald's wrappers, and sugar-laden drinks bottles. He looked at Dougie's narrow face, thin beyond belief, and his filthy beard full of food and grease. He wondered if they were really asleep – perhaps they were pretending, hoping he would go away so they could get their stash out behind his back. The stash he had paid for, that they had bought with his stolen money!

He stood up and went into the kitchen. Holding open the heavy door was a rusty old iron. It had once been a lovely piece of metalwork, burnished black, and it had probably ironed ladies' lawn handkerchiefs, or their knickerbockers; he smiled at the thought.

Picking it up, he walked back into the room and, raising the iron above his head, he brought it down with all the force he could muster on to Dougie's face.

Dougie, so full of heroin he couldn't feel a thing, was knocked out cold by the first blow. Ten blows later his face was gone and, placing the iron carefully on to the floor by the body, James Tailor methodically searched the man's clothes for anything of value – he wouldn't miss it now, after all – before leaving the flat. He had to get away. Far away.

Chapter One Hundred
and Twenty-Three

'But it's my scan, you said you'd come with me.'

At the other end of the line, Vincent could hear the disappointment in Gabby's voice.

'Look, babe, I can't do anything about it now.' He sighed. 'I have to go to this meet, it's important, OK?' A few minutes later he put the phone down, and turned back to his two comrades. 'So are you in then?'

They both nodded. Geoff Gold was clearly thrilled, but his brother Micky was not as easily pleased.

'Hang on a minute, who told you all about this place?'

Vincent smiled; he had expected this question before now and, in hindsight, he would realise that it should have bothered him. He tapped his nose. 'Never you mind. It's enough that I trust the bloke. The fewer people who know our business the better, don't you think?'

The two men nodded, but he could see that Micky Gold was not that impressed, which annoyed him. The Golds were from Canning Town and they were a pair of blond Adonises. Both were tall, had thick wavy blond hair and dark blue eyes framed by long black lashes. Derek Greene said they attracted too much attention to be villains of any real note – women took too much notice of them for a start – but they would not be put off by that. Their father had been some Scandinavian seaman and their mother was a good-looking local girl who had often moonlighted as a brass in the various pubs of East London during the sixties and seventies. They loved their old mum and would do anything for her. She, in turn, supplied them with food, did their washing, and lied to everyone for them, from girlfriends to judges. They had a good little rep, but had never done the big one.

'Look, Micky, if you don't want in just fucking tell me and I'll stop wasting me breath.'

Geoff looked at his younger brother and said hastily, 'Shut the fuck up! This is all kosher, and I want in.'

Micky shrugged but he was still chary and it showed.

Vincent wasn't bothered. If nothing else, this job would appeal to their greedy natures; after all, that's what had made *him* so interested. He poured the Scotch out and they sat down in his office at the garage he was beginning to make such a success of. Then he took them through the robbery that was being planned for a bank in Borough Green, Kent. By the time he had finished outlining the proposition, both were smiling widely, as he had known they would be.

'This, my friends, is what is known as a piece of piss.'

The Gold brothers were only too happy to drink to that.

Chapter One Hundred and Twenty-Four

Cynthia Callahan was looking at the two policemen in complete shock.

'He what!'

The elder of the two men took her gently by the arm and walked her through to her kitchen where he helped her into a chair at the scrubbed pine table. The younger man put the kettle on, knowing this was a cup of tea and a chat scenario; the poor woman looked mortified.

'I'm sorry to be the harbinger of such distressing news, but we feel we have to warn you. Your son has murdered a man called Dougie McManus, and we believe he may come here at some point. In the squat where he was living we found exercise books that were your son's, in which he detailed how he was going to harm you. Burn you out, in fact. So we need you to be on your guard.'

Cynthia nodded, but her mind was whirling. 'He's killed someone. He has finally killed someone.'

The policeman looked at his young counterpart to see how he was getting on with the pot of tea.

'I'm afraid that's true, Mrs Tailor—'

She interrupted him. 'I'm Callahan – Miss Callahan. I reverted to my maiden name after my husband's death.'

He made a note of that in his little book. 'Now, has he approached you?'

She shook her head. 'No, but I think he's been stalking me for a while. My daughter warned me about him the other day, funnily enough. You know he has severe mental problems?'

The policeman said he did.

'He was diagnosed schizophrenic at a very young age, after his father committed suicide. It's very sad. I need to know, have you any idea where he could be?'

'Well, Miss Callahan, I was going to ask you that very same thing.'

She shook her head again. 'I avoid him like the plague, to be honest. He's a very difficult person to deal with. He believes he is being watched by government forces. If you talk to his doctors they will explain it to you.'

He nodded – he had spoken to the doctors already.

'My daughter might know something, but I doubt it – same with my parents. He's not someone you encourage into your life, if you get my drift. Very violent, and very easily riled up. He cut a neighbour's cat's throat when he was just coming up to nine.'

The policemen were surprised to note that, as she described her son's problems, there was no real emotion there at all for him.

'My daughter seemed to think he was on drugs. She said he looked like he was on something when she saw him just down the road from my house. She stopped the car and spoke with him. I had her little daughter staying with me at the time so naturally she was worried in case he came here in front of the child . . .'

He waited until the teas were placed before them all, before saying gently, 'We believe he is on heroin – a lot of the mentally disturbed take that drug on the streets. We also found a crack pipe, and evidence that he'd used it, at the murder scene. Is there anyone you can think of that he might go to? Any friends?'

She shook her head. 'No, nobody. He's a loner, a strange boy. I wish I could help you more.'

Five minutes later they were ushered out of the front door and, seeing the number of locks she had on it, they realised that she had been preparing for her son coming for her long before they had arrived on the scene.

'You keep yourself safe now, Miss Callahan, and, if he comes near you, ring the police immediately. All the forces are looking for him, so try not to worry.'

Cynthia closed the door and locked it, every bolt and chain, then she went around the house making sure everywhere was secure.

In the kitchen she poured herself a large vodka and tonic and then, smiling slightly, she wondered if he would have the guts to turn up here. Burn her out! She'd like to see the little fucker try.

Picking up the phone she rang her daughter. If he went near her grandchild, she'd skin him alive. The only good bit of all this aggravation was that they'd have to lock him up again and, hopefully, this time, they would throw away the bastard key.

Chapter One Hundred
and Twenty-Five

'Look, Gabby, all men are the same, they get you pregnant but they have no real interest in the actual pregnancy – it's only the baby they are interested in, and even that wanes after a while.'

Gabby sighed. Did her mother really think she was helping? The worst thing of all was she had a feeling that what she was saying was true. She was heavily pregnant and Vincent was never in the house for any length of time. The garage was doing well, and that pleased her; they were beginning to save some money, and they were moving to a new council house before the baby was born. But he was out from early morning till late at night.

Cynthia looked at her daughter and felt the urge to shake her. What was it with this girl? She couldn't see what was under her nose – she had bagged herself a blagger, and blaggers were not known for their homing instincts. She should think herself lucky she had a man out grafting for her – not that she was that enamoured of her daughter's 'partner' as they called them nowadays. He looked down his nose at her, and did not bother to hide his indifference. Dislike she could cope with because it meant she'd made an impact at least. Indifference, on the other hand, meant she had not had any effect on the idiot in any way. He ignored her completely, which really pissed her off, and the fact that her daughter didn't even defend her to him really annoyed her as well.

'Any news on Nutty?'

Gabby rolled her eyes and said huffily, 'Will you stop referring to James like that? They haven't found him yet. God knows where he is by now.'

Cynthia snorted then. 'Fucking Broadmoor is where he should be, locked away for good.'

'He's your son, Mum!'

Cynthia snorted again. 'Stop fucking saying that, he's nothing to do with me! Anyway, he's over eighteen – he's his own person now, responsible for his own actions.'

Gabby didn't answer; it always amazed her that her mother could just push the blame away from herself without a second's thought. She rubbed her belly – she was feeling awful today.

Seeing her daughter's discomfort Cynthia said, 'Get your stuff, Cherie, you're coming home with Nanny.' She held a finger up to her daughter in protest. 'Not a word, you need your rest. Now, I've put a lasagne in the fridge, and I've got your ironing. So stop panicking and put your feet up.'

Gabby felt a rush of gratitude to this woman who she alternately loved and hated. Since Cynthia had seen how ill she had been with this baby she had been a diamond. She even talked about the baby as if she was looking forward to it, which Gabby thought she secretly was. Cynthia was buying little bits for it, and she had got out Cherie's old cot, so she must be expecting the child to stay there on occasion.

For the first time in years, Gabby felt a modicum of contentment in her mother's company as they chatted and laughed. It was as if the heavier she got with this baby the better her mum liked her. Her nana Mary thought she was mad, but they didn't see this side of Cynthia – so few people ever did. There was no doubt about it – as her mother got older, she was becoming more like a mother should be. OK, not where James was concerned maybe, but then he'd always been difficult, to say the least. Gabby hoped none of her kids inherited his mental illness, that would be too cruel. Whereas her mother had never been a loving mother exactly, Gabby was – she loved her family with all her heart.

She had tried to tell her nana and granddad about how her mum was behaving these days, but they both dismissed it out of hand, saying she was after something, just as she had been before. Gabby understood that they didn't trust Cynthia, but even if she was after Cherie, now that Vincent was back he would never let anything happen to them.

Having him there made her so happy – she just wished he was home more. She knew that it had taken lot of work to get the garage off the ground, and he wanted to make a success of it. It was all for them so she shouldn't really moan too much.

Cherie had her little bag packed, and was impatient to go with her nanny Cynthia now. She had brought all her drawing books with her; she loved drawing, and her nanny Cynthia had got her an easel which she loved painting on. She had a white smock just like the real painters in a book her nanny showed her.

Cynthia really thought the child had a talent, and she was determined to see her make the best of it. She could be the next Tracey Emin, that was Cynthia's belief. She knew with certainty that this little girl had a brilliant future ahead of her, and she would move the heavens to see she got the chances Cynthia felt had been denied to her. She saw herself in little Cherie, saw her as she would have been with different parents, with people who could have given her a proper start in life. Cynthia blamed her parents for the way her whole life had turned out, and her son's life as well. She believed with all her heart that her mother had had more say in James Junior's upbringing than she did and, consequently, the blame for his condition lay at her mother's door.

It never occurred to her that dumping her children at will, not loving either of them, and placing impossible demands on them might have had something to do with her son's illness and her daughter's desperate craving for love. In fact, Cynthia was proud of her Gabriella; she was doing all right, and so long as she let her have Cherie she would remain in her good books.

It was Vincent that Cynthia had the main problem with these days. He didn't like her having too much to do with the child. She knew she had to sort something out there. He needed taking down a peg or two. Since he had been released he thought he was the dog's gonads – well, what man didn't?

She smiled at the thought of bringing him down, and she drove back to her house lighter in spirit, with her little Cherie chattering away beside her.

Chapter One Hundred
and Twenty-Six

The Golds had been watching the bank in Borough Green for the last few weeks and they knew down to the last detail who went in and who went out, at what times the bank was quiet, and when it was busy. On one specific day in every month, the bank held over one hundred thousand pounds before it was taken away by guards. Today they were sitting in a small coffee bar, watching the handover with interest.

There were three men outside the vehicle, and two inside – one driving, the other riding shotgun – so they were going to need to get the safety deposit box *before* they hit the inside of the back doors. It seemed to be a doddle.

The guards appeared very complacent, joking with the manager, and acting very relaxed. That was the beauty of carrying out robberies in small villages; they looked sleepy, and no one thought anything bad could happen in them. With sawn-off shotguns and the element of surprise to their advantage, this would be over in minutes.

Pleased with the day's findings, the Golds got into their nondescript car and drove away sedately, sure that this was going to go without a hitch.

Chapter One Hundred
and Twenty-Seven

'Well, she's asleep. Surely you don't expect me to wake her up!' Cynthia's voice was low, but full of contempt. Vincent was on the phone asking why she had not brought his daughter back as arranged.

She had not said when she would be bringing her back for definite, she had just said maybe Sunday night. Anyway, she had rung her daughter earlier and left a message to say that Cherie was a bit under the weather and then she had put her to bed. It wasn't her fault that Gabriella had not checked her messages and she said as much. But Vincent was not a happy bunny.

'You know she should be here, Cynthia, she's got school tomorrow.'

Cynthia snapped right back at him, 'Not with a cold, she isn't. Plus, poor Gabby's just about ready to drop, she can't be running around after that lively little mare. Unless you're staying home, of course.' She knew she had him then and she smiled down the phone imagining how angry he was.

'Well, I want her back tomorrow, all right? She spends far too much time at your drum for my liking.'

Cynthia didn't answer him; she had won this battle and if it was left to her she would soon be winning the war.

When she put the phone down she went back into her kitchen and looked through Cherie's drawing case. She had found a piece of paper earlier, and on it, written in pencil, were the plans to rob a security van for a bank in a place called Borough Green, which was apparently in Kent.

Cherie had drawn a picture of a nice house, and she had been admiring it when she had spotted the little diagram on the back. This was how you planned any robbery, Cynthia knew, from her time in Jonny's circle. You used Ordnance Survey maps and you always used pencil – never pen. Then, once the route was established, the map was destroyed, along with anything else incriminating. Cynthia knew that this would have been destroyed eventually, but Little Miss Trouble had got to it first, unaware that it was her father's blueprint for his next job. She laughed with glee. That Vincent really should be more careful about what he left in his office at the garage.

She hugged the paper to her chest. Oh, the old saying was right: God really did pay back debts without money; of that she was now sure. In her hands was the fate of Cherie's interfering fuck of a father, and she knew *exactly* what she was going to do with it.

Chapter One Hundred
and Twenty-Eight

Mary Callahan wasn't well, and Jack knew it. She was having trouble breathing, and she seemed to spend longer and longer having a 'bit of a lie down', as she called it.

He looked at her now as she slept next to him in their bed. Her face still held some of the beauty that had attracted him all those years ago. In repose, the lines were not so harsh, and she seemed younger somehow, more how he liked to think of her. She had been an eyeful all right, like their Celeste. Hers had been an understated beauty, as opposed to Cynthia's in-your-face sexuality. Mary had aged prematurely; all the trouble that Cynthia had brought to their door over the years had certainly taken its toll on her as, he supposed, it had on him too. But, for all their trials, he still loved this woman, and he hoped to God that he died first, because he didn't think he would cope without her.

He decided to make her an appointment at the doctor's, but tell her it was for him – she would accompany him then to make sure he went. It was the only way he'd get her there – she spent so much time worrying over everyone else, but not a second did she waste on herself.

She had never been the same since their Celeste went. He knew that she blamed herself for her daughter's eventual decline but it wasn't her fault. Celeste, unlike her sister and indeed her own mother, hadn't had the strength of mind needed to cope with what life had thrown at her. It had finally worn this wife of his down too; she was losing weight by the day, and she had no appetite.

He was suddenly assailed by a memory of her having their Cynthia. She had given birth at home and he had been angry because his racing paper had been used to mop up after her waters had broken. It had made him feel slightly sick. Then, after what seemed like ages, he was presented with his little daughter. Even then, as a newborn, Cynthia had been absolutely gorgeous – everyone said so. And he remembered saying to his exhausted wife, 'She'll break some hearts, this one!'

If only he had known then that she would break not only hearts but also whole families apart, he would have drowned the evil cunt there and then. He remembered his Mary, tired but triumphant, looking down at that child as if she was the most precious thing in the world. Where had it all gone so wrong?

He felt near to tears, and told himself it was just his age creeping up on him. If truth be told, he wouldn't be too trashed about shaking off this mortal coil, and going for the long sleep. In fact, he would rather enjoy it.

He laid his wrinkled hand on to his wife's hair, and it was only then that he realised she was cold. His Mary had died in her sleep. She was past all the hurts that life had thrown at her. For the first time in years, Mary Callahan was really at peace.

Sitting up in bed, Jack Callahan held his wife's hand and cried bitter tears. He blamed Cynthia for this; Mary should have had years left to her. They should have had years left *together*. If Mary had not taken on the burden of her daughter's children and all their combined problems, they could have lived out their twilight years in peace and companionship. His Mary was but another casualty in the war that was Cynthia Callahan. She had never really stood a chance.

Chapter One Hundred and Twenty-Nine

Vincent held Gabby while she cried, and he knew it couldn't be good for her or the baby. Mary's passing had hit her badly, very badly. She had been the only real mother she had ever known, and he had a lot to thank her for, he knew. Without Mary and Jack, his Gabs would have been alone in the world with his daughter and completely at the mercy of Cynthia Callahan. Things had been bad enough as it was, and the guilt he felt at leaving her was ever present. As was Cynthia. It felt like she was always round, helping out.

All he needed was a couple of robberies under his belt and he could get them a decent house of their own, bought and paid for, and then get on with his legit businesses. He would only go out for a drive every year or so. It was a foolproof plan, and he wanted to make sure that this girl of his – and the children, of course – had everything they needed for the rest of their lives. It was important to him that they were all well set up.

He wanted his Gabby in their own little house, his kids at the best schools available, and a place in the sun. That had been his dream throughout his prison sentence, and now he would make it all come true.

Fuck Greene and Warner, with their 'be patient' and 'bide your time' nonsense. He was a fucking shrewdie and he knew what he was doing. He was looking after his family; after all, that was a man's job.

Cynthia brought in a tray with tea for her and Vincent and a small brandy for Gabby.

'She can't have alcohol, she's pregnant.'

'One little shot won't hurt her, and it will make her sleep, calm her down. All this crying can't be good for her or the baby.'

He could see the sense in what she was saying.

Cynthia took Gabby from his arms and, holding her close, said gently, 'Come on, love, drink this up, eh? It'll make you feel better.'

Gabby did as she was told, and drank the brandy, coughing at the raw taste.

'There, that will make you feel better, love. Now come on, put your feet on the couch, darling. I'll make you some hot milk with honey in it, like my mum used to make for me when I was feeling ill. I bet she did it for you too, eh?'

Gabby smiled brokenly and nodded her head.

Twenty minutes later the milk had been drunk and she was asleep. Cynthia looked at Vincent and sighed. 'She's taken it bad, Vincent, but it's to be expected – my mum was more of a mother to her than I ever was.'

Vincent stayed silent; he didn't know how to answer that statement.

'Do you want me to take Cherie with me? I can take her to school, the usual – it's best to keep to a routine with kids. There's going to be a lot of running about with the funeral to arrange and everything. And, well, my dad isn't going to be much use, is he? My mother did everything – he can't even boil an egg.'

It was strange talking to Cynthia like this, she seemed almost normal, caring even. Vincent knew she loved his daughter, of that there could be no doubt. It was just a pity she had never felt like that about either of her own kids.

As if reading his mind, she said, 'I was never a good mother. I found the kids got on my nerves a lot of the time. I suppose being lumbered with James didn't help – he was hard work, Vincent. Not that he meant to be, but he was so weak. I had to sort out everything, from the bills to the washing and the cooking. Everything. I think I just wanted to be free, you know? Free of all the responsibilities. And my mum, well, she wanted the kids there all the time, and I got into the habit of letting her have them.' She smiled and her whole face was transformed. 'I suppose that's where Gabby gets her mothering skills from – she certainly didn't get them from me!'

For the first time ever, Vincent felt himself warming to Cynthia, disarmed by her honesty.

But Cynthia on full charm offensive was hard to resist; many men had found that out to their cost. She saw him softening towards her. Well, when she was finished with him, he would be her best mate, she would see to that. Although he might not be around too long if she had anything to do with it. At least this way it would allay any suspicions he might have about her. She wanted him to believe that she had his Gabby's best interests at heart, that she had simply found her maternal instinct later than most women, and that she would always be there for his children, as well as Gabby.

It was so easy. Men were such fucking children – all you had to do was tell them what they wanted to hear, act the little housewife, and Bob really was your uncle and Fanny your aunt.

Chapter One Hundred and Thirty

'It's a lovely day – cold but sunny. A fine day to have a baby!'

The Jamaican midwife was trying to make Gabby laugh and, to be nice, she smiled weakly. But she had only just buried her nana Mary, and now the pains were ripping her to pieces. She knew it would be worth it, that her baby would be born perfect, and she would have a proper little family. She wished her nana was here though; it was hard without her.

She saw Vincent walk into the room, and she smiled tragically. Then another pain gripped her and she grimaced as the noise of the air leaving her body sounded like a loud fart and she laughed with him, as he said, 'Fuck me, Gabs, what hole's this baby coming out of!'

She bore down, and felt the baby crowning, watching Vincent as the miracle of birth was revealed to him. She hoped he wouldn't be put off with all the blood. But far from being repulsed, he was entranced. Pleased as punch to be there and, as their second child, and their first son, slid into the world, she saw only pure joy and amazement on his face.

As he cradled their little boy in his huge arms, she was happier than she had ever been in her life. She finally had what she had always craved. Now she had a real family, and it felt good.

Chapter One Hundred and Thirty-One

As Cynthia held Vincent Mark Two, as his father referred to him, she was once again overwhelmed with the feeling of belonging he engendered in her. It was as if he was her child, the same emotion she had experienced when she had first seen little Cherie five years before. That her Gabriella could produce such perfect children with that dolt she had lumbered herself with was, in itself, amazing. But, once again, this child looked like her. It had her eyes and the same shaped face as her, as well as that sovereign-coloured hair – blond with red streaks – which had always made her stand out from the crowd.

'He's stunning, Gabriella, absolutely beautiful. Well done, you two.' She aimed her smile at Vincent and she saw the delight on his face at her words. Like his genes alone could have presented her with a grandson like this! It would take her time to stamp out the O'Casey traits, she was sure. This little boy would be someone, a banker, or a doctor; he was like a blank canvas waiting for her to colour him in. One thing was for sure – he wouldn't be a fucking bank robber like his old man, she would see to that. Her smile widened as she thought of what she had done. She had made sure that his father would not be around to interfere in his little life. It was her secret gift to her new grandson.

She smiled at Vincent Senior once more, aware that she

would have to put up with it until he was captured trying to rob a bank in Borough Green. The police were watching them all, and she knew that the conspiracy to rob charge would keep him out of their lives for at least seven years.

Gabriella would be heartbroken, which was to be expected; after all, the girl loved him. Cynthia understood that, but she was more concerned that, if left with these two people, her grandchildren would never have anything in their lives, not anything worth having anyway. They would end up labelled blaggers' kids, and they would go the way of all thieves' children, embracing that life as all that would be open to them. So she was pleased with herself, pleased at what she had done.

As Vincent took his son from her, and gazed down into his perfect little face, she did not feel an ounce of shame. She was saving these kids from a fate worse than death.

'He'll be someone this little lad, Gabby, I can feel it in my bones.'

Cynthia laughed with her daughter at the words and, looking at Vincent, she winked happily at him.

He winked back, oblivious that his fate, like that of his little family, was well and truly sealed.

Chapter One Hundred
and Thirty-Two

'What a fucking mug! But would he listen to anyone?'

Bertie Warner was incensed at the news young Vincent O'Casey had been captured as he and the Gold brothers were about to enter a bank in Kent. They were caught with guns, balaclavas, the works. A whisper had got out, and somehow the Filth had got wind of it. How, he didn't know, because it was the first *he* had heard about any of it. In fact, it seemed that no one had any idea about the fucking robbery at all. So either one of the Golds had become loose-lipped, which was very doubtful, or Vincent had mentioned it to someone. Not a chance of that; knowing how Bertie felt about him going back into the game too soon he would have kept it quiet. No, this had to be close to home. Micky Gold had just dumped his wife for a seventeen-year-old blonde, but then would he mention a piece of work to his old woman? It was a melon scratcher all right.

But they were bang to rights now, and they would be looking at a good few years behind the fucking door, before they would be out celebrating Christmas with their families. Stupid, stupid fuckers. Especially that young Vincent. Bertie had had such high hopes for him.

He thought about that girl of his. She had not long had her second baby – a lovely little boy – and she would be devastated by this news; after all, it was not the first time Vincent had left her literally holding the baby. The poor little whore. Some girls really were unlucky. Still, what was done was done, and life on the outside continued.

But all day he kept thinking about young Vincent and about what a waste of a life it was. The second stretch was always worse than the first – for a start, you knew what to expect. Bertie would grease a few palms, make it easier for him, pay out and get him his own cell, a bit of snout and a few luxuries. Vincent would be out one day, and Bertie wanted him to remember that they had not forgotten him. He would slip that little bird a few quid too, tide her over till she was sorted out. It was the least he could do.

Chapter One Hundred and Thirty-Three

Vincent O'Casey sat in Brixton on remand and listened to the sounds that were once more his background music. Prisons were really noisy at night. Snoring, arguing, laughter, and often the sound of muffled sobs from the men who were desperately missing their families. The sound of the POs walking up and down, hearing the loud sliding noises of the slats opening and closing as they checked to make sure no one had topped themselves or were up to some kind of skulduggery such as digging their way out or making a shiv. This was to be his life again, and it would be his life for years and years.

He wished he had listened to Bertie and Derek, but it was too late. It was way too late for everything and anything now; his little lad would grow up without him like little Cherie had done. His poor Gabby would be left with two kids, and no visible means of employment – without him the garage would need to be sold, he knew that. Why had he been so determined to do it? If he had listened to men older and wiser than himself, he would be at home now holding his little son and, later on, holding his lovely Gabby in his arms. Instead all he had to look forward to was absolutely nothing. Nothing worth anything anyway. He hoped Gabby would be OK, but at least she had her mother. Love or loathe Cynthia, she adored those kids, and she wouldn't let anything happen to them.

He would kill the fucking Gold brothers! One of them must have had a loose lip, because he had told no one, absolutely no one, about the blag. So it *had* to have been one of them. The worst of it was they had been nabbed before they had even got out of the fucking car. How humiliating was that?

Lying down, he put his face into the pillow and, like many a man before him, he cried like a baby; he cried for his family, for the life he had lost, and for the life he would now be living. But mostly he cried for Gabby and the knowledge he had left her high and dry for the second time in six years. That was what really hurt. Her world as she knew it was gone. The life they had planned was not to be. She had a baby less than three weeks old, and no one to tell her they loved her late at night. That, he knew, would be the hardest for her to bear.

Chapter One Hundred and Thirty-Four

2008

Cynthia was tired but pleasantly so. At three years old, little Vincent was a real handful, but she had enjoyed the day at the zoo as much as he had. With his sister Cherie loving the bones of him, and his nanny Cynthia treating him like a king, he was a very contented little boy.

As she put the pushchair away in her hall cupboard, and walked through to the lounge, she saw the children dutifully taking their coats off and removing their shoes. They were such good kids, did anything at all she asked without her having to yell or bully them into it. So different to her own son and daughter. The thought brought her back to Gabriella, and the news she had imparted earlier that day. It seemed that '*her* Vincent', as she sickeningly referred to him, might get early parole. A bit too bloody early for Cynthia's liking.

Cynthia had enjoyed three years of more or less complete autonomy over the children, but now her daughter, with the help of her antidepressants, was finally getting herself back on her feet. She had taken Vincent's departure very badly, and lost interest in everything and everyone – even her little boy. As Cynthia had pointed out, that ponce had left her holding the baby *twice*; any other woman would have legged it, but not her Gabriella. Cynthia conveniently ignored her own part in

386

Vincent's arrest – she had long ago convinced herself she did everything for her daughter's own good. Gabriella would never have understood that it was for the best. She had taken losing Vincent very badly indeed. The doctors had blamed it on postnatal depression, and she had not disputed that.

Then, when little Vincent was five months old, Gabriella had had a complete nervous breakdown. She had needed to be hospitalised, and she had stayed there for eight months. Those had been the happiest eight months of Cynthia's life. She had moved into a house closer to Gabriella's and she had taken the children. She had made herself a lovely little family and, on top of all that, she had been given benefits, actual *money*, to look after them! This country was wonderful really, with its welfare state – she got more than her daughter would have, what with Carer's Allowance, and all the other perks. A right little scam if truth be known and it was easily abused – they even paid for her car! But, more than that, the money made them even more hers – she had the Child Benefit book, *everything* in her name. Legally, that was worth a fortune to her as they were in her custody. Possession, as they say, is nine tenths of the law.

Now Gabriella was being difficult, wanting them back home with her. Cynthia intended to make sure that didn't happen – these were *her* babies now, and she would fight to the death to keep them.

'Why are you scowling, Nanny?' This from nine-year-old Cherie who was very observant.

Cynthia forced a smile on her face as she said quietly, 'I was just wondering how you would both cope if you had to go back to your poor mummy.' Her voice sounded as if that was inevitable, and she was gratified to see the alarm in the child's eyes.

'They won't make us, will they, Nanny?'

Cynthia shrugged, as if it was in the hands of the fates, and walked out of the room, knowing she was leaving a very troubled and worried little girl behind her. It was exactly the kind of reaction she was hoping for. If the kids didn't *want* to go home, she knew that her daughter would not be the one to force them. Also, the social workers would not be too hard on them either – she had made sure that they knew the score – or her side of it anyway. After all, mental illness ran in the family, didn't it? Her son James was as mad as a box of frogs, and her sister Celeste had not been the full fucking shilling either. Then her daughter, the mother of these beautiful children, was not exactly a shining example of motherhood or normality. She had become hooked on the very pills that were meant to be helping her! She didn't eat, sleep or shit at regular intervals without them – she was basically a mess. Maybe she *was* trying to sort herself out, but Cynthia had told the appropriate authorities that, while her daughter could visit her children here as often as she liked, she despaired of their lives if forced to go back to their mother's home full time. It seemed that they agreed with her. They bloody better had in any case, or she would want to know the reason why.

Gabriella had been allowed to have them next weekend for a trial period, so Cynthia had until then to devise a plan to make sure that they never let her daughter within five foot of these kids in the future. She was doing this for the benefit of the children. At least that is what she told herself. Without her, the kids would not be able to cope, and Gabriella needed to accept that the children were no longer hers. The sooner she accepted that the better. She could start another family with that fucking oik Vincent O'Casey when they finally let him back out on the street but, as far as these two were concerned, there was no way Cynthia was giving them up.

Chapter One Hundred
and Thirty-Five

Gabby spent the day cleaning and polishing the house; she had got in all the treats that kids loved, and she had rented a couple of Disney DVDs. Their rooms looked lovely, and she had also made sure she had lots of drawing paper for Cherie – she was showing a talent for art that made her really stand out at school. At least that's what her mother told her anyway.

She sighed as she thought of her mother. Cynthia, she knew, loved the kids – it was in a way her only saving grace – but she had moved heaven and earth to stop Gabby, their own mother, from being any part of their lives. Gabby blamed herself of course. After Vincent had been captured yet again, and she had seen herself once more on her own with another child, she had hit rock bottom. Coming so quickly after her nana's death, it had all but destroyed her. It had taken her three long years to get herself back on her feet, and she was determined to make sure that her children came back to her where they belonged. She had promised Vincent that she would get them back, and she intended to keep that promise. He had been a great help to her even though he was far away, and he gave her the confidence she needed to fight her mother. It was so hard fighting Cynthia because she always, *always*, seemed to be in the right.

Cynthia didn't seem to be particularly worried about her daughter's problems. She was so tied up with her grandchildren,

she didn't have the time or inclination to care about her relationship with her own child – the very same child who had borne
the only two people Cynthia loved. Gabby appreciated all that
her mother had done, but then surely any mother would have
done that for her daughter? So why couldn't Cynthia go the
whole hog, and let her have the kids back? Why was she so
determined to make sure that they had the least possible contact
with her? It felt personal, as if her mother was punishing her for
wrongs, real or imagined.

When she had spoken to her psychiatrist, something he had
said had rung very true with Gabby. 'Psychopathic personalities
can emulate the emotions and actions of the people around
them, even though they could never experience those actual
emotions for themselves.' He had been talking about her
brother but, for some reason, it had made her think of her
mother. She had felt a deep disloyalty at that because, when all
was said and done, her mother had stepped into the breech
when she had been needed. But now she was no longer needed.
It wasn't as if Gabby would stop Cynthia seeing them ever again
– she knew how close they were to their nanny. She could only
dream that one day they would love *her* that much. But for now
she would be content to be a part of their lives. She wanted
them back home with her and, eventually, with their father
Vincent. Her mother was making it all so difficult, and that was
what hurt her the most.

Gabby could not even risk arguing with her – if she did, her
mother told the social workers that she had been 'aggressive',
that she had 'frightened the children' and, as the social workers
knew that her children were not exactly enamoured of Gabby,
she had to tread very carefully indeed. Cynthia was ruthless and
she would do anything in her power to keep these kids as she
was demonstrating daily. No one else knew exactly what her
mother was really capable of – especially the goody two-shoes
social workers. They thought she was wonderful; a fucking

martyr. Well, they obviously didn't spend much time with her, or they would have seen her other side by now.

Thankfully Vincent would be back soon, and he would not take any nonsense from her mother or anybody else. She had that much to look forward to at least. Her mother was wary of her Vincent, and so she should be – he was stronger than she realised. Strong enough for both of them and together they would face her down once and for all.

Gabby glanced at the clock and stopped her cleaning; she had to be around her granddad's at six to make sure he had something to eat, and have a bit of a chat with him. He was still missing her nana Mary and she knew that without her in his life he would just give up.

She would pop the kids round there – that's what she would do. They could all stay there Saturday night, and it would give him a thrill to see them. He loved it when they came round, which wasn't very often thanks to her mother. Her nana Mary had warned her years ago that Cynthia wanted her children. Gabby wished now that she had listened to her.

Chapter One Hundred and Thirty-Six

'I love you too, Vincent. I'll be up the weekend, OK?' Gabby replaced the receiver and turned to Cherie and little Vince, who were looking at her as if waiting for her to do something. She had picked them up an hour ago from her mother's – not that they had been very enthusiastic about coming with her. Now they both seemed so uncomfortable around her it was breaking her heart.

'Did you like talking to your daddy?' She had hoped it would be a treat for them to speak to him.

Cherie shrugged. 'It was all right.'

'He'll be home soon, and you'll be able to see him all the time.'

Cherie gazed at her with her big, wide-spaced blue eyes, and the expression in them told her that was *not* something she was looking forward to.

Smiling with difficulty, she said gaily, 'So, what do you want to do?'

Cherie looked at her brother and they both said in unison, 'Go home.'

Gabby swallowed her disappointment; she knew she had to give it time, once they realised they could have fun with her as well as their nanny they would come round. But she could feel the ache of tears in her eyes and throat. 'Well, you can go,' she nearly said 'home', but quickly replaced it with, 'back to Nanny's soon. Now, who wants to go in the car?' She knew little Vince would want that; he loved cars, he had inherited that from his father all right.

When they arrived at her granddad's she saw Cherie sigh heavily. 'I don't like Great-Granddad Jack. He smells and so does his house.'

Gabby had had enough and, before she could stop herself, she said quietly but with emphasis, 'You know that's not true – that's just what Nanny Cynthia says. My advice to you is get out of the car now, and keep your opinions to yourself in future. I really can't believe some of the things you say, Cherie. You're nine now, not four. Stop parroting my mother.'

'I'm not parroting anyone. He smokes like you do and it stinks.' She curled her lip in disdain as she spoke.

Gabby replied angrily, 'Your nanny smokes.'

'Not near us, she don't. She knows it's bad for us to breathe in all that crud and toxic fumes.' The inference being that her mother didn't care if she was poisoning them, because she didn't care, period.

'You keep your opinions to yourself, young lady. You are going in there and you are going to be a good girl. Do you hear me, madam? You will do what you are told for once in your life.'

If she had taken back her arm and beaten the child to the floor the effect could not have been more extreme. Cherie's eyes filled with tears and she started to shake and, as Gabby looked at her in alarm, it brought back a memory. That was how her mother would act when she didn't get what she wanted. She had seen her father buckle down at that stance, and she felt a chill of fear that this child was already too far gone from her. She emulated her nanny Cynthia in everything, and the poor thing believed that was right.

Gabby fought the panic she felt rising in her chest and, taking little Vince out of his car seat, she said as nonchalantly as possible, 'Now out of the car, and not another word, OK?'

She was dreading telling the child they were staying the night. Little Vince went into his great-granddad's happily but Cherie trailed behind. It occurred to Gabby that she *had* done the right thing; she spent too much time trying to please the child when she should be making her see who was the parent.

Chapter One Hundred and Thirty-Seven

Cynthia had got herself sorted early, and now she was ready to go. She wondered briefly if she was taking things too far, but she knew that if she didn't go far enough, it would be overlooked. Gabriella was gradually winning the social workers round to her side and, if that happened, Cynthia would be left with nothing. Surely they could see how well those children had blossomed under her care? So what if she was the grandparent? Their own mother couldn't have done a better job of raising them. In fact, she had all but deserted them and now Gabriella expected to walk in and take them back, as if all Cynthia had done was for nothing. The thought of those kids stuck in that place with her and Vincent made her blood boil. They would never have a chance at anything.

She understood then that she had to do what she had planned. It was for the good of the children and, at the end of the day, they were what really mattered. She would do anything, literally *anything*, to see that one day she would have them for ever. All she had needed was an opening and today it had come. She had had a phone call from her granddaughter saying that her mother was making them stay at her great-granddad Jack's and she wanted to come home.

As she had spoken to the child, Cynthia knew this was the

perfect opportunity to prove her daughter's uselessness as a parent. This was like a gift from the gods, and she intended to take full advantage of it.

Chapter One Hundred
and Thirty-Eight

Jack Callahan watched as his great-granddaughter turned her pretty little nose up at everything in his home. He was glad, for the first time, that Mary wasn't here to witness this; it would have broken her heart. Cherie had been a sweet little thing when she was born, but now she was Cynthia's spawn, there was no doubt of that. He was sorry that he could find nothing to like about the child – even her beauty wasn't enough to make up for her natural air of superiority over everyone around. Like Cynthia before her, she already thought she was the dog's gonads, and he was itching to put his hand across that spoilt face. The worst thing of all was seeing poor Gabby trying her hardest to win the spoilt little mare over and only managing to make the child respect her even less. It was obvious the child knew the state of play, and was happily making her poor mother jump through hoops.

The little boy, however, was too young for Cynthia to have done much damage. Either that or the lad had more of his father in him, and wasn't so easily swayed. Jack hoped so, because if not, a few years down the line, there was going to be another troubled boy, like that fucking looney James Junior. Jack watched a lot of daytime TV these days and he knew all the psychobabble, and the words 'mother-damaged' always sprang to mind where that boy was concerned. Cynthia was like a disease, a cancer which invaded everyone around her until they were all infected with her spite and hatred. Now Jack could see her all over again, reincarnated in this little girl before him. He wasn't sure he could take it any more and his plea to her was heartfelt.

'Please, Cherie, will you just for once stop your yammering! Let's all sit together in peace.'

Little Vince was watching in fascination; he always did what his sister wanted – it was easier that way. But he didn't want to watch a film about Barbie, he wanted to watch Buzz Lightyear. He liked him, he was funny. He wondered if his sister would get her own way – she usually did where their mummy was concerned. He liked his mummy, and he liked his great-granddad Jack, but he knew that his nanny Cynthia didn't like them, so that could be difficult sometimes. He had learned at a young age never to let his feelings show; it caused too much trouble.

'I don't want to watch that film, it's for boys.'

Jack decided he had really had enough of this one's attitude. He leant forward from his armchair then, and said firmly, 'Well, that's what is known as tough shit. *I* want to watch Buzz Lightyear, so does your mum, and so does your brother. Look up the word "democracy" in your dictionary, love. It means that the people with the most votes win! Now, put a sock in it, and let's get this show on the road.'

Vincent, thrilled at the turn of events, climbed on to his great-granddad's lap happily. But his enjoyment was short-lived. As the film began, his sister unleashed a tantrum which was, without doubt, her biggest and loudest to date. In short, pandemonium broke out.

They were back at their mother's by five past eight.

Chapter One Hundred
and Thirty-Nine

Cynthia was nervous, but she felt sure she was doing the right thing. She had everything she needed to hand and all she had to do now was wait until it was late enough, and she could put her plan into action. As she waited patiently until she could safely leave her flat, she daydreamed of the life she would have with the kids she adored. And adore them she did, especially her Cherie, but then her little Vincent, though she hated the name the child bore, had stolen her heart as only a boy can. When she recalled the way he would climb up on to her lap and put his chubby little arms around her neck, she felt justified what she was doing for them was right. Anyone would do the same to save their grandchildren from a life of misery and degradation, she was sure of that.

Their father was a bloody blagger for starters! And, as she was always pointing out to the social services, caught not once but twice! She conveniently forgot her own past associations with the criminal classes and her part in them. She was good at rewriting history – she could wipe out anything that did not fit in with her version of events.

But now, thanks to Cherie, and the training she had been given to update her nanny on what they were doing with her mother, Cynthia had the opportunity to prove once and for all to the powers-that-be that her daughter was not fit to look after her own children.

Then they would be hers, and they would *stay* hers. Let Gabriella and Vincent make a new family, because there was no way they were going to get these kiddies. She would do whatever it took to get what she wanted. A little voice reminded her it wouldn't be the first time but, as always, she forced the thoughts away. Over the years she had become very good at that.

Chapter One Hundred and Forty

'No, Cherie, you can't go back to your nanny's. Look, you got what you wanted – we came back to my house. Your brother is asleep in the other room, and I'm very tired too. So come on, honey, you can sleep in here with me tonight.'

Cherie looked at her mother and decided that she had better do what she was told; after all, she had won the fight about staying at Great-Granddad Jack's. It wasn't really that he smelled – she didn't like it there because her great-granddad was all over little Vince. She used to be his favourite but that all changed when her brother came along. These days he hardly took *any* notice of her, except to say she was 'too much like Cynthia', and he said it as if it was a *bad* thing. Now she was lying in bed with her mummy, and she was feeling quite tired. Getting her own way could be exhausting.

'Can I have a story, Mummy?'

Gabby pulled her close, and said happily, ''Course you can, darling. What story do you want?'

'Little Red Riding Hood, please. The *long* version.'

Gabby laughed and started telling her the story. Cherie was asleep in no time and, holding her daughter to her own body, Gabby felt close to her for the first time. She couldn't wait for this to be her normal life. Soon she would have her babies back, and she would have her Vincent home. He had sworn he would go straight this time, that he would not do anything that would part him from his family. She knew that everyone thought she was mad, but she loved him, and she had to believe what he told her. It had been even harder when he had gone away this time and she had not coped well at all. And poor Vincent had been stuck on the island again, and unable to do anything to help her. She knew how hard that must have been for him, but that was all in the past now. She was on the mend, and he would be home at some point. All she could do was look to the future. She would not keep the kids away from her mum; after all, she had been there for them for a long time. But she wouldn't lose them to her. She would show them all that *she* was the best thing that could happen to her kids.

Gabby fell asleep smiling, thinking of how lovely it would be to have her family back together. Her, the kids, and her Vincent. It was the stuff that dreams were made of.

Three hours later, she awoke to a room full of smoke.

Chapter One Hundred and Forty-One

Cynthia let herself into her daughter's home and stood in the darkness of the kitchen, looking around her in the gloom. It was clean, she would give her daughter that, but it was still shabby. It was still council in her eyes. It broke her heart that her grandchildren would be reduced to this. Well, not for long.

She knew the best way to cause the fire was to start it from the front door, and let it take its own course, so that is exactly what she did. As she set to work, it did not cross her mind that she was destroying everything her daughter owned in the world – her photos, her clothes, all her personal effects. All she had to do was start the fire and then the Calor Gas heaters her daughter used for warmth would do the majority of the damage for her. She was grateful for the light from the street-lamp outside – she daren't put a light on, or make a noise. These places were like rabbit hutches, even a toilet flushing next door could be heard by all and sundry. She was smiling as she lit the match, and she slipped out as quietly as she had come in.

On the way home she was playing ABBA on her car stereo and singing at the top of her voice. This really was her Waterloo; she would play up her daughter's dangerous stupidity for all it was worth. A lit cigarette could cause untold damage – ten lit simultaneously could do even more! She guessed the washing basket full of clothes would be the first to really ignite, but the bin in the kitchen would also be a big help.

She would explain away the petrol by saying it was an insurance scam, that her daughter had hinted at money to come. She had covered all bases, and now she would have those kids until they sorted out accommodation and all the other shite that went with a major fire. Either way, this was a win-win situation for her.

Chapter One Hundred
and Forty-Two

Cherie was shaking Gabby, screaming at her to wake up.

'Mummy, Mummy, the house is on fire!'

Gabby could barely breathe; the bedroom was engulfed in smoke. Coughing, she jumped out of the bed. Vincent, the only thing she could think about was her baby Vincent, alone and afraid in his room.

She phoned the fire brigade in a panic and then, taking her daughter by the hand, she did the worst thing possible; she opened her bedroom door.

Chapter One Hundred
and Forty-Three

'Are you Cynthia Callahan?'

Cynthia, who had partaken of a few drinks to celebrate her late-night excursion, was bleary-eyed as she looked at the policeman and woman at her door.

'Yes, I am. What's going on? What's happened?'

Sergeant Proctor could hear a rising panic in her voice. He walked her through to her kitchen and, sitting her down, he nodded to the policewoman, who looked through Cynthia's cupboards until she found a bottle of brandy. Pouring out a large one, she placed it in front of the frightened woman.

All the time this was going on there was a panic rising inside Cynthia. This wasn't just about a burnt-out house. This was too ominous.

'Please, tell me! What's happened?'

Sergeant Proctor took her trembling hand in his and said gently, 'There's been a fire at your daughter's house. I'm very sorry to have to tell you that your grandson Vincent O'Casey died in it. The fire was too fierce for anyone to get to him and, believe me, your daughter tried. She's suffered third-degree burns on her hands as a result. Both she and your granddaughter are in the Old London. Your granddaughter is unharmed though – she's just being treated for smoke inhalation.'

Cynthia could hear the Sergeant's words, but she couldn't

take in what he was saying. 'But they weren't in the house! *Why* were they in the house? They were staying at my dad's. Cherie told me on the phone that they were staying at my dad's . . .' She was shaking with shock. She looked into the Sergeant's eyes, pleading with him to tell her that none of it was true. When she had sneaked into the house, no one had been there – the house had been *empty*. She knew that because they were supposed to be at her fucking dad's! Oh, why could her daughter *never* do what she was supposed to! Now look what had happened. If that girl could only do what she was supposed to . . .

'You're wrong. You *must* be wrong. My daughter and my grandkids are at my dad's. You've got the wrong house, the wrong people . . .' Cynthia started to cry then. 'Please . . . Please tell me you've got the wrong people, please . . .'

Sergeant Proctor held her while she cried and, as he would say later back at the station, never had he heard crying like it. She had sounded like a wounded animal. It was only when the doctor finally arrived and sedated her that her raving abated and she dropped into a deep, troubled sleep.

Chapter One Hundred and Forty-Four

'It's like I'm cursed, Granddad. The first night they stay with me, and my little boy gets burned to death. My mum was right, I should never have been allowed to have them on my own – look what happened. Cherie had been on at me about smoking, she said she hated the smell of it. It's why I came home from your house. Why didn't I just stay at yours?'

Jack Callahan wished to God that he could ease his grand-daughter's pain, but he knew no one could do that for her. Still, he hoped that what he had to tell her would relieve her of some of her guilt.

'Look, Gabby, there's something you should know. The police think the fire was started deliberately, and they think it was James who did it. Someone got into your house and lit cigarettes all over the place. It wasn't you. Whoever it was had placed piles of clothes under the fags, and your wastepaper basket and bin. I wasn't supposed to tell you this – they didn't want you to know until they thought you could cope with it, but your mother thinks it was James and so do the Old Bill now. She said he had turned up at her house a few days before and demanded money. I rarely agree with her, but I think this time Cynthia is right. It was James – it *had* to be. Who else would do something so fucking wicked?'

Gabby was thunderstruck. 'James? But why would James hurt me and my kids? It don't make sense!'

Jack shrugged. 'Why does that mad bastard do anything? There's no sense to be had out of this, and you'll drive yourself crazy trying to make some. He's a fucking nut-bag, always was, and always will be. So stop beating yourself up, love. I'll tell the police I've told you. Will you believe it if you hear it from them too?'

Gabby was numb; of all the explanations for what might have happened that night, her brother being the culprit was not one of them. But she supposed it had to be true – maybe he had thought they were out?

She felt the tears streaming down her face once more, and she looked at her heavily bandaged hands that had been burned down to the bone with her efforts to open her son's door. Her baby boy, her Vince, was dead, and it was her own brother who had killed him. There was no doubt about it – they were cursed, the whole family was cursed.

Chapter One Hundred and Forty-Five

Cynthia was not herself and everyone remarked on it. In the week following little Vincent's death the weight dropped off her and she looked older. People talked about how good she had been with those kids; she was hailed as a wonderful grandmother who had given up her life to raise her daughter's children. But she knew the truth, and it was eating at her like a cancer.

It had been quick thinking on her part, even in her distress, to say her son must have done it, and that had seemed to ring true. After all, *they* were the ones who'd told her about his threat to burn her out. He would eventually turn up like a bad penny, and they would charge him. It would do some good anyway; this time they would lock him up and throw away the key. They should have done that years ago.

It was the nights that were the worst for Cynthia. She thought she could hear little Vincent calling for her. And he would have called for *her* not his mum – it was Cynthia he would have wanted. She felt the sweat as it suffused her body, and the shortening of her breath that always accompanied it. Why had she done it? She had just wanted to make it seem as if her daughter was trying to fiddle the insurance and get herself a better house to live in into the bargain. Why had she not checked the bedrooms? She felt the tears once more, the tears that were never far from the surface. That little boy, that dear, handsome little boy . . .

As Cherie came and placed herself on her nanny's lap, Cynthia held her tightly, loving the feel of her small body, and remembering little Vince as he snuggled into her, his sweet baby smell of Johnson's powder. Now he was gone, burned to death, bless him, though the fireman said the smoke was what finished him off. He would have been lying in that cot, choking, and calling for his nanny Cynthia. He would have expected her to come and save him, she who had loved and cared for him all his life.

She leant forward and took a large swig of her whisky; it was the only thing that afforded her even a modicum of peace. She drank it whenever she needed solace, and that was all too often this past week. She needed its strength to help her forget for a few hours what she had done. Nothing in the world could ever wipe it out completely, but the Scotch helped and she drank it like water.

All she had left was her Cherie, and she could not lose her as well.

Chapter One Hundred
and Forty-Six

Vincent was devastated, and he knew that whatever he was feeling, his Gabby would be feeling it a hundredfold. Little Vincent, his namesake, was gone. It was hard to believe, because he had never really known him. But he had still been his son, the boy he watched being brought into the world, the boy he had such hopes and dreams for. His heart bled for Gabby, facing the worst that life could throw at a woman, and facing it alone, without him. It was like a nightmare.

Everyone in nick was being fantastic – even the POs had been sympathetic. One had even brought him in a bottle of Courvoisier brandy, courtesy of Bertie Warner and Derek Greene, and he had appreciated that. It was good of them to think of him, and he had been told they would stand the money for the funeral for which he was grateful. But he would pay them back every penny; the least a man could do was bury his own.

He was getting a day release to go to his son's funeral, how fucking fucked-up was that? Well, he would go and support his Gabby, then he would work at getting out of this dump and, when he did, he was going to hunt down that mad slag of a brother of hers, James fucking dead man Tailor, and he was going to kill him. He would kill him slowly and painfully; he would burn that skank alive, and let him know just how it felt, how his little lad had felt, choking and coughing, the room filling with black smoke and that cunt laughing about it. Because he would surely laugh about it would James, just like he apparently had when he had killed that poor fucking kitten.

Vincent poured himself another drink, and swallowed it quickly. He would give ten years off his life to be with poor Gabby now, holding her, and comforting her. They said her hands were very badly burned from trying to open the metal doorknob; burnt down to the bone. She was an incredible woman. She had taken their daughter to safety first, and then gone back inside to try and get her boy. She had done everything in her power to save him. Vincent couldn't hold back the tears then. He felt the uselessness of his life, and the complete waste of these years he had spent away from his family. He could have been with them every day if he had just used his loaf. It was too late for recriminations now, all he had left inside him was a thirst for revenge.

He knelt down in his cell and, placing his hands together, he made a pledge to God; he was going to find James Tailor and he was going to kill him. That was the only thing keeping him sane.

Chapter One Hundred and Forty-Seven

Cynthia was awake. She knew she should at least try to sleep, but it was the child's funeral tomorrow and she couldn't stop thinking about it. She wondered if she would be able to face it. She knew she had to go, if for no other reason than to allay suspicion, but she was dreading standing at the grave, knowing that the little boy being buried was there through her fault alone.

She wondered at life and how it could sometimes hold up a mirror and make you see yourself as others see you. It could hurt more than any physical injury. If she could, she would do anything in her power to change the last few weeks.

She had always been faithless; the nuns, priests, all the people who believed in God were nothing more than fools to her. Now, though, she wondered if she had been too hasty in blowing *Him* off. God, her mother used to say, paid back debts without money, and she must owe *Him* more than most people.

She knew she had to face her daughter, and make her believe that she was only interested in what was good for her and the child. She would let Gabriella see Cherie often, she could not be any fairer than that. But, after this, she knew more than ever that she could not live alone now. She could not be without her Cherie – she was all that she had left.

Chapter One Hundred and Forty-Eight

Gabby was pleased it was a cold and grey day – it would have felt wrong to have been burying her baby in the sunshine. She knew that she would never feel any warmth again; it was as if a lump of ice had settled in her chest, and it would never budge.

She glanced at his little white coffin, and wondered at a god who could take away a child from its mother. What really hurt was that she had had him for only one night and now he was dead. It didn't matter that it was her brother not her who had burned them out – it had still happened on her watch, as her mother had so succinctly put it.

Maybe her mother was right. Gabby's life was a shambles in many respects, and that had been driven home to her more and more lately. The only man she had ever loved had been twice banged up for armed robbery – hardly a good role model in the eyes of the courts, or anyone else for that matter. She was not allowed access to her kids unless her mother deemed it OK, and *she* had the legal rights that should have been Gabby's. Life was unfair, but she had to accept the blame for a lot of what had happened to her and her children. She had been too young, too stupid to have a child alone the first time round, and with little Vince fate had interfered once more, and she had been left holding the baby again.

She saw her Vincent walking towards her, flanked by and handcuffed to two prison officers. She stepped towards him, the sight of him opening the floodgates, and she heard herself sobbing as if from a distance.

Chapter One Hundred
and Forty-Nine

Cynthia was amazed at the reaction of the people at the funeral. She had been hugged and given condolences by people who would normally cross the road to avoid her.

She could see Gabriella, a beautiful name she had always felt was wasted on her daughter, standing with Vincent. The two POs with him looked suitably solemn and out of place at a child's funeral.

The sight of Vincent O'Casey in handcuffs angered her; he was bringing this lovely child's funeral down to the level of his family. They were there as well, though standing apart from everyone else, all looking like rejects from *The Jeremy Kyle Show*. They were just using the boy's death to worm their way back into Vincent's good books. She could easily walk over there and fell each and every one of them, punch and kick them to make them leave this place that was not supposed to be soiled by the likes of them. But she would leave that to Vincent; his opinion of his family was just about the only thing they could agree on. The irony was not lost on her.

Cherie was holding her hand tightly and, even though she knew she should make the child go to her mother and father, her innate cunning told her to keep her there. People would see that the child preferred her and that was the main thing. She had made a terrible mistake with little Vince, and she had paid dearly, but it had just made her all the more determined not to let this little one go from her. Without Cherie she had nothing, and that was wrong; after all, Gabriella could have more kids. She should have looked after the children she already had, not succumbed to her depressions and her pills. She was not fit to look after a child as intelligent and special as Cherie. She was wholly Cynthia's child, and that, she was determined, was never going to change.

Chapter One Hundred and Fifty

As Vincent listened to his Gabby sobbing, watched that piece of shite Cynthia keeping his daughter by her side, and saw poor old Jack Callahan aged and broken, he swore there and then that this was all going to change.

He had caught Cherie's eye and she had looked away, then up at her nanny Cynthia, as if asking permission to go to him. He allowed for the fact he was in handcuffs, but it wasn't as if she didn't know he was banged up – she had been to visit him. He knew it was Cynthia who had poisoned her, but he also accepted that Cynthia, whatever she was or she wasn't, had been there for the kids when poor Gabby couldn't be. He blamed himself for that; he had left her twice on her Jack Jones, twice holding the baby, *literally*.

He hadn't been there for either of his kids for any length of time, so was it any wonder his daughter didn't beat a path to his door? She was nervous of him and, from what Gabby had said, her mother had made them both out to be the bastards of the universe. They couldn't blame the child for that, though, in his heart, he hated Cynthia for the way she had manipulated them all, even him. At one time it was either Cynthia or care, and Cynthia was preferable to those kiddies being in the system. It was a fucking abortion and it was his fault.

That moron James had always been a few chips short of a McDonald's and, as Cynthia had been the cause of his fruit-caking, he was not impressed with her having too much authority over his daughter.

He felt powerless. He would never get used to it, yet he had been experiencing it for far too long. All he could think about was wiping out that bastard James; after that, everything else would fall into place, of that much he was sure. If he went away again, at least this time it would be for a good reason.

As the thoughts of revenge swirled around his head he held his Gabby as best he could under the circumstances.

Chapter One Hundred and Fifty-One

Jack Callahan had never felt so old and weak. He could not believe they were burying that lovely boy. Why had he let them go home that night? Why had fate chosen that night for James to have one of his rampages? And why couldn't the police find him? That's what he asked himself day and night – where could he be? If Jack had an inkling he would go and take the fucker out himself. It was as if James had disappeared off the face of the earth. Cynthia had said that when he had come to her house he had been high on drugs, accusing them all of ruining his life, accusing her of loving his sister's kids more than her own, a truth that must have hit home even to someone as thick-skinned as Cynthia.

He glanced at her and wondered how someone like her and her son could be allowed to roam the earth, when such a lovely little boy had died. It was all wrong.

Poor Gabby was beside herself with grief, and Jack was glad his Mary wasn't here to see this. As the priest himself had said to him, this would surely have killed her. It was a wrong day, in so many ways.

Chapter One Hundred and Fifty-Two

Bertie Warner stood in the cemetery and watched the proceedings with a suitably respectful expression. He didn't like things like this at all; he saw death as an inevitable thing, but he hoped that he would go naturally when the time came and not by the hand of someone else. In his opinion, cancer was preferable to a bullet in the brain – at least then you had the opportunity to tie up loose ends and say your goodbyes.

A child's funeral was a bastard; it was the wrong order, and it made everyone who attended feel they were blessed because it wasn't *their* child who had died. There were times when he could launch his lot into the atmosphere, but he wouldn't part with them for the world. If one of them died he would be distraught, and that was exactly how poor young Vincent and Gabriella looked.

Truth be told, though, it was Cynthia who was the star turn at this funeral, stealing all the attention. She looked like something from an American mini-series; black fitted suit, high-heeled shoes, and a small hat with a lacey bit hiding her boat race from the world. She still had the looks, he had to admit – not that he would touch her if she begged him. Well, he might if she begged him *really* nicely.

It was a sad day and no mistake. So why did he feel that there was something awry – he liked that word, it was something an old-fashioned Filth would use. But his shit detector, and he prided himself on his shit detector, was telling him there was something fishy about all this. It *smelt* wrong and, even though that nutter James was capable of something this heinous, it all felt a bit too convenient for his liking.

Now, it was common knowledge that he hated Cynthia; she had outed a close friend of his, even if he couldn't fault her actions at the time. But that hatred he had for her also made him suspicious of her, and what she was capable of. Though, from what he could gather, she loved those kids, so he was most probably barking up the wrong tree.

Still, he liked a nice little snoop occasionally, and he had plenty of Filth who owed him favours. If nothing else he would be able to give Vincent a proper update on his son's murder case, because this was murder, whichever way you looked at it.

Chapter One Hundred and Fifty-Three

As they lowered little Vincent's coffin into the grave, Cynthia's crying could be heard above everyone else's, and that only proved to the onlookers how much she had loved that child. The gossips speculated how that boy would still be alive if he had been at his nanny's where, in fairness, he had lived most of his life.

Gabriella was a lovely girl but she had been incapable of taking proper care of those children. She was like that Celeste and everyone knew *she* hadn't been the full shilling. No, the general consensus was that Cynthia, whatever people might think of her in the past, had proved herself in the end.

Cynthia felt the tide of good wishes and basked in their warmth and, as she stood by her daughter, hand on her arm, her granddaughter clutching her other hand, she knew that she had won, at least where public opinion was concerned.

Everyone watched her pull Gabby into her arms, and they said afterwards that when it came down to it, no matter what, you always wanted your mum when things were bad.

Chapter One Hundred and Fifty-Four

It was almost nine months since the funeral of little Vince, and Gabby was finally getting back to some kind of normality. It had not been the greatest of times, and she knew it would take a long while before she felt strong enough to feel anything close to happiness again.

Vincent was home, working at a garage in East London and they were gradually getting things together. It had been hard for them; he had never really known his son, but he had grieved for him as they both had. Cherie wasn't living with them, but they saw her a lot, and that was enough for Gabby these days. As Vincent said, it was a shame to take the child away from her nanny until they had replaced everything and had a proper home for her. But Gabby knew it was because Cherie didn't really bother with him. He had been away for so much of her life, she just didn't know him any more. It was sad but it was a fact of life.

Now she was pregnant again, although she was too frightened to get excited about it. Vincent was over the moon; he saw it as a chance for them to start again with the family they both had always longed for. Gabby wouldn't allow herself to get too caught up in his dreams. She had never been lucky in that way – every time she had believed her life was back on track it had been destroyed.

She had a lot of trouble with her hands still. It didn't bother her that they were scarred, but it was difficult to pick up small things, like pins or stamps. Even a knife could be quite difficult for her, but she was doing a lot of physio, and soon she would have another skin graft and then things would be even easier. She supposed they might put that off now until after the baby was born.

She hoped it was a girl; she didn't want to replace little Vince with another boy, but she knew that Vincent was hoping for a son he could take to the park and play football with. He wanted a little lad he could lavish all his time and energy on. She wouldn't begrudge him that – he had been her rock in so many ways, helping her through her grief and her guilt. Because she did feel guilty about what had happened, and would bear that guilt for the rest of her life.

It hurt that her own brother hated her so much he was willing to do that to them all, was capable of setting fire to her home, when she was the only one who had always tried to do what she could for him. In her own way she had kept in contact with him and, consequently, she had brought him into her children's lives. What a price they had paid for her stupidity!

It was hard getting through the days, and she still had very black moods when she wondered at what was going on with the world and she questioned everything. Why had this happened to her? Why she had been singled out for so much heartache? She had no answer. But it meant she would not celebrate this new baby until it was born – anything could happen between then and now.

As she combed her thick hair into place, the phone rang and she answered it carefully, making sure not to drop the receiver. It was the police. She listened for a few moments, before asking, 'Is this about James?'

She hoped they had found him; the thought of him out there after what he had done was worse than anything. Supposing he came back to finish the job? That was her nightmare – him sneaking back to burn them to death in their beds. He was capable of murder as they all knew – look at that Dougie person he had killed. She shuddered at the thought. Plus, if they caught him, then that meant her Vincent could not get his hands on him. Revenge wasn't worth doing life over. Her greatest fear was that Vincent would be banged up for the rest of his days. She knew he spent hours trying to track James down and had put a price on his head. Anyone with information could get twenty-five grand if it led to him being found. That was a big incentive, and she knew it.

'I beg your pardon, are you sure?' She listened for a few more seconds then she said in a dazed voice, 'No, I'll tell my mother, I don't think she should hear this over the phone.'

She put the receiver back in its cradle and went into her kitchen. Sitting at the kitchen table, she looked around her for a few moments, unable to get to grips with what she had just been told.

James was dead. He had been dead for over a year, although he had only just been found in a squat in Leicester. He had died of a heroin overdose, and he had been lying there all that time, undiscovered. They had deduced that it was James through his belongings, despite the body being in a state of decay. They would confirm with a DNA test, but they were more or less certain it was him.

If James was dead, then who had tried to burn her house down? Who had killed her little boy? And, more to the point, who had been at her mother's a few days before the fire? None of it made any sense. The person they had found could not have been James, surely? She decided to ring Vincent. He would know what to do.

Chapter One Hundred
and Fifty-Five

Cynthia was happier than she had been for a long while. She was finally getting over losing that little child and his awful death. She still needed a drink to get her through the day – and especially the nights – but she was beginning to feel she had it all under control.

Vincent had not taken to his daughter, and she had not taken to him, thank God. Cherie looked down her nose at him, and so she should. Cynthia had drummed into the child to expect better in life and she would make sure she got it. It had worked out quite well for her. Well, it had worked out as well as could be expected, all things considered. At least she had Cherie who, at ten, was so like her at the same age it was uncanny.

Now that silly cow was pregnant again. Didn't she ever learn? The girl was a total bloody idiot where Vincent was concerned. She could not see further than his dick, and that was about the strength of their relationship. He fucked her, he got her in the club, and then he left her. Gabriella believed it was third time a charm. As if that oik would be able to keep out of prison long enough to fucking see it born! If only he could find James before the police did – that would make sure Vincent wasn't around to interfere for a *very* long time. Even if her daughter *was* once more pregnant by him, she would happily see him put

428

away for good – especially if it meant James was out of the picture too.

She had made up her mind that she wasn't going to have too much to do with this new grandchild. She decided that, if she used her loaf, this would be the perfect opportunity to get Cherie away from them both for ever, and keep her for herself.

As she poured herself another of her 'black' teas – her euphemism for whisky and water – she pondered on how she could talk them into letting her move right away with Cherie. She couldn't stand to be in London any more – everywhere she looked she was haunted by memories of baby Vince. Every road, park and zoo reminded her of him and she could hear his voice asking her things, making her laugh. Oh, how he had made her laugh – he had been such a dear little fellow. She realised she needed to get as far away from those memories as possible.

Gabriella had phoned to say she would be here soon. She wondered what she had to talk to her about? Probably wanting help with that baby she had on the way.

Chapter One Hundred
and Fifty-Six

Gabby had parked her car by the new Somerfield's at Chrisp Street Market; she needed to pick up a few bits for Vincent's dinner, before calling at her mother's. She couldn't drive for long with her hands as they were but she could manage the automatic Vincent had got for her to get around locally. Vincent was as mystified as she was about the news about James. He said he'd dig around a bit for some more information. As she walked out with the trolley, she was startled from her thoughts when she heard someone call her name.

'Is that you, Gabby?'

Gabby looked into the woman's face, unable to place her. She grinned at her before saying in a friendly manner, 'Sorry, do I know you?'

The woman smiled; she was in her late forties and she had kind eyes and heavy legs. 'I'm Jeannie Proctor. I lived next door to you in Ilford when you were a nipper.'

Gabby smiled back. 'Oh, really? I'm sorry, I don't remember.'

The woman looked her over, and she said in wonderment, 'You are the living image of your mother – that's what made me recognise you. Beautiful, just like her. How is Cynth these days?'

Gabby nearly said, 'Well, she would not be happy to be referred to as "Cynth"!' Instead she said, 'She's fine, you know me mum!'

It was meant in jest, but the woman nodded, then said seriously, 'Oh, I know Cynthia all right! Tell her she still owes me for the dry cleaning bill.'

Gabby laughed then. 'What dry cleaning bill?'

Jeannie Proctor paused for a few seconds as if she was wondering if she should speak, then she said candidly, 'It was a long time ago, so I don't suppose it matters now. She torched the house – for the insurance, like. She had spent so much on it that they could never get the price it was worth, so she torched it. Left fags all over the place, she did, and open cans of paint and turps. Looked like she was decorating, see. She was a fucking girl, her. Mind you, in those days you could get away with murder with insurance companies. Can't any more, they're wise to everything now.'

The woman was laughing, but Gabby could feel herself going cold.

'I had my bedroom windows open, and the smoke damage was atrocious, as you can imagine . . . Here, where you going?'

Jeannie Proctor watched as the girl hurried away from her. 'Well, what on earth rattled her cage?'

Chapter One Hundred and Fifty-Seven

Gabby sat in her car and thought back to what Jeannie Proctor had said to her. Somehow she knew that the woman was telling her the truth. But did that mean her mother had burned *her* house down too? Had killed her baby boy? Somewhere inside she knew that was what had happened.

It was all falling into place now. She had been on the verge of getting the kids back, she had straightened herself out. In her heart she should have known her mother would not have countenanced that. Her mother had always wanted those children more than she had ever wanted anything in her life. Gabby had actually deemed that at one time her mother's saving grace – the undeniable love she had for those two little mites. It was the love she had never had for her own kids, but she had lavished it on her grandchildren. Gabby had been so grateful to her, had felt so indebted to her for all her help. She recalled how badly her mother had taken little Vince's death; Gabby had assumed, like everyone else, that it was because she had loved him and cared for him. But it had been guilt. The wicked bitch had been consumed with guilt.

Even as Gabby's heart was trying to deny what she was telling herself, her brain was telling her that it couldn't have been her brother who started the fire. The brother who her mother had said had visited her a few days before, and who she subsequently admitted had threatened them all with death, pain, torture and destruction, was well and truly dead by then.

Gabby remembered her mother's devastation at the kids having to leave her to go home to their terrible mummy. How she had kept saying Gabby wasn't ready to have the kids back yet, that she still needed to sort herself out. It was exactly what she had said about Cherie coming back to her after the fire. Gabby had believed her mother was doing her a favour by keeping Cherie with her then. Cherie, who could have died as well if she had not slept in her bed that night, who would have been in the same room as little Vince, who had been so determined to leave her great-granddad's house because of Cynthia's bad mouthing.

She could see that her mother hadn't intended to kill them. She had believed they were at her granddad's that night. Cynthia had burned the place down thinking it was empty, but she had done it to make it look like Gabby was incapable of looking after her own children. A big fire would make them think twice about letting the children come back home, especially when there was no fucking home for them to go to. Gabby could almost hear her mother saying to the social workers how irresponsible she was to have left a fag burning, and imagine if the children had been in there with her.

Well, they *were* in there with her. While her mother was creeping around her house with every intention of burning it down, she had been asleep upstairs with her babies. It all made perfect sense now – her mother would have had to keep the children at least until she was re-housed, and back on her feet. And that would have been months, if not years.

Cynthia had done it deliberately, and she had done it for no other reason than to get what she wanted, as she had always got what she wanted. Gabby had lost not only her little boy in that fire, but all her photos, the memorabilia of her life, of her kids' lives, of her nana Mary and her all-too-little time with Vincent.

Her mother had been willing to leave her with *nothing* in her determination to keep those kids, and instead she had murdered her little boy.

Gabby thought back to how her mother had always made sure she got whatever or whoever she wanted – by hook or by crook. Cynthia had taken Jonny from poor Celeste, she had taken the kids from her own daughter, and she had been the reason her husband had killed himself. She had murdered in cold blood once – to save her sister she claimed, but she had done that to save herself too. It would always be about *her*, and what *she* wanted. It would *never*, could never, be about anyone else.

And what about poor James Junior? Cynthia had blamed James from the get-go. She had put him in the frame with her lies about him going round there and threatening all sorts. Was there nothing she wasn't capable of?

Gabby was outside her mother's flat, parked up all neat and tidy, but she had no memory of driving there. She got out of the car, and she felt as if she was walking through water, so heavy and awkward did her limbs feel.

Chapter One Hundred and Fifty-Eight

Gabby was throwing up in her mother's toilet, and all she could hear was her mother's voice going on and on and on.

'I don't feel well, Mum. I feel ill and out of sorts.'

'Well, whose fault's that then? Pregnant again, aren't you? He'll leave you like he did the last two times. He won't keep out of the nick, love – it's all he's fucking fit for. And I can tell you now, I'm not looking after any more kids either. You're on your own this time, lady. I told you when you met that idiot Vincent O'Casey, I said then, and I stand by my words, he has the brains of a fucking rocking horse and the face of a Tonka toy. But would you listen to me? You should get shot of that baby. How can you have another one? I mean, I ask you, how long before he'll be banged up again?'

Gabby was frightened of the hate spiralling inside her. She was terrified of the feelings consuming her, and the thoughts that were spinning out of control inside her head. She didn't want to hurt her mother, she *mustn't* hurt her – not yet anyway, not until she had found out the truth, no matter how painful it might be. But she had to know.

She took a deep breath and said calmly, 'Have the police spoken to you yet?'

Her mother went quiet at that, and then she asked warily, 'What about? Why would they want to speak to me? More likely they were after your old man. What's he gone and done this time?'

'*Vincent*? My Vincent ain't done nothing, but it seems they have found James.' She saw her mother's face pale, and she wanted to smile.

'Where? Where did they find him? Have they charged him? The murdering little fucker.'

She was good, Gabby would give her that. What was it the psychiatrist had said about mimicking emotions? Oh, that was her mother all over.

'Well, where is he? Is he in custody? Have they collared him or what?'

Gabby could almost feel the panic emanating from her mother, and she knew then that she would enjoy bringing her down, she would love every second of exposing her for the liar she was. 'He's in a morgue up in Leicester. He's been dead for over a year, Mum. You do realise what that means, don't you?' She saw Cynthia trying to take onboard what she had said to her. 'It means he couldn't have been the one who set fire to my house, and it also means that you couldn't have spoken to him a few days before like you said you did. Because he was dead then. Unless you saw him through a fucking medium, you lying, treacherous, fucking whore of a woman.'

Cynthia was taken aback by the vehemence of her daughter's accusations. She knew only too well that her daughter was telling the truth. Now she had to find a way out of her lies and subterfuge. Trust that fucking James to be dead! That was so like her kids – they always let her down.

'I know what I saw, and it was not long before the fire, but it might have been a few weeks before – I was confused, I was upset. For fuck's sake, Gabriella, it was a terrible time. What are you trying to prove here?'

Gabby laughed harshly. Oh, she was really good. Her acting was of Oscar standard. Move over, Dame Judi Dench, you are an amateur in comparison with Cynthia Callahan. 'What *I* am trying to prove? I am trying to prove who was responsible for the death of my little boy, Mum, that's what I am trying to prove. And, by all accounts, it wasn't my brother, your son, James, so who does *that* leave?'

Cynthia just shook her head in utter disbelief, stalling for time. She was thinking on her feet now, trying to work out how she was going to explain it all away. 'I don't know, darling – maybe he got someone else to do it, or it was someone after your Vincent. You know what villains are like – he probably fucked someone over in stir, and that door of yours was never safe, was it? One good push and it was open.'

Gabby just stared at her mother, the woman who had carried her in her belly, and who had never in her life given her a thing that was worth having. The very same woman who was now trying her hardest to talk her into believing that her house burning down and her son dying was all some kind of conspiracy by persons unknown, as the police would put it. *She* had burned that house down to stop Gabby having access to her own children. That was the truth of it all. Cynthia had done it to get what she wanted, Just as she had always got what she wanted all her life, no matter who suffered because of it. It was a wicked, calculated act that had been the cause of her little son dying, choking to death in thick black smoke. She could hear his voice calling for his nanny over and over – that made it even worse. He hadn't called for his mummy – only his nanny who had made sure he wanted her over his own mother. Even Cherie didn't want her, or her father either, come to that. She was a spoiled, rude and arrogant little girl who, if she had not been so fucking ruined, would not have made them all leave her granddad's house.

'It was Cherie, you know, who made us come back that night. She didn't like it at your dad's – she said it *stank*. You have always drummed into her how your mum and dad smelt, and were not nice people, and that I can't be trusted to take care of them. And so, to please her, to make her happy, I brought them back to my house. The house where her brother died, because her adored nanny tried to burn the place down while we were sleeping in our beds. How the fuck do you sleep at night! Knowing what you did, how the fuck do you sleep a wink? Is that why you went on the drink? Because you drink a lot now, Mum, don't you? Does it drown out the knowledge that you fried your grandson in his cot?'

Cynthia tried not to react to that; it was a truth which ate away at her every day. She *had* to get Gabriella onside again. 'What would I know about starting fires, you silly girl. You're overwrought, Gabriella, listen to yourself, for fuck's sake! You haven't been right since that child died, and I understand that, babe, I feel the same way . . .'

It was 'babe' now; Gabby could see she was really pulling out all the stops. 'No, you don't, Mum. You've never cared about anyone or anything in your life. You're a fucking leech. You take everything from people. You pretend you care, but you don't, you don't know how to. You'd even blame poor James – James who you sent off his fucking rocker in the first place . . .'

'You are not going to make me listen to this shit, Gabriella. You are wrong, *very* wrong. Use your bloody head, girl! I loved that little boy with all my heart . . . and, as for your brother . . . I don't believe a word of it – they must have the wrong person.'

But Gabby could see the fear in her mother's eyes and she knew that it was true. Every word of it.

'I met your old mate, Jeannie, today. That's how I know everything – she told me *all* about the house in Ilford.' She could see her mother's head working, trying to figure out exactly what she was saying, could almost hear her brain whirring as she tried to lie her way out of what they both knew was the truth.

'What the hell have you been taking this time, eh? What the fuck are you on, Gabriella, to make you come out with this shit?'

Gabby found she'd picked up a large bronze statue of a cat. As she held it in her scarred hands she felt the weight of it. Her mother kept talking. The world according to Cynthia Tailor who, along with God Himself, was almost omnipotent in the lives of her family, who ruled everyone around her with a rod of iron. She could see her mother's mouth moving constantly, but she couldn't hear what she was saying any more; all she was conscious of was a rushing noise in her ears. Then she struck her.

She lifted the bronze statue back over her head and hit her mother across the face with it, using all the force she could muster, and enjoying the feeling of total retaliation. For once it was her doing the hurting, and that felt good. She hit her over and over again, watching the spray of blood as it spurted from her mother's head, enjoying her mother's pain, and her mother's suffering.

She knew that this had been a long time coming, and that she should have done it years ago, should have done it when she was a young girl. She could have saved so many people so much heartache. She was determined now, determined to shut her mother up once and for all. Shut her up for good.

Cynthia fell sideways on to the white leather sofa. She could hear a gurgling noise that was almost comical. The blood was still spraying out everywhere like a crimson mist, and she was glad, glad the lying, two-faced, murdering whore was finally shutting her big, filthy mouth up. She hoped she was in as much pain and terror as her little boy had been when he was fighting for his last breath, expecting to be saved by this woman who had started the fire in the first place so she could get what she wanted.

Gabby hit her mother again and again, each blow easing the knot inside her, each blow easing the hate she had inside her for this woman who had been the bane of her whole life.

She looked down at the bloodied form and, for the first time in years, she felt almost at peace. Her mother's face was unrecognisable, a deep red gash that was pumping out blood at an alarming rate.

Gabby looked at the woman she had hated nearly all her life. Then she sat down on the ladder-backed chair her mother was convinced was an antique, put her face into her bloodied hands and cried.

Chapter One Hundred
and Fifty-Nine

'Fucking hell, Vince, when your lot go they don't muck about, I'll give them that!' Bertie Warner's voice held a tinge of admiration in it. 'Maybe I should give her a job on the firm!' Bertie laughed at his own joke.

Vincent looked around the room, and shook his head in amazement that his Gabby was capable of this kind of violence. But then, after what she had told him, he understood it to an extent. All her life Cynthia had done everything possible to destroy those around her, and it seemed that now, finally, one of those people had retaliated and in a spectacular fashion.

Gabby was still sitting on the ladder-backed chair. Her face and hair and clothes were sprayed with blood, but the strangest thing was, for the first time in years, she actually looked at peace.

'She did it, Vince, she fucking killed our baby. She torched our home so she could keep our kids with her. Keep them in her power. Everyone had to be in her power, had to do what she wanted; she would never be happy with anything else.'

Vincent went over and held her gently. She felt so frail, her body was so slender still, even with the pregnancy, and he knew that this had been coming for a long time. He blamed himself – if he had not been away so long, none of this would have happened. He should have been there for her and for his kids, instead of rotting away in prison. But that was the chance you took in his game, and you had to accept that or you would go off your head. His old cellmate used to say hindsight is a wonderful thing, but it was fucking foresight that people needed.

Bertie looked at young Vincent, as he still thought of him, and wondered at a man who could be so calm in the face of such carnage. Gabby had literally taken her mother's face off – this was the act of someone who had reached the end of their tether.

He nudged Cynthia's body with his foot none too gently; if she groaned he would finish the slag off himself. He smiled. Just as he thought – as dead as the proverbial dodo. Good riddance to bad rubbish, he was glad she was gone. He had had his own axe to grind with her; after all, she had taken out one of his closest friends. He cleared his throat noisily and said, 'We better get this place cleared up before Lily Law comes a-snooping! You take her home and sort her out, son. I'll deal with this little lot.' He sighed theatrically. 'Thank fuck she lived in this end house – bit more privacy, if you know what I mean!'

Chapter One Hundred and Sixty

Gabby was lying on the bed; such was her relief at the knowledge her mother could never interfere in her life again she almost felt lighter in her body. Even the pain of her hands couldn't bother her. It was as if the heavy weight she had carried all her life had been taken away from her and, consequently, she felt better than ever, mentally as well as physically. She felt no remorse for what she had done. Thank God that Cherie was having a sleepover at her friend's house; she was going straight from school, so no one would be any the wiser about Cynthia's disappearance until tomorrow when she didn't pick up Cherie from school. Vincent said it would all be sorted; all she had to say was that she went round there and she wasn't in, so she had left her a voicemail message and then come home again.

She pulled herself on to her back, and stretched her arms above her head. She felt a luxuriousness overwhelming her, as if she had finally found the secret to eternal happiness. Knowing that Cynthia was gone was like receiving the greatest gift ever. It meant that her life would change drastically in every way. She could do *what* she wanted, *when* she wanted; there would be no Cynthia to stick a spoke in the wheel, no Cynthia to shoot down her hopes and her aspirations, no Cynthia to make her feel inadequate any more. And no Cynthia to burn her children to death or turn them against her.

Her granddad Jack came in to the room with two cups of tea, and she smiled at him dreamily, 'She's gone, Granddad, and I don't feel an ounce of guilt.'

Jack sat on the bed carefully and, taking her hands very gently in his, he said seriously, 'Listen to me, love, you will. When this sinks in you will realise the enormity of what you have done. Now, I'm not saying that what you did was bad but, love her or loathe her, and I certainly loathed her, she was still your mother when all was said and done. That will be the thing that will play on your mind.'

Neither of them spoke for a while. Then Gabby said honestly, 'I won't let her ruin the rest of my life, Granddad. She's ruined so much of it already, I can't let her ruin the rest. I'm glad I did what I did; it's just a shame that someone didn't do it to her earlier, then my little boy would still be alive, and I wouldn't have her blood on my hands. She was not a person who had any right to decency or kindness, she was not a person to aspire to be. She was cruel, and she was evil in many ways. She took what she wanted from anyone, she was nasty, vindictive and she never threw me a kind word. She was the reason my dad killed himself, why Auntie Celeste went off her head, and why my brother never knew a happy day in his life. I don't feel a second's guilt over that bitch, so don't worry about me, OK? I'm fine, better in fact than I have been for many a long year. Me and Vince have a chance now, we can be a real family and Cherie won't have her dripping her poison in her ears at every available opportunity. I am actually looking forward to the future now, and that is something I could never say before today.'

Jack picked up his tea from the bedside table and drank it quickly. He heard the truth in the girl's words. 'I'm glad to hear it, love, I just don't want her on your mind.'

Gabby laughed softly. 'No fear of that, Granddad. I feel free, really *free* for the first time in my life. It's as if I can finally breathe again. I paid her back for my boy, and for everyone she ever contaminated by her touch. So don't worry about me, mate, I have never felt better.'

Chapter One Hundred
and Sixty-One

'"No, officer, I haven't seen or heard from her for days."' Detective Sergeant Smith laughed as he spoke. 'That's all we hear, sir. It's as if Cynthia Tailor has dropped off the face of the earth. There's nothing at her house – she's gone, lock, stock and barrel. The neighbours said a moving van turned up and was gone within an hour. It's as if she never existed.'

Dectective Inspector Williams nodded. This was a really strange affair; he knew there was skulduggery afoot but actually proving it would be impossible.

DS Smith continued, 'It seemed she had scammed quite a few men over the years, sir – it could have been one of them she was running from. A David Duggan made a criminal complaint against her but she seemed to have swerved that with ease. But, on closer inspection, she wasn't what you would call a model citizen, if you know what I mean?'

DI Williams shook his head. 'I know exactly what you mean. Cynthia Tailor, Callahan that was, could start a fight in an empty house. But the point is now, where the fuck is she?'

DS Smith laughed then as he answered. 'Your guess, sir, is as good as mine.

'What about the daughter? Didn't she have her children at one point?'

DS Smith nodded. 'From what we can gather, sir, the

daughter is as baffled and bewildered as we are. Heavily pregnant now and lost her little boy in a fire. She seems to think her mother has done a moonlight flit. Her expression, not mine. She doesn't seem unduly worried about her and, as for Cynthia Tailor's father, he thinks she will turn up, as he said in his own words, like the proverbial bad penny.'

DI Williams sighed. 'Leave it with missing persons then, we've done all we can.'

DS Smith nodded once more and left the office of his superior. He was in line for a forty-grand bonus for this little piece of work, and he was absolutely thrilled about it. He wondered what part of the new M25 Cynthia was now resting in. He would put his money on a slip road, but she might be holding up a flyover. Either way, there was no way she was ever coming back, of that much he was sure.

Chapter One Hundred
and Sixty-Two

Vincent looked around his new house and smiled in satisfaction. It was lovely, and he knew that they would be very happy here. It was a new start for them, and that was something they needed desperately.

As he looked at Cherie's pretty face he smiled at her, and she tentatively smiled back. 'You can decorate your room any way you like, sweetheart.' She was only happy when she was getting something – mainly her own way. She was related to Cynthia all right. 'Go and help Mummy with the bags, would you?'

She skipped off to do as she was told. Since she had been away from Cynthia she was becoming easier to handle, but it was the change in his Gabby that was the real eye opener. She was like a young girl, laughing, easy with herself and everyone around her. It was as if Cynthia's death had unleashed the real Gabriella Tailor. He hoped that she stayed this happy always, because although he loved the old Gabby – always had and always would – now he felt as though he had been given another woman to love alongside the old one. This one made plans, had ideas, was sure of herself, whereas the old one had always been frightened to be happy because it had never lasted for her. Now she was strong, strong in every way. And he loved her with all his heart and soul. This was the beginning of the rest of their lives, lives without the burden of Cynthia Tailor and what she entailed.

Picking up Gabby, he carried her across the threshold and her high laughter drew the attention of the passers-by who could not help but smile at such complete and utter happiness.

Epilogue

Richard O'Casey, known affectionately as Ricky, was laughing his head off, and he was obviously enjoying his day out. His older sister Cherie was grinning at him, and he was grinning back. As they ran back to their parents, they were holding hands.

Richard had the unmistakable Callahan eyes, and the sovereign-coloured hair. He was a good-looking and a happy boy. Cherie was growing up and she could easily pass for older than she was, with the unmistakable Callahan femininity she exuded. Vincent watched her like a hawk, as did Gabby. Cherie knew all this and she had made sure that she acted how they wanted her to act; that way she got a lot more leeway, but she was already a terrible liar, who had an eye for the men, not boys, *men*. Gabby feared there was far too much of Cynthia in the girl, but that was to be expected – she had been her role model for so long. Gabby suspected she was a lost cause, but they were determined to do the best they could for her, and make her into a better person because they loved her in spite of everything. It was hard work though – if Vincent had not been as strong-minded as he was, Cherie would have been walking all over him by now. She already knew how to captivate any males in her vicinity.

Ricky, on the other hand, was a wonderful little boy, who enjoyed life, and understood the word 'no'. As he looked at the gravestone, he said sweetly, 'Great-Granddad Jack's down there.'

They smiled at his words. 'That he is, my little lovely. He's with your great-nana Mary – she would have loved you!' Gabby wished her grandparents could see them now.

Vincent held Gabby's hand, and he squeezed it affectionately as she looked down at the grave of the only two people who had ever cared about her when she was growing up.

Cherie watched them both warily; she hated the way they were always hanging off each other. And how could her dad hold her mother's *hands*? They were awful – all scarred and deformed. If *she* had those hands she would wear gloves all the time.

She glanced across the cemetery at her uncle James's grave. They put flowers there as well, though why they would acknowledge a nutter like that she didn't know. She would never understand her family, not if she lived for a thousand years. Since her nanny Cynthia had gone on the trot they had all acted like it was Christmas every day. Well, *she* missed her nanny and she couldn't understand why she not taken her with her. She said to her mum then, 'I wonder if we'll hear from Nanny Cynthia this year?'

Gabby shrugged. 'You never know, she could turn up out of the blue. I wouldn't put it past her.'

Vincent O'Casey looked at his family and felt that, after everything, they were finally getting on track. He had bought his garage back now, courtesy of Derek and Bertie. He tuned up certain motors for certain people for certain jobs; it was very lucrative, but nothing that could put him back in the nick. He loved his freedom too much to do anything to jeopardise it, and he loved his family too much to leave them ever again. As he looked at his wife, because they were married now, and saw the little bump under her coat he felt a great wave of happiness. He hoped this baby was a girl. They were still young and they had their whole lives ahead of them.

Cynthia Callahan was dead and gone, buried all alone and far away from the people she was supposed to love. Her days of dictating other people's lives were past. It was just them now, and they were happy, really happy. Unlike Cynthia Callahan, they knew the value of love, and they knew the value of loyalty. And they were determined that they would be happy despite everything and everyone who had tried to destroy them. After all, as Mary Callahan had always said, what can't kill you can only make you stronger. They had faith in each other and in their ability to live a happy life, and that wasn't bad for starters, was it?

'Who fancies fish and chips?'

Richard was jumping up and down with sheer excitement and even Cherie looked keen. They walked away together as a family.

As they neared the cemetery gates, Gabby looked back to where her brother lay alone. Just for a few seconds in the autumn sunshine she thought she saw her, Cynthia, standing by his grave. She looked lost, unhappy, sorry. Gabby knew it was a trick of the light, but somehow it made her feel better. So she closed her eyes and said quietly, 'Goodbye, Mum.'

Then, smiling, she followed her husband and kids to the car.